What Others Have Said About:

The Art of Herbal Healing: A Guide to Health and Wholeness

"Since publication of the first edition of Nicholas Culpeper's *English Physician* in 1652, each generation in the modern era has seen publication of an accessible, comprehensive herbal that stands as a testament to herbalism for that time period for future generations. Susan Clearwater's *The Art of Herbal Healing: A Guide to Health and Wholeness* is one of those herbal touchstones that defines a generation. The book delivers a deep perspective on the fundamentals of herbal medicine, covering the roots of herbal healing traditions, along with clear, concise foundations for understanding where herbs come from — the botany, rarity, cultivation and sustainable harvest of medicinal herbs. Detailed information infused with experience guides the reader through the broad-ranging practical guidance on herb preservation and preparations, along with details on herbal combinations. Additional topics include dosage calculations, guidance on discerning quality, and a frank, clear discussion on herbal safety, pros and cons. An essential explanation and pathway to understanding chemical constituents of herbs and their relevance to herbal healing is a welcome primer to what can be an intimidating subject. An excellent narrative on defining commonly used terms on the qualities of herbs provides more detail to help decipher how herbs work and heal. Next, the heart of the book, a materia medica of fifty common herbs, which includes the full range of topics outlined above for each of the herbs.

Susan embraces tradition with heart and delivers science with compassion. A single word comes to mind as I peruse and mingle my thoughts with the information and ideas within these pages, and that word is comfort. The book invites you to become confident with understanding and experiencing herbs to integrate your own health into nature herself. It is a practical guide for herbalism today. It doesn't shy away from philosophical and spiritual underpinnings that might make some scientists squirm in their lab coats, yet at the same time, Susan blends traditional wisdom with scientific understanding in a comprehensive and practical style. It provides a thorough deep-dive into each herb, leading one to explore further. An important feature of the book is that it is fully referenced throughout. This is a book I wish I had at the beginning of my herbal interests over four decades ago."

—**Steven Foster,** Author of *Herbal Renaissance*, and international herbal photographer

"I know that Susan with her life's experience as a mother, teacher, holistic nurse, and clinical herbalist is a person to be honored for this chosen path and vast accumulated knowledge. Susan certainly welds the power of the green spark. It took 25 years to write *The Art of Herbal Healing*, but that's what it takes to give the world such an amazingly complete herbal. *The Art of Herbal Healing* is an engaging and well-thought out great green treasure-trove, much more than just a materia medica. It is a vast herbal text that can be used by herb schools and all plant people and their families. This book gives all a path to further our direct relationship with plants, important since there would be no humans or animals without them. Even with so much information available here, it is presented in an easy to understand and interesting format with great illustrations.

All throughout *The Art of Herbal Healing*, I found information I needed to know or topics I needed to think about. I have never seen or delved into such a clear picture of herbal history and early medicine. It is a perfect way to start this book. The section of herbal medicine of indigenous people contains a fascinating and enlightening interview with Dark Rain Thom. It's all here – herbal botany, endangered medicinal herbs, botanical sanctuaries, cultivating, harvesting, drying, herbal preparations, formulations, dosage, safety, chemical constituents and, of course, excellent coverage of using herbs for healing and the materia medica.

I consider this book an herbal bible that will stand the test of time."

—**Paul Strauss,** Equinox Botanicals, sanctuary steward, author of *The Big Herbs*

The Art of Herbal Healing

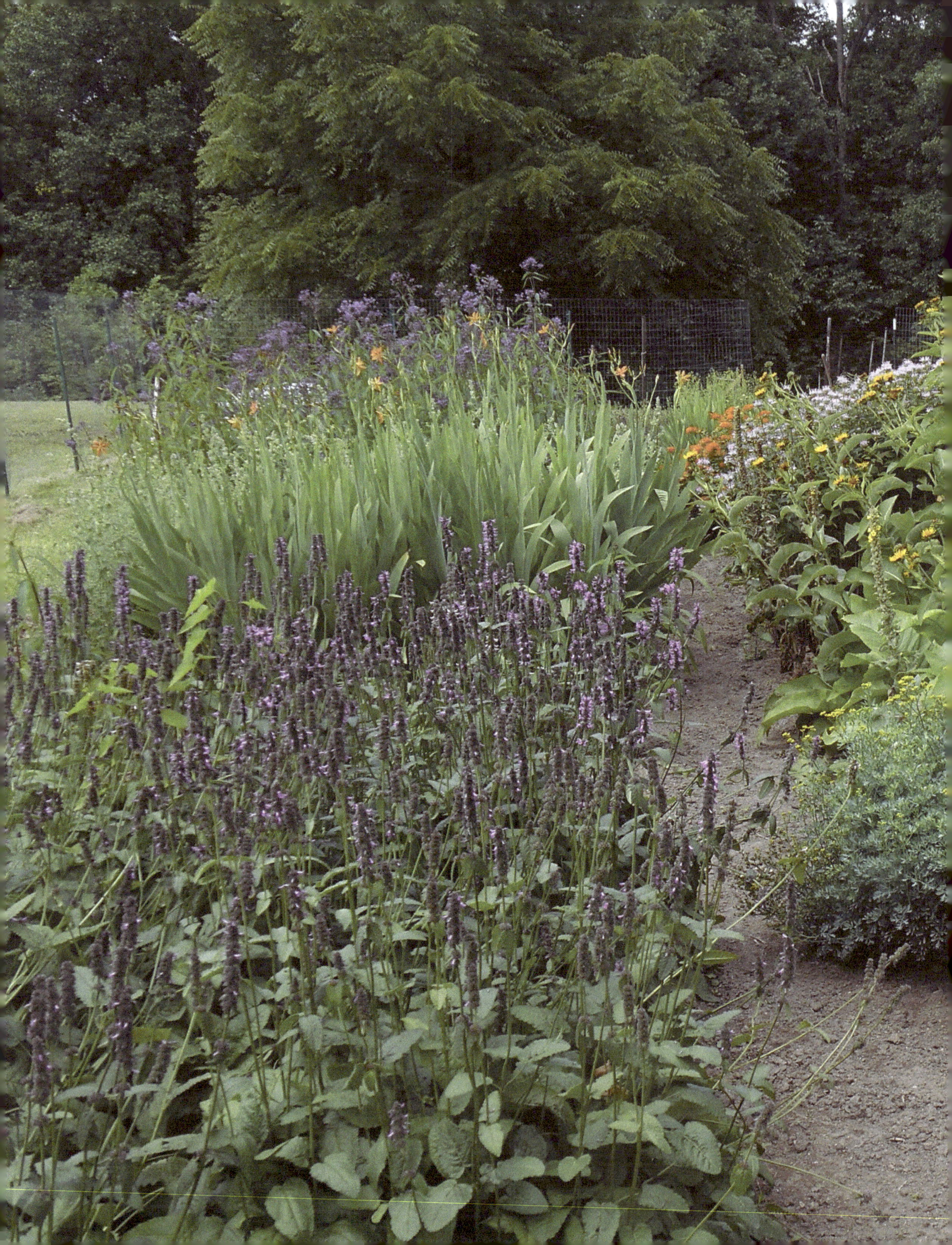

The Art of Herbal Healing

A Guide to Health and Wholeness

Susan Clearwater, RN, BSN
Holistic Nurse & Clinical Herbalist

Green Turtle Publishing
Nashville, Indiana

Manufactured on acid-free paper in the United States of America

ISBN 978-0-692-10575-7-Paperback
ISBN 978-0-692-18452-3-Hardcover

Front cover plant photographs: American Centaury (*Sabatia angularis*), Passion Flower (*Passiflora incarnata*), and Goldenrod (*Solidago odora*)
Title page photograph is the main garden Green Turtle Botanical Sanctuary, Nashville, Indiana

Photo of Pleurisy Root (*Asclepias tuberosa*) on page xx;27862, ©2018 Steven Foster, used with permission.
Photo of Baical Scullcap (*Scutellaria baicalensis*) on page 551;86246, ©2018 Steven Foster, used with permission.
Photo of Blue Vervain (*Verbena hastata*) on page 614;81816141, ©2018 Steven Foster, used with permission.

Disclaimer

The herbal remedies and health suggestions offered in this book are gathered from collective knowledge of herbalists around the world and from my personal experience as a medicinal herb grower, private practice registered nurse, and clinical herbalist. The treatments and recommendations in this book are generally regarded to be safe. However, the author is not liable for the reader's misunderstanding or incorrect application of the information and cannot predict or be responsible for individual responses. Information about medicinal herbs continues to change and expand due to ongoing scientific research, clinical data, and differing opinions among authorities. Therefore, it is the responsibility of the reader to be informed and make wise personal health care choices.

The information in this book is intended to supplement rather than be a substitute for professional medical care. Consulting and working with a team of physicians and other healthcare practitioners for health issues are always recommended.

How to Order Additional Copies of *The Art of Herbal Healing*

Please consider supporting the author by buying directly from her website **GreenTurtleBotanicals.com.**

Green Turtle Publishing
Green Turtle Botanical Sanctuary
4830 Dove Bill Lane
Nashville, Indiana 47448

Table of Contents

SECTION ONE
Fundamentals of Medicinal Herbalism

SECTION TWO
The Materia Medica

SECTION THREE

APPENDICES

Dedication

This book is dedicated to the plants that give us life, beauty, and healing medicine,
and to the people who love and tend them.
Thank you for your gifts.

May this book be a worthy voice of the plants
to connect and empower us with the healing potential within Nature and ourselves.

Acknowledgments

My sincere gratitude and thanks to all who helped in the creation of this book:

Dale Edson, who made writing this book possible with his valuable support, computer expertise, and patience in teaching me how to format the book and use Adobe Indesign; and for his love of Nature and help when we cultivated large herb gardens and established a botanical sanctuary together.

Sarah Torbeck, my primary editor, friend, apprentice and fellow plant-lover, whose amazingly astute editing skills and insightful perspective have been indispensable in writing and preparing this book. You will always have my sincere appreciation.

Anne Steigerwald, for beginning the editing process and guiding me with her wise suggestions.

Dark Rain Thom of the Shawnee Nation, United Remnant Band, for sharing her herbal wisdom and healing perspectives, which have been passed down through generations of her Native American ancestors.

The United Plant Savers organization of dedicated herbalists, for their commitment to preserve medicinal herbs, seek solutions for overharvesting, and for their support in education, cultivation, and promoting a North American botanical sanctuary network, which includes my own Green Turtle Botanical Sanctuary. Thank you also for permission to use Kevin Morgan's etching, "If you listen, they will teach you."

Mike Kelsey of Inari Information Services in Bloomington, Indiana, for his professional expertise and kind assistance in helping with the Adobe Indesign program and patiently solving many formatting issues.

Stephen Williams, for being an incredible project manager, designing the book cover, and directing the final stages of completing this book.

Steven Foster, herbalist and photographer, for permission to reproduce three of his photographs.

Graciela Randall, Jennet Walker, and Ingrid Fox at Pfizer Corporation, for permission to reproduce 15 paintings of Robert Thom from two books published by Parke, Davis and Company, *Great Moments in Pharmacy* and *Great Moments in Medicine*.

The Lloyd Library and Museum in Cincinnati, Ohio, for permission to take photographs.

Herbalist Paul Bergner, for permission to quote from his clinical newsletter, *Medicinal Herbalism.*

Marie Romo at New World Library, for permission to quote from Eckhart Tolle's book *Stillness Speaks.*

Rosemarie Cerminaro at Simon & Schuster Publishing, for permission to quote from the book *Lame Deer Seeker of Visions* by John Lame Deer and Richard Erdoes

Andrea Wollitz at National Geographic Society for permission to quote from *Nature's Medicine* by Joel Swerdlow.

Heartfelt thanks to my sons Scott and Noah (you have always taken my herbal medicines, even the most bitter-tasting), family, friends, and students for your patience, love, and support during the lengthy process of writing this book, and to all who have offered suggestions, pointed out errors, and assisted with editing.

Acknowledged with great respect are past and present herbalists, wise women, healers, researchers, authors, and all others whose experience and wisdom have contributed to the global wealth of herbal knowledge and healing practices and have greatly enriched this book.

Introduction

My Life with the Plants

Nature has always been a place of refuge for me. Being among the trees and plants in woodlands and meadows, even as a child, has always been a source of deep stillness. In the graceful beauty of Nature, I was able to intuitively and physically feel that deep well of peace and calm within myself. Nature and the plants became, and continue to be, the great teachers of the "way of life," reflecting the creative forces of life that, when we are observant and pay attention, reveal the wonder and magnificence of the universe within a single flower, and within our own heart. Many years ago, on my 18th birthday, I took an early walk on a cold, crisp morning in late November. As I watched a leaf slowly drop from a tall tree and silently glide to the earth, time became eternal without beginning or end, and all life, like the leaf from that tree, existed in a continual flow of birthing, living, and dying; everything completely connected and interdependent within the hugely diverse web of life. In the few seconds it took for that leaf to fall, I became filled with an understanding of existence and my place of belonging within it. This insight has sustained and inspired me throughout life. Thank you to that tree and leaf and moment in time for such a revelation and life-enhancing teaching!

Soon after this experience, I moved into a rustic cabin with some friends, enjoying a quiet and serene existence of simplicity and close connection with the earth. My interest in medicinal herbs began when I developed a bad head cold and my friend Jeffrey offered me a cup of Goldenseal tea. Although it was quite bitter, I drank it and woke up the next morning surprised to be feeling so much better. From that initial spark, I was "hooked" and began a passionate study of medicinal herbs: drinking herbal teas, using herbal preparations when I got sick, reading all the books and magazines about herbalism that I could find, and writing and accumulating massive pages of notes that became the beginning of this book.

Over the years, I have become acquainted with many healing plants through practical experience. In 1980, I moved into my log cabin home in the hilly woodlands of southern Indiana with my sons, Scott and Noah. It was heaven! As a hiker, I loved roaming the countryside and discovering the abundance of medicinal herbs populating the area. With the guidance of several herb identification books, I slowly and methodically began identifying, collecting, and recording all the local plants with healing ability and historic medicinal uses. I cultivated medicinal plants in my gardens and discovered the joy of having beautiful annual and perennial herbs close to home, within easy reach for harvesting. I grew to know the plants more intimately by observing their life cycles, touching and smelling them, tasting their flavors, and experiencing their healing qualities. Herbalist Paul Strauss of Equinox Botanicals, who I call my "salve mentor," taught a class in which I learned how to make salve and tinctures (alcohol extracts of plants). I became enthralled with the art of creating herbal teas, salves, tinctures, poultices, eyewashes, and many other types of preparations. After gathering plants from the fields, woodlands and gardens, I cleaned, chopped, and processed roots, leaves, and flowers into wonderful medicines in my kitchen. As my experience with herbs evolved, friends and neighbors started asking for herbal advice and preparations, and my sons and family also provided opportunities for learning and healing.

My career in teaching about medicinal herbs and holistic healing began with an invitation to speak at a large gathering in the early 1980s. Since then, I have been blessed with the opportunity to offer many classes, and teaching about the plants and sharing their healing gifts with others is one of my favorite and most rewarding activities. As I look back at this special time, I see that it had a magical quality. The medicinal herbs were continually becoming a more intimate part of my life, not only in their healing ways but by sharing their beauty and bringing balance, meaning, financial support, and good people into my life.

Motivated by the vision to become a registered nurse and develop a private practice in which I could incorporate holistic healing and medicinal herbalism, I returned to college and graduated from Indiana University School of Nursing with a Bachelor of Science degree in Nursing in 1988. After almost four years of working at Bloomington Hospital as a medical/surgical charge nurse, I took a leap of faith and left the hospital to manifest my vision. Everything fell into place and I quickly developed a successful holistic nursing practice in Bloomington, Indiana, with clients of all ages seeking help for a wide variety of health issues and health maintenance.

Becoming involved in Traditional Chinese Medicine (TCM), I visited China in 1995 with a delegation of nurses to study TCM. We were instructed in basic TCM theory, Chinese herbalism, Tuina (traditional Chinese massage), Qi Gong, and Tai Chi. After returning from China, I completed a year-long program of TCM and oriental massage through the New York College for Holistic Health, Education and Research. In 1999, I was certified as a Holistic Nurse Practitioner by the American Holistic Nursing Association. In my nursing practice, the holistic perspective of healing and herbalism is blended with the Western allopathic medical model and Traditional Chinese Medicine (TCM) to evaluate clients and provide them with a comprehensive health care program. Nutritional food and herbal therapies are typically recommended as a foundation to promote strong, healthy minds and bodies. I am grateful for my nursing practice because it is constantly exciting and fulfilling to help people be empowered by participating in their own healing journey and witnessing the healing potential of the plants and the human body.

While enjoying my nursing practice, I became a member of United Plant Savers (UpS), a grassroots organization of herbalists dedicated to herbal research and education; cultivating and preserving medicinal plants, especially endangered species; and helping people develop botanical sanctuaries on their property. Sharing the same dedication and responsibility of stewardship towards the land and plants, I established my property and gardens as Green Turtle Botanical Sanctuary under the umbrella of UpS. My one-day herb workshops evolved into six-month medicinal herb apprenticeship and intern programs. The herb gardens, meadows, and woodlands were the main "classrooms" and provided abundant plant material to make teas and other herbal preparations. Students learned about the herbs through study and personal experience, including their history, healing properties, how to identify, cultivate and harvest them, and how to create teas, tinctures, salves, poultices, and other remedies. Apprentices and interns participated in all the projects and activities at Green Turtle Botanical Sanctuary, established their own herb gardens at home using Sanctuary seeds and plants, and developed an extensive pharmacy of herbal preparations. We grew together in the spirit of friendship and love of the herbs as we played in the dirt, planted seeds, chopped roots, drank tea, shared our dreams and insights when the plants spoke to us, and immersed ourselves in the wonders, beauty, and healing gifts of the plants. The medicinal herbs have been a constant source of inspiration and fulfillment throughout my life. I am grateful for the gracious bounty of healing gifts they shower on me and so many others.

This book arises from the hearts and voices of the plants and from the place within myself that abides in their healing ways. It is offered to you as a guide and companion for healing and restoring balance in your life and, hopefully, in the lives of others. It is my sincere wish that this book serves you well, that the pages become worn and tattered over time as you explore and experience the healing potential of the magnificent plants.

May you feel the heartbeat of Mother Earth within your own heart, and may the beauty, wisdom, and healing gifts of the plants enrich your life and make you whole.

Susan Clearwater, RN, BSN

March 21, 2018

The Holistic Perspective

Living and Healing in Holism

My perspective of life, the foundation of my nursing and herbal practices, and *The Art of Herbal Healing: A Guide to Health and Wholeness* are all inherently rooted in holism. The word "holism" comes from the Greek *holos,* meaning "all, whole, entire." Holism is the fundamental condition in which all parts and individual units make up the whole of creation; all parts are inseparably contained within wholeness. The whole is always greater than the sum of its parts, and each part or individual unit can be fully understood only by looking at its function and relationship to the whole.

When applying holism in medicine and healing, all aspects of the individual are taken into consideration, including the physical body, food and nutrition, psychological thought patterns and beliefs, emotions, and social relationships with family and friends. In the holistic model of the human body, all cells, tissues, glands, and organs are understood to be related, interdependent units that influence each other and make up the whole body. When using medicinal herbs in health care, the holistic view helps us understand that the healing capacity of a plant comes from the synergistic combination of hundreds of chemical constituents within each plant. The biological effects from ingesting a whole plant preparation will be different than taking one chemical by itself.

A core foundation of holism is an intuitive understanding that the smallest known particles and the essence of everything – rocks, plants, animals, humans, and even plastic – is light. Sages and ancient teachings spoke of this truth and regarded people as emerging from light, as children of light. Modern science and breakthroughs in quantum physics demonstrate that all matter, including the human body, is composed of particles of light. Light is a wave or stream of energy, and the higher the wave frequency, the more energy it carries. These discoveries bring awareness that light is the thread of life that connects and unites each individual with the whole of existence, making everything related and interdependent. The essence of everyone and everything is light, and each one of us is part of the boundless wholeness of the universe and never separate from it.

Within the light that permeates all matter dwells pure consciousness, also called divine presence or innate intelligence, manifesting in the DNA encoded in the cells of every plant and animal, and in the universal patterns and organization of Nature from the tiniest atom to the vast bodies of planets, stars, and suns throughout our universe. Every human being is an inseparable part of Nature. The intelligence that sustains Nature is the same innate intelligence of the body that makes our hearts beat, our lungs breathe, our immune systems fight infections, and infants grow and develop within the womb – all without conscious awareness or directive from the human mind. By recognizing the miraculous unfolding and interdependence of all life, we are better able to trust and abide in the intelligence of Nature, the body's intelligence and ability to heal, and in the intelligence and medicine of the healing plants growing from the earth.

Nature is the universal teacher and healer because it is the pure manifestation and natural outflow of the creative force known as God, the Great Mystery, supreme universal intelligence, and space of limitless creative potential from which the universe and all life arise. Everyone has access to Nature, which is all-inclusive and not segmented or diminished by national borders, cultural bias, and religious differences. Plants are teachers that can guide us to greater balance and more vibrant health because they embody the wholeness and abundance of life. Developing a relationship and connection with Nature through the plants is a life-transforming experience that continually brings new awareness, peace, joy, and vitality into one's existence. Experiencing the peaceful quiet of Nature helps us feel that same stillness within ourselves. In this stillness of being dwells the heart of compassion, clear awareness, and potential to heal at the deepest levels.

In his book *Stillness Speaks,* Eckhart Tolle beautifully elaborates:

> The moment you become aware of a plant's emanation of stillness and peace, that plant becomes your teacher. Watch an animal, a flower, a tree, and see how it rests in Being. It *is* itself. It has enormous dignity, innocence, and holiness. However, for you to see that, you need to go beyond the mental habit of naming and labeling. The moment you look beyond mental labels, you feel that ineffable dimension of nature that cannot be understood by thought or perceived through the senses. It is a harmony, a sacredness that permeates not only the whole of nature but is also within you. (Tolle, 2003)

It is vital for our individual health and the environment of the earth that we understand the holism within Nature and ourselves and that we learn to live in this balance of wholeness. The segmented view that our body and the world are a conglomeration of separate, unrelated parts creates disruption in the human psyche and body, resulting in experiences of isolation, fear, and "dis-ease." When we take the great leap in identifying ourselves as the beings of light we actually are, we more easily tap into our inner source of peace, wisdom, compassion, and healing potential.

Maintaining a *dynamic state of balance* in all aspects of our life is essential for optimal health of both mind and body. This includes balance within the individual and between the individual and the environment. From a purely energetic viewpoint, *a simple definition of individual health is the balanced flow of energy throughout the body*, which nourishes and vitalizes cells and organs to function harmoniously within the whole system. *Pain and illness arise when the flow of energy is disturbed, blocked, excessive, or deficient.* A balanced flow of energy throughout the body is always enhanced by emotional and psychological peace and well-being, substantial nutrients, clean air and water, adequate activity and rest, time spent in Nature, and life-affirming choices. Balance between the individual and environment refers to the environment of our relationships with the people we live, work, and spend time with and to the physical environment we live in, whether a city, suburbia, or country setting.

It is essential to realize that the *underlying cause of most disease, especially chronic degenerative conditions, is disruption in the flow of energy within the body*. This disruption of energy originates from 1) being out of touch and unconnected with our inner being, the space of stillness and access to compassion, innate intelligence, and healing potential; 2) discord from erroneous perceptions and misinterpretations of ourself and the world; and 3) reinforcing and habitually clinging to harmful, disturbing thoughts and emotions based in fear, anger, isolation, and the assortment of other psychological sufferings that plague humanity. When using herbs and other healing modalities, it is imperative that we pay attention to our thoughts and emotions with the intention of bringing them into a calm and dynamic balance. By reducing anxiety brought about by disturbing, harmful thoughts and emotions, our life force, rather than being disrupted and dissipated, is focused on the innate impulse of the body to heal physically and psychologically. Addressing illness from these causal levels is a source of true healing that goes beyond symptomatic relief. Even natural remedies like herbs, vitamins, and healthy foods can be insufficient if these basic holistic principles are not understood and utilized.

Embracing the enlightened attitude that *illness and pain are opportunities for transformation, wholeness, and healing* gives meaning and purpose to difficult situations. By releasing the energies of guilt, shame, and belief that illness is punishment, we mobilize our restorative healing abilities. *Sickness is a profound teacher*, urging us to dive deep within to explore the inner universe of our body and the nature of our thoughts and emotions. Sickness and pain invite us to courageously examine, forgive, and release old patterns and ways of thinking and acting that no longer serve us, and to nurture our life force by connecting with our inner wisdom and healing potential.

Rather than fighting our physical imperfections and infirmities as an enemy, *the experience of suffering eases when we accept and embrace the reality of life* – that we are born into a body for a temporary amount of time, we live in our body and experience life, the body ages, weakens, illness occurs as a normal event of life, and eventually the body dies from accidents, illness, or deterioration from old age (notice that I did not say *you* die). Rather than ignoring or fearing these conditions of human existence, *empower yourself and harness your healing potential by being radically accepting and grateful for your body and the circumstances of your life*. To a great extent, it is our response to life's difficulties that determine the outcome rather than the difficulty itself. Problems appearing to be unworkable are often solved not by attacking the problem, but by changing our attitudes and interpretation of the situation. We usually have no control over other people or situations external to ourselves, but we can be empowered to promote positive change by observing and adjusting our own attitudes and behaviors.

Do not be diminished or limited by identifying yourself as your body, thoughts, emotions, or illness. The truth is that you reside in your body and experience thoughts, emotions and sickness, but you are much more than these. How can we rely on our thoughts and emotions for stability and security when they can easily change from one extreme to another in a short time, creating constant ups and downs in our moods and experience of happiness? It has been said that "thoughts and emotions have as much substance as clouds in the sky." Lack of control over random thoughts and disturbing emotions creates chaos and imbalance in the flow of energy throughout the body's tissues, fluids, and nerves. It is well known that feelings and expressions of love and joy create a movement of energy radiating outward that relaxes the body, increases life force and vitality, and promotes life-enhancing chemicals, immunity, and feelings of well-being. The opposite occurs when fear, anger, hatred or grief consume us, which distorts and restricts the flow of energy and life force through the body, causing rigidity, anxiety, weakened life force and immunity, and greater tendency towards physical and psychological illness and suffering.

Although we reside in our body for a length of time and all of our choices and actions are directed by our thoughts and emotions, how much time do we actually spend examining our physical body and the thoughts, concepts, and feelings of our daily experiences? How often do we feel controlled and powerless by incessant disturbing thoughts, raging emotions, or destabilizing anxiety? We live in such a chaotic and often cruel world, and it can easily feel like we are alone and adrift in a turbulent, stormy sea with no life-jacket for stability.

Understanding that our thoughts and emotions have an extremely powerful influence in either promoting or diminishing health and well-being illustrates the importance of using our conscious intent to bring balance to these aspects of ourself. Remember that whatever we focus our attention on grows because our attention is a force of energy moving from our mind out to the point of focus. In the same way, "e-motions" are "energy in motion." So it is vital to put attention into inspiring and directing our minds to understand and engage in holism as a model for health and opportunity to enjoy a more fulfilling, active life.

To expand the understanding and experience of holism and to tap into the healing potential of Nature, the medicinal herbs, and your own body, I sincerely encourage you to 1) spend as much time as possible in Nature with the plants, and 2) engage in a daily exploration into the "universe of you." Spend as much time as possible outside in Nature to more easily relax by feeling the peaceful calm inherent in plants and the land itself. Commit to developing a daily routine of sitting quietly in a peaceful place to relax, bring your focus of attention to yourself, and courageously explore your thoughts, feelings, and the physical sensations within your body. Spend time every day, whether ten minutes or one hour, to relax, breathe, and pay attention to what is going on within yourself. Early mornings are often the best time for these sessions and are a peaceful yet powerful way to start the day. Before settling down, some people benefit from gentle, centering movements such as Tai Chi, Qi Gong, and Hatha Yoga. When ready to sit and focus your mind and develop intention, it is helpful to read something inspirational, ask for help through prayer, or sing and use the power of sound to balance and heal. If discomfort or pain is felt in your body, if grief is felt in your heart or anger in your gut, explore and embrace these with kindness as you would a hurt child or animal. As you inhale, draw your breath to your heart, acknowledging the life-giving, healing energy in each breath you take. From your heart, as you exhale, use your breath to push the energy to any area of discomfort. Examine your thoughts, attitudes, and feelings about yourself and the world – these direct and dictate our actions. Allowing misguided, incorrect ideas to "pilot" our life eventually causes the suffering of physical and psychological illness. Developing some control over the mind and emotions enables us to have more control over our physical body and inner life. Over time, as you practice this process, your body and mind will respond by naturally relaxing, opening and healing, allowing greater connection with the calm center of innate intelligence within you. You are invited to experience several beautiful healing meditations that come directly from the plants that are in the deva readings from the Materia Medica section of this book (see Deva Meditations in the index).

A quiet time of daily reflection and inner discovery can become the "life-jacket" in the stormy sea of life, the anchor connecting us to the inner calm and intelligence of creation that is the essential core of light within each human being. Embarking on this journey of discovery through our inner landscape is challenging and rewarding in countless ways. Feeling connected with our inner being opens us to feel the same connection with other people, animals, the plants, and all of Nature. The connection we feel for the wholeness of life brings freedom from the bondage of feeling separated and isolated. As we connect and identify with the inner light of which the ancients and quantum physicists have spoken, we tap into the essence of healing.

Plants provide humankind with indigenous medicines brought forth from the innate intelligence of Nature and the earth. Medicinal herbs work with the natural functions and forces of the body to promote balance and enhance the inherent ability to heal. As you develop a relationship with the herbs and use them in your health care, remember to empower yourself and harness your healing potential by trusting in the innate intelligence of Nature, the plants, and your own body. Speak to the plants from your heart, open yourself to their healing potential with gratitude, and allow them to bring greater beauty, health, joy, and peace into your life and touch your heart to the core.

A human being is part of the whole, called by us 'Universe,'
a part limited in time and space.
He experiences himself, his thoughts and
feelings as something separated from the rest,
a kind of optical delusion of his consciousness.

This delusion is a kind of prison for us,
restricting us to our personal desires and
affection for a few persons nearest us.

Our task must be to free ourselves from this prison
by widening our circle of compassion
to embrace all living creatures
and the whole of nature in its beauty.

Albert Einstein

How To Use This Book

The Art of Herbal Healing: A Guide to Health and Wholeness is a comprehensive guide and reference for wise and responsible health care. In addressing the multiple aspects of medicinal herbalism and its application in healing, the book is broad in scope and covers a vast expanse of time and perspective, from the mythology and wisdom of ancient cultures and traditions to modern times with advanced scientific research, technology, and new discoveries and applications. The subtle yet powerful intrinsic energies of plants and the healing process are explored and revealed, adding a beautiful and enlightened dimension to our understanding and relationship with Nature and the medicinal herbs. You, the reader, are invited to participate in the wondrous world of the healing herbs through experiential interaction with living plants in the wilds and gardens. Within these pages, you are provided with thorough instructions and visual guides to enable you to interact with medicinal herbs at whatever level you choose — from gardening, harvesting, and creating herbal teas and other preparations to deciding which herbs are helpful for specific conditions.

Since the herbs are the main characters in the book, their common names are respectfully capitalized. And because I discourage the harvesting and medicinal use of endangered plant species (unless they come from renewable cultivated sources), they are not recommended and are only mentioned for historical reference. Every attempt has been made to create a user-friendly book allowing fast and easy access to information and references. The book is divided into three sections.

Section One, *Fundamentals of Medicinal Herbalism*, offers basic information to provide the reader with a strong foundation for thorough study and safe, intelligent use of medicinal herbs in health care. Familiarity with the material in Section One will greatly benefit the reader in understanding and applying the information given in the *Materia Medica* and the rest of the book. The chapter titled "The History of Herbalism and Early Medicine" explores the beginning of herbal healing and early history of modern medicine, which emerged from plant and other natural therapies. The healing traditions of Native Americans, Europeans, Traditional Chinese Medicine, Ayurvedic medicine from India, and Unani medicine from the Islamic culture are the primary focus. "Nomenclature and Classification of Plants" explains the Latin binomial system of naming and classifying plants. The physical structure of plants and the miraculous ways they exist and function in Nature are described in "Botany for Herbalists." The chapter "Endangered Medicinal Herbs ~ Botanical Sanctuaries to the Rescue" addresses the dilemma of the continuing popularity and rising demand for medicinal herbs, which is causing reduced plant populations and dangers of extinction. In response, botanical sanctuaries throughout North America are being developed as workable solutions to this problem. Active participation in cultivating and harvesting herbs is an increasingly necessary aspect of herbalism and a primary focus of this book. Two chapters, "Cultivating Medicinal Herbs" and "Sustainable Harvesting of Medicinal Herbs," are dedicated to this and bring the process to life in the garden and wild-growth areas. "Drying and Storing Medicinal Herbs" and "Creating Herbal Preparations" provide detailed instructions with pictures for preparing a wide variety of herbal remedies including teas, tinctures, salves, poultices, eye washes, and flower essences. Three chapters, "Creating Herbal Formulas," "How to Calculate Dosages" and "Weights and Measures for the Herbalist," contain helpful information and charts to use when preparing and administering herbal remedies. The chapter on "The Safety of Medicinal Herbs" explores the issues of herbal safety, contraindications, and drug interactions. In "Chemical Constituents in Plants," the primary compounds, or phytochemicals, in plants that are responsible for their healing actions are examined. The final chapter in Section One, "Healing Qualities of Herbs," can be used as an additional index when choosing herbs that are appropriate for treating specific health issues.

Section Two consists of *The Materia Medica,* which contains comprehensive information on 50 medicinal herbs. The material on each herb is arranged in a specific sequence of topic headings that are reviewed in the first chapter, "How to Use the Materia Medica." Brief explanations of Traditional Chinese Medicine and the plant devas and their teachings are provided at the end of this chapter. The second chapter, "How to Use Herbs for Healing and Daily Health Care," offers basic suggestions and considerations when incorporating medicinal herbs into one's lifestyle. The remaining chapters are the Materia Medica.

Section Three consists of two references. ***The Art of Herbal Healing* contains two primary indexes**. The *General Index* appears at the end of the book. In Section Three, the "Index of Health Issues and Herbal Recommendations" is an extensive index of health problems with listings of appropriate herbs to address each condition. This index is intended to be a primary reference tool to use when choosing appropriate herbs to maintain optimum health and vitality, build immunity, and prevent and treat specific health issues. The second reference in Section Three, "Herbs for Pregnancy, Childbirth and Lactation," discusses how to use specific nutritious and medicinal herbs that have an extensive history of safe use during these sensitive times in a woman's and infant's life.

Three Appendices include the "Glossary" for easy reference, a "Cross-Reference of Common and Botanical Plant Names," and a list of "Media Sources for Herbal Research."

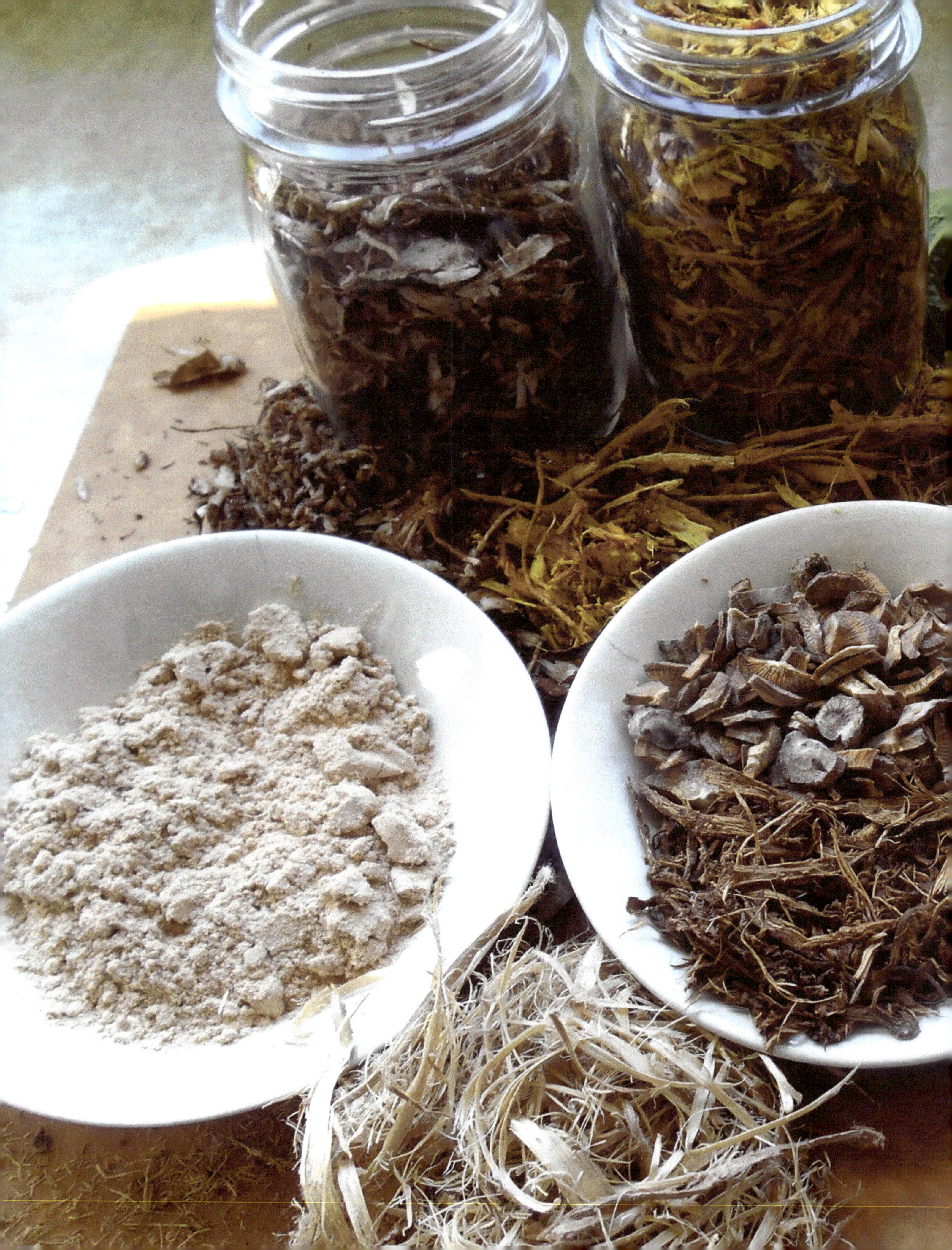

SECTION ONE

Fundamentals of Medicinal Herbalism

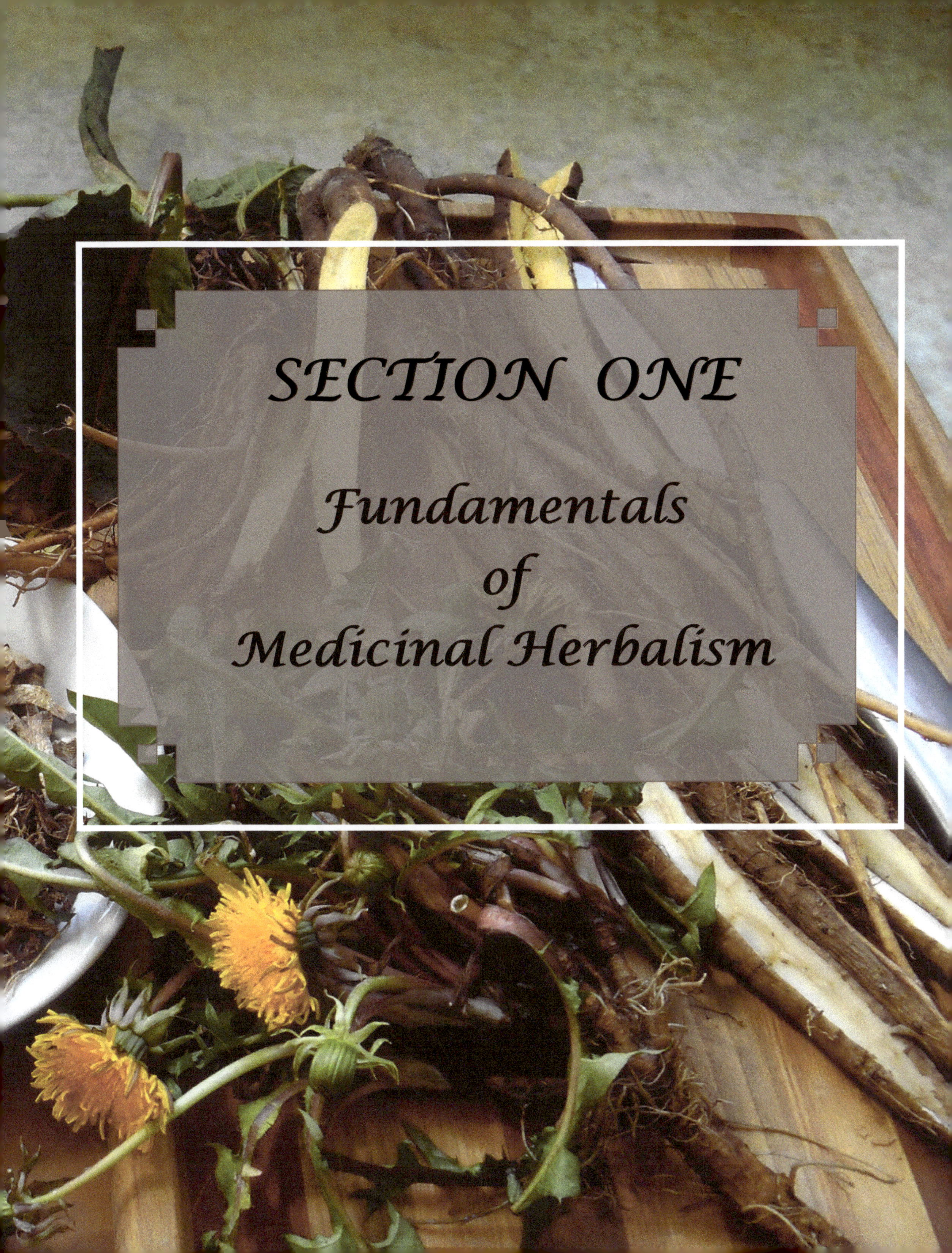

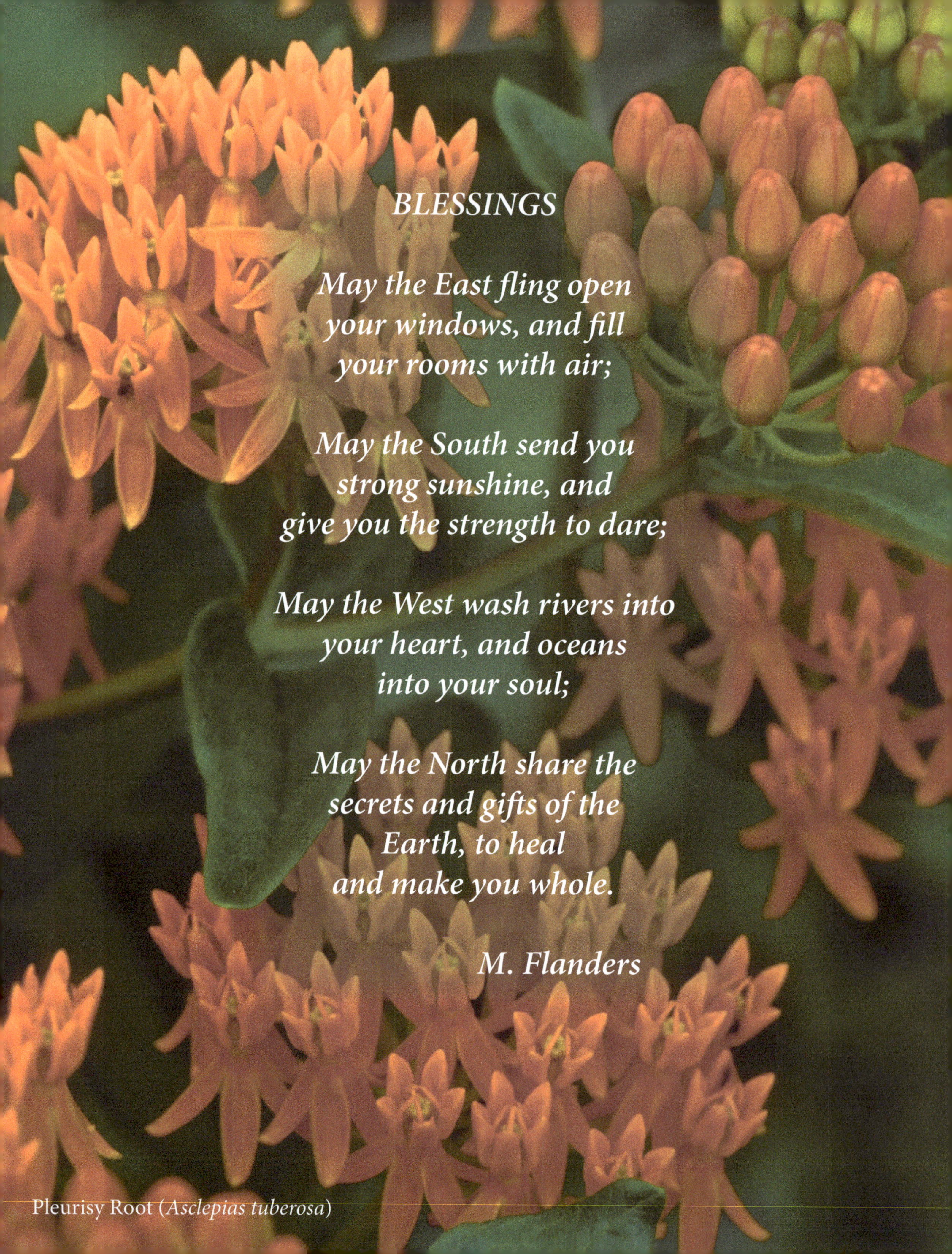

BLESSINGS

May the East fling open
your windows, and fill
your rooms with air;

May the South send you
strong sunshine, and
give you the strength to dare;

May the West wash rivers into
your heart, and oceans
into your soul;

May the North share the
secrets and gifts of the
Earth, to heal
and make you whole.

M. Flanders

Pleurisy Root (*Asclepias tuberosa*)

The History of Herbalism and Early Medicine

Since the emergence of humanity, the plant kingdom has abundantly provided us with a multitude of blessings. All animal and human life depends on plants as our source of food and fundamental necessities for existence. Our prehistoric ancestors learned to use plants for shelter, clothing, dyes, cosmetics, weapons, magical charms, and protective amulets. Herbal plants and ornamental flowers adorned people and buildings, and were used in religious rituals, celebrations, rites of passage, and to celebrate births and honor the dead. Herbs were valued for incense, embalming, and to flavor and preserve foods. The most significant use of herbs throughout history, however, has been for medicinal healing.

Most people suffer from illness during their lifetime. In response to this universal need to heal disease and reduce suffering, ancient people turned to the materials in their immediate environment in their quest to find remedies. No one knows how long it took them to uncover the healing power of plants and develop the art of herbalism. We can only imagine how humankind's knowledge of medicinal herbs evolved over time. Our ancestors learned by instinct and intuitive wisdom, by "listening" to the natural world around them, by observing which plants sick or injured animals ate, and through generations of trial and error and clinical observations.

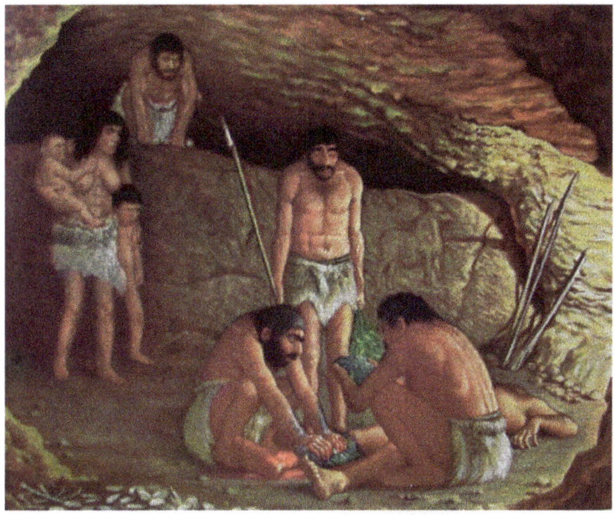

Before the Dawn of History

Image by Robert Thom. Courtesy of Pfizer Inc.

Folk medicine is the oldest tradition of herbal healing, originating in prehistoric times. Based on word-of-mouth transmission of knowledge, it was passed on by the common people, from mother to daughter and master to student over many generations. As time passed and people grew more sophisticated in discovering and implementing the healing properties of plants, the wealth of herbal knowledge evolved into rich and practical folk medicine traditions. All ancient cultures and civilizations engaged in a common quest to learn the secrets of healing and relied on plants to treat illness. Although cultures used different plants according to their geographical locations, they all developed herbal folk traditions. Herbal manuscripts were hand-written until the invention of the printing press greatly augmented the cross-cultural exchange of knowledge and development of herbal medicine. As the science of botany evolved and systems of naming and classifying plants were established, philosophies and techniques of herbal healing developed. Advances in chemistry and technology resulted in a continual expanse of scientific information about the medicinal properties of plants and their applications in healing.

Herbs were the primary substance of medical treatment worldwide from prehistoric times until the 1800s, when advances in Western technology enabled scientists to isolate chemicals from plants to make standardized medicine and produce synthetic drugs. As these "new age" synthetic medicines became more popular, university-trained doctors, who established the new and increasingly dominant **Western allopathic medical system**, incorporated these drugs into their practice. Most doctors eventually stopped prescribing herbal preparations, considering them inferior and old-fashioned. Not only were herbal medicines dismissed, but the **holistic philosophy of healing**, fundamental to the art of herbalism, was also forsaken. This ancient philosophy views health as a dynamic balance within the body and between the individual and the environment. Nature is the great healer, and by living a life in balance with nature and natural laws, optimal health might be achieved. The ancient focus on the integrated healing of body, emotions, mind, and spirit was replaced by the reductionistic reliance on chemical and synthetic drugs, rather than nature, to heal. Over time, allopathic medicine came to be viewed as the most sophisticated and advanced form of medicine throughout most of the world, and eventually nations in South and Central America, Africa, the Middle East, and Asia followed the trend of the Western world in adopting allopathic medicine. Many professionally trained doctors abandoned their traditional herbal healing systems. However, while most allopathic physicians disregarded the healing benefits of herbs, the knowledge and art of herbalism was kept alive by many of the common people. In remote areas like the American Appalachian Mountains, the Amazon jungle, and villages in Africa and Asia where herbal healers and shamans were the only available doctors, the traditional folk practice of herbalism quietly, and sometimes secretly, coexisted with the modern medical world.

A change of consciousness, rippling through America and Europe during the late 1960s and 1970s, resulted in an herbal renaissance that spread throughout the world. Today, more people actively take responsibility for their health through improved lifestyle, spiritual and religious practice, and the use of vitamins, minerals, and herbal preparations. The ancient philosophy that "nature heals" is returning to mainstream awareness. Many people in the general population, including naturopathic doctors, chiropractors, holistic nurses and medical physicians, are embracing this more enlightened perspective.

The predominant allopathic medical system provides important drugs, technology, and incredibly effective diagnostic and surgical techniques to relieve human suffering. However, a significant and growing portion of the population is demanding that more medicinal herbs and other holistic therapies be incorporated into our mainstream medical system. Consequently, there is renewed scientific research to determine the chemical properties and biological activities of many plants and their appropriate uses in medicine. Interestingly, this research tends to validate the ancient uses of many herbs. It is, in fact, these venerable folk medicine traditions that form the basis of modern herbal knowledge and application, as well as the development of pharmaceutical drugs.

The history of herbalism is intimately intertwined with the early history of medicine. Both emerged from the beliefs, theology, and philosophy of different cultures throughout time, and were regulated by the ruling powers that controlled the political, religious, educational, and healing systems of the people. It is a complex and interesting history. This chapter focuses on the evolution of herbs in Western medicine and includes examination of Native North American healing traditions, Islamic Unani herbalism, Chinese medicine, and India's Ayurvedic system. The following is a condensed glimpse and interpretation of the history of herbalism, a vast and intricate aspect of the human experience.

The Great Mother/Goddess Traditions

As prehistoric people evolved from a nomadic hunter-gatherer existence into a more settled agricultural lifestyle, ancient civilizations acknowledged the nurturing, feminine qualities of the earth, which provided them with boundless vegetation, animals, and life itself. People expressed their love and reverence for this feminine life-giving power by worshiping her personification as the Great Mother or Goddess. Her attributes were expressed and given form through art and sculpture. Numerous pictographs, pieces of pottery, and sculptures portraying women in stone, clay, and bone have been discovered throughout Europe and the Middle East, and are the most tangible evidence of this ancient Goddess culture.

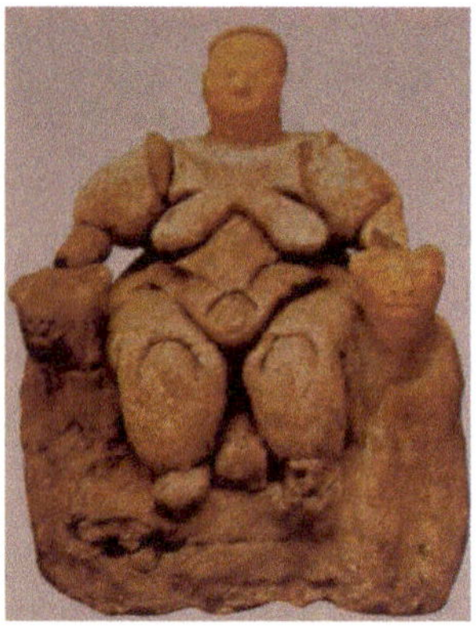

Statue of a fertility goddess giving birth *circa* 5700–6500 B.C.

The Great Mother/Goddess is usually portrayed as a rotund, fertile woman with a large pregnant belly and full breasts exemplifying the archetypal female qualities of nurturing, fertility, abundance, and benevolent compassion. The Goddess is the personification of nature, the earth and feminine aspect of life, and she is the provider of food and herbal medicine. She is the Great Mother of all life and creatures. As Mother Nature, the Goddess embodies the living biosphere of the earth and the elemental forces of fire, air, earth, and water. She embodies the emotions and intuition, birth, death, and the "mysteries of life."

The Goddess religion evolved over time. Worshipers bestowed offerings and held ceremonies to honor her. The blessings of the Goddess were invoked when fields were planted and harvested, when young women passed into puberty, when babies were born, and during other celebrations and passages of life.

Different cultural expressions of this feminine earth-based religion flourished in ancient Mesopotamia, Egypt, Europe, Asia, and the Americas. Historians estimate that the Goddess religion originated with the nomadic hunters in Paleolithic times over 35,000 years ago. Over time, the Goddess has been adorned with many names and forms. In the ancient Sumerian culture she was called Inanna, Eriskegan, Irnini, and eventually evolved into the Babylonian Goddess, Ishtar. Prehistoric Egyptians worshiped several of her forms culminating in Isis, whose following continued in Rome until A.D. 394, when the last of her temples closed. Images of the Goddess as the Queen of Heaven, dating back to 7000 B.C., have been found along the eastern Mediterranean coast. The healing system of the Goddess religion was based on herbal medicines and the art of living in balance with nature. Hippocrates, who is considered to be the "father of medicine," practiced the Asclepian medical tradition, which was an extension of the Goddess religion.

Over time, many of these ancient matriarchal cultures practicing the Great Mother/Goddess religion were invaded and dominated by more powerful and aggressive people. These conquerors replaced the Goddess with their own masculine warrior gods. In ancient Greece, all the personifications of the Goddess were married to these new warrior gods, resulting in the Olympic Pantheon. The Goddess religion, also known as the Old Religion, was incorporated into the ancient Druid culture in the British Isles. Fragments of the Goddess religion survived in Europe until the advent of the Christian church and the Inquisition, when it was replaced by the masculine image of God promoted by Christianity. During this time, the Church fought hard to suppress and root out all Goddess worship. In modern times, veneration of Mary, the mother of Jesus, has replaced devotion to the Goddess, but Mary continues to embody the classic feminine qualities of nurturing, love, and compassion that rest at the heart of the Earth Mother/Goddess traditions.

Ancient Mesopotamian and Egyptian Herbal and Medical Traditions

The earliest evidence and accounts of herbal healing extend far back into antiquity. Ancient writings and pictographs from Mesopotamia, Egypt, India, and China confirm that these civilizations, quite knowledgeable about the medicinal qualities and cultivation of many plants, established sophisticated and skilled healing traditions. One of the oldest specimens providing proof of early man's use of healing plants was discovered inside a cave in northern Iraq during an archeological dig in 1960. Scientists believed the cave was the burial site of a Neanderthal man whose remains are estimated to be around 60,000 years old. An analysis of the soil around the bone remnants revealed pollen and fragments of at least eight species of medicinal plants that had been placed around the body, indicating early use of herbs at burial sites.

The oldest known written records of herbal medicine are clay tablets of the Sumerians of Mesopotamia, an ancient civilization that encompassed the Tigris and Euphrates river basin and what is now eastern Syria, southeastern Turkey, and most of Iraq. Many consider Mesopotamia to be the "cradle of civilization." These clay tablets were written between 5000–3000 B.C. and describe well-established uses for Poppy, Belladonna, Mandrake, Henbane, Hemp, Senna, Garlic, Licorice, Myrrh, Thyme, Cumin, Sage, Laurel, Saffron, Caraway, and many other herbs commonly used today. On the clay tablets, ancient physicians recorded symptoms of diseases, herbal prescriptions and directions for their preparation, and an invocation to the gods used during healing ceremonies.

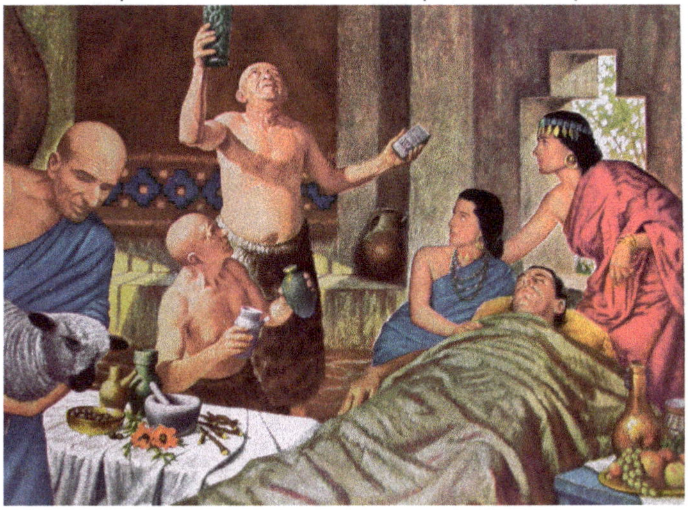

Pharmacy in Ancient Babylonia
Image by Robert Thom. Courtesy of Pfizer Inc.

The religion and mythology of ancient Persia emerged from the belief in two creators and two creations that existed simultaneously. Ahura Mazda was the god of light and creator of all goodness, who was assisted by lesser deities. Opposing them was Angra Mayniu, the god of evil, ignorance and darkness, who struggled for possession of the world. Medicine played an important role in this mythology. The art of healing was said to have originated in the garden of Ameretat, the goddess of long life. Thousands of herbal plants grew in her garden, including a tree that cured all sickness and bestowed immortality. The sick prayed to Mithra, the god of health.

In ancient Persia and other old civilizations, the art of healing and use of medicinal plants were often associated with the mysterious and supernatural. Healers were believed to have special knowledge and connection with the spirit world. As time progressed, medical practitioners became associated with priestly functions and the priest-magician became the healer of both body and soul. Prayers, incantations, and herbal preparations were the treatments used to purge the body from the demons of disease.

Stone artifacts indicate that hunters, gatherers, and fishermen inhabited the Nile River basin in Egypt over 12,000 years ago. As populations became less nomadic, agriculture developed and grains, vegetables, and fruit became primary food crops. Healers wildcrafted herbs and the cultivation of medicinal plants evolved. The Egyptian civilization, like the Sumerians and other ancient Mesopotamians, believed in supernatural forces. Deities and demons influenced their world, controlling daily life, health, and disease. Most illness not caused by obvious reasons was believed to be the work of evil spirits and wrath of malevolent gods. Thus magic, religion, and medicine were inseparably intertwined. Ancient Egypt was a repository of occult knowledge, particularly in the field of medicine and the priesthood. Evoking the supernatural to drive out evil entities was part of the cure for disease. Herbal preparations, magic, incantations, amulets, and appealing for favors from the multitude of Egyptian gods and goddesses were important aspects of healing performed by the priest, magician, and physician. Ancient Mesopotamians and Egyptians also used astrology to determine the influence of the planets and constellations on human life and health. This close association between medicine, magic, nature, and religion has remained in human consciousness for thousands of years, continuing through the Roman Empire into the Middle Ages, the Renaissance, and into modern times.

Physical evidence of Egyptian herbal medicine dates back to 10,000–5000 B.C., revealing that medical practice and herbal remedies were very advanced. A basic knowledge of anatomy was probably obtained from the practice of embalming the dead. Reading the pulse played an important part in medical assessment. Physicians knew how to make herbal dressings for wounds and perform surgery. Advanced levels of personal and social hygiene were practiced. Early Egyptian physicians kept detailed accounts describing culinary and medicinal uses for plants, recording prevalent diseases and their treatments on scrolls of papyrus (crude paper) that were several yards long. The oldest papyrus yet discovered is the *Kahun Gynecology Papyrus* dating back to 1825 B.C. It describes methods of diagnosing pregnancy, diseases of women, and medical treatments, including herbal preparations and vaginal medications. The *Ebers Papyrus,* written *circa* 1500 B.C., is the most famous and lengthy collection of ancient Egyptian medical writing. It is a collection of 811 prescriptions composed of 700 drugs with directions for their preparation. The prescriptions were composed primarily of herbs in addition to some animal parts and minerals. Some of the plants mentioned are Aniseed, Cinnamon, Dill, Fenugreek, Flaxseed, Garlic, Licorice, Sesame, Myrrh, Parsley, Thyme, Turmeric, Basil, Bayberry, Mandrake, Castor bean oil, Opium Poppy, Cannabis, Willow, Frankincense, Fennel, Senna, Juniper, Aloe, Coriander, and Cumin. The *Ebers Papyrus* includes formulas for teas, pills, lotions, ointments, salves, suppositories, enemas, inhalants, snuffs, gargles, eye drops, and poultices. It describes how active ingredients of herbs were extracted in water, milk, honey, beer, wine or oil, and how polypharmacy (combining several herbs) was practiced. The *Ebers Papyrus* was a reference for internal medicine as well as diseases of the eyes, skin, and reproductive organs. It included knowledge about the position of the heart, blood circulation, and human anatomy and physiology. Magical incantations, spells, and remedies reputed to have originated and been used by various gods were also mentioned. Many remedies in the *Ebers Papyrus* are thought to come from a time of remote antiquity, and the dates and authors of the *Papyrus* remain unknown.

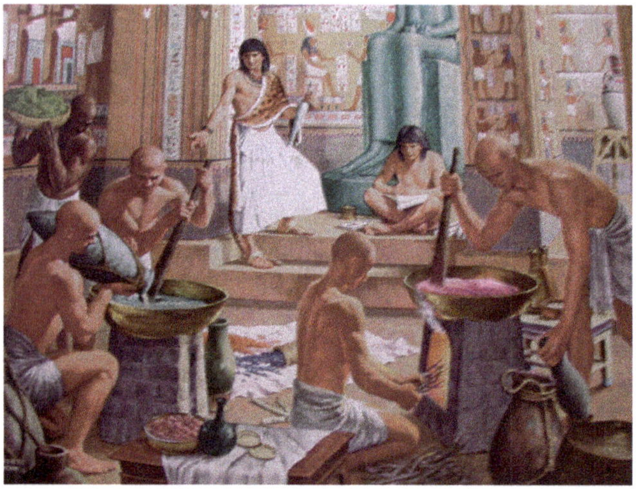

Days of the *Papyrus Ebers*
Image by Robert Thom. Courtesy of Pfizer Inc.

The *Edwin Smith Papyrus,* named after the American who purchased it in 1862, is an older document believed to have been written between 1700–1550 B.C., although it may be based on more antiquated texts written about 2640 B.C. This papyrus is second to the *Ebers Papyrus* in length and describes 48 surgical cases involving wounds of the head, neck, shoulders, and chest. It includes instructions of diagnostic procedures, examinations, herbal treatments, and surgical techniques.

Scholars believe that the Egyptian medical system consisted of an elite group of specialists. Included were the physicians who directly cared for the sick and administered medicines, and the pharmacists who prepared the medicinal preparations. Herb gatherers traveled within and outside Egypt to gather plants for the pharmacists, while the "conservators" properly prepared and stored the herbs.

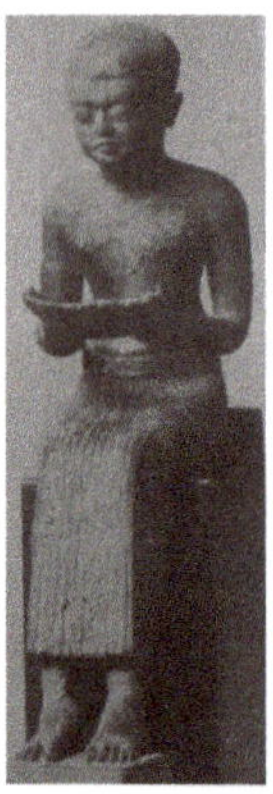

Imhotep

Many Egyptian gods and goddesses were attributed with healing powers. Among mortals, **Imhotep** was one of the most renowned figures and is honored as the first physician in recorded history. He was a famous physician to a pharaoh around 3000 B.C. and was deified as the god of Egyptian medicine about 2,500 years after his death. The ancient Greeks later adopted him into their tradition and associated him with their god of healing, Asclepius.

Isis was perhaps the most important goddess in Egyptian mythology. Her primary functions included healing the sick, supporting motherhood, and working magical spells and charms. **Sekhmet**, the lioness goddess of healing who also punished mortals for their sins, eventually transformed into Hathor, a peaceful goddess of pleasure and happiness. **Serget**, a scorpion goddess, was petitioned to save the lives of those bitten by scorpions and to assist women during childbirth.

Around 330 B.C., Alexander the Great invaded Persia, India and Egypt, and founded the city of Alexandria in northern Egypt. Alexandria became a primary center of cultural exchange in the European and Middle Eastern worlds. Great philosophers attended the temple-schools in Alexandria to study philosophy, medicine, surgery, anatomy, botany, astronomy, and alchemy. The schools included botanical gardens of medicinal herbs. The Temple of Zeus was a famous medical school established around 300 B.C. in Alexandria. It contained a huge library of 700,000 books, including many herbal texts and most of the accumulated knowledge of the ancient world. Alexandria became a center of Greek culture, and the temple-school of Zeus continued as a center of medical teaching even after the Roman invasion in 31 B.C. Under Roman rule, Christianity was established in Egypt until the Arab conquest in A.D. 640. By the end of the fourth century, Christians destroyed many cultural treasures and burned the Temple of Zeus medical school and library. After conquest by other nations, the Egyptian language fell into disuse and became a dead language. Reading ancient Egyptian medical texts was nearly impossible until the 1800s and 1900s, when scholars were able to translate some of the remaining scrolls. Although this ancient civilization has vanished, the Egyptians contributed significant medical knowledge and a sophisticated herbal pharmacy to the development of Indian, Islamic, and Western medical traditions.

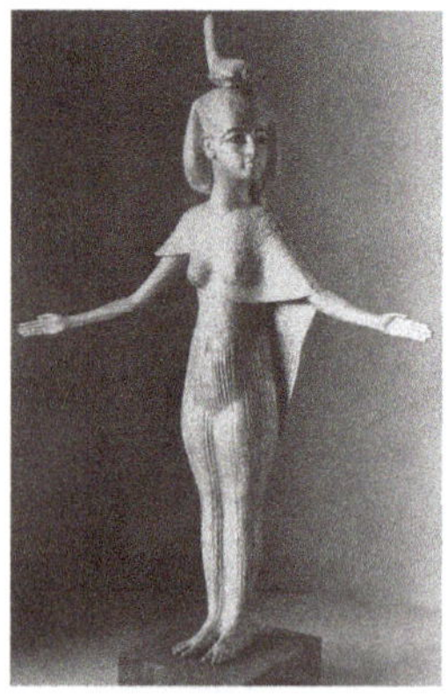

Serget the scorpion goddess

European Healing Traditions

Mythological Beginnings

The ancient Greeks and Romans derived much of their herbal knowledge from the ancient civilizations of Mesopotamia, Egypt, India, and China. Like the Sumerians and Egyptians, the Greeks and Romans believed that the gods were the original herbalists and physicians who taught humans the art of healing. Sickness and disease, linked to supernatural forces, were believed to be curses from the wrathful gods. People prayed to Apollo, their god of medicine, for healing.

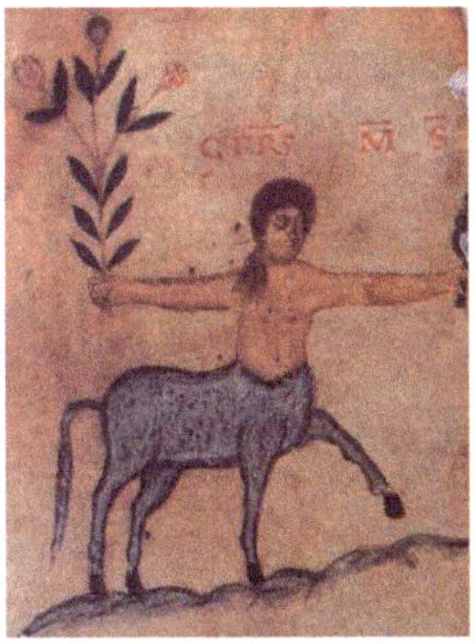

Chiron the centaur, half man and half horse

Asclepius (also known as Aesculapius in Latin) was a demigod born to the god Apollo and Coronis, a mortal woman and princess of Thessaly in Greece. According to mythology, Coronis betrayed Apollo when she married Ischys while pregnant with Apollo's child. Apollo condemned the lovers to death, and as Coronis lay burning on the funeral pyre, Apollo snatched his unborn son from her womb. Apollo sent his son, Asclepius, to the centaur Chiron, who was a master of medicine with vast wisdom of the healing arts. Chiron taught Asclepius to become a brilliantly skilled healer who performed miraculous cures. Eventually, Asclepius had a family of healers. His wife was Epione, who soothed pain. His daughters were Hygeia (where we get the word "hygiene"), the goddess of health and healthy living, and Panacea (meaning "curing all"), the goddess of medical therapy. His son, Telesphoros, helped people recuperate after illness or injury. Asclepius' skill at saving lives became so great that Hades, ruler of the dead, feared the underworld would become empty. He complained to Zeus, who was also angered by Asclepius' healing power. Zeus struck Asclepius down with a thunderbolt, but allowed him to ascend into the heavens to become the deity of healing and medicine.

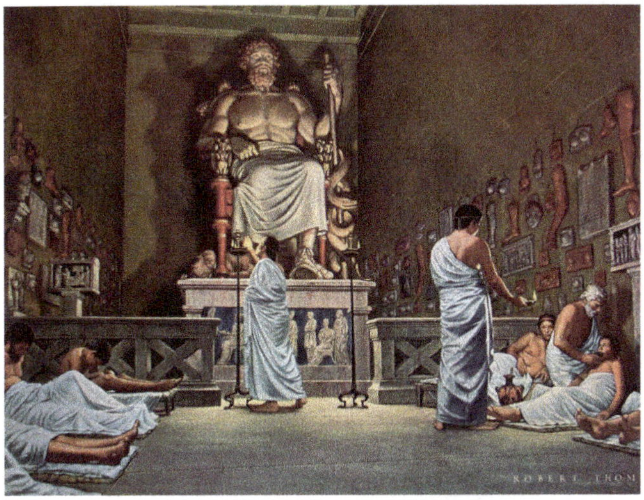

The Temple and Cult of Asclepius
Image by Robert Thom. Courtesy of Pfizer Inc.

Separating fact from myth, historians believe that Asclepius was an actual physician who lived around 1200 B.C. He became immortalized and regarded as a deity between the eighth and fifth centuries B.C., when he replaced Apollo as the god of healing. Asclepius became the personified symbol of healing and medicine in Greek and Roman mythology and eventually throughout Europe. By the fourth century B.C., the Asclepian tradition of healing was established in Thessaly, where the oldest known temple honoring Asclepius was erected. Over time, more than 200 temples were built throughout ancient Greece, Italy, and Asia Minor to perpetuate his medical model. The temples, called Asclepia, were teaching institutions and repositories of medical knowledge that served as hospitals to treat the sick and dispense herbal medicines. The sick underwent a healing ritual called incubation, or temple sleep, and as they slept, Asclepius or one of his priests visited them in their dreams to offer advice and healing. The patients often left the temple the following day, having been cured.

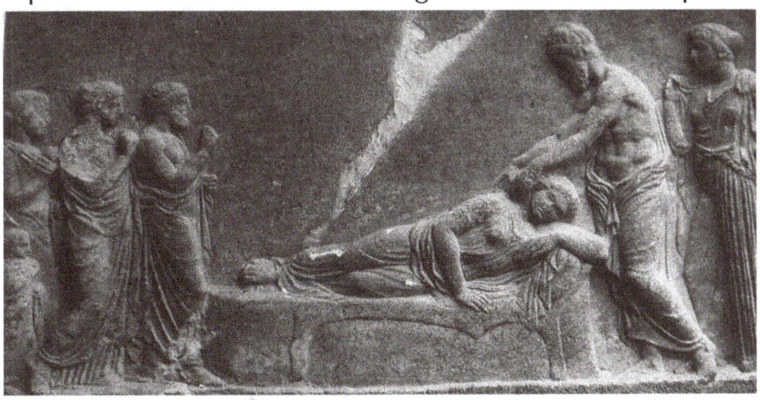

Asclepius healing a sleeping patient

Many ancient people believed that humanity originated from divinity. They also associated the healing of human suffering with divine intervention, and healers were often religious leaders. Priests were regarded as physicians, prophets, and diviners. They incorporated the healing powers of the earth and nature, herbal plants, baths, recreation and worship, all in the Asclepian model of gentle balance and harmony, dignity, and compassion. Asclepian temples existed for centuries under the guidance of the priest-physicians, who passed their knowledge down from father to son and master to student, continuing into the Christian era. The Asclepian temple on the island of Cos (the birthplace of Hippocrates) was the most famous of these temples.

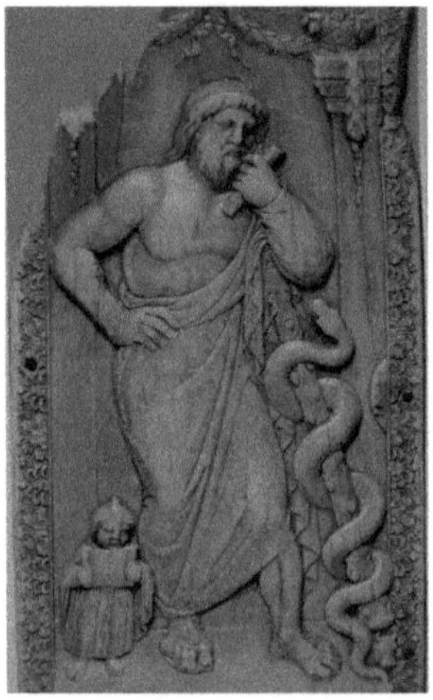

Asclepius with his staff

Many statues and pictographs of Asclepius still exist. They show him carrying a wooden staff embellished with a large serpent wrapped along its entire length, the serpent holding a plant in its mouth. The serpent was believed to possess knowledge of herbs and medicine, and was regarded as a sacred and universal symbol of healing in many cultures. The Greeks, Egyptians, Mayans, Incas, and Hindus venerated snakes as agents of wisdom, renewal and immortality, and believed that they possessed the power to discover healing herbs. Asclepius, the ancient patron deity of physicians, remains the symbol of healing and medicine throughout the modern Western world.

The official insignia of medical physicians and the American Medical Association (AMA) originated from the **staff of Asclepius** with a snake wrapped around it. The most popular insignia of the AMA, as well as that of the U.S. Army Medical Corps, is a similar emblem called the **caduceus**. The caduceus was originally seen in the hand of Thoth, the Egyptian god of knowledge. The Greeks adopted the caduceus and associated it with Hermes, the analogous god in their pantheon who also ruled over scientific and occult knowledge. The caduceus is a winged wand or staff intertwined by two serpents representing the magic wand and wings of Hermes (known as Mercury in ancient Rome), who was the messenger of the gods. According to one legend, Apollo gave his staff to Hermes, telling him that it had the power to unite all beings divided by hate, and when Hermes saw two snakes fighting, he threw the staff down between them and they wound around it in friendship. Hermes carried the caduceus as a symbol of peace.

Another more esoteric interpretation of the caduceus involves the chakras, or energy centers of the human body. The staff represents the central spinal cord and flow of energy within it. The two snakes portray the dualistic and polarizing energies of life, the positive and negative, which constantly circulate throughout the body. The seven spaces formed by the intertwining serpents symbolize the seven chakras of the body. According to ancient view, the chakras or energy centers are seven distinct areas around the spinal cord and head that absorb universal energies to nourish and maintain the body. The human body is understood to be an energetic system, and health results when the energies flow in a dynamic balance. The wings at the crown of the staff represent an evolved or "enlightened" state of being arising from equilibrium between the dualities of positive and negative, and from the harmony resulting from balance within the seven chakras. This profound understanding of energetic harmony and balance is at the heart of many traditional healing systems worldwide and is fundamental to holistic healing. It is interesting that the staff of Asclepius and the caduceus, both rooted in ancient legends and concepts, continue to be the symbols of medicine in modern times.

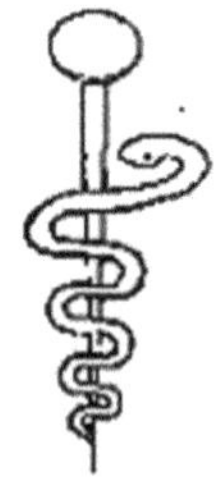

Staff of Asclepius

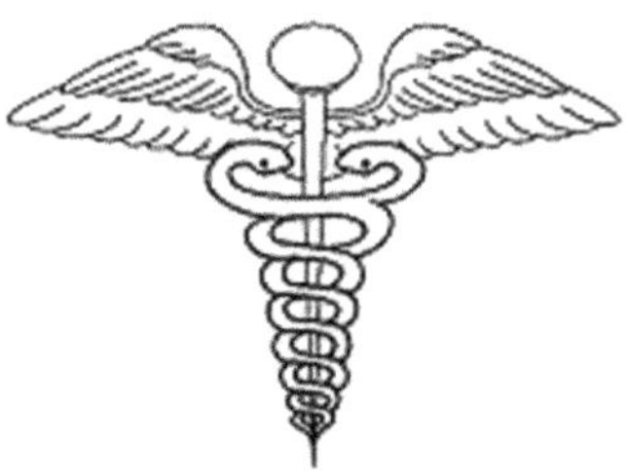

The Caduceus

The Roman Empire

The Roman Empire was a huge domain stretching throughout Europe, Asia Minor, and northern Africa. The ruling power was seated in Rome, held by a succession of emperors and maintained by a powerful army. The building of Rome started about 753 B.C., and the invasion and acquisition of foreign lands into its vast empire began around 264 B.C. The Roman Empire flourished until its armies were overcome by invading tribes and fell between A.D. 400 and 500.

The ancient Greeks and Romans believed that herbal plants were gifts from the gods and goddesses given to humans to cure illness and bestow beauty. Herbs were employed in everyday life to flavor and preserve food that would spoil without refrigeration. When people did not have access to abundant water or bathing was difficult, herbs served as perfumes and deodorants. Aromatic herbs were burned as incense to please the gods and invoke their protection and blessings. Freshly picked leaves and flowers were placed on floors of homes and temples to pleasantly scent the air when walked upon. The Asclepian healing tradition and philosophy dominated medicine during the entire Greek and Roman period. Herbal plants were used in most medical preparations and the healing arts flourished.

The peak of Greek and Roman civilization were times of relative stability and wealth. Such luxury enabled privileged people to focus on the finer aspects of life, including the observation and study of the natural world. The ancient Greeks developed rational systems of medicine based on natural causes rather than magical and supernatural elements. They introduced the study of botany and herbology to the Western world. A multitude of common people also contributed to the development of herbal traditions within their villages, and those who became skilled in the harvesting, preparation, and medicinal applications of plants eventually gained honor as healers in their communities.

Hippocrates (*c.* 460–*c.* 377 B.C.) was a famous Greek physician who initiated the classical period of Greek medicine. He is known as the "father of medicine" and is considered to be the first person in the Western world to establish and document a scientific medical system. His medical philosophy differed from the predominant belief of his era that illness was caused by magic and malevolent actions of the gods. He perceived wellness and disease to be determined by natural laws, defining health as a state of dynamic equilibrium between body, mind, and environment. He established diagnostic methods and herbal treatments based on this holistic view.

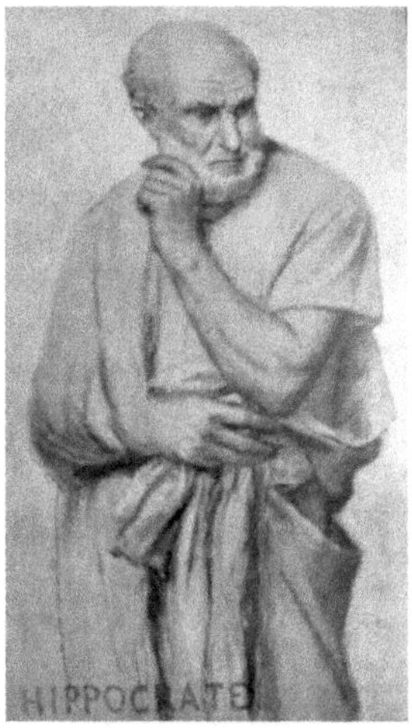

Hippocrates: A portrait designed from ancient medals and coins

Hippocrates was born on the island of Cos in the Aegean Sea. Little is known about his life or written work except what was passed on by authors who lived at least 200 years after his death. His father's family name was Asclepiadae and historians have traced his ancestry back to Asclepius, the physician who was deified as the god of healing. Hippocrates' family had long been trained in the Asclepian healing tradition. His father and grandfather were physicians and his mother a midwife. Hippocrates followed the Asclepian model and developed an extensive pharmacopoeia of herbs to treat his patients. His successful healing practices brought him much fame. He eventually became a traveling physician throughout Greece and Asia Minor; practicing, writing, and teaching medicine. Later in his life he moved to Thessaly in Greece.

Hippocrates initiated a transition in medical practice from invoking mystical spells and superstitious magic to observing laws of nature and the human body, and applying these natural laws to healing. He comprehended the body's inherent tendency to self-heal when provided the necessary conditions. He embraced philosophies from Arabian, Chinese, and Ayurvedic Indian physicians who understood the natural world and human body to be composed of **four basic elements: earth, water, fire,** and **air**. Hippocrates recognized that health is determined by a dynamic and balanced equilibrium between these four elements. In the human body, these elements were expressed as the **four humors**, or liquids, which included blood, bile (black bile), choler (yellow bile), and phlegm. The word "humor" is derived from the Latin *humere,* meaning "to be moist." **Blood** was associated with the heart and air element, and was warm and moist. **Black bile**, associated with the spleen and earth element, was cold and dry. **Choler**, or **yellow bile**, was associated with the liver and fire, and was warm and dry. **Phlegm**, associated with the brain and water, was cold and moist.

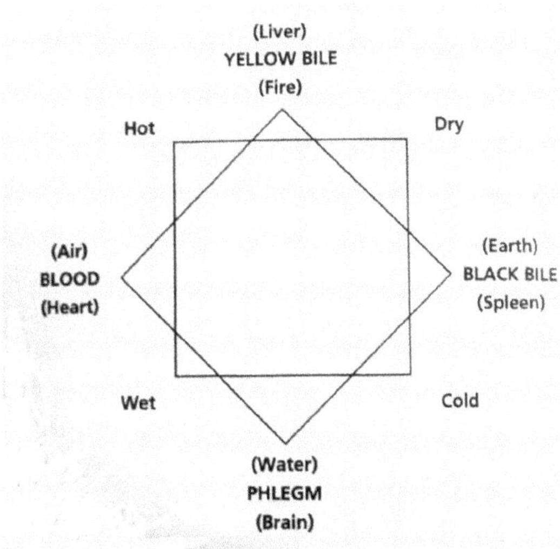

Hippocrates' humoral system from his book *On the Nature of Man*

People were typed according to these **four constitutional humors** or **elements**. Hippocrates classified the nature of diseases and the energetic qualities of plants into the four categories of hot or cold, and wet or dry. He believed that balancing these opposites promoted health, although in most people one humor was thought to dominate. The correct humoral balance was maintained by a vital force or energy in the body. To strengthen this vital force, Hippocrates prescribed the Asclepian model of nourishing food, healthy lifestyle, ample activity and rest, and herbal therapies when necessary. Long ago he advised, "Let your food be your medicine, and let your medicine be your food." According to the model of the four humors, conditions involving heat, fever, or inflammation were treated with cooling foods and herbs. Conditions of excess dryness were treated with moisturizing foods and herbs. Problems caused by coolness or stagnation were healed by balancing with warming and stimulating plants. Excess wetness, such as bleeding, phlegm or diarrhea, was treated with drying or astringent herbs.

The **humoral philosophy** was the foundation of Western medicine until the late 19th and early 20th centuries. The first known written version of the four humors philosophy in Europe predates Hippocrates and is credited to **Empedocles**, a Sicilian philosopher who lived from 490–430 B.C. The system of healing based on this philosophy was then further developed by Hippocrates. Interestingly, recognition of the elemental forces of nature and their relationship to health and disease is inherent in most ancient and indigenous cultures. Aspects of this view was, and continues to be, the foundation of the Indian Ayurvedic and Traditional Chinese Medicinal systems, as well as the current Western holistic model that many respected herbalists still employ when treating imbalance and disease.

Hippocrates wrote about 60 manuscripts explaining his healing philosophy and remedies, which have been compiled and are collectively called the *Hippocratic Corpus*. He was well-known and respected during his lifetime, and he profoundly influenced the development and application of herbal medicine and the ethics of physicians in Europe and North America. He believed the role of a physician was to understand and assist nature to heal, and is quoted as saying that "nature is the healer of disease." He instituted ethical principles defining ideal physicians as modest, incorruptible, and compassionate. Even today, American physicians take the Hippocratic Oath, which is the ethical code of honor for practicing medicine. It begins, "I swear by Apollo the Physician, by Asclepius, by Hygeia and Panacea and by all the gods and goddesses, making them my witness, that I will fulfill according to my ability and judgment this oath and covenant." The Asclepian tradition of healing that Hippocrates firmly established in ancient Greece dominated European and Islamic medicine for another 1,000 years until the rise of Christianity in A.D. 300.

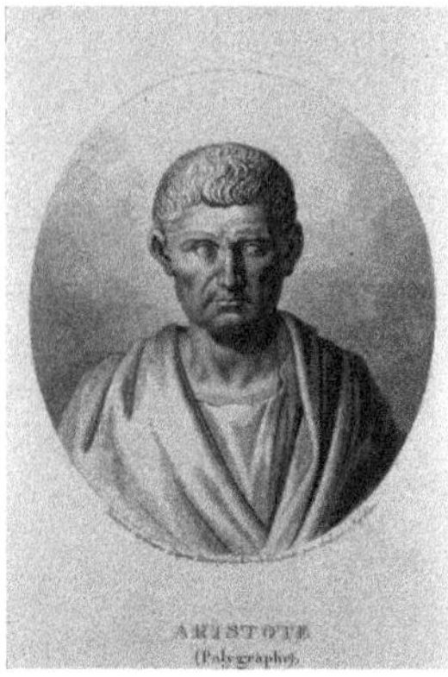

Aristotle

The Western world was also fortunate for the genius of two outstanding men, Aristotle and Theophrastus, whose enduring influence directly followed on the heels of Hippocrates. The famous Greek philosopher **Aristotle** (384–322 B.C.) was another shining light of philosophical thought who influenced healing and herbal medicine in Europe and the Muslim world for centuries. His father was a physician and author of several books on medicine and natural history. Aristotle moved to Athens when he was 17 years old and became one of Plato's favorite students. He adhered to the Asclepian philosophy of balancing the four humors and elements of air, earth, fire and water within the body, and based his herbal healing on these principles. His special interest was in morphology, the science of plant form and structure, and how it related to the evolution of plants. He kept an apothecary (drugstore) in Athens and wrote 50 books on anatomy, natural science and medicinal plants, none of which remain today.

Theophrastus of Eresus (*c.* 370–*c.* 287 B.C.) is known as the "father of botany" and regarded as one of the greatest Greek philosophers and natural scientists. He studied philosophy in Athens under Plato and later became the favorite student of Aristotle, who chose him to be his successor in governing the medical school in Athens. Scholars believe that the written history of Western botany began with Theophrastus and his book, *De Historia Plantarum (The History of Plants)*, in which he accurately classified and described the distribution, structure, behavior, and medicinal properties of about 500 food and herbal plants. This work consisted of nine books that were the compilation of botanical knowledge of that era. In the ninth book, he specifically addressed the medicinal properties of herbs and their preparations and uses in healing. His accurate documentation of the medical qualities of herbs was based on Aristotle's accounts, his own exchanges with foreign travelers, and his observations and logical inferences. Drawing from personal experience in cultivating herbs and developing the art of grafting and propagation, Theophrastus authored *De Causis Plantarum (The Causes of Plants),* which described plant physiology and methods of agriculture and cultivation. His writings were honored as important and reliable herbal references for over 2,000 years.

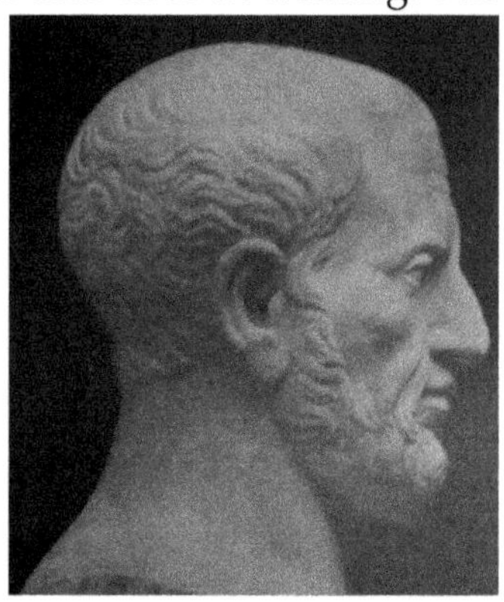

Theophrastus

Pliny the Elder was a famous Roman author and naturalist living from A.D. 23–79. He was born to a wealthy family, enabling him to receive a formal education and travel throughout Europe. Pliny was very knowledgeable about gardening, and his extensive travels allowed him direct contact with many new plant species, some of which he introduced into Roman gardens. He believed in magic, charms, and incantations. Pliny was another major source of early botanical writings and authored a multitude of books and manuscripts, but he is best remembered for *Historia Naturalis (Natural History)*, a 37-volume encyclopedia of natural history and science. It contained manuscripts on botany, drugs, and medicine that were influential until the Middle Ages and could be found in many of the larger monastic libraries. However, his books were based on many superstitions and fabrications, containing so many errors that they have been called "a repository for all the errors of antiquity" and are no longer regarded as reliable texts.

The **Doctrine of Signatures** is an interesting perspective that was popular and endorsed by many herbalists during the time of the Roman Empire and into the Renaissance period. The doctrine originated as a spiritual philosophy in which God marks all plants with a sign or signature indicating their uses for healing. In 1664, the European herbalist Robert Turner wrote, "God hath imprinted upon the plants, herbs and flowers, as it were in hieroglyphics, the very signature of their virtues." According to the doctrine, plants express their healing qualities by various signatures, or characteristics, such as their shape, texture, color, odor, flavor, or growing habits. For example, the shape of the three-lobed Hepatica leaf resembles the lobes of the liver and was given for liver afflictions. Yellow-flowered plants like Goldenrod and Dandelion were thought to be good for treating jaundice (which turns the skin yellow), urinary problems (because urine is yellow), and liver problems (because bile is yellow). Red plants like Cayenne Pepper were used as medicines for the blood, and because Cayenne Peppers have four inner chambers like the human heart, they were recognized as a beneficial heart remedy. When flowers and leaves of St. John's Wort are placed in oil or alcohol, the

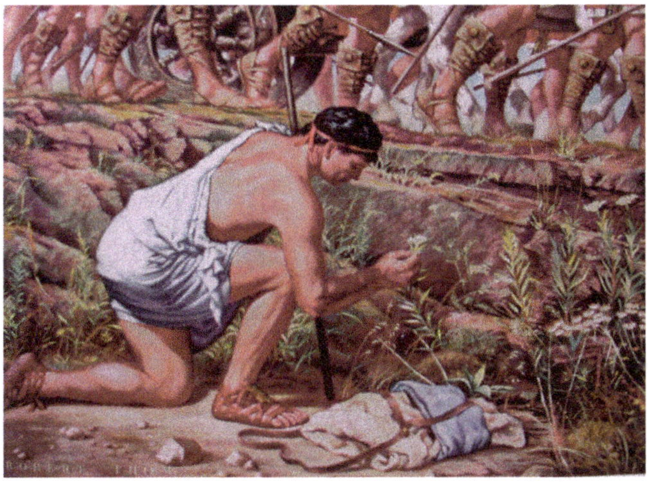

Dioscorides: A Scientist Looks at Drugs
Image by Robert Thom. Courtesy of Pfizer Inc.

liquid turns red, indicating its use for blood disorders. Because the leaves of St. John's Wort contain glands that look like tiny pinpricks, they were employed to heal holes or cuts in the skin. The brightly colored yellow and orange flowers of Calendula indicated their use in treating depression and melancholy. Many common names of herbs such as Boneset, Liverwort, Eyebright, and Toothwort reveal their medicinal uses as suggested by the Doctrine of Signatures. Boneset has pairs of leaves fused across the stem, hinting at its use for fusing broken bones together. Eyebright flowers have brightly colored centers, which suggest their use for clearing the eyes and improving vision. Since ancient times in many parts of the world and in different healing systems, the Doctrine of Signatures has been one of the principle methods used by common people and folk doctors to help them recognize medicinal plants and their uses.

One of the most important, influential contributors to the development of European and Islamic herbalism was **Pedanius Dioscorides,** a famous Greek physician, botanist, and pharmacologist born in what is now Turkey. Living around A.D. 40–90 during the time of the Roman Empire, he obtained much of his knowledge by traveling as a surgeon with the armies of the Roman emperor Nero throughout Italy, Europe, and Asia Minor. This position allowed Dioscorides the opportunity to study the features, distribution, and medicinal properties of many plants and minerals, and to exchange herbal knowledge and experience with other physicians. He employed herbs in his practice, recorded his studies and observations, and wrote about the medicinal uses of hundreds of plants. Originally written in Greek, his herbal writings were later translated into Latin and compiled into his major work, *De Materia Medica*. This series of five books on herbal healing is one of the oldest surviving Western texts on herbal medicines. Written around A.D. 60–78, *De Materia Medica* is a treatise on the properties and applications of 600-700 plants and many animal and mineral substances. The most notable aspects of the text are the accurate descriptions of herbal plants based on his personal and methodical observations. It provides information on the preparation, dosage, and administration of herbs, and their therapeutic benefit for specific diseases. For more than 1,500 years, *De Materia Medica* was the standard herbal text and authoritative reference on medicinal plants, influencing the study and practice of medical herbalism in Europe and the Islamic world throughout the Middle Ages and Renaissance. Galen praised Dioscorides' work, and the herbal physician John Gerard (1564–1637) said of him, "He wrote not only of plants, but a total materia medica, to which study he was addicted even from his childhood, which made him travel much ground, and lead a military life, the better to accomplish his ends. And in this he attained to that perfection, that few or none since his time has attained to, of the excellence of his work, which is . . . the foundation of all that has since been delivered in this nature."

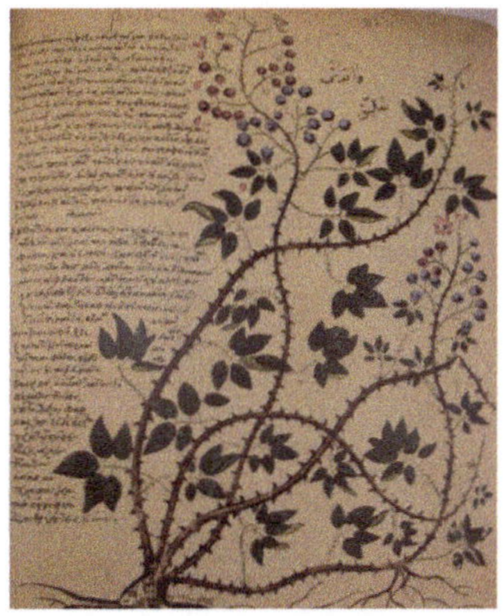

A page from *De Materia Medica,* printed *c.* A.D. 512

Claudius Galenus, known as **Galen** (*c.* A.D. 131–*c.* 200), was one of the most famous people in the history of medicine. He was a Greek physician and pharmacist, and one of the most advanced anatomy and physiology scholars of his time. He traveled for 12 years, spending much time studying at the renowned medical school in Alexandria, Egypt, where he was trained in the Asclepian and Hippocratic traditions of the four humors. Galen returned to Greece in A.D. 157 and was appointed physician to the gladiators, providing him with an excellent opportunity to study anatomy, physiology, herbology, and surgery. In A.D. 162, he went to Rome to be a physician and surgeon to the emperor Marcus Aurelius, wealthy aristocrats, and the common people.

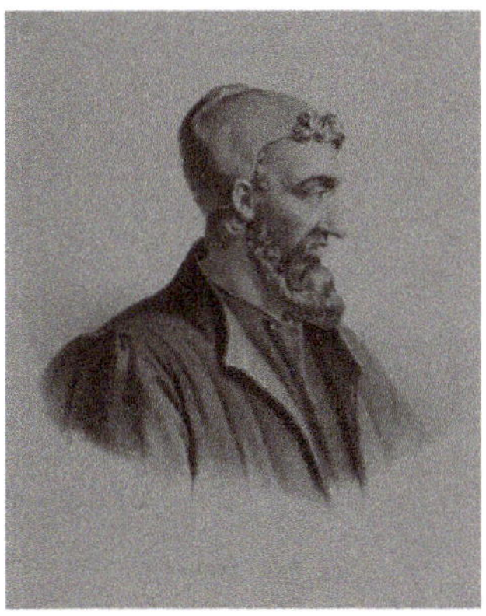

Galen

Galen practiced, taught, and wrote about diet, hygiene, herbal pharmacology and healing, and was committed to integrating philosophy with medicine. As a man of science, he excluded magic and superstition from his medical system. He advocated that balancing the four humors promoted health, and in A.D. 180 wrote *De Simplicibus*, his herbal materia medica based on the philosophy of the four humors. Galen developed a vast and sophisticated body of knowledge on plant and mineral remedies, and is credited with establishing an elaborate classification system for Western herbs. During this time, most herbalists used single herbs or simple formulas with only a few ingredients, but Galen introduced **polypharmacy**, the system that combines several herbs into one specific formula. He established principles and methods of preparing, extracting, mixing, refining, and combining herbs and minerals. His medicinal formulas containing several ingredients were called "galenicals" and were a major contribution to the development of medical herbalism. He wrote about 500 books and treatises on all aspects of medical science, pharmacy, and herbalism. In addition, he established a thriving medical practice plus his own pharmacy that he stocked with hundreds of plant- and animal-based medicines.

Galen devised a system of medical philosophy, therapeutics, and pharmacology that became the embodiment of Greek and Roman medical knowledge. His system and medical texts dominated European medicine throughout the Middle Ages and into the Renaissance, and were employed and refined by physicians for 1,500 years after his death. Arabian herbalists and physicians read his written works and adopted his system of medicine. Medical schools were established in Europe and the Middle East to teach Galen's system of healing. Ultimately, his galenic medicines, philosophy, and writings provided an important foundation for the evolution of herbalism and modern medicine.

The Middle Ages

When the Roman Empire crumbled a few centuries following Galen's death, Europe plunged into the Dark Ages. The Dark Ages (A.D. 400–1000) spanned the first six centuries of the Middle Ages and were a dismal time in human history. Also known as the medieval period, the Middle Ages lasted 1,000 years after the fall of the Roman Empire in A.D. 400–500 until the advent of the Renaissance in the 1300s.

The Dark Ages were a period of tremendous social and political upheaval initiated by the fall of the Roman Empire to invading tribes, and eventually by the domination of the Catholic Church. The common people suffered many physical hardships, including insufficient food, poor sanitation, and constant warfare, disease, and terrible plagues. Fear abounded during this period of history, as did superstitious notions and belief in magic and malevolent forces. Religion, magic, and medicine were often inseparable, and herbal preparations continued to be the primary form of medical treatment.

Throughout the early Middle Ages, constant fighting between Romans, Christians, Muslims, and invaders from the north resulted in the destruction of numerous libraries and schools, which were filled with thousands of irreplaceable manuscripts containing the repository of accumulated knowledge from earlier civilizations. As the Catholic Church established itself and gained authority throughout Europe and Asia Minor, it attempted to exert strict control over religion, education, and the practice of medicine. The Church discarded the Roman Empire's medical system based on the ancient Goddess religion, the Asclepian tradition of healing arts practiced by Hippocrates, and Galen's system. Experimentation and original ideas were discouraged and punished, and science and the study of plants came to a near halt. The Church held secular knowledge and learning in low esteem, and no professional medical education or universities existed in Europe until the later period of the Middle Ages.

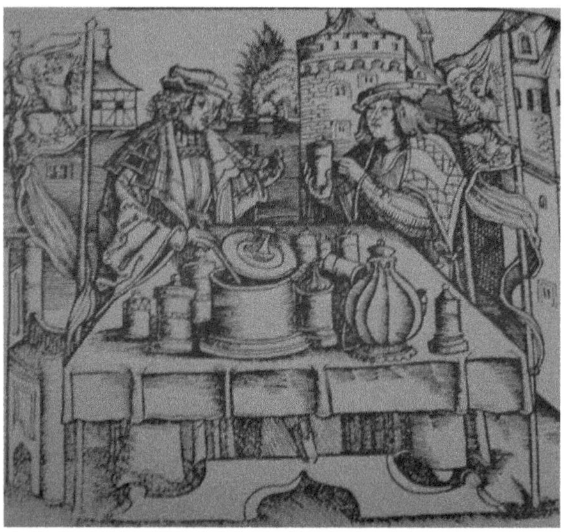

16th-century woodcut showing the preparation of herbal medicines

During the Dark Ages, until the Inquisition ignited in a frenzy in the 1500s, traditional herbal folk medicine continued as it had for centuries in the homes and villages of rural peasants, who wildcrafted medicinal herbs or grew them in their gardens as part of daily life. Most healers acquired their art as a practical craft handed down over the generations from parent to child or master to apprentice. In the British Isles, knowledge of healing within this folk tradition dates back to the Druids, an ancient culture that enjoyed an extensive herbal and medical system for at least 1,000 years before Christianity arrived, beginning in the 500s. The Druids incorporated the ancient Great Mother/Earth Goddess religion, which was a major aspect of the European folk medicine tradition. Eventually, an Anglo-Saxon herbal healing system developed throughout Europe combining the Druid, Goddess, and Asclepian tradition of the Greeks and Romans that was kept alive by many of the common people. Among these people were the **wise women**. Communities often had a wise woman, well-versed in the art of herbalism, who helped heal the sick, assisted in childbirth, offered blessings for bountiful harvests, and served as priestess for rituals, ceremonies, funerals, and other needs of the people. The wise women, sometimes called "**wicca**," received extensive training from their mothers, aunts, grandmothers, or a master, and over time they developed a skillful and refined herbal healing tradition that was an honored and intricate aspect of village life.

While traditions of the wise women and herbal folk healers continued, Catholic monasteries eventually became the Church-sanctioned and formally accepted local centers of medical knowledge and herbal healing from about A.D. 400–1100. During this period, the Catholic Church controlled medicine and imposed strict regulations on the medical profession, allowing it to develop only within the parameters of Catholic doctrine. According to the Church, God determined health and disease, and to interfere with God's will was a serious transgression. Disease was caused by sin, and the Church was responsible for all medical treatment. Priests and monks resorted to prayers and holy water, invoked the aid of saints, advised the sick to visit holy shrines, and used holy relics and superstitious practices to cure illness. The casting out of demons for diseases like epilepsy and mental illness was common practice among the priests. The policy of the Catholic Church was the regressive, pre-Hippocratic belief that illness was God's punishment for mortal sins and only curable through prayer, purification, penance, and religious faith. Science and all other doctrines that contradicted the Church's views were regarded as heresy, and repressive and negative attitudes about the human body and women were embraced. The glorified perspective of the human body as sacred that was once held by the traditions of Hippocrates, Aristotle, and the Goddess religion became distorted, deteriorating into the belief that the human body, especially the female body, was vile and unclean. Holy people did not wash or touch themselves, since to do so was sinful. Women were regarded as tempters who provoked God-fearing men to engage in carnal sexual encounters, and like Eve in the Garden of Eden, women were thought to entice men into evil misconduct.

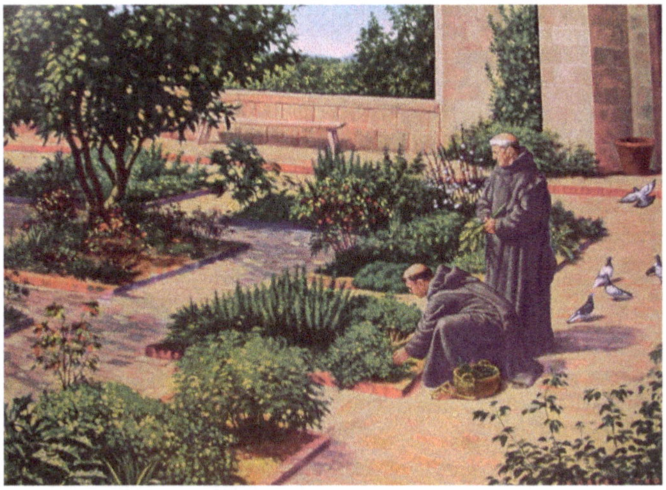

Monastic Pharmacy
The herbal or "physic" gardens
Image by Robert Thom. Courtesy of Pfizer Inc.

During this time, Catholic monasteries and convents had a major impact on herbal medicine and healing. When they were unable to cure themselves from illness, local people living close to monasteries sought the help of priests or nuns to provide herbal remedies and perform religious divinations. Monks and nuns cultivated medicinal herb gardens, called "physic" gardens, and wildcrafted plants from the countryside to provide people with medicines. Monastic infirmaries housed the sick and comforted the dying. Beginning in the 400–500s, the Catholic Church established some of the first European hospitals. The monks of the Benedictine order were the most progressive monastic herbalists. St. Benedict encouraged his monks to care for the sick with herbs and prayer, but forbade the study of medicine because he believed cures were only possible through divine intervention. The Benedictines were the first Europeans to make alcohol extracts from herbs, known as **tinctures**, which was a practice learned from the Arabs. The Roman emperor Charlemagne (742–814) was so impressed by the herb gardens of the Benedictine monks and their practice of herbal medicine that he ordered all monasteries in his kingdom to plant herbal gardens to ensure an adequate supply of medicines throughout his realm. Monks were responsible for keeping the traditions of Greek and Roman herbalism alive during the Dark and Middle Ages. Prior to the invention of the printing press, all books and manuscripts were hand-written. Monks spent countless hours tediously translating and transcribing numerous old medical texts from the works of Hippocrates, Dioscorides, Galen, and eventually Arabian scholars and physicians. These transcribed texts preserved valuable treasuries of knowledge and provided original manuscripts that were eventually mass-produced with the invention of the printing press during the Renaissance.

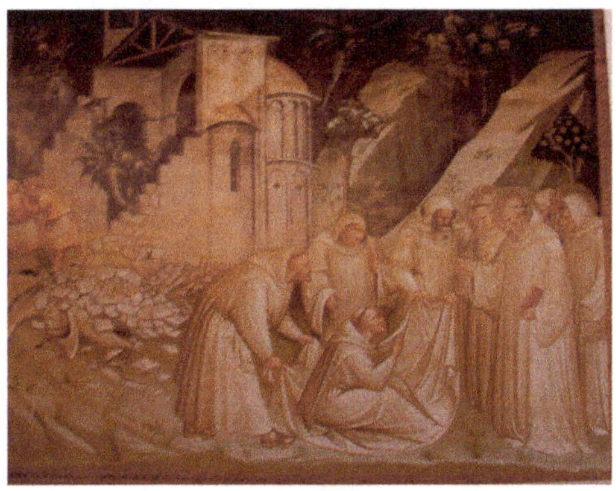

St. Benedict healing a monk in a fresco (*circa* 1387)

Very few women herbalists and healers are known from this period because Church doctrine dictated that medicine be under the exclusive control of men. However, German Benedictine nun **Hildegard of Bingen** (1098–1179) was the founder and Abbess of a German convent who became a well-known and respected herbal healer in her time. After experiencing visions of God commanding her to heal the sick and share her medicines, she wrote *Hildegard's Medicine*, a compilation of her personal work with herbs combined with mystic Catholicism, traditional German folk medicine, and the ancient doctrine of the four humors. She was the only medieval woman known to have documented any of the wise woman healing practices. She was supposedly very intuitive and had visions of luminous objects as a young child. Hildegard wrote treatises about natural history and instructions for employing the curative powers of natural objects such as plants, animals, trees, and stones for healing. Many bishops, popes, and kings requested her medical advice.

Towards the end of the Middle Ages, from 1095–1295, Christian crusades invaded the Muslim world and early trade routes to the Far East developed. These became avenues of opportunity for trading herbs and spices, and for exchanging knowledge about medicinal herbs and healing systems. When the Muslims swept across the continent and conquered northern Africa, Spain, and southern France, they introduced their advanced herbal and medical traditions, which were eventually absorbed into the western European healing system. Herbal and medical traditions from Greece and Rome, the Arab world, India, and the Far East became available to share and assimilate. Many old Latin and Islamic herbal and medical texts were translated, allowing greater accessibility to medical knowledge and catalyzing a revival of learning.

As the Middle Ages drew to a close, the Church enforced strict adherence to Catholic doctrine by establishing a judicial system in which the pope assigned men, usually Franciscan or Dominican monks, to investigate the "heretical depravity" of questionable people. By the end of the 1200s, inquisitors were assigned to work in most European communities in cooperation with local bishops. The inquisitors' job was to identify heretics and force them to confess and repent their sins to regain approval from the Church. Those who refused were persecuted and often burned at the stake after suffering torture. Church councils required secular rulers to prosecute heretics, and manuals were published as instruction guides for the inquisitors. During the Inquisition, which continued through the 1600s, the inquisitors' focus turned to the women healers.

While the Church weeded out and executed all perceived heretics, European medicine became established as a secular science and profession of university-trained male doctors toward the end of the Middle Ages. In the 900s, a medical school was established in Salerno, Italy that became the primary center of medical education in Europe for about 200 years. During the 1200s and 1300s, more universities with standardized curriculums and graduation requirements were established throughout Europe, teaching liberal arts, law, theology, and medicine. During this period, the schism between the two prevailing systems of healing deepened. While the ancient herbal folk tradition was still practiced and embraced by much of the peasant population, the developing medical profession of wealthy and educated university-trained physicians gained dominance. State authorities and the Church regarded it as the superior healing system. However, the Church retained tight control and final authority over medical practice, demanding that physicians only treat patients in the presence of a priest. The patients first had to confess their sins, which the Church blamed as the ultimate cause of illness. Women were excluded from universities and banned from all formal medical practice except midwifery. Physicians once again embraced the Hippocratic regimen of good diet and healthy lifestyle, as well as the philosophies of Galen and other Greek physicians. Standard medical treatments included drugs made from herbs, minerals and animals, surgery, bloodletting and the use of leaches, incantations, and superstitious rituals. The Church accepted the Doctrine of Signatures and permitted physicians to include astrology and alchemy in their medical practice. The period of monastic medicine officially ended in 1130, when the Council of Clermont prohibited monks from practicing medicine.

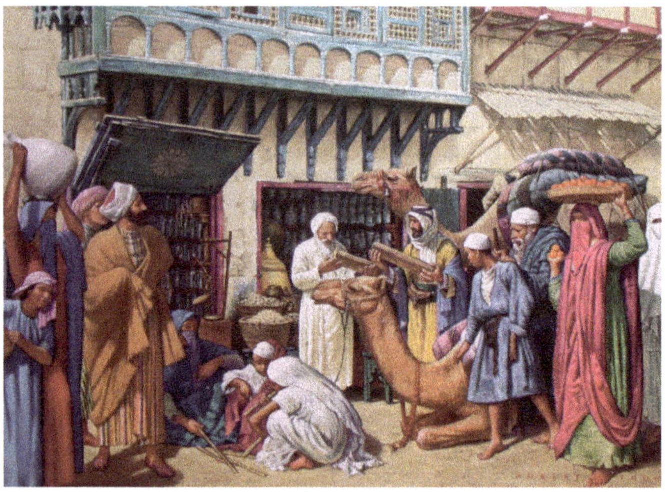

The First Apothecary Shops Established in Baghdad

Image by Robert Thom. Courtesy of Pfizer Inc.

During the 700s, the Arabs established apothecaries as the original drug stores for preparing and selling herbal and mineral medicines. These became the models for apothecaries that later developed in Europe. European countries exposed to Arabic influence instituted public pharmacies around the 11th century.

Towards the end of the Middle Ages, medical theory, education, and practice were primarily based on Galen's healing system and on the *Articella Medica* (also called the *Ars Medica*) Greek-Arabic medical texts that physicians owned and studied. The *Articella Medica* were comprised of the writings and herbal medicines of Hippocrates, Galen and Arabic physicians, and became the established body of Greek and Arabic medical literature. Galen's philosophy and medical system based on the four humors and elements of hot, cold, dry, and damp regained popularity. His views of God, nature, and medicine were sanctioned by the Catholic Church and regarded as absolute and infallible during the Middle Ages and Renaissance. Those who dared to question or disagree with Galen's theories were punished as heretics. The *Articella Medica* and Galenic philosophy became the predominant foundation of the professional medical system, which contributed to standardizing medical practice and education in Europe. The most dramatic advances in European medicine during the Middle Ages occurred during this latter period when universities and townships established institutional, legal, and social frameworks that determined the study and practice of medicine for the next 500 years.

The Renaissance

Beginning in Italy in the 1300s, this "period of enlightenment" slowly spread throughout Europe during the 14th–16th centuries. The study of utilizing plants for food and medicine once again flourished, and many herbal books were written during this era. Botanical gardens became increasingly popular in universities and medical schools. There was a great deal of continuity between medieval and Renaissance medicine. Herbal preparations continued to be the mainstay of medical treatment until the end of the 1500s, when new chemical medicines became popular among professional physicians all over Europe. Although the Renaissance was a period of cultural progress, it was overshadowed by severe restrictions and repression by the Catholic Church, stifling the folk herbalists and healers. This was also the time of deadly famines, devastating plagues, outbreaks of syphilis, and the Inquisition, when thousands of female herbalists were killed by Church decree.

During the Middle Ages and into the Renaissance, herbs and medical practice were surrounded by pagan and Christian superstition. Many plants such as St. John's Wort (*Hypericum perforatum*), Vervain (*Verbena officinalis*), and Yarrow (*Achillea millefolium*) were used in magical amulets and talismans to protect the wearer from evil. Fear of the devil and evil forces, perpetuated by the powerful Church, was widespread. Within the tradition of folk herbalists were the well-respected woman healers and midwives, called "**wise women**" by the common people, and "witches" and "heretics" by the Church. Springing from the ancient lineage of herbal practitioners, the wise women preserved the Goddess and Druid traditions. They were shamanic in their view of the unity and spark of light within all life, and in their use of nature's elemental forces for healing. They were expert herbalists who refined the chemistry, combinations, and administration of medicinal plants to a precise and exquisite art. The wise women used natural anesthetics derived from plants for childbirth and painful conditions. In 1527, Paracelsus, the "father of modern chemistry," recorded that much of his understanding about herbalism and the natural laws and practices of healing developed from conversations with these female healers. Since the Church forbade priests to assist mothers giving birth, women were allowed to be midwives during the Middle Ages until university-trained male physicians took control of this role during the 1600s and 1700s. Eventually, the esteemed reputation of the wise women was obliterated by male physicians and by the fear and deluded view of the "evil witch" promoted by the Church. This resulted in an atmosphere of terror that permeated the hearts and minds of many people.

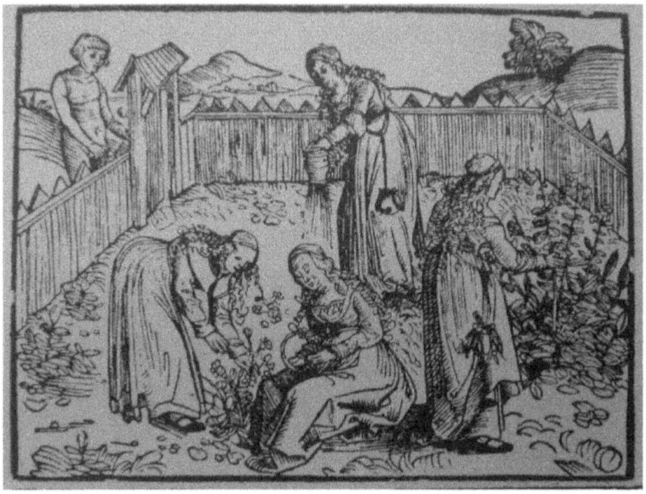

Wise women in their herbal gardens

Physicians in England feared losing their monopoly on medicine, and in 1511 their influence drove King Henry VIII to decree that the practice of medicine was reserved for physicians graduating from medical schools and for barber-surgeons who had completed apprenticeships. Anyone else had to pass a test given in Latin. As few folk herbalists and common people could read Latin, many were forced to stop practicing herbalism or go underground to practice in secret and risk severe punishment. In 1518, English physicians and surgeons organized themselves and established the College of Physicians. They determined who could legally practice medicine, excluding all women and practitioners of "sorcery and witchcraft."

The Church and state were the dominant rulers throughout Europe, and they smashed a perceived threat to their power by turning against the revered wise women healers and folk herbalists, accusing them of witchcraft and performing the work of the devil. Women were prohibited from practicing medicine and any form of healing other than midwifery. The once-honored archetypical female virtues of nurturing, intuition and empathy, embraced by Hippocrates and the Goddess and Asclepian traditions, became threats and impediments to the progress of the Church and the prevailing medical system. A new objective to displace all "pagan" traditions was set in motion by the Church. Anything related to the supernatural was declared heresy and punishable by the most brutal methods. The resulting Inquisition and witch hunts against accused heretics and herbal healers endured for more than 300 years during the 1300s–1600s, and are a sad and startling commentary on the cruelty and persecution aimed against the peasant population, especially women. Witch hunts began in France and Germany, spreading throughout Europe into England and eventually to colonial America. Various historical accounts estimate that between a few hundred thousand to five million people (primarily women but also children and men) were killed in Europe for allegedly practicing witchcraft. A much over-looked historical event! During this time of slaughter, any evidence of herbal healing could be interpreted as proof of witchcraft. Consequently, wise women and other folk herbalists were forced to end their healing practice or work in secrecy with the dreaded possibility of discovery and punishment. Inevitably, much of the ancient herbal tradition was lost. Some of the attitudes born during that period continue to persist in our modern world. Today, many people retain a deeply ingrained cultural fear and suspicion of powerful folk healers, the use of herbal plants for healing, and any reliance on nature's provisions to promote balance and health.

While the Inquisition persisted throughout the Renaissance, tremendous social change and expanded knowledge also highlighted this period. The invention of the printing press in the 1440s allowed mass production of herbal manuscripts written by Theophrastus, Dioscorides, Galen and Avicenna (a leading Arab pharmacist and physician), making medical knowledge more accessible to people. Extensive European exploration, discovery of the Americas, and the establishment of new trade routes stimulated a revival of innovative experiences and ideas. Explorers discovered many unique plant species that they brought home to be cultivated, and many were incorporated into European herbalism. From the early 1500s to the mid-1600s, the Protestant Reformation, led by Martin Luther, opposed the doctrines and absolute control of the Catholic Church. By the end of the 1600s, when the European Inquisition declined, folk healers had been forced out of work. Medical practice was exclusively the domain of the new class of university-trained male physicians. Apothecaries (a term referring to pharmacists and their drugstores) and physicians became the sole distributors of herbal and chemical medicines. As the medical profession grew, physicians continued to exert their elevated status and authority over barber-surgeons and apothecaries, demanding exclusive rights to practice medicine in their concerted efforts to drive out non-professional practitioners.

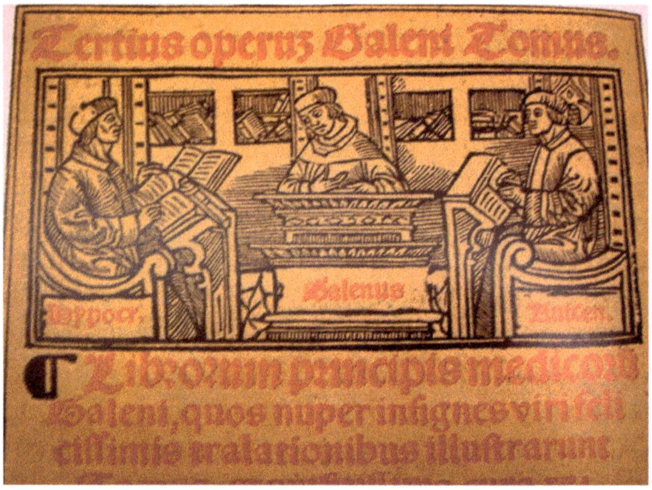

A manuscript illustration showing Hippocrates, Galen, and Avicenna as leaders of medical knowledge

Later, during the 17th century, which was known as the "age of scientific revolution," advances in technology and science promoted new medical philosophies and chemical drugs. These new drugs, which were gaining popularity among physicians, began to replace herbalism as the mainstay of medical treatment. Physicians and surgeons challenged and rejected many of Galen's concepts that were based on ancient Asclepian and Hippocratic traditions dominating medical philosophy and practice up to this time. The medical profession also became self-regulated and independent of the authority of the Catholic and Protestant Churches.

In the standard medical practice during the Renaissance, the physician's role was to diagnose and prescribe treatment, while the apothecary dispensed medicine and attended the patient. Originally, apothecaries only sold drugs, but eventually their skill and knowledge expanded, enabling them to prepare their own drugs and formulate remedies. They purchased herbs and roots collected in the countryside by "green people" (a name given to rural herb collectors) and imported exotic plants and spices from abroad. The apothecaries also established their own medicinal herb gardens, which became very popular and were commonly referred to as "physic" gardens. As the science of botany continued to develop and medical science advanced, physicians continued to rely on apothecaries to supply their herbal medicines.

Astrology played a big role in medical herbalism during this time. According to the various characteristics and properties of plants, astrological herbalists assigned them different signs of the zodiac. Illness was treated by determining the sign and planet that ruled over the ailing part of the body, and herbs were prescribed according to their appropriate astrological sign.

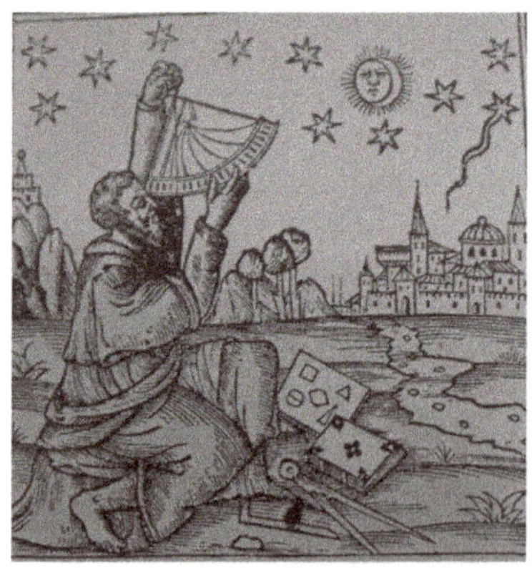
An astrologer making calculations

Many practitioners contributed to the development of medical herbalism during the Renaissance. **Paracelsus** (1493–1541) was a famous Swiss physician and alchemist who lived during the time of the Inquisition. He initiated the study and practice of mineral and chemical pharmacology and the scientific method, which were fundamental to modern medical practice. His birth name was Theophrastus Bombastus von Hohenheim, but later in life he arrogantly named himself Paracelsus, Latin for "greater than Celsus," who was a famous Roman medical writer in the first century A.D. Paracelsus' father was a chemist and physician who taught his son the medical theory and practice of their time that was still based on the writings and philosophy of Hippocrates, Galen, and the famous Arab physician, Avicenna. Plant-based remedies were the primary treatments for illness during this period. Paracelsus was a precocious youth, and at age 19 he entered the University at Basel in Switzerland. His restless and rebellious nature enticed him to travel throughout Europe, where he studied at various universities and under the tutelage of many scholars, apothecaries, and physicians. Paracelsus was a metaphysical mystic as well as a scientist, and he took the opportunity during his travels to meet and exchange knowledge with herbalists, alchemists, astrologers, gypsies, wise women, magicians, and sorcerers. In Constantinople, he studied under advanced Muslim physicians and learned the art of alchemy, which involved the process of transforming minerals into pharmaceutical drugs. Although he focused on science and chemistry, he also searched the invisible side of nature to understand metaphysical causes of disease and health. Paracelsus believed that knowledge is attained through intuition and experience, and he perceived that all beings derive life from the radiant light of a universal life force. He advocated the theory that disease arises from five basic causes: 1) sidereal and astral influences of the earth's magnetic field and planetary bodies; 2) impure, toxic, and harmful substances entering the body; 3) unhealthy physical habits; 4) psychological imbalances, harmful emotions and thoughts; and 5) spiritual causes, including deviation from the divine order of natural laws. He emphasized hygiene and sanitation, nutritious diet, and harmonious balance with nature. In his medical practice, he used talismans made of specific metals according to astrological influences.

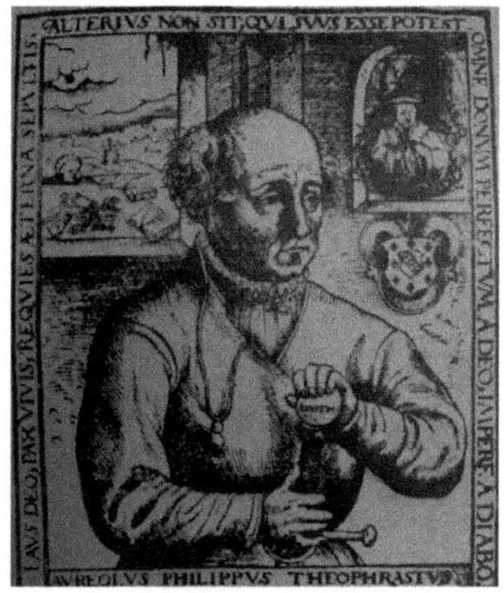

Paracelsus preparing medicines

Paracelsus' profound dissatisfaction with the medical philosophy of his contemporaries led to his association with the peasant population and his appreciation of their folk wisdom. His success in healing was well known during his lifetime, and he was loved and appreciated by the common people. Historic references report that he employed herbs for healing and encouraged the use of locally grown herbs rather than expensive plants from foreign countries. He harvested herbs with utmost care, acknowledging that growing location and harvesting time affected their potency. Paracelsus advocated the ancient **Doctrine of Signatures**, which stated that a plant's structure, appearance, color, smell, and other qualities reveal its healing attributes. He wrote:

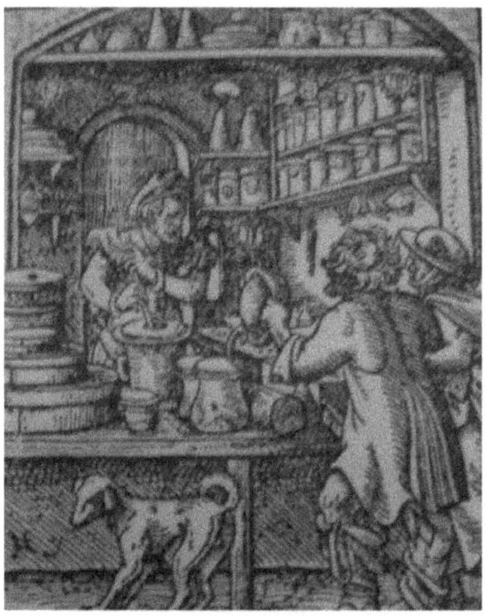

European apothecary selling herbal remedies

> The soul does not perceive the external or internal physical construction of herbs and roots, but it intuitively perceives their powers and virtues, and recognizes at once their *signatum*. This *signatum*, or signature, is a certain vital organic activity, giving to each natural object a certain similarity with a certain condition produced by disease. This signature is often expressed even in the exterior form of things, and by observing the form we may learn something in regard to their interior qualities, even without using our interior sight. We see that the internal character of a man is often expressed in his exterior appearance, even in the manner of his walking and in the sound of his voice. Likewise the hidden character of things is to a certain extent expressed in their outward forms. As long as man remained in a natural state, he recognized the signature of things and knew their true character; but the more he diverged from the path of Nature, and the more his mind became captivated by illusive external appearances, the more this power became lost. (Hartman, 1985)

After serving as an army surgeon in Italy, Paracelsus returned to Switzerland in 1526 and taught physics, medicine, and surgery at the University at Basel. He argued that the medicinal properties in plants are derived from the chemicals they contain, and promoted the use of concentrated plant extracts called **tinctures** rather than using crude roots, leaves, or flowers as remedies. His pharmacy was based on isolating specific chemicals in herbs to treat illness, whereas previous herbal therapy had employed the entire plant part containing a multitude of chemical components. He developed laudanum (tincture of opium), which became a popular and approved narcotic in Europe for many years.

However, as his knowledge and use of minerals increased, Paracelsus eventually abandoned the socially accepted philosophies of Hippocrates, Galen, and Arab physicians, which focused on humoral imbalances and adjusting the qualities of hot, cold, wet, and dry. No longer relying on herbal remedies, he introduced mineral-based preparations and a medical model based on alchemical principles to heal disease, in which minerals such as sodium, sulfur, and mercury were believed to be both the cause and cure for disease. Many of his chemical remedies were derived from minerals such as arsenic, copper sulfate, iron, mercury, and sulfur.

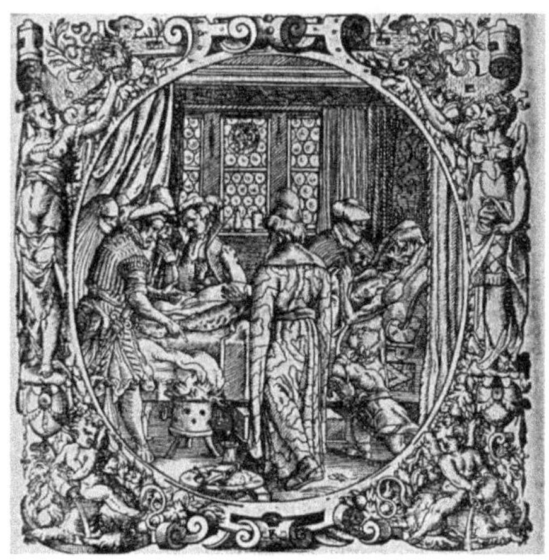

Physicians discuss treatment at the bedside of a dying man

Paracelsus was considered to be a defiant and arrogant heretic who practiced unorthodox medicine for his time. His original ideas and condemnation of traditional medical philosophies and herbal therapies often got him into trouble with the medical profession. In his lectures at the university, he boldly criticized the use of "old-fashioned" herbal remedies and denounced the popular theories of Dioscorides, Galen, and Avicenna. He even resorted to burning books authored by these famous herbalists in his classrooms and in the marketplace of Basel. He constantly and brazenly attacked the medical profession, and many of his contemporaries considered him to be a heretic.

During this period of history, there was a notable distinction between physicians and surgeons. Surgeons evolved from the barber's trade and originally used similar tools and knives as barbers. Barber-surgeons were considered to be mere craftsmen rather than respected medical professionals. While physicians enjoyed the privileges of upper-class scholars, active participation at the patient's bedside was considered to be beneath their dignity. Paracelsus was very vocal in his stand to incorporate surgeons into the medical profession, further arousing the hostility of physicians. His introduction of the systematic use of metals and isolated chemicals for healing created a major schism in the evolution of medicine. This resulted in one discipline that continued using herbal therapies, while another branch favored the approach of alchemy that relied on metals. Paracelsus is often considered to be the originator of modern allopathic (pharmaceutical) medicine. Over the next hundred years, his theories and techniques were taught and implemented, eventually replacing the once-predominant model of Galen.

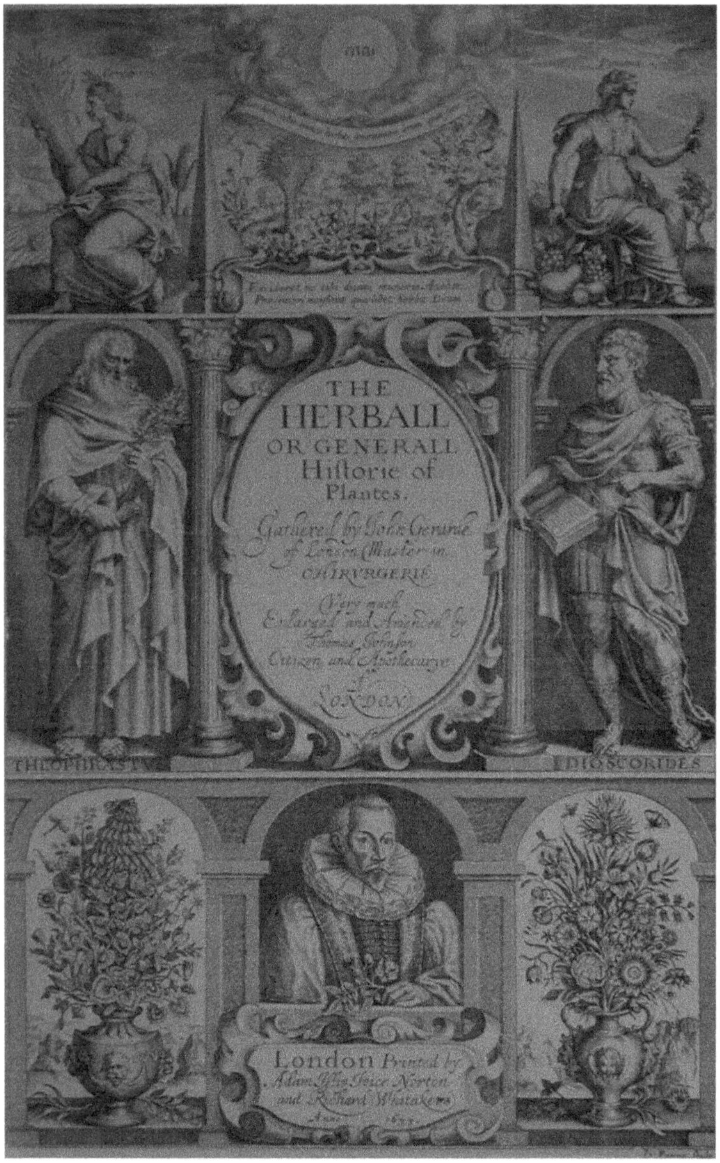

Title page of John Gerard's *The Herball or General Historie of Plantes.* Theophrastus is pictured on the middle left and Dioscorides is on the middle right. John Gerard is pictured at the bottom of the page.

Medical practice among physicians was changing during this time, and men like Francis Bacon (1561–1626) and William Harvey (1578–1657) were influential in transforming science from speculation into an experimental process. The new emphasis on science-based experimentation and the creation of chemical medicines that evolved did not blend well with the revival of the Doctrine of Signatures and astrology, increasing the conflict and division between herbalist apothecaries and university-trained medical physicians.

Two famous English herbalists, John Gerard and Nicholas Culpeper, exerted a lasting influence on medicine. **John Gerard** (1545–1612) was a renowned herbalist, gardener, apothecary, and barber-surgeon in London who slowly rose to the top of his profession. He is best known for his major work, a catalogue of plants called *The Herball or General Historie of Plantes*, first published in 1597. This was one of the first English herbals (an antiquated term given to books and manuscripts dedicated solely to the subject of medicinal plants) and it contained information on more than 1,000 plant species. The text was largely based on a 1583 herbal written by Belgian botanist Rembert Dodoens. Gerard combined Dodoens' knowledge with his own experience. He wrote *The Herball* during the period of incredible exploration when Europeans were discovering new lands, cultures, plants, and animals. In *The Herball*, Gerard compared new plant species with what was already known, categorizing and assigning qualities and virtues according to the humoral theory and the Doctrine of Signatures.

An excerpt from an edition of Gerard's *Herball* states, "Gerard was drawn to medicine at an early age and superintended botanical gardens (owned by Lord Burghley in London and Hertfordshire) for about 20 years, growing a huge variety of herbs. Apparently he traveled abroad, and became knowledgeable about foreign rare and exotic medicinal herbs, and grew them in his garden. During his lifetime he was greatly respected for his wide knowledge" (Woodward, 1927). Gerard had an outstanding

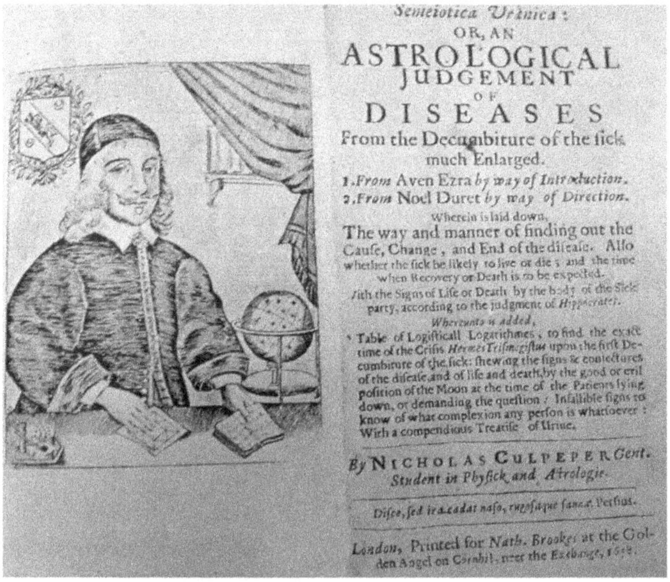

Culpeper pictured on the title page of one of his books

practical knowledge of plants, and his work gave an impetus to botanical study unparalleled by previous writers. His *Herball* was unrivaled in popularity in England and considered a classic in herbal literature for generations. Even today, modern herbal texts often refer to information from *The Herball*.

Nicholas Culpeper (1616–1654) was another of England's most influential herbalists and a proponent of the Doctrine of Signatures and astrological herbalism. He wrote *The English Physician* in 1652, which was later renamed *The Complete Herbal*. After studying at Cambridge University, Culpeper moved to London and apprenticed with a master apothecary (pharmacist). He eventually became a knowledgeable herbalist and very popular apothecary among the common people, although he was not licensed. He rebelled against university education and was considered a radical by his contemporaries, who were angered by his attitudes and practice of combining astrology and the Doctrine of Signatures with herbal remedies.

Culpeper blatantly criticized the superior attitude and snobbery of doctors towards folk healers and their herbal remedies. He condemned their use of toxic substances like arsenic and mercury, and the practice of bloodletting in which patients were cut and bled to "discharge disease." During this era, medical texts were still written in Latin, which most people could not read, and this served to keep information only in the hands of the educated and wealthy. To bridge this gap between the elite physicians and ordinary people, Culpeper translated and printed the College of Physicians' Latin manual into English and named it *The London Dispensatory and Physical Directory*. This was a huge step in making medical and herbal knowledge more accessible to everyone, regardless of social status. Culpeper incurred the wrath of physicians for these efforts, but he earned the respect and appreciation of apothecaries, midwives, and the common people. He was one of the foremost and radical figures in herbal medicine during his lifetime, and his work remains a popular reference for modern herbalists.

During the 1700s, the Swedish botanist and physician **Carolus Linnaeus** (1707–1778) designed the system of **binomial nomenclature** in which plants are assigned a generic and specific name known as genus and species. His method of plant classification created a universal language and system that provided a uniform framework to classify, identify, and name specific plants. This enabled more exact communication between herbalists and botanists. Linnaeus introduced this system in a two-volume work called *Species Plantarum (Kinds of Plants)*, published in 1753. Although best known for this great contribution, a few years earlier in 1749 he had published *Materia Medica*, an herbal reference for physicians. It included information on illness, appropriate treatments, and the pharmaceutical effects, dosage, and country of origin of medicinal plants. Over time, botanists accepted Linnaeus' binomial system of nomenclature, and *Species Plantarum* continues to be the starting point for identifying and naming plants. Linnaeus' great innovation eliminated much confusion in plant identification. Read more about Linnaeus in the "Nomenclature and Classification" chapter.

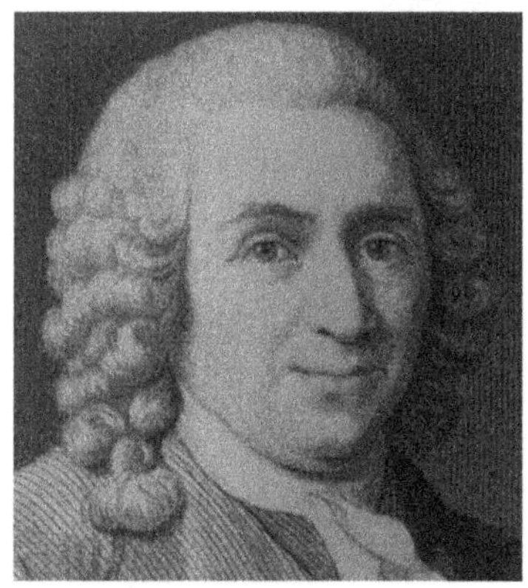

Carolus Linnaeus

Prior to the Industrial Revolution in Europe, most people lived in agricultural communities in the countryside, growing their own food and treating illness with herbal remedies. Knowledge of healing herbs remained deeply ingrained in the culture, and for many centuries householders continued growing and wildcrafting herbs for their families. After the Industrial Revolution (1760–1840) erupted in Great Britain, there was a tremendous population shift out of rural areas and into cities, forcing urban dwellers to rely more on herbal practitioners, apothecaries, and physicians for their medicines instead of growing or collecting plants themselves.

The Development of Medicine and Herbalism in Modern Europe

During the 1700s and 1800s, many professional physicians continued to administer herbal preparations. However, drugs containing mercury, iron, sulfur, copper and arsenic, which were introduced by Paracelsus, became increasingly popular and were embraced by the medical profession. The rapid growth of the Industrial Revolution and science of chemistry allowed for more precise measurement, uniformity, standardization, and improved testing of medicines for purity. Rather than using traditional whole plant remedies, scientists started focusing on the isolated chemicals that give herbs their specific medicinal properties. Advanced technology and laboratory techniques enabled scientists to isolate chemicals from herbs and manufacture chemical substances previously administered in crude plant form. Drugs were initially developed by modifying chemicals extracted from herbs. Aspirin was refined from Willow bark, quinine from the Peruvian Cinchona plant, caffeine from coffee beans, digitalis from Foxglove, menthol from Peppermint, and morphine was produced from the flowers of the Poppy plant.

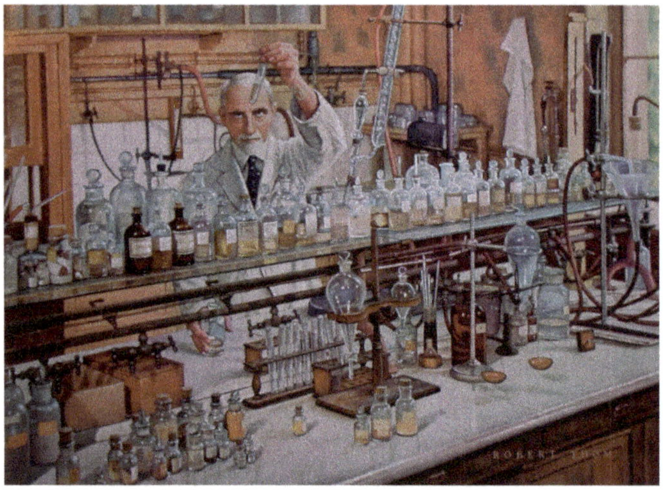

The Development of Chemotherapy; Producing drugs for standardized medicine
Image by Robert Thom. Courtesy of Pfizer Inc.

Allopathic medicine promoted pharmaceutically-manufactured drugs, medical technology, and surgery for the treatment of disease and injury. It became the established and dominant medical system in the Western world during the 20th century. Although the American medical profession abandoned herbal therapies, the practice of herbalism continued in the folk traditions and conventional medical institutions of Europe, where pharmaceutical drugs and botanical medicines are mutually accepted and continue to peacefully coexist today. Europeans generally consider herbalism to be conventional medicine rather than an alternative therapy.

There is currently renewed interest in herbs and the rapidly expanding body of scientific research and documentation continues to accelerate in Europe. According to the late Dr. Varro Tyler, Ph.D., Distinguished Professor Emeritus in the School of Pharmacology at Purdue University, "Herbal medicines have been successfully integrated into health care systems in countries like Germany, France, England and Italy." Many medical doctors in Europe are trained in herbalism during their medical education and prescribe herbal medications as well as pharmaceutical drugs. Since 1993, medical students in Germany are required to complete a section of their board examinations in the area of phytotherapy as a prerequisite to practicing medicine. *Phyto* comes from Latin meaning "plant," and the European terms for plant-based medicines are **phytomedicines, phytotherapy,** or **phytopharmaceuticals.** During the 1990s, approximately 70 percent of German physicians prescribed herbal medicines, but in 2004, the German government discontinued payment reimbursement for herbal medicine, causing a decline in sales. Despite this, herbal medicines are still commonly used and sometimes prescribed by physicians.

Germany is recognized as a world leader in financing extensive scientific research and clinical trials to identify chemical constituents in plants and to determine their biological effects and safety. In 1978, the German Federal Health Agency established an expert committee composed of physicians, toxicologists, members of the pharmaceutical industry, and laypersons. The main task of this herbal regulatory committee, known as the **German Commission E**, was to examine the safety and efficacy of botanical medicines. The German Commission E evaluated the effectiveness of over 380 botanical medicines using a standard of "reasonable certainty," which is very different from America's Food and Drug Agency's (FDA) standard of "full certainty" required for approval of new drugs. The Commission's approval of herbal medicines was determined by considering their traditional and historical uses, chemical analysis, laboratory research, clinical and epidemiological studies, and unpublished data. These standards were more complex than those in other European countries like France and the United Kingdom, where the traditional use of herbs has generally been considered to be ample proof of their safety and efficacy.

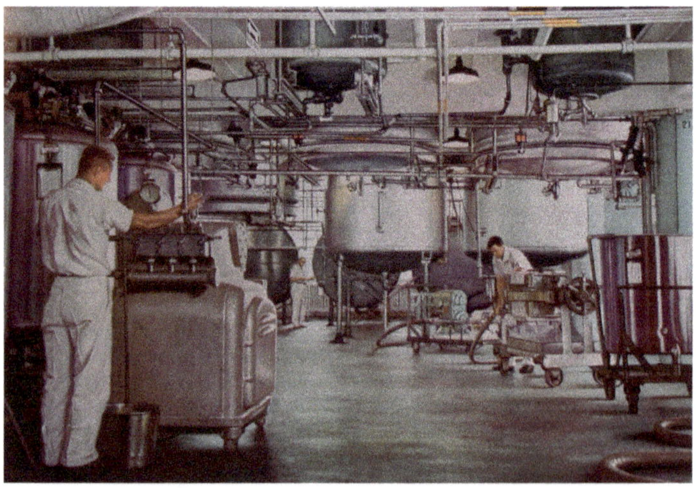

Pharmaceutical Manufacturing Comes of Age
Image by Robert Thom. Courtesy of Pfizer Inc.

European appreciation and reliance on herbal remedies has created a huge commercial market that continues to grow. Countries belonging to the European Union regulate phytomedicines according to the **European Directive** and legally classify botanicals as drugs. Herbal medicines are generally sold in pharmacies as licensed nonprescription or prescription medicines, and are required to meet the same criteria as pharmaceutical drugs. Most countries incorporate a regulation system in which herbal medicines can be approved based on their long historic use, sufficient data supporting specific therapeutic claims, and adherence to quality control guidelines.

Each nation includes botanical monographs in its official **pharmacopoeia**, a book that specifies official drug standards. An **herbal monograph** is a scientific treatise about a plant genus or a particular species. Monographs are valuable and reliable sources of information based on scientific research and technological data. They provide information on the identification of a plant genus and species, taxonomy (classification of living organisms) and nomenclature (Latin names), a botanical description of the entire plant, microscopic descriptions of the cellular structure, and various chemical tests to determine identity and purity of plant constituents.

The **European Scientific Cooperative for Phytotherapy (ESCOP)** is an affiliation of scientific and phytotherapy organizations in Western Europe. It was founded in 1989 in response to the increasing popularity of medicinal herbs and the need to standardize and regulate them. ESCOP aims to support scientific research, develop a coordinated scientific framework to establish criteria for the assessment of phytomedicines, and to promote acceptance of phytotherapy in Europe. ESCOP reflects collaboration of European scientists in researching and gathering data to expand herbal knowledge, and in developing therapeutic monographs to establish uniform regulations and policies for phytomedicines throughout the European community. ESCOP reviews hundreds of herbs and prepares monographs to provide valuable information and guidelines for physicians, pharmacists, and consumers.

The art of herbalism and use of phytomedicines continues to be a vital part of European medical care. European regulations foster greater acceptance and use of herbal medicines among the mainstream population, and continuing research and clinical trials will help ensure that Europe's ancient and rich traditions of herbal healing thrive and remain intact for many years to come.

Unani: Islamic Herbalism and Medicine

Islamic culture, philosophy, and medicine were greatly influenced by the civilizations of ancient Mesopotamia, Persia, Egypt, India, China, and later by the Greeks and Romans. These civilizations established healing systems primarily based on herbal medicines and the philosophy of balancing the four humors and the natural elements of earth, water, fire, and air. Ancient trade routes and the exchange of medicinal herbs, seeds, and spices became a vast international commerce that promoted much sharing of knowledge between these cultures.

Islamic history began in Arabia with the prophet Muhammad (A.D. 570–632), who was born in the city of Mecca. Like other ancient people, the Arabs were polytheistic, believing in many gods that were both good and evil. In A.D. 610, Muhammad declared a new religion called Islam that upheld the belief in only one god, Allah. In the name of Allah, Muhammad united the nomadic and warlike Arab tribes to produce a strong nation embracing the Islamic religion. Muhammad and his Muslim followers invaded and conquered neighboring nations to create a huge Islamic Empire. After only three years of conquest they controlled most of the Middle East. They conquered Egypt, Armenia, and Persia (present day Iran), and by the year 711, the Islamic Empire occupied Spain, ruling for over 700 years. In 831, the Muslims occupying North Africa invaded Sicily and controlled parts of southern Italy for 200 years.

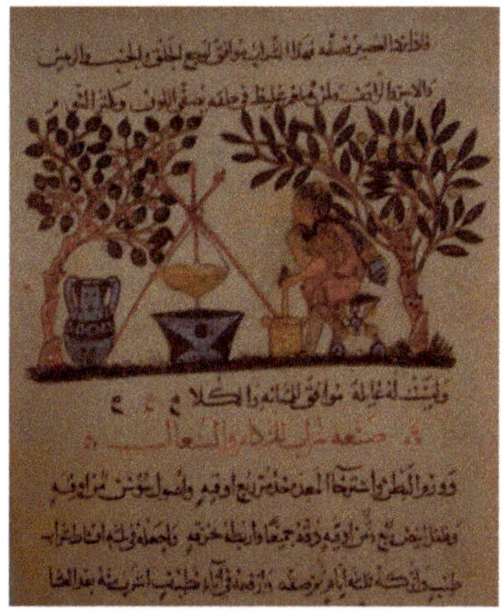

A page from an Islamic herbal book

Muslims often respected and preserved the science and medicine of the people they conquered. The tremendous exchange of knowledge during the Middle Ages was assimilated into each culture's philosophy and medical traditions. Arab physicians acquired many Greek and Roman texts on herbalism, astrology, alchemy and medicine, and they especially favored the writings and philosophy of Hippocrates, Aristotle, Dioscorides, and Galen. The systemized classification of medicinal plants that Dioscorides described in his *Materia Medica* became the foundation of Islamic pharmacology, and many herbal medicines employed by Arabian physicians were added to Dioscorides' work. By the 10th century, all major Greek herbal and medical texts had been translated into Arabic, and Muslim scholars added their own discoveries, observations, and traditions. The accumulation of herbal and medical knowledge was expounded, assimilated, and systematically codified into a flourishing Islamic medical system.

Islam was a religious lifestyle embracing a code of personal ethics that greatly influenced medical philosophy and practice. Sickness was cured only by the will of Allah, and practitioners and their medicines were considered agents through which Allah healed. Healers developed a sophisticated medical system based on disease prevention that emphasized healthy lifestyle, diet, moderation, fasting, and the use of a vast pharmacy of medicinal plants, including Cedar, Thyme, Ginger, Cumin, Cardamom, Rue, Camphor, Cloves, Myrrh, Senna, Saffron, Aniseed, and Sandalwood from India. Like the Europeans, Chinese, and Asian Indians, Islamic healers classified diseases and plants according to the qualities of hot or cold, wet or dry, and medical treatment aimed to balance the elements and humors within patients.

In contrast to the dismal Dark and Middle Ages in Europe, the Islamic world was far advanced in many areas, including education, mathematics, science, and sanitation. The Arabs taught geography from a globe when the Catholic Church insisted that the earth was flat. Arabian cities implemented high standards of sanitation while filth and excrement littered the streets of Europe, contributing to the plagues that swept through towns killing thousands. At a time when the Church and Christian monarchs in Europe punished heretics and fought to dominate all education, science and medicine, many Islamic rulers respected physicians and philosophers of other cultures, encouraging learning and expansive thought. In the field of medicine, the Arabs excelled in compiling and expanding upon all current knowledge, resulting in a systematic healing system and herbal pharmacy that eventually became the cornerstone of European medicine. The Islamic people established botanical gardens and a rich herbal tradition incorporating many new and highly valued species of medicinal and culinary herbs from the Middle East and Asia that were eventually introduced into Europe. Muslims were advanced in the study of chemistry (alchemy) and the art of pharmacy, and greatly contributed to the European development of these sciences. New types of Islamic herbal preparations were developed, including syrups and confections (remedies made with sugar or honey). The Arabic discovery of distillation led to the production of **tinctures**, which are herbal medicines prepared with varying proportions of alcohol and water. Alcohol is a sterile and stable preservative for herbal extracts, so European herbalists enthusiastically adopted this superior method of preserving herbs, called "tincturing." Muslims established the original apothecaries, or drugstores, which eventually became the model for apothecaries developed in Europe. The first recorded privately owned apothecary was established in Baghdad late in the 700s. Arab physicians had an extensive knowledge of diseases and their therapies, and employed examination of the pulse and urinalysis for diagnosis. Like the Europeans, they embraced astrology for diagnosis of illness and choice of herbal treatment.

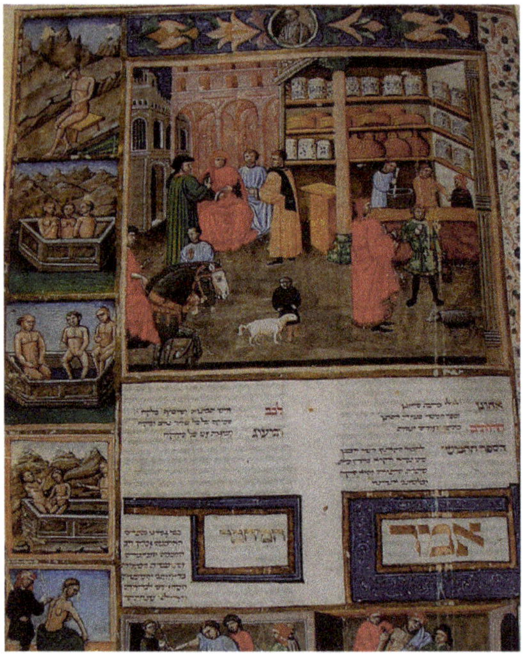

A 15th-century Italian manuscript of the text of Avicenna. The main scene shows a physician (on the right in red) in a walk-in pharmacy.

Libraries, schools, and hospitals were built and flourished during the early years of Islam. The first Islamic school of medicine was established in Baghdad in 765. Physicians became educated and certified by schools and hospitals. Many non-Islamic practitioners living in the Islamic world, including Christians and Jews, were respected and allowed to practice medicine. Untrained and self-proclaimed healers practiced medicine until the early 900s, when they were required to take exams. Midwives were allowed to practice obstetrics and gynecology due to the Islamic taboo against men touching female genitalia. Hospitals provided service to all people regardless of their finances, race, or religion. The first recorded Islamic hospital was founded in Damascus in the year 707. Another was established in Cairo in 874 and two in Baghdad in 918. By the 10th century, Arab physicians performed complex surgeries with advanced instruments and techniques, and used anesthetics to render patients unconscious. Baghdad is reported to have had 60 hospitals by 1160. Although monastic and church hospitals existed in Europe, they were inferior to Islamic hospitals in terms of sanitation, care, and facilities. Muslims were much more compassionate than Europeans in their treatment of the poor and mentally ill. Christians emphasized the salvation of the soul to promote healing, while Muslims focused on restoring the body. The highly developed Muslim hospitals became a model for professional hospitals established later in Europe, and Islamic medicine, with its hygiene, preventative medicine, pharmacy, surgery, and universities, set advanced standards for the Western world.

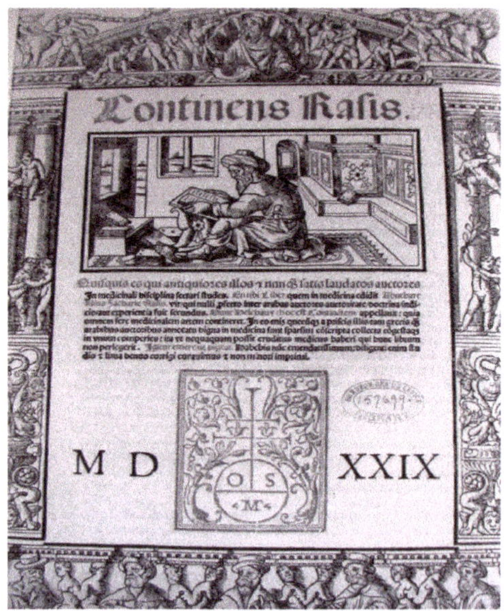

Title page of Rhazes' *Comprehensive Book of Medicine*

Many Islamic herbalists, physicians, philosophers, writers, and scientists contributed to their culture's herbal and medical traditions, but Rhazes and Avicenna stand out for their excellence. **Rhazes** (*c.* 865–*c.* 925), one of the most famous and influential Persian physicians, wrote over 200 books on medicine, philosophy, theology, natural science, alchemy, and astronomy. He attended medical school in Baghdad and was educated in Arabic, Hindu, and Greek herbalism and medicine. He implemented the perspective of Hippocrates and followed Galen's humoral theory. While Rhazes served

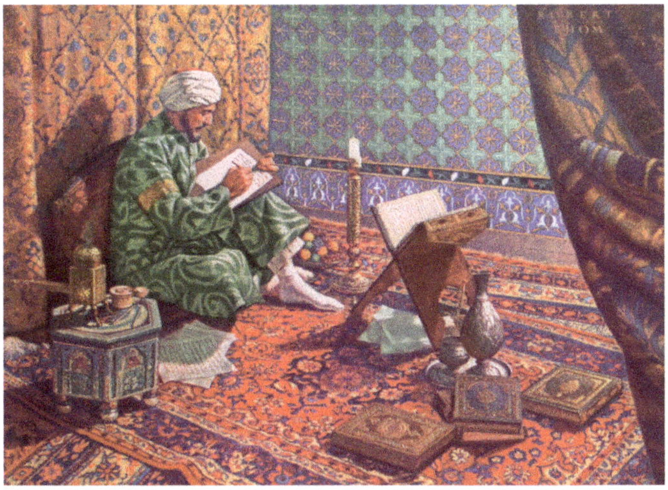

Avicenna: The "Persian Galen"
Image by Robert Thom. Courtesy of Pfizer Inc.

as director and chief physician of a large hospital in Baghdad, he wrote books on children's diseases and gave the first accurate medical descriptions of measles and smallpox. His encyclopedic manual summarizing Islamic medicine, known as the *Liber Continens,* was translated into Latin for European physicians. His focus on hygiene helped improve European medicine during the Renaissance, and his medical system and written works continue to be valued by traditional Islamic healers.

One of the most brilliant men to contribute to the science of pharmacology and medicine was **Abu Ali al-Husayn Ibn Sina** (c. 980–1037), called **Avicenna** in the Western world. He was a famous Persian pharmacist, scientist, physician, philosopher, poet, and diplomat. Like European herbalists, he studied astrology and applied it to herbalism and medicine. He traveled extensively, studied, wrote 200 books and treatises, taught a multitude of students, and was the companion of Persian rulers who supported his scientific and medical work. His major medical work, *Al-Qanun fi al-Tibb (The Canon of Medicine)*, is regarded as a valuable, comprehensive, and well-organized compilation of all Greek and Arabic medicine. In it he combined the herbal traditions of Hippocrates, Dioscorides, and Galen with the herbal and medical practice of his culture. He advocated the philosophy of the four humors and the holistic approach encompassing pure air, healthy diet, adequate rest, activity and elimination, and healthy emotions. He taught and practiced the principles of chemistry, botany and pharmacy, founded hospitals, and developed the process of distilling plant oils and alcohol. Avicenna expanded the science of urinalysis and pulse diagnosis, and developed a pharmacy containing hundreds of medicinal plants and their preparations. His medicines were primarily herbal but also included drugs derived from minerals and animals. His *Canon of Medicine* was one of the most influential medical texts ever written and was translated into most languages of the civilized world, including 28 editions in Latin. It was popular throughout Europe during the 11th–17th centuries and provided a foundation for the medical curriculum taught by European universities. It was the primary source of medical information during the Renaissance and the accepted authority on pharmaceutical knowledge in the Western world until the 1600s. Avicenna's medical system, and Islamic medicine in general, is known as **Unani**.

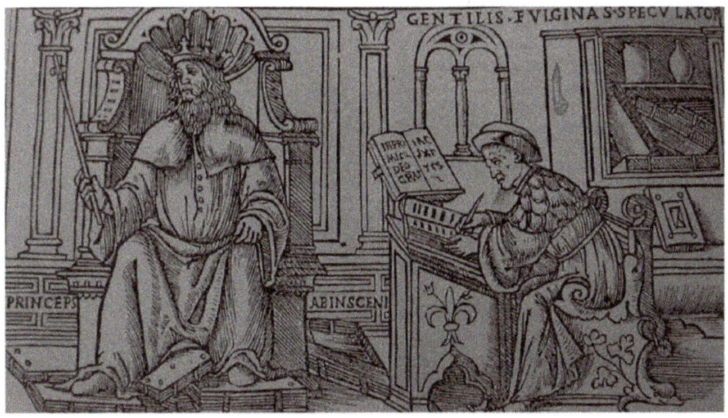

Avicenna, the "prince of physicians," is pictured wearing a crown in this 1522 Venetian edition of *The Canon of Medicine*

Islamic medicine advanced rapidly for several centuries following Avicenna's valuable contributions. Baghdad, the capital of the Islamic world, became a universal center of knowledge renown for cultural exchange, universities, and hospitals where many physicians received training and taught. Throughout the Renaissance period, Islamic medicine, surgery, herbal and medical texts, especially the works of Rhazes and Avicenna, were highly esteemed by the Western world and became the basis of medicine taught in all European universities. The Islamic system requiring standardized medical training became a model adopted by European universities in educating their professional physicians. Eventually, Baghdad and other Islamic centers of learning became places of refuge for persecuted scholars and healers from Europe who were forced to flee from the Inquisition and the Church's tight restrictions during the Middle Ages and Renaissance.

As science and technology advanced in Europe during the 1860s and early 1900s, Western allopathic philosophy and drugs became more widely accepted and were considered superior and more sophisticated than herbal medicines from older traditions. Western medicine became more dominant in Islamic countries, and although the Unani system declined in popularity, it continued to be taught in some Islamic and Indian schools. Currently in the Islamic world, Unani traditional medicine and herbal therapies are regaining popularity and continue to coexist alongside modern allopathic medicine. Contemporary Unani practitioners utilize a blend of herbal and nutritional knowledge, psychological insight, and spiritual understanding and discipline. Unani practitioners, schools, research institutions, and hospitals exist throughout the world and continue to contribute to the global wisdom and practice of herbal and holistic medicine.

Herbal Medicine in North American History

The Indigenous People of North America

Indigenous people throughout North America developed sophisticated healing traditions centuries before the arrival of Europeans. Like most cultures throughout the world, Native American Indians utilized an elaborate pharmacopoeia of medicinal plants and practiced an energetic and spiritual approach to healing. Medicine always implied power to native people. It is estimated that they used over 2,000 different plant species in their healing practices. Most indigenous people possessed a basic knowledge of common herbs growing in their localities and used plants on a daily basis for both food and medicine. Women traditionally gathered culinary and medicinal plants to meet the needs of their families.

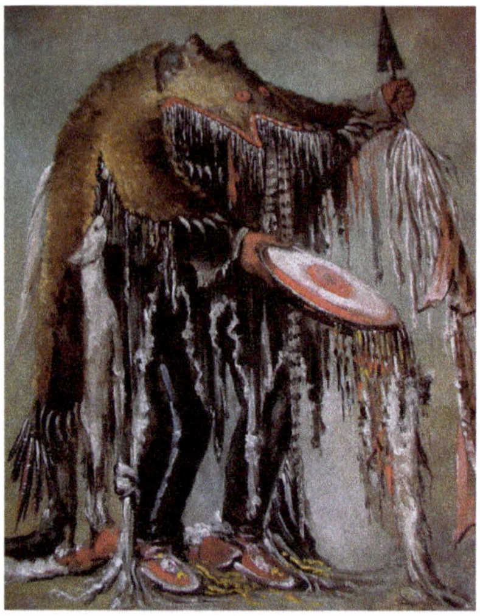

Medicine Man, Performing His Mysteries Over a Dying Man
by George Catlin

Many tribes had specialized medicine societies consisting of a shaman or chief medicine man, seers and prophets possessing expanded vision and clairvoyant abilities, and herbalists who were both men and women. The chief medicine men were highly influential and respected community leaders who helped keep the tribal healing traditions, ceremonies, mythology, and way of life vibrant and alive.

Healing the sick or injured usually involved plant remedies and a ceremony in which the forces of nature were summoned and prayers were made. Woodland tribes purified themselves by sweating in small lodges as water was poured over hot rocks to produce steam. Often the water contained herbs, creating a medicinal steam. Sometimes sacred Tobacco was added to the water. The use of herbs to purge was also common.

Healing ceremonies varied according to different tribal groups and medicine people, and often included fasting, songs and chants, drumming, rattles, and the use of stones, bones, feathers, and other natural items. **Shamans** were summoned for difficult cases. They understood and interacted with the elemental forces and the unseen spirit world to restore balance in their patients and their environment. Shamans listened to the wisdom of the rocks, plants, and animals. When treating sickness in a patient, the shaman typically called upon and entered the spirit world to seek wisdom and healing through prayer and the use of plants and animal helpers. Specific rituals were performed and herbs were employed to promote healing.

Shamanism transcends limitations of time and space, involving the ability to move between different states of consciousness and the invisible realms of the spirit world. Shamans perceive the connection of all life and the spiritual essence at the heart of life. Shamans are the original priests and healers. In ancient times, training required many years of apprenticeship under a master and was an extremely honored position in the community.

In his book, *Lame Deer Seeker of Visions*, the Lakota Sioux healer and holy man writes:

Medicine man - that's a white man's word like squaw, papoose, Sioux, tomahawk - words that don't exist in the Indian language. We have different names for different men who do different things for which you have only that one puny name. First, we distinguish the healer – *pejuta wicasa* – the man of herbs. He does not cure with the herbs alone; he must also have the *wakan* (Creator) power to heal. Then we have the *yuwipi*, the tied-one, the man who uses the power of the rawhide and the stones to find and to cure. We also speak of the *waayatan* – the man of vision who can foretell events which will happen in the future. Then there is the *wapiya* – the conjurer – what you might call a witch doctor. If he is a good man he does the *waanazin* – the shooting at the disease, the drawing up and the sucking out of your body evil things which have been put into a person by a bad spirit. If such a conjurer is bad, he himself will put a sickness into you which only he can cure - for a price. Another kind of medicine man is the *heyoka* – the sacred clown who uses his thunder to cure some people. But the more I think about it, the more I believe that the only real medicine man is the *wicasa waken* – holy man. Such a one can cure, prophesy, talk to the herbs, command the stones, conduct the sun dance or even change the weather. The *wicasa waken* . . . likes to meditate, leaning against a tree or rock, feeling the earth move beneath him. The *wicasa wakan* loves the silence, wrapping it around himself like a blanket. Such a man likes to be in a place where there is no sound but the humming of insects. He sits facing the west, asking for help. He talks to the plants and they answer him. He listens to the voices of the *wama kaskan* – all those who move upon the earth, the animals. He is as one of them. From all living beings something flows into him all the time, and something flows from him. Medicine men – the herb healers as well as our holy men - all have their own personal ways of healing according to their visions. I believe that being a medicine man, more than anything else, is a state of mind, a way of looking at and understanding this earth, a sense of what it is all about. You become a *pejuta wicasa*, a medicine man and healer, through one's own vision, or because a dream tells you to do this. A medicine man, when he's old, tries to pass his vision and knowledge to his son. (Lame Deer, 1972)

Medicines of the Native American people primarily consisted of plants prepared as tea or simply chewed and swallowed. Roots and leaves were pulverized into a mash or powder and applied on wounds as an external poultice. The roots, bark, leaves, gums, and resins of trees such as Cherry, Oak, Walnut, Dogwood, Maple, Birch, Slippery Elm, Persimmon, Pine, Hemlock, and Spruce were used for healing. Sassafras was a popular remedy for wound healing. Native Americans were experts in treating wounds, fractures and dislocations, and employed remarkable herbal remedies for snakebites and other venomous injuries. They honored the gifts of nature and treated herbal plants with great respect, taking only what they needed and never being wasteful. When harvesting medicinal herbs, it was standard practice to make an offering gift of Tobacco or cornmeal to the Earth in gratitude.

Native American Indians, like the ancient Europeans, Chinese, and Asian Indians, recognized that plants give clues about their medicinal properties by their appearance, taste, smell, color, and other characteristics. This perspective, corresponding to the Doctrine of Signatures, was another integral aspect of Native American herbalism.

Native Americans maintained a high level of cleanliness and sanitation. They bathed frequently, quarantined those who were sick or feverish, and often burned the clothes and bedding of people who died of illness. European physicians did not recognize the value of quarantine to prevent the spread of disease until the mid-1800s. When the Europeans arrived in North America, they were amazed at the overall vitality, endurance, and physical beauty of the indigenous people.

The generally excellent health of native people before the arrival of the Europeans, and their ability to live without polluting or destroying their environment, serves as an excellent example for those of us who now populate this land. Modern man's widespread pollution and desecration of life is shameful and self-destructive. We would do well to listen to the wisdom of our geographical ancestors and to follow their example of living in health and balance. Their wisdom enabled them to live in the Americas for centuries without damaging and poisoning the environment, our life-source. It is tragic that the wisdom of Native Americans is not honored as one of our most valuable and indispensable national resources!

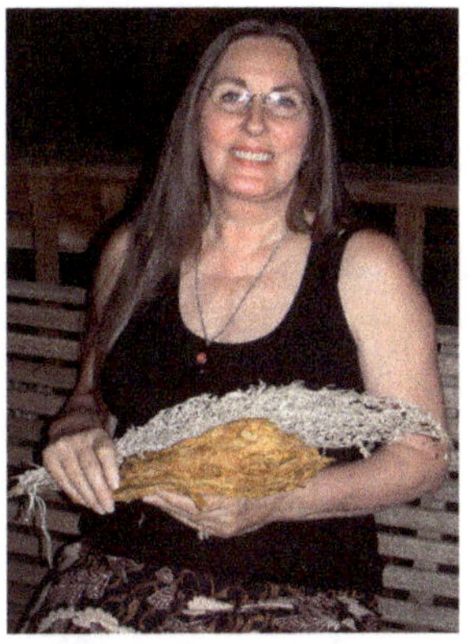

Dark Rain Thom holding bundles of Sage and Tobacco

When writing this section on Native American herbalism, I asked my friend, Dark Rain Thom, to speak about the medicine ways of her people, and she kindly agreed to two interviews. Of Shawnee descent, Dark Rain is also part Wyandotte and Cherokee. She is the Water Panther Clan Mother of the Shawnee Nation, United Remnant Band of Ohio. Dark Rain serves as a council member of the Shawnees in Ohio, some of whom are descendants of the warriors of Tecumseh, the revered Shawnee leader, wise man, visionary, and warrior. Her knowledge comes from the eastern woodland tribes and other native healers, including Mayan and Aztec medicine people. Throughout her life, Dark Rain has been taught by many Shawnee, Wyandotte, Cherokee, Potawatomi, Ojibwa, Creek, and Abenaki traditional healers. Many of the herbal and medical teachings she learned from these different nations are similar, although some are quite different. She was taught not only about herbal medicines, but also the philosophy and psychology of healing and treating the whole patient. She has studied with botanists, medical physicians, and pharmacists. Dark Rain is a teacher of the ancient Shawnee oral and historical traditions, has given traditional presentations on behalf of her people for over 45 years, and is the author of *Kohkumthena's Grandchildren ~ The Shawnee*. She is highly respected and continues to serve her people and their traditions by voicing the truth and wisdom of the ancient ways. Dark Rain is a powerful, kind-spirited woman who loves the plants and nature, and remains firmly rooted in the ways of her ancestors. The following is an account of what she shared during our conversations about the healing ways of her people.

Teachings from Dark Rain Thom

"Native American healers had their different specialties, knowledge, and skills. Herbal gatherers knew exactly where the medicine plants grew and collected them, but they may not have been a good preparer, so someone else may have had this job. Medicine people administered roots and herbs to their patients, reset bones, and stitched wounds together. Some even performed surgeries. But they may not have known how to deal with chronic illness or treat the external forces that caused some people to be ill. So we had varying degrees of healers and types of medicine people.

"Healers may study a lifetime and be 60 years old before they were recognized by their communities to be healers. It was not uncommon to have more than one healer or medicine person within our communities. But there would only be one who was called the shaman. The shaman was the ultimate healer and medicine man who knew all there is to know. He worked with the spirit world and the psychology of the mind, and with root and herbal medicines. The medicine people assisted the shaman, and the herbalists assisted the medicine people. So they had a medicine hierarchy. The large communities had the shaman, and smaller villages would go to the larger ones for ceremonies and healing serious illness. But every little village of 20 families or more would have one person specialized in medicinal roots and herbs, and in healing practices and procedures. Many women were trained in the use of common herbs to provide for their families, and about 150-200 herbs were commonly known and used by most everyone. There were always midwives in every community. The women taught their daughters and each other the procedures of normal and breech births, and the medicines to staunch bleeding and to speed up or slow down labor.

"Cleanliness had a great deal to do with our health and medicine. Indian people looked at water as a gift and took great care not to pollute it, even though it was abundant. People did not go out to the creek to get rid of their bodily waste. They were taught to go into the woods and cover it with soil. We bathed once a day minimum, and in warm weather often twice a day. This practice was based on need because the animals we hunted could smell us and be scared away. Daily bathing kept our disease at a true minimum, and when we experienced the great filth of the Europeans, it was appalling.

"Historically, more than 80 percent of our captives did not want to go back to white life because their lives were so much easier being Indian. We had more food and better medicines. We enjoyed a sense of community and belonging rather than the loneliness of frontier life. The humor within our communities was medicine for the psyche in itself. Oh, we were constantly fighting bugs and fleas, but the Indian people were not infested with lice and ringworm. We rubbed our bodies with herbs like Elderberry leaves in bear fat or weak Bloodroot to deter bugs and lice. Our beds were lined with Cedar, which bugs shun. We rubbed our bodies with herbs to mask our human smell when hunting animals, and because we took pleasure in the pleasant aromas of the plants.

"When Europeans came to this land their life span was only between 32-38 years of age, while the Native American typically lived at least 45 years, and many grew much older. During times of peace, it was not uncommon for people to live to be as old as 68 or even over 100 years of age. Warfare was our biggest mortality problem. We had an active and rigorous life, which helped to keep us healthy and probably was part of the reason for living longer. Unlike the Europeans, our people guarded against incest and marriage within families, and this prevented many deformities, congenital defects, and diseases that were common among the Europeans.

"We had very few diseases caused by nutritional deficiencies, like rickets or scurvy, because our diet was abundant and varied. It consisted of meat, nuts and seeds, berries, greens, and vegetables we grew and wildcrafted. Our seasonal diets were supplemented in winter with well-preserved foods that were dried in summer and autumn, including things we added that contained vitamin C, although I am sure we never knew that term. In summer, when people came to visit from another place, they usually walked and lost a lot of body fluids from sweating. We offered them a revitalizing drink of corn juice broth prepared from fresh cut corn that is naturally sweet and full of the mineral salts that people lose from sweating. We considered this a healthy drink as well as good hospitality.

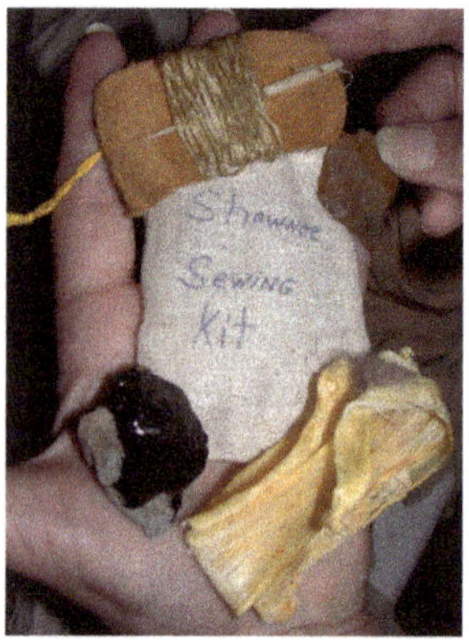

Dark Rain's suture kit with sinew thread, a bone needle, and sharp flint for cutting

"Healers also knew how to deal with the psychology of healing and the patient. A good example of this can be seen in the process that warriors went through before and after battles to heal the psychological trauma of war and killing. Before men went off to war, the medicine man made a healing hut, or sweat lodge, five to ten miles outside the village. The medicine man had the sweat lodge ready for the warriors to enter and purify themselves to become spiritually, emotionally, and mentally ready for battles. Then the war chief took over and built their blood lust up to go into battle. After the fighting was over, the medicine man, usually with the help of the shaman, had to bring the warriors back to reality and heal their spirit after violating Creator's law that you do not kill. The shaman attended to their psychological healing by having the warriors do their war dances and brag about their accomplishments in the battle field until they were exhausted and got the blood lust out of their system. Warriors were allowed the privacy to weep and mourn for the dead and for damages they may have done to other living beings who were innocent victims. All warriors need private grief time to help their minds heal. Without this healing process, the spirit suffers and people become ill or unable to return to their community in a healthy way. Without spiritual and mental health, no herbal remedies or anything else will really heal people.

"The medicine man also treated wounds and injuries. We had particular plants or pieces of plants that were used as bandages, and plants that produced resins were used to glue wounds shut or hold them together until they healed. We had needles and sutures, and we never amputated because we had enough knowledge of herbs and cleanliness to avoid gangrene and heal infections. Some medicine people even performed surgeries as delicate as trepanning [an ancient art of drilling a small hole in the skull bone] to relieve pressure and swelling from brain injuries. The people knew where the heart was and what it did, and they knew other organs and their functions. With the taboo against violating the bodies of the dead, it is interesting to contemplate how they knew these things without dissecting cadavers like Europeans had to do. Perhaps they really did remember all that Creator taught them in the beginning.

"Injured warriors were kept out of the village until they were healed. This was for the psychological welfare and morale of the tribe as well as the warriors, so that they could return walking rather than being carried with open wounds. The warriors would hear cheers instead of sorrowful sounds as they returned to their villages. Our dead were buried near the battlefields or put into the rivers, but were not brought back to the villages, where putrefaction of their wounded flesh might cause illness among the people. This system and psychological process provided the tools that prepared the warriors for the jobs they had to do during warfare. When battles were over, warriors were assisted in assimilating the experience in their mind, heart, and spirit to heal from battle so they could fully assimilate back into their community in a peaceful way, and without being damaged people.

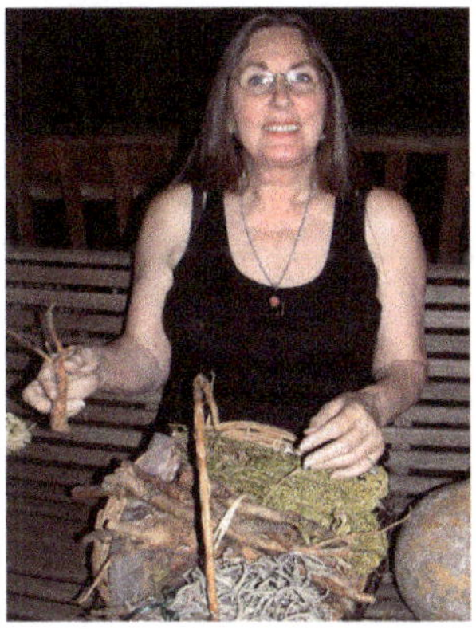

Dark Rain holding her basket of medicinal herbs

"Native people also had very specific practices when gathering and preparing their herbal medicines. We had songs that were made up of words and sounds with feelings attached to them. When collecting herbs for medicine, we had our songs, our digging tools, and our containers of Tobacco and other herbs. And we would be clean. We would go with a clean heart, clean mind, clean spirit, clean utensils, and be respectful like a visitor who is begging. We would know when we were in the neighborhood of the right medicines when we saw the first plants that we were searching out. The first four plants were like grandfathers and we honored them and did not pick them. We acknowledged them, gave them a pinch of Tobacco in appreciation of their healing gifts, and thanked them for their presence. But the collector of herbs would keep walking without taking those first plants. They would go to the main colony and walk to the largest plant, offer it Tobacco, then take what was needed, and no more. Some people sang to the plants throughout the entire harvesting and preparation process.

"We believe that everything is alive and has some form of intelligence. Everything has purpose and everything can communicate. It is for us to learn the language of the plants, the rocks, and the animals. We are the dumb ones because we only know our own language. They not only know their own language, but they also know our language and how to communicate with us if we just respect them, and listen or observe.

"When collecting and preparing herbal medicines, the plants need to know what we need from them. Many plants can provide more than one type of healing, and they need to know exactly what we need so they give us healing that is useful. We come to them as beggars, begging for their help. There is so much to healing, and it is not just the herbs. We have to know what these herbs are for; we have to talk to them about it and ask them to help us. We were not created to be little dictators here, but partners and friends, a part of creation. We are the pitiful ones and every time we pray, Shawnee are taught to ask Creator for pity; please take pity on us. We cannot survive without the help of Creator and the plants. We must not have the sin of arrogance within ourselves when we are sick. If we have done unkindness towards another, towards the earth, towards Creator or towards ourselves, we must go back to our relationship with Creator and ask forgiveness.

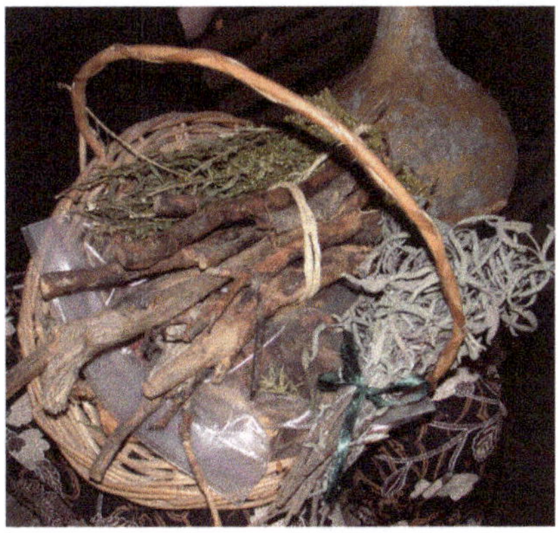

Dark Rain's basket of Sage, Sassafras root, and Sweet Annie

"The main forms of herbal preparations used by the people were teas, salves, and poultices. Many plants were used fresh immediately after harvesting. Some plants like Jewelweed lose their ability to soothe and heal unless they are used fresh, so we do not preserve them. We would dry some plants outside in the sun, which was the quickest way, so they would not lose too much of their strength and could be stored and used in the future. Herbs were often ground between stones like a mortar and pestle. We had flat stones with small holes or round grooves in them that were filled with the herbs and ground with a small pestle made from stone, horn, or wood.

"Teas were prepared by steeping or soaking plants in hot water for about 20 minutes and no more than an hour. Water was not always boiled to make tea. The most efficient way to heat water and make tea was to heat stones in a fire pit and then place them in a gourd, clay pot, or pouch of water. Six or seven red-hot stones, usually the size of a small child's fist, would bring the water to a boil within minutes, if not immediately. Remember that we always had a fire going for cooking food, even in the summer, so we did not have to start a fire each time it was needed. Women usually kept a few small stones to be ready for heating water. Fire is another sacred thing that we consider to be alive. It has intelligence and gifts to give us but we must have great respect for it. It is a tool for our benefit. We never poke it or stir it, and we never spit in it or burn trash.

"Salves were created by combining animal fat with different herbs, and occasionally nut or corn oils were used. Bear fat was most often used, but raccoon, goose, and groundhog fat were other options. There is also oily fat in the hump of a buffalo that was occasionally used for medicine. Because bears eat herbs, we believe that strong medicinal properties are stored in their fat. Animal fat was first rendered, which means it was heated over a fire and melted down into liquid. Then we would add herbs that had been dried and powdered, or harvested fresh and cut into small pieces or mashed. Animal fat was usually stored in deerskin, which did not leak. Sometimes the fat would get rancid and then we would put pieces of Box Elder in the container to sweeten it, especially if we needed the fat for cooking. Bear fat smells mild like bacon fat when it is rendered, and I have had some for over eight years and it has not spoiled. You only need a little bear fat for healing because it liquefies into oil and covers a large area when it is warmed by body temperature.

"The herbalist would sometimes sing or talk to the herbs to advise them what was needed for healing because most things have more than one medicinal purpose. Then the herbal salve was applied to the skin for wound healing and to deter flies, fleas, lice, and other bugs.

"A poultice or paste was prepared by mixing water or fat with powdered or mashed herbs, and applied to the skin. Mosses were also used as a poultice. Roots or bark were shredded with a knife, soaked in hot water to soften them, and applied to the skin. Herbalists often combined two to five herbs together rather than using only one herb. Herbalists had their own methods of preparing plants, so there was some variation.

"The herbalist would harvest the herbs, make the preparations, and give them to the official medicine person with instructions for application to the patient. The medicine person would always ingest the medicine first or apply the herbs to their skin as a poultice or salve before giving it to the patient. We were frugal, and because we lacked refrigeration, we only prepared medicines that were needed for a person's immediate healing rather than ahead of time. If medicine was administered two or three times a day, it was often prepared each time rather than all at once.

"We had all kinds of containers for dried herbs, teas and salves, including gourds, turtle shells, shells from rivers and oceans, clay pots with lids, leather pouches, and the dried hollow organs of animals like the stomach or bladder. Gourds were made into containers by cleaning them, drying them out, and cutting around the stem to create a lid. Herbs were put inside and the lid and exterior of the gourd might be sealed with yucca glue or fish glue, which kept out moisture, insects, and mice. Sometimes the end of the neck of a small gourd was cut so that tea could be poured into it and the patient could suck the tea out through the cut end. There were underground storage pits for things that needed to be preserved with some moisture, like pumpkins, but most pit storage places were very dry and lined with grasses that drew away any moisture to help keep the foods and herbs from spoiling.

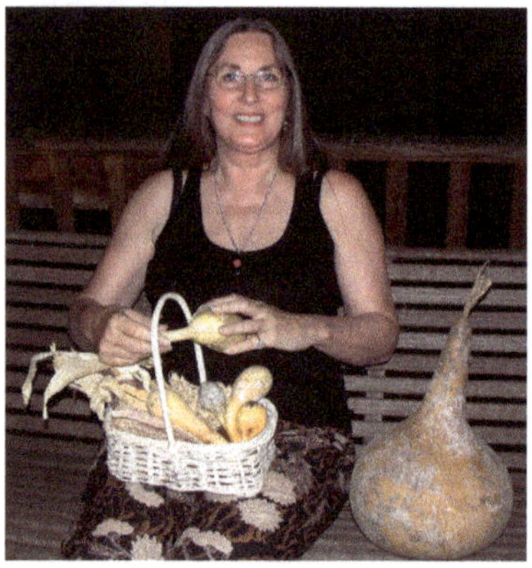

Dark Rain with her basket of gourds

"Echinacea was used to get the attention of the immune system for quicker healing, but the mechanism that medicine healers used was even quicker than Echinacea. In many indigenous cultures, the medicine man or woman would chew or take the very first dose of whatever medicine was given to the patient. The patient would lay down to rest and the medicine person would spit out the herb or tea on the belly of the patient about one to three inches below the belly button. This shocks a bundle of nerve endings and shouts 'wake up, you've got work to do!' And then the body goes into a healing mode immediately so the herbal medicines start to work as soon as they are ingested. Many North American Indian healers used this method.

"Over time we have learned much about medicine from the animals. Everything the deer eat can be used for medicine, so we would watch them and learn. The bear also taught the people which plants to use, and the mother bears teach us how to be good parents. A common method of treating children or adults with an upset stomach and uncontrollable vomiting and diarrhea was to capture and kill a buzzard and empty out its stomach contents. Then they would make a lukewarm soup or broth in the stomach of the buzzard because its stomach is so full of digestive enzymes that it kills bacteria. This was considered a reliable remedy for people with extreme vomiting and diarrhea.

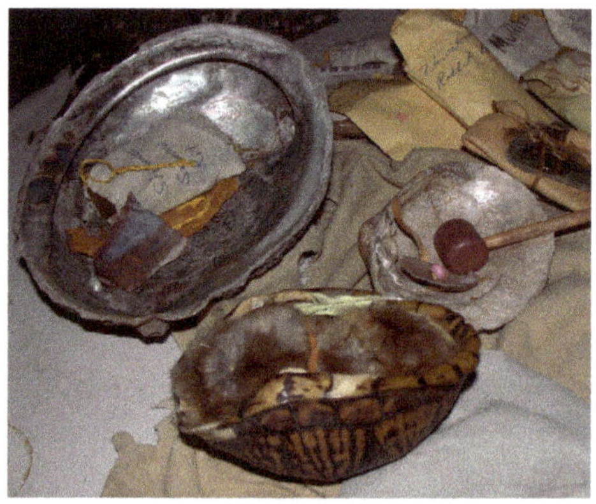

Abalone, mussel, and turtle shells used as containers for herbs

"Through the eons, the elders learned the differences between medicinal requirements and dosages for men, women, and children. There was women's medicine that was not just for menstrual cramps or birthing. There was men's medicine that was not just for war wounds. And there was children's medicine that wouldn't harm anybody, but might not help someone who is not a child.

"Different tribes had different uses for the same medicines, and the differences were often in the dosage. So dosage is extremely important, as is the cooperation of the patient. We learned the combinations and doses of herbs and roots, and what to use them for. When making a batch of herbs, healers knew how much ingredient to use per dose, with how much water or oil, and this was taught by the traditional teacher. Children learned much by watching their mothers and grandmothers, and were eventually called upon to make remedies themselves. They were taught how to find and harvest medicinal plants from the time they were about nine years of age, or younger if they were interested in medicine. The young healers would also learn at their elder's elbows, and then they would have to do it themselves with the assistance of the elder until they could work independently. If the medicine didn't work, the patient would be told, 'I'm sorry my medicine doesn't work with your illness, but there is another person who may help you.'

"Creator gave Native Americans instructions for living on the earth. He told us how to use plants and animals, water, soil, air, and fire. He gave us all the instructions. People naturally migrated, and when they went to a new place, they explored new plants and experimented with them. According to oral tradition, there was a time when the plants and animals spoke to us and we all communicated with each other. Many of our oral traditions that we used to teach our children moral standards and how to behave and interact together come from the time when we all spoke with one another and understood each other. Europeans have a difficult time understanding this because there have been so many different civilizations occupying the same space in Europe, compared to people like the Hopi, who have oral traditions of astronomical occurrences that happened thousands of years ago. So if a people have been there that long, what have they not explored and experimented with and learned how to use?

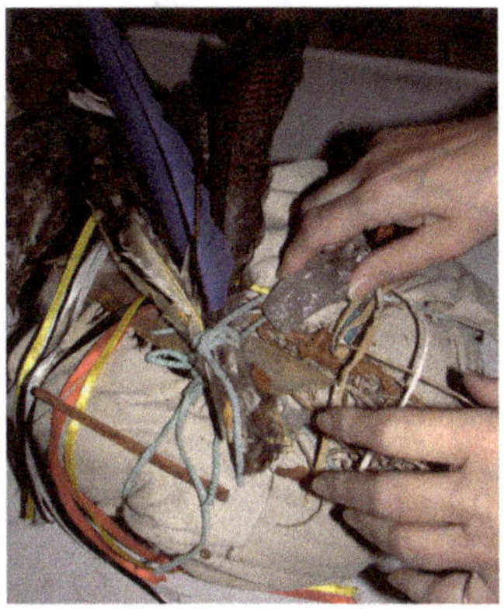

Dark Rain's medicine bundle of deer skin adorned with ribbon, feathers, and a quartz crystal

"There were countries in Europe that had a great deal of herbal knowledge, but people lost and suppressed that knowledge. We feel this happened when men took away the God-given right and natural ability of women to heal and kept it for their own. They did not have a lifetime of training, but rather than going and asking the old women who knew, they killed off the women and their knowledge. Now many nations are trying to recapture their old medicine ways and knowledge. There is honor in everyone when you live with kindness and respect, and you don't need to be jealous or fearful that someone seems to have more power than you. None of us have power, only Creator has power. We just need to learn to live well together and help carry each other along rather than being mean-spirited. There are so many things in human beings that need to be healed: their relationship with themselves, their relationship with the universe, their relationship with Creator, and with all other nations that share this planet. Indian people acknowledge other nations such as the birds, animals, trees, plants, stones, water, air, clouds, and fire. Without a good spiritual relationship with Creator, everything in our life is a mess, including our body, our attitude, and our friendships. It is good to know our place in the universe and on earth, what we are here for, what's expected of us, and how we are to interact with others.

"Plants that provide food and medicine were placed here for all of us long before we were brought to earth. Our spirit was created where Creator lives and He said, 'I will create a place for you to live.' And so He made the earth and everything we need to survive and thrive, to be healthy and raise our young. Then He brought us down and put us here. He had already made clean water, rich earth, trees with fruit and nuts to feed and shelter us. He provided roots, shrubs, plants, and grasses to heal and feed us, and creatures to help take care of us, to clothe us, give us tools, teach us how to take care of the young, and show us our medicines.

"If you have not had an elder to teach you about the medicine or if you are in a strange place, you can stop where there are many plants and make a Tobacco offering. You can say to the plants, 'I am sick, I am a stranger here, I don't know which of you are supposed to help me with this illness. Will you please let me know who you are, that I may take you to make me well, to make my family well?' One of the plants will acknowledge you; they will be the only one to wiggle or they will bend over when everything else is standing straight. Something will happen that the plant will identify itself to you and tell you, 'You may take me and I will help you. That is what I am here for.' When we go into the fields and woods, we make a Tobacco offering in a grateful and humble way. We explain to the plants why we are there. We don't take the first ones we see, or the biggest or the best or the oldest plants. We leave plenty for everyone else. The plants do have intelligence and make better medicine when we approach them in a respectful way.

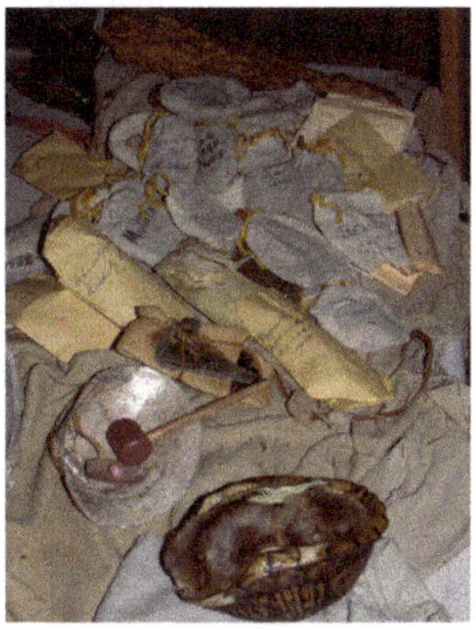

Contents of the medicine bundle: packets of herbs, stone pipe, abalone, and turtle shell

"Not all Indian ways are extinct, but the American government did so much to destroy our culture. The government forced Indian children to live away from their parents and community in Christian boarding schools, where they learned English and the white man's ways. The children were forbidden to speak their own language and severely punished if they did so. In almost every tribal society, it is the grandparents who teach the children. When these children returned home after several years in boarding schools, they only spoke English. Some could speak a pidgin language with their parents, but their grandparents didn't speak English. So within one generation, all the traditional and generational knowledge that had accumulated for 10,000-30,000 years by being passed on from grandparent to parent and grandchild, was broken. There was so much that was not translated over to the children's generation that when they had children, the knowledge and many of the old ways were forgotten. So much of what goes on now is not the full body of traditional healing. There are very, very few medicinal healers in the tribes who learned the healing ways from their grandparents because it was against American law to practice our medicine or religion. Offenders would be thrown off the reservation with no way to survive. Or they'd be put into prison or killed. And the last option is what usually happened.

"So people did not openly practice our healing ways. Many elders went into the woods and secretly practiced their medicine and healing ceremonies, but they could not teach or let the children take part because of the danger. Children did not understand that kind of danger and might speak about the ancient

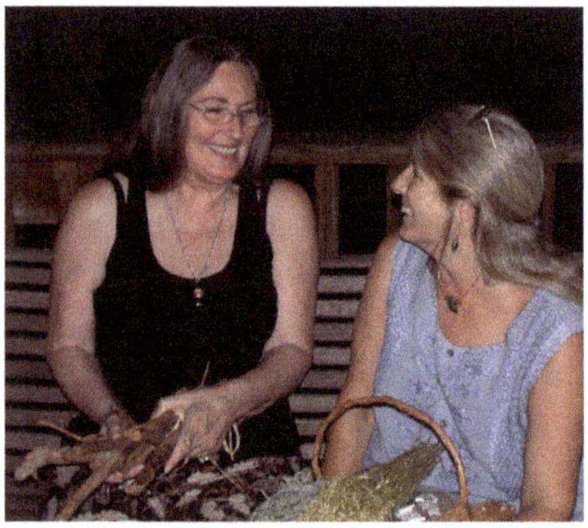

Dark Rain conversing with with Susan Clearwater

ways to the wrong people, which would bring hardships and even death to the family. So much was lost long ago. We could not legally even practice our religion in this country until 1974!

"There is so much to healing, and I assure you that I don't know one to two percent of what my grandmother knew. And my grandmother felt that she knew less than her mother and grandmother. The loss of so much knowledge and the ancient healing ways over the past several generations is very sad. I wish many of my relatives were back to teach me, and I wish I had paid better attention to them in my younger years."

Dark Rain's generous and eloquent teachings provide an authentic glimpse into the rich herbal traditions and spiritual perspective of Native American life and medical systems prior to the devastation of their culture. The huge herbal pharmacy and robust health of the indigenous people are testimonies to the wisdom and value of their medicine and lifestyle. May their intrinsic wisdom and connection with nature always be present on the earth!

Herbal Medicine in Colonial America

Many of the first Europeans to arrive in North America respected and became friends with the indigenous people. These explorers, traders, and trappers were able to survive in the wilderness by learning native skills and knowledge of medicinal plants. Stories of sick immigrants who were saved by herbal remedies abound, and many immigrants owed their lives to Native American healers and herbalists. There are numerous written accounts of native healers who treated Europeans suffering from injuries and illness, but most were unwilling to divulge their herbal remedies to white men. However, knowledge was exchanged over time, and much of our information on native herbs and healing techniques comes from the journals of these early Europeans. They acknowledged the large herbal pharmacy, the amazing herbal cures, the robust health, and strong, handsome bodies of the Native American people. Indigenous people did not suffer from the diseases and plagues that erupted in crowded, filthy European towns and cities.

When the colonists migrated across the Atlantic Ocean in the early 1600s, they brought important items from their homelands necessary for survival in the new world, including tools and seeds for cultivating food and herbal medicine. Over the years, many medicinal herbs planted in colonial gardens escaped cultivation and eventually became naturalized in the new world. Native Americans adopted many of these European herbs into their own healing traditions. In this way, an exchange of herbal medicines naturally occurred.

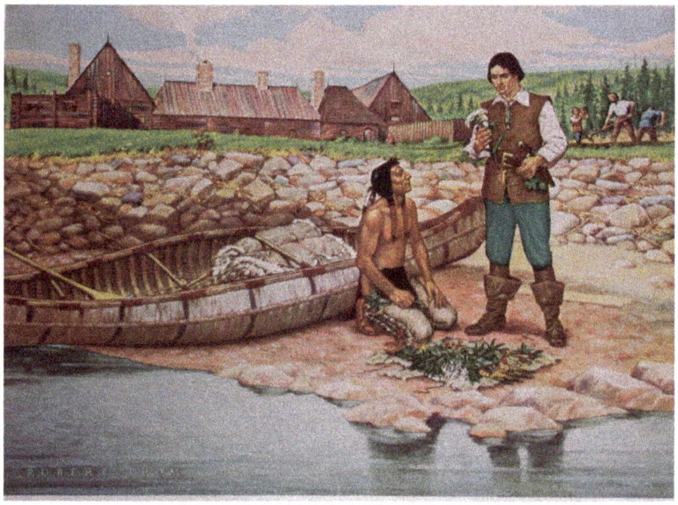

Louis Herbert: Apothecary to New France (Canada) Cultural exchange of herbal knowledge

Image by Robert Thom. Courtesy of Pfizer Inc.

Attitudes toward accepting Native American herbal medicine reflected the diversity of European settlers. Native medicine and indigenous herbs were more accepted by laymen than by missionaries, priests, or physicians. Settlers living in isolated rural areas and in the South embraced native medicine more readily than the puritanical New Englanders. Although some of the early Europeans respected and befriended the indigenous people, the majority of colonists regarded them as "savages and heathens," and held fast to the belief that their European herbal medicines were superior to the roots, bark, leaves, and flowers of the Native American pharmacy. This ethnocentric arrogance was especially obvious in their rejection of Native American healing ceremonies, which many missionaries and common people regarded as "devil worship and witchcraft." The Europeans had come from a culture immersed in the religious dogma of the Church during a time when herbalists were burned at the stake for practicing witchcraft. They came to the new land obsessed with beliefs in white supremacy and fear of the devil, and looked upon the Native American people with puritanical eyes. When Europeans witnessed Native American healing ceremonies using drums, rattles, songs, and natural objects such as feathers, rocks and herbs, they perceived them as savagery and superstitious rites when, in fact, these were used as tools to align the healers' consciousness with the healing powers of the four elements, Mother Earth, and the Creator. Most Europeans were unable to fathom the wisdom, spirituality, and devotion to the Creator at the heart of Native American healing traditions and culture.

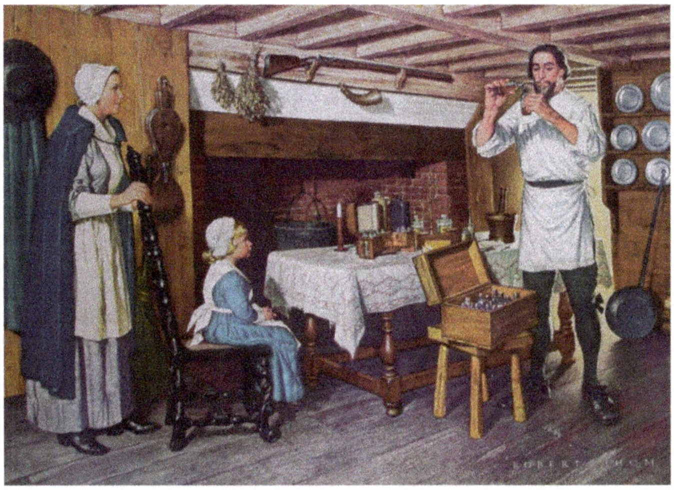

The Governor Who Healed the Sick: Medicine in Colonial America John Winthrop, Governor of Massachusetts Bay Colony Practicing Medicine
Image by Robert Thom. Courtesy of Pfizer Inc.

Few physicians emigrated from Europe, and there was a general lack of medical knowledge or adequate training on the American frontier. The colonists suffered from poor hygiene and sanitation. During the 1600s and 1700s, medical practice in colonial America was open to almost anyone who could demonstrate healing skills. Medical services and remedies were provided by governors, churchmen, educators, self-appointed doctors, and housewives. Initially, colonists relied on importing plant and mineral medicines from Europe while ignoring the rich array of herbal medicine in the new land. Most colonial women grew herbs from their homelands. All efficiently run homes had medicinal and culinary herb gardens, with racks of drying herbs hanging in barns and attics to be stored for later use. John Gerard's *Herball*, which listed many European herbs for treating various illnesses, and *The English Physician* by Nicholas Culpeper were popular herbals and medical references during the colonial period. There were no hospitals in America until 1751, when one was established in Philadelphia, and the first hospital pharmacy was established there one year later.

Eventually, out of necessity, more colonists and healers relied on the medicinal herbs employed and introduced by Native Americans. Part of the colonists' new reliance on indigenous plants stemmed from a nationalistic spirit and desire to be independent from England and Europe in all ways. But because of their ethnic arrogance, most colonists lacked any respect for native wisdom, and Native American herbalism only survived in very fragmented pieces. Constantine Rafinesque (1783–1840), a botanist who recognized the valuable contributions of Native Americans, once said, "When America was settled, the native tribes were in possession of many valuable vegetable remedies discovered by long experience, the knowledge of which they gradually imparted to their neighbors. This knowledge was partly adopted even as far as Europe, and partly rejected by medical skeptics, and became scattered through our country in the hands of country practitioners, herbalists, and botanists." During the first half of the 1800s, the title of "Indian doctor" became popular, especially on the frontier. These "Indian doctors" were actually white men claiming to be tutored in native herbalism by Indians. For a period of time in American history, the "Indian doctors" and the herbs they sold were held in fairly high esteem.

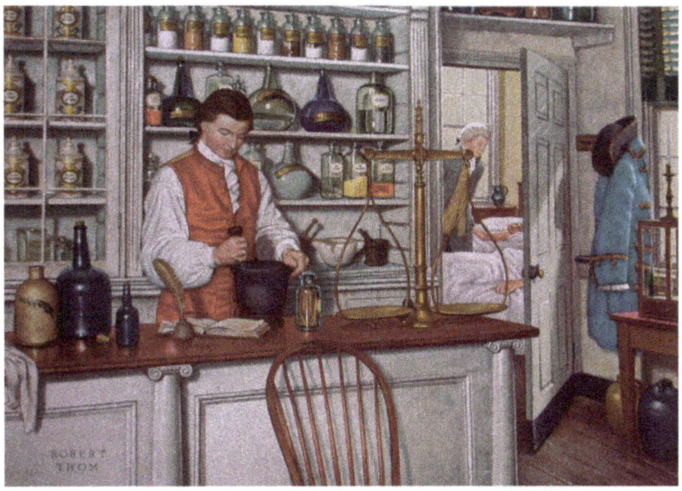

The First Hospital Pharmacy in Colonial America Established in Philadelphia in 1752
Image by Robert Thom. Courtesy of Pfizer Inc.

Although Native Americans and their healing traditions were not generally respected by the colonists, many of their herbal medicines were eventually adopted by physicians and listed in the two primary drug references of that era. Over 200 indigenous herbs used by Native American Indians have been listed as official drugs in the *United States Pharmacopoeia* since it was first published in 1820 and in the *National Formulary* since it originated in 1888. In most cases, Native American uses of the herbs corresponded with those approved in these reference manuals. Of the 212 plants listed in the 1820 edition of the *U.S. Pharmacopoeia*, nearly 100 plants were used by Native Americans. However, the book's explanations and directions for medicinal uses of the herbs were based on European perspectives and the four humors theory, without any reference to Native American knowledge or healing practices.

During the time when Native American herbalism interfaced with the medical practices of the colonists, life for the indigenous people was forever changed. Although Native Americans greatly contributed to colonial survival and medicine in the new land, the Europeans, who desired freedom and had fled from Europe because of religious and political persecution, in turn persecuted the people whose land they invaded. The United States government initiated a full-scale and long-term plan to annihilate Native American culture, and thousands of men, women, and children were massacred. The ravages of disease brought from European cities killed huge populations of native people, whose immune systems had no defense against alien diseases like typhus, scarlet fever, influenza, measles, venereal diseases, or cholera. Soldiers deliberately gave blankets belonging to people dying of small pox as "gifts" to Indian villages. Native culture and traditions were further destroyed by forcing the remaining people to live in guarded reservations, and by declaring the practice of their religion, customs, and lifestyle illegal. Indian children were taken from their parents at a very young age and sent to boarding schools where they were taught English and Christianity. They were often severely beaten and even killed if they disobeyed or spoke their own language. After several years they returned to their families on the reservations, and they no longer remembered their own language or tribal ways. Over the next 100 years, the white man's shameful near-annihilation of the Native American population eroded and nearly destroyed their rich culture and healing ways. The elders alive today tend to protect the remnants of their traditions and, understandably, are not always willing to share their healing plants and ceremonies with those whose forefathers took their land and ended their way of life. Fortunately, some Native American medicine people are willing to share their herbal and healing knowledge. They should be greatly appreciated and generously compensated for their willingness to do so, and hopefully their wisdom will be treasured for future generations!

American Medicine and Popular Health Movements of the 1800s

As the richness of Native American life and healing traditions declined on destitute reservations, the medical movement in America moved forward. The University of Pennsylvania established the first School of Medicine in North America in 1765. Columbia University College of Physicians and Surgeons was founded in 1767, followed by Harvard Medical School in 1782. Initially, medical training consisted of only two months to two years of education, and high school diplomas were not required for college admission. Many early medical schools lacked clinical facilities, and students received no practical experience with patients.

During this era in American and European history, the principles and practice of medicine diverged into two distinct disciplines. In the early 1800s, university-trained doctors began to establish a professional medical organization and distinguished themselves from herbalists and lay practitioners by calling themselves **"regular" doctors**. Over time, the new European medical system, based on chemical and mineral drugs administered by "regular" doctors, was incorporated into the developing American medical system. Medicines made from refined chemicals and minerals were called **allopathic drugs**. The medical treatments employed by the "regulars" were called "heroic," referring to the powerful and invasive methods of bloodletting, excessive purging, and the use of strong and sometimes toxic substances such as mercury, arsenic, sulfur, and opium. By 1830, 13 states had passed medical licensing laws forbidding herbal and lay practitioners from practicing medicine, establishing the "regular" doctors as the only legal healers. In 1847, the first national medical organization of professional physicians was established as the **American Medical Association (AMA)**.

> *University-trained "regular" doctors used allopathic (chemical) drugs, while the "irregular" physicians relied on herbal medicines from nature.*

In response to the laws that established and controlled medicine as an elite profession, the **Popular Health Movement** emerged during the 1830s and 1840s. It was driven by dissatisfaction with the harsh heroic therapies and by a patriotic fervor against the "regular" allopathic doctors representing European aristocracy. The Popular Health Movement held to the ancient belief that "Mother Nature heals" and supported traditional folk and plant medicine provided by lay people, female healers, midwives, and herbalists. Many women endorsed and fought for this old healing tradition, and the Women's Rights Movement played an active part in the Popular Health Movement. Many holistically oriented methods of healing, such as hydrotherapy (water cure), vegetarianism, homeopathy, naturopathy and herbalism, became popular during this time, offering an alternative to the heroic cures of the allopathic physicians. The Popular Health Movement was so strong that, by the 1840s, the medical licensing laws had been repealed in most of the 13 states. Throughout the 1800s, "regular" physicians and the **"irregular" physicians** of the Popular Health Movement attacked each other and fought for control of the American medical system.

Early regulation of medicinal preparations was initiated in 1820 when a group of 11 physicians published the first edition of the ***United States Pharmacopoeia (USP)***. The *USP* was the first book designed to create professional standards for official medical drugs, specifying tests for their identity, quality, and purity. It was an authoritative guide to ensure uniformity in medicines for apothecaries, who collected and dispensed medicinal herbs, and for physicians, who at that time did some of their own compounding. The United States Food and Drug Act of 1906 recognized the *USP* as the official drug standard in the country, enforceable by law. It contains monographs that describe drugs and is the most authoritative source of information for safe drug dosages.

The original medicines listed in the *USP* were mostly herbs and minerals. Out of the 650 original medicines, 70 percent were derived from plants. In 1880, the number of herbal preparations rose to almost 75 percent. The development of organic chemistry and rise of pharmacology occurred toward the end of the 1800s as production of synthetic medicines evolved, and by the early 1900s, the use of herbs greatly declined among physicians. Between 1920 and 1936, many plant-based medicines were regarded as ineffective and replaced by synthetic drugs, including antibiotics that were available by the early 1940s. In the 11th edition of the *USP* released in 1936, only 40 percent of the listings were derived from plants, and by 1990, fewer than two percent of the entries were plant-based, a decline that continues today. In comparison, although European pharmacopoeias also excluded plants from their listings, they did so to a lesser degree.

The ***National Formulary*** is another official listing of pharmaceutical formulas and preparations that documents legally enforced drug standards. The first edition, produced by the American Pharmaceutical Association in 1888, was a recognized authority for physicians and pharmacists. In 1980, the *USP* and the *National Formulary* were merged into one book, which continues to be periodically revised.

Thomsonian Medicine, Physiomedicalists, Eclectic Physicians, and Naturopaths

Several important healing modalities and organizations that evolved from the **Popular Health Movement** greatly contributed to the continuation of medical herbalism in North America. One of America's most famous herbalists during this era was **Samuel Thomson** (1769–1843), an outspoken leader of the Popular Health Movement who developed his system of **Thomsonian medicine**. He was very sickly as a child, but recovered his health after receiving herbal treatments from an elderly woman who was taught by Native American healers, and practiced as a "root and herb" doctor. The herbal medicines were successful after the "regular" allopathic physicians' heroic treatments had failed, and this made a lasting impression on young Thomson. He eventually became a self-trained healer who incorporated the ancient philosophies of Hippocrates, Galen, and North American Indians to balance and restore the four humors and promote health. Thomson realized that most illness results from a diminished life force in the body, and his treatments were aimed at restoring this vital energy through healthy lifestyle, diet, and remedies prepared from herbs indigenous to North America. He advocated simple herbal remedies and steam baths derived from Native American healing traditions. His well-known treatment of purging and cleansing the body with Cayenne and Lobelia stimulated vital energy and eliminated toxins. In 1813, Thomson received a patent for his herbal formulas that he packaged and sold. His successful herbal healing practice became quite popular among the general public, and the **Thomsonian Medical Reform Movement** peaked during the 1840s as botanical medicines grew in popularity throughout the United States. Thomson publicly denounced the American allopathic medical physicians and their profession, condemning their use of chemical drugs and their heroic, and sometimes dangerous, treatments. He constantly incurred the wrath of the medical community, which unsuccessfully attempted to prosecute him in court for his criticisms and outspoken advocacy of herbalists.

Alva Curtis (1797–1881), one of Thomson's medical assistants, established a professional group of "irregular" physicians called the **Physiomedicalists**. They founded their own sectarian medical schools and embraced a more holistic view of health and disease, relying on herbal medications rather than the allopathic drugs of the "regular" doctors. The Physiomedicalists incorporated the humoral philosophy of Hippocrates along with the Chinese concepts of balancing the polarities of Yin (female), Yang (male), and the natural elements of water, earth, fire, and air. Their physical exams, which included a pulse and tongue assessment, determined which herbs were prescribed. The Physiomedicalists were most popular in the 1880s, and although they never gained significant momentum in the United States, their healing system was accepted in England and taught at the College of Herbal Medicine until the 1970s.

> *The Eclectics were a large group of professional medical physicians who used indigenous herb plants as their primary tools of healing.*
>
> *They were very influential from the 1880s through the 1930s.*

The **Eclectics** were an influential group of professional physicians who broke away from mainstream medicine and were also known as "irregular" doctors. Emerging during the Popular Health Movement, they were an active force from the 1880s through the 1930s. The Eclectics offered an alternative to allopathic medicine by advocating the superiority of plant-based medicines over those derived from minerals and synthetic chemicals. They introduced a distinctive pharmacy based on plant preparations, employing many herbal remedies of Native American and old European traditions. Like the Physiomedicalists, the Eclectics practiced medical herbalism according to holistic philosophy and the doctrine of the four humors, similar to the ancient European, Arabic, Chinese, and Indian Ayurvedic systems. Eclectic physicians prescribed herbal remedies to balance excess hot, cold, wet, and dry conditions that promote illness. As strong proponents of formal medical training, they established their own medical institutions in the United States.

The Eclectic medical system primarily evolved from the work of **Wooster Beach, M.D.** (1794–1868). He initiated a sectarian group of herbal practitioners called the **Medical Reform Movement** (sometimes referred to as the **Reformed Botanical Movement**). He renounced allopathic medicine after graduating from medical school in New York, determining that herbal medicines were superior. He credited "root and Indian doctors" as possessing valuable remedies and actively collected information from Native healers, herbalists, and female practitioners. Beach founded the Reformed Botânic College in New York in 1829, which later relocated to Cincinnati, Ohio. In 1845, Beach founded the Eclectic Medical Institute in Cincinnati, and by the 1850s, this had progressed into the primary Eclectic school and was one of the largest medical schools in the country, graduating over a quarter of Ohio's physicians. By the mid-1800s, the Medical Reform Movement became known as Eclectic medicine, adopting "sustain the vital forces" as its credo. Eclectics were "vitalists" who acknowledged that the vital energies of food, herbs, the human body, and the environment must all be kept in a dynamic balance for optimal health. The Eclectic physicians observed the pulse, tongue, complexion, and mental attitude of their patients in order to correctly prescribe herbal therapies. Their vitalist doctrine asserted that "man assists but Nature heals."

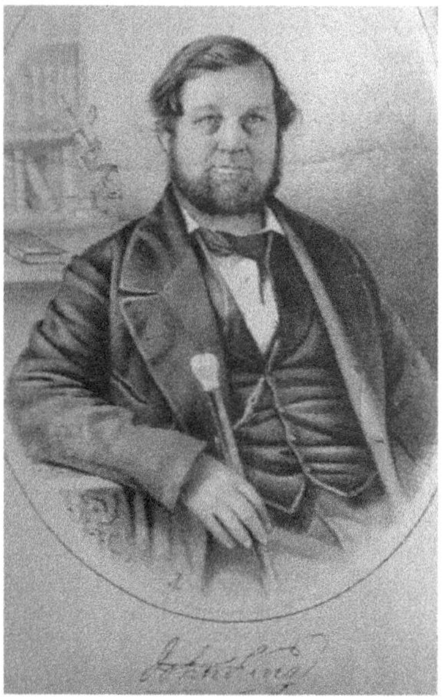

John King, M.D., Eclectic physician

The Eclectic physicians developed extensive monographs of individual herbs that included information about their morphology (form and structure), chemistry, toxicology, physiologic and therapeutic actions, forms of preparations, and dosages. They valued using whole plant preparations rather than isolated extracts of specific chemical constituents. By 1860, 13 Eclectic medical colleges were in operation in the eastern United States, and by the late 1800s, there were more than 10,000 practicing Eclectic physicians in the United States, compared to over 72,000 allopathic doctors and 8,640 homeopaths.

John King, M.D. (1813–1893) was another primary force in the development of the Eclectic schools. A prominent doctor, pharmacist, and medical author, he joined the faculty of the Eclectic Medical Institute in Cincinnati in 1851. He became one of the most prominent Eclectic medical practitioners and is renowned for his major works, including *The American Family Physician* and *King's Eclectic Dispensatory*, which describe his clinical use of herbs. **John Milton Scudder, M.D.** (1829–1894), a colleague at the Institute, devised a method of prescribing single herbal medicines in small amounts according to specific medical indications. John King introduced **John Uri Lloyd** (1849–1936) to the professional Eclectic medical community in the September 1870 issue of the *Eclectic Medical Journal*. He and Scudder convinced Lloyd, a brilliant young pharmacist, to develop premium quality botanical preparations for the Eclectic physicians.

John Uri Lloyd became the famous herbal pharmacist of the Eclectics. As a leading proponent of herbal medicine, his work greatly contributed to the development of medicinal herbalism in America. Lloyd was a respected pharmacist, scientist, and herbal product manufacturer who taught chemistry at the Eclectic Medical College and the Cincinnati College of Pharmacy. Working closely with the Eclectics during the 1890s, his work was accepted by all medical schools due to his scientific approach of researching medicinal plants, and to his great contribution in the study and development of pharmacy. He devised new and improved methods of herbal extraction and made standardized preparations for distribution exclusively to physicians rather than the general public. His formulas and methods of preparing herbal medicines, called "Specific Medicines," were the most popular of his time, and some herbalists continue to use them today. His widely read book, *The Chemistry of Medicines* (1881), was among the first medical chemistry texts published in the United States. In recognition of his professional leadership, Lloyd served as president of the American Pharmaceutical Association from 1887–1888. His research and documentation of herbal elixirs helped in the development of the first *National Formulary* published in 1888.

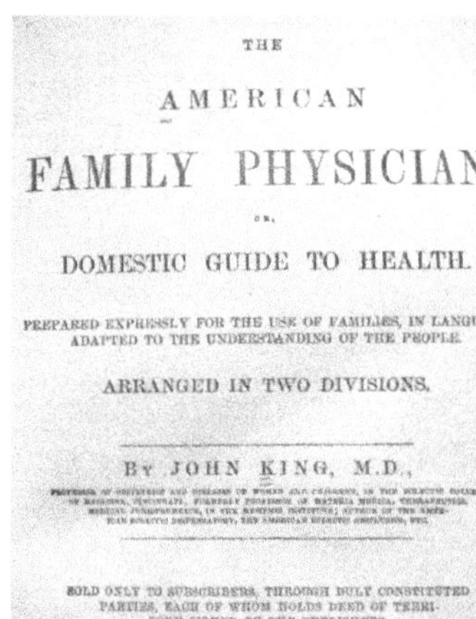

THE

AMERICAN

FAMILY PHYSICIAN;

OR,

DOMESTIC GUIDE TO HEALTH.

PREPARED EXPRESSLY FOR THE USE OF FAMILIES, IN LANGUAGE ADAPTED TO THE UNDERSTANDING OF THE PEOPLE.

ARRANGED IN TWO DIVISIONS.

BY JOHN KING, M.D.,

SOLD ONLY TO SUBSCRIBERS, THROUGH DULY CONSTITUTED PARTIES, EACH OF WHOM HOLDS DEED OF TERRITORY SIGNED BY THE PUBLISHERS.

DIVISION I.

INDIANAPOLIS, IND.:
A. D. STREIGHT, PUBLISHER.
N. E. COR. WASHINGTON AND MERIDIAN STREETS.
1864.

Title page of the famous manual by John King, MD

Lloyd and his Eclectic colleagues believed in the superiority of natural botanical medicines over mineral or synthetic drugs. They prepared herbs as whole plant extracts, although as time passed, the Eclectics became more interested in isolated plant alkaloids that commercial manufacturers aggressively promoted. Lloyd and his brother developed their own company called the Lloyd Brothers Pharmacists in Cincinnati, Ohio, specializing in preparations derived from North American plants and producing 379 Specific Medicine herbals. He also established the Lloyd Library and Museum in Cincinnati, considered the world's most important pharmacognosy library, which contains written works of the Eclectic physicians and other very old herbal manuscripts. Lloyd supported standardized regulation of the pharmaceutical manufacturing industry and was a major player in the enactment of the first Pure Food and Drug Act in 1906. The publication of *King's American Dispensatory* in 1897, revised by Lloyd and **Harvey Wickes Felter, M.D.** (1865–1927), became a milestone in supporting scientific and clinical scrutiny of indigenous North American medicinal plants. Lloyd's contributions were in large part responsible for the development and acceptance of an American herbal materia medica. King, Scudder, and the Lloyd brothers combined forces to become the leading manufacturers of Eclectic herbal preparations, producing botanical drugs that supplied physicians throughout the United States.

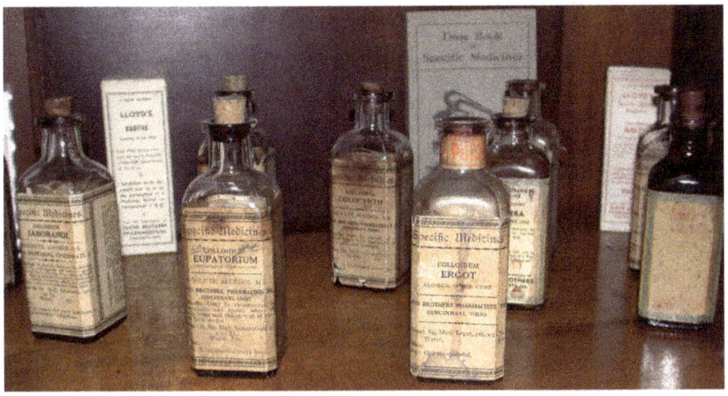

Eclectic herbal preparations manufactured by the Lloyd Brothers Pharmaceutical Company (photo taken in the Lloyd Library, Cincinnati)

Most allopathic doctors belonging to the American Medical Association considered Eclectic physicians to be quacks for using herbal medicines and regarded them as competitors in the medical profession. The Eclectics constantly criticized the "regulars" for their use of dangerous mineral remedies like mercury and heroic methods like bloodletting. During the 1800s, the development of systematic pharmacognostic (the branch of pharmacology dealing with natural plant medicines) and botanical studies by the Eclectics were important components of the American medical system. The Eclectic's use of herbal therapy coexisted with the allopathic medicine of the "regular" physicians until the 1880s, when production of synthetic drugs increased and became widely available through the rapidly expanding pharmaceutical industry. By the early 1900s, plant medicines were being replaced by synthetic compounds produced in research laboratories and manufactured for national markets. Pharmaceutical companies produced drugs from one chemical compound that could be precisely analyzed, standardized, and measured in exact dosages, allowing for more reliable and consistent biological effects in patients. The demise of herbal medicine was reflected in the *U.S. Pharmacopoeia,* where synthetic drugs replaced many herbal preparations. Whereas European countries incorporated pharmaceutical and synthetic drugs into their health care systems while continuing the practice of herbalism, herbal medicine in America became regarded as old-fashioned and inferior, and was almost completely replaced by pharmaceutical drugs. The art of healing was largely displaced by the science of medicine.

Scudder, King, Felter, William Cook, and **Finley Ellingwood** (1852–1920) were university-trained medical doctors of the Eclectic school who established a profoundly valuable legacy by recording their herbal therapies, holistic philosophies, and clinical experiences in several books. Their works are the most massive and important documents of early American medical herbalism, and they continue to be reliable sources of information validated by years of clinical experience and by chemical analysis performed by the Lloyd brothers. Most of these books are housed in the **Lloyd Library and Museum** in Cincinnati, Ohio, which is open to the public. The library contains John Uri Lloyd's research, the entire personal library of John King, MD, and an extensive collection of recent and rare old herbal manuscripts. In the words of Michael Flannery, the director of Lloyd Library, "this library could be considered the mother-lode of 19th century American medicinal plant information." Much of the Eclectic documentation is also available on the Internet.

The demise of the Eclectic movement accelerated in 1907 when Andrew Carnegie and John Rockefeller commissioned Abraham Flexner to investigate hospitals and medical schools and to advise them on the best investments in American medicine. The Flexner Report was issued in 1910 by the American Medical Association, recommending that only medical schools committed to scientific research based on models developed in the 19th century should receive financial support. Flexner reported that the "regular" physicians using surgery and pharmaceutical medicine would provide the greatest development of industrial technology and profit. He depicted the Eclectic physicians as "drug mad" due to their emphasis on botanical therapies. Endorsed by the financial support of Carnegie and Rockefeller, allopathic medicine flourished. The well-established Eclectic medical schools, promoting herbal remedies and holistic philosophy, disappeared due to lack of funding and political harassment encouraged by the harsh criticism contained in the Flexner report.

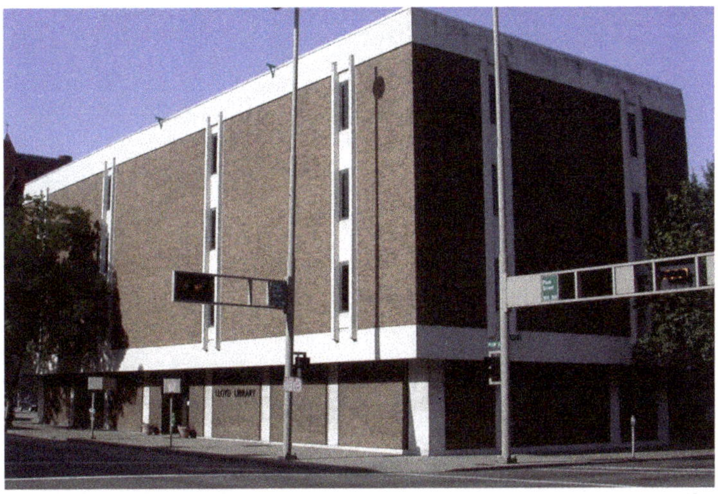

The Lloyd Library and Museum in Cincinnati, Ohio

All of the Eclectic colleges were closed by 1939. Researchers were no longer interested in studying whole plants for medicine, focusing instead on single active constituents and synthetic chemicals. Plant medicine research in the United States came to a virtual standstill as doctors and scientists became more interested in potent medicines produced in the laboratory. The use of herbal medicines declined, and drug companies focused on developing synthetic drugs that would provide profit through patent protection. Many people believe that the production of safer and more effective drugs caused the decline of herbal medicine, but synthetic pharmaceutical medicines also replaced herbal remedies because of laws and money. Medical schools in the United States excluded botany and herbalism from their curriculums in favor of pharmacology. Naturopathy, homeopathy, and herbalism were forced out of the mainstream medical system and relegated to the status of folk medicine and quackery.

After the Eclectic tradition was replaced by modern allopathic medicine, the practice of medical herbalism almost disappeared in the United States. It was preserved by a few unique individuals and people in rural communities who, isolated by geography and poverty, were forced to rely on herbal healers and plant remedies handed down through their families for generations. These individuals and a few exceptional herbal books kept the flame of herbalism alive.

Dr. Benedict Lust (1872–1945) is considered to be the "father of modern naturopathy." He came to America from Germany in 1896 after being cured of tuberculosis by Sebastian Kniepp, a German physician and priest. Kniepp taught his natural healing techniques to Lust and commissioned him to promote the program of hydrotherapy (water) treatments, herbs, and simple lifestyle that had cured his tuberculosis. Lust earned an osteopathic degree in 1898 and a medical degree from the Eclectic Medical College of New York in 1914.

Lust called his healing methods "**naturopathy**." Naturopathy uses simple elements of nature to cure disease and strengthen the body, similar to the Hippocratic, Asclepian, and Eclectic models. Naturopathy offers a basic philosophy for living and acknowledges that the body is capable of self-healing when given the right environment. Diet, stress reduction, cleansing, immune system enhancement, the use of herbs and homeopathic remedies, and a holistic view are all part of naturopathic therapy. Naturopaths learned by apprenticeship and formal education, and many were educated in osteopathy and chiropractic medicine.

By 1902, Lust had established a naturopathic sanatorium, the American School of Naturopathy, and a Naturopathic magazine. He founded the Naturopathic Society of America, which was eventually reorganized as the American Naturopathic Association (ANA) in 1919. He also opened the first health food store in the United States. In 1953, the ANA published *Natural Medicine and Naturopathic Dispensatory*, a landmark work presenting the application of natural therapies, naturopathic philosophy, and many botanicals employed by the Eclectics. The popularity of naturopathic medicine has waxed and waned in North America, but continues to thrive as an alternative approach in the American health care system.

Another exceptional clinical herbalist was **Jethro Kloss**, who ran a sanitarium where he employed the herbal therapies described in his well-known 1971 classic herbal, *Back to Eden*. **John Lust**, an herbal clinician and nephew of Dr. Benedict Lust, wrote *The Herb Book* in 1974, which continues to be a popular reference guide for North American medicinal herbs.

American Herbalism and Modern Medicine

American herbalism had thrived as a well-established medical system from the colonial period until the early 20th century. However, a shift occurred when the last of the Eclectic medical schools were forced to close in the 1930s, resulting in the "herbal dark ages" of disrepute and almost total abandonment. The modern industrial era was the only time in human history when plants were abandoned as the primary source of medicine.

Finally, during the late 1960s and early 1970s, the dawn of the "herbal renaissance" began to flicker as the emerging counter-culture and back-to-the-land movements embraced the wisdom and natural inclination to partake in Nature's offerings of healing plants. Many Americans shifted their fundamental attitudes, feeling empowered to manage their health care by incorporating herbal remedies into their lifestyles. This renewed appreciation of botanical medicine evolved in conjunction with increased scientific and clinical research on herbs, popular self-help psychologies, and consumer disappointment with limitations of the medical establishment and health care system. Some people felt discouraged and overburdened with the constantly rising cost of prescription drugs produced by a multi-million dollar industry. Although industrialized nations have invested huge amounts of money in the development of pharmaceutical drugs, many of these have proved ineffective against viruses, influenza, cancer, and chronic conditions like hypertension, asthma, and arthritis. Numerous drugs originally endorsed by the Food and Drug Administration (FDA) have been recalled from the market due to toxicity or dangerous side effects. These issues have prompted many people to seek alternative sources of medicine.

> *Disillusioned by limitations of the medical system and the side effects and rising cost of drugs, many Americans have enthusiastically embraced the "herbal renaissance."*

Acknowledging the dramatic popularity of herbs and other supplements, Congress mandated the establishment of the **Office of Alternative Medicine (OAM)** at the **National Institutes of Health (NIH)** in 1992, reflecting Congressional support for legitimizing alternative therapies. Congress gave OAM the mission to evaluate medicinal herbs and other alternative medical modalities for their effectiveness and safety, and to help integrate reliable treatments into mainstream medical practice. In response to this mandate, OAM researches and compiles data on alternative medicines to determine and report their safety and efficacy.

OAM sponsors conferences on a wide variety of topics about holistic medicine, and issues research grants to universities, hospitals, and foundations.

Although public demand grows for more acceptance and incorporation of herbal supplements into our health care system, the American Medical Association (AMA) is much more reserved about allowing the entry of medicinal herbs into its domain. Plant-based medicines are under critical scrutiny by the medical and pharmaceutical communities, and are cautiously being incorporated under the umbrella of **Complementary and Alternative Medicine (CAM)**. Supported by the endorsement of CAM, more physicians are receiving training in botanical medicine as the number of medical colleges offering classes in herbology, nutrition, and complementary modalities gradually increases. Continuing education courses in botanical medicines and their interactions with prescription drugs are being offered in response to requests by pharmacists, nurses, and physicians. Many prestigious medical schools and universities, including Harvard, Columbia, Duke, Stanford, California University in San Francisco, Jefferson Medical College and the University of Arizona, have established departments of Alternative Medicine and offer courses in Integrative Medicine.

> *The most progressive health care systems combine allopathic medicine with the ever-expanding menu of complementary therapies, enabling people to participate in freedom of choice and individualized health care.*

Accredited Naturopathic Colleges specialize in teaching holistic and clinical applications of herbal therapies with other models of alternative medicine. Such colleges currently include Bastyr University in Seattle, Washington, the National College of Naturopathic Medicine in Portland, Oregon, and the Southwest College of Naturopathic Medicine in Scottsdale, Arizona. Each offers a complete curriculum in botanical medicine.

Of all the alternative therapies, herbalism seems to be the most difficult to incorporate into mainstream medicine. This is in part because medical school curriculums have neglected to include herbal medicine or nutrition classes until recently. It also reflects the absolute reliance on pharmaceutical drugs that we, as a nation, have developed. Although the process is just beginning, herbal medicine will hopefully be incorporated into a national health care system. The most progressive and competent health care system is one that includes the Western allopathic tradition with the constantly expanding menu of alternative modalities, enabling people to participate in freedom of choice and individualized health care.

Herb Regulation in the United States

The dynamic increase in consumer use of botanical preparations has necessitated new laws and adjustments of older drug laws regarding safety regulations and the provision of guidelines for manufacturing and marketing industries. Federal laws and agencies regulate the production and marketing of all drugs, medicinal herbs, and dietary supplements. The **Food and Drug Act of 1906** was the first attempt by the United States government to regulate herbal and pharmaceutical medicines. This Act prohibited the adulteration and faulty labeling of drugs, and focused primarily on the quality of drugs being marketed rather than their safety or effectiveness.

The **Food and Drug Administration (FDA)**, an agency of the Department of Health and Human Services, was established by Congress in 1928 to regulate and enforce laws requiring all drugs to meet specific standards. The FDA regulates the pharmaceutical industry by requiring manufacturers of new products to file a New Drug Application, an expensive pre-market testing and approval process. Applications must specify scientifically proven laboratory and clinical trials demonstrating the safety and effectiveness of new drugs. These trials typically require 5-12 years of research and can cost millions of dollars for each new drug. The pharmaceutical industry primarily focuses only on products they can patent, which excludes naturally occurring products like herbs because the manufacturer does not profit without a patent.

In 1938, the **Federal Food, Drug, and Cosmetic Act (FD&C Act)** was established to ensure that all drugs sold in the United States are proven safe before reaching the market. This law mandated that manufacturers perform toxicity tests on laboratory animals before seeking FDA approval to market a drug. This act was later amended to require any drug produced after 1962 to be scientifically proven safe and effective before reaching the marketplace. Products that had been approved prior to 1962, demonstrating evidence of safety but lacking proof of efficacy, were "grandfathered" in and allowed to remain on the market as long as the producers made no efficacy claims. Then in the 1980s, the FDA decided to examine these grandfathered products and commissioned a study of over-the-counter (non-prescription) drugs, including many herbal preparations, to determine if there was valid scientific evidence to support claims of safety and effectiveness. Many herbs failed to pass this examination.

The **Nutrition Labeling and Education Act (NLEA)** of 1990 required packaged foods to state their ingredients on labels, and health claims had to be consistent with FDA standards. Although the FDA lists many herbs as safe, herbal manufacturers were not legally allowed to claim therapeutic benefits of their products without the support of scientific evidence. This created a huge debate between the FDA, the herbal industry, and concerned consumers. In response to this controversy, Congress unanimously passed the **Dietary Supplement and Health Education Act (DSHEA)** in 1994, a major victory for the interests of herbal consumers, producers, and merchants. The Act stated, "Consumers should be empowered to make choices about preventative health care programs based on data from scientific studies of health benefits related to particular dietary supplements."

The purpose of DSHEA was to ensure consumer access to herbs and other supplements, and to construct a framework for the regulation of dietary supplements and the supplement industry. Prior to the establishment of DSHEA, herbs and other dietary supplements were regulated as either foods or drugs, depending on their intended use. Products used for taste, fragrance, or nutrition were regulated as foods and subject to the "food additive" provisions of the FD&C Act. A product was regulated as a drug if it made therapeutic claims of affecting the structure or function of the body, and had to conform to the drug safety and efficacy requirements of the FD&C Act.

A monumental shift occurred when DSHEA ruled to regulate herbs as dietary supplements, forbidding the FDA from treating them as food chemicals or drugs. This protected herbal products from the FDA's very expensive pre-market testing and approval requirements. Shortly after the passage of DSHEA, manufacturers who had previously ignored herbal remedies due to patent laws and lack of financial incentive quickly developed herbal preparations that started flooding the commercial market. Manufacturers had to be responsible for validating the safety of their products. Under DSHEA, the FDA was granted authority to establish proper manufacturing practice regulations and to take action against products that present safety problems or are improperly labeled. Herbs and other supplements marketed prior to the passage of DSHEA are not required to demonstrate safety or efficacy due to an assumed degree of safety, since these products were already being marketed to the public.

DSHEA classifies herbs as dietary supplements.

The purpose of DSHEA is to regulate dietary supplements and the supplement industry, and to ensure consumer access to herbs and other supplements.

DSHEA specifically addressed labeling and health claims on supplement containers, requiring that the term "dietary supplement" appears on labels and ingredients are disclosed. Manufacturers were allowed to provide warnings, recommended use, and contraindications on labels. For the first time, information from books and scientific literature was provided with the sale of dietary supplements as long as the information was not false or misleading, did not promote a brand or company, and was not displayed in the immediate vicinity of the supplements.

DSHEA allowed dietary supplement labels to state health benefit claims called "statements of nutritional support," which are commonly referred to as structure/function claims because they describe the effect of the supplement on the structure or function of the body, and on general well-being. The claims must be supported by scientific evidence and accompanied by a disclaimer that the product is not intended for treating or preventing symptoms or diseases. According to DSHEA, herbal dietary supplements cannot make health claims about a specific disease or health-related condition. Labels can say, for example, that a botanical preparation "promotes healthy circulation and heart function," but are not allowed to state that it "prevents cardiovascular disease."

DSHEA also required the formation of an executive level Commission on Dietary Supplement Labels and authorized $5 million to establish an **Office of Dietary Supplements** in the **National Institutes of Health**. Its purpose was to conduct and compile scientific research on dietary supplements. This office acts as the principle advisor on supplements to the Secretary of the Department of Health and Human Services, the National Institutes of Health, the Center for Disease Control, and the FDA.

Good Manufacturing Practices (GMPs) for herbs and other dietary supplements were established in 2007 by the FDA under mandate of DHSEA. Compliance with GMPs helps ensure that manufacturers are producing unadulterated and properly labeled supplements using a consistent and reliable process.

The American Herb Market

In recent years, the new industry of herbal manufacturing has emerged, creating a huge selection of crude herbs, herbal formulations, and standardized extracts that are readily available to consumers. When popularity of medicinal herbalism was on the upswing during the 1960s and 1970s, a handful of dedicated people started producing and selling herbal products, paving the path for the evolution of the current herb industry. What started out as a few privately-owned small businesses committed to producing superior quality herbal preparations has evolved into a huge corporate marketing arena. Botanical preparations are now available in almost any retail outlet, from health food and grocery stores to discount department stores, health professional offices, mail order catalogues, Internet sales, and multi-level marketing. When DSHEA classified medicinal herbs as "food supplements" in 1994, herbs were exempted from official FDA drug standards. Consequently, herbal sales increased at most major retail stores. To some extent, this widespread availability seems to have increased consumer appeal and confidence in using herbs for health care.

One problematic outcome of the increasing popularity of medicinal herbs and the resulting multi-million dollar herb industry is the production, by some manufacturers, of herbal preparations made from poor quality, low-potency plant material providing minimal therapeutic effects. The preparation of top quality and therapeutically potent herbs depends on many factors, including correct identification of the herb, proper cultivation methods that address the specific needs of each plant species, proper harvesting and handling, and special considerations and selection of techniques necessary to stabilize plant constituents. The fine art of herbal preparation is often neglected and the quality of the product is compromised when new players of mass production are primarily motivated by profit gain and lack basic herbal knowledge. The current practice by many manufacturers of adding sugar, artificial colors, flavors, fillers, and other unnecessary additives counter-productive to health is a travesty to the fundamental art of preparing pure, organic herbal remedies. Many of these less expensive but inferior herbal products are available in bargain discount stores and grocery stores, so buyer beware! Be sure to read product labels to avoid preparations containing unnecessary ingredients. There are many ethical and knowledgeable herbal manufacturers creating quality preparations that are usually more expensive, but just as with most things, you get what you pay for. When comparing a $4 bottle of Echinacea pills sold in a discount store to a $14 bottle of Echinacea tincture in a reputable health food store, it is likely that the $14 preparation has been produced with better quality control standards and has greater therapeutic value than the cheaper brand. It is always wise and economically prudent to buy top quality herbs and other supplements from reliable health food stores or health care practitioners who purchase their products from reputable companies.

Buyer beware of cheaply produced herbal preparations!

Always buy herbs and other supplements from health food stores or health professionals offering high quality and potent products.

Another recent market development is the appearance of medicinal herbs in conventional foods that lure consumers with advertised "healthy ingredients." This new category of "nutraceuticals" includes Ginkgo potato chips and breakfast cereals, Echinacea fruit drinks, and Ginseng candy bars. When the food industry adds herbs to foods, it tends to mislead consumers who expect increased health benefits when it is unlikely that these foods contain the necessary amounts or potency of herbal ingredients to provide significant effects. The industry's decision to add medicinal herbs to processed foods is alarming to consumers and herbalists concerned with misrepresentation and exploitation of medicinal herbs, especially rare and endangered plants like Ginseng. Although this may be considered free marketing, it reflects the industry's attempt to profit from the growing popularity of herbs, and its disregard of the ecological impact on some of our "at risk" herbs. It also creates the potential problem of confusing food with medicine. Although many herbs are medicinal as well as culinary, such as Basil and Cayenne in tomato and pesto sauce, Garlic and Ginger in salad dressings, or Dill in pickles, adding medicinal herbs to processed foods can be an indiscriminate use of valuable resources.

Although herb sales fluctuate with the changing tides of public opinion, media coverage, and product availability, the market for medicinal herbs continues to grow. In 2004, the World Health Organization (WHO) estimated the global market for medicinal plants at about $14 billion, and projected herb sales to rise to $5 trillion by the year 2050.

As the market and herbal industry continue to expand and create a global impact, it is paramount that balance be maintained and wise choices implemented. For the market to continue providing herbal medicines to the public, several considerations require attention. Rising demand necessitates increased cultivation and preservation of land where plants grow. Increased cultivation necessitates the need for clean, unpolluted air, water, and soil for plant proliferation. Problems that must be addressed and rectified include deforestation, land misuse, and the exploitation of indigenous people's knowledge of herbs without appropriate appreciation or compensation.

Herbal Research

The purpose of botanical research is to understand the chemistry and therapeutic activities of plants and their constituents. Research plays a vital role in the continuing practice of medicinal herbalism, especially as it exists alongside the conventional medical and pharmaceutical industries.

Most of the significant studies on the clinical uses of herbs come from Europe and China, thanks to their regulations supporting scientific and clinical research. Only a small fraction of money allocated for medical research in the United States is focused on traditional uses of plant remedies. The **National Center for Complementary and Alternative Medicine (NCCAM)**, a branch of the **National Institutes of Health**, spends a significant portion of its funds on researching herbal medicines. In 1999, approximately $60 million was funded for this purpose, increasing to $89 million in 2001.

The majority of research in the United States has focused on analyzing plants for their biological activity by identifying and isolating one or a few specific chemical compounds exerting the most noticeable and influential activity. These isolated chemicals are measured, concentrated, and prepared as drugs, or they are synthetically manipulated and replicated into pharmaceutical medicines that can be patented by drug manufacturers for huge profits. American pharmaceutical companies and other research institutions invest millions of dollars to discover single active compounds. Since research is so expensive and herbs cannot be patented unless their chemical structure is altered, large pharmaceutical companies typically do not research whole plant extracts. The chemical diversity and variability of herbs certainly presents a major challenge to the scientific and medical communities, and researchers may be making a fundamental mistake by only focusing on one or a few active chemical constituents in plants. The American medical system will never utilize the full medicinal power of plants unless it moves beyond its strong reliance on a single active compound.

A plant is composed of hundreds of naturally occurring chemical components that interact synergistically and exert activity in the human body.

Focus and research on only one component does not reveal or represent the activity of the whole plant, and can lead to incorrect conclusions about herbal toxicity and efficacy.

In contrast, European policies make it economically feasible for manufacturers to research and develop herbal medicines. A major difference between American, European, and Chinese herbal research is the basic principle of European and Chinese drug regulations that regard the entire herb as the active ingredient. There are no requirements to isolate and demonstrate activity of specific chemicals since they occur naturally, and the combination of all the constituents is recognized as producing the biological effects.

Modern scientific research of medicinal plants provides extremely valuable information. This is paramount to the continued understanding and application of medicinal herbs for appropriate herbal regulation, and for the benefit of the herb industry and general public. However, herbal research often lacks uniform evaluation criteria, and it must be regulated by reliable and consistent methods to ensure accuracy. Valid research must be designed with consideration of the unique characteristics of each herb, and must test plant material that is correctly identified, cultivated, harvested, handled, processed, and stored using quality control standards. Standardized guidelines need to be established to regulate testing procedures, evaluation, and reporting. Information about the herb being researched should include the correct species identification given in Latin nomenclature, the part of the herb being tested, the form of preparation (powdered crude herb, water extract, or alcohol extract with ratio of water-to-alcohol content), and its exact concentration and quantity. Valid research outcomes can be highly variable depending on all these factors, and are certainly dependent on the age, shelf life, quality, and potency of the herb being tested. Herbal pills or capsules made from old, poor quality material will demonstrate very different activity and outcomes compared to a concentrated tincture extract produced from high quality, freshly harvested plant material.

Researchers test and analyze herbs according to the scientific method, a powerful tool that is nonetheless susceptible to personal and professional bias, political and economic manipulation, and conflict of interests. One major research flaw in Western methods arises from analyzing herbal medicines in the same way synthetic drugs are evaluated, which comes from a reductionistic model. Herbs and whole plant medicines, by their very nature, are not pure compounds like pharmaceutical drugs. They consist of hundreds of naturally occurring chemical components interacting synergistically to exert pharmacological activities. Yet scientists often extract and analyze one plant chemical that is tested for biological activity. The outcome is recorded and conclusions are determined. Research on only one chemical component will not reveal or represent the activity of the whole plant, and can lead to incorrect assumptions and hypothetical statements about herbal toxicity and efficacy, often conflicting with centuries of anecdotal folk use and empirical evidence. While such statements are often clinically unsubstantiated, they are publicized and become "locked" into the media pool of misinformation. The current popularity or decline of many herbs is often largely determined by this type of faulty research and resulting media coverage, which can mislead and confuse health care providers and the general public.

When evaluating research, remember that any chemical isolated from a food or herb, if ingested in excessive amounts over a period of time, can cause imbalance that leads to disease.

When evaluating research methods and outcomes, it is important to remember that any chemical isolated from a food or plant and ingested in excessive amounts will, in all likelihood, create imbalance within the system that can cause side effects or eventually lead to disease. To accurately investigate herbs, laboratory research techniques must reflect their real-life application.

Herbal research using the scientific method consists of two primary tests, ***in vitro*** (Latin meaning "in glass") and ***in vivo*** (Latin for "within the living"). *In vitro* studies are test tube or petri dish experiments that often investigate a whole plant or an isolated chemical extracted from a plant to observe and analyze its activity or toxicity. Animal testing and human clinical trials are the two forms of *in vivo* research, and are better suited for observing the overall effects of a phytochemical or whole plant on a living subject. Although using animals for research provides important information and is legally sanctioned, many people do not endorse inflicting pain or suffering on any creature. It is unfortunate that so many animals are sacrificed in research labs, including those that investigate plants.

> *The scientific method of botanical research involves two primary tests.*
>
> *In vitro tests are done with petri dishes and test tubes.*
>
> *In vivo research involves testing with animals and human clinical trials.*

In vitro studies may be limited since isolated chemicals do not necessarily reflect the complex biological activity of the whole plant when ingested by people or animals. A good example of this type of misrepresentation can be seen in a Loma Linda University study on the effects of St. John's Wort, Echinacea (*E. purpurea*), Ginkgo, and Saw Palmetto on human reproduction (Ondrizek, 1999). In the study, extracts of these four herbs were tested to evaluate their effects on hamster eggs stripped of their protective coating. Live sperm and ova were soaked in liquid solutions of each herb. Sperm were incubated in the herbal extracts for seven days, and the ova were incubated for one hour. Results showed that Saw Palmetto had no effect on fertilization, but high concentrations of the other three herbs reduced sperm mobility, and St. John's Wort caused sperm mutation. Although there are major errors in the methodology and unsupportable conclusions of this research, several misleading articles appeared in prestigious medical journals and many newspapers, including *The New York Times*, cautioning people against the potential danger of St. John's Wort, Echinacea, and Gingko causing infertility. The actual results of this study indicate that sperm and eggs can be damaged by soaking in herbal extracts. The obvious flaw is that this study is completely unrealistic and misrepresents the effects of these herbs when they are ingested by people. Herbs must pass through the digestive system into the bloodstream and do not have direct contact with eggs or sperm. The researchers also failed to mention any details about the source or preparation of the herbal extracts that were tested. These herbs have been used extensively in the United States and Europe for many years with no epidemiological or clinical evidence of reproductive damage. Regardless of the unscientific nature of this research, the outcomes and bizarre conclusions were highly publicized.

It is also important to note that the type of herbal preparation and production methods can alter research outcomes. For example, a liquid extract or tincture made with 40 percent alcohol may have different biological effects than one made with 80 percent alcohol. Water extracts contain different chemical constituents than alcohol extracts, so teas may have different therapeutic value than alcohol tinctures. The age of the herb material is another consideration. Alcohol tinctures have a long shelf life, while dried plant material in pills, capsules, or tea bags deteriorates within one to three years. The time of harvest effects chemical quantity and potency, and a one-year-old root will have different chemical properties and quantities than a five-year-old root. All these issues must be taken into account and documented to provide accurate and reliable tests and outcomes.

> *Modern scientific research and identification of plant constituents often confirm what indigenous people discovered about herbs over the millennia.*

Another example of flawed testing occurred when American researchers conducted a study of 30 HIV-infected people to investigate the safety and antiviral activity of St. John's Wort (Gulick, 1999). Rather than using the traditional whole plant extract consisting of the upper leaves and flowers containing all the chemical constituents, researchers used synthetic hypericin. The synthetic version yielded disappointing results by causing severe phototoxicity (sensitivity to sunlight) in 48 percent of participants and showing no antiviral activity. Although researchers singled out hypericin to be one of the most active ingredients in St. John's Wort, the test was flawed at the onset by using a synthetic form that is biologically much different than the naturally occurring extract of the whole plant.

Valid scientific research will continue to be an indispensable tool for assessing therapeutic benefits or dangers of medicinal herbs. But rather than allowing research to be the sole criteria, herbs should also be evaluated according to their historic use in traditional healing systems. From ancient times, herbalists have relied on their instincts and intuition, word-of-mouth, and trial-and-error to determine which plants are healing and which are harmful. It is very interesting that most of the modern research on botanical medicine tends to confirm what indigenous cultures discovered about herbs over the millennia. A valuable outcome of scientific research and identification of plant chemicals is this validation of many historic folk remedies and explanations as to why and how medicinal herbs work. When determining the health benefits and safety of herbs, it is always important to review research that is scrutinized for accuracy and validity in the context of the herb's historical applications and anecdotal evidence.

Traditional Chinese Medicine (TCM)

China's expertise in the healing arts and application of medicinal herbs is respected by many medical systems and herbalists throughout the world. Early Chinese civilization and medical arts were incredibly advanced long before Western medicine became established. Archeological discoveries trace the origins of China's herbal tradition back 5,000 years. Traditional Chinese Medicine (TCM) has been refined and extremely well-documented over time. Over 2,000 herbal texts have been written by about 330 herbalists and physicians during the span of Chinese history. TCM offers a rich and vast treasure of herbal therapeutics developed from empirical observation of the experiences of millions of Chinese people.

Chinese medicine evolved from **Taoist philosophy** formulated by the master **Lao-Tzu** around the fifth century B.C. According to this ancient holistic view, the universe and all of life arises from the formless and eternal Tao. From the Tao arises the dynamic force or power that envelops and flows through all things to maintain life. It regulates the order and harmony of nature, the natural processes of life, and provides the life force of plants, animals, and humans. Taoism perceives all life to be a dynamic flow of energies that are inseparably interrelated. Taoism is called the "way of life" and is a timeless model for living in balance. In applying Taoist philosophy to the healing arts, nature was revered as the manifestation of the balance and harmony of the Tao. By following natural laws, people could enjoy health and well-being, and a peaceful social order could prevail. Herbs, nutritious foods, and massage were employed to restore harmony when the body became imbalanced. From about 200 B.C. through A.D. 1000, records indicate that Taoists were accomplished in testing, applying, and compiling knowledge of herbal remedies, and they played a major role in the development of Chinese herbalism and medicine.

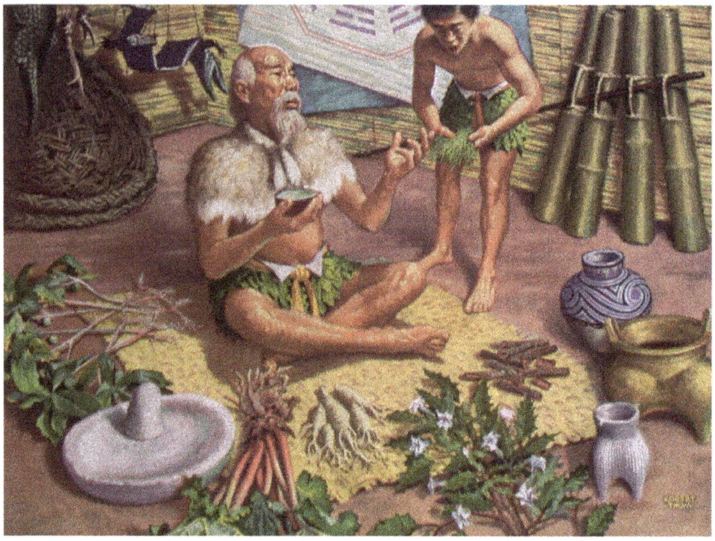

Pharmacy in Ancient China
Image by Robert Thom. Courtesy of Pfizer Inc.

The origins of Chinese herbalism are also credited to three legendary Chinese emperors: Fu Hsi, Shen Nong, and Huang Ti. **Fu Hsi**, also known as **Pao Hsi**, lived about 4,000 years ago. He developed the *Pa Kau* or *Eight Diagrams*, which established principles of TCM and is the basis of the classic *I Ching* or *Book of Changes*. The oldest known Chinese herbal on treating disease was written sometime between 1065 and 771 B.C. and is called the *Wu Shi Er Bing Fang (Prescriptions for Fifty-Two Diseases)*. It included 283 prescriptions containing herbs, foods, minerals, and animal parts. Ancient belief in malevolent spirits as the cause of disease is evident in the magical rituals described throughout the text. This herbal was discovered in 1973 during an excavation of a tomb in the Hunan providence, which archeologists date back to 168 B.C. Before this discovery, China's oldest known herbal materia medica was the *Shen Nong Ben Cao Jing (Divine Husbandman's Classic of the Materia Medica)*, attributed to the legendary emperor and sage **Shen Nong**, who lived around 2700 B.C. Actual dates vary among authors, and the true origin of this work is lost in antiquity, probably representing the works of several herbal practitioners. Shen Nong is remembered as the "Divine Plowman or Farmer" and is venerated as the "father of Chinese medicine." According to ancient legends, he developed agriculture and taught people how to cultivate grains for food, discovered the medicinal virtues of many plants, and established the art of medicine. He determined the medicinal qualities of herbs by ingesting the plants himself to test their effect, and died from eating one that was poisonous. Historians believe that the *Shen Nong* herbal was compiled sometime between 2600 B.C. and A.D. 100, and published around the year A.D. 500. The herbal refers to Taoist philosophy, the concepts of Yin and Yang, and describes over 365 Chinese medicines composed primarily of plants with some animal and mineral substances. A few of the plants mentioned include Ginseng, Licorice, Gotu Kola, Astragalus, Sesame seeds, Ginger, Ephedra, Coltsfoot, and Rhubarb root. Most of the plants included in the *Shen Nong* herbal continue to play an important role in modern Chinese medicine. This book remains one of the most important TCM classics of materia medica and is one of ten ancient classics still used in modern TCM.

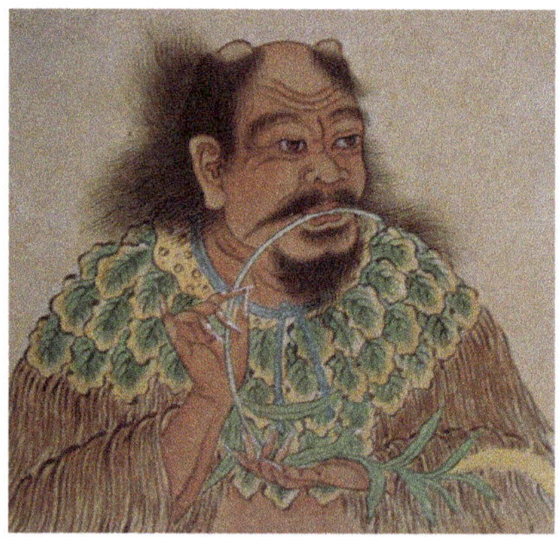

Shen Nong
Wellcome Library, London

The other legendary emperor who contributed to the origins of Chinese herbalism was **Huang Ti** (2698–

2598 B.C.), also known as the **Yellow Emperor**. He is accredited with writing *Huang-Ti Nei Ching* (*Yellow Emperor's Inner Classic*), but scholars believe it was compiled by unknown authors much later between 200 B.C. and A.D. 100. The *Inner Classic* provides the philosophical foundation of TCM, including the concepts of Yin and Yang, the five elements (fire, earth, air, water, and wood), the humoral system, and energetic forces of the cosmos and human body. Therapies include herbal medicine, acupuncture, diet, and exercise. The *Inner Classic* has remained a standard reference of Chinese medicine over thousands of years.

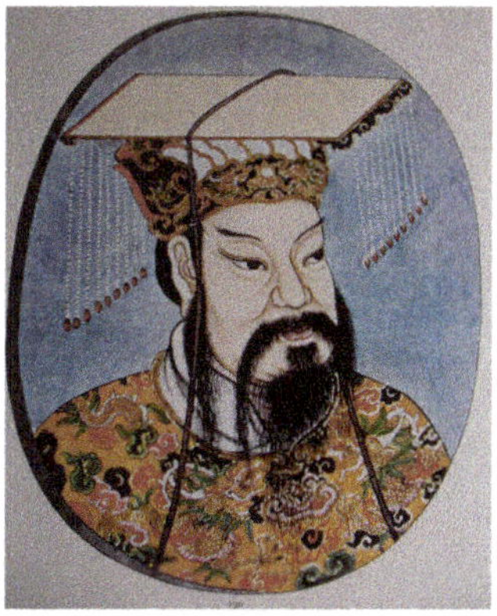

Huang Ti
Wellcome Library, London

The ancient doctrines of Confucius forbid any violation of the body, so early medical knowledge was based on experimentation, observation, and reasoning rather than on anatomical dissection. During China's long history, great healers wrote many manuscripts and passed on their herbal wisdom, each one contributing to the existing repository of herbal knowledge. Although China's development was relatively isolated, early trade routes established contact with India, Tibet, Persia, and Europe. During the second century B.C., a Chinese ambassador spent more than 20 years studying medicine in Mesopotamia, Syria and Egypt, and returned with medical knowledge and herbal remedies that greatly influenced Chinese medicine. In the fifth century A.D., trade routes through India, Japan, Korea, and Arabian countries allowed a wide dissemination of knowledge. Islamic medicine and Ayurvedic medicine from India also made an impact on Chinese medicine. Chinese medicine was established long before the Christian era and its influence spread into Korea, Japan and Tibet, becoming a foundation for their healing systems.

The first formal Chinese medical school was founded in A.D. 443, and eventually many more were established. Medical knowledge was also passed down to family members and from master to student. The *Tang Ben Cao* (the *Tang Herbal*), completed in A.D. 659 by 22 physicians, is considered the first official Chinese pharmacopoeia. It describes 850 drugs and includes many more herbs than the previous herbal by Shen Nong, along with new applications and greater detail. The most famous Chinese herbal, *Ben Cao Gang Mu*, was written by **Li Shi-Zhen** (1518–1593). It is considered the most extensive herbal materia medica ever compiled by one author, taking him more than 27 years to write the 52 volumes. Based on his herbal experience and information from earlier herbals, it summarized what was known of herbal medicine up to his time. The book describes 1,892 drugs and 11,096 prescriptions for treating hundreds of different illnesses, and includes treatises on botany, zoology, and mineralogy. By the 1600s, it was translated into Latin, English, French, German, Russian, Japanese, and Korean.

TCM flourished as the only medical system in China until the gradual spread of European influence during the 1800s. Beginning in 1842, foreign missionaries and doctors introduced European medicines and established hospitals in China, in addition to translating their medical books into Chinese. More Chinese interacted with Westerners, as did Sun Yat-sen (1866–1925), who lived in the West for part of his life and received a medical degree in Hong Kong. He was greatly influenced by Christianity and allopathic medicine, and after founding the Koumintang Nationalist government in 1911, Sun Yat-sen advocated establishing Western medicine as China's primary health care system. Acting on the assumption that modern allopathic drugs were superior to "backwards and superstitious" herbal remedies, Chinese doctors were encouraged to become educated in Western medicine, and many were sent abroad to study. In an effort to encourage the implementation of modern medicine in China, the Koumintang government attempted to eliminate TCM by outlawing traditional medicine in 1929. Even though it was declared illegal, TCM and herbal practices were so deeply entrenched in China's culture and daily lives of the people that these practices continued to be used as they had for centuries, especially in remote villages.

Shortly after the establishment of the People's Republic of China in 1949, the Communist government was faced with the choice of adopting Western medicine and either eliminating or keeping their traditional medicine. To make this decision, extensive scientific research and clinical studies were conducted on Chinese herbs during the 1950s to compare allopathic drugs with Traditional Chinese herbal medicines. These studies provided extensive documentation supporting the effectiveness of TCM, herbal therapies, and acupuncture. Mao Tse-tung restored traditional medicine to official status, declaring TCM a national treasure. In 1958, the government adopted a policy to integrate and implement both Western allopathic medicine and TCM. Consequently, government-approved medical colleges were established to teach TCM.

In the 1985 *Chinese Pharmacopoeia,* more than 500 herbs were listed as "official drugs," although over 5,000 medicinal plants are currently recognized and used in China. By the end of 1995, there were 1,020 medicinal herb enterprises in China. Chinese scientists are skilled in researching traditional herbs using modern technology and have provided a steady flow of scientific documentation. In fact, China has produced more extensive documentation of their herbal remedies than any other country.

Over hundreds of years, the Chinese have developed a system of using herbal plants according to balance and relationship. Herbs are classified according to their properties of hot or cool, moistening or drying, and also according to their taste of sweet, sour, bitter, or pungent. Medicinal plants are processed according to special methods designed to alter and enhance their chemical and energetic properties. The processed herbs are then combined into formulas for specific therapeutic effects on patients. Most Chinese herbs are prepared in combinations rather than used singly. Some ingredients treat the illness directly, others support the immune system and help reduce side effects of other ingredients, and some are added to improve flavor. Herbal formulas are always specifically designed to restore balance. Medicines are prepared as teas, liquid extracts, liniments, ointments, capsules, or tablets.

Careful study and close observation reveals the ancient wisdom and common sense of the TCM perspective and methodology. It is based on the energies and elements of people and the natural world, and on their relationships with each other. The forces and elements of nature and life are never stagnant, and the human body is also in a perpetual flux of change. TCM has devised a language to describe the processes and continual transformation of the forces and natural elements that make up our world and our bodies, offering therapies that strive to keep these in a dynamic state of harmonious equilibrium.

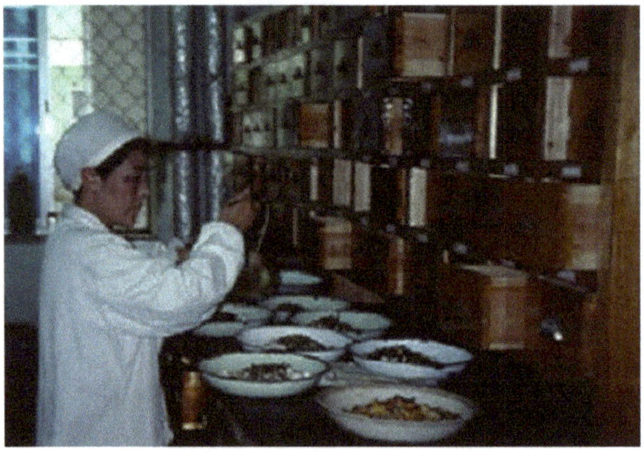

Chinese pharmacist measuring herbs to fill prescriptions

Currently in modern China, TCM is taught and practiced alongside allopathic Western medicine. Physicians and patients decide which system they want to use, or elect to combine both. This has proved to be a successful approach, allowing people to receive the best of both systems. Herbal medicine accounts for 30-50 percent of China's annual medical consumption. Herbs are integrated into the daily diet, and they are also considered to be drugs that are dispensed by health care practitioners or sold from stores. A study determined that China had 3,785 TCM hospitals in 2004, in addition to most regular hospitals having a TCM department. There were 97 TCM research institutes located at 30 colleges and universities, employing 12,901 researchers and educating 234,558 students. TCM generated $8.8 billion in industry sales in 2004, while the TCM hospitals reported $410 million in revenue (Liu, 2010).

China continues to be a world leader in the use, research, and manufacture of herbal medicines. Western interest and acceptance of TCM and Chinese herbs continues to grow. Many physicians and holistic and naturopathic practitioners in Europe and the United States have incorporated TCM theory, pulse and tongue diagnosis, acupuncture/acupressure, and medicinal herbs into their practice, finding them to be extremely valuable in helping clients stay healthy.

In 1995, I visited China with a delegation of nurses to study TCM. It was an extraordinary and exciting experience! We had an opportunity to study at a modern teaching hospital in the city of Hangzhou, where both Western allopathic medicine and TCM are practiced. Our delegation observed Chinese doctors interviewing patients, using tongue and pulse diagnosis, and practicing acupuncture, moxabustion, Tuina massage, and Qigong. Following the medical examination, most patients were given a prescription for herbs that they took to the hospital herb pharmacy, which contained thousands of medicinal plants. Pharmacists filled each patient's prescription by getting a big piece of paper and going to large wooden drawers containing specific herbs, weighing out the correct amounts, and piling them on the paper. Most TCM doctors prescribe a combination of several botanicals, so the piles were an interesting mass of roots, twigs, berries, leaves, flowers, and sometimes minerals and animal parts. The paper was then folded up, and several were tied together into a large bundle. Patients were instructed to boil the herbs in water and drink the thick, dark tea over a period of several days or weeks.

After returning from China and pursuing more extensive studies in Chinese medical perspective, application and herbology, I have integrated TCM into my nursing practice and find it is an invaluable and skillful tool that effectively blends with Western medical training and holistic modalities. Clients respond well to this approach and can easily comprehend the common sense language and philosophy of TCM. For a more complete explanation about the basic principles of Chinese medicine and herbal applications in healing, please refer to "Traditional Chinese Medicine (TCM) Perspectives" in the Section Two chapter titled "How to Use the Materia Medica."

It should be noted that when purchasing Chinese herbal products, it is important to buy from well-known and reputable companies that maintain high standards of quality control. Unfortunately, much of the water and soil in China have become quite polluted and can contaminate plants. There have also been problems with mislabeling and cases where pharmaceutical and other ingredients were added to TCM formulas but omitted from labels. Fortunately, several excellent American-based companies produce and market TCM herbal formulas that are scrutinized according to American "quality controls" and are much safer to use.

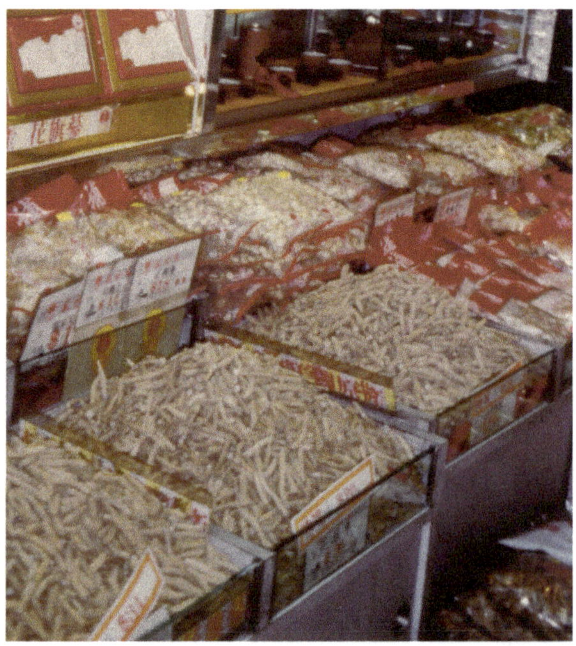

Herbalism in the Ayurvedic Medical System of India

Plants, which as receptacles of light were born three ages before the Gods,
I honor your myriad colors and your seven hundred natures.
A hymn to the plants from the *Rig Veda* (1500 B.C.)

Indian culture and medicine evolved from the prehistoric Indus Valley civilization in what is today Pakistan and western India. This civilization flourished during the time of ancient Mesopotamia and Egypt around 3000–1500 B.C., and is often referred to as the Harappan civilization, after the first discovery of the city of Harappa. Archaeological excavations have unearthed remains of carefully planned cities with advanced architecture and plumbing, indicating a culture well-versed in engineering, mathematics, and geometry. Latrines and drains emptied into community sewers, and elaborate bath houses indicated emphasis on hygiene. Large granaries and pictographs of domesticated animals are evidence of a peaceful culture engaged in agriculture and trade rather than warfare. These excavated cities and remnants of human bones, tools, clay pottery, and tablets are the only remaining artifacts. Many clay seals and statues of female figures indicate the existence of a goddess religion. Since the Harappans were an agricultural people conscious of good hygiene and advanced in the sciences, it is very probable that they developed a system of healing using herbal remedies.

When the Harappan civilization appeared to have been in decline, some historians think that a dominant people known as Aryans migrated from the north to the Indus and Ganges river area about 2000–1500 B.C. They were a fair-skinned race who thought themselves superior to the darker-skinned Harappans and other indigenous people they encountered as they moved southeast through Persia and India. As they migrated, the powerful Aryans gradually assimilated other cultures into their own, and maintained control throughout their domain.

The only records and source of information from this era are the *Vedas*, named for the Sanskrit word meaning "knowledge." Composed between 3000–1000 B.C. (known as the Vedic Period), they were written in the Sanskrit language of the Aryans after being passed down through oral tradition by the Brahmic or priestly caste for about 1,000 years. Ancient hymns in the *Rig Veda* tell of the Aryans from the north conquering the native people of India and driving the indigenous Dravidian culture into southern India. Aryans are described as enlightened people with a brilliant understanding of the cosmology and their place in it. The *Vedas* describe them as war-like with masculine warrior gods, chariots, and weapons. The roots of Ayurvedic herbalism and medicine trace back to this Vedic period in ancient India. All the science, medicine, and knowledge of ancient India originated from the four *Vedas*, which explain the origins of life and contain the songs, prayers, and knowledge of the Aryans. The *Rig Veda,* a compilation of verses or hymns on the nature of existence, is considered to be the original Vedic text and the oldest surviving book in Indian literature. Many great yogis and scholars who understand the astrological references in the hymns date the *Rig Veda* back to 4000 B.C. and perhaps as early as 12,000 B.C. Modern Western scholars tend to estimate that it was written around 1500 B.C.

All four of the *Vedas* mention Ayurvedic medicine, especially the *Atharva-Veda* (written between 1000–800 B.C.), which contains hymns, prayers, charms, and incantations offered to a pantheon of Aryan gods for treating a wide variety of diseases and injuries. Amulets, talismans, and plants were used for protection and healing. The Aryans and Hindus, like other ancient people, believed disease was punishment from the gods for human transgressions. Herbs were praised as a gift from the god Soma to free people from curses, sin, and disease. In the Vedic hymns, the power and blessings of the gods were invoked to protect people from harm and to exorcise demons believed to cause illness. One hymn was dedicated to magic and all medicinal plants, and was used as a universal remedy. A translation of this hymn reads:

> The plants we do invoke. May they protect this man from the disease sent by the gods, the herbs whose father is the sky, whose mother is the earth, whose root is the ocean. The waters and the heavenly plants are foremost, they have driven out from every limb thy disease, consequent upon sin. I call on thy behalf, the plants derived from all the gods that furnish life to man. (*Atharva-Veda*, 1000–800 B.C.)

The *Vedas* list the divisions of Ayurveda as internal medicine, surgery, treatment of the eyes, ears and nose, toxicology, psychiatry, pediatrics, gerontology, and gynecology. The *Vedas* contain some of the oldest records of medicinal plant use, and include information on over 400 medicinal plants. The ancients also used purified minerals by reducing them to ash as a remedy for disease. The *Vedas* make references to many important medicines that are still used today.

The Aryans believed that the universe has a creator who is eternal, all-knowing, and without cause. Life arises from the pure consciousness of this one absolute source. The traditional Indian medical system of Ayurveda is believed to have originated from the wisdom of this creator who revealed it to the gods, and eventually people recorded this wisdom in the *Vedas*. Although the Vedic pantheon of gods and goddesses is complex, they are all manifestations of the one universal power and spirit of the cosmos called Brahma. In classical Hinduism, the primary trinity is Brahma the Creator, Vishnu the Preserver, and Shiva the Destroyer. Shiva often appears with his consort Kali, who personifies death and destruction of all that lives. Vishnu preserves and sustains the world, and his consort is Lakshmi, the goddess of life, beauty, and good fortune.

All the gods influence health and illness, but Dhanvantari was the deity of medicine who taught the art of healing to humankind. A popular myth states that it was Brahma who first perceived the principles and philosophy of Ayurveda. He taught Ayurveda to Dakshprajapati, who passed it on to the Ashvini Kumars. They were twin brothers and celestial physicians to the gods who wrote important manuscripts on medicine and surgery. Many hymns in the *Rig Veda* are addressed to these twin gods credited with teaching people advanced levels of medicine and surgery. Another version of mythology involves the Aryan god Indra, who learned Ayurveda from the Ashvini twins and taught it to Dhanvantari, who taught it to men.

Most scholars agree that knowledge of the *Vedas* was systematized and Ayurvedic medicine was advanced and firmly established in India by 1000 B.C. The development of Buddhism in India began around 500 B.C. and exerted a powerful influence on medicine. Due to Buddhist doctrines, anatomy and surgery declined, but hospitals and schools were established and flourished, especially around 250 B.C. when India was united under the rule of the benevolent Buddhist king Asoka (273–232 B.C.). During his reign, a well-organized Ayurvedic medical system thrived, hospitals were built long before they appeared in Europe, and gardens of medicinal trees and herbs were cultivated throughout the country to supply raw materials for a sophisticated and extensive pharmacy.

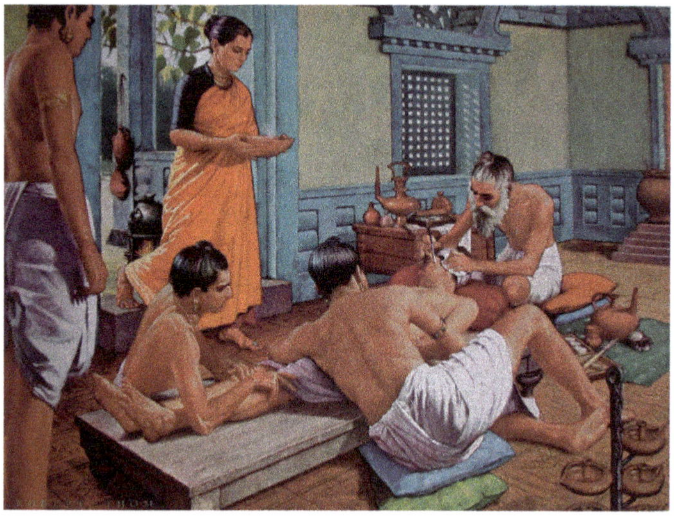

Sushruta: Surgeon of Old India
Image by Robert Thom. Courtesy of Pfizer Inc.

The "golden age" of Indian medicine spanned a period of 2,000 years from about 1000 B.C. through A.D. 1000. This age was highlighted by medical textbooks known as the *Charaka-Samhita*, attributed to a physician named **Charaka**, and the *Sushruta-Samhita* written by the surgeon **Sushruta**. These treatises offered monumental contributions to the development of Ayurvedic medicine. Historians estimate that Charaka lived and wrote sometime between 320 B.C. and A.D. 100. He was the most renowned physician of his time and was believed to be the incarnation of Shesha, the Serpent-god with 1,000 heads who held the repository of all science and medicine. The *Charaka-Samhita*, one of the oldest treatises on medical science, is a systematic presentation of internal medical therapies and describes 580 herbs. It discusses the tridosha (the elements of earth, water, fire, and air similar to the four humors system), methods of examination, embryological development, different types and classifications of herbal therapies, daily regimens of healthy lifestyle, dietary advice, and discourses on the soul, mind, and salvation.

Sushruta, the other great physician of India's golden age, lived sometime between 500 B.C. and A.D. 300. He studied Ayurvedic medicine with Devodasa, the king of Banares, who was believed to be the incarnation of the divine physician, Dhanvantari. Sushruta returned home after completing his studies and wrote the *Sushruta-Samhita*, which contained extensive discussions of many diseases, their causes, symptoms, instructions in pulse and urine diagnosis, and treatments using foods and about 760 herbs. The text was primarily devoted to writings on sophisticated surgical techniques practiced in the 400s B.C. and described over 120 surgical instruments. Accurate descriptions and classification of diseases, anatomy, pathology, biology, medicine, and midwifery were included, and attention was devoted to hygiene, massage, exercise, and disease prevention. Disease was explained as a disturbance in the balance of the humors, a view that was adopted by Greek and Roman physicians several centuries later. Disease was also believed to be caused by evil demons and transgressions committed in former lives. The *Sushruta-Samhita* mentioned the influence of soil and seasons upon herbs, described the structure (morphology) of plants, and classified herbs according to their taste, therapeutic properties, and the five elements. Sushruta's herbal materia medica was extensive and mainly consisted of elaborate methods of preparing herbs derived from indigenous plants, including instructions for making decoctions, paste, extracts, and powders.

During this time, physicians collected and prepared their own herbal preparations. Many herbs were combined into formulas and used in teas, ointments, and poultices. Medicines also contained animal parts and minerals such as sulfur, arsenic, lead, copper, and gold. Physicians excelled in treating poisonous bites and stings, and wrote excellent descriptions of the circulatory and digestive systems, fetal development, anatomy, physiology, physics, and chemistry. The Ayurvedic *Samhitas* of Charaka and Sushruta were translated into Arabic by the late A.D. 700s and were mentioned in the writings of the famous Persian herbal physicians, Avicenna and Razes. The *Samhitas* were later translated into Latin and German, greatly influencing the European medical system.

Ayurveda is a Sanskrit word derived from *ayur* meaning "life" and *veda* meaning "knowledge." Although Ayurveda is an ancient science and holistic system of healing that evolved among the Brahmin priests and sages of India 3,000–5,000 years ago, it is still practiced today with renewed interest. According to Ayurveda, the entire creation and the human body exist from the blending of spirit, or pure consciousness, with matter. The human body is seen as a microcosm of the universe. Above all, the aim of Ayurveda is the attainment of the ultimate truth by which the human mind realizes the identity of the individual soul with the Universal Soul (the Supreme Consciousness), and can thus rise above unhappiness, disease, and pain. Ayurveda is a complete medical system postulating that health manifests by the grace of the Absolute acting through the laws of nature, which is similar to the Asclepian view of the ancient Europeans and to the Traditional Chinese medical system originating from the Tao.

The Ayurvedic perspective honors all of creation and views the entire universe as a divine union. The delicate balance between the elemental forces of nature and the mutual existence of humans and nature is acknowledged and serves as the model for healing illness. Ayurvedic medicine assists nature by promoting and maintaining dynamic equilibrium of life energies within the body, recognizing that each person has a unique constitution requiring individualized remedies. It focuses on healing the fragmentation and disorder of the body, mind, and emotions to restore harmony and wholeness. Ayurveda asserts that every living being has an inherent tendency to move in the direction of self-healing and balance when provided with a natural, simple, healthy lifestyle and diet.

According to Ayurvedic philosophy, all forms of life are composed of varying combinations of the five basic elements of creation: **earth, water, fire, air,** and **ether** or **space**. These five elements blend into three energies or humors, known as the **tridosha**, that regulate all life processes. The three doshas or body types are known as vata, pitta, and kapha. Each person is born with a genetically determined and permanent constitutional blend of all three doshas.

Vata is the air or wind element formed from the combination of ether and air, and is the most subtle of the elements. All matter is composed of atoms that consist of electrons revolving around the inner neutrons and protons. Ether is the empty space between the mass of electrons and protons in the atom. Thus, ether surrounds and encloses all form, even the hardest rocks and metals that are composed of atoms. Vata is also the power or force of movement. It creates all movement throughout the body, including the flow of oxygen and the breath, circulation of blood and lymphatic fluid, movement of food through the digestive and eliminative system, movement of nutrients into cells, movement of nerve impulses, and the flow of thoughts through the mind. People with a strong vata constitution tend to be thin and exhibit the ether and air qualities of being light, dry, cool, active, clear, and dispersing.

The **pitta** dosha is formed from the combination of fire and water, but is typically thought of as fire and heat. Pitta is the stimulating fire within the body that produces warmth and the energy that makes everything function. Pitta regulates the process of metabolism and transformation of food into nutrients and nutrients into energy. This includes the heat and energy needed for digestion, metabolism, and nervous system function. People with a strong pitta constitution tend to have a medium build and exhibit the properties of fire which are hot, sharp, fast-moving, light, and oily.

The **kapha** dosha is the combination of water and earth elements. Water represents all the fluids in the body, and earth represents the minerals, proteins, vitamins, and other substances that form the structure of the body. The earth element within kapha provides structure for tissues and bones, supporting growth, maturation, strength, stability, and endurance. The water element of kapha provides all the body fluids, lubricates the joints, and moisturizes the skin and tissues. People with strong kapha constitutions tend to be heavier and stockier, and exhibit the qualities of water and earth, which are heavy, slow, cool, liquid and oily, dense, thick, and static or concentrated.

The biological, emotional, and psychological life of a person is governed by the tridosha elements. Every person is composed of a unique combination of these three doshas, which accounts for individual diversity. Usually one of the three doshas is more prominent in each person. When the doshas are in balance, the person experiences good physical and mental health. Temporary imbalance of the doshas creates acute illness, and chronic imbalance eventually manifests as disease. The goal of Ayurvedic medicine is to promote balance of the doshas for optimal health.

Ayurvedic medical diagnosis included extensive inquiry and observation of the tongue, pulse, face, eyes, nails, lips, and urine. Ancient physicians were trained in the arts of healthy diet, detoxification, massage, yoga, water treatments, breathing, meditation, and herbal remedies to help people achieve balance and treat disease. Cleansing, balancing, and rejuvenation were emphasized and implemented with herbs, fasting, exercise, and peaceful, harmonious thoughts and emotions. Astrology was also used for medical purposes. Just as with Traditional Chinese Medicine, an Ayurvedic healer matched a person's constitution and symptoms of illness with the energetic properties of specific herbs and foods to restore harmony. Herbs were sometimes added to oils for massage and to water for steam to stimulate and remove toxins. Plants were considered to be composed of the five elements and expressed their various properties such as hot or cool, wet or dry, stimulating or sedating. In applying Ayurveda to a person with strong pitta qualities who is very active and prone to conditions of excess heat such as acid stomach, high fevers, flushed skin, and itchy, eruptive skin rashes, the Ayurvedic practitioner would promote balance by recommending foods and herbs that are cooling and calming. For a kapha person suffering from excess phlegm, recurrent respiratory infections, constipation or slow metabolism, a regime of warming and stimulating herbs such as Cayenne, Cumin, Cinnamon, Garlic, and Ginger would be advised.

The Ayurvedic medical system had a huge impact on the development of medicine worldwide. Many Ayurvedic herbs and the philosophy of the four/five elements and four humors were adopted by healers in ancient Egypt, Persia, Greece and Rome, Tibet, China, Indonesia, and Japan. Hippocrates recommended several Indian plants in his materia medica that were mentioned in earlier Sanskrit works. Dioscorides, the first century Greek physician and botanist, investigated the medicinal properties of Indian plants available in European markets and incorporated them into his materia medica. In the second century, Galen incorporated Indian herbs and endorsed the humoral philosophy in his system, which became the cornerstone of European medicine until the close of the Renaissance. Indian philosophy also influenced Chinese medicine and herbalism. By A.D. 400, Ayurvedic works were translated into the Chinese language, and by A.D. 700, Chinese physicians and scholars were studying medicine at Nalanda University in India.

Ayurvedic and Islamic medicine greatly influenced each other. During the 700s, many Ayurvedic Hindu physicians practiced in Baghdad, and Ayurvedic works were translated into Arabic. Ayurvedic medicine was in its prime during this period, and Hindu kings encouraged and funded medical schools and herbal research. During the 10th century, when Islamic warriors invaded and conquered India, Ayurvedic practitioners were overshadowed by Islamic physicians, known as Hakims, who practiced their traditional Unani medicine and controlled much of India's medical practice. Islamic rule was uprooted when the British colonized India and established themselves as the ruling class during the 1700s. They imported their own European medicines and doctors, built hospitals, and promoted Western medicine that eventually became the established medical system. Ayurvedic herbal medicines were regarded as inferior, and this ancient medical system suffered decline. However, after India established its independence from Great Britain in 1947, Ayurvedic medicine resumed its popularity, and it is currently estimated that 70 percent of the Indian population still rely on Ayurvedic doctors and herbs. Like Chinese medicine, Ayurveda is experiencing a renaissance and many medicinal herbs are being researched and utilized by Westerners.

Currently, Ayurveda and Western allopathic medicine coexist in the Indian medical system. In 1970, the Indian Parliament recognized the legitimacy of Ayurvedic medicine, created a central council for Ayurveda, and provided accredited colleges with standardized certifications. In modern India, Ayurvedic physicians complete a five-and-a-half-year post-graduate degree program from state or government-supported Ayurvedic colleges and hospitals throughout India. The Ayurvedic pharmaceutical industry that manufactures and markets herbals is also thriving. In 2004, it was estimated that India had about 500,000 medical doctors. Of these, nearly 60 percent were involved in non-allopathic systems of medicine, including Ayurveda and homeopathy. The World Health Organization (WHO) recognizes Ayurveda as an effective traditional medical system that will continue to thrive and expand into the Western world.

Parting Thoughts on the History of Herbalism

Modern herbalism emerges from a diverse blend of cultures, folk traditions, anecdotal evidence, scientific research, and clinical experience. The ancient healing traditions of Old European herbalists, Traditional Chinese Medicine, India's Ayurvedic system, Islamic Unani medicine, Native American Indians, and other indigenous people throughout the world offer an amazingly rich and diverse wealth of herbal wisdom and expertise. It is interesting to note the undeniable similarities among various cultures in their understanding of the vital forces and elements of nature, and their application of medicinal herbs for healing. The ancients understood the art of balancing and harmonizing these forces and elements to promote health, and they worked with the inherent healing qualities of nature and the medicinal plants. Most ancient people shared similar concepts about the humoral and four elements philosophy. Many old civilizations had mythologies in which medical knowledge and herbal plants were given to humans by the gods, and all strongly believed in the existence of unseen forces that were both helpful and malicious. These civilizations developed sophisticated healing systems that, to varying degrees, still exist today. Old trade routes allowed much dissemination of knowledge among ancient civilizations. And even with oceans and great distances separating them, indigenous people of numerous diverse cultures have been able to tap into and acquire similar perspectives and innate knowledge of herbal plants, and have created healing rituals and medical systems that overlap in philosophy and treatment. Now, modern scientific and botanical researchers are able to identify the bioactive chemical constituents in herbs, often validating the ancient folk wisdom and utilization of many medicinal plants.

The common thread weaving its way through herbal traditions of all cultures is the universal wisdom of our connection with the earth and plants. Through this intimate relationship, an inherent perceptual reality emerges, helping us view ourselves and all of creation as interrelated and interdependent parts of the entire universe. Through this intuitive experience, we "re-member" and become one with the whole of life.

In reviewing this condensed synopsis of herbal history, it is apparent how massive and ancient our global accumulation of herbal knowledge and application really is. Humanity has always depended on plants for healing our afflictions. Herbal therapy is intricately woven into the fabric of daily life for people in many cultures and countries, providing an abiding source of medicine since antiquity. And today herbal preparations and therapies continue to coexist alongside the established medical and pharmaceutical industries.

In 1976, the World Health Organization (WHO) acknowledged that 1) the majority of the global population depends on traditional medicine for primary health care; 2) the manpower represented by traditional medical practitioners is an important resource for the delivery of health care; and 3) medicinal plants are of great importance to the health of individuals and communities. WHO emphasizes the importance of traditional medical practitioners, urges countries to use traditional health care systems, and supports a comprehensive global approach to medicinal herb use. In 1985, WHO estimated that 80 percent of the world's population depends on herbs for their primary health care, and plant extracts or their active constituents are a major part of traditional healing therapies. WHO promotes the development of worldwide integration of botanical medicine with the Western allopathic medical system. Proponents point out that phytomedicines can be employed for health maintenance, disease prevention, and reduce skyrocketing health care costs for all nations.

It will be interesting to observe and experience the herbal movement in this country and globally as time passes. Whatever direction it takes, hopefully the true art of herbal healing will never be lost to human understanding and application. For many people, relying on nature's medicines to promote health and treat illness may seem very distant from the technology and drugs provided by modern medicine, which are often based on the assumption that technology can surpass the ability of Nature to make potent medicines. Using herbs encourages us to trust Nature and the plants that the earth provides for us. Ultimately there is no separation between the earth, the plants, and people. We are totally dependent on the plants for life; they are the ground substance of our physical bodies and our very existence. It is only our perception that unites us or separates us from life's wholeness and blessings. Most certainly, the continuing history of the medicinal plants, and humanity itself, will reflect our ability to be co-creative partners with Nature and to live in a gentle, harmless way with the plants, ensuring their proliferation and our own survival as well.

A comical but thought-provoking reflection on the world history of herbal medicine has become popular these days.

Doc, I have an earache!

2000 B.C. Here, eat this root.
1000 B.C. Using that root is heathen, say this prayer.
1850 Prayer is superstition and unscientific, drink this potion.
1930 That potion is snake oil, take this pill.
1970 That pill is ineffective, take this antibiotic.
2000 That antibiotic is artificial, here, eat this root.

Author unknown

Nomenclature and Classification of Plants

Human dependency on plants has naturally inspired the development of systems to name and classify them. It is estimated that more than five million different kinds of living organisms inhabit the earth, including more than 550,000 species of plants. Approximately 257,000 of these are flowering plants, trees, shrubs, and herbs. The remaining species consist of ferns, mosses, liverworts, algae, and fungi.

The branch of botany concerned with classification is called "taxonomy," derived from the Greek word *taxis* or *taxo*, meaning "to put in order or arrangement," and *nomos*, "the law." **Plant taxonomy** is the science of identifying, naming, and classifying the huge biodiversity of plants by using a methodical hierarchy of groupings that have an orderly relationship to each other. **Botanical nomenclature** is the formal scientific naming of plants and is an integral part of taxonomy. Plant taxonomy and nomenclature enable people to organize their studies and use a universal botanical language agreed upon by scientists. Plant taxonomy and nomenclature are not fixed systems because they constantly evolve as people continue to learn more about the plant kingdom.

Assigning scientific and common names to plants is an ancient practice, and plants have been classified in diverse ways throughout history. Theophrastus (*circa* 370–*c.* 287 B.C.) was a student of Aristotle's who wrote *History of Plants*, one of the first botanical manuscripts in the Western world to initiate the process of plant classification. Later, the Roman writer Pliny (A.D. 23–79) used the size and form of plants as criteria to establish three primary groups of classification: herbs, shrubs, and trees. During the Middle Ages, herbalists in Europe classified plants according to their uses and formulated three categories of plants: edible, medicinal, and poisonous.

During this era, ordinary people living in towns and the countryside throughout Europe identified plants by many simple names varying from one locality to the next and from one language to another. Latin was the language used exclusively by the upper classes of scholars and educated priests in the Catholic Church. In addition to common names known by the general population, scholars assigned scientific names to plants and animals by using long descriptive Latin phrases called **polynomials**, meaning "many names." For example, the polynomial for Catnip was *Nepeta floribus interrupte spicatus pedunculatis*, which describes the plant's appearance and translates as "*Nepeta* with flowers in an interrupted pedunculate spike." The first word of polynomials named the genus to which the plant belongs. For example, all varieties of Pine trees were given polynomials starting with the genus name *Pinus* and all species of Ginseng began with their genus name *Panax*.

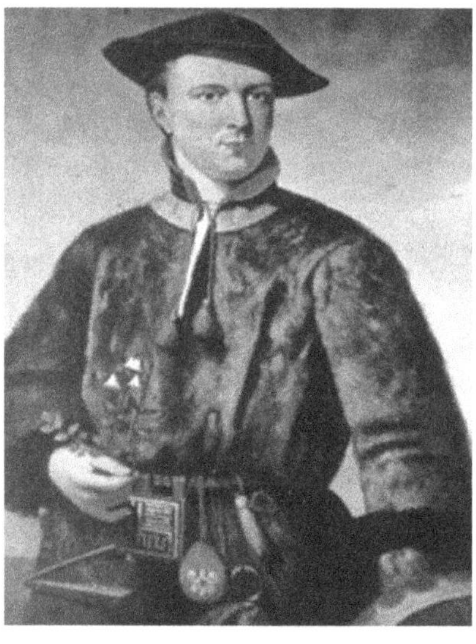

Carolus Linnaeus, Father of the Binomial System

The modern binomial system for identifying plants and animals was devised by the Swedish naturalist and professor of medicine and botany, Carl von Linné (1707–1778), better known by his Latinized name, **Carolus Linnaeus**. He believed that every form of life exists within patterns and organized relationships corresponding to an ideal model, and that by classifying them he was discovering and revealing the grand pattern of creation. With great motivation, he attempted to name and classify all known species of animals and plants in his lifetime. An ambitious man!

As an experienced botanist and physician, Linnaeus had firsthand knowledge of hundreds of plants and probably became frustrated by their tiresome and lengthy polynomials. He began developing a convenient shorthand method of nomenclature in 1741 when he made a list of plants and animals he observed while exploring two Baltic islands. In 1753, he revolutionized the scientific system of naming plants by publishing a two-volume book called *Species Plantarum* (*Species of Plants*) in which he introduced his binomial system. In his book, he divided all the flowering plants into 24 classes based on their **morphology** (form and structure), which included the number and arrangement of their flower parts, and specifically the number of their stamens and pistils. He wrote the description of each species in the traditional polynomial fashion using no more than 12 Latin words to describe each plant. However, in the book margins next to the polynomial names of each species, he wrote one word that became the species name. For example, he abbreviated the polynomial for Catnip from *Nepeta floribus interrupte spicatis pedunculatis* to *Nepeta cataria* to reflect cats' attraction to this herb. Linnaeus shortened the polynomial for Belladonna, *Atropa caule herbaceo foliis ovatus integris* ("the atropa with herbaceous stems and leaves that are oval and entire"), to the binomial *Atropa belladonna*. His system established organized guidelines and a universal language to identify and classify plants in a scientific manner.

The Binomial System of Naming Plants

According to Linnaeus' binomial system, scientific names of plants include the generic or **genus** name and the **species** name, both derived from Latin. The genus name appears first and is always capitalized. The genus name is determined by the morphology, or common structural characteristics, of each plant. The second name of a binomial identifies the individual species that distinguishes the plant from others in the same genus. For example, all Scullcaps have the genus name *Scutellaria* but each variety has its own species name. *Scutellaria lateriflora* is the species most often sold commercially, while *Scutellaria incana* is a North American woodland variety. Two Chinese species are called *Scutellaria baicalensis* and *Scutellaria barbata*. All Ginseng plants have the genus name *Panax*. Different species include *Panax ginseng* (Asian Ginseng), *Panax quinquefolius* (American Ginseng), and *Panax trifolium* (Dwarf Ginseng). The species name is often descriptive of the plant. For instance, *quinquefolius* is the Latin word meaning "five-leaves," which is the number of leaflets on all adult members of this species. *Trifolium* means "three-leaves" and describes the number of leaflets on the Dwarf Ginseng.

Modern scientists and botanists around the globe agree upon Linnaeus' brilliant concepts as the standard model for uniform methods of naming and classifying plants. Although a plant species may be known by a variety of common names among different people, each plant generally has one Latin binomial that is universally used to provide exact identification and eliminate confusion. Latin is used as the language of scientific terminology for biology and medicine because it is a dead language that remains consistent, and it poses no bias in favor of one currently used language over another. Every six years, botanists from all over the world meet in an International Botanical Congress to examine, establish, or revise the rules of nomenclature. The results are published in the International Code of Botanical Nomenclature, the standard guide for assigning plants Latin names that are both universal and specific.

International Standards of Taxonomic Names and Abbreviations

The International Botanical Congress has determined the following "rules and regulations" for writing the Latin names of plants and classification groupings.

❖ All taxonomic names, including the division, class, order, family, genus and species, are written in italics and the first letter of all names is capitalized, except for names of species and sub-species. An example of a taxonomical classification of Calendula is:

Division or Phylum: *Tracheophyta* (vascular plants)

Subdivision: *Euphyllophytina*

Class: *Angiospermae*

Subclass: *Dicotyledonae*

Order: *Campanulates (Asterales)*

Family: *Compositae (Asteraceae)*

Genus: *Calendula*

Species: *officinalis*

❖ Throughout the ages, botanists have sometimes assigned different names to the same plant family. As an example, the family *Compositae* was recently renamed *Asteraceae* because the International Botanical Congress agreed that all names of plant families should now end in "*-aceae*." When referring to plant families with two names, the older name appears first and the newer name follows in parentheses. For instance, since *Compositae* is the older name for the Aster Family and *Asteraceae* is the newer name, the family name is written as *Compositae (Asteraceae)*.

❖ The genus of the plant is the first name in its Latin binomial and is capitalized. The species name is second and written in lower case letters. For example, the scientific name or binomial for Mugwort is *Artemisia vulgaris*. *Artemisia* is also the genus name for other species such as *Artemisia absinthium* (Wormwood) and *Artemisia annua* (Sweet Annie).

❖ The abbreviation "**sp.**" means "one **sp**ecies" and is used when the actual specific name cannot or need not be specified. The abbreviation "**spp.**" ("**sp**ecies **p**lural") refers to several or all species of a genus. For instance, *Echinacea* spp. refers to all species in the genus Echinacea, including *E. purpurea, E. angustifolia, E. pallida*, and *E. paradoxica*.

❖ After the genus name is first mentioned in a written text, it may be abbreviated to a single letter in later references. For example, *Artemisia vulgaris* is abbreviated to *A. vulgaris* and *Echinacea purpurea* is abbreviated to *E. purpurea.*

❖ Sometimes Latin binomials include an abbreviation for the botanist who named the plant. Thus, *Nepeta cataria* L. means that the botanist Linnaeus named Catnip. *Ulmus fulva* Michx. refers to the Latin name of Slippery Elm provided by the French botanist Andre Michaux. *Ulmus rubra* Muhl. refers to the original Latin name given to Slippery Elm by Gotthilf Muhlenberg. Botanists occasionally change the genus and species names of plants as their knowledge increases, and sometimes one plant species has two different Latin names. When the name of a plant has been changed, the name of the original author is placed in parentheses followed by the name of the most recent author. An example is *Angelica sinensis* (Oliv.) Diels.

❖ A multiplication sign (x) appearing in the Latin name means the plant is a hybrid of two species. As an example, *Mentha x piperita* (Peppermint) is a hybrid species developed by cross-pollinating *Mentha spicata* (Spearmint) and *Mentha aquatica* (Watermint).

❖ A plant variety that is developed by cultivation has a common **cultivar** name (meaning **culti**vated **var**iety). The cultivar name appears in single quotes after the name of the species. For example, a cultivar of Purple Basil is called *Ocimum basilicum 'Purpurascens.'* A Lemon Basil cultivar is called *O. basilicum 'Citriodora'* and as its cultivar name implies, it has a citrus scent.

❖ Binomial names of plants belonging to a specific subspecies or variety may consist of three parts that include the name of the variety, written as "**var**." For example, the complete binomial of the Flowering Dogwood tree is *Cornus florida* var. *rubra*, the peach tree is *Prunus persica* var. *persica*, and the nectarine tree is *Prunus persica* var. *nectarina*. Subspecies is written as "**ssp.**" or "**subsp.**"

Classifications of the Plant Kingdom

Linnaeus also introduced plant taxonomy and classified plant life according to a systematic hierarchy of related groups known as **kingdom, division** or **phylum, class, order, family, genus,** and **species**. These classifications are determined by a plant's genetic relationships, structure, appearance, and reproductive organs. Sometimes sub-groups occur in each of these categories, such as a subdivision, subclass, or subspecies. The most important groups for herbalists to be aware of are the family, genus, and species. However, the entire spectrum is interesting to look at and offers a clearer perspective of the evolution of the plant kingdom, showing the intricate and interwoven relationships between plant families and species.

The taxonomy of a plant is similar to a person's "family tree." Each individual plant descends from a long lineage of genetic ancestors and is a member of a family containing many relatives, some close and some distant. A plant division can be compared to the ethnic group to which a person belongs. The plant class, order, and family are like a family tree of ancestors with great-grandparents, grandparents, aunts and uncles. The genus is similar to a person's family name, like Smith, and the species is an individual name, like Laura. All the species of a genus can be seen as the siblings of the parent genus.

Although the purpose of classification is to create a clear and universal language, scholars do not always unanimously agree, so there are some variations in classification systems and terminology. The following descriptions of plant groups focus on divisions or phyla of medicinal herbs, and serve as a basic foundation for understanding the intricate and complicated science of taxonomy.

KINGDOM

A kingdom is the largest unit of biological classification. All living organisms belong to a kingdom. In the past, all life forms were divided into the animal, plant, or mineral kingdoms. But with more scientific technology and knowledge, scientists now group life forms into five primary kingdoms:

Monera or *Prokaryotae* (prokaryotes) are simple, one-celled organisms that are visible only under a microscope and include bacteria, blue-green algae, and archaea. They have genetic material but no nucleus. This is the oldest kingdom, probably originating three to four billion years ago.

Protista (protists) are primarily microscopic, single-cell organisms such as algae and protozoa that often live in colonies. These cells contain a nucleus and are divided into groups based on their mobility. For example, *ciliates* move by wave-like action of their hair-like cilia, and *zooflagellates* propel themselves with a long tail called a flagellum. *Protista* also include slime molds, water molds, and algae.

Fungi (common fungi) are multi-cellular, plant-like organisms that live off dead or living organic matter, and include yeast, molds, slime molds, mushrooms, and lichens.

Plantae (plants) include trees, shrubs, grasses, and flowering plants.

Animalia (animals) include multi-cellular organisms that are mobile and eat and digest their food.

DIVISION OR PHLYUM

The plant kingdom is divided into two large groups of non-vascular and vascular plants. **Non-vascular** plants lack true leaves, stems, roots, or vascular tissues to circulate water and nutrients. They reproduce by spores and most live in moist areas, although some can survive in extremely dry or cold regions.

Vascular plants (called *Tracheophyta* or tracheophytes) are a much larger group with specialized transporting vessels called the xylem and phloem, which circulate nutrients and water throughout the plant body. This advantage allows these plants to grow much larger than non-vascular plants. The vascular group includes spore-producing plants and the more highly evolved seed-bearing and flowering plants.

Names of the many divisions or phyla (plural of phylum) within the plant kingdom vary according to different scientific groups and botanical reference books. The following is a traditional classification that divides the plant kingdom into four primary phyla.

Division *Thallophyta* contains the most primitive and simplest one-celled and multi-celled plants originating in oceans and fresh waters. These include non-vascular fungi, mushrooms, bacteria, and molds that all lack chlorophyll and depend on other plants or animals for their food source. Green thallophytes include algae, seaweeds, slime molds, and riverweeds. These contain chlorophyll and are primarily aquatic.

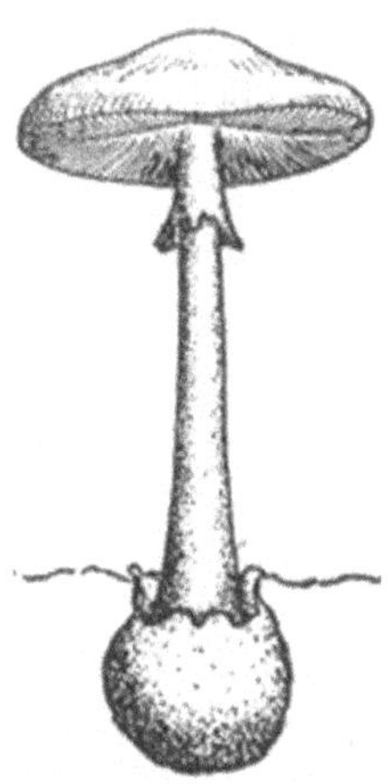

Mushroom

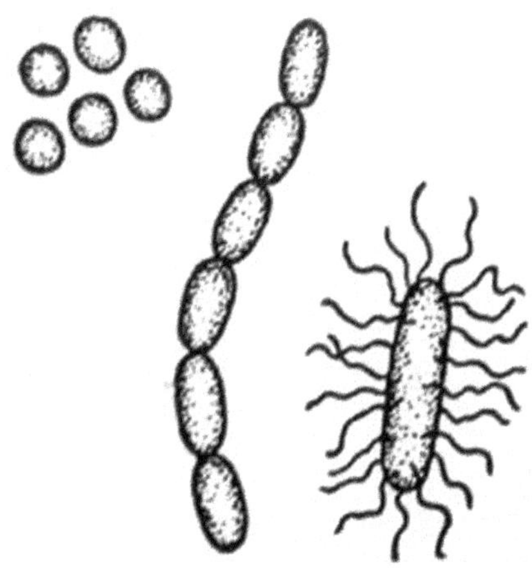

Bacteria

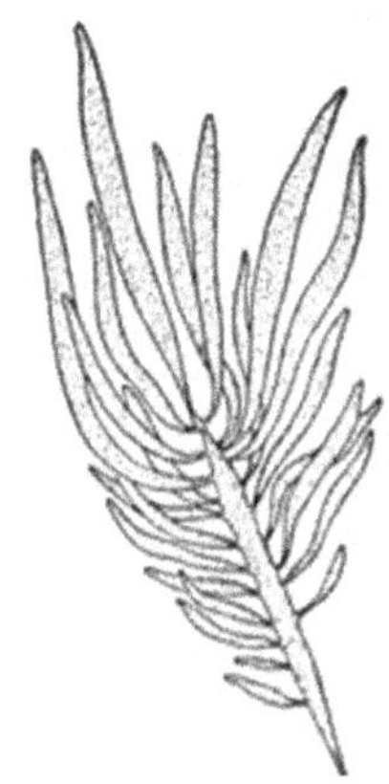

Algae

Division *Bryophyta* includes soft-bodied plants that contain chlorophyll, green leaves and stems, but no true roots. Their roots serve as anchorage but cannot transport water or nutrients. Members of this division have a primitive reproductive system and reproduce by spores rather than seeds. Bryophytes were probably the first plants to grow on land and include the mosses, liverworts, and hornworts.

Division *Pteridophyta* consists of seedless vascular plants having roots and stems with primitive veins, but no true leaves. Members of this division reproduce by spores and include ferns, horsetails, and club mosses that prefer damp, shady habitats. The Pteridophytes were the earliest type of vascular plants to evolve and possess stems that conduct water from their roots to the leaves. Ferns have green leaf-like structures called fronds. Male Horsetail plants have primitive leaves that look like long pine needles.

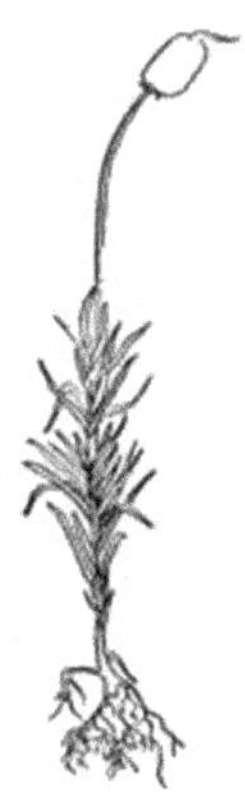

Moss

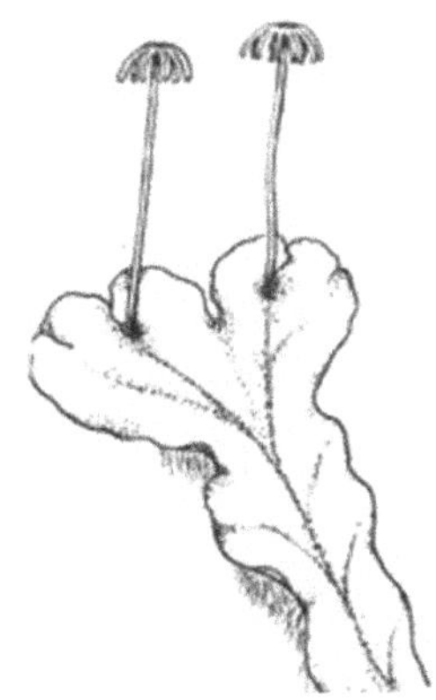

Liverwort

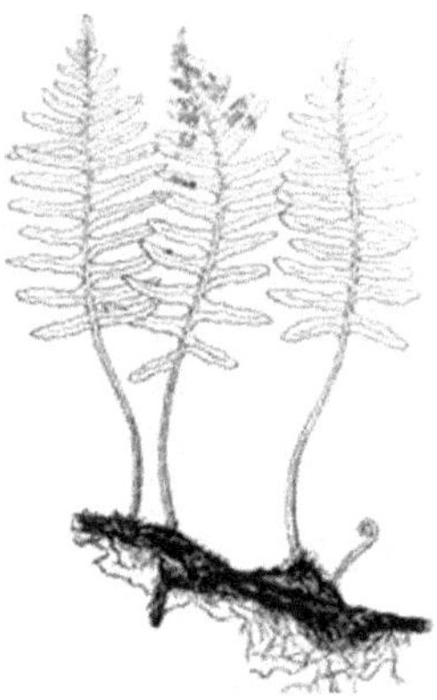

Fern

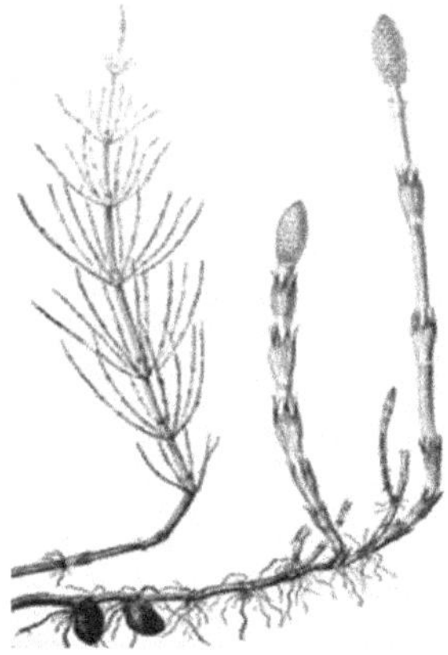

Horsetail

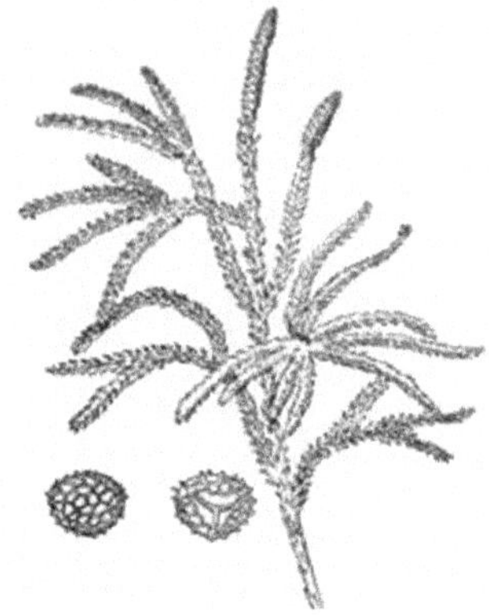

Club Moss

Division *Spermatophyta* contains the most highly evolved plants that are seed-bearing and possess true roots, stems, leaves, and flowers that bear fruit. The Spermatophytes are divided into two classes, the gymnosperms and angiosperms, which include the medicinal herbs.

CLASS

For herbalists, the most important classes of vascular plants are the gymnosperms (also known as *Gymnospermopsida* or *Gymnospermae*) and the angiosperms (known as *Anthopsida, Angiospermae,* or *Anthophyta*).

Gymnosperms are non-flowering plants and include the cone-bearing evergreens. *Gymnospermopsida* translates as "naked seed" because their seeds are not enclosed in fruits or pods, as happens in flowering plants. Instead, pollen from male cones is carried by the wind directly to the ovules, or unfertilized seeds, produced on the scales of female cones. Gymnosperms that bear their seeds in cones are called conifers. They have green, needle-like leaves and include Fir, Pine, Juniper, Spruce, Cedar, Sequoias, and the giant Redwood trees. The well-known *Gingko biloba* tree is a member of the *Gymnospermopsida,* but its unique fan-shaped leaves are blades rather than needles.

Angiosperms are flowering plants that produce seeds enclosed in fruit or a pod. To a great extent, their classification is based on the structure of their flowers and fruits. They are the dominant land plants and include all the herbaceous plants. Angiosperms are the most recent group to evolve and represent the pinnacle of evolutionary development. We cannot know exactly how long flowering plants have existed on the planet, but by analyzing fossils, geologists estimate that they evolved over 120 million years ago.

SUBCLASS

The flowering angiosperms are further divided into two subclasses: *Monocotyledonae* and *Dicotyledonae*. Plants belonging to the subclass ***Monocotyledonae*** are also known as **monocotyledons** or **monocots**. Monocots have only one leaf emerging from their germinating seed (*mono* means "one" and *cotyledon* means "seed leaves"). Plants classified as ***dicotyledonae*** are also known as **dicotyledons** or **dicots**. Dicots (*di* means "two") have two leaves called cotyledons that first grow from their seeds.

The similarities between these two subclasses far exceed their differences, although there are obvious structural variations. Monocots are thought to be the most recent products of plant evolution and include the grasses, cereal grains (wheat, corn, oat, barley, rice, rye, millet, buckwheat), irises, lilies, orchids, palms, sugar cane, bamboo, and cattails. The dicots are a much larger class and include almost all the familiar trees and shrubs (with the exception of the evergreen conifers), flowering plants, vegetables, and the medicinal herbs.

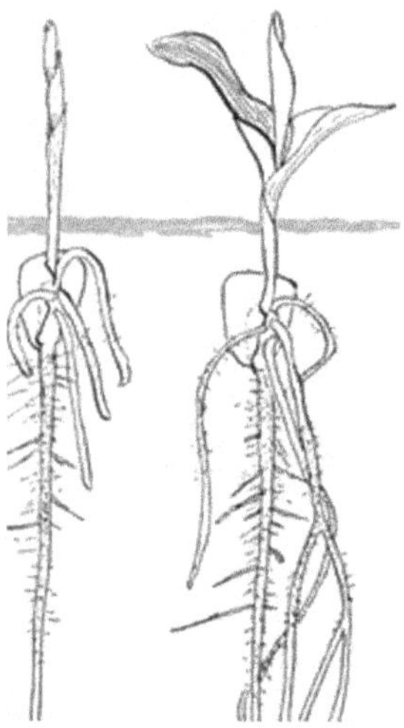

Monocot
Corn Seed

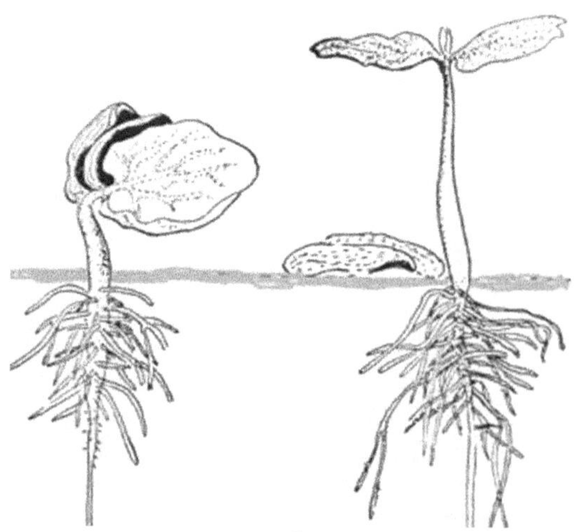

Dicot
Castor Oil Bean Seed

ORDER

An order is a further division of a plant class or subclass. Orders can contain several families. Names of orders generally end in "*–ales*." For example, the order Rosales includes the family *Rosaceae* (Rose), which is representative of the order, and also the family *Hamamelidaceae* (Witch Hazel) and *Leguminosae* (Pea).

FAMILY

A family is a group of genetically related genera (plural of genus). Plants in the same family share fundamental and structural characteristics that are helpful for identification. For example, members of the Pea family share a similar shape of flowers and seedpods. Members of a plant family often have similar growing requirements or similar mechanisms for pollination and seed dispersal. They can also harbor the same diseases and pests. The names of plant families usually end in "*–aceae*." Older family names such as *Leguminosae* (Pea family) are sometimes changed to newer names ending in "*–aceae*," and the most recent name for the Pea family is *Fabaceae*. The Pea family name is written as *Leguminosae* (*Fabaceae*).

GENUS AND SPECIES

Families are further divided into genera containing one or many related groups called species. Plants within the same genus share kinship through ancestry and have similar structural and genetic characteristics. Plants of the same species have an even closer genetic relationship and can cross-pollinate to interbreed among themselves. Despite their vast variety and numbers, classifying plants down to the species provides a convenient way to identify and catalog all plants. New plant species resulting from cross-pollination and hybridization are discovered or developed every year, and are appropriately named.

The species name often describes distinguishing plant characteristics such as the color of the flower, odor, texture, growing habitat, or medicinal uses. Familiarity with commonly used Latin terms helps in understanding a plant's name and characteristics, and the following often appear as species names:

alba (white)
angularis (angular)
angustifolia (narrow-leaved)
aqua (water)
arbor (tree)
aureus, chryso (golden yellow)
bi (two)
biloba (two-lobed)
californicus (indigenous to California)
campanulata (bell-shaped)
canadensis (indigenous to Canada)
cardiaca (relating to the heart)
communis (common)
crispus (curled)
diphylla (two-leaved)
ellipticus (oval)
filiformis (thread-shaped)
flavescens (yellow)
floridus (bearing abundant flowers)
foetida (emitting a stinking odor)
frutescens (having shrubby growth)
hispida (covered with coarse, erect hairs)
lanceolata (having a pointed, lance-shaped leaf)
latifolia (broad-leaved)
linearis (long and narrow)
luteus (yellow)
millifolium (possessing many leaves)
montana (indigenous to mountainous areas)
multi (many)
nigra, niger (black)
ob (reversed)
occidentalis (from the West; Europe and Americas)
odorata (pleasantly sweet-smelling)
officinalis (an historically official medicine)
ovatus (oval-shaped)
pendulus (hanging down)
perforatum (perforate or cut through)
purpurea (purple)
quinquefolius (five-leaved)
racemosa (a spike-like flower stalk)
radicans (having aerial roots)
reptans (creeping)
rhodo, roseus (rosy red)
rubra, ruber, and *erythro* (red)
sanguinia (blood-red)
sinensis (indigenous to China)
spicata (spiked)
tormentosa (covered with short, matted hairs)
triloba/trifolia (three lobes/three leaves)
viridis, chloro (green)
vulgaris (common)

VARIETY OR SUBSPECIES

Some species of plants contain two or more **varieties** or **subspecies** that bear an overall resemblance to each other, but exhibit at least one important variation such as the color of the flower or shape of the leaf. Hybrids are new varieties of plants developed by human manipulation from plants of the same species. Seeds produced by hybrid plants will not necessarily develop into duplicates of the parent plant, so hybrids must usually be propagated by root divisions or stem cuttings to reproduce a replica of the parent plant.

When plants of the same species are bred to produce a distinct variation having specific desirable characteristics (like a large bloom or specific color), the resulting plant is called a **cultivar**, another variety engineered by humans. Seeds produced from cultivar plants usually do not grow into a duplicate of the parent plant, and like hybrids, cultivars must be propagated by root division or stem cuttings.

Examples of Plant Classification

When writing the taxonomy of plants, the divisions descend from the most general group characteristics to the most specific. The names of each group traditionally end in distinct suffixes that are shown in parentheses.

Division (-phyta)
Class (-aea, opsida)
Subclass (-ae)
Order (-ales)
Family (-aceae)
Genus
Species

The scientific classification of the common Dandelion is written as follows:

Division *Spermatophyta*
Class *Anthopsida*
Order *Asterales*
Family *Asteraceae*
Genus *Taraxacum*
Species *officinalis*

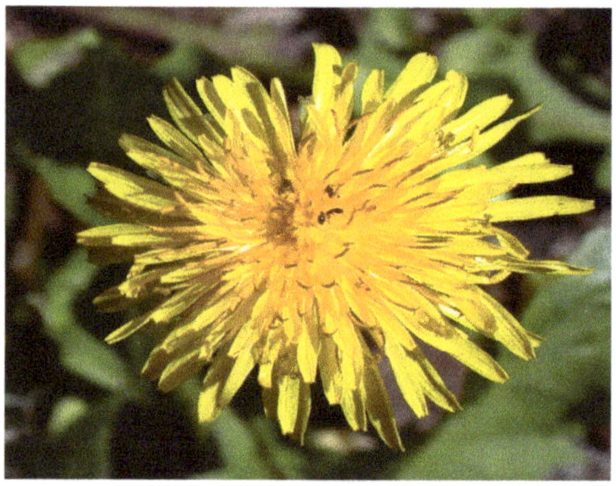

Dandelion
Taraxacum officinalis

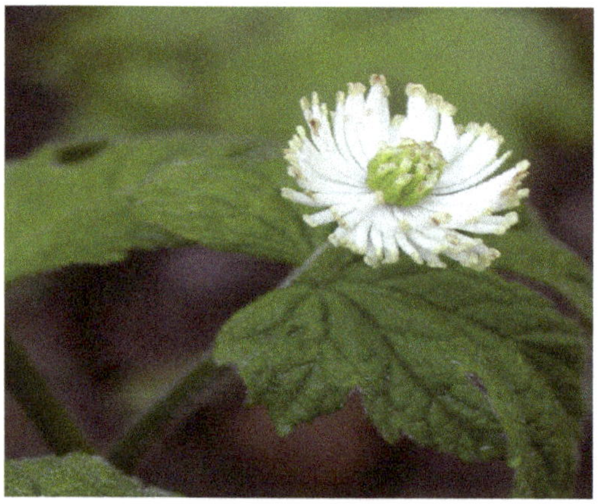

Goldenseal
Hydrastis canadensis

Goldenseal is classified as:

Division *Magnoliophyta*
Class *Magnoliosida*
Order *Ranunculales*
Family *Ranunculaceae*
Genus *Hydrastis*
Species *canandensis*

Balloon Flower is written as:

Division *Spermatophyta*
Class *Anthopsida*
Order *Asterales*
Family *Campanulaceae*
Genus *Platycodon*
Species *grandiflorus*

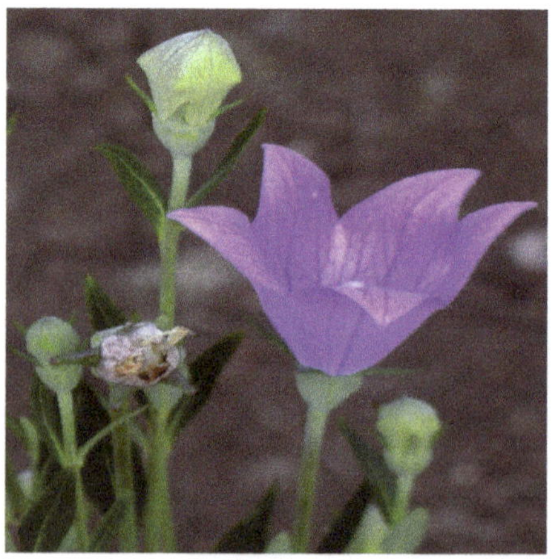

Balloon Flower
Platycodon grandiflorus

Botany for Herbalists

Every plant is a member of a collective group and exists, in part, to preserve the species. The roots, stems, and leaves provide anchorage, nutrients, and energy to sustain the individual plant. To ensure continued survival, plants are also sexual beings that display their reproductive organs in the most efficient ways to attract pollinators. These sexual organs have evolved over time as flowers, which often appear in bright colors, intriguing shapes, and alluring aromas to entice birds and insects.

Over the centuries, people have attempted to understand, define, and label plants and their life cycles, and the resulting synthesis of observation and knowledge gave birth to the science of botany. The term "botany" originates from the Greek word *botane* meaning "plant." **Botany** is the branch of biology dealing with plant life and is a universally accepted scientific language that provides accurate descriptions of plants. Botanical studies typically include the cellular and gross physical structure of plants, and how they live and function in nature.

The botanical scope offered in this chapter pertains to the needs of herbalists for plant identification and learning terminology used for botanical descriptions. A good foundation of plant anatomy is provided, and the basic parts and types of plants are introduced and described, as well as special features. Acquiring basic knowledge and using this chapter as a reference guide will help you to correctly identify medicinal plants. It will also come in handy when reading descriptions of herbs in this and other botanical books.

Bring this chapter to life by taking it with you into the garden, field, and forest when observing plants. Your perspective, understanding, and appreciation of plants will evolve as you look at them through the eyes of a botanist. It is especially fun to purchase a 16X loupe magnifying glass for a fascinating and intricate view into another dimension of roots, stems, leaves, and flowers. Botany can "open our doors of perception" to behold the amazing organization and patterns of Nature that manifest in the beauty of plants and flowers.

Classification of Plants According to Life Span

Annual plants live for only one year. They complete their entire life cycle in this time by germinating from seed to develop roots, leaves, and flowers. The flowers mature into seeds that ensure future generations of plants for the continuation of the species. Annual plants die after their seeds mature.

Biennials have a two-year life span. Their roots and leaves develop in the first year, and flowers and seeds appear during the second year. When seeds have matured, the plant dies.

Perennial plants survive for many years, flowering and producing new seeds each year. In temperate regions, stems and leaves usually die back during cold weather, and roots stay dormant over the winter. In spring, warmth and increased light stimulate roots to develop stems and leaves, and the cycle continues. Evergreens are perennials with leaves that stay green during the winter and remain on the plant for more than a year. In tropical climates, perennials simply keep growing until their life span eventually ends. **Deciduous** trees and shrubs have leaves that die and fall off over winter and sprout again in spring.

Classification of Plants According to Water Requirements

Mesophyte plants require moderate amounts of moisture in the soil and atmosphere.

Hydrophyte plants depend on an abundance of water. They grow in wet soils and in water, either totally or partially submerged. Examples are Cattails, Blue Flag, Seaweeds, pond Lilies and marsh-loving plants.

Xerophyte plants are adapted to dry habitats and have resistance to drought. Cactus and other desert plants are xerophytes.

The Cellular Structure of Plants

The basic structure of all plants, animals, and humans is the cell. Primitive plants like algae may only consist of one cell, but the vast majority of plants contain millions of cells that are specialized for different functions. Cells in plants, animals, and humans are amazingly alike. They are composed of similar materials arranged in organized patterns and structures to maintain all the functions that sustain life.

All cells have a nucleus containing chromosomes encoded with the specific genetic blueprint of the plant, animal, or person. Some plant and human cells contain the same organelles (tiny bodies within cells) which reflect the biological similarities and relationships between all forms of life.

Chloroplasts are organelles unique to plants because they contain the green pigment called chlorophyll, and photosynthesis occurs in chloroplasts. Chlorophyll is like the life blood of plants and, like hemoglobin in human blood, both are indispensable to life. Chlorophyll enables photosynthesis and hemoglobin transports oxygen to all cells. Interestingly, they share a similar chemical structure. Both

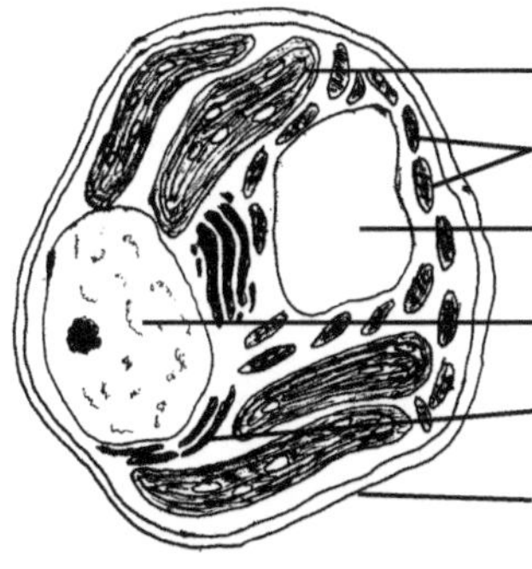

Typical Plant Cell

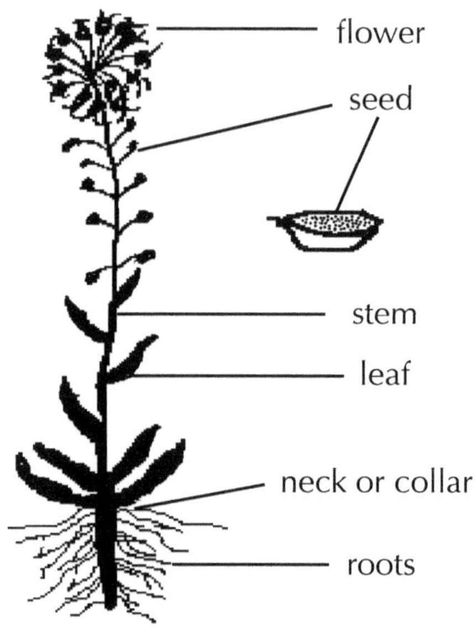

Plant parts

are built upon a porphyrin ring containing four nitrogen molecules. In hemoglobin an iron ion is bonded to nitrogen, while a magnesium ion binds nitrogen in chlorophyll.

Mitochondria, another type of organelle, are the source of cellular energy for both plants and animals. Vacuoles are filled with water and contribute to structural support of plants. Ribosomes synthesize chains of amino acids to form protein molecules.

Primary Parts of Plants

The primary parts of a typical plant are the roots, stems, leaves, and the flowers that eventually mature into seeds. **Roots** anchor plants in the ground, absorbing and storing minerals and water from soil. The point at ground level where the root connects with the aerial parts is called the **neck** or **collar**. **Stems** provide structural support and transport nutrients and water to leaves and flowers. **Leaves** transform soil nutrients and sunlight into energy necessary for plant survival and growth. **Flowers** are the reproductive organs that eventually mature into **fruit** and **seeds**.

The Growth Process of Plants

Like animals, plants grow by cell division during the process of mitosis. During mitosis, the nuclear DNA in one cell becomes organized into two sets of thread-like chromosomes that divide into two cells. Following the germination and initial development of seedlings, growth of new plant cells occurs almost entirely in the **meristems**, which are localized areas where cells divide and are capable of indefinitely adding new cells to the plant body. The two primary types of meristems are apical and lateral. **Apical meristems** are located at the tips of roots and stems, and are involved in the extension and lengthening of the root and plant body. The roots continually grow out and down towards minerals and water, while stems, leaves, and flowers grow up toward sunlight. This type of growth is called **primary growth**. When roots and stems reach a certain length and height, they start thickening to provide strength and stability to the plant. This is called **secondary growth** and is accomplished by **lateral meristems** residing inside along the length of stems and roots of larger plants, woody shrubs, and trees. These meristem cells divide laterally, resulting in stronger and more massive stems and roots.

The Vascular Transport System of Plants

Most plants have a circulatory system with similarities to our own. Vascular plants were specifically named because they contain a system of vessels that transport nutrients and water through their roots, stems and leaves, just as our blood vessels carry fluids, nutrients, and other components to our cells. Vascular plants include ferns, horsetails, club mosses, conifers and cycads, and all the flowering plants. Most plants are vascular except those in the Thallophyta division that includes fungi, mushrooms, mold, bacteria, algae and seaweeds, and in the Bryophyta division composed of the liverworts, hornworts, and mosses.

After water and nutrients pass into the root hairs of vascular plants, they flow to the center of the root into specialized transporting cells. Transport cells start at the root tip and extend up the stem and into the leaves, where they are visible as **veins**. Transport cells are hollow cylinders stacked vertically on top of each other to form a long, continuous column or tube called a vessel. The two types of transporting tissues are the xylem and phloem. **Xylem** tissues conduct water and dissolved mineral salts in an upward direction through the plant body. **Phloem** tissues transport food nutrients produced by photosynthesis both upward and downward between the leaves, stems, and roots. These two types of vascular tissues occur together to form a continuous and efficient circulatory system throughout the plant. Xylem and phloem tissues are involved in food distribution, food storage, and plant growth. They also contribute to the structural integrity and rigidity of the plant.

Plants obtain all water by root absorption from moisture in soil. Leaves typically do not absorb water. However, up to 97 percent of the water that plants absorb through their roots is lost to evaporation from their leaf surfaces. Dry, sunny days and high winds greatly contribute to water loss from leaves. Water is necessary for photosynthesis to occur, and during this process, pores on leaf surfaces, which are called **stomata**, must be open to allow for evaporation. In plant bodies, water only moves in an upward direction. Water transpires, or is pulled up, from the roots into stems by the draw created from water evaporation through the leaf pores. This pull of water keeps plant cells hydrated, creating a pressure or turgor that enables plants to stand upright. Insufficient water slows down the transpiration process and reduces photosynthesis. Plants naturally respond to dehydration by closing their stomata in order to retain water, and leaves droop and curl inward.

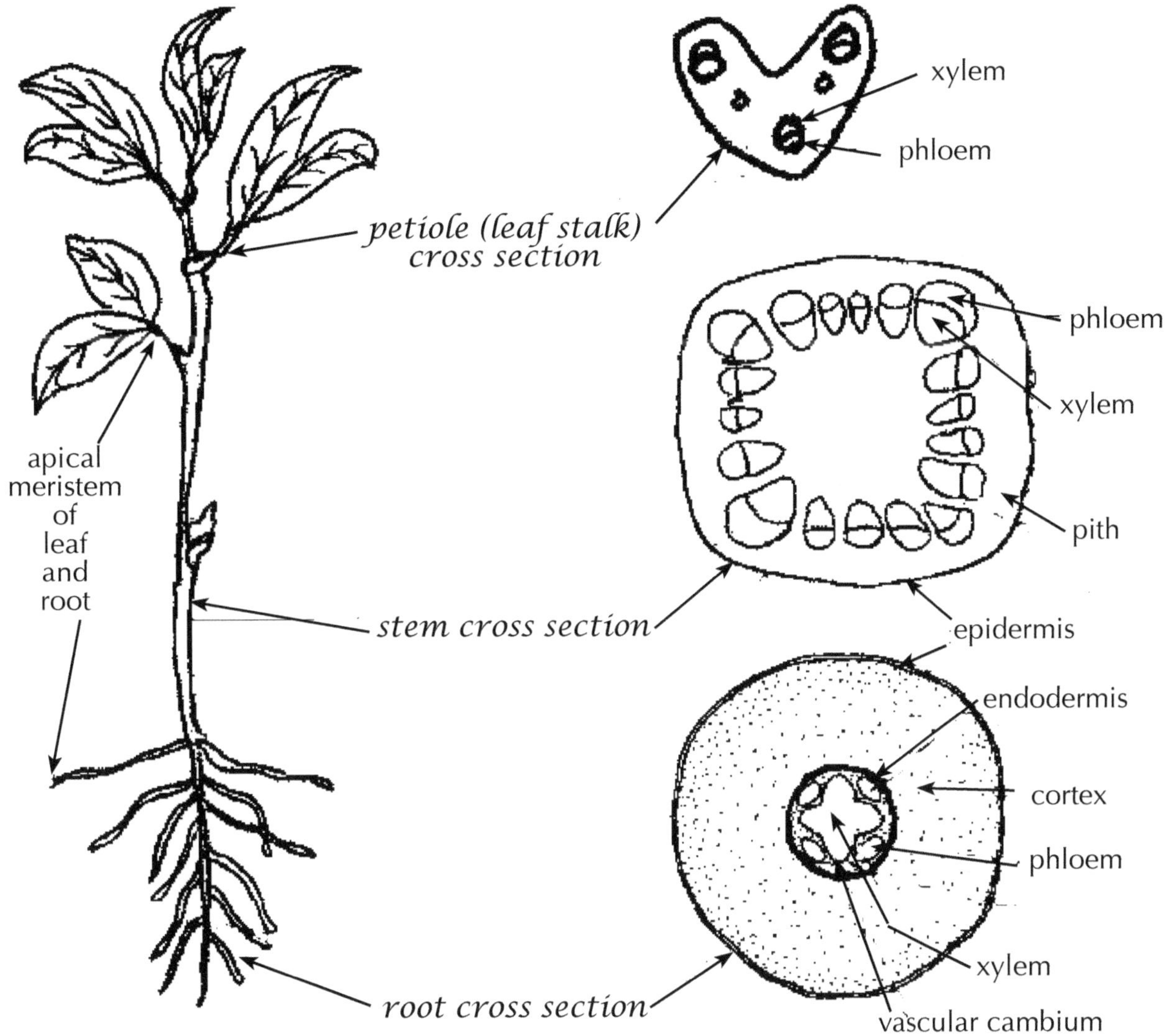

Three cross-sections showing the inner tissues of a typical root, stem, and leaf stalk.

Roots and stems have an outer protective covering called the **epidermis**. The phloem and xylem are bundles of vascular transporting tissues held in place by the surrounding **cortex** in roots and by **pith** in stems. Reserve food is stored in the root cortex. Pith in stems provides flexibility, allowing them to bend without snapping or breaking.

ROOTS

Roots are the underground portion of plants. Their three primary functions are: 1) anchoring the plant in soil; 2) absorbing water and minerals from soil; and 3) storing food nutrients for future use. Some taproots and tuberous roots like Yam, Comfrey, Dandelion, and Burdock are specifically designed to store large amounts of vitamins, minerals, and starches. Since there is a large concentration of nutrients and other constituents in the roots, they often provide a potent source of medicinal components or food, depending on the plant.

Roots have a symbiotic relationship with bacteria and fungi that naturally exist in the soil around them. They mutually feed each other. Bacteria and fungi grow on plant roots and increase the plant's ability to absorb minerals and water from soil. These beneficial bacteria and fungi are abundant in humus, which is nutrient-rich soil consisting of decomposing plant and animal material.

When germination occurs in seeds, the tiny **radicle** or **embryonic root** is usually the first structure to emerge, eventually developing into the **main** or **primary root**. In many plants, **secondary** or **lateral roots** grow off the larger primary root. Roots are typically covered with multiple thread-like **root hairs** that are extensions of the outer root cells, and are vital for absorbing water and soil minerals. The walls of root hairs act like a membrane that allows water and mineral salts to pass through by the process of osmosis, when water and nutrients move from an area of high concentration in the surrounding soil to an area of lower concentration in the roots.

Root growth occurs behind the tips of roots in the area of the **apical meristem**, where the process of cell division produces new layers of root tissue. All growth responsible for lengthening roots takes place in the apical meristem. The root tip is protected by the **root cap** as it pushes its way through soil. Although root tips look fragile, their power to push through hard soil and even rocks is an impressive example of their force and tenacious nature to continually grow. Roots increase in thickness due to cell division taking place in **lateral meristems** located inside roots throughout their length.

The two basic types of roots are fibrous roots and taproots. Most plant roots fall into one of these categories, but some roots are a combination of both. **Fibrous roots** consist of many thin, profusely branching roots that are relatively equal in size and extend out fairly evenly from the stem in all directions. There is no obvious dominant root. A **taproot** is a single, well-defined root growing downward into the earth. Taproots sometimes branch or divide into two or three large roots, and they often have thread-like hairs growing off their sides. Taproots are much thicker than fibrous roots. They provide sturdy anchorage and greater storage capacity for nutrients and starch to feed the plant. When leaves and stems of biennial and perennial plants die back in winter, nutrients stored in the roots sustain them through the winter months and enable regeneration of new foliage the following spring.

There are several distinctive types of taproots. A **conical taproot** tapers from a thickened crown to a thinner apex (bottom of root). Carrot, Burdock, Yellow Dock, Dandelion and *Echinacea angustifolia* roots are examples. A **fusiform root** tapers up and down symmetrically like a radish. **Napiform roots** are swollen at the base so they are wider than they are long, like beets and turnips. **Fasciculated roots** have thick fibers like Comfrey and Marshmallow roots.

Adventitious roots grow off of stems and leaves that are placed in soil or water instead of developing from seeds. Strawberries and Raspberries have this specialized type of root.

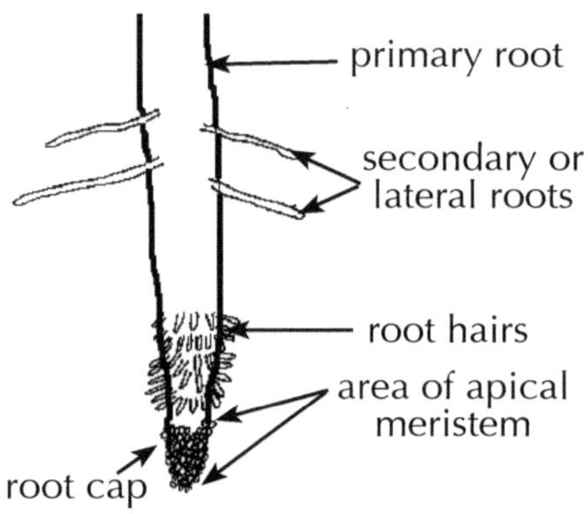

Radicle or embryonic root

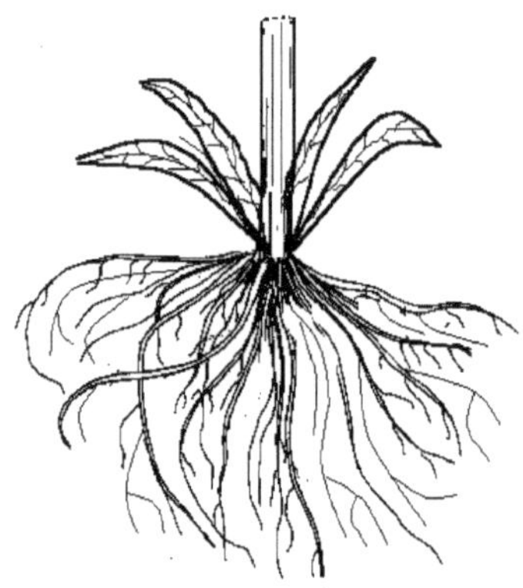

Fibrous root

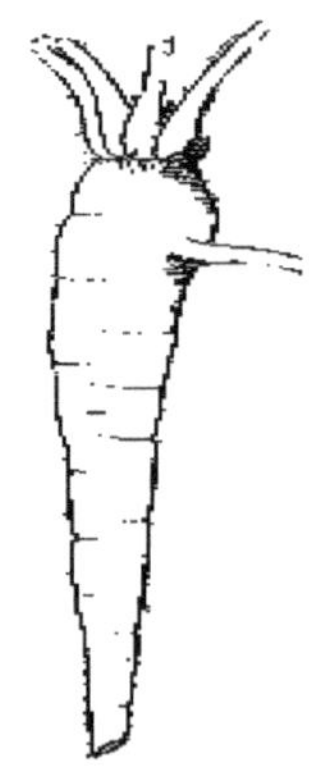

Taproot (conical)

STEMS

Stems are the structural "backbone" of plants because they support the leaves, flowers, fruits, and seeds. They raise leaves towards the sun to facilitate photosynthesis. The stem is a main pathway of the circulatory or vascular system as it transports fluids and nutrients from the roots up to the leaves and flowers. It also moves hormones, food produced by photosynthesis in the leaves, and other metabolites to different parts of the plant. Stems produce new living tissue and store food and water.

The stem is the aerial portion of a plant that rises upward from the germinating seed at the same time as the root tip grows down into the soil. The growing stem with its branches and leaves is collectively called the **shoot**. These all develop from the apical meristem or bud located in the uppermost stem tip, where cells divide and growth occurs. Stems have two primary types of buds called apical and axillary. The **apical** or **terminal bud** sits at the tip of stems and is responsible for cell divisions that 1) make the stems grow longer; 2) provide leaf growth; and 3) develop branches. On herbaceous, non-woody stems, **axillary** or **lateral buds** usually appear along the stem at the base of each leaf in the leaf axil. Axillary buds remain dormant until they are stimulated to grow into secondary branches, leaves, and/or flowers. Occasionally,

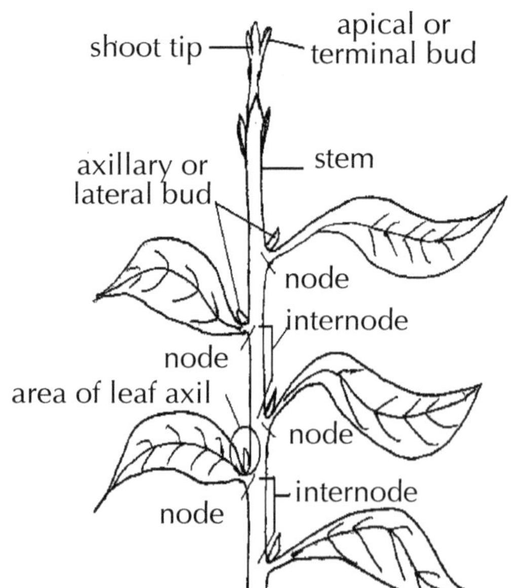

Stem nodes and internodes on a shoot

adventitious buds arise in unusual places, such as the site of an injury.

The areas along stems where leaf and flower buds attach are called **nodes**. **Internodes** are the spaces or segments between the nodes. As the stem grows, the internodes lengthen and spread the leaves apart, allowing more exposure to sunlight and air circulation. The area where an angle is formed between each leaf stalk and the stem is called the **leaf axil**.

The outer surface of stems is formed by a single layer of cells called the **epidermis**. The **cuticle** is a layer of waxy cutin on the surface of epidermal cells that helps prevent water loss and protects the stem against molds and other infections. Herbaceous stems can be smooth and **glaucous** (lacking hairs) or **pubescent** (hairy). The word "pubescent" comes from Latin and means "downy." Hairs often deter insects from eating plants. Stems can be round, square, or angular in shape. They may be smooth or lined with groves or furrows.

Plant Classification According to Stems

The size and type of stem is an easy way to classify plants into one of the four major groups consisting of herbs, vines, shrubs, and trees. **Herbs** have soft tissue stems and typically die down to the ground over winter. **Shrubs** and **trees** have woody stems and branches that live year after year, becoming bigger and thicker each successive year. A **shrub** is different than a tree because it has many branches growing off the roots and is usually less than 10 feet tall. **Trees** are typically more than 10 feet tall and grow only one main trunk that divides into many branches. **Vines** are long stems that trail, twine, or climb with the assistance of tendrils or suckers. Vines can have either soft tissue or woody stems. Some shrubs with woody stems that climb or twine are also considered to be vines. Vines are usually perennials, and although the stem and leaf may die back over winter, new foliage emerges from the dormant roots in spring.

Specialized Types of Stems

Some plant parts that are commonly considered to be roots are actually underground sections of the stem. Rhizomes (or rootstocks), tubers, bulbs, and corms are underground stems adapted to store adequate quantities of starch and other nutrients between growing seasons to ensure the plant's survival. Runners (or stolons), suckers, tendrils, and thorns are specialized stems growing above ground that serve other functions, including propagation, support, and protection.

A **rhizome** or **rootstock** is an underground stem that grows horizontally. Typical of all stems, rhizomes have nodes bearing leaves, axillary buds, and internodes. Rhizomes are anchored in soil by adventitious roots arising from nodes along the bottom of the rhizome, while erect stems and leaves grow from the upper side. One characteristic that separates rhizomes from true roots is the presence of scaly leaves at regular intervals along its length, at buds, and at nodes. Nodes typically occur on the rhizome ends. Plants with rhizomes are perennials, and each year rhizomes grow a new section and send up at least one stem or leaf. The age of many rhizomes can be determined by counting the number of longitudinal segments they contain, counting one segment for each year of life. Rhizomes reflect the climate and amount of rainfall during previous years, since times of drought limit growth, making short and thin sections along the rhizome. Most rhizomes are rather thick and fleshy. Rhizome plants can be propagated asexually by dividing the rootstock into pieces, making sure each piece contains a bud, and then planting each one. Examples are Bloodroot (*Sanguinaria canadensis*), Wild Ginger (*Asarum canadense*), Solomon's Seal (*Polygonatum multiflorum*), and Goldenseal.

Tubers are enlarged, fleshy, horizontal underground stems. They arise from the swollen tips of rhizomes. Tubers grow adventitious roots that produce more tubers. Like rhizomes, tubers are easy to propagate into new plants by dividing them into sections, making sure each one contains a bud. Once planted, the buds develop into stems. The Potato, Yam, Sweet Potato, and Jerusalem Artichoke are examples of tubers.

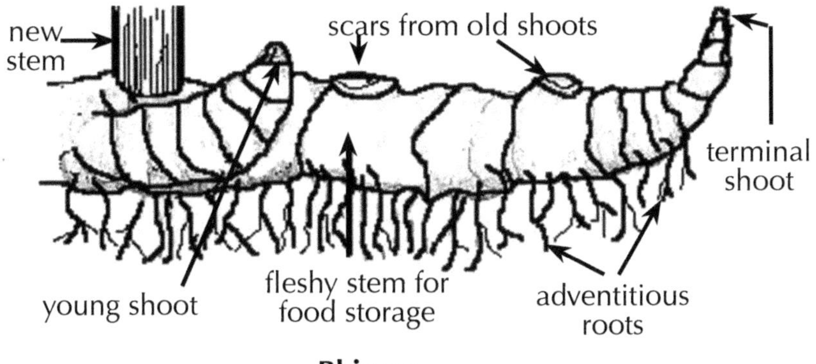

Rhizome

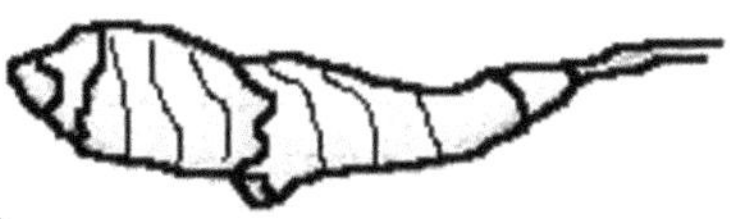

Tuber

Bulbs are large buds consisting of a small, erect, conical stem enclosed by numerous layers of enlarged, fleshy, scale-like leaf bases mounted on a small, disk-shaped stem. The outermost scale leaves are thin and brown, serving to protect the bulb against invasion by soil microorganisms and insects. Adventitious roots grow out from the bottom of bulbs. Bulbs differ from corms because food is stored in the leafy scales rather than the stem. Bulbs can be annuals or perennials, and include Onions, Garlic, and Daffodils. Bulbs and corms are always monocot plants.

Corms are shortened, swollen, fleshy, underground stems. They grow vertically and typically live for several years. Many plants that people call bulbs, such as Gladiolus, Crocus and Cyclamen, are actually corms. Although corms often resemble bulbs, they are formed differently. Like bulbs, they consist of stem and leaf tissue, but most of the corm is a thickened stem. The leaves are usually thin, dry scales and much smaller than bulb leaves. Most of the food stored in corms is a form of starch found in the fleshy stem.

Corms go into dormancy during the winter, and then produce new foliage and more corms each growing season. New corms develop from axillary buds. In addition, short underground stems may form with a single small corm developing from the tip. In its second year of growth, the new corm produces at least one stem and more new corms.

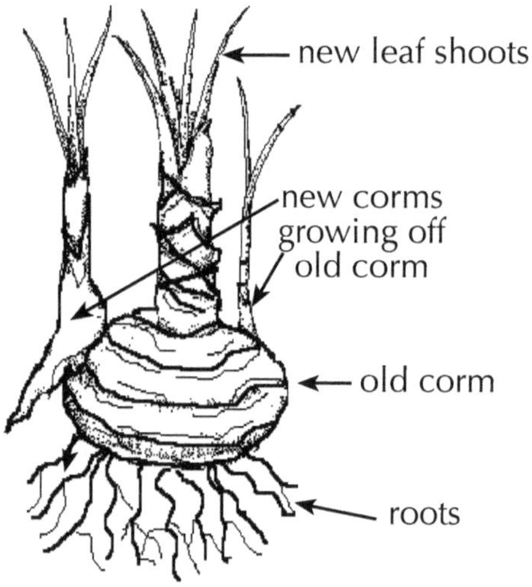

Corm

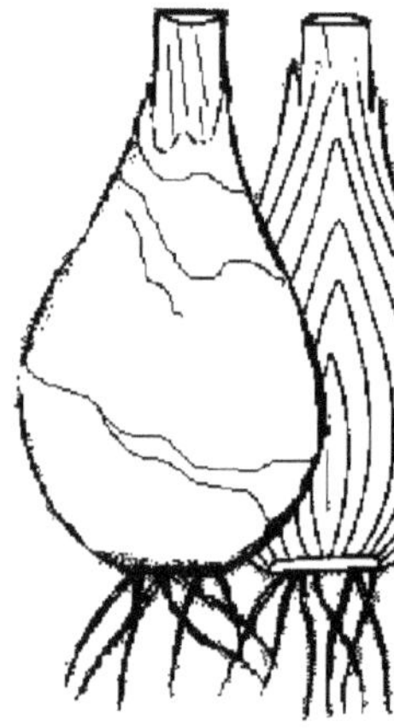

Bulb

Runners or **stolons** are long, slender stems that grow horizontally along the soil surface. Runners emerge from the base of the plant to grow and lengthen over the ground. When the stem node or terminal bud at the tip of a stem touches the soil, it takes root to produce a new plant. This type of root is called **adventitious** because it grows from unusual places, like stems and leaves. Some runners are covered with leaves along their entire length, and others only have leaves at their tips. After runners propagate new plants, they often dry up and die. The remaining plant can be left alone or transplanted to another location. The Strawberry family is a classic example of natural propagation by runners. White Clover and some Roses also produce and multiply by runners.

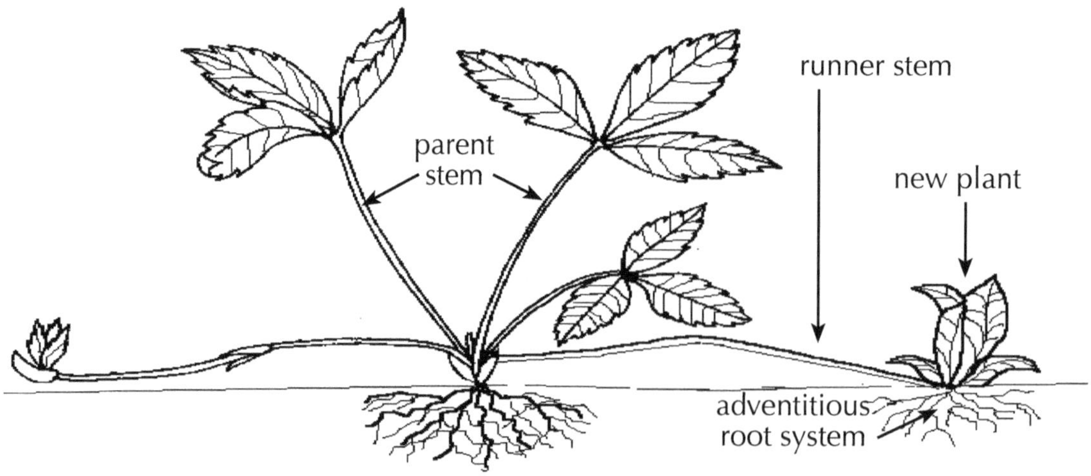

Runner stem taking root on a Strawberry plant

Suckers are adventitious upright shoots growing from roots, horizontal rhizomes, or lower stems of a plant. The shoot then develops as an independent plant. Many fruit trees and Lilacs grow suckers from their roots and from buds on the base of their trunks. Suckers often emerge from the stumps of trees that have been cut down, especially fruit trees. Blackberries, Raspberries, and Roses multiply by suckers.

Tendrils are slender, leafless stems on vine plants that are sensitive to contact stimuli and coil in a spiral to wrap themselves around objects for support. Tendrils are considered to be stem or leaf modifications. Passion Flower vines, Pea vines, and Grape vines all produce tendrils.

Thorns are modified stems or outgrowths of stems. They grow from axillary buds and terminate in sharp, hard points. Thorns are a protective mechanism developed to help plants survive animal predators.

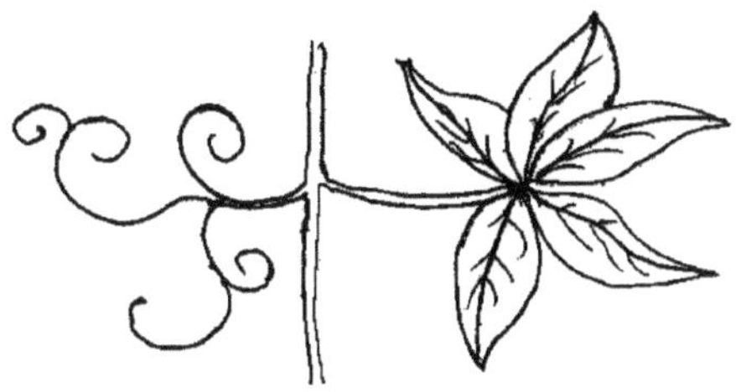

Tendril stem

Direction of the Stem

Erect stems stand upright vertically.
Declining stems bend over toward the earth.
Diffuse stems spread outward in all directions from the center of the plant.
Decumbent stems lay on the ground except at the tip, where the minimal weight of the flower allows it to grow upright. These are more delicate stems that lack the structural strength to stand erect.
Procumbent or **prostrate** stems lay completely on the ground.
Creeping stems branch out and grow along the ground surface, or use other plants for support.

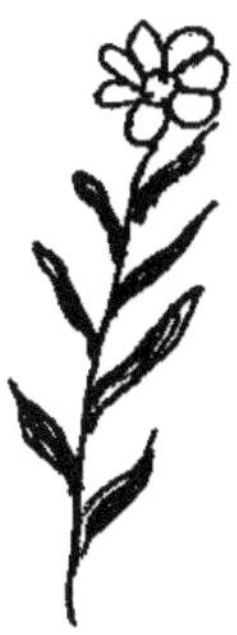

Erect stem

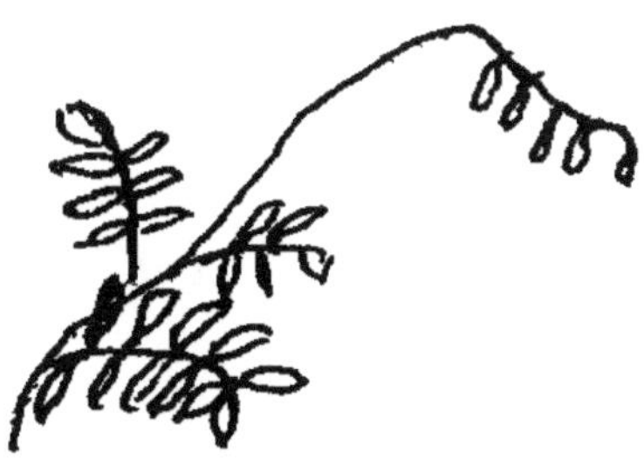

Declining stem

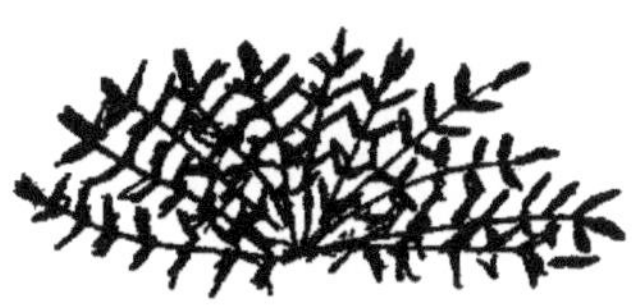

Diffuse stem

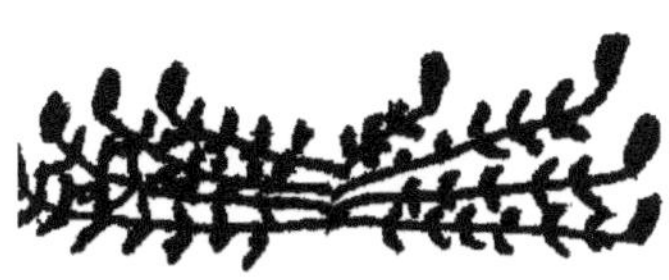

Decumbent stem

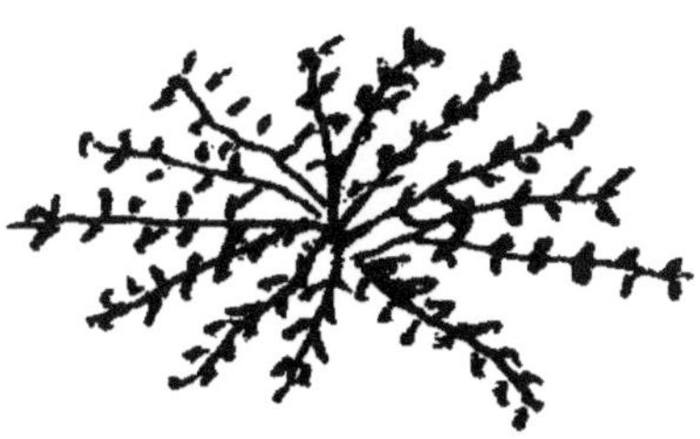

Procumbent stem

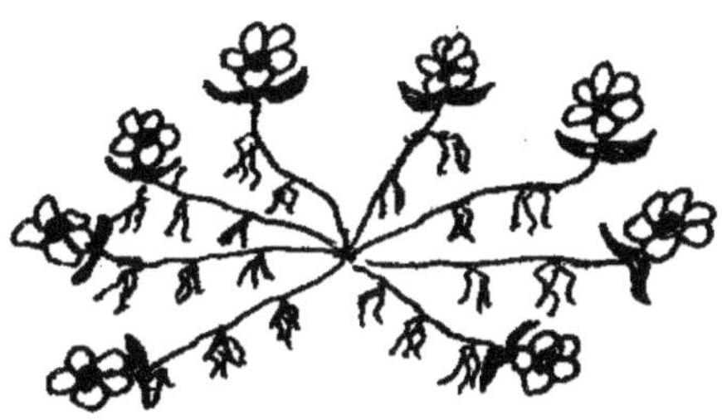

Creeping stem

LEAVES

Leaves appear in a multitude of shapes and sizes, including some that resemble stems or flowers. Leaves grow directly from roots or stems. Their primary purpose is to manufacture energy and nutrients for the entire plant by **photosynthesis**. This amazing process takes place within specialized leaf cells called **chloroplasts**. These chloroplasts contain **chlorophyll**, the green pigment giving plants their green color.

Photosynthesis occurs when energy from sunlight is absorbed by chlorophyll, allowing carbon dioxide and water to form glucose (sugar), which is the energy source for plants. During this transformation, leaves absorb carbon dioxide and release oxygen produced as a by-product. Photosynthesis maintains oxygen levels in the air, and is the source of energy for almost all life on the planet. In this regard, plants, animals, and humans have a symbiotic relationship. People and animals need oxygen and release carbon dioxide into the atmosphere as a waste product. Plants depend on carbon dioxide for their life and release oxygen.

EQUATION FOR PHOTOSYNTHESIS: CO2 (carbon dioxide) + H2O (water) + sunlight = CH2O (glucose) + O2 (oxygen)

Leaves are the sites of photosynthesis and they have evolved various adaptations for this purpose. Most have a large, flat surface area well-suited to absorb sunlight and carbon dioxide from the air. The outermost layer of cells on leaves and stems is the **epidermis**, which is involved in photosynthesis and is protected by a waxy covering that retards water loss. The underside of leaves contains multiple small openings called **stomata** (one opening is a **stoma**) that allow carbon dioxide and oxygen gases to pass in and out. **Guard cells** are specialized epidermal cells that regulate the opening and closing of stomata. Responding to environmental and physiological changes, the stomata open to "inhale" carbon dioxide and to "exhale" water and oxygen. Stomata usually close at night, during strong winds, and on hot, dry days to retain water. It is crucial for leaves to restrict water loss and avoid dehydration or eventual death. Some leaves are covered with dense mats of hairs that reduce evaporation from stoma pores, and also deter insects from eating and damaging the plant. An extensive network of veins brings water and nutrients into the leaves, and transports glucose produced by photosynthesis to the rest of the plant.

Leaf Anatomy

Cotyledons are the first leaves to appear on the stem of newly germinated seedlings. They store food for the developing plant, and as other leaves mature, cotyledons decrease in size and eventually drop off. The typical dicot leaf is flat, and the main body is called a **leaf blade** or **lamina**. The lower portion of the blade called the **leaf base** is thickened and elongated. The blade tip is the **apex**, and the **margin** is the leaf edge. The **midrib vein** runs through the center of the leaf and many **side** or **lateral veins** branch off from it. Leaves are often attached to the stem by a miniature stalk called the **petiole**. The **axillary bud** emerges from the notch formed by the stem and petiole stalk. Buds are small shoots with scale-like leaves that grow into mature leaves under suitable conditions. Some leaves have two small leaf-like outgrowths known as **stipules** at the base of their petioles. Often they protect the buds and developing leaves before falling off. They are typically paired in some dicot species and are absent in monocots. Stipules are basal appendages to the petiole and can appear as hairs, tendrils, spines, or leaves.

Monocot leaves do not have distinct petioles. Instead, the leaf is composed of two parts: the **sheath** and **blade**. The sheath is the bottom portion that is typically green and completely envelopes or sheathes the stem. The upper blade has a more leaf-like appearance.

A **bract** is a very small, modified leaf at the base of some flowers. There are usually two or more bracts that surround the stem at the flower base, and are collectively called the **involucre**.

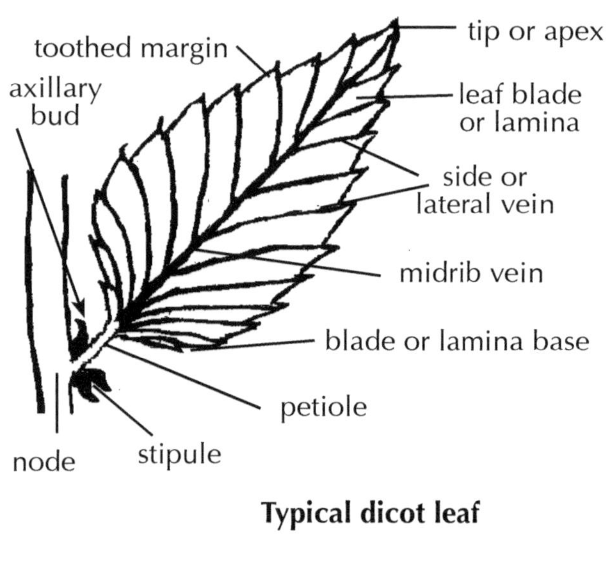

Typical dicot leaf

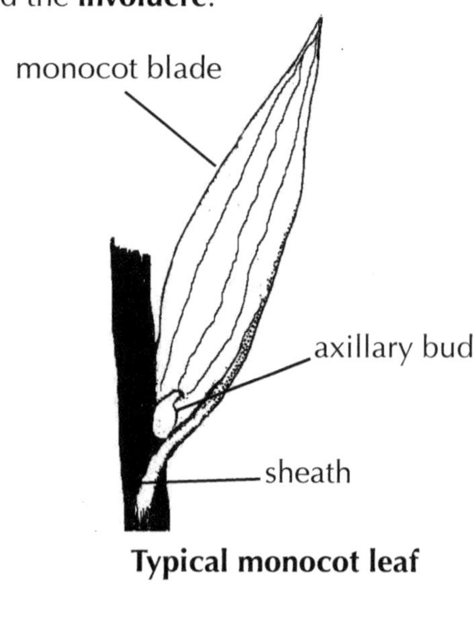

Typical monocot leaf

Petiolate and Sessile Leaves

Petiolate leaves are attached to the stem by a small petiole stalk. The petiole allows leaf blades to move in the direction of the sun to optimize the process of photosynthesis, and to provide greater flexibility during strong winds and heavy rains. **Sessile** leaves attach directly to the stem and lack a connecting stalk. *Petiolus* is a Latin word meaning "stalk" and *sessile* means "sitting on."

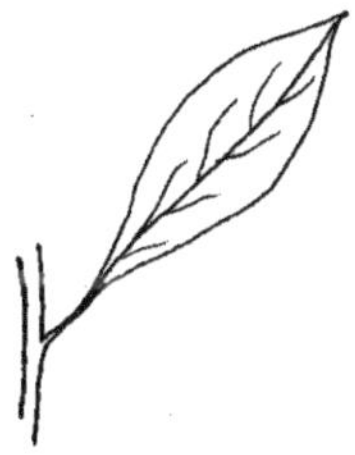

Petiole leaf
(has a stalk)

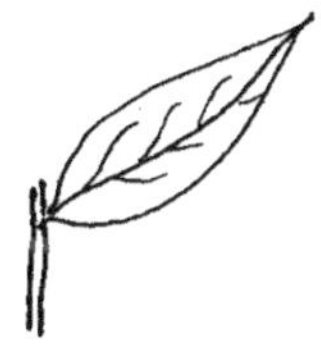

Sessile leaf
(has no stalk)

Simple and Compound Leaves

Leaves are classified as either simple or compound. A **simple** leaf has one single blade that is not divided into distinct parts, although it may be deeply lobed. **Compound** leaves have two or more blades that are separate **leaflets**, which are actually one leaf divided into many sections. A compound leaf can be mistaken for a stem with many leaves on it, but it is actually considered to be one very divided leaf. A few differences that are helpful in distinguishing between a leaf and leaflet are: 1) buds and stipules appear in the axils (the base) of simple and compound leaves, but not in the axils of leaflets; 2) leaves emerge from the stem in different planes, while leaflets are usually organized symmetrically, all laying on the same plane so the entire leaf forms a flat surface; and 3) most leaflets have their own small petiole, they all look alike, and do not bear flowers like stems do.

A **simple leaf** is **lobed** when it has several deep indentations dividing it into sections. **Palmately lobed** leaves look like an outstretched palm. **Pinnately lobed** leaves have indented sections that are symmetrically opposite each other and resemble the shape of a feather.

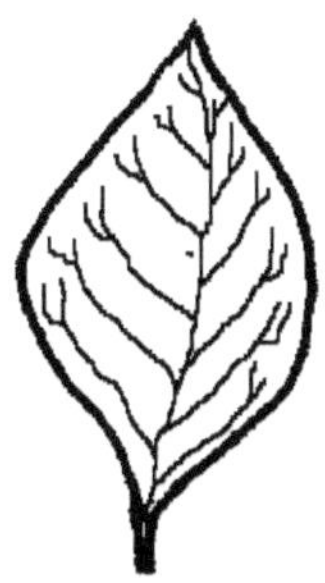

Simple leaf without lobes

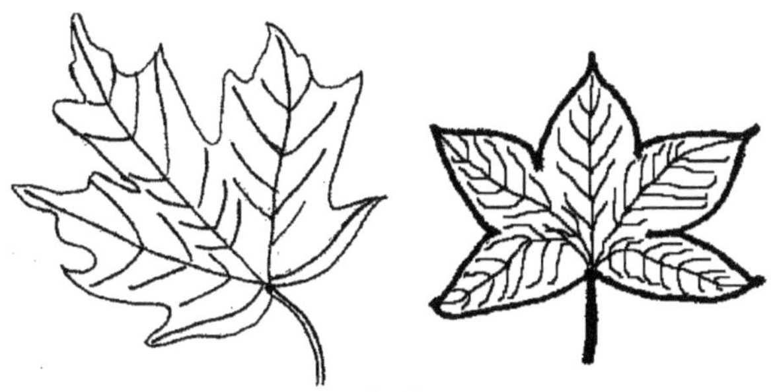

Simple leaves palmately lobed

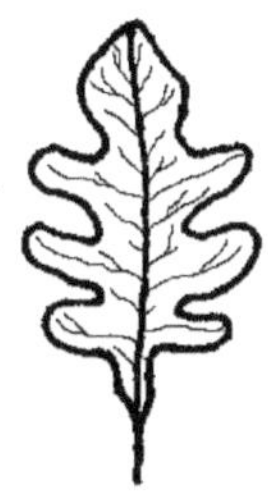

Simple leaf pinnately lobed

Compound leaves are either palmate or pinnate. **Palmately compound** leaves consist of individual leaflets that grow from a single point at the tip of the petiole and radiate outward like an outstretched hand. A palmately compound leaf with three leaflets is called **ternate**.

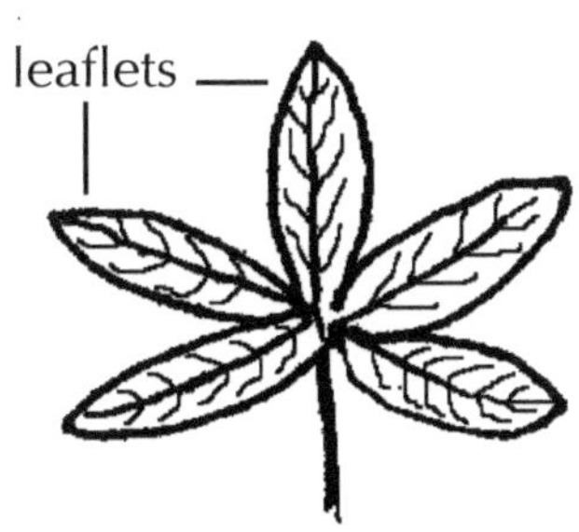

Palmately compound

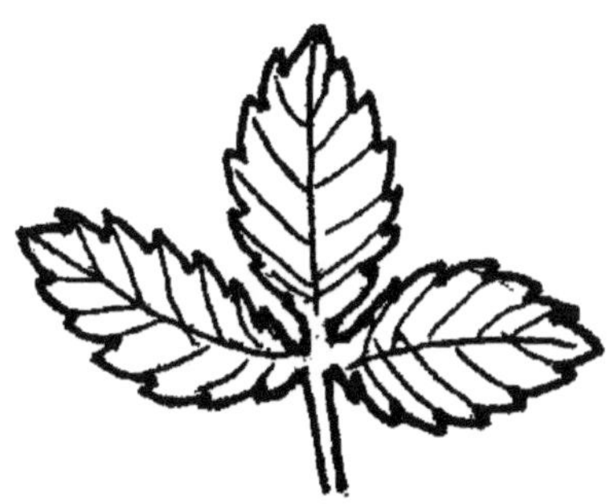

Palmately ternate

In **pinnately compound** leaves, the individual leaflets are arranged in two symmetrical rows on opposite sides of the **midrib** or **rachis**, which is an extension of the petiole. Leaflets often have a small petiole or stem stalk attaching them to the midrib. Pinnate means "resembles a feather." Pinnately compound leaves may have one rachis or branch out into more. In **bipinnately compound** leaves, each leaflet is subdivided into smaller leaflets, and two midribs branch off the petiole in opposite directions.

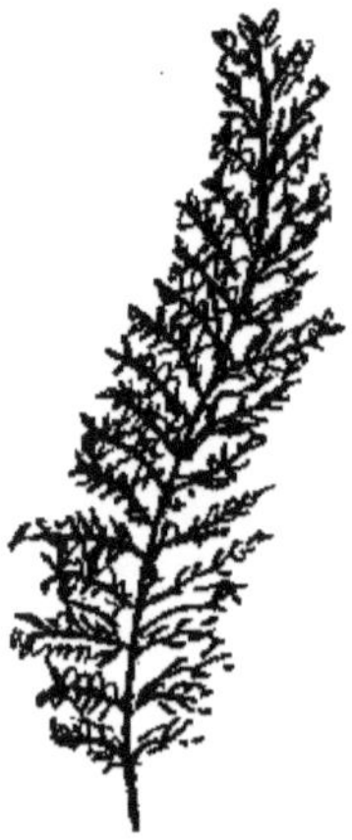

Pinnately compound

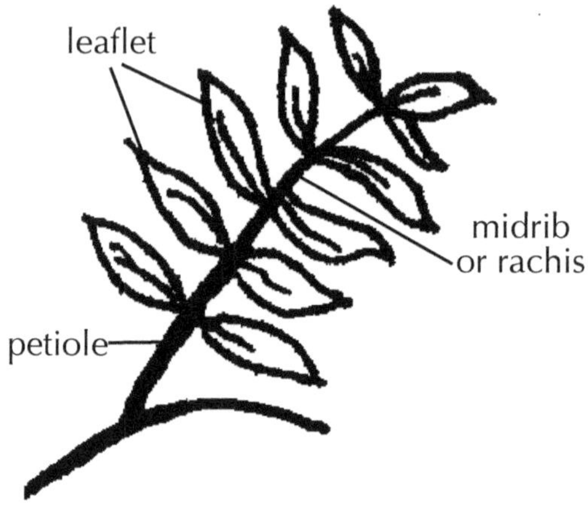

Pinnately compound

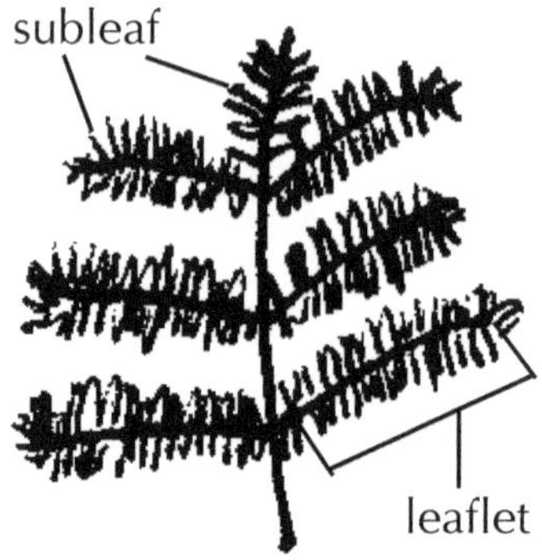

Bipinnately compound

Leaf Lobes

Leaves can have shallow or deep indentations that form lobes. Some of the most common types of lobes include the following:

Incised leaf margins are cut sharply and deeply, usually into symmetrically shaped lobes.
Lacerate lobes are deeply incised but are not symmetrical and appear to be randomly torn.
Laciniate lobes are deeply slashed, similar to incised, but the cuts are more sharply angled.

Venation (Vein) Patterns

A patterned network of **veins** support and nourish leaf blades. Veins are part of the vascular transport system of the roots and stems that carry water, mineral salts, and other nutrients to and from the leaves. **Venation** refers to the pattern or arrangement of veins on leaves, which is typically either netted or parallel.

Most dicot plants have **netted (reticulate) venation** with a net-like appearance. Netted venation is usually classified as pinnate or palmate. Leaves with **pinnate venation** have veins arranged in a branching pattern with a larger longitudinal vein, called the **midrib** or **midvein**, which extends through the center of the blade from the middle of the leaf base to the leaf tip. Many smaller veins branch off from the midrib in the typical pinnate feather pattern. In **palmate venation,** all the veins arise from one point at the leaf base and branch out in a relatively symmetrical pattern. Some dicots and most monocot plants have **parallel venation**, in which many veins that are fairly equal in size run parallel along the length of the leaf.

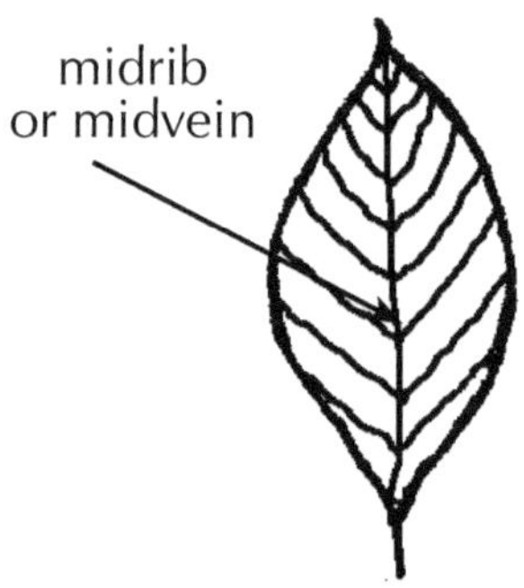

Pinnate veins

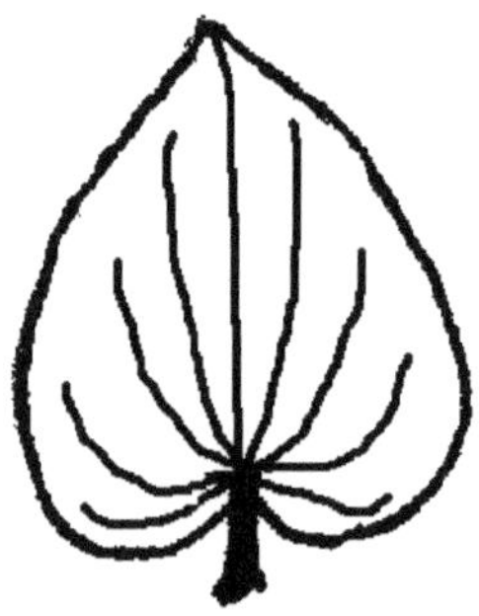

Palmate veins

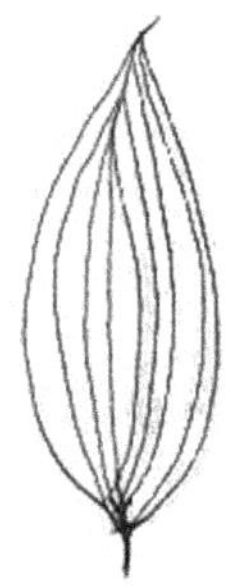

Parallel veins

Leaf Texture and Surface Features

Leaves may be thin or thick. **Succulent** leaves are thick because they contain large amounts of water. A protective cuticle layer of **cutin**, which is a wax, covers the surface of many leaves to restrict water loss.

Hairs often cover leaves to help reduce water loss from evaporation, and to inhibit herbaceous nibblers from eating them. Hairs can be present on any part of a plant, including the leaves, stems, and rarely the flowers.

The following terms describe common textures and surface features of leaves, flowers, and stems:
Glabrous is a smooth texture lacking hairs.
Pubescent is a downy texture with fine, short, soft hairs.
Pilose surfaces have scattered hairs.
Hispid means having stiff, thick, coarse hairs.
Hirsute surfaces have rough, coarse hairs.
Tormentose is a smooth texture composed of woolly, long, soft, matted hairs.
Glacous surfaces have a thin, waxy, or whitish powdery coating.
Viscid means the surface of the plant is sticky.

Leaf Margins: Entire or Toothed

The margin or edge of a leaf can be straight and smooth or have various sizes and shapes of indentations called **teeth**. The leaf is **entire** when the margin is smooth, unbroken, and without indentations. The margin of a **toothed** leaf has a more-or-less regular pattern of shallow indentations. The indented margins may be sharp and pointed or wavy and scalloped. All the myriad types of leaf margins are variations of these two major characteristics.

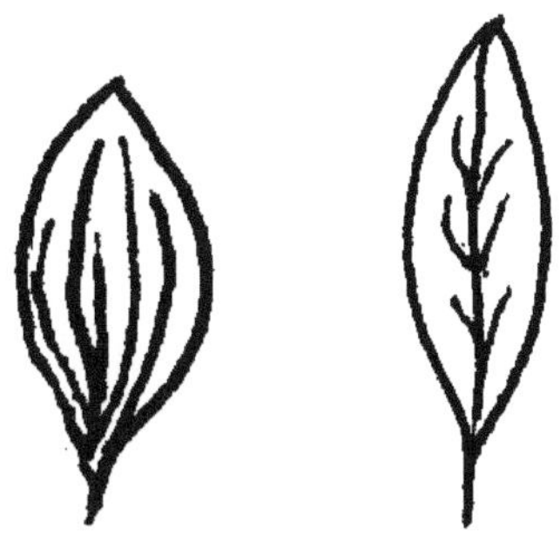

Leaves with entire margins

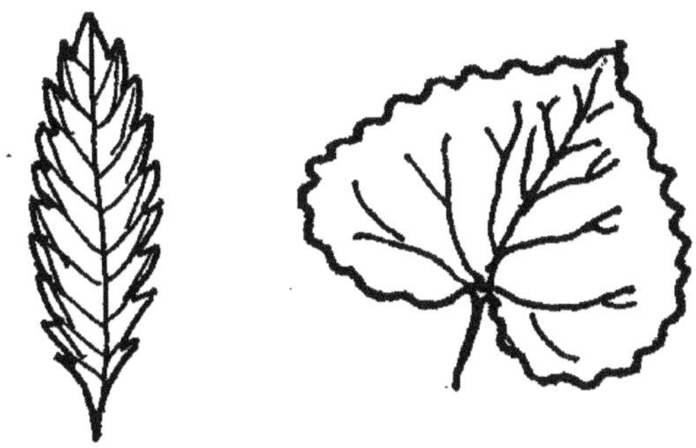

Leaves with toothed margins

There are many variations of teeth shapes and sizes along leaf margins.
Serrate leaves have margins with sharp teeth that all point upwards toward the apex or leaf tip. A leaf is **double serrated** when small teeth occur along the margins of larger serrated teeth.
Dentate leaves have sharp teeth that point outward, but they do not all point upwards towards the apex.
Crenate leaves have rounded teeth.
Sinuate leaves have alternating concavities and convexities creating pointed peaks and valleys along the margin.
Pectinate leaves have very close, narrow divisions like the teeth of a comb. Yarrow leaves are an example.
Undulate leaves have wavy margins. Yellow Dock and Burdock leaves are examples.
Ciliate margins are covered with fine, tiny hairs.

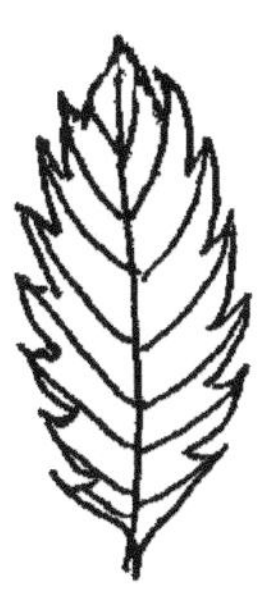

Serrate

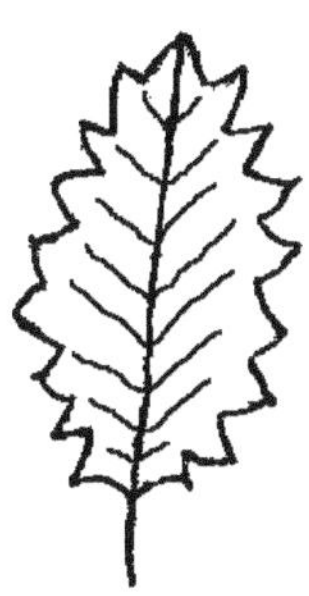

Dentate

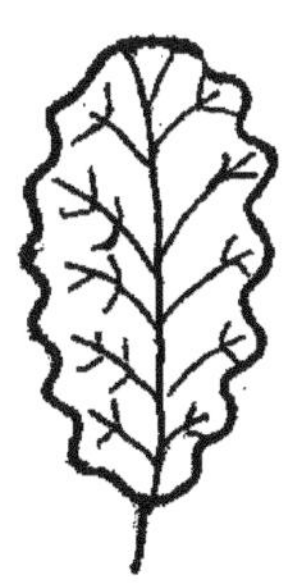

Crenate

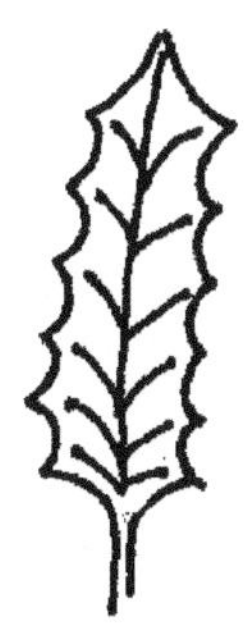

Sinuate

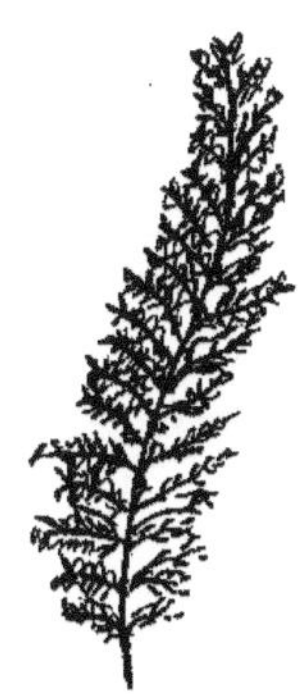

Pectinate

Shapes of the Whole Leaf

The following is a list of the different terms used to describe and identify the many shapes of leaves:

Cordate leaves are shaped like a heart.

Cuneate leaves are narrow and elongated with a rounded tip and a pointed base that attaches to the stem.

Deltoid leaves have a triangular shape with a broad base and pointed tip.

Obdeltoid is the reverse of deltoid. The leaf base is pointed and the tip is broad.

Elliptic leaves are shaped like an ellipse. They are widest in the middle and taper equally towards both ends, so the leaf tip and base are symmetrically shaped.

Hastate leaves are triangular. The wide base is perpendicular to the stem and tapers to form a narrow tip.

Lanceolate leaves are shaped like a long, narrow lance or spear. The margins are symmetrically curved and taper to a distinct point at the tip. The leaf base is somewhat rounded.

Oblanceolate is the reverse of lanceolate. The most distinct point is at the leaf base, not the tip.

Linear leaves are long and narrow with sides that are parallel.

Oblong leaves are elongated with a non-pointed, rounded tip and base. The shape is similar to elliptic, but margins are parallel rather than curved.

Orbiculate or **orbicular** is an orbital or circular-shaped leaf.

Ovate leaves are somewhat oval or egg-shaped with a pointed narrow tip.

Obovate is the reverse of the ovate shape. Obovate leaves are oval with a pointed narrow stem base and a more rounded tip.

Peltate leaves are shaped like a round shield, and stems are attached to the under-side rather than to the base or margin of the leaf.

Reniform leaves are shaped like a kidney.

Rhombic or **rhomboidal** leaves are somewhat diamond-shaped.

Sagittate leaves are similar to hastate, but the spreading lobes at the base point downward rather than perpendicular. Sagittate leaves are shaped like an arrowhead.

Spatulate leaves are shaped like a spatula. They have a wide, rounded leaf tip and a narrower but rounded base that attaches to the stem.

Fronds are fern leaves.

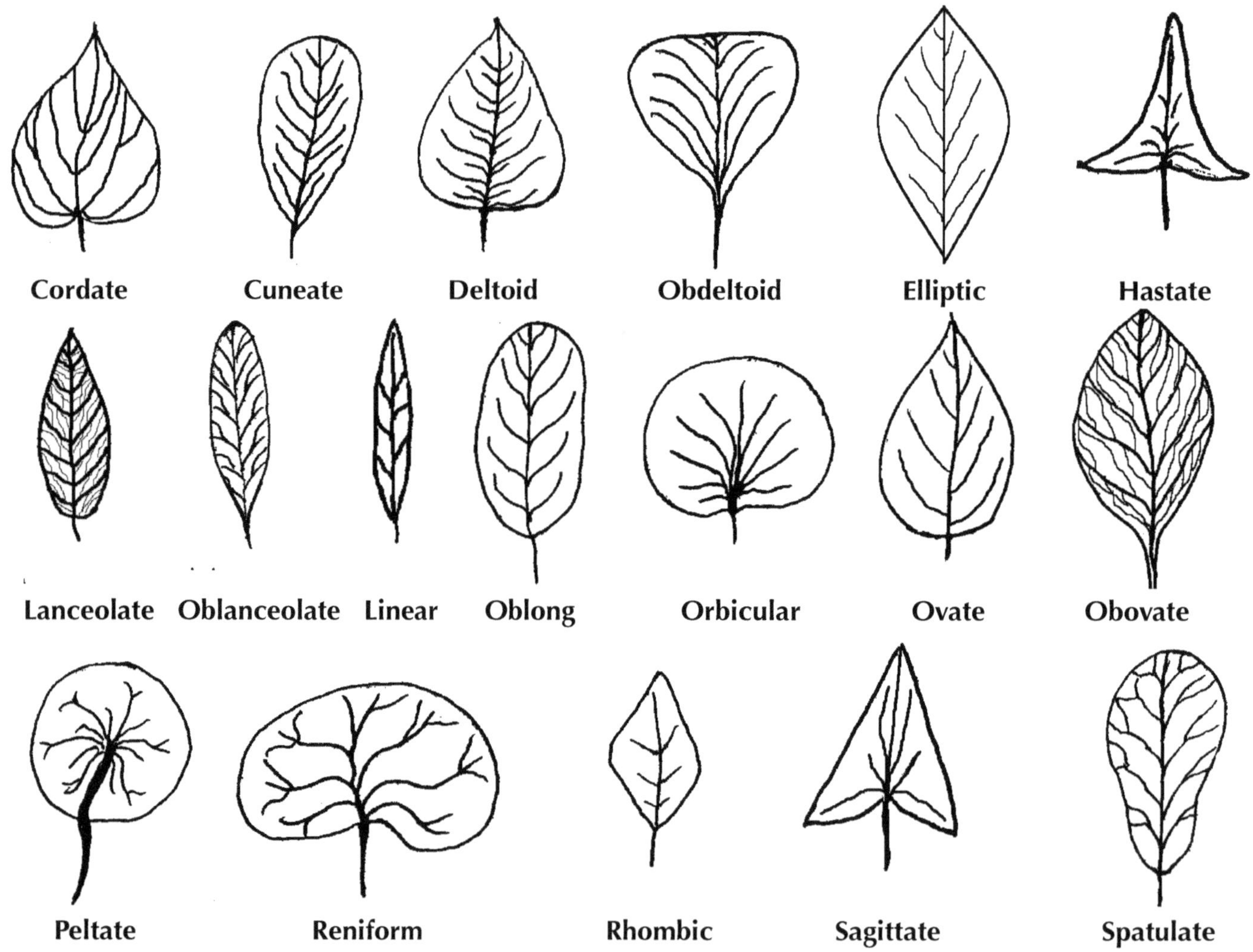

Shapes of Leaf Tips

The tips of leaves are called the **apex** and they appear in a wide variety of shapes that are characteristic of different plant species. The following are some of the most common shapes of leaf tips:

Acute leaves have an angled, pointed tip and the margins of the leaf are straight or convex.
Acuminate leaves have a more sharply defined tip point than acute leaves, but the leaf tapers gradually to a longer point at the tip. The sides or margins of acuminate leaf tips are concave.
Aristate leaf tips end in an elongated, sharp spike that is hard and bristle-shaped.
Caudate leaf tips are similar in appearance to acuminate leaves, but their sharp tip tapers into a long tail.
Cuspidate tips are similar in appearance to acuminate, but are narrower and gradually taper to a point.
Emarginate leaf tips are very broad and flat rather than pointed.
Mucronate tips have an abrupt, small, narrow projecting point that is a continuation of the midvein.
Obtuse leaves are rounded and blunt at the tips.
Obcordate leaves are notched at their tip like the shape of a heart.
Retuse tips look like an obtuse tip that is slightly notched or depressed at the apex.

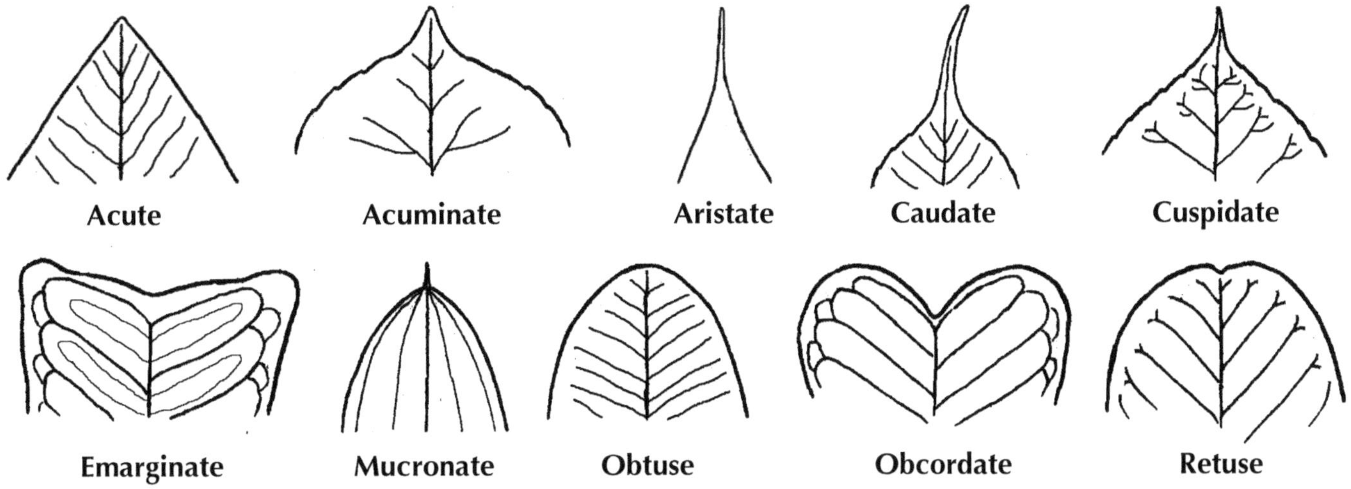

Shapes of Leaf Bases

Like leaf tips, the bases of leaves also appear in a variety of shapes.

Acute leaf bases taper to a sharp point, and the sides or the margins of the leaf are convex.
Auriculate or **clasping** bases have rounded projections that hug and surround much of the stem.
Cordate leaf bases are heart-shaped.
Cuneate bases taper to a sharp point and look similar to acute bases except the leaf margins are straight rather than convex.
Hastate bases have long lobes pointing outward on a horizontal plane.
Oblique bases are not symmetrical on both sides.
Obtuse bases are blunt and rounded.
Sagittate bases have long lobes jutting downward that give the entire leaf a distinct arrow shape.
Truncate leaf bases form a straight transverse line with a square appearance.

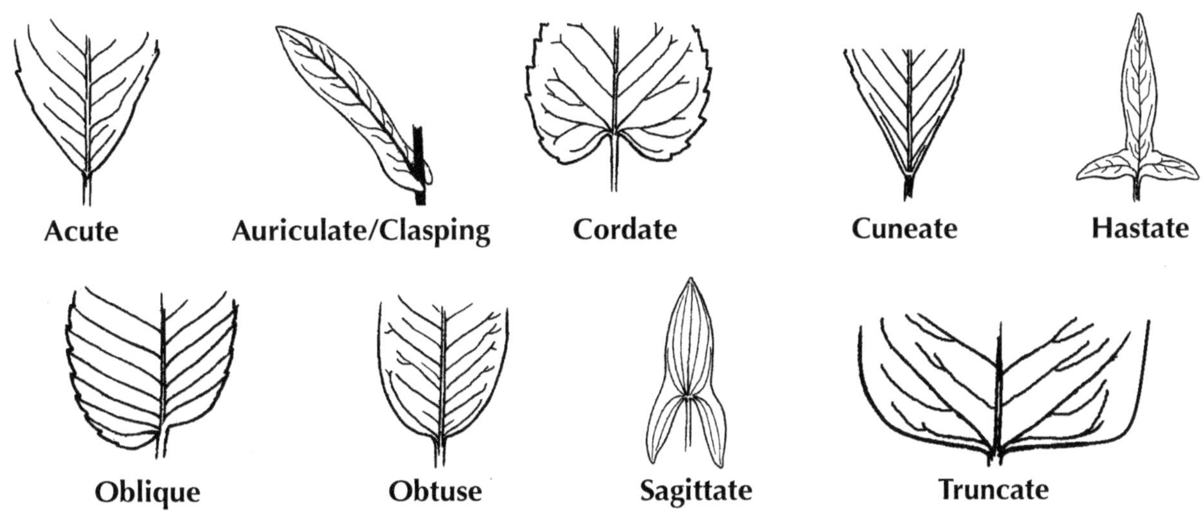

Position of Leaves on the Stem

Leaves are positioned in different places along stems, which is another distinguishing characteristic of plant species.

Basal leaves or **rosettes** grow directly from the base or root crown of a plant.

Stem leaves are also called **cauline, lateral,** or **axillary** leaves and grow above the plant base along the stem. Many plants have both basal and stem leaves.

Radical leaves are a type of basal leaf without stems that grow directly from a root or rhizome.

Terminal leaves grow at the very end of a stalk.

Bracts are modified leaves growing directly below individual or clustered flower heads. Bracts are usually small and look different from foliage leaves.

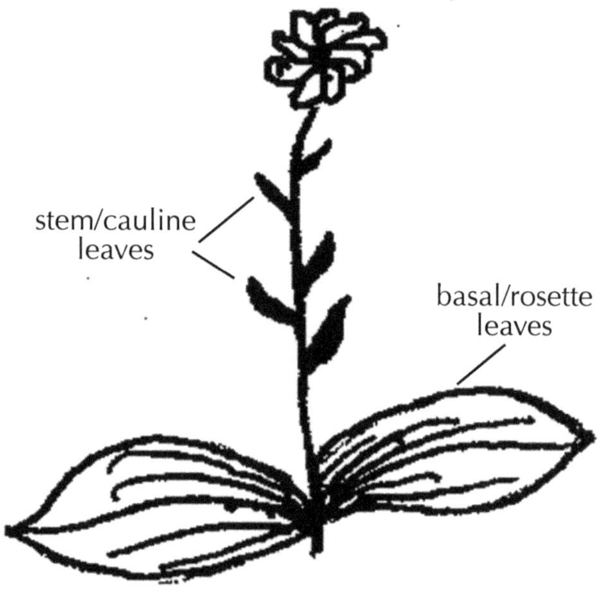

Basal and stem leaves

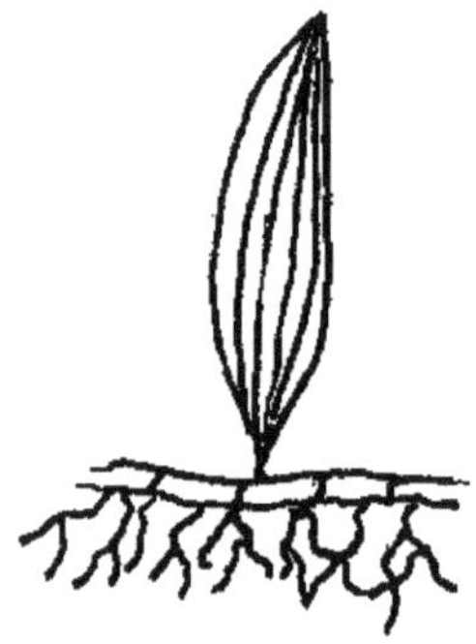

Radical leaf

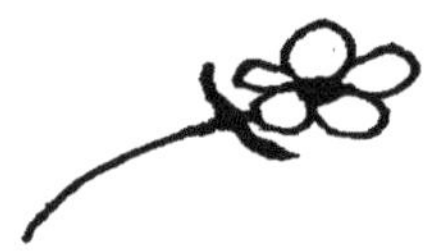

Bract leaf

Leaf Attachment to the Stem

The patterns in which leaves are arranged on a stem are other distinctions helpful for plant identification.

Opposite leaves grow directly across from each other in pairs and originate from the same stem node.

Alternate or **spiral** leaves grow on opposite sides of the stem but are arranged singly, one after another, with only one leaf emerging from each stem node.

Whorled leaf arrangements grow from one stem node and are clumped together in swirls of three or more.

Perfoliate leaves are perforated by the stem, which passes directly through the leaf.

Clasping or **auriculate** leaves wrap themselves around the stem. In most monocots and some dicots, the leaf base is expanded into a **sheath** that wraps around the stem.

Imbricate leaves overlap each other and have a pine cone appearance.

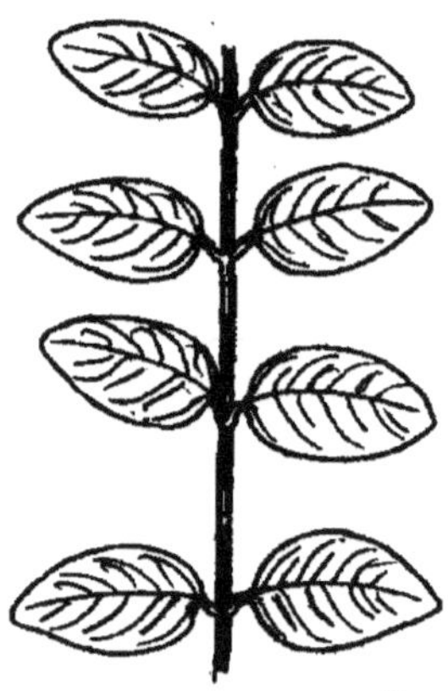

Opposite

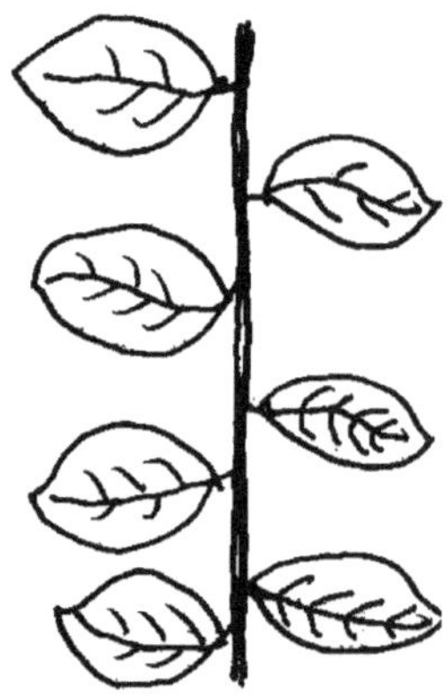

Alternate

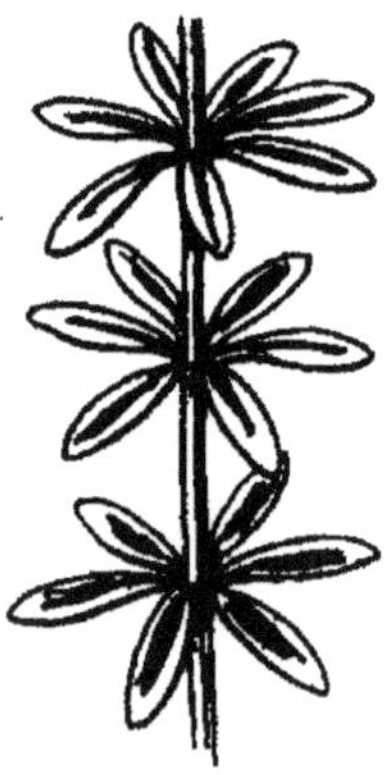

Whorled

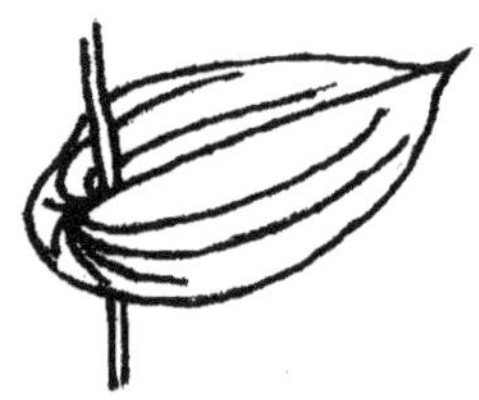

Perfoliate

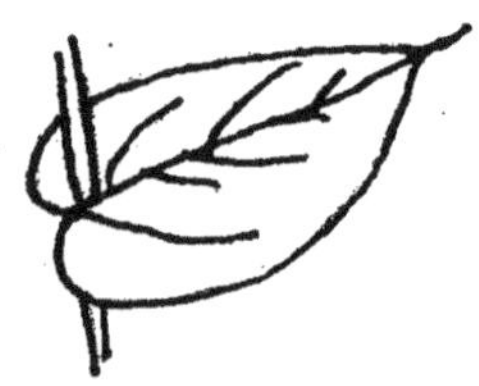

Clasping/Auriculate

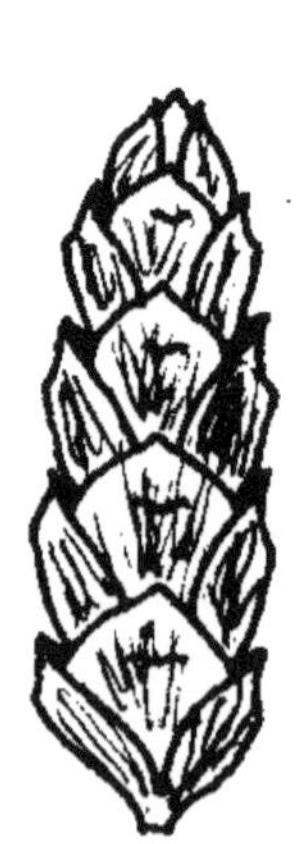

Imbricate

FLOWERS

Flowers are usually the most beautiful parts of plants and contain the reproductive organs vital for the continuity of the species. The vibrant colors, intriguing shapes, and fragrant aromas of many flowers attract insects and birds needed to assist in the process of pollination.

Flower Parts

The typical flower consists of the sepals, petals, stamen, pistil, receptacle, and stem. **Sepals** are modified leaves at the base of the flower. They are the outermost aspect of the flower and cling to the stalk. Having the appearance of miniature leaves or scales, sepals are typically green but can also be brown, colorful, or blend in with the color of the petals. Sometimes the sepals have a petal-like appearance and true petals are absent. The entire cluster of sepals surrounding the flower is collectively called the **calyx**. The main job of the calyx is to cover and protect the flower bud before it opens. As the flower blooms, the surrounding calyx opens up into individual sepals. Do not confuse sepals with bracts, which do not cover flower buds.

Petals are the showy, colorful parts of flowers that are the crowning glory of the plant. The main job of the petals is to attract pollinating insects and birds by their bright colors and alluring fragrance. The petals of some flowers have very tiny glands called **nectaries**, which produce sweet and fragrant nectar to attract pollinators. Nectaries may be simple sac-like structures on the surface of the petals or much more complex structures like spurs or spikes. The entire cluster of flower petals is collectively called the **corolla**. The corolla and calyx are collectively called the **perianth**. Sepals and petals that look alike and are difficult to differentiate are collectively called the **tepal**.

Stamens are the male organs of a flower. In perfect flowers, which contain both the male stamen and female pistil, all the stamens typically surround the pistil and appear in a ring or whorl in the center of the flower. A group of stamens is collectively called the **androecium**, which means "house of men." A stamen usually consists of a pronounced slender stalk or **filament** that ends in a two-lobed **anther**. The anther typically contains four **pollen sacs** for reproduction. **Pollen** consists of a multitude of tiny grains containing cells that hold the male genetics of the plant species. When the anther breaks open to release pollen, wind and animals assist pollination by carrying the tiny grains to the tip of a pistil, and fertilization or "plant sex" happens!

The **pistil** is the female seed-bearing organ. It typically emerges from the center of flowers and is surrounded by a ring of stamens. The parts of the pistil are collectively called the **gynoecium**, meaning "house of women." The pistil consists of one or more **carpels**, which bear and enclose one or more female eggs, called **ovules**. A carpel is made up of three segments consisting of the stigma, style, and ovary. The **stigma** is a sticky area on the tip of each carpel that captures pollen for fertilization. The stalk or neck portion is the **style**, an elongated column connecting the stigma to a bulbous lower portion called the **ovary**. The ovary contains tiny **ovules** or eggs that transform into viable seeds when fertilized with pollen from the male stamen. Following fertilization, the ovary matures into a dry or fleshy fruit containing new seeds.

The entire flower sits on top of a **receptacle** or **torus**, which is the enlarged end of a stem where the flower base joins the apex of the stem. There are two primary types of flower stems. A **peduncle** is the stem of an individual flower or a flower cluster that connects to the main stalk. A **pedicel** is the stem of an individual flower within a cluster.

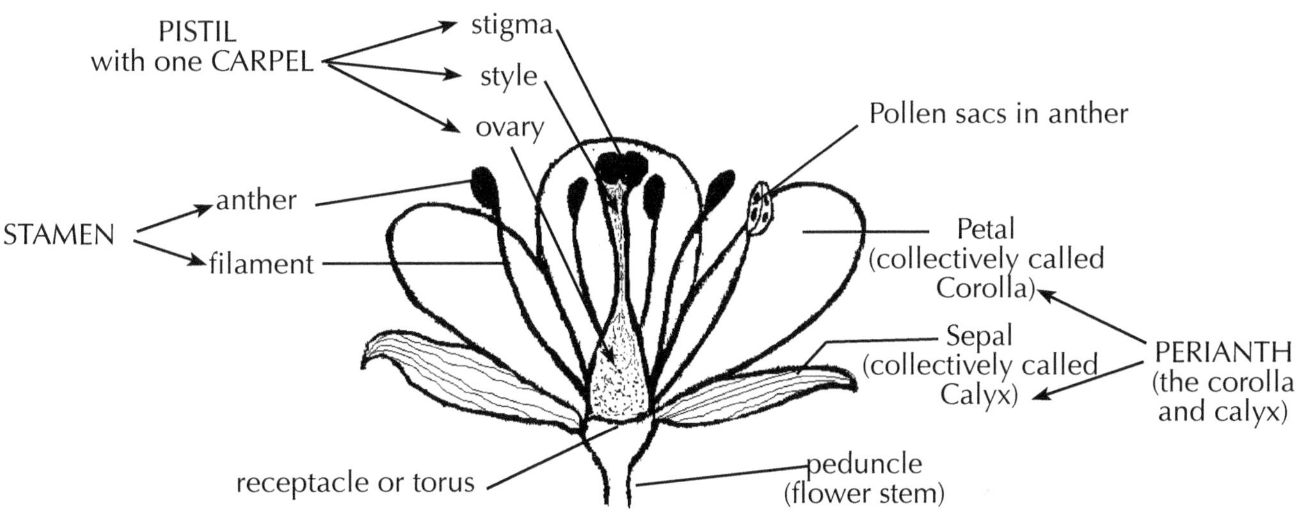

Typical Flower

Sexuality of Flowers: Complete and Incomplete Flowers

The majority of flowers are **bisexual** and capable of reproducing themselves. Bisexual flowers are called **perfect** or **complete**, and possess the four primary flower parts, including sepals (the calyx), petals (the corolla), male stamens, and at least one female pistil. Perfect flowers are capable of self-pollination (fertilizing themselves or other flowers on the same plant) and cross-pollination (fertilizing flowers on different plants).

Unisexual flowers have only one sexual organ, either the stamen or pistil, and are called **imperfect** or **incomplete**. Imperfect flowers are either **staminate** (male) if they only have stamens or **pistillate/carpellate** (female) if they only have pistils. There are two other commonly used terms when describing imperfect staminate and pistillate flowers. **Monoecious** (*mono* means "one" and *oikos* means "household") plants have both male and female flowers on the same plant. Corn is a good example, as the tassel is composed of male (staminate) flowers and the ears are composed of female (pistillate) flowers. In **dioecious** (*di* means "two") species, the male and female flowers are on separate plants, so all the flowers on each plant are either male or female. Dioecious plants include Hops, Ginkgo, Horsetail, and Hemp (*Cannabis sativa*). **Polygamous** plants have stamens and pistils that are separate in some flowers and united in others, either on the same plant or on two or three different plants.

Distinct and Coalescent Flowers

When parts of a flower are physically separate from each other they are called **distinct**. When they are connected or joined together they are called **coalescent**.

Position of the Flower Ovary

The level where the sepals, petals, and stamens join at the flower base can vary in relation to the position of the ovary. The sepals, petals, and stamens may be attached at the top of the ovary, at its base, or on an equal level. If these flower parts are attached to the receptacle below the ovary, the ovary is said to be **superior** and the flower is **hypogynous.** When flower parts are attached above the ovary, the ovary is labeled **inferior** and the flower is **epigynous**. A flower is **perigynous** when its sepals, petals, and stamens emerge at an equal level around the ovary. In perigynous flowers, the sepals, petals, and stamen can fuse together, forming a cup-shaped extension of the receptacle called the **hypanthium**.

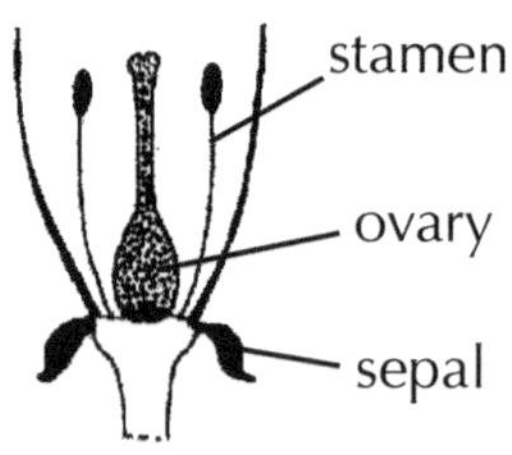

Hypogynous flower with superior ovary

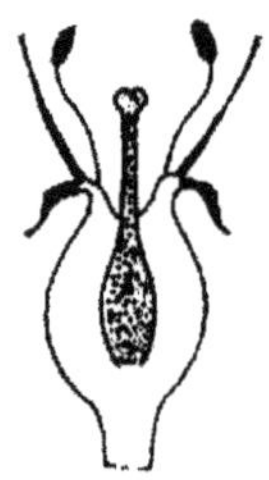

Epigynous flower with inferior ovary

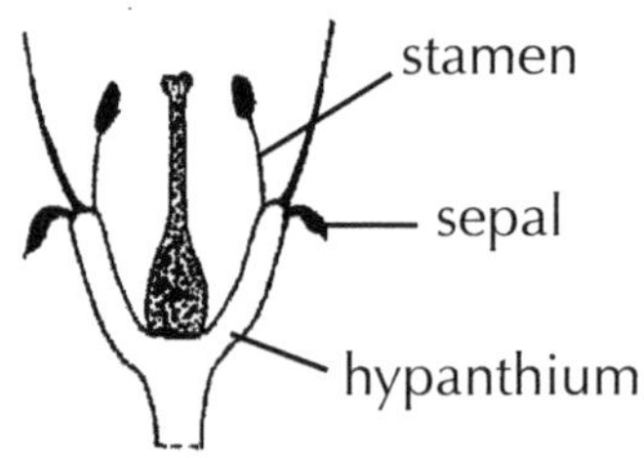

Perigynous flower

Types of Flowers

The general pattern and symmetry of a flower are evident when looking directly at its face.

Regular or **radially symmetrical** flowers have four or more petals radiating from a center like the spokes of a wheel. Each petal is similar in size, shape, and color to the others. If divided in half, the flower separates into two equally symmetrical parts. Regular flowers are also called **actinomorphic**.

Irregular or **bilaterally symmetrical** flowers lack a symmetrical pattern and often have a lip and lower and upper parts. The flower parts vary in size, shape, or color. Irregular flowers are also called **zygomorphic.**

Regular or radially symmetrical flower

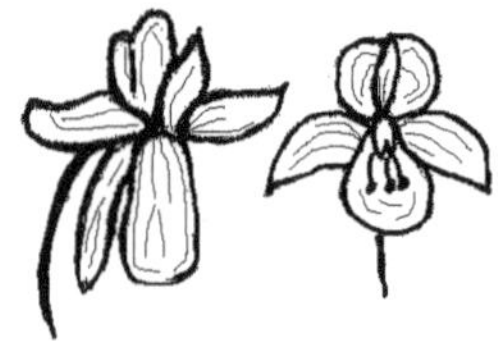

Irregular or bilaterally symmetrical flower

Different Types of Flower Arrangements

Flowers appear in a multitude of displays ranging from a single flower to massive clusters.
Terminal flowers grow at the ends of stems or shoots.
Axillary flowers emerge from leaf axils along the stems.
Solitary flowers occur singly rather than in groups or clusters.
Whorled flowers are clumped together in a symmetrical cluster around the stem and emerge from the same stem node.

An **inflorescence** is a cluster of flowers. There are many variations of inflorescent flowers, including those in the *Compositae* (Daisy) family called heads, determinate flowers, and indeterminate flowers.

A **head** is a disc-shaped inflorescence of small flowers lacking pedicels that are tightly crowded on the surface of a flattened or convex disc-shaped receptacle. Heads are the characteristic flower of the *Compositae* (Daisy) family in which the central **disc flowers** produce seed. The larger **ray flowers** are sterile and surround the center of disc flowers. The Sunflower is not one flower, but a flower-cluster bearing many tiny flowers. In some Composites, like Dandelions, the flower head is made up entirely of ray flowers. In others, like Blazing Star (*Liatris*) and Ageratum, the head is made exclusively of disc flowers.

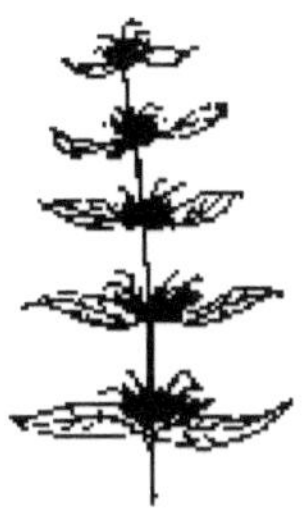

Whorled flower

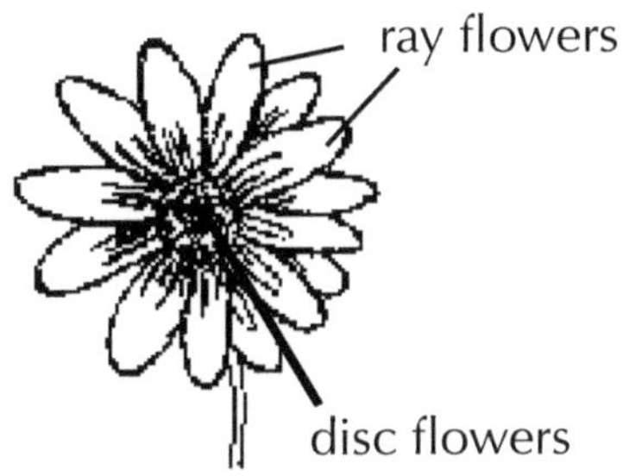

Composite flower head

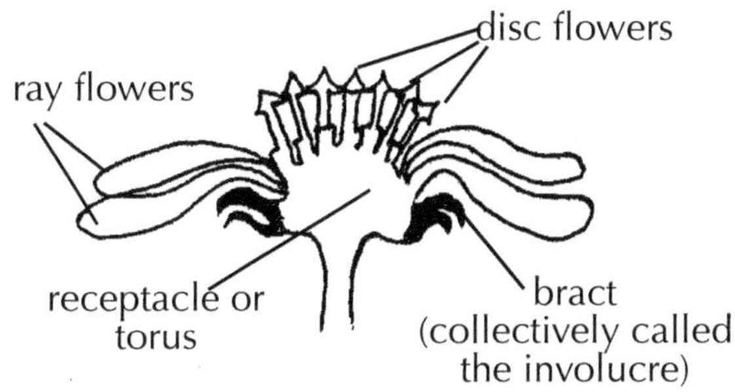

Composite flower head side view

Determinate inflorescence flower heads do not grow in length, so their growth is regarded as "pre-determined." When these flower heads appear in an elongated spike, the buds on top of the cluster flower first. When flower heads form more of an umbrella shape, flowers in the center bloom first. Determinate inflorescences include umbels and cymes.

Umbels are umbrella-shaped flower heads in which all the flower stems (pedicels) grow from one point on the top of the main stem. The pedicels are equal in length. Virtually all flowers of the *Umbelliferae* family display this form of inflorescence, hence the name of the family. **Compound umbels** have several umbel flower heads growing from the stem

Cyme flower heads are a broad class of inflorescences with many branching stems that all end in a flower. The main stem, or rachis, also ends in a flower with numerous flowering branches surrounding it.

Indeterminate inflorescences are flower clusters that continue to grow as they bloom. When this type of flower head grows in a spike, the lower buds bloom first. Upper flowers continue growing for an indefinite time and form new flowers in succession. Indeterminate inflorescence flowers include spikes, racemes, corymbs, and panicles.

A **spike** is a cluster of flowers arranged on a long stem called the **rachis**. The flowers are sessile (they lack stalks connecting them to the stem) and attach directly to the rachis. Spike flowers mature from the bottom of the rachis, where they begin blooming and gradually bloom further up the spike. Usually there is a leaf bract at the base of each flower. A **catkin** is a specialized type of spike in which the flowers are unisexual and have either a pistol or stamen, but not both. Catkins only occur on woody plants such as Black Locust, Willow, Oak, and Birch trees. This pendulous spike hangs down from branches and blows in the wind, allowing its pollen to be dispersed. The **spadix** and **spathe** flowers found in the *Araceae* (Jack-in-the-pulpit) family are modified spikes that have small flowers crowded on a fleshy tube.

A **raceme** is a long cluster of flowers growing on a stem (rachis) just like a spike, except the flowers have a pedicel stalk attaching them to the rachis. In a raceme, the rachis continues to grow in length with the oldest flowers at the base and the youngest at the tip of the stalk.

A **corymb** is a slightly rounded or flat top inflorescence. The outer and lower flower stems (pedicels) are longer than the upper ones, so all the flowers are on the same level plane in an umbrella shape. The outer flowers always bloom and bear fruit first, while the center flowers may only be in the budding stage.

A **panicle** is a compound or highly branched inflorescence describing a cluster of racemes, spikes, cymes, or corymbs.

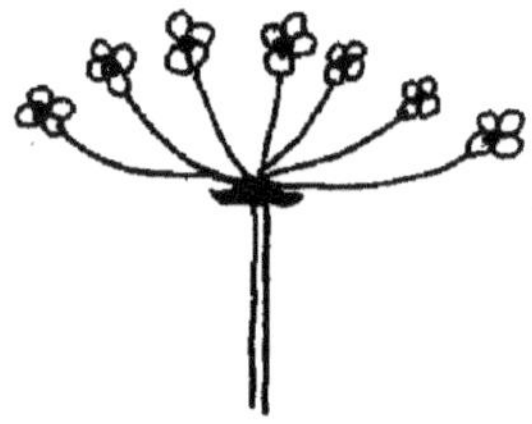

Umbel flower

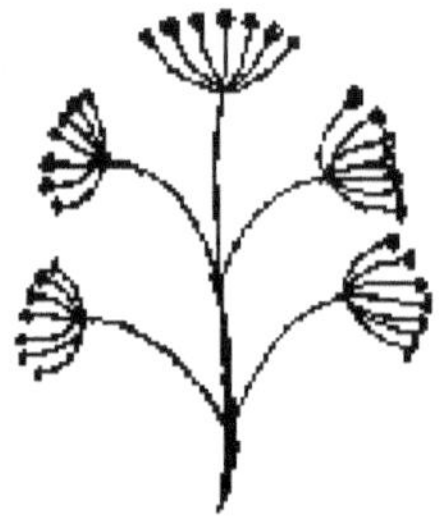

Compound Umbel

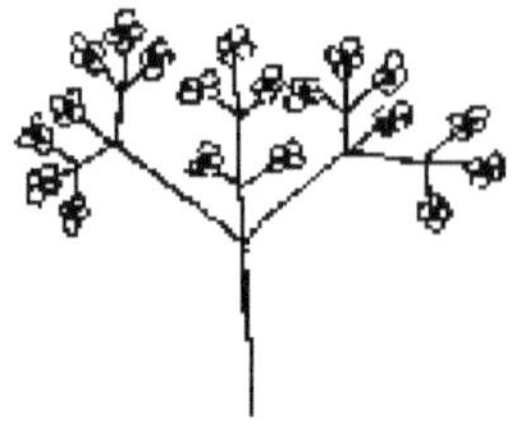

Cyme flower head

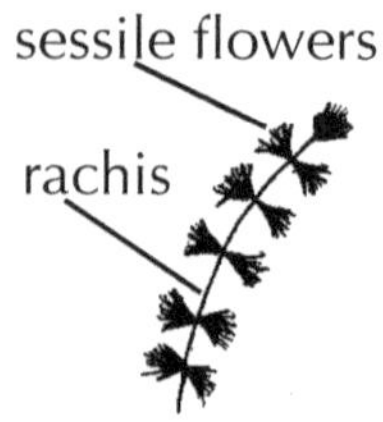

Spike flower

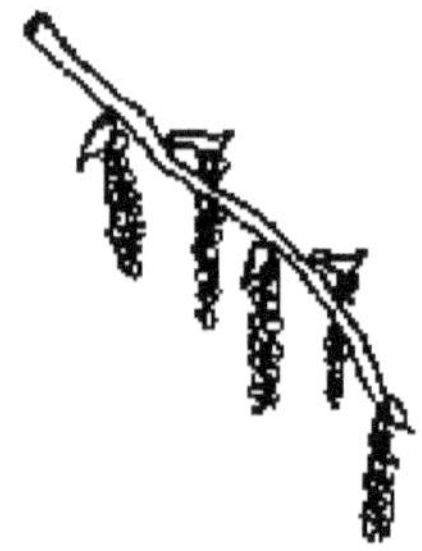

Catkin

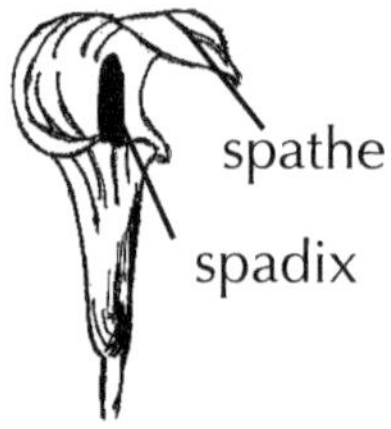

Spathe flower

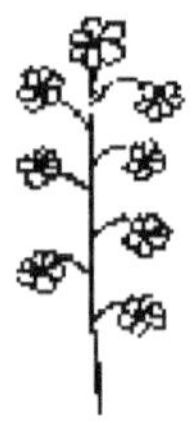

Raceme

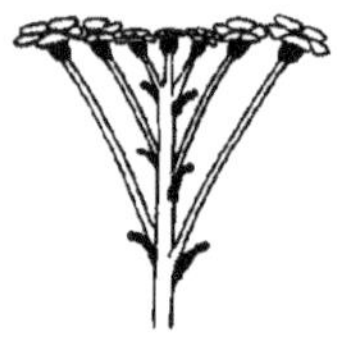

Corymb

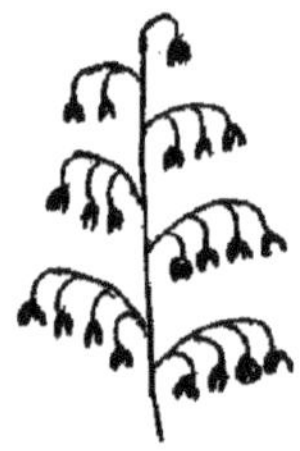

Panicle of racemes

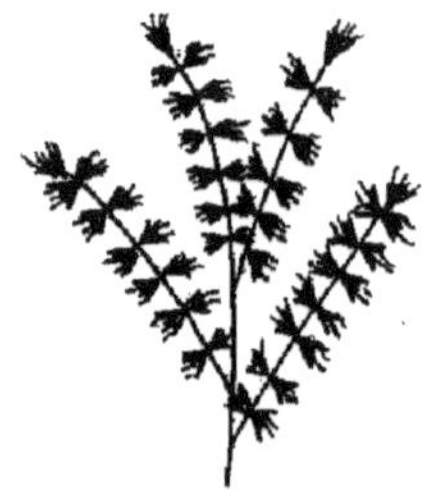

Panicle of spikes

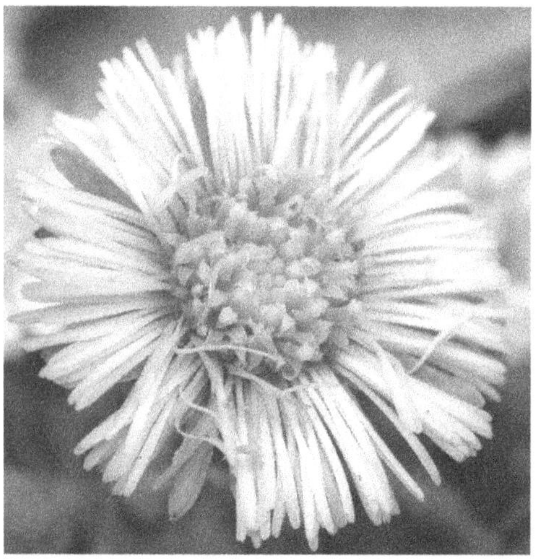

Composite flower head
Coltsfoot (*Tussilago farfara*)

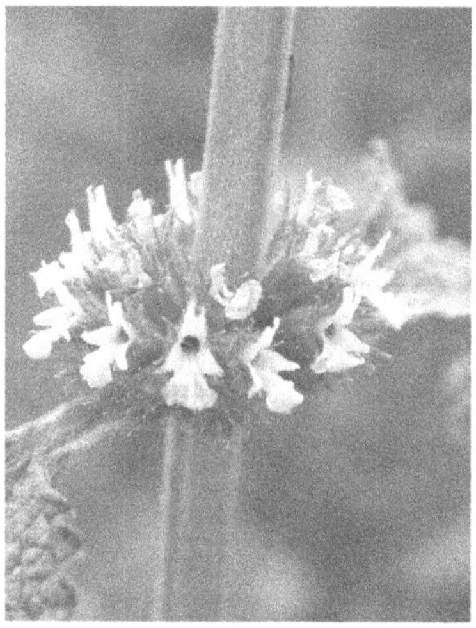

Whorled flower
Horehound (*Marrubium vulgaris*)

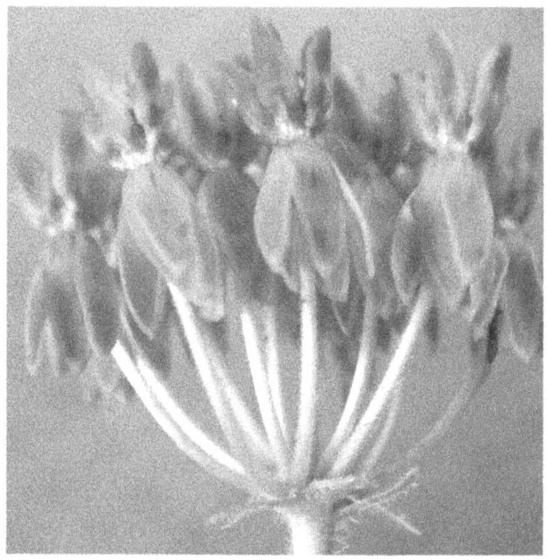

Umbel flower head
Pleurisy Root (*Asclepias tuberosa*)

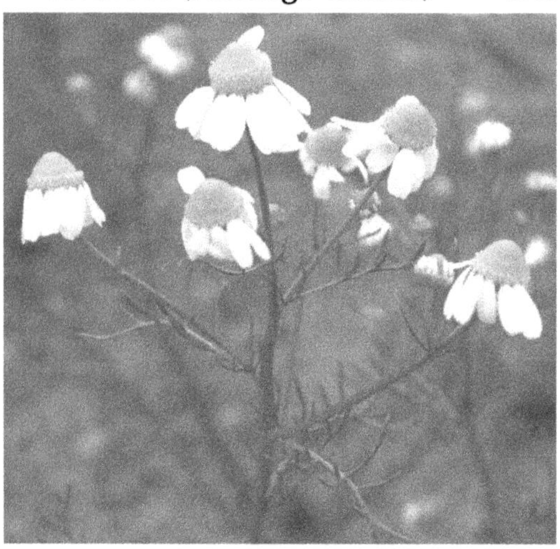

Cyme flower head
Chamomile (*Matricaria recutita*)

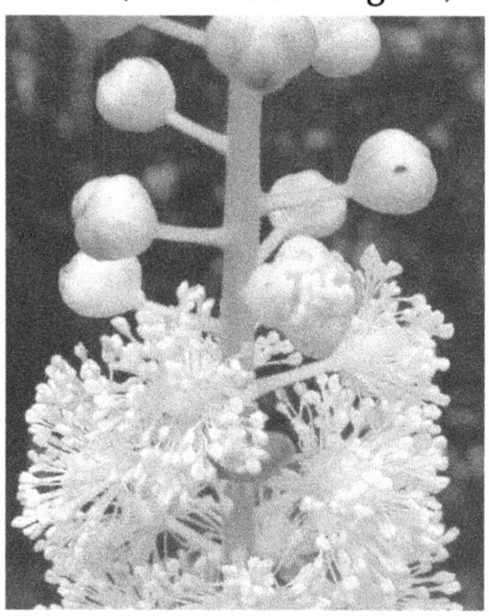

Raceme flower head
Black Cohosh (*Cimicifuga racemosa*)

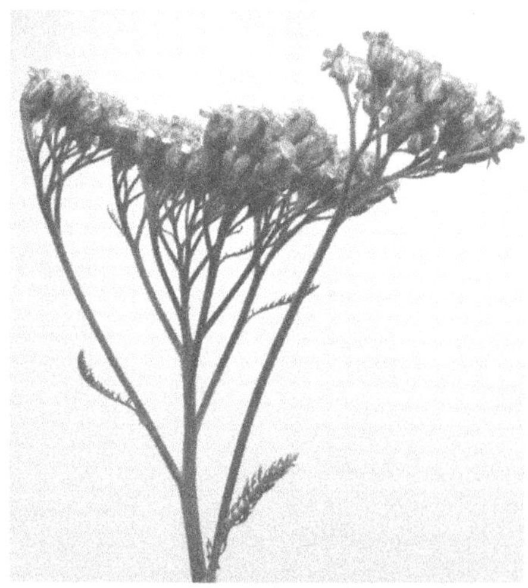

Corymb flower head
Yarrow (*Achillea millefolium*)

Pollination

A primary function of flowers is to produce seeds for reproduction, ensuring continuity of the species. In simple terms, pollination is plant sex leading to fertilization of the egg, and is necessary for the development of all plant seeds. Pollination involves the transfer of pollen from the anther on the male stamen to the stigma on the female pistil. After landing on the pistil, sperm cells from pollen grains begin their journey into the ovary and unite with female eggs to form zygotes, or rudimentary seeds.

There are essentially two kinds of pollination. **Self-pollination** occurs in perfect flowers containing both male and female parts, when the pollen of a flower fertilizes the same flower or another flower on the same plant. **Cross-pollination** occurs when the pollen from one flower fertilizes a flower on another plant. Cross-pollination can happen between separate plants of the same or different species.

Pollination occurs in a variety of ways depending on different plants and physical circumstances. The most common ways involve direct contact between stamen and stigma with the assistance of wind, insects, birds, and other animals. Flowers that rely on wind for pollination tend to lack fragrance and may be smaller in size with an inconspicuous appearance. But they can possess large anthers and feathery, extended, or well-developed stigmas. Plants depending on animals for pollination have evolved alluring features such as large, brightly colored and fragrant flowers, sweet and sticky nectar, and specific flower shapes for insects and birds to rub against. Flower pollens may be heavy, waxy, or sticky to optimize their adherence to the pollinator's body. In these ways, many plants and animals maintain a symbiotic relationship ensuring mutual survival.

Pollen is composed of tiny particles called **pollen grains** with each grain containing two specialized cells. The alluring surface of the female stigma is often moist and sticky, and is coated with sugars, proteins, and growth hormones. When pollen grains from a compatible species land on a stigma, these nutrients and growth hormones stimulate the pollen to germinate. One specialized cell of the pollen grain causes a bulge to develop in the outer wall of the grain, which becomes the **pollen tube** or **germ tube**. This is a tube that lengthens and penetrates down through the cells of the stigma and style into the ovary, where it locates and travels through a microscopic opening into one of the ovules. The pollen tube eventually reaches the egg cell inside the ovule. One flower ovary can be impregnated by several pollen tubes that grow into different ovules. While the pollen tube develops and grows towards the ovary, the other specialized cell in the pollen grain divides into two sperm cells that travel through the pollen tube. When the tip of the tube finally reaches the female egg cell, the tube opens to release the two sperm cells. One of the sperm cells fuses with the egg cell to create a single-celled zygote, which is the rudimentary seed. This fusion completes fertilization and the zygote starts to divide into many cells. The other sperm cell moves further into the embryo sac to create endosperm tissue, which is a vital layer of fats, starches, proteins, vitamins, and minerals needed to sustain life in the seeds during dormancy and germination.

After pollination and fertilization are complete, the flower petals and sepals have fulfilled their purpose and begin to wither. Germ tubes develop towards the ovary as flowers die off, and the ovary continually grows larger as the fertilized egg, or **zygote,** matures. The zygote goes through countless cell divisions until a mature seed is formed.

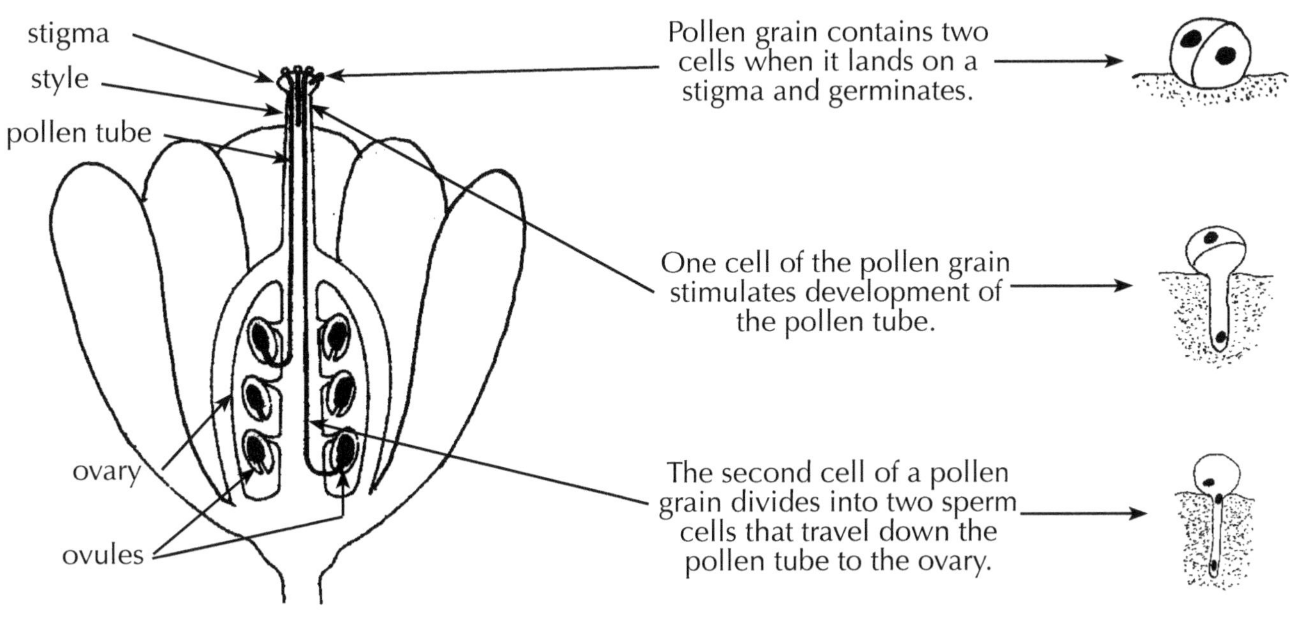

The Process of Pollination

Fruit and Seeds of Angiosperms ~ The Flowering Plants

Unlike human and many animal infants that remain with their parents as they mature, seeds are ejected from their parent plants and left to survive in a rather harsh world. Seeds may have to endure a variety of environments and weather conditions before germinating. Some travel many miles by wind or water before landing in soils that are suitable for germination to occur. Others are scorched by fires or endure drought and freezing. Some are eaten and pass through the digestive systems of animals before being deposited into soil. Many seeds lay on soil or are buried in the earth, but do not germinate for many years until favorable conditions arise. Nature has equipped seeds with a life support system that includes a hard, protective coating and a supply of stored food. Plants, like humans, carry the essence for the continuity of life within their genetic coding. Seeds contain genetic information from the parent plant that maintains each offspring's connection with the collective species. The embryo within each viable seed holds this genetic "template" or blueprint that determines the appearance, structure, and biological activity of the mature plant.

A **fruit** is the ripened ovary of a flower. People usually think of "fruit" as something edible like an apple or grape, but botanically speaking, it is actually a capsule that encloses one or more seeds. The fruit protects and incubates the inner seeds while they mature, and typically assists in the dissemination of the seeds at the appropriate time and season. The fruit may be a fleshy berry like a tomato, blueberry or mulberry, or a drupe like a cherry, apricot, olive, or walnut.

A **seed** is a ripened ovule that is an embryonic plant in a dormant stage. Far from being lifeless, seeds are actually living (viable) and maintain slow metabolic activity while dormant. Seeds contain an embryo, endosperm, and a protective coating. An **embryo** is the undeveloped plant formed from the union of a male and female cell during fertilization. The embryo consists of a rudimentary bud, stem, leaf, and root. The **endosperm** is plant tissue that stores nutrients necessary to keep seeds viable and contains proteins, fats, sugars, vitamins, and minerals. The fact that seeds are little powerhouses of stored nutrients is the reason why larger nuts and seeds are an excellent food source for animals and people, especially when eaten raw. The **seed coat** protects the embryo from damage, holds in necessary moisture and nutrients, and keeps seeds safely dormant until environmental conditions stimulate germination.

Germination

Germination occurs when seeds are in a suitable growing environment with favorable weather conditions. Adequate light, warmth, nutrients, air, and moisture are the necessary requirements. Enough water must be absorbed into seeds to make them swell and soften their protective coat, which eventually ruptures. Water also activates enzymes that stimulate the embryo to digest stored nutrients for further growth and development. When the seed coat ruptures, rudimentary root shoots become hydrated and emerge to provide initial anchorage. **Cotyledons** are the first green leaf-like structures to sprout from newly germinated seeds. Often the cotyledon has a completely different shape than leaves that the plant develops later. At the stage when seeds germinate and root and leaf shoots emerge, the transformed seed is called a **seedling**. During this initial growth phase, seedlings are nourished by nutrients stored in the seed endosperm and cotyledons.

The Two Classes of Angiosperm Seedlings: Monocots and Dicots

Seeds of the flowering Angiosperms contain either one or two cotyledons. **Dicot** plants have two cotyledons (*di* means "two") and **monocots** only have one (mono) cotyledon. Although the seeds of flowering plants vary in size, shape, texture and hardness, most of them follow the two basic structural designs of monocot or dicot.

Differences Between Monocots and Dicots

Characteristics	Monocots	Dicots
Cotyledon (first leaf)	Consists of one leaf	Consists of two leaves
Leaf venation	Usually parallel	Usually palmate or pinnate
Flower parts	Typically in threes	Typically in fours or fives
Root system	Fibrous roots	Taproot or fibrous roots
Secondary growth with vascular cambium	Absent	Often present

Dicot plants usually have palmate or pinnate venation, while monocots typically have parallel veins. There are very few exceptions to this rule, so it is a good way to distinguish between the two groups. Some dicots appear to have parallel venation because they are narrow and thick, which obscures their netted venation.

Flowers of monocot plants typically produce three petals or multiples of three, while the majority of dicot flowers have parts in fours or fives. Most monocots and some dicots have leaves that wrap around the stem at the leaf base (called sheathing or clasping bases). Both monocot and dicot plants contain many vascular tubes (the xylem and phloem) that transport fluids and nutrients throughout plants. These vascular tubes are scattered in the stems of monocots, but in dicot stems they are arranged in a ring. Monocots are herbaceous because they have green, fleshy, non-woody stems. They lack the vascular tubes that produce secondary growth leading to the formation of wood and bark. Many dicots do have stems containing the vascular cambium, which are the actively dividing cells that produce wood, so they can be woody or herbaceous.

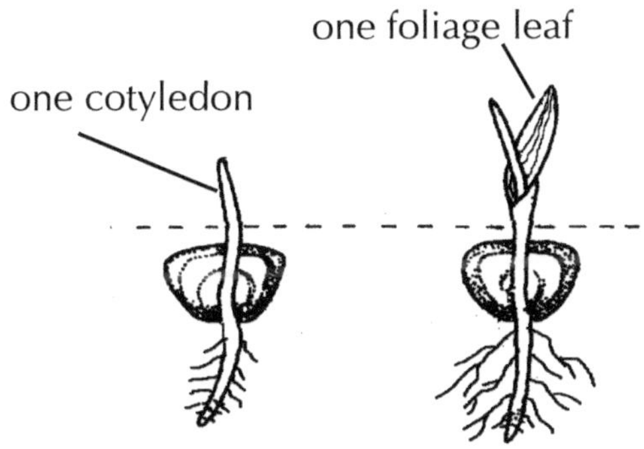

Monocot Seedling

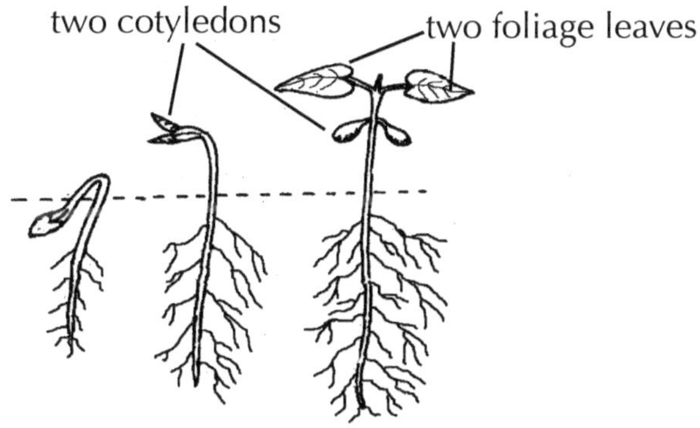

Dicot Seedling

Ways Plants Disperse Their Seeds

Mother Nature has provided many methods for plants to scatter their seeds in order to optimize their chances of germinating and preserving the species. Some seeds simply drop off the parent plant and land close by, while others are travelers that have been provided with specialized wings, feathery parachutes, or burrs that help them travel a distance away from the parent plant before making contact with soil.

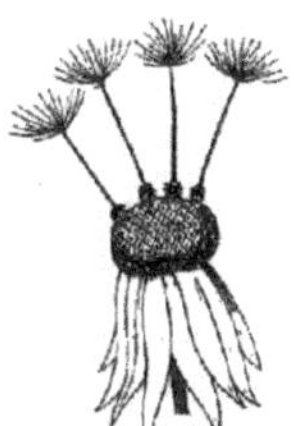

Dandelion seeds

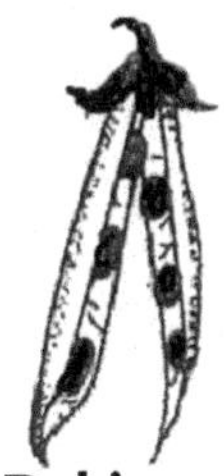

Dehiscent

❖ The process some plants use to scatter their seeds is called "dehiscence." **Dehiscent** fruits dry out and split open when they ripen in order to free their inner seeds. Beans, Peas, Bloodroot, Astragalus, Pleurisy Root, Senna, and Jewelweed all have dehiscent fruits. **Indehiscent** fruits do not split open.

❖ Some seeds cling to the parent plant until they are pulled out or dislodged. Others simply fall to the ground when ripe.

❖ Many plants like Dandelion, Elecampane, Boneset, and Pleurisy Root have feathery, hair-like fibers attached to their seeds that act like parachutes to help the seeds ride the wind and scatter a distance away from the parent plant.

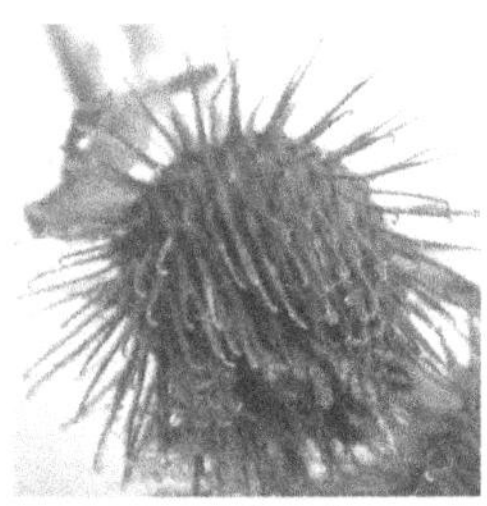

Burdock seed

❖ Seed pods on plants like Burdock, Cleavers, and Wild Carrot are covered with hairs, Velcro-like burrs, spikes, or barbs that cling and attach to clothes or fur of creatures that brush past the plant and serve as carriers.

❖ Plants like Goldenseal, Ginseng, Elderberry, and Raspberries display brightly colored, pleasant-tasting berries that attract birds and other animals to eat them. As berries pass through an animal's digestive system, the seeds are freed from the fleshy fruit, the protective seed coat is broken down by digestive enzymes, and then the animal excretes the prepared seed in a little pile of fertilizer a distance away from the parent plant.

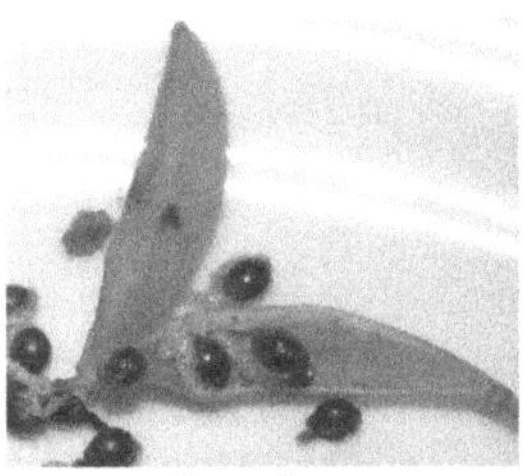

Bloodroot seeds with aril

❖ Some seeds like coconuts are dispersed by water.

❖ **Myrmecochory** refers to dispersal of seeds by ants. Violets, Bloodroot, Celandine, and other spring wildflowers have a small amount of sweet carbohydrates attached to their seeds on an appendage called the aril. Ants carry the appetizing sweet seeds back to their nest as a food source and disperse the seeds in the process.

Types of Fruit

There are several types of fruit. Some develop only from the ovary, and others are formed from the ovary and additional flower parts. **Perocarpium** fruits are formed from an ovary. **Anthocarp** fruits develop from the ovary and have floral parts that grow after fertilization to help disseminate the seeds.

Achene or **nutlet** is a simple, dry, indehiscent, one-seeded fruit in which the seed is attached to the fruit wall. It develops from one ovary. Sunflower seeds, Dandelion seeds, and Strawberries are examples.

Berry or **bacca** is a simple, fleshy fruit that is indehiscent (it does not dry and break open). It develops from

a compound ovary and contains many seeds. Examples are Grape, Goldenseal, and Ginseng.
Capsule is a dehiscent fruit formed from more than one ovary, and usually contains many seeds. Bloodroot, Astragalus, Senna, and Poppies are examples.
Caryopsis or **grain** is a fruit that only contains one seed and is indehiscent. Examples are Corn, Grass seeds, Oats, Rice, Wheat, Barley and other grains.
Cypsela is a fruit having wings, bristles, or plumes attached at its tip that carry the small seeds in the wind. Examples are Dandelion, Elecampane, and Boneset.
Drupes develop from one ovary. This is a fleshy, indehiscent fruit with one or more internal stones or pits that usually contain one seed, and occasionally two or three seeds. The stone protects the seed when traveling through animals' digestive systems. Drupes include the Peach, Mango, Plum, Apricot, Cherry, Olive, Almond, and Walnut.
Follicle is a dry dehiscent fruit that develops from one ovary and opens through only one slit to allow seed dispersal. Members of the Milkweed family, including Pleurisy Root, have follicle fruits.
Glans is a fruit having an enlarged receptacle, pedicel, or peduncle. Acorns are a type of glans.
Legumes or **pods** are dry dehiscent fruits formed from a single ovary that usually open along two longitudinal seams. Legume fruits are characteristic of the Pea and Bean families.
Pome is a fruit that is enlarged and fleshy with a central seed-bearing core like an Apple, Persimmon, and Paw Paw.
Samara is a simple, dry dehiscent fruit with one or two seeds and wings that disperse seeds by wind. The wings are outgrowths of the ovary wall and each winged portion is called a fruitlet. Maple and Elm trees have samara fruits.
Schizocarp is a dry fruit with two carpels that split along the midline into two one-seeded indehiscent halves when mature. They are characteristic of the *Apiaceae (Umbelliferae)* or Carrot family.

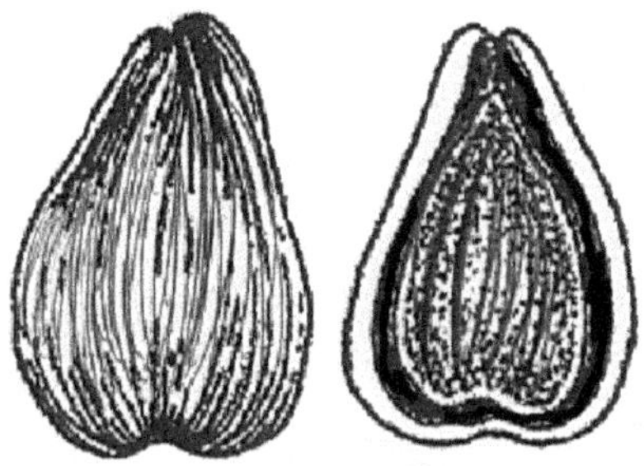

Achene or Nutlet

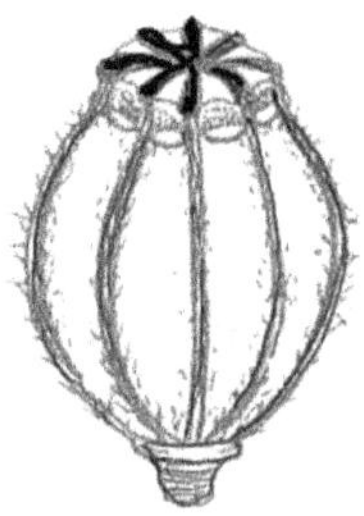

Capsule

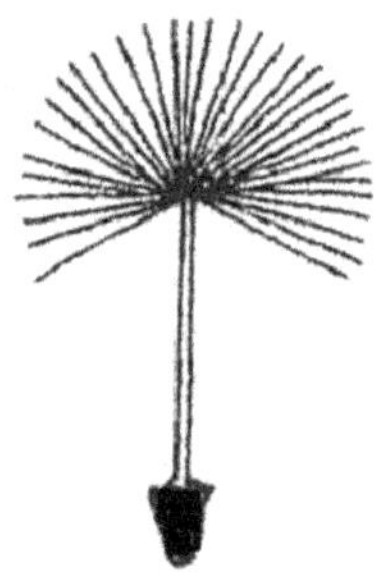

Cypsela

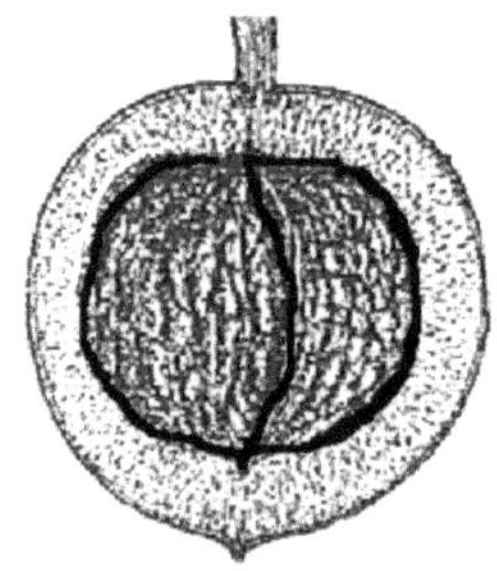

Drupe

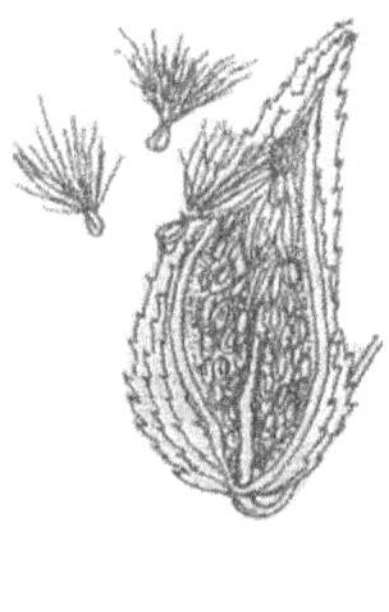

Follicle

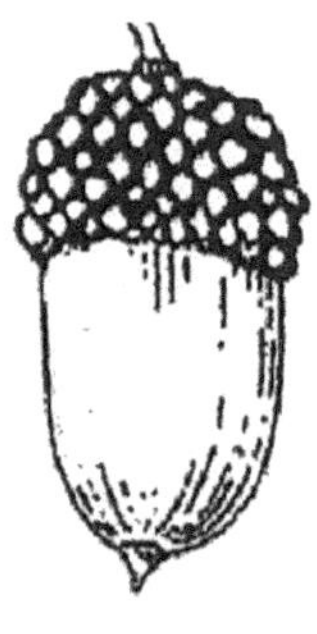

Glans

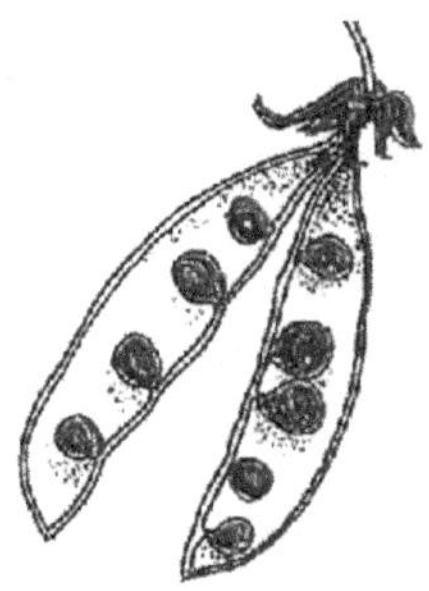

Legume or Pod

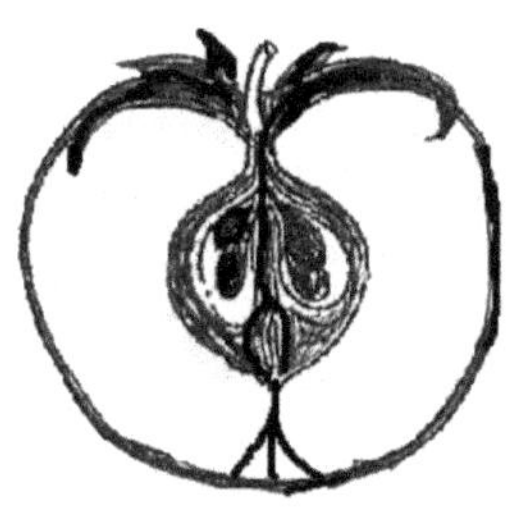

Pome

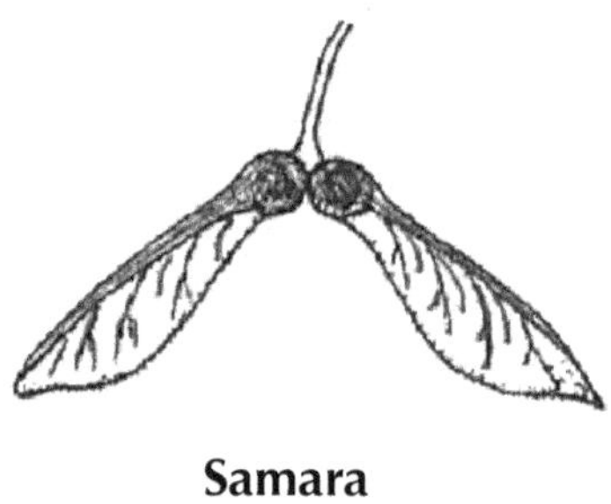

Samara

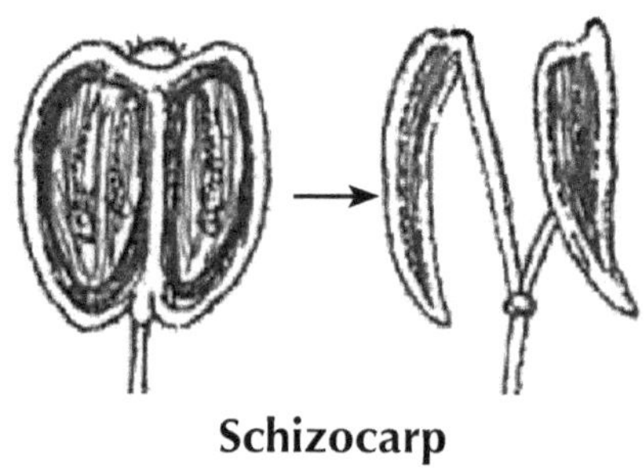

Schizocarp

Endangered Medicinal Herbs ~ Botanical Sanctuaries to the Rescue

While the herbal renaissance is flourishing around the world, many plant populations that once grew abundantly in their native habitats are disappearing. The revival of interest in medicinal herbs is increasing demand on the world market and threatening plant populations required to sustain the herbal industry. Motivated by rising market prices, increased numbers of wildcrafters who gather non-cultivated plants from the wild have over-harvested many native plant stands at a rate that exceeds their ability to reproduce. Consequently, increasing numbers of our most valuable medicinal plants have disappeared or are becoming rare to the point of extinction. In November 2004, the World Conservation Union convened its Third World Conservation Congress in Bangkok, Thailand, attended by 10,000 experts from 181 countries. The Congress reported that over 15,589 plant and animal species are facing extinction, and these species are recorded in the Union's 2004 Red List of Threatened Species. The leading cause of plant extinction is habitat destruction due to human over-population resulting in road intrusion and industrial, commercial, agricultural, and housing development. Additional causes include exploitation for plant medicine, the lumber industry, environmental pollution, plant disease, climate changes, and introduction of invasive species that overrun indigenous plants (American Herb Association Quarterly Newsletter, 2005).

It is important to remember that plants have a unique and valuable role in the grand scheme of life, and saving them just so we can use them for our own benefit is missing the point. Not only do plants provide food, medicine and shelter, they are the lungs of the world, exhaling oxygen into the atmosphere. Plants are irreplaceable in the web of life, and the earth is diminished by their disappearance. Plants are here not only to serve our needs, they also sustain and regulate the balance of life and health of the planet.

> *The logic and greed propelling the global momentum of plant and forest destruction is alarming and even suicidal.*

The prevailing global attitude is focused primarily on grasping and taking as much of the earth's natural resources as possible to benefit ourselves, without acknowledging the age-old law of reciprocity and balance. Indigenous people all over the world understood this natural law and were able to live in relative harmony with their environment without destroying it. They understood how to plant seeds and propagate roots, and to take only as much as they needed when harvesting so that next time someone needed the plant medicine or food, it would be there. By continually taking from the earth without re-establishing plant and forest populations, we are destroying a crucial resource necessary for our survival. This lack of consciousness and imbalance between the earth and ourselves also creates imbalance in our own bodies. After all, health is a state of dynamic balance. Since we are completely dependent on the plants and animals for our life, the logic propelling the global momentum of plant and forest destruction is alarming, even suicidal!

In 1973, the United States Congress passed the Endangered Species Act, directing the Secretary of the Interior to protect plants and animals threatened by extinction based on scientific evidence. The U.S. Fish and Wildlife Service is responsible for recommending a species to be listed as "endangered" if it is in danger of extinction throughout all or most of its range. Plants are classified as "threatened" if the species is likely to become endangered in the near future. Once a species has been designated as endangered or threatened, the Endangered Species Act prohibits people from collecting or destroying plants on federal land. The act also mandates that plans be made to aid the species' recovery. An initial list of endangered plants was established in 1977 and new plant species are usually added to the list each year.

Several international groups are responding to the global threat and loss of valuable medicinal plants. The Convention on International Trade in Endangered Species of Wild Flora and Fauna (CITES), an international treaty involving over 100 nations, regulates international commerce of endangered plants and animals through a system of permits and certificates. Implemented in 1975, CITES protects plant species from the trade market by listing them in Appendix I, which prohibits trade, or in Appendix II and III, which protect and regulate plants in foreign trade.

The Medicinal Plant Specialist Group of the International Union for the Conservation of Nature (IUCN) consists of scientists and specialists in the global herb trade. Its mission is to monitor endangered plant species, publish a directory and bibliography for medicinal plant conservation organizations and publications, and establish programs to reduce pressure on threatened species. The IUCN has created the Red List, the world's most comprehensive inventory of the global conservation status of plant and animal species. The IUCN has a strong scientific foundation, and the Red List is recognized as the most authoritative guide to the status of biological diversity. The purpose of the Red List is to convey the urgency and rate of extinction of plant and animal species to the public and policy makers, and to encourage the global community to protect all species with special focus on endangered populations.

The IUCN and several other organizations worked on a 20-year survey showing that habitat destruction and introduction of non-native species have caused approximately 34,000 species worldwide to become extremely rare, at the brink of extinction. It is estimated that the survival of one out of every eight plant species on the planet is currently threatened. In 1998, the IUCN speculated that 29 percent of the 16,000 plant species growing in the United States have become so rare that they could easily disappear.

TRAFFIC North America is the wildlife trade monitoring program of the World Wildlife Fund-US that is based in Washington, D.C. TRAFFIC monitors the effects of commercial trade on plants with the intention of halting their unsustainable harvest and exploitation, and has issued reports on threatened medicinal species. The Nature Conservancy in the United States does an admirable job of obtaining parcels of land to become wildlife preserves, and working with TRAFFIC to monitor and analyze domestic and foreign trade impacts on North American medicinal plants.

Botanical Sanctuaries for the Preservation of Medicinal Herbs and the United Plant Savers (UpS) Organization

A **botanical sanctuary** is land designated as a place of safety and refuge where medicinal plants are grown and protected, while ensuring their abundant, renewable supply for future generations. The establishment of botanical sanctuaries by individual landowners is an exciting and successful response to the dilemma of endangered plant species. Sanctuaries restore and preserve habitat for all wildlife, both plants and animals.

Solutions to dwindling herb stands and excessive wildcrafting involve the promotion and organization of herbal cultivation. Extensive research is currently being conducted to understand and develop the most efficient methods of cultivating rare and endangered plant species. **United Plant Savers (UpS)** is an exceptional group of dedicated people working for the continued survival of our native medicinal plants. This grassroots nonprofit organization is a coalition of herbalists, botanists, herbal manufacturers, researchers, and other organizations, including the American Botanical Council and Herb Research Foundation.

> *Designating your property as a botanical sanctuary is an empowering, individual response to the threat of endangered plant species.*

Founded in the early 1990s, UpS is dedicated to the preservation, organic cultivation, and survival of medicinal plants and the land they grow on, with special concern for endangered species. To protect native plant populations from extinction, UpS encourages cooperation from all segments of the herbal industry, including growers, wildcrafters, manufacturers, health practitioners, and consumers. UpS is not calling for a moratorium on herbal use or wildcrafting, but instead encourages people to cultivate rather than wildcraft endangered herbs. The organization initiates educational and cultivation programs designed to raise public awareness and preserve medicinal herbs.

With appropriate research and techniques, the quality of organically cultivated herbs can meet and even exceed the quality of wild herbs. UpS offers involvement at a very personal level by encouraging and assisting property owners to designate their land as a privately-owned botanical sanctuary where native medicinal plants can grow and prosper. Botanical sanctuaries serve as educational and research centers, propagation facilities, and models for sustainable land use. Anyone with even a small amount of property is encouraged to become part of this sanctuary network steadily creeping across the country, creating corridors of protected land where medicinal plants can grow undisturbed.

UpS has developed a 650-acre model botanical sanctuary in Meigs County in southeastern Ohio, which serves as an educational facility and testing ground for researching propagation, cultivation, and re-introduction of native species back into the wild. UpS holds yearly conferences and gatherings, offers membership, provides seeds and live medicinal plants to establish in gardens, issues a newsletter, and provides support to anyone wishing to develop a sanctuary or help the cause in other ways. It is a wonderful organization and network to help people become involved in planting and sustaining medicinal herbs.

Several UpS members are developing a general census of herb populations throughout the country, and have compiled a list of plants that are at risk of extinction and a list of plants to closely watch. As you read these lists, remember that some of these plants may be abundant in some areas and rare in others.

UpS "At Risk" Plant List

American Ginseng (*Panax quinquefolius*)
Black Cohosh (*Cimicifuga racemosa*)
Bloodroot (*Sanguinaria canadensis*)
Blue Cohosh (*Caulophyllum thalictroides*)
Echinacea (*Echinacea* spp.)
Eyebright (*Euphrasia* spp.)
False Unicorn Root, Helonias Root (*Chamaelirium luteum*)
Goldenseal (*Hydrastis canadensis*)
Lady's Slipper Orchid (*Cypripedium* spp.)
Lomatium (*Lomatium dissectum*)
Osha (*Ligusticum porteri*, spp.)
Peyote (*Lophophora williamsii*)
Slippery Elm (*Ulmus rubra*)
Sundew (*Drosera* spp.)
Trillium, Beth Root (*Trillium* spp.)
True Unicorn (*Aletris farinosa*)
Venus Fly Trap (*Dionaea muscipula*)
Virginia Snakeroot (*Aristolochia serpentaria*)
Wild Yam (*Dioscorea villosa*, spp.)

UpS "To Watch" Plant List

Arnica (*Arnica* spp.)
Butterfly Weed, Pleurisy Root (*Asclepias tuberosa*)
Cascara Sagrada (*Rhamnus purshiana*)
Chaparro (*Castela emoryi*)
Elephant Tree (*Bursera microphylla*)
Gentian (*Gentiana* spp.)
Goldthread (*Coptis* spp.)
Kava (*Piper methysticum*)
Lobelia (*Lobelia* spp.)
Maidenhair Fern (*Adiantum pedatum*)
Mayapple (*Podophyllum peltatum*)
Oregon Grape (*Mahonia* spp.)
Partridgeberry (*Mitchella repens*)
Pink Root (*Spigelia marilandica*)
Pipsissewa (*Chimaphila umbellata*)
Spikenard (*Aralia racemosa, A. californica*)
Stillingia (*Stillingia sylvatica*)
Stone Root (*Collinsonia canadensis*)
Stream Orchid (*Epipactis gigantea*)
Turkey Corn (*Dicentra canadensis*)
White Sage (*Salvia apiana*)
Wild Indigo (*Baptisia tinctoria*)
Yerba Mansa (*Anemopsis californica*)
Yerba Santa (*Eriodictyon californicum*)

What You Can Do to Help Endangered Herb Populations

As individual citizens, we can make many effective choices to reduce the destruction of plant populations and contribute to their continued survival. Here are several suggestions:

❖ Designate your property as a botanical sanctuary whether you own a city lot, an acre, or 100 acres. A sanctuary is a sacred space of refuge and protection, a reserve for people, animals, and plants. Here we can feel peaceful and experience the abundance and renewal of nature. Be a good caretaker of the land you live on by treating it as a sanctuary, and understand that we are part of a long line of stewards who come and go as time passes. Help restore the biodiversity of your area by re-introducing native plants that used to grow there. Often the consciousness and activities of one person rouses the interest of neighbors, inspiring others to follow a splendid example. Contact the United Plant Savers organization (www.UnitedPlantSavers.org) to connect with like-minded people, receive helpful support and information, attend educational gatherings, and participate in plant giveaways to help establish your own sanctuary.

❖ Educate yourself with classes, books, and magazines. Many herbalists and sanctuary stewards offer hands-on classes on herbal cultivation, making herbal preparations, and learning the medicinal properties of the plants. A wealth of herbal literature and internet information is available to everyone. An excellent magazine is *HerbalGram,* published by the American Botanical Council (ABC), an important and successful organization dedicated to "provide education using science-based and traditional information to promote responsible use of herbal medicine." *HerbalGram* is a highly respected journal because it is global in its perspective and focuses on all aspects of medicinal herbalism ranging from current research to historical traditions. By becoming a member of ABC, you will receive issues of *HerbalGram,* have access to a wealth of information on the ABC website, and stay up-to-date with the latest information on herbs around the world and in your backyard.

❖ Treat yourself to the joys and empowerment of gardening! Plant seeds and roots to create your own medicinal herb gardens. If you have access to woodlands, prepare beds for planting forest herbs such as Goldenseal, American Ginseng, Blue Cohosh, Black Cohosh, and Wild Yam. Gardening allows you to harvest your own plants for medicine rather than depending on the market. And by gathering seeds from your own gardens, more plants can be propagated without extra expense.

❖ Share and exchange the seeds and plants you cultivate with friends and other growers to perpetuate the herb species and expand your own gardens.

❖ People who wildcraft herbs are asked to consider the ecological impact of collecting "at risk" and endangered plants from the wild, and are encouraged to practice sustainable wildcrafting. This involves waiting until seeds mature before harvesting the plant and replanting seeds back into their natural environment. When roots such as Goldenseal, Bloodroot, and Black Cohosh are collected, they can be divided to provide some for harvest and the remainder for replanting to maintain the plant population. Never "clear-cut" a stand of herbs! Sustainable wildcrafting involves harvesting only a small percentage of a patch, allowing plants to reproduce and continue to survive. Plant stands of rare and endangered species should not be harvested at all, but left to mature and expand.

❖ Herbalists, clinical practitioners, and authors of herb books and journals are encouraged to avoid promoting or recommending endangered herbs unless they have been cultivated rather than wildcrafted.

❖ Be a conscious and responsible consumer when purchasing herbs. If a choice is available between wildcrafted or cultivated herbs, purchase the cultivated herb if it is a rare or endangered plant. More growers are producing certified organic herbs. Support these growers and ask your local health food stores to supply cultivated "at risk" and endangered herbs rather than wildcrafted.

❖ Use herbs that are not endangered to replace those that are threatened. For example, *Echinacea angustifolia* grows very slowly and is becoming scarce due to excessive wildcrafting, but *Echinacea purpurea* can be used instead because it exerts similar healing action, grows much faster, and is easier to cultivate. Oregon Grape Root contains berberine, the same medicinal chemical constituent found in Goldenseal, and can be substituted for this endangered herb. Marshmallow root can be substituted for Slippery Elm, which is endangered due to the epidemic Dutch Elm disease. Marshmallow is easy to cultivate and contains similar medicinal mucilage as Slippery Elm.

❖ Make use of all the herbs that grow in abundance and can be harvested without threatening their survival such as Chickweed, Dandelion, Burdock, Stinging Nettle, Red Clover, Mullein, Mints, and Yellow Dock.

❖ Get political in your community and state! Write letters and meet with your state legislators to support clean environment and protect forests and wilderness areas. Join an organization that works to preserve our native herbal resources. Help to eliminate forest clear-cutting and other practices destructive to plant and animal habitats. When areas are destined to be developed or clear-cut despite all efforts to the contrary, plants can be rescued by transplanting them to safe ground. Many property owners will allow people to do this, and it can be a productive way to ease tension between environmentalists and developers.

❖ Educate people and talk about wildcrafting, over-harvesting, and solutions for protecting our herbal medicines. If you are an herbal educator, it is imperative to address these issues and advocate herbal propagation and conservation. United Plant Savers provides an educational package and slide show presentation of "at risk" plants.

❖ If you want to be able to purchase organic herbs and foods free of dangerous pesticides and herbicides, *please* do not use these toxins yourself. Toxic chemicals spread on lawns and gardens contaminate water levels in the earth and kill not only insects and weeds but also earthworms, toads, frogs, birds, pollinators, and other creatures that are vital to the cycle of life on our planet. Rather than spraying Dandelions in your yard, take advantage of Nature's free bounty and eat the nutritious flowers and leaves in salads or stir-fries and make tea with the roots to support your liver and kidneys! As an organic herb and vegetable gardener for over 45 years, I can honestly say that organic gardening and lawn care are effective and not difficult. We all must assess how important it is to keep our environment clean for ourselves and future generations, and what we are willing to do in our personal lives to facilitate this. Is a weed-free lawn and garden laden with toxic chemicals worth the resulting contamination and hazardous health risks, which include cancer?

❖ Live a healthy lifestyle and eat a nourishing diet as a basic foundation for good health. Please do not live on soda, hot dogs, sugar and "junk food," and use herbs with the expectation that they will counteract such abuse and keep you healthy. It is ethically irresponsible to contaminate our bodies with devitalized food and then waste precious herbs attempting to regain balance. Please be respectful of the herbs, and if you choose to use them for your healing, do your part by eating wisely and living a health-promoting lifestyle.

On a Personal Note . . .

In my private practice as a registered nurse and clinical herbalist, I have chosen not to recommend herbs that fall into the "at risk" category unless they can be obtained from cultivated and renewable sources rather than wildcrafted. Throughout this book, I discourage the use of non-renewable rare and endangered herbs for medicinal uses, and I encourage other herbalists to do the same. It is important to note the valuable historic applications of these herbs, but to deter their continued use unless they are cultivated.

For many years, I have designated my five-acre property in Nashville, Indiana, as Green Turtle Botanical Sanctuary under the wings of United Plant Savers (UpS). If you own even a small amount of land, I encourage you to establish your property as a botanical sanctuary and become a sanctuary member. Joining UpS connects us with a large network of dedicated people striving to ensure the protection of our precious plants. Creating a sanctuary is a wonderful way to promote stewardship of the earth on a personal level, making a tangible difference to the survival of the medicinal herbs.

It is satisfying to cultivate plants and to enjoy their beauty and healing gifts. Interacting with Nature in this way helps us understand and be at peace with our place in the world, and to experience our deep connection with all of life. Nature instills calm hearts and wise minds. In a world engulfed in so much insanity and destruction, the gift of working with the plants offers a wealth of beauty, abundance, and purpose. Designating properties as botanical sanctuaries helps us remember that we are, after all, stewards of the land for a short time. May we all be inspired to care for the earth as she cares for us!

Cultivating Medicinal Herbs

Gardening offers a unique opportunity to participate in the miraculous process of life from growth through decay and eventual renewal and regeneration. Herbal **cultivation** is the process of planting seeds, roots, or whole plants in prepared soil and coaxing them into vigorous growth by watering, mulching, weeding, and tending with the intention of producing potent, healing medicine.

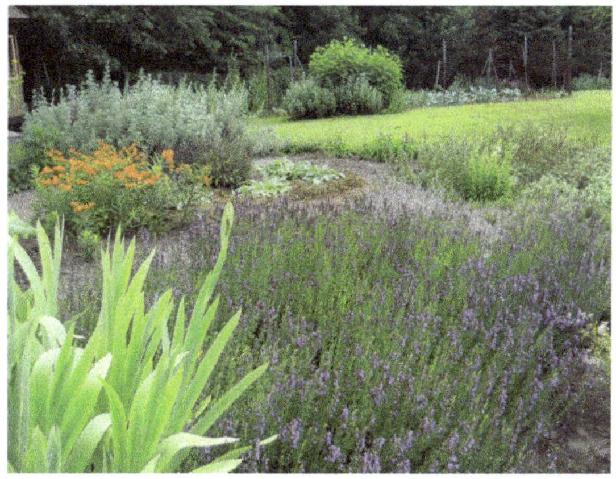

The garden is an exciting place to play, experiment, marvel, and co-create with Nature, the great Mother of all life. Gardening in partnership with Nature helps us develop a personal and experiential relationship with the plants. Growing herbal medicines and interacting with the elements in the garden expands our perspective of life, inviting us to be more conscious of our impact on our environment, to live in greater harmony with our surroundings, and to move and flow with the cycles of the seasons. Cultivating plants in our gardens helps us cultivate beauty, balance, joy, and abundance in our personal life, connecting us with the earth and plants in a profound and fulfilling way!

Medicinal herbs naturally grow in the wilds, tended by Nature, the master gardener. When we bring plants into our gardens and exert our influence on them, we can help them achieve optimal growth, vitality, and potency. When the gardener is attuned to the needs of plants and works with Nature and the cycles of life, a special alchemy occurs between people and plants. In my long-time experience of cultivating plants and using them for herbal medicines, I have found that when they are grown with the loving intentions and caring attention of people, plants have an increased potential for healing that can be quite exceptional.

The Importance and Necessity of Growing Your Own Medicinal Herbs

Until fairly recently, a large portion of the global supply of medicinal herbs has been obtained from **wildcrafting**, which is the practice of harvesting naturally occurring, non-cultivated herbs growing in the wilds. As human populations grow and housing, business and agriculture expand, many plant species that were once abundant are becoming increasingly scarce or extinct. The increased popularity of medicinal herbs and a rapidly expanding market has created the need to cultivate many herbs to keep up with consumer demand. The continued survival of many endangered species now primarily depends on their cultivation.

Adding to the necessity of cultivating our own herbs are the legalities determining how herbs are manufactured, marketed, and distributed to consumers. Laws in the United States are determined and regulated by the government and the Food and Drug Administration (FDA). They determine which herbs are allowed on the market. Creating an herb garden provides personal access to the plant medicines of your choice. No matter what happens with legal regulations or the economy, gardening is a wonderful survival skill providing a fundamental and satisfying sense of security and empowerment.

Nature is the most majestic cathedral. The sacred space of a garden offers refuge from the chaos and stress of life, where inner peace and our connection with the earth and her plants are restored.

There are other advantages to cultivating herbs. As a gardener, your choices and personal attention to plants assures the creation of good quality medicine. Careful selection of seeds and live plants guarantees the correct species required for medicinal purposes. You can grow herbs organically in fertile soil under the best possible conditions. And you can harvest and process the herbs using optimal methods to enhance freshness and potency.

Compared to many vegetables, herbs have less stringent growing requirements and tend to be much easier to cultivate. Herbs have a stronger genetic resistance to animal and insect predators due to their strong and sometimes bitter flavors, pungent odors, and hairy stems and leaves. They are also less prone to plant diseases. Herbs do not require as fertile a soil as vegetables, and they tend to be hardier in harsh environmental conditions such as drought or freezing. For people lacking access to outdoor gardens, some medicinal herbs can be grown on porches, patios, or indoors in large pots and containers. Many medicinal herbs are beautiful to have growing around your home. They attract birds and butterflies and can be brought indoors for flower arrangements. The joy of stepping into your garden to harvest herbs for culinary or medicinal purposes is delightfully satisfying!

The experience of gardening also offers possibilities for profound personal transformation on many different levels. Being healthy implies a dynamic state of harmony and equilibrium within our bodies and our environment. Maintaining this balance ultimately lies at the heart of all healing. Many people tend to focus only on acquiring as much as possible from the earth, harvesting excessive amounts of herbs and disregarding the need for their continual survival. People often ignore the perspective of balance and reciprocity, taking resources from the earth without restoring or giving anything back. Planting seeds and cultivating herbs is a wonderful opportunity to help restore this balance, guiding us in cultivating balance within our own lives and bodies. Gardening, at its deepest level, is a healing act of reverence, cooperation, and gratitude to Mother Earth and to the creative and sustaining source of all life.

Alienating ourselves from nature severs us from our source of physical existence and our inner being.

The act of gardening can heal this separation and is a gentle and delightful pathway back home.

Interacting with the elements of earth, water, sun, and air draws us into greater connection with Nature. Working in the soil reminds us of our roots and complete dependency on the earth, minerals, and plants for our survival. The garden, like life itself, is a continual process of birth, life, decay, renewal, and evolutionary change. Working intimately with plants moves us to acknowledge the power and forces of Nature, and to participate in the continual dance and rhythmic cycles of the gardens, seasons, and life. Growing plants and working with Nature brings greater meaning and purpose to our lives, helping us feel a part of the whole rather than isolated individuals. Honoring and co-creating with Nature produces good herbal medicines and happy gardeners!

The practical experience of growing your own medicinal herbs is the best way to become familiar with their appearance, texture, odor, taste, life cycles, and individual qualities. This depth of familiarity allows a more intimate relationship and guides us to greater understanding of the healing qualities and opportunities each herb offers. Joyfully working and caring for your plants, fulfilling their needs, and enjoying their beauty and healing gifts are all ingredients in creating abundant and vibrant gardens, potent medicines, and a more peaceful, contented life.

In many ways, being in an herb garden can be as healing as ingesting medicinal herbs. Standing quietly in the garden, it is restoring and nurturing to feel the powerful presence of the plants, to experience their unconditionally beneficent healing essence. It is delightful to be in their presence, to enjoy their profound grace and beauty. As you weed around your green friends, you may experience the "weeding out" of your own worries, resentments, and other disturbing thoughts and emotions arising from deep within. Our own inner "weeds" can be naturally released while digging around in the dirt. Being in the presence of the plants helps us feel more centered and calm. Their kind and nurturing essence can feel like Mother Nature's kind hands soothing the soul. The beautiful colors, shapes, and patterns of flowering plants, and the birds and butterflies they attract, help ease our weary minds. The garden is a safe and peaceful sanctuary to retreat from the chaos and stress of the world, to be quiet, sing, pray and meditate, to listen, and to be with our plant friends.

The garden is a portal into the creative forces and mystery of life.

Grow Organically

Please grow herbs and foods organically for your own sake and in consideration of the fragile nature and preciousness of all life. Save yourself, your family, animals, and our environment from the frightfully destructive effects of toxic chemical fertilizers, herbicides, and pesticides that continuously build up in the soil, water and air, and in animal and human tissues. Toxic chemicals have a domino effect, disrupting the delicate balance within the entire ecosystem. When applied to lawns, gardens and fields, these chemicals leach deep down into soil and ground water to contaminate drinking water, lakes, rivers, and eventually the oceans. Toxic chemicals mutate and kill fish, worms, toads and frogs, insects, birds, and other animals that eat fish and insects. Transmission of these toxins filters into the human food chain. Children and pets are detrimentally affected when they play in lawns, parks, and school playgrounds where toxic chemicals have been sprayed. Blood tests and tissue samples document that the toxic chemicals prevalent in our environment are finding their way into our bodies in increasing amounts. This is a frightening trend contributing to many serious health problems and degenerative diseases, including allergies, skin diseases, respiratory problems, sterility, birth defects, weak immune systems, neurotoxicity and nerve pain, cysts, tumors, and cancers.

Honor the delicate balance of life.

Grow organic.

Live organic!

There is really no reason *not* to grow herbs organically. Their requirements for moderate fertility can be fulfilled by applying organic materials and fertilizers. Most herbs are not threatened by insect and animal predators, but if the need arises, eco-friendly organic pesticides are available. Mulch and cultivation can greatly reduce the amount of weeds, eliminating the need for toxic herbicides.

Your property and gardens can be certified as organic if they have not been contaminated with chemicals over a specific period of time, depending upon the regulations of your county. Your local County Farm Extension offices, Cooperative Extension Service, or Soil Conservation District can help you locate certifying agencies, and they provide valuable soil and gardening information and education.

Step One: Preparing the Garden

The Initial Planning Stage

This is the opportunity to sit down with pen and paper to reflect on your dreams and visions for a garden. Spending ample time developing ideas, researching and collecting information, and establishing well-thought-out plans is vital. Your efforts will ensure productive and enjoyable gardening.

Consider the following questions:

- *What herbs do I want to grow? Which ones do I need for medicine?*
- *Am I choosing herbs that are native to my region and growing zone?* Unless you are willing to spend a lot of extra time and energy, it is best to grow herbs in their native habitats. Do not try growing alpine plants in damp lowlands, or desert plants in wet or humid areas.
- *Are the herbs I want to grow invasive varieties?* Avoid invasive plants that tend to crowd out and reduce native plant populations, and potentially create a lot work for the gardener trying to control them.
- *Am I choosing varieties that are easy to grow or more difficult?* Start simply.
- *Are they sun-loving or shade plants?*
- *What are their growing requirements, soil fertility, pH and moisture needs?*
- *What quantities of herbs do I need, and how large a garden space is necessary to provide this?*
- *How does the size and terrain of my property lend itself to gardening?*
- *What are the financial considerations?*
- *What are my expectations, abilities, and goals for the first and following years?*

When deciding which herbs you want to grow, be sure to research their uses and cultivation requirements. Take advantage of the vast wealth of resources available through books, magazines, multimedia and Internet, garden clubs, libraries, universities, seed and live plant companies, county extension offices, classes, and apprenticeship programs. Enlist the aid of other gardeners and herbalists to benefit from their expertise.

Choosing the Location for Your Herb Garden

The next step is to choose the optimal spot for your garden. Walk around and look at your property. Get a feel of the land. Winter months are the best time to view slopes and valleys of wooded areas hidden by foliage during the warm seasons. Pay attention to the surrounding land and be sure that water run-off flowing in your direction is not a potential problem, especially if your neighbors use toxic chemicals on their lawns or fields. Think about your water sources and options for watering or irrigating a garden. Consider water drainage by observing the lay and slope of the land. A gentle, 5-10% slope will assure good drainage so plants do not stand in water and become overly saturated. Avoid steeper slopes that encourage erosion and possibilities of flooding. Plants that like continual moisture, such as Boneset, Marshmallow, Coltsfoot, and Skunk Cabbage, will need a different growing environment than Yarrow, Echinacea or St. John's Wort, which like drier and well-drained soil.

Deciding between a sun or shade garden depends on the requirements of the herbs you intend to grow. Sun-loving herbs need an open space with access to a full day of sun. Shade-loving plants can be situated in a shaded garden, in prepared soil under large trees, along the northern side of a house or garage, or in clearings in the woods. Observe the path of the sun throughout the day at the site of the future garden to get an idea of how much or how little sunlight the area will get from spring through fall. Check for established plants already growing on your potential garden site that you may want to save by transplanting. Animals living in the area also require consideration.

Soil fertility and structure are important factors in determining garden location. Always test the soil and choose the most fertile areas when possible. Soil testing kits can be purchased from nurseries. And very importantly, be sure to avoid areas close to power lines, roads, railroads, and other sources of pollution.

Keep a Garden Log

Maintaining well-organized and updated garden logs provides convenient reference guides. This is a great way to record all kinds of information and observations from your own gardening experiences and to keep track of gardening projects, including the successes and failures. This documentation can also be important for personal research. A yearly garden log makes gardening more interesting, and it is especially important for larger gardens and growing operations. When growing perennial herbs, it is especially helpful to record the year they are planted to keep track of optimal harvest times – unless your memory is impeccable, it is easy to forget exactly when certain herbs were planted. To create a garden log, map out your property and draw in buildings, gardens, shrubs, fruit trees, etc. Use a big sheet of paper if you have a large piece of land. Write the names of all plants in the gardens. Update your log each year by sketching new beds, plants, shrubs and trees, and make a key for each year. At the end of every growing season, sit down to mentally review and list all your gardening activities and projects for the year. Include general weather conditions during the growing season and any other pertinent information. Then take a stroll around the property to help yourself remember anything you may have forgotten.

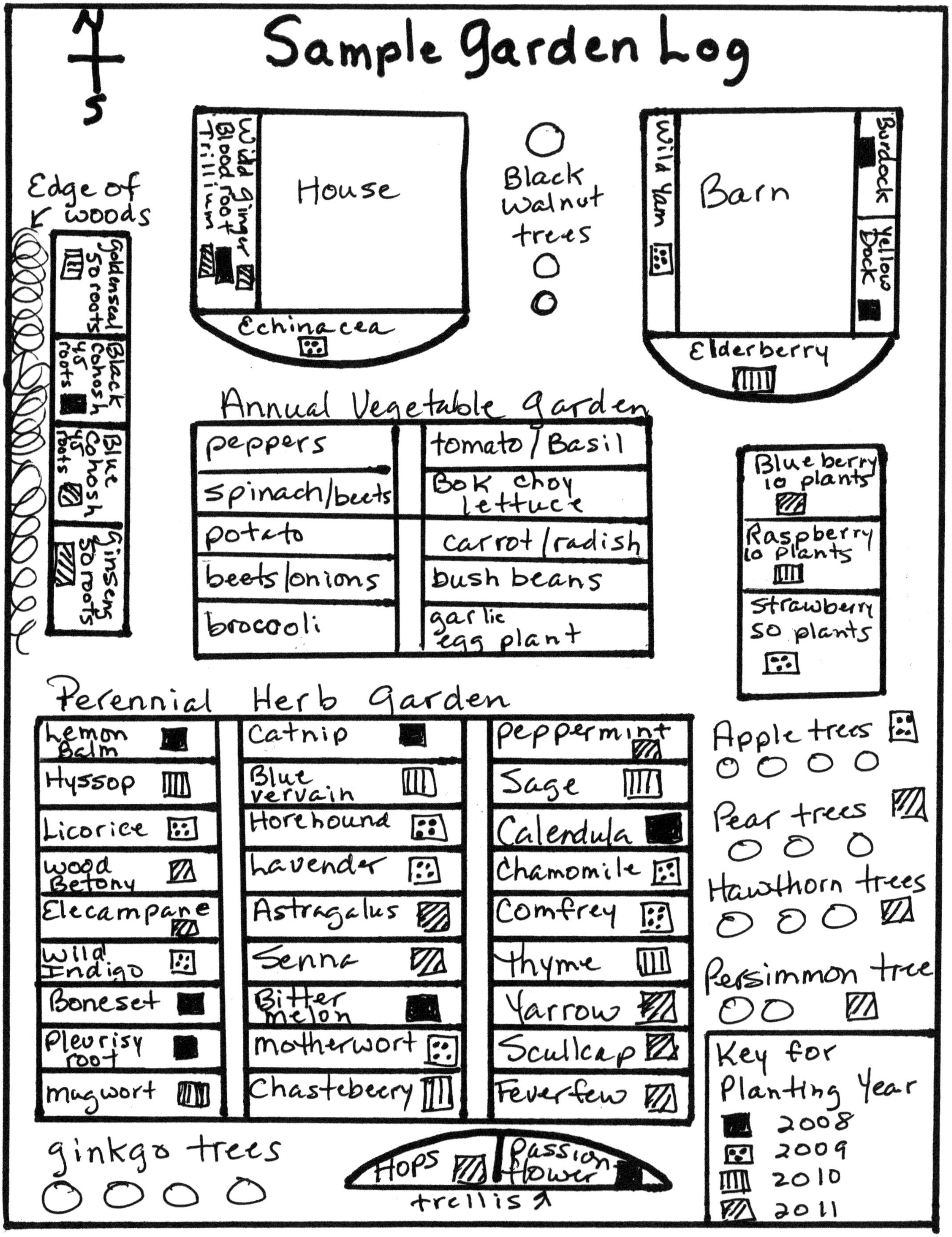
Sample Garden Log
N
S
Edge of woods
Goldenseal 50 roots
Black Cohosh 45 roots
Blue Cohosh 45 roots
Ginseng 50 roots
Wild Ginger
Blood root
Trillium
House
Echinacea
Black Walnut trees
Wild Yam
Barn
Burdock
Yellow Dock
Elderberry
Annual Vegetable Garden
peppers
spinach/beets
potato
beets/onions
brocooli
tomato/Basil
Bok choy lettuce
carrot/radish
bush beans
garlic egg plant
Blueberry 10 plants
Raspberry 10 plants
Strawberry 50 plants
Perennial Herb Garden
Lemon Balm
Hyssop
Licorice
Wood Betony
Elecampane
Wild Indigo
Boneset
Pleurisy root
mugwort
Catnip
Blue vervain
Horehound
lavender
Astragalus
Senna
Bitter melon
motherwort
Chasteberry
peppermint
Sage
Calendula
Chamomile
Comfrey
Thyme
Yarrow
Scullcap
Feverfew
Apple trees
Pear trees
Hawthorn trees
Persimmon tree
Key for Planting Year
2008
2009
2010
2011
ginkgo trees
Hops
Passion flower
trellis

Sample of written garden log for a year

Spring came early with lots of rain. August and September were dry.
Tested garden soils with tester kit and applied aged horse manure and grass clippings to vegetable garden, herb gardens, and around fruit trees in spring after first mowing.
Second and third grass clipping applications done in mid-summer and early autumn.
Poor year for strawberries with low yield, probably from so much rain during blooming season.
Woodland plant additions for April: 45 Black Cohosh roots and 45 Blue Cohosh roots.
Collected 132 Goldenseal berries and 59 Ginseng berries. Planted 75% of the seeds in nursery beds and gave 25% to other growers.
Boneset and Burdock seed collected from wild plants last fall were planted in greenhouse March 10th and transplanted into garden bed the second week in May.
Additions to the herb garden:
Lemon Balm, Catnip, Bitter Melon, and Scullcap seeds were planted in greenhouse on April 1st and transplanted into garden beds by the end of June.
Peppermint roots were transplanted from neighbor's garden.
Calendula seeds collected last autumn were directly sown in garden bed May 1st.
Hops roots were dug up, divided, and planted in new bed in June.
Good growth year for all herbs. The only insect problem was Japanese beetles, so collection bags were put up and captured massive amounts of beetles.
At the end of the season 28 gallons of tincture and 5 gallons of salve were processed from herbs.
Two Persimmon trees were planted and are doing well.
Apple and Pear trees had lots of blossoms in spring and high yield of fruit in summer.
Started peppers, tomatoes, eggplant, broccoli, and cauliflower seeds in greenhouse by April 1st.
Annual vegetable garden successful with bumper crops of red peppers and broccoli.
Started 15 new Raspberry plants and 10 new Elderberry plants by stem cuttings – all doing well.
Late summer and autumn seed collection done and seeds prepared for storage till spring.

Soil ~ the Ground Substance of Life

Thoughtful planning for soil preparation is absolutely essential for growing vigorous, healthy plants and well worth all the necessary time and effort. In the long run, it is much easier, faster, and more productive to take plenty of time preparing your garden space before herbs are planted. However, well-established perennial gardens can also be improved and fertilized by top dressings that leach into underlying soil, breaking down into rich humus. An in-depth understanding about the nature of soil and how it fulfills the needs of plants provides gardeners with an expanded appreciation of this element that is so basic to all life on earth. This knowledge can guide gardeners to successful methods of amending and improving soil to provide plants with all their growth requirements.

Soil is the ground substance of life. All living things come from the soil and all life returns to it, becoming soil once again. As we walk upon the earth, we tread on our ancestors and all that have existed before us. It is a sacred walk. Tread gently…

Soil is typically regarded as mere "dirt." But by taking a closer look, we can glimpse the patterns and order within nature, and the astounding processes of life, death, and transformation occurring at every moment around us in the soil we simply take for granted. Soil is indeed the ground substance and source of all plant, animal, and human life. Soil and minerals are recognized by many cultures as the "earth element" that provides structure to plants and animals. Inorganic minerals in rocks are broken down into tiny particles of soil that plants are able to absorb and transform into organic (living) plant matter. When humans and animals eat plants, the minerals they contain provide structure to tissues and bones. Through this process, inorganic minerals originating in soil provide this important "earth element" basic to life on the planet.

Components of Soil: Mineral Particles, Organic Matter, Air, and Water

Soil is a complex living entity composed of mineral particles, organic matter, water, air, and billions of microorganisms. It is formed on the outer portion of the earth's crust. **Topsoil** is the outer surface of this crust and contains organic matter with the greatest fertility. Depth of topsoil varies considerably from less than an inch to several inches. Below this layer lies subsoil, which usually contains more rocks and very little organic matter, and is affected less by climate. Solid bedrock is the deepest layer. Soil mechanically supports plant roots and provides access to nutrients, air, and water. The texture and structure of soil determine how readily water and air move through it. The chemical properties in soil, including the pH, also regulate the availability of nutrients to plant roots.

Mineral Particles

Soil is composed of rock that is slowly broken down into small mineral particles of varying sizes. This is accomplished by millennia of erosive and transformative natural forces, including water, wind, pressure, heating and freezing temperatures, and chemicals and gases like carbon dioxide that dissolve limestone. The type of soil is determined and named by the predominate type of rock it contains. Mineral particles generally comprise about 45-50% of soil structure and include sand, silt, and clay. Loam is a relatively equal mixture of sand, silt, and clay particles, and the dominate particle would be expressed as a sandy loam, silty loam, or clay loam.

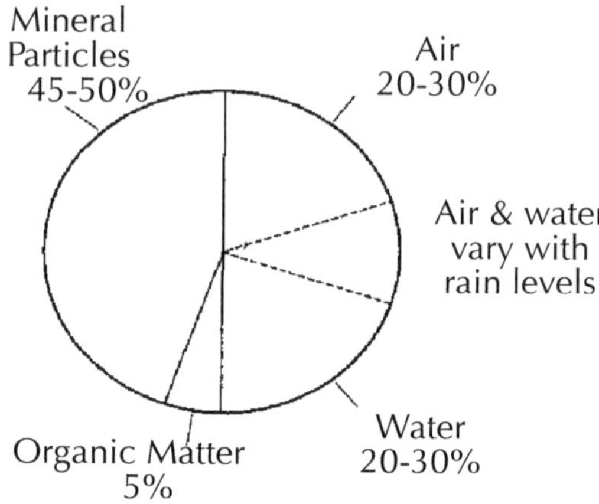

Components of Ideal Soil

Organic Matter, Microorganisms, and Humus

Organic matter is a broad term referring to plant and animal residue at various stages of decomposition and includes beneficial microorganisms called microbes. Organic matter is vital for fertile soil and healthy plants, serving as food for microorganisms and larger creatures (macroorganisms) like earthworms, beetles, bugs, and other insects. These creatures constantly transform soil by digesting organic matter and releasing residues that are eventually converted into a dark-brown or black, porous, spongy substance called **humus**. Humus is a form of organic matter that has undergone some degree of decomposition and emits a pleasant, earthy fragrance. Rich humus usually contains earthworms that increase fertility by tunneling through soil, aerating and loosening it, and digesting dirt and rock particles that are excreted as rich castings. A fistful of healthy soil contains millions of microorganisms that can include bacteria, algae, molds, fungi, actinomycetes, viruses, protozoa, yeasts, and nematode worms. These all break down decomposing plant and animal matter to make fertile humus. Microorganisms and decaying organic matter release acids that break down minerals, and they also add nitrogen and other nutrients to soil. Plants have a symbiotic relationship with microorganisms growing on their roots. These microbes release acids and enzymes into the surrounding soil, which dissolve and break down rocks, dirt particles, and minerals into usable nutrients that can be absorbed into plant roots. Due to its biochemical nature, humus can balance or buffer excessively acidic or alkaline conditions in soil, making it ideal for all gardens.

When soil temperatures fall below 60° Fahrenheit, microorganism activity slows down, stopping entirely when soil freezes. Soil moisture and adequate aeration for gas exchange are also necessary for their survival. Without microorganisms, soil would be an inert mass incapable of growing any vegetation. Healthy soils contain about 5% organic matter, although undisturbed, damp woodlands can contain much more. Increasing the organic matter in soil by adding compost, animal manure, leaves, grass clippings, and straw is an excellent way to increase soil fertility, vigorous plant growth, and high yields.

Humus makes overly light, sandy soil heavier and makes compact clay soil lighter. Decomposed components of organic matter are sticky, acting like a beneficial "glue" that binds fine clay particles together into small clumps, while also loosening clay soil. Wind erosion can be a big problem if fine soil particles are not held together by organic matter. Humus naturally holds 80-90% of its weight in water, so adding it to excessively porous, sandy soils helps improve water retention. When organic matter is added to soil, it creates more air space between the particles, allowing soil to heat up faster and respond quicker to temperature changes. Increased air space also improves water drainage, and humus reduces the tendency of water to puddle on the surface of compact clay soils. Remember, smart humans make humus!

Air

Healthy soil contains equal proportions of air and water, about 25% of each. Air circulates in soil through the pores or spaces between mineral particles by the process of aeration. Air in soil is vital for plant roots, microbial, worm and insect life, decomposition of organic matter, and for the oxidative breakdown of minerals into plant nutrients. Soil that is porous (allowing air movement) will support optimal fertility, microbial life, and plant vegetation. Plant roots absorb oxygen and release carbon dioxide into the soil. The reverse occurs in leaves, which absorb carbon dioxide and release oxygen as a waste product. Poorly aerated soil is considerably higher in carbon dioxide content and lower in oxygen. Nitrogen is another gas that enters through soil pores and is absorbed into roots to be transformed into plant proteins. Air in soil is displaced by water saturation during rains, and returns as rainwater recedes.

Due to the tiny size of their particles, heavy clay and silt soils are very compact, causing inadequate aeration, especially when wet. This can encourage root rot or stunted growth. Two of the best ways to maintain adequate soil aeration is to add sand and organic material on a regular basis. Legume crops like clover and alfalfa are excellent ground covers to increase soil porosity due to their deep-growing, nitrogen-fixing roots. Double digging and tilling also improve soil aeration.

Water

Plants are composed of approximately 90% water. Ideal soil contains about 25% water, which fluctuates with rain levels. Water is vital for delivering food to plants. All soil nutrients must be dissolved and suspended in water to be absorbed through roots. Microbes attached to plant roots will only release acids into moist soil, and then the acids dissolve soil minerals into usable plant food.

In poorly drained soils saturated with water, soil pores are all filled with water, making oxygen unavailable to plant roots. Water also affects soil temperature. Poorly drained soils lack air and do not warm up as quickly as soils that drain well.

Soil Structure

Soil structure is determined by the way particles of sand, silt, clay, and organic matter aggregate or bind together into clumps. A loamy blend of these particles with plenty of humus provides the best soil structure. Soil with good structure is aerated, has good drainage, and crumbles apart rather than sticking together. It can be readily penetrated by plant roots and is easy to cultivate. There are several ways to describe soil structure:

Friable soil crumbles readily rather than being dense and compact. It is easy for gardeners to cultivate and a pleasure to work.

Tilth of soil refers to its texture (fine to coarse), structure, aggregation (tendency to clump together), density, drainage, and ability to hold water. Soil with good tilth has a loose, friable structure allowing aeration and good drainage. This soil is easy to work and crumbles apart rather than clumping together.

Porosity refers to the tiny spaces or pores between soil particles. It affects both structure and texture of soil. Good porosity means that there is adequate space between particles to allow water drainage and air flow. Soil with good structure and porosity consists of about 50% pore space, which is filled with equal amounts of air and water. Pore spaces are large in sandy soil and extremely small in clay.

Permeability is the ability of air and water to move through porous space between soil particles. Permeability is determined by the structure, porosity, and texture of soil.

Soil Types and Textures

The **three primary types of soil are sand, silt**, and **clay**. Most soils consist of varying combinations of these types. Soil type refers to the relative proportions of sand, silt, and clay particles. A **loamy soil** contains relatively equal amounts of these particles. Soil texture is determined by the qualities and feel of these different sized particles. The ability of soil to absorb and drain water, porosity, and tilth all depend on the size of soil particles.

RELATIVE SIZE AND TEXTURE OF SOIL PARTICLES

Coarse sand	0.5-2 millimeters in diameter	Gritty
Medium sand	0.25-0.5	Coarse
Fine sand	0.1-0.25	Less coarse
Silt	0.002-0.05	Powdery
Clay	less than 0.002	Fine and hard when dry, slippery when wet

Sandy Soil

Sandy soil is composed of large, irregular particles ranging in texture from coarse to fine. Sandy soil is at least 75-85% sand, with no more than 10% clay and 15% silt. The large-sized particles allow good drainage and aeration, increasing soil capacity to warm up in spring or cool down in cold weather. However, the large particles also make water retention difficult, so sandy soils tend to be dry and deficient in organic matter and vegetation.

Soils with high sand content are light, coarse, gritty, and are generally pale in color. They need a lot of humus and organic matter to increase fertility. Adding clay or silt soil in addition to compost helps hold sand particles together to improve water retention, and contributes nutrients and beneficial microorganisms.

Silty Soil

Silty soil contains 80% or more silt, less than 10% clay, and 20% or less sand. It has medium-sized particles and greater fertility compared to sand and clay. Silt particles are fine, and the soil is dusty and feels like smooth, fine powder.

Clay Soil

Clay soil typically contains about 60% actual clay, 10-20% sand, and 20-30% silt. Clay particles are so microscopically tiny that there is little space between them for air and water circulation. Additionally, the tight bonds that "glue" the tiny particles together cause them to clump into a heavy, compact mass rather than crumble apart. This stunts root growth and causes poor drainage, reducing nutrient absorption due to inadequate oxygen and water availability to roots and microbial life. Water tends to run off the surface rather than leaching into the soil, but with enough water, clay eventually becomes saturated and puddles. Thus, roots can suffocate from lack of air or drown from too much water. Lacking air space, clay soil is slow to warm up in spring. When wet, clay soil holds its shape and feels very smooth and slippery. It dries into a hard, compact mass.

Clay particles are slightly acidic and negatively charged. They attract positively charged minerals and form strong, tight bonds. Clay provides a storehouse of mineral nutrients, but they are not accessible for root absorption without microbes and humus, which exert chemical changes that break these bonds. Predominantly clay soil inherently lacks sufficient organic matter, making soil amendments mandatory for successful gardening. Increase microbial life and fertility by adding large sand particles to improve soil aeration and drainage. Also include ample quantities of organic matter such as leaves, grass clippings, sawdust, manure, and compost.

Clay soil is beneficial when used to amend sandy soil. The addition of microscopically fine clay particles fills in spaces between the large particles of sand to improve soil texture and fertility. Clay provides minerals that increase soil nutrients and it improves the ability of sand to retain water.

Loamy Soil

Loam is a relatively balanced mix of sand, silt and clay, and is the most ideal soil for gardening. It is high in organic matter and humus which encourages microbial activity and provides ideal water retention and nutrient availability. Loamy soils contain 10-25% clay, 30-50% silt, 25-50% sand, and 5-15% organic matter. Ideally, loam contains about 50% solid matter and 50% space (between particles) that should be filled with half water and half air for optimal plant growth. If the mineral content of loam is more than half sand, it is called a sandy loam. If clay predominates, it is a clay loam, or if it contains mostly silt, it is called a silty loam. Loam has a dark, rich color, an earthy smell, good tilth (workability), and is friable (crumbles easily). Most herbs prefer soils somewhere between a loamy sand and loamy clay.

Water Holding Capacity of Soil Types

Sand is like a sieve that allows water to run through it and dries out quickly.
Silt has moderately sized particles that are larger than clay and smaller than sand. This makes it ideal for holding water while also allowing good permeability and adequate drainage.
Clay is the most compact soil type and prohibits optimal water penetration, circulation, or good drainage. Clay soil has the tendency to crack in dry weather. Rainwater often pools on the surface rather than leaching into the soil.
Loam is a balanced mix of particles with a high content of organic matter and humus, which greatly improves its ability to hold water and allow adequate drainage.

Soil Analysis

Knowing the type of soil you have to work with is an important part of garden preparation. Soil tests will determine what amendments are necessary and in what amounts. Professional soil testing is available by many state universities, independent laboratories, and county cooperative extension offices. If you want to test soil yourself, which can be a lot of fun, simple and inexpensive soil test kits can be purchased from nurseries.

Soil analysis includes assessment of:

- soil type (sand, silt, clay, or loam)
- soil structure (tilth, friability, porosity, and permeability)
- mineral, macronutrient, and organic matter content
- concentration of potassium, phosphorus and nitrogen, which are the primary plant nutrients in soil
- pH value of soil

These are a few easy soil tests you can do yourself:

- A **squeeze test** helps determine the type of soil and its structure. Squeeze a handful of moist soil. It should not form into a compact ball or be so powdery that it falls apart too easily. If it clumps into a solid ball it probably contains excess clay, which holds its shape and feels slippery. Preferred silty and loamy soils will be crumbly and loose, only partially holding their shape. Sandy soil feels gritty and does not hold its shape at all, even when wet.
- Do an **earthworm count** to get an idea of the amount of organic matter in the soil. On a warm day, select a square foot of moist soil, and dig down 6-7 inches. Carefully sift through the soil. If there are 5-10 earthworms, the soil probably contains ample amounts of humus.
- **Test water drainage of soil** by digging a hole 1 foot deep and filling it with water. If it does not completely drain after 5 hours, the soil is too compact and will probably be too wet for plants requiring good drainage. If the hole empties quickly in less than 20-30 minutes, the soil is probably too sandy and requires extra clay or silt.

❖ Test for **soil type and texture** by digging soil samples from the ground surface down to 5-6 inches. Put 2 cups of the soil sample in a glass quart jar, fill it with water to the top, cover with a lid, and shake vigorously. After 24 hours, observe how the soil sample has separated into layers revealing the soil profile. The largest and heaviest sand particles settle on the bottom, followed by silt, and then clay with the smallest and lightest particles. Organic matter will float on the surface. Roughly calculate the percentage of each layer.

❖ In the past, farmers used to taste their soil to determine its **fertility**. Excessively acidic soils tend to taste sour and overly alkaline soils taste bitter. Neutral soils high in organic humus have a sweet taste.

Soil pH is the measure of its acid or alkaline content. The symbol pH means "potential hydrogen" and is a measurement of the amount and type of hydrogen ions in soil. The pH scale ranges from 1 (most acidic) to 14 (most alkaline). A pH of 7.0 is neutral, a pH of 6.0 or under is acidic, and 8.0 and above is alkaline. Soil pH generally ranges between 4.0 and 9.0.

pH CHART

1	2	3	4	5	6	7	8	9	10	11	12	13	14
(most acidic and negatively charged)						(6.5-7.5 optimal range for herbs)							(most alkaline and positively charged)

Most herbs prefer soil with a pH between 6.5 and 7.5. Food crops like slightly more acidic soils with a pH between 6.0 and 7.0. Soils that are excessively acid or alkaline do not support most plants because beneficial microorganisms thrive in a neutral pH range of 6.0 to 7.5 and cannot exist in extreme acid or alkaline environments. Soil pH also affects the ability of minerals to dissolve in water so they can be available for root absorption. Excessively acidic soils undergo chemical reactions creating tight bonds between major nutrients like phosphorus, calcium and magnesium, making them insoluble and unavailable to plants. Soils that are too alkaline have poor structure and are usually low in organic matter and nitrogen. Dry, sandy desert soils can be very alkaline, reaching pH values up to 9.0 or 10. Regions of heavy rainfall that support more vegetation tend to have richer soil with more humus, which is acidic. Peat bogs are very acidic and can have pH values as low as 3.0.

Compost Is "Black Gold" for Gardeners

Composting is a method of mixing different organic materials in a pile and providing moisture and air to transform them into fertile humus. Composting is an accelerated version of nature's own process of decay and transmutation to create fertile soil. All topsoil originates from millennia of rotted vegetation, dead animals, and animal waste. Everything that once lived and died is eventually transformed into rich soil, becoming the ground substance for all continuing life. What an amazing, life-sustaining process occurring almost everywhere on the planet!

One of the most satisfying benefits of composting is the awareness it evokes of cooperatively working with Nature and utilizing, rather than wasting, our valuable resources. Composting offers an efficient and responsible way of managing home and garden waste. Recycling these reusable materials is a much better alternative than throwing them in kitchen garbage disposals or dumping them in landfills that are filling at alarming rates.

Composting is an easy way to recycle yard trimmings, grass clippings, leaves, weeds, kitchen waste, and other organic materials by encouraging decomposition through microbial action. A healthy compost pile is loaded with microbial life. Beneficial microorganisms such as bacteria, fungi and protozoa digest, break down, and transform organic materials into rich humus. Larger creatures (macroorganisms) such as earthworms, mites, grubs, beetles, centipedes, snails, spiders, ants, and flies are also important in the decomposition process.

Microorganisms and larger insects need air, moisture, carbon, and nitrogen to do their work. As these microorganisms consume organic materials, they break down sugars and starches, proteins, fats and cellulose, and convert them into simple molecules. In the process, carbon (present in all organic material) is converted into energy and burned, creating heat. This is why active compost piles are very hot inside. Nitrogen from decaying plants, air, and surrounding soil is also necessary to sustain microbial life and activity. Compost material containing large amounts of nitrogen generates more heat and tends to break down rapidly. When composting is complete, the organic materials are transformed into rich, dark-colored humus. Humus typically contains about 5% nitrogen and 60% carbon.

Compost is one of the best organic fertilizers. It improves soil texture and structure through its ability to retain nutrients and moisture, provide aeration, and moderate pH levels. Compost breaks up and aerates clay soil and increases water retention in sandy soil. It reduces soil erosion and compaction, holds moisture in soil while improving drainage, and moderates soil temperature. It supports populations of beneficial earthworms and microorganisms, and it provides slow release of nutrients for plants. Compost can be applied around plants as fertilizer and mulch to keep the soil and roots moist and cool and discourage weed growth. Backyard composting is an easy and economical way for gardeners to maintain a continual source of nutrient-rich organic mulch and fertilizer.

Composting Techniques

There are several ways to compost common household and yard materials. Find the method that works best for you.

❖ Small quantities of compost can be processed in large **garbage cans or bins**, which require little space and are neat and tidy. This works well for city living and people with small yards.

❖ For those with large yards providing greater quantities of organic material, **compost piles** are the way to go. Decide on an area large enough to contain the amount of composted material to suit your needs. Remember that the pile should ideally be turned over and mixed, so digging a hole that requires bending over may put an unnecessary strain on your back. It is better to pile the compost on the ground. To improve the appearance of your pile and deter animals from getting into it, contain the pile within a barrier by making a boxed structure from scrap lumber, logs, fencing, rocks, bricks, cement blocks, chicken wire, or other appropriate material. Build the structure so that it opens on one side to facilitate adding organic material, mixing, and removing the finished product.

❖ Another method is to bury yard material and chopped up kitchen wastes in **underground trenches or pits** in established gardens. Cover each addition of materials with a shovel of soil. Allow at least 4 months before harvesting the compost or planting in it. This is a good way to fertilize new garden space.

❖ **Sheet composting** utilizes yard waste such as leaves, grass clippings, or pulled weeds. These are evenly spread directly on the garden during fallow (empty) periods or placed around plants as mulch. The compost can be dug in or tilled directly into planting beds in autumn or a few months before planting. If weeds are used for composting, be sure they have not gone to seed to avoid adding lots of unwanted weed seeds to your garden.

Always put your compost piles or bins in full sun because heat increases the breakdown process. Simply add food waste from your kitchen, yard clippings, and other organic material as it becomes available. Chopping and shredding materials into small pieces greatly speeds up decomposition. It works well to layer different materials on top of each other. Remember that microorganisms require plenty of nitrogen. If nitrogen-deficient compost is added to soil, microorganisms have to get the nitrogen from the dirt, which creates a temporary nitrogen loss in the soil and depletes available nitrogen needed by the plants. So it is important to use organic matter containing enough nitrogen necessary for its own decay.

A RECIPE FOR RICH COMPOST

1 part nitrogen-rich material + 30 parts carbon-rich material + water + air = **compost**

High nitrogen materials are green and moist, and include manure, urine, kitchen scraps, coffee grounds, tea bags, grass clippings, weeds, hair, feathers, alfalfa, cottonseed, and fish meals.
High carbon materials are brown and dry, and include leaves, tree bark, wood chips, sawdust, hay, and straw.
To produce the best compost, combine and layer these different nitrogen and carbon materials:

Common nitrogen-rich materials:	**Carbon: Nitrogen ratio**
Human feces (humanure)	5-10:1
Human urine	0.08:1
Cow manure (aged)	20-30:1
Horse manure (aged)	22-50:1
Poultry manure (fresh)	3-10:1
Poultry manure with bedding straw	13-18:1
Vegetable waste	12-20:1
Coffee grounds	20:1
Seaweed	17:1
Grass clippings	12-25:1
Hay	15-80:1
Common carbon-rich materials:	
Horse manure with straw or sawdust bedding	30-60:1
Leaves	40-80:1
Shrub and tree trimmings	50-70:1
Straw	40-100:1
Tree bark	100-130:1
Sawdust	200-750:1

Keep your compost pile organic and avoid adding man-made chemicals, insecticides, pesticides, treated wood, or other toxic materials. If grazing dogs, deer, raccoons, or other animals are a problem, do not attract them by throwing dairy products or meat scraps on the pile, and cover your compost with a lid or screen.

The amount of effort put into tending a compost pile will determine the time it takes to decompose and the quality of the final product. The key to successful composting is to provide warmth, moisture, air, and nutrients for valuable microorganisms and earthworms. Most decomposition in natural habitats and compost piles occurs during the warmth of late spring, summer, and early autumn. Cold temperatures halt microbial activity, but the process resumes with warm weather. Painting the compost container black or covering the pile with a black tarp will capture solar heat. Heat inside the pile increases as microorganisms digest plant material. The inner area of an actively decomposing pile can reach temperatures between 130-170°F. These high temperatures encourage faster composting and can kill many infectious pathogens and weed seeds. Larger piles that are at least 3′x 3′ hold heat better than smaller ones.

Fulfill microbial moisture requirements by keeping the pile moist with rain or an occasional sprinkling with a hose or watering can. Dry compost piles break down slowly, and overly wet piles lack oxygen and are forced to decompose anaerobically (without oxygen), making them slimy and stinky. Either way, microbial activity decreases. If your pile gets too wet or odor is a problem, simply mix in high-carbon materials like leaves, straw, or sawdust. To aerate the pile and encourage uniform breakdown, mix it and turn it over with a pitchfork or shovel every 1-2 weeks. These are the ideal ways to compost, but remember that all organic material will eventually rot and decompose regardless of how it is arranged or worked.

As compost heats up and materials decompose, the pile will shrink in size. The composting process proceeds slowly, taking from 3 months to 1-2 years for complete breakdown, depending on the methods employed. Eventually the finished compost is transformed into dark, crumbly, earthy-smelling soil that is a marvelous fertilizer.

For many years, I have thrown lawn clippings, leaves, pulled weeds, and kitchen scraps into a big pile in full sun. Without any maintenance or tending, the compost breaks down into dark, loamy soil after 1-2 years. Putting more effort into your compost pile allows for faster breakdown, but if you have patience, lazy gardening works just fine. Back in the 1980s, the bathroom for my log cabin home was an outhouse (once deemed the "most beautiful outhouse in Brown County, Indiana" by friends). After each "deposit," a handful of wood ashes or sawdust was sprinkled down the hole, and all kitchen scraps were dumped on the pile. After about 4 years, I decided to empty out the oldest material underneath the back wall of the outhouse, and I was amazed how it had completely decomposed into a dark, rich, crumbly soil that smelled pleasant and earthy. Although some sources say not to use human waste as compost because of the danger of pathogens, I have never experienced problems when applying completely "cooked" outhouse compost around fruit trees, shrubs, and plants whose edible parts grow above ground. Using human manure (**humanure**) as fertilizer is an age-old practice in many countries, especially in the developing world, and is also implemented in some areas of the United States. Human waste is a valuable resource when correctly processed.

Organic Fertilizers and Soil Conditioners

To maintain life, plant roots must absorb specific nutrients that can only be derived from the earth. Soil nutrients come from several sources. Minerals in rocks and soil particles are broken down and dissolved in water, enabling their entry into roots. Microorganisms, larger insects, and worms release nitrogen and other nutrients as they decompose organic matter. Nitrogen and oxygen are also delivered to plant roots by air in soil and through rainwater, which contains gases from the atmosphere.

Assessing your soil will determine what amendments (changes and improvements) are necessary. Gardeners can work cooperatively with Nature, improving even the poorest soil over time with the addition of the appropriate organic fertilizers and soil conditioners. Applying organic matter on a regular basis continually replenishes nutrients and, when combined with tilling, the layer of topsoil can be substantially increased and enriched.

Primary fertilizers used by organic gardeners include animal manure and by-products, compost, rock powders, and plant vegetation called "green manure." To avoid confusion, realize that one meaning of "organic" applies to materials derived from natural sources rather than highly concentrated man-made chemical fertilizers. A different meaning of "organic" and "inorganic" relates to plant and rock fertilizers. All plant and animal fertilizes are considered "organic" because they contain carbon, a primary component of their structure. Rock fertilizers are called "inorganic" because they lack carbon in their molecular structure, but they are excellent and commonly used for organic gardening.

Fertile soil contains all the minerals essential for plant growth along with an abundance of organic matter and humus. The **primary nutrients** in soil that are required for plant growth include nitrogen, phosphorus, and potassium. These are absorbed rapidly by plants and depleted from soil, and must be supplied at regular intervals to maintain soil fertility. These three essential plant nutrients are sold as commercial fertilizers and are commonly known as N-P-K. ("N" is the chemical symbol for nitrogen, "P" the symbol for phosphorous, and "K" for potassium.) **Secondary nutrients** required for plant growth include calcium, magnesium, sulfur, and sodium. **Macronutrients** are needed in trace amounts and include zinc, manganese, iron, copper (all these are alkaline and positively charged), and boron, molybdenum, and chlorine (all are acidic and negatively charged).

The Primary Nutrients

Nitrogen gives plants their green color and is the primary component of plant proteins, genetic material, and chlorophyll. It promotes the growth of leaves, stems and flowers, and a deficiency causes yellow leaves, spindly stems, and stunted growth. Excess nitrogen creates an overabundance of foliage with delayed flowering. Some of the best nitrogen sources are blood meal, fish meal, cottonseed meal, clover, alfalfa, grass, animal and human urine, worm castings, and manure. Nitrogen dissolves easily in water and tends to quickly leach out of soil, so it should be added frequently to gardens. When organic matter decomposes, nitrogen and carbon are necessary to dissolve and release phosphorus and potassium for plant use.

Phosphorus is vital for healthy root development, especially in young plants, and promotes flowering and seed formation. A deficiency causes stunted growth, premature dropping of flowers and fruits, and seed sterility. It is less water-soluble than nitrogen and tends to stay in soil longer. The best sources include rock phosphate, bone meal, blood meal, and poultry manure.

Potassium is often called **potash** by farmers and gardeners. It encourages strong, vigorous root and stem development, and improves disease resistance in plants. It is especially necessary for tuber and root crops. Potassium is required for cell division and the formation of starch and proteins. It regulates absorption of calcium, sodium and nitrogen, and activates many enzymes essential for photosynthesis and respiration. Potassium has a positive charge that draws water movement through plants and regulates the opening and closing of leaf pores. Signs of potassium deficiency on leaves are yellow streaks or spots (called chlorosis), burning and curling, and poorly developed root systems. Leaf tips often die first. Sources of potassium include wood ashes, manure, compost, granite dust, potash rock, and basalt rock.

Approximate Percentage Composition of Common Organic Materials

	Nitrogen	Phosphorus	Potassium
Alfalfa hay	2.45	0.5	2
Blood meal	13-15	1.3-2	0.6-1.0
Bone meal	2-4	15-25	0.2
Clover hay	2.1-2.5	0.5	2
Cocoa shells	1	1.5	2.7
Coffee grounds	2	0.35	0.65
Compost (dry)	1.5-3.5	1	1-2
Cow manure	0.3-2.4	0.17-1.11	0.35-0.56
Dried blood	12-15	3	0
Egg shells	1.2	0.4	0.14
Feathers	12-15	0	0
Fish meal	10-14	4-6	0
Granite dust	0	0	3-5
Grass clippings	1.2-2.4	0.3	2
Greensand	0	1-2	5-7
Hair	12-16	0	0
Horse manure	0.45-2.3	0.17-1.25	0.35-1.4
Human manure (humanure)	5-7	3-5.4	1-2.5
Human urine	15-18	2.5-5	3-4.5
Leaves	0.7-1	0.1-0.5	0.15-0.6
Phosphate rock	0	30-32	0
Pine needles	0.46	0.12	0.03
Poultry manure	2	1.9	1.85
Rabbit manure	2.4	0.62	0.05
Red clover	0.55	0.13	0.5
Seaweed	1.7	0.75	5
Wood ash	0	1.5	1-10

Plant- and Animal-Based Fertilizers and Conditioners

An abundance of plant and animal materials containing the necessary nutrients required for plant growth can be added to compost piles or directly applied to the garden. Organic fertilizers and soil conditioners derived from plants and animals include the following:

❖ **Compost** is one of the best organic fertilizers and soil conditioners that improves all types of soil. It contains substantial amounts of phosphorus, potassium, and nitrogen.

❖ **Grass clippings** are a rich source of nitrogen, phosphorus and potassium, along with many trace minerals. Soil containing high concentrations of minerals produces grass with greater amounts of these nutrients. Grass clippings are usually readily accessible, easy to handle, and are a favorite fertilizer and mulch for many gardeners. Be sure to cut grass before it goes to seed to avoid loading your garden with grass seed. As a fertilizer, grass clippings can be used as green manure when applied as a top-dressing or tilled into garden soil. They can also be added to compost piles where they easily break down and create the heat necessary for optimal decomposition.

To use grass as mulch, place dry grass clippings around plants and on empty spaces in the garden. Grass clippings are excellent to keep soil and plant roots damp and cool, discourage weed growth, and quickly break down into humus that enriches soil. Grass clippings give gardens a neatly manicured appearance. Freshly cut grass may temporarily rob the soil of available nitrogen as it breaks down, but this condition is so short-lived that it will not damage or stunt the rapid growth of plants.

❖ **Leaves, pine needles, and shredded tree bark** can be applied as mulch around plants and will eventually break down to fertilize the soil. When preparing a garden bed, place the mulch on the ground as a top-dressing and till it in or allow it to decompose over winter. Leaves are excellent for making humus but need materials high in nitrogen, such as manure, for faster breakdown. Remember that oak leaves, pine bark, and pine needles have a lower pH that makes them more acidic. They are excellent mulch and fertilizer for acid-loving plants like Strawberries and Blueberries.

❖ **Sawdust** is a good natural mulch and soil conditioner. It aerates clay soils and increases the moisture-holding capacity of sandy soils. Sawdust contains mostly carbon and its major drawback is its low nitrogen content. Excessive amounts can cause a nitrogen deficiency in soil, so it should be applied with high-nitrogen materials like manure and grass clippings.

Although sawdust is generally regarded as slightly acidic, a comprehensive study conducted from 1949-1954 by the Connecticut Experiment Station never showed sawdust to cause an increase in soil acidity. The pH of sawdust really depends on the wood from which it derives. Sawdust from hardwood trees will have a more alkaline pH than acidic pine trees.

❖ **Peat moss and sphagnum moss** are naturally occurring, partially decomposed remnants of plants that have accumulated over many centuries under cool, moist conditions. They are lightweight particles that are slightly acidic and have natural anti-fungal properties that inhibit damping-off disease. Many gardeners use these mosses for potting mix and soil conditioning because they loosen heavy soils and bind light soils, increase aeration, hold large amounts of water yet drain well, and allow easy root development. Both types of mosses are harvested from wetlands and natural bogs that have evolved over millennia and are not quickly renewable resources. To help decrease the harvest of mosses which destroys wetlands, bogs, and the plants and wildlife they support, please do not purchase peat or sphagnum moss. For potting mixes, perlite and vermiculite are good alternatives to mosses.

❖ **Cover crops and green manure** include grains or legumes that are planted in fallow ground in late summer or early fall, allowed to grow over winter, and are then tilled under the following spring before they mature and disperse seeds. The cover crop then becomes green manure as it decomposes, adding nutrients and creating humus. When gardens are fallow, cover crops replenish soil and protect topsoil from wind and water erosion. Cover crops are tilled in before going to seed to obtain the greatest amount of nitrogen and to prevent seeding the garden. They can be tilled 2-3 weeks before spring planting to allow the green manure to start breaking down. Chopping vegetation into smaller particles with a mower or disk before tilling speeds up decomposition and makes the soil more workable.

Legumes such as clover, alfalfa, peas, beans, and vetches are widely used cover crops because their long root systems help loosen soil to improve aeration and drainage, and they add substantial amounts of nitrogen to soil. Grasses and grains such as Winter Rye, Rye grass, Millet, Buckwheat, and Oats are also used, but they lack the large amounts of nitrogen contributed by legumes. Cover crops should be sown from mid-August to mid-September so they are well-established before frosts begin.

Even weeds can be allowed to grow and then tilled under as a cover crop. Some gardens have naturally occurring outbursts of seasonal weeds like Chickweed (*Stellaria* spp.) or Purslane (*Portulaca oleracea*), which can form a thick blanket of green foliage. Rather than viewing them as useless, treat them as voluntary cover crops to be tilled in to nourish the soil. Some garden weeds, including Chickweed, Purslane, Dandelion and Violets, are edible and have medicinal value.

❖ **Coffee grounds** are easily collected from coffee shops and added to soil as a rich source of nitrogen.

❖ **Cottonseed meal** is a by-product of cottonseed and contains substantial amounts of nitrogen. It would be an excellent fertilizer, but commercially produced cotton is grown with toxic chemicals.

❖ **Seaweeds** are exceptional fertilizers offering abundant minerals. However, due to radioactive nuclear waste, mercury, and other toxins in the ocean, most seaweeds can no longer be considered safe or organic.

❖ **Wood ashes**, especially from hardwood trees, are a rich source of potassium plus some phosphorous, magnesium, and trace minerals. In fact, when plants are burned, the only residues are the minerals remaining in the ashes. In this form, they readily dissolve in rainwater and absorb into soil as available plant nutrients. Wood ashes are very alkaline and should be spread thinly.

❖ **Animal manures** include cow, horse, goat, rabbit, poultry, pig, and sheep. As some of the oldest and most effective fertilizers, animal manures provide a perfectly efficient way to recycle animal waste. Manure supplies significant amounts of nitrogen, phosphorus, potassium, trace minerals, bacteria, and organic matter to enrich soil. Composted manure has a neutral or slightly alkaline pH. When applied with rock fertilizers, the acids in manure dissolve rock minerals to make them more available for plant absorption. The high nitrogen content in manure is more easily absorbed by plants in the presence of phosphorus. However, never mix raw manure with lime because it releases ammonia and nitrogen is lost. Avoid placing fresh manure around plants because the heat during decomposition may damage or kill them. Manures should be aged 4-6 months before application around plants. Poultry manure is very hot and needs to be aged 6 months. When preparing a garden bed in autumn, apply fresh manure and dig or till it into the soil before the ground freezes, allowing it to decompose over winter. Fresh manure is an important addition to compost piles because it provides lots of nitrogen that creates heat and catalyzes decomposition. Manure "tea" is an excellent fertilizer that can be made by soaking manure in a bucket of water for 1-2 days. Dilute the resulting manure tea with water until it turns light brown and pour small amounts of it around plants.

❖ **Human manure (humanure)** is a valuable resource when decomposed with adequate moisture and heat to destroy potential pathogens. It is safest to use humanure to fertilize plants used for their leaves, flowers, and above-ground food or medicinal sources, but not for root crops. The collection of humanure and urine into centralized processing centers to be chemically treated and dumped into bodies of water not only creates pollution, but impoverishes the soil and creates dependency on harmful artificial fertilizers.

❖ **Worm castings** are the end-product of the breakdown of organic matter by earthworms (*Eisinea foetida*). Earthworms eat and digest dirt as they tunnel through soil, leaving behind nutrient-rich organic fertilizer and soil conditioner. Castings boost microbial activity and contain nitrogen, potassium, phosphorus, and trace minerals. As worms eat dirt, their tunnels increase aeration and water drainage.

❖ **Human and animal urine** are excellent sources of nitrogen and potassium. The minerals in urine are dissolved in a water solution making them available for easy and fast absorption by plant roots. Urine should always be diluted with 50-60% water when it is directly applied around plants to prevent "burning" the roots. Urine is a safe organic fertilizer because it is almost always sterile and free of pathogens.

❖ **Blood meal and dried blood** are by-products of the meat industry and are not organic because of the antibiotics, synthetic hormones, and chemicals that are typically given to animals. Products from organically raised animals are an excellent source of nitrogen and are suitable for gardening.

❖ **Bone meal** is another by-product of the meat industry and its organic status is questionable unless animals were fed organically. Bone meal is rich in nitrogen, phosphorous and calcium, and reduces soil acidity.

❖ **Fish emulsion** is very high in nitrogen. It may be diluted and applied as a liquid to soil around plants.

❖ **Hair and feathers** contain substantial amounts of nitrogen. They can be added to compost piles or mixed into soil where they will decompose and improve fertility. Collect hair from your local barbers and hairdressers, but beware of chemicals in hair products.

Mineral-Based Fertilizers and Soil Conditioners

Fertilizers and soil conditioners are also available from various types of rocks that have been crushed and ground into granules or powders. These contain minerals necessary for good soil structure, fertility and healthy plants, and provide an important option for organic gardeners. Remember that rock is dense because rock minerals are bound together by extremely strong positive and negative ionic (atomic) charges. Minerals from rock become available as plant nutrients only when their bonds are broken by chemical reactions requiring the presence of water and weak acids. This reaction dissolves mineral nutrients and suspends them in water, which plant roots are then able to absorb.

Rock minerals with an alkaline pH and positive charge (such as rock phosphate, basalt, potash, and limestone) are broken down through contact with water and the negatively charged acidic materials in manure and humus. Be sure to add these organic materials when applying rock powders to your soil to stimulate decomposition. An ideal and balanced mix consists of rock phosphate (which provides phosphorus), granite dust (containing potassium), and compost with animal manure and grass clippings (to supply nitrogen and humus).

Large rock granules require more time to break down in soil and are considered to be slow inoculators. However, rock that has been pulverized into powder breaks down and releases nutrients into moist soil at a faster rate, and is typically applied in smaller amounts. All meals, powders, and granulates are applied by broadcasting (sprinkling) over the garden as a top-dressing and are then tilled into soil. Apply fine powders on a day that is not windy and wear a protective mask to avoid inhalation.

Rock fertilizers and soil conditioners that are recommended for organic gardening include the following:

❖ **Rock phosphate** is one of the best sources of phosphorus. It generally contains 65% calcium phosphate and several trace minerals that fertilize soil and increase its porosity, which is especially important for clay soils. The rock is pulverized into powder and added to soil where it slowly releases over time. Rock phosphate is slightly alkaline and barely soluble in water. To be accessible to plant roots, it must be dissolved by acids in the process of ionic exchange between roots and soil. This lasts over a period of several years until the phosphorus is depleted. Applying slightly acidic materials such as compost, leaves, grass, and manure along with rock phosphate increases the breakdown of phosphorus into usable plant food. It is also dissolved by microbes in humus and by carbon dioxide released from plant roots.

❖ **Crushed granite dust** is an excellent source of slow-releasing potassium. It has a neutral pH and typically contains 3-5% potassium and many trace minerals. It may be used as a top dressing or worked directly into soil.
❖ **Basalt rock** contains significant amounts of phosphorus, potassium, calcium, magnesium and iron, and can be applied directly to soil for slow release. It is slightly alkaline.
❖ **Potash rock** is one of the most effective potassium fertilizers that also contains many trace minerals. It is slightly alkaline, and when finely ground, its nutrients are readily available to plant roots.
❖ **Limestone,** which contains calcium carbonate, is alkaline and used primarily to neutralize excessively acid soils. Ground limestone is the best form to apply on gardens because it breaks down slowly, making it available to plants over several years. When added to clay soils, it causes the microscopic particles to clump together, creating space for better aeration and water flow. In sandy soil, limestone draws the particles together, which improves water retention. Lime in soil also releases phosphorus and potassium from insoluble rock, providing more plant food. Lime is considered to be more of a soil conditioner than fertilizer, but its ability to condition and improve the quality of soil has the effect of increasing soil fertility.
❖ **Dolomite** is a type of limestone that is particularly valuable to gardeners because it contains magnesium, an important trace mineral needed by plants. Specifically, dolomite is a combination of calcium and magnesium carbonate. It is quarried and pulverized into powder that slowly breaks down into usable plant nutrients over 3-4 years.
❖ **Gypsum** is a naturally occurring mineral containing about 20% calcium oxide and 65% calcium sulfate. The sulfur content tends to acidify soil, so its effect is opposite that of limestone. The acidity helps break down and liberate potassium and other minerals for plant use. Gypsum is a wonderful soil conditioner that loosens and aerates clay soils, and improves water drainage.
❖ **Greensand** is pulverized rock derived from ancient oceans. It contains many minerals naturally occurring in salt water, including large amounts of potassium, magnesium, silica, iron, and other trace minerals. Greensand absorbs and holds water well, stimulates the growth of beneficial soil organisms, and never burns plants. It is an excellent soil builder and is good for conditioning hard clay and sandy soils.
❖ **Perlite** is volcanic rock that has been expanded by heat and ground up (pulverized). It looks like small, crumbly white pebbles and comes in various sizes. Perlite breaks up and lightens heavy soil, creates air space, helps prevent water loss while improving drainage, and promotes root development. Perlite is often added to potting soil because it promotes seed germination. It offers a good alternative to peat moss and sphagnum moss, which are less renewable resources from endangered wetlands and bogs.
❖ **Vermiculite** is made from heating the shiny, silvery-gray mineral known as mica. This causes the mica to expand into small, light, spongy particles capable of soaking up and holding large amounts of water. Vermiculite lightens heavy soils, increases aeration and water retention, and improves drainage. Like perlite, it is more expensive that other rock fertilizers and conditioners, and small amounts are commonly used in potting soil mixes for seed germination. Use vermiculite as a good alternative to peat moss or sphagnum moss.

Balancing Soil pH

To determine if soil amendments are necessary, it is helpful to test the pH of your garden soil. The acid-alkaline balance is an important consideration because excessive acid or alkaline pH will block the release of plant nutrients from soil, reduce microbial activity, and severely deter plant growth. Most herbs and vegetables require a pH level between 6.5-7.0 or 6.5-7.5. Always be aware of the pH value of materials that are added to compost piles and gardens in order to maintain the desired soil balance. If soil testing indicates a pH imbalance, use natural materials to amend the soil. Altering soil pH takes time, so do not expect rapid changes. Instead, work steadily towards providing plants with ideal conditions. Remember that compost is one of the best ways to amend excessively acid or alkaline soil because it tends to neutralize both.

TIPS TO CORRECT SOIL pH

Alkaline materials are positively charged and include potassium, calcium, magnesium, sodium, many trace minerals, and wood ashes. Manure is neutral or slightly alkaline.

Acidic materials are negatively charged and include phosphorus, sulfur, manganese, and organic matter such as straw, hay, grass clippings, sawdust, leaves, and compost.

For excessively acidic soils add limestone, dolomite, oyster shell and bone meal (these contain calcium and lime, which are alkaline), wood ashes, compost, and manure.

For excessively alkaline soils, add all types of organic matter, including compost, pine needles and oak leaves (which are especially acidic), grass clippings, blood meal, and gypsum. Any kind of sulfur will acidify the soil, but some sulfates (like aluminum sulfate) can cause toxicity. Gypsum (calcium sulfate) adds calcium to soil and improves drainage and aeration.

Basic Gardening Tools

The primary hand tools for gardening are fairly simple: a hoe, a rake for leaves, a metal dirt rake, trowel, spade with a flat-edged blade, a shovel with a rounded and tipped blade, spade fork, pruner, and clippers. Ample lengths of hoses and sprinklers for watering are important, and rain barrels and watering cans are handy. Compost piles or bins can be set up to recycle weeds and other organic waste.

Larger, more expensive but back-saving equipment includes a tractor for big gardens or a rototiller for smaller ones. These cultivators are efficient in turning over cover crops or heavy grass, creating new garden plots, and maintaining old ones. They till in weeds and dead plants while breaking up and aerating soil. Of all the implements, tillers do the best job of preparing your soil for planting, saving hours of shoveling and hoeing.

Protective gear for gardeners includes gloves, hat, sun protection, and natural insect repellents like citronella oil. Rubbing alcohol is wonderful to splash on skin that is irritated by poison ivy, poison oak, or rough, scratchy plants. People with more sensitive skin may find that after a few hours of brushing against plants in the garden, their arms can get red and irritated with a hive-like rash. Apply a few washes of rubbing alcohol on the irritated skin for almost instant relief, and watch the hives fade away. Immediate application after contact with poison ivy neutralizes the irritants in the ivy oil and can actually prevent the itchy rash.

Step Two:
Designing the Garden and Establishing Beds

After all the preliminaries of planning, research, deciding on the garden site, and soil testing have been completed, the next steps are to design the garden, establish beds, and make any necessary soil amendments. Take plenty of planning time to design and arrange placement of beds and individual plants. Play with all your different ideas and sketch them out on graph paper. To get accurate measurements and proportions, let each square box on the graph paper represent 1-2 square feet of garden space. Start with a rough draft of your basic ideas, and consider various possibilities as you research. Look at the pros and cons of your options, and refine your plans until you are satisfied.

Remember that gardens are always a "work-in-progress" and usually change with each season. Even the best intentions and well-thought-out plans can fall short, and weather, animal pests, and other elements of nature can bring unexpected surprises. Most importantly, have fun and enjoy being outdoors under the sun and blue sky with the birds singing and the wind blowing through your hair. Relax. Be present. Embrace trial and error. Gardening beckons you to a miraculous, creative, and fulfilling experience!

Deciding the Shape of the Garden

You have the pleasure of choosing the shape you want for your garden at this stage. Different shapes that can add to the beauty of gardens and create interesting and pleasantly comfortable spaces include:

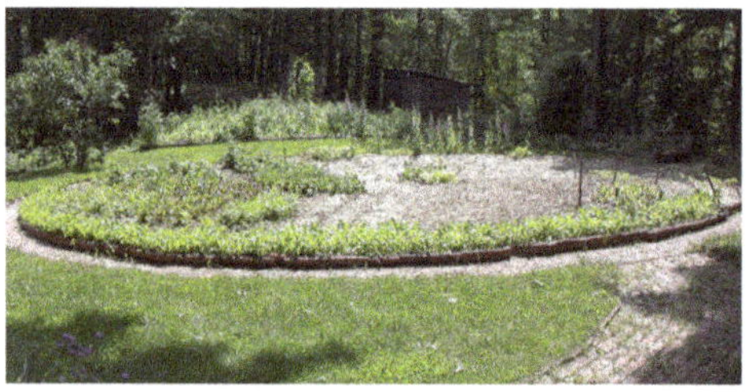

Round garden

- ❖ **Square and rectangular plots** are often preferred because the linear edges simplify cultivation, especially when the plots are rototilled.
- ❖ **Round and oval gardens** may require more creativity in arranging walkways and beds, but they have a unique charm of their own.
- ❖ **Terraced gardens** are perfect for slopes and hillsides, and offer attractive landscaping options.

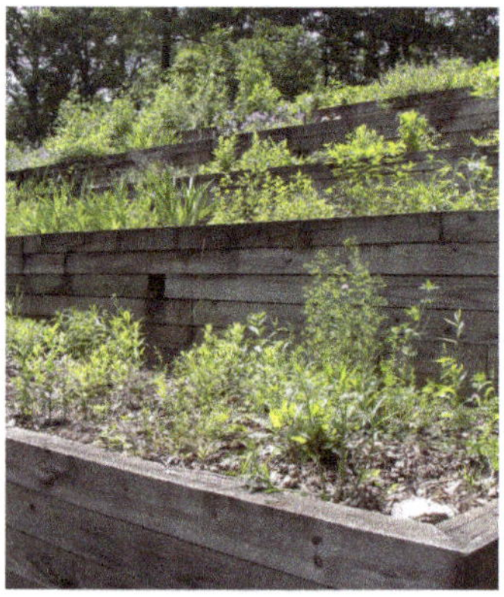

Terrace garden

Stake off the shape of the future garden to make the boundaries visible. Simply stake off the four corners of a square or rectangular plot. If the garden is to be round, pound a stake into the middle of the circle and tie a string around it. Walk to the edge of your future garden and cut the string. Pound another stake in the ground at the point where the string ends. Then hold the string while walking around the center stake, and every several feet, mark the boundary of the circle by putting a stake where the string ends. This is an easy way to lay out a perfectly round garden space.

Breaking Ground

After the garden plot has been selected and staked off, preparing the ground is the next project. First, it must be cleared of all debris and vegetation. Remove all rocks, brush, dead tree branches, and other debris. Mow grass and weeds, burn or compost dead material, and remove or kill grass and other plant roots (without herbicides). There are several ways to clear ground that include the following:

❖ Cover the designated garden area with old rugs, a tarp, or cardboard for several weeks to block light and eventually kill all plants underneath. When the covering is removed, the dead plant material can be rototilled in or dug into the topsoil to create more humus.

❖ Cover the area with several layers (10-15 sheets) of black and white newspaper, and then add layers of organic material such as grass clippings, leaves, manure, sawdust, or straw. Eventually all grass and weeds will die and decompose. Then the plot can be dug up or rototilled. If the layer of fully decomposed humus is deep enough (6-8″), a hole can be dug through it and plants put directly into the soil without any digging or rototilling. Most black newspaper ink is soy-based and is safe to use in organic gardens. Do not use paper with colored ink because it contains toxic materials detrimental to health.

❖ Grass can be removed by using a spade to dig it out below the root level. The grass clods can be put in a pile and allowed to decompose into soil.

❖ A tractor or rototiller can be used to break up the soil. This should be done several times over a period of 2-4 months to allow grass and other plant roots to completely die and decompose into the topsoil.

Soil Cultivation

Building fertile soil is an important long-term project. **Cultivation** refers to digging or tilling soil in order to loosen it and improve aeration, and includes the addition of organic fertilizers and soil conditioners. Good cultivation methods can improve soil structure and drainage, making it more friable (workable) and hospitable to plant roots. Well-cultivated soil is a vital preparation before seeds and live herbs are planted. Once vegetation is cleared from the garden plot to expose the underlying soil, organic fertilizers and soil conditioners may be applied as a top dressing and tilled in. Allow 1-4 months for them to break down before planting anything. Early spring or late fall are good times to apply fertilizers and soil conditioners. Cover crops can be planted in late summer and tilled in spring. Allowing weed seeds to germinate and tilling them under helps eliminate them and fertilize soil with green manure.

Soil should be cultivated when it has adequate but not excessive moisture. To determine this, squeeze a handful of soil into a ball. When you open your hand, the soil should crumble apart fairly easily. If it clings together in a ball, it is too wet and you must wait until it dries out. If it crumbles too easily, it is too dry and should be watered. (In your assessment, take into account that clay soil sticks together in a hard clump and extra sandy soil always falls apart). After grass and other vegetation have been removed and soil moisture is appropriate, the exposed soil needs to be cultivated by double digging, rototilling, or disking with a tractor.

Double digging is strenuous work that requires only a shovel and strong back. This is a method of preparing a garden plot by digging about 1′ deep and setting this dirt aside. Then a spade fork is used to loosen soil another 1′ deep. This process continues until the desired bed is formed.

To begin, mark off the designated garden area and divide it into foot-wide sections using string or stakes. Then dig a foot-wide trench across one end of the plot, about 1′ deep. Put the topsoil from this trench in a wheelbarrow or on ground cloth. Loosen the subsoil at the bottom of the trench by inserting the tines of a spade fork to a depth of 1′ and gently rocking the handle back and forth. This dislodges the soil and aerates it at deeper levels. The exposed, loosened subsoil can be covered with a layer of compost.

Continue by digging the topsoil out of the next trench and putting it back into the first trench on top of the compost layer. This method keeps topsoil on the soil surface, where it best nourishes plant roots. When the topsoil is removed from the second trench, use the spading fork again to loosen the subsoil. Continue in this way, putting topsoil from the third trench into the second, and so on until the end of the plot is reached. The last trench is then filled with topsoil taken out of the first trench. Although double digging requires time and intensive labor, there are benefits. Hand digging spares many earthworms that are normally killed by rototilling. It also keeps topsoil on the surface where it provides nutrients to plant roots.

Rototilling is another cultivation method that is very popular. It is much easier, faster, and less labor-intensive than double digging. Owning a rototiller is a major luxury for gardening ease. Rototilling thoroughly breaks up and aerates soil, and tills in compost, weeds, old growth, and other organic materials to decompose in soil. Unfortunately, these machines do kill earthworms and other beneficial garden creatures. Excessive tilling can break soil particles into fine dust, which weakens soil structure and promotes wind and water erosion. Adding organic materials like grass clippings and manure to rototilled gardens helps repair damage caused by rototilling.

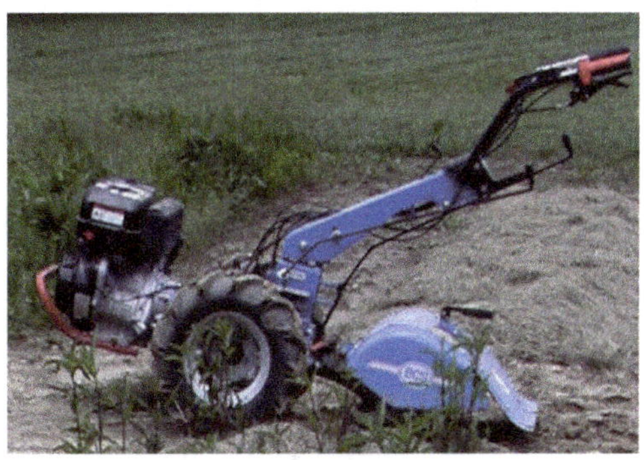

Rototiller

Lasagna gardening is an interesting technique of fertilizing soil and creating beds that can eliminate the need for digging or tilling. Several layers of newspaper are placed on the ground, and in the same way lasagna is prepared, different types of organic materials and soil conditioners are multi-layered in a pile and allowed to decompose over a period of 5-12 months. Large piles that are stacked high with organic materials will eventually make several inches of topsoil and create fertile beds. Plants can be placed directly into the "lasagna" bed.

Making Beds and Arranging Plants

After the garden plot has been fertilized and conditioned with the necessary amendments, cultivated, and the organic materials have had adequate opportunity to decompose, it is time to design the interior of the garden to create spaces for the plants to grow. Be sure to lay out rows and beds according to the slope of the land to prevent soil erosion and maximize drainage. Consider the path of the sun across the sky throughout the day and how this affects shade and available sunlight.

There are several ways to create planting beds.

❖ **Long rectangular rows** can be made along the entire length or width of the garden. A width of 4′ is recommended for beds because this allows easy reach into the center from both sides. Walkways between long rows can be mulched or tilled to deter weeds and to create attractive borders. Herbs can be arranged in evenly spaced plantings or grown in thick clumps.

❖ **Various shapes** for beds are possible. Some people like square or circular plots. Round gardens can be sectioned off into pie-slice shapes. Combinations of shapes in a garden can create beautiful symmetrical mandala patterns that are especially attractive.

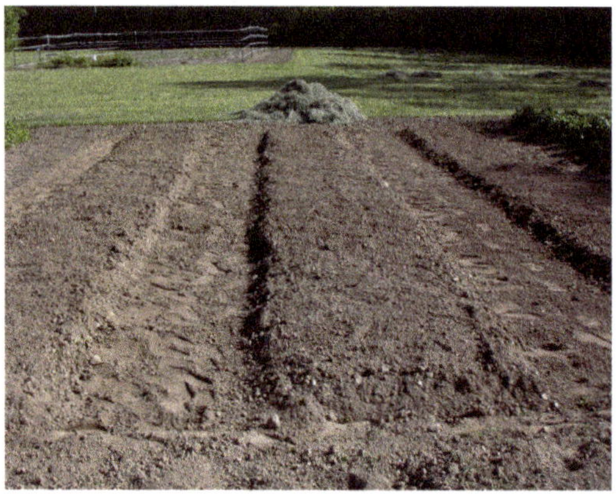

Raised beds

❖ **Raised beds** are a favorite style of many gardeners. They can be made with or without holding containers. Simple raised beds can be constructed by shoveling dirt from the walkways surrounding a bed onto the top of the bed. This lowers the walkway path and heightens the bed. The sides or edges of the raised bed can be tapped down or supported with an application of grass clippings, straw, mulch, or shredded bark. Permanent raised beds can be framed with stones, bricks, cement blocks, used wood, barn boards, or untreated lumber. (Remember that treated wood contains arsenic that leaches into the soil.) Make a container box with these materials and fill it with soil. Upon completion, the raised bed should be 4-12″ higher than the walkways. Raised beds can be rectangular, square or round, but should be no wider than 4′ to allow easy access to the center from both sides. When beds are mulched with organic materials on a regular basis to enrich the soil, the beds will continually remain elevated. There are several benefits to growing herbs in raised beds. They provide roots with good air circulation and drainage, and the soil is not compacted by foot traffic. Raised beds are attractive, they warm up faster in spring, and they make gardening easier with less bending over.

❖ **Garden pathways** can be left in dirt, which can be periodically tilled to reduce weeds, or pathways may be covered with thick layers of grass clippings, sawdust, wood chips, straw, bricks, or stone.

After the beds are prepared, consider the best locations and arrangements for placing specific herbs.

❖ It is usually best to separate annual, biennial, and perennial herbs because they have different cultivation requirements. Annual herbs can be planted in areas where the soil can be tilled each year. Biennial plants must be left undisturbed for two years before completing their growth cycle, and soil holding perennial herbs must be left undisturbed.

❖ Consider the growing conditions and requirements of each species. Herbs requiring extra moisture can be planted in low-lying areas, while those needing drier soil with better drainage are placed on higher ground. Plants sharing similar pH requirements should be grouped together.

❖ Consider the colors of the flowers you want to grow and the seasons when they bloom. Try creating splashes of color that occur throughout the growing season for a beautiful garden.

❖ Research the mature size and shape of the herbs you intend to grow. Tall or bushy plants can block out light from short ones if planted too close. Large herbs look best in the middle of a plot, with smaller and shorter plants surrounding them. If the garden borders a wall or fence, large plants look most attractive planted against these barriers with smaller plants placed in front of them.

❖ Consider which herbs are good growing companions and which are not. Strong-smelling Garlic can help keep insects away from surrounding plants. Some plants like Wormwood, Rue, and Black Walnut trees have strong oils that can leach into soil during heavy rains, adversely affecting other herbs growing nearby.

❖ Fast-growing plants like the Mints or vigorous self-seeders like Chickweed and German Chamomile that spread out quickly should be separated or contained to prevent them from crowding out other herbs.

❖ A trellis must be provided for vines and climbing herbs like Passion Flower, Wild Yam, Hops, and Bitter Melon. Fencing material, chicken wire, and the sides of a house, garage, or barn may be used as a trellis.

❖ If more than one species of a genus are grown, they should be planted at least 3 miles away from each other to avoid cross-pollination. For example, if *Echinacea purpurea* and *Echinacea angustifolia* are grown close together, they can cross-pollinate and their seeds will be a combination of both, rather than true *purpurea* and *angustifolia*. Sometimes this presents a challenge, so do the best you can to keep different species of a genus apart.

❖ **Create a border for the garden.** Create a visually appealing border around the garden with attractive rocks, logs, bricks, or other available materials. Maintaining a tilled "weed-free" zone of soil between the garden and lawn is another good border and an easy way to prevent grass from creeping into the garden.

Woodland Gardens

Woodland gardens provide the ideal natural habitat for shade-loving herbs like Black Cohosh, Blue Cohosh, Bloodroot, Ginseng, Goldenseal, Trillium, Wild Ginger, and Wild Yam. Making woodland garden beds can be more challenging than the usual lawn or field gardens in full sun, but it is a worthwhile and interesting project. If you do not have access to wooded areas, the north or east sides of a house, garage, or barn can provide the necessary shade for a woodland type of garden. Many shade-loving plants grow well, or even thrive, on eastern sides of buildings where they receive morning sunlight and are shaded from the more intense afternoon heat as the sun moves across the western sky. Shaded areas under big trees offer another good possibility. Adequate amounts of compost and humus can be added to make garden soil comparable to the rich humus naturally occurring in forests.

If you do own or have access to woodlands, walk through the property to assess areas with the best garden potential. Notice how the tree canopy will affect lighting for understory plants in spring and summer. Look at the lay of the land and observe how water flows during big rains. Avoid putting a garden where it can get washed out or be too damp from inadequate drainage. Check the soil fertility and structure in different areas of your woodlands to find the most suitable garden site for specific plants. Most woodland plants like a rich, loose, loamy soil that is both damp and well-drained. Slightly sloping low areas in valleys and land by creeks and ponds often provide these requirements. Find areas where there is enough space between trees that you can either hand dig or rototill a bed. Look around for naturally occurring medicinal herbs. You may want to make a garden around them, protect them, or even transplant them.

After selecting the site for your garden, cut down or weed whip all standing plants and bushes, and then rake debris off the site. Double dig or rototill the area thoroughly so the soil is loose and breaks apart into small particles. Then rake out all debris from the soil again, including old roots and stones. Be very careful not to damage tree roots while digging or rototilling. Long-range planning works well when selected plots can be prepared, fertilized if necessary, and allowed to sit several weeks. This way, fertilizers and soil conditioners can decompose and disturbed weed seeds can germinate. The bed is dug or rototilled and weeded several times during this preparation phase to create a more weed-free and workable bed. The prepared soil can then be raked out flat, or even better, raised beds can be made. Simply rake or dig out pathways between the beds, placing the extra soil on top of the bed to elevate it. Herb seeds, roots, or live plants can then be planted in the well-prepared beds.

Aside from gardening, if you own wooded areas, you may want to do some cleaning up and restoration. Check your area for invasive plants. Grape vines that wrap around trees and choke them can be cut at ground level with a saw or hatchet. The tenaciously invasive Multiflora Rose can be eradicated successfully by cutting it at ground level with pruning shears or a metal-blade weed whip. Do this once or twice every year until their roots eventually give up and die. Buy a tree identification book and explore which species of trees grow in your area. You may want to watch over some special ones you've discovered. Thinning out over-crowded areas can help trees grow more vigorously (do *not* cut down mature trees). Always remove diseased plants and burn them if possible. Sometimes tree and shrub pruning can help to encourage growth. Be a good steward of the land and take periodic walks through your woodlands to monitor for plant diseases, make improvements, and to enjoy the beauty and observe the miracles Nature has to offer.

Step Three: Propagating Herbs

Propagation is the process of growing and producing a plant from an original parent plant. The most commonly used methods of herb propagation include seed planting, root division, stem cuttings, and stem layering. Starting plants from seed is a type of sexual propagation because all seeds originate from the union of male and female flower parts. Root division, stem cutting, and stem layering are all asexual or non-sexual propagation because new plants are started by dividing roots or encouraging root growth from stems of existing plants and do not depend on male and female union. Asexual propagation ensures exact genetic duplication and appearance of the parent plant, and new plants are usually produced faster than those originating by seed germination. Asexual propagation works well with plants producing seeds that have short viability such as Blue Cohosh, Black Cohosh, Bloodroot, and Goldenseal, or with Comfrey that produces non-viable seeds. Asexual propagation is best to start hybrid species like Peppermint (*Mentha x piperita*), which is a cross between Spearmint (*Mentha spicata*) and Watermint (*Mentha aquatica*). Remember that hybrid seeds will not necessarily mature into plants that are identical to the parent, because their genetics will often take a turn in the direction of one parent species or the other.

After researching and deciding which herbs you want to grow, it is time to obtain the seeds, live roots, or entire plants. Purchasing these from nurseries and production companies is always an option. Many gardeners enjoy exchanging their herb seeds or plants with each other. Herbs that grow abundantly in the wild can be transplanted into the garden. But please *do not* remove endangered or small populations of plants from their natural environments! This is an unethical practice at a time when so many plant species are threatened by scarcity and extinction. There are still vast amounts of commonly found wild herbs that can be transplanted into home gardens without endangering their survival, or their seeds and stem cuttings can be harvested and propagated.

When purchasing seeds and live plants, always buy from reputable companies that offer catalogues listing plants according to their Latin botanical names. This provides better chances of obtaining the exact species you want. Choose herbs that thrive in your climate and growing zone. Starting from seed is usually the least expensive way to get plants going, and most herbs can be propagated from seed quite well when their growing needs are met. Once established, many herbs self-sow by dropping their seeds, which sprout close to the parent plant later in the season or the following year. Or gardeners can harvest seeds to plant.

Many perennial herbs propagate easily by root division, and live roots are available through retail merchants. For many first-time gardeners, it is most rewarding to start easily and quickly by purchasing live plants and putting them directly into a garden bed. Live plants are more expensive, but they provide an instant garden! After your plants mature and develop seeds, be sure to harvest them to plant at the appropriate time and increase your number of plants. (For specific information about harvesting and preparing seeds for cultivation, refer to the chapters on "Sustainable Harvesting" and "Drying and Storing.") In many cases, original plants that were started from seed can be used for root divisions and stem cuttings when they are large enough. These first plants can become the "mother stock" of many future generations!

Starting from Seed

Seeds possess the mystifying ability to contain the energy, life force, and nutrients necessary to nurture themselves during dormancy. **Viability** is the capacity of seeds to maintain this life force and eventually germinate into a plant when conditions are favorable. Some seeds remain viable for a few weeks or years, while others (like grains found buried in ancient Egyptian tombs) are miraculously viable for hundreds and even thousands of years! Every seed is like a womb holding potential life, and is the vehicle through which plant species continue and evolve through eons of time.

Understanding seed botany helps gardeners be more successful when working with seeds and attending to their needs. Most seeds have a hard protective outer coat. The embryo inside is a miniature plant containing a rudimentary root and one or two leaves. Nutrients stored inside the embryo provide food for the dormant seed. All seeds need oxygen, moisture, and warmth to germinate. When seeds are exposed to water, their protective coat expands and ruptures. As water moves into the seed, it activates the breakdown of complex starch molecules that provide more nutrients to the embryo. Hormones that trigger growth and tissue development are also released. The rudimentary root tip emerges from the embryo and grows downward, absorbing water and providing anchorage. From the other end of the seed, one or two rudimentary leaves called the **cotyledon** emerge, which store nutrients for the growing seedling but are not true leaves. At this stage of development the plant is called a **seedling**. Planting seeds in early spring and watching them germinate into delicate little seedlings is an exciting harbinger of warm weather and a pleasant way to get your own creative juices flowing. The following steps are important to consider when planting seeds.

Deciding Whether to Plant Seeds Indoors or Outdoors

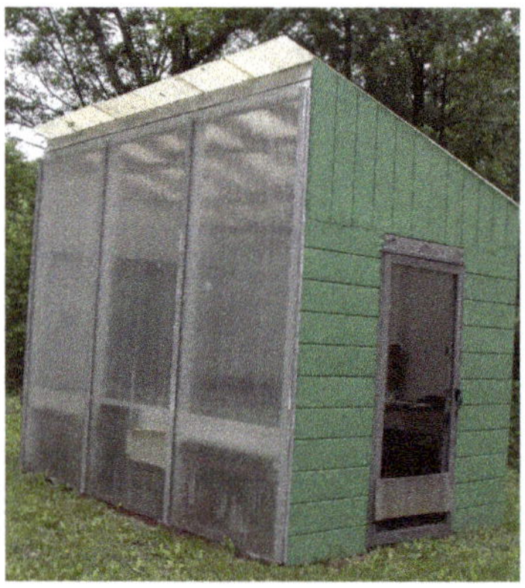

Greenhouse

Planting seeds indoors or in a greenhouse is usually more productive than planting them outdoors directly into garden soil because it allows more control over the environment. Seedlings are protected from harsh weather and heavy rains. Gardeners can get a head start planting indoors in early spring when temperatures are too frigid to plant outdoors. Maintaining constant warm temperatures, providing adequate light, and watering with a gentle spray are more easily accomplished indoors. Most gardeners enjoy keeping a watchful eye on developing seedlings that indoor planting allows. If a greenhouse is not available for early planting, seed trays can be placed by a sunny, south-facing window or put under fluorescent lights in the home.

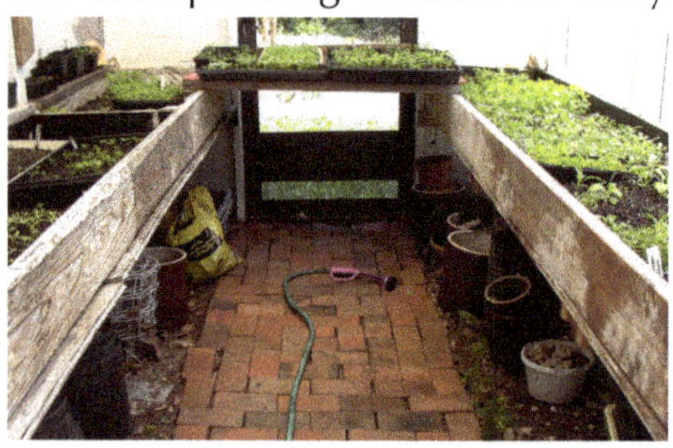

Inside greenhouse

Sowing seeds directly into permanent garden beds means relinquishing these "environmental controls." Birds and other creatures may eat seeds or seedlings. Although the seedbed may be weed-free when seeds are sown, weed seeds already in the soil will inevitably germinate with the seeds you planted, causing potential confusion over whether seedlings are herbs or weeds. It is also more difficult to keep outdoor soil constantly moist for germinating seeds. Exceptions include some of the perennial woodland herbs like Goldenseal, Ginseng, Black Cohosh, Blue Cohosh and Bloodroot, which do best when seeds are planted immediately after harvesting. Place these seeds in outdoor shaded nursery beds or around the parent plant, because they must remain moist to be viable and need an extended period of 1-2 years to germinate.

Potting Containers for Indoor or Greenhouse Planting

Before planting seeds, decide what you want to use for potting containers. Here are some helpful suggestions for obtaining potting containers:

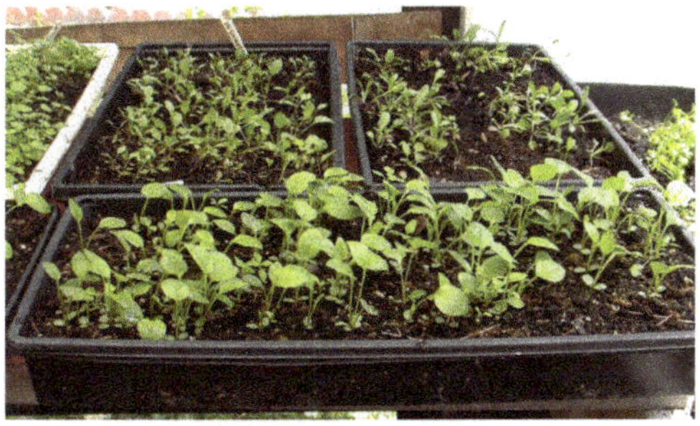

Planting trays

❖ Clay flowerpots, wooden flats, and plastic trays make good containers. Large rectangular plastic flats or trays are more space-efficient than round pots. Deep containers allow longer root growth.

❖ Market packs are sold by seed companies and garden centers. These are cardboard trays consisting of small individualized potting containers. One or two seeds are put in each small container. When seedlings are mature, each individual container is torn off the tray and planted in soil. Seedlings do not have to be removed from this type of container before planting, because their roots are able to grow through the paper sides, and the paper naturally decomposes into soil. This system allows easy handling and prevents shock or damage to the roots.

❖ An inexpensive seed tray can be created using a cardboard box. Simply cut down the sides so the box is about 5″ deep. Line the inside of the box with plastic to prevent deterioration of the cardboard from soil moisture and watering. Always poke holes through the bottom of the box and plastic to allow for drainage. Homemade box containers work well because they are deeper than plastic trays and allow deeper taproot growth. Carefully remove mature seedlings from the box and plant them in a permanent garden.

❖ Pots can also be made from recycled food containers such as plastic milk jugs, yogurt and cottage cheese containers, or juice cartons. Poke holes in the bottom of all types of containers for drainage.

❖ If you reuse plant containers or trays, be sure they are clean and not contaminated by fungi or other plant diseases. Washing with a solution of 9 parts water to 1 part chlorine bleach kills these pathogens.

Potting Mixes for Starting Seeds

Potting mixes are special blends of organic material that provide the required nutrients and soil environment to encourage seed germination. Seeds will germinate in many types of soil, but providing optimal conditions is always more productive and rewarding. Several types of potting mixes sold in bags can be purchased from nurseries and gardening, hardware, or discount stores. Many gardeners like to make their own potting mix by combining equal amounts of perlite, vermiculite, sand, and compost or humus from woodland soil. Commercial potting soil may be added to this mix. A potting mix should be lightweight to provide plenty of air space and moisture, allowing unrestricted root growth. Perlite and vermiculite are especially beneficial additions to potting mixes because they help to fulfill these specific requirements. Remember that growing mediums lacking compost or potting soil tend to be nutrient deficient.

Many vegetable gardeners buy sterilized potting soil that has been exposed to heat in order to kill potential weed seeds. Sterilization can be done at home by spreading soil in pans or cookie sheets and baking it at 140-200°F for 30-40 minutes. Although sterilization kills unwanted weed seeds, it also kills important microorganisms in the soil. These microorganisms form a symbiotic relationship with plants, feeding their roots and protecting them from disease. Herb seeds typically germinate best in non-sterilized soil alive with microbial life. The seeds of some plants like Pleurisy Root, Gentian, Lobelia, Ginseng, Lady's Slipper, and Trillium actually require non-sterile soil because they rely on soil enzymes to soften their seed coats and initiate germination. Follow nature's example and use non-sterile potting soil for herb seeds.

When your potting soil is prepared, fill your containers with the mixture. Be sure the potting mix is damp before sowing any seeds.

Pretreating Seeds to Aid Germination

Seeds have an internal survival mechanism called **dormancy**, which protects them from germinating under adverse conditions in which they would die. Seeds generally require a period of dormancy before they germinate, and this trait contributes to their survival. Some seeds have very hard outer coats that keep moisture out and prevent germination until they are gradually worn down by the elements, eaten away by microorganisms in the soil, or dissolved by digestive enzymes when they are eaten by birds and other animals.

When attempting to germinate seeds with hard coats, here are a few tricks to coax them along:

❖ **Scarification** is a method of nicking or scratching hard, thick seed coats to enhance water absorption. Seeds can be nicked with a knife or file, or placed between two sheets of sandpaper and rubbed. Be careful not to damage or break the seed. Without human intervention, thick seed coats are slowly broken down over time by temperature changes, erosion, and fungi and bacteria in soil.

❖ **Soaking seeds in water** for 2-24 hours before planting accelerates the rate of water uptake and speeds the germination process. This is especially helpful when seeds are large or have a very hard, thick coat. Some seeds can be scarified before soaking.

❖ **Stratification** is the practice of exposing seeds to alternating cold and warm temperatures for a period of time to stimulate germination. This process requires growers to work with the seasons and be aware of the incubation and germination requirements of medicinal herbs. Perennial herbs drop their seeds in late summer and autumn. Alternating freezing and thawing temperatures during winter and spring naturally stratify these seeds. By observing and mimicking these natural cycles, we can participate in Nature's creative patterns.

These are a few ways to stratify perennial seeds:

❖ Gardeners can plant seeds outdoors in prepared nursery beds in late autumn or very early spring, allowing alternating temperatures to naturally stratify the seeds. The beds should be sheltered from wind and can simply be a fallow garden area. Beds are kept moist, mulched, and weeded. Winter weather usually provides constant moisture in the soil without requiring extra watering. Germination should start with warm weather, although some perennials take more than a year before seedlings appear. Seedlings are thinned to 1½-2" spacing and transplanted to a permanent bed when they are 2-4" tall.

❖ Seeds may be planted in an unheated greenhouse in late autumn or late winter, but must be kept moist.

❖ Artificial stratification can be accomplished by placing seeds in a plastic bag with a little moistened sand or wrapped in a slightly damp cloth. Put the bag in a refrigerator (33–38°F) for a couple weeks or months. Taking the seeds out a few times to warm up helps mimic Nature's fluctuating temperatures. Seeds are planted when stratification is complete.

Light Requirements and Depth for Planting Seeds

The size of seeds usually determines their light requirements and optimal depth of planting. Smaller seeds tend to need light for germination, while larger seeds prefer darkness and should be buried deeper. Sunlight penetrates through porous soil to a depth of ¼-½". A good rule is to bury seeds about 1½-3 times the depth of their widest diameter. Very tiny seeds tend to be **light-dependent germinators**, meaning that they need the stimulus of light to germinate. These seeds should be gently pressed into the soil rather than being buried under it. Larger seeds germinate in complete darkness but need plenty of light as soon as the first leaves (cotyledons) appear. Deficient light causes plant stems to grow long and leggy in search of light, which weakens stems and makes the seedlings top-heavy.

If there is not enough natural light available, seed trays can be placed directly under 40 watt fluorescent lights. The lights can be hung about 3-6" above seedlings and raised as plants grow taller. Keep plants under light for 12-16 hours a day. Seeds grown under lights dry out quickly and need more watering than those grown in natural light.

Heat and Temperature Requirements for Seed Germination

Most seeds germinate between temperatures of 60-75°F within 2-4 weeks. If planting indoors, the seed tray may be placed on top of a refrigerator, furnace, or radiator for consistent bottom heat, or placed under a lamp.

Planting Times for Seeds

When deciding the optimal time to plant seeds, it is helpful to research the needs of each herb. Observe and consider how and when Mother Nature plants her seeds, and follow this example.

Spring sowing: Annuals and other fast germinating seeds tend to do best with spring planting in warm soil. Perennial seeds sown in spring will often flower in late summer or fall, and at least get their root systems established before winter approaches. Seeds of biennial plants are sown in spring and develop roots and leaves the first year and flowers the second year. Seeds may be planted in early spring 4-6 weeks before the last frost date if they are started indoors or in a heated greenhouse.

Summer sowing: Heat-dependent germinators like Poke, Passion Flower, and many tropical plants germinate best when planted in very warm soil after all cool spring weather passes. Many woodland herbs such as Goldenseal, Ginseng, Blue Cohosh, and Black Cohosh develop mature seeds in summer. These can be harvested and immediately planted around the parent plant or in outdoor nursery beds. In this way, the seeds are stratified over the winter months and will germinate the following spring, or they may require an entire year to develop roots before the first leaves (cotyledons) of the seedlings appear.

Autumn and very early spring sowing: Perennial herb seeds requiring a period of stratification over winter months are sown in outdoor beds or unheated greenhouses during cool weather in autumn or very early spring. Soil must be kept moist, and seeds will germinate as the soil warms up in spring.

Gardening according to astrology: Planting and harvesting according to astrological considerations offers fun and interesting perspectives when working with herbs. The most "fertile" signs for planting and germination occur when the moon passes through the astrological signs of Taurus, Cancer, Scorpio, and Pisces. Taurus is an earth sign and the other three are water signs. Ancient European herbalists often planted their seeds when the moon was in one of these fertile signs. If this intrigues you, find some good astrology books for more information on this ancient art. I have planted seeds according to astrological signs for many years, and find that planting during "fertile" Moon signs does result in better germination.

Handling Seeds in a Conscious Way

Doing a little energy work with seeds before placing them in soil is a wonderful and enlightened practice to increase seed germination and strengthen our bonds of cooperation with Nature. Before planting seeds, hold them in the palm of one hand and cover them with your other hand. Take a moment to be quiet and aware of what you are doing. You are putting dormant seeds into the earth and, by the miracle of life, they transform into vibrant plants. Realize that all animal and human life depends on the plant kingdom for survival. Take a deep breath and spend a moment to thank the plants for sustaining your life. As you inhale the sacred breath of life into your lungs, imagine it moving into your heart and showering you with light. Then inhale again, and as you exhale, push the breath from your heart through your arms and hands into the seeds you hold. Envision the spark of life contained within your breath stimulating the seeds to burst open, germinate, and grow into healthy, vigorous plants. Invite the plants to live in your garden. Promise to take good care of them and get to know them. Many gardeners have discovered from personal experience that growing plants with gratitude and consciousness deepens our connection and understanding of the herbs. This relationship has the potential to deepen our sense of joy and love of life, and also creates noticeably potent and superior herbal medicines. In this age, when the predominant attitude and activity of so many people is to take from the earth in a greedy and careless way, it is an act of responsible stewardship to give something back to the earth in the form of awareness and gratitude. Working with nature in this cooperative way will nurture the earth, the plants, and ourselves!

How to Plant Seeds in Containers and Greenhouse Beds

After all the preliminaries have been completed, follow this step-by-step method of planting seeds in containers and indoor beds:

❖ Prepare potting mix and fill containers with as much mix as possible, allowing enough depth for root growth.

❖ Add enough water to thoroughly dampen, but not saturate, the potting soil.

❖ Gently press on the potting mix and level the surface with your hands.

❖ Always label your potting containers and greenhouse trays with the name of the herb and planting date. Use waterproof ink.

❖ When planting tiny light-dependent seeds, simply sprinkle them in rows or broadcast (sow over the entire surface rather than in rows). Gently press the soil without covering the seeds.

❖ Larger seeds can be planted in straight, shallow furrows. Planting in straight rows makes it easier to distinguish weed seedlings from the ones you planted. Use a stick, pencil, or your fingertip to carve out shallow furrows. Space furrows 1-2″ apart. Place seeds about 1″ apart in the furrows and gently cover with soil.

❖ Water seeds with a mist sprayer. Watering with a strong spray can easily dislodge and damage delicate seedlings, so misting them with a gentle spray is important.

❖ Check the seeds and seedlings on a daily basis. Keep soil consistently moist by misting but do not over-water. If the soil is allowed to dry out before the seeds germinate, they will die. Newly planted seeds can be covered with a few sheets of newspaper to keep moisture in the soil. Light-dependent germinators can be covered with plastic to allow in light, but space must be provided for airflow. Remove newspaper or plastic covering as soon as seeds start to germinate.

❖ **Damping-off** is a soil-borne fungal disease that rots the roots and stems of young seedlings. It causes stems to shrivel, turn dark, and collapse at soil level while the leaves initially stay green. Fungi thrive in stagnant air, excess soil moisture, and high humidity. Therefore, be sure seeds are planted in moist, well-drained potting mix in well-ventilated areas. Fans can be used to circulate air if humidity gets too high. Remove all seedlings that exhibit signs of damping-off to avoid contaminating other plants.

❖ Pull out all weeds and thin out the weakest seedlings if necessary. When thinning or weeding around delicate seedlings, simply snip off the unwanted plant at soil level rather than pulling out the whole plant, which may disturb neighboring roots.

❖ Some gardeners transplant very young seedlings into larger containers before planting them in a permanent garden bed. However, this step can usually be eliminated by planting in containers with enough soil depth to allow roots plenty of growing room. This avoids shock that transplanting may cause.

❖ Keep in mind that many herb species do not all germinate at the same time. This is a genetically programmed ability that protects plants from extinction. **Multi-cycle germinators** are seeds that require a number of seasons to germinate. These are obviously slow and more difficult to germinate, sometimes taking a few years to appear. They include Hawthorn, Eleuthero (Siberian Ginseng), Gentian, Goldenseal, Uva Ursi, Blue Cohosh, and Blue Flag. Multi-cycle germinators can be planted in clay pots buried in soil to absorb moisture. Check them periodically, making sure they are moist enough, and wait patiently for seedlings to appear.

❖ **Fresh seed requirements**: Some seeds like Goldenseal, American Ginseng, Ginkgo, Blue Cohosh, Black Cohosh, and Bloodroot do not tolerate dry storage and lose their viability if dehydrated. They require moist, cool conditions for storage, but have much better survival rates if planted immediately after harvesting. If the ground is excessively wet or dry, seeds may be planted temporarily in pots or flats so they can sprout, and later transplanted into a permanent bed. Or they may be stored in a plastic bag filled with a little moist sand and refrigerated until outside weather and growing conditions are acceptable.

Hardening Off and Transplanting Seedlings into Permanent Beds

Seedlings can be transplanted into a permanent garden bed when they have developed several leaves and are 2-4″ tall. They can be planted outdoors after the last expected frost date. For more sensitive plants, wait until the soil is thoroughly warm. These are basic guidelines for transplanting seedlings:

❖ Seedlings started indoors need to be "hardened off" or acclimated prior to being planted in a garden. This is the process of gradually exposing young, tender plants to the more extreme outdoor environment in order to reduce transplant shock. Take them outside in their container on a mild, windless day and place them in a sheltered area where they will receive only filtered, partial light. Or place them outside on an overcast, cloudy day. Bring them in at night or, if temperatures are warm enough, leave them outside in a sheltered area for a few days before planting in a permanent bed.

❖ Always transplant seedlings and mature plants in the early morning, evening, or on cloudy days because bright sunlight can shock delicate roots and cause leaves to wilt.

❖ Water the seedlings an hour or two before transplanting. This helps plants stay hydrated and makes it easier to keep dirt clumped around the roots when handling them. Always keep dirt around the roots when transplanting to avoid shock and root damage.

❖ Be sure the soil in the permanent bed is adequately moist before planting seedlings. If necessary, water the bed a few hours before planting, or allow it to dry out if the soil is too wet.

❖ Use a large spoon or a trowel to gently scoop the seedlings out of their containers, or turn individual containers upside down and coax seedlings out. Always attempt to keep dirt around the delicate roots to protect them and avoid shock during transplanting.

❖ Dig a hole using a trowel in the prepared bed and plant the seedlings. Cover the roots with soil and gently press the dirt around each stem.

❖ Water each seedling liberally to soak the roots. Then mulch around the plant with dry straw or grass clippings. Keep plants watered, especially until they have established themselves.

❖ Keep a watchful eye on your transplants and tend to them like babies!

Sowing Seeds Outdoors

Seeds can be directly sown into a prepared nursery bed, permanent garden bed, outdoor flats and clay pots, or cold frames. Sowing seeds outdoors is ideal for perennial herbs that require stratification and for hardy annuals and biennials. Seeds sown outdoors must always be kept moist until germination occurs.

Steps for Planting Seeds in a Prepared Nursery Bed

❖ Prepare a nursery bed with fertile soil that contains plenty of humus and has good drainage. Soil should be free of large clumps, and the surface of the bed smoothed out and leveled.

❖ Soil should have adequate but not excessive moisture. To determine moisture content, take a handful of soil and squeeze it into a ball. When you open your hand, the soil should crumble apart fairly easily. It is too wet if clings together in a ball, and too dry if it crumbles easily.

❖ Nursery beds do not need to be large if seedlings are to be transplanted to a permanent bed.

❖ Make straight furrows in the soil, spacing them 2-3″ apart. Make straight lines for long rows by putting two sticks at each end of the row. Tie a string to each stick and, with the end of a hoe or rake, make a straight line in the soil by following the string. Plant seeds in furrows according to their depth requirements, allowing enough space between each seed to avoid crowding. When seeds are planted in rows it is much easier to distinguish the emerging seedlings from weeds. This is especially beneficial in outdoor beds that have greater potential for lots of weed seeds.

❖ Label rows with names of the plants and the planting date.

❖ Seeds can also be broadcast. Do this by holding a handful of seeds and use a broad, sweeping motion with the arm to throw and scatter them as evenly as possible onto prepared soil.

❖ Rake soil over the seeds so they are covered with as much dirt as the seeds are wide. Seeds that are light-dependent germinators should be pressed into soil rather than buried.

❖ Water with a gentle spray to settle and soak the soil. Germination is stimulated by this first application of water, along with soil and light contact.

❖ Be sure to keep the bed constantly moist. Allowing the seeds or seedlings to dry up can kill them. Watering can be reduced as plants become established.

❖ Keep continual vigilance over the seed babies. Thin out plants and weed as necessary.

❖ Transplant seedlings into a permanent bed when they are 2-4″ tall.

Steps for Planting Seeds into Permanent Beds

Follow the same instructions given above for planting in nursery beds. There is no need to transplant seedlings since they are in their permanent beds. However, they may need to be thinned out or moved around within their permanent bed for uniform plant arrangement.

Planting Seeds in Outdoor Flats and Clay Pots

Seeds can be planted in flats and pots that are deep enough to allow ample space for root growth. They are planted either in straight rows or broadcast, and are left outdoors to germinate. Always label the tray or pot with the plant name and planting date. Soil in containers can dry out quickly on sunny days, so soil must be checked regularly for adequate moisture. When seeds requiring stratification are planted in autumn, they can be sown in clay pots that are then buried in soil. This allows water to absorb through the clay pot so watering over winter months is not necessary.

Planting Seeds in a Cold Frame

A cold frame is a four-sided structure that is usually made of wood and covered with a sloping lid made of a transparent material (plastic or glass) to allow sunlight in and capture its warmth. The cold frame is partially buried in the ground for better insulation and faces south to maximize thermal warmth. Potting soil is dumped inside the frame and leveled out. Provide good drainage by using good quality potting soil, and by placing the cold frame on a slight slope or by putting a layer of small stones under the potting soil in the same way stones are placed in the bottom of flowerpots. Seeds are planted and the emerging seedlings are kept warm under the glass. On cold nights the frame can be covered with blankets to hold heat inside. During the heat of the day, the glass top is propped open to allow for air circulation. Cold frames are easy to make and offer plants protection against cold, harsh weather, and damaging rain or frost. They can be used to sow early spring seeds, provide edible greens during late autumn and early winter months, or house perennial seeds needing winter stratification.

Propagation by Root Division

Many perennial plants with large root systems tolerate root division, which is usually an easy and reliable method of propagating several plants from a larger one. To reduce shock to the plant, it is always best to divide roots when the plant is in dormancy or going into dormancy. Early spring or late autumn are the best dormancy periods for root division, allowing the divided roots to become established during the warm season. The cool soil of autumn and warming soils of early spring stimulate the development of root systems and their symbiotic interaction with soil microorganisms. Root divisions and plantings must always be done when the soil contains adequate but not excessive moisture. Protect the roots by working out of direct sunlight in early morning, evening, or on cloudy days.

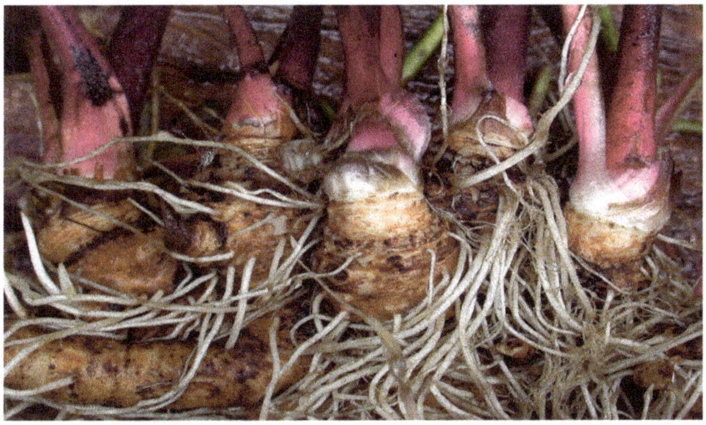

Elecampane root (*Inula helenium*)

Keep in mind that roots can often be divided when they are harvested for herbal medicine. Many plants have a dormant bud at their base where the stem connects to the root. Simply cut off the stem just above the bud and leave ½-1″ of root attached to the bud. This is usually enough rootstock to grow into a new plant. The bud and root are planted and the remaining root can be taken for medicinal purposes. This environmentally ethical and sustainable method of combining harvest with propagation provides a wonderful way to enlarge your gardens while enjoying continual harvests.

Steps for Propagation by Root Division:

❖ Dig up the root to be divided and gently shake off the loose soil.

❖ Remove stems and any dead growth with pruning shears or a hatchet.

❖ When dividing fibrous roots, try to divide the crown (the top of the root system that connects to the stem) and adjoining roots into equal parts.

❖ Some plants have multiple crowns that are clumped together. These can be pried apart by hand or carefully chopped apart with a knife or hatchet.

❖ Tuberous roots such as Elecampane are divided into pieces that often contain one bud or eye, and are usually planted 1-2″ deep.

❖ Rhizomes like Goldenseal and Bloodroot are cut into 1-2″ pieces. Pieces of root containing a bud do best at sprouting a new plant. Many pieces without buds also do well but take longer to sprout.

❖ After dividing the roots, immediately replant them in a prepared bed of fertile, loamy soil with good drainage. They can also be placed in pots, deep flats, or greenhouse beds.

❖ Always plant root divisions in the same orientation as they naturally grow. Horizontally growing roots like Goldenseal and Solomon's Seal should be planted in this same direction. Lay the root cuttings horizontally in the soil at a depth of 1-3″. Fibrous roots attached to a crown should be planted vertically in the same direction or orientation as they were growing. Cover these roots with dirt to the same depth they were at originally.

❖ Always water and mulch the newly planted root divisions. Check them frequently to monitor their progress and check for adequate soil moisture.

Propagation by Stem Cuttings

Another asexual method of creating new plants involves cutting stems off healthy plants and putting them in a moist soil mix that will stimulate roots to sprout. This is an easy way to propagate woody and herbaceous plants. Take cuttings in late spring or early summer after new growth is firmly established, or early in autumn. Always take stems from young plants that are vigorous and free of disease. Water the plant well for a few days before taking cuttings.

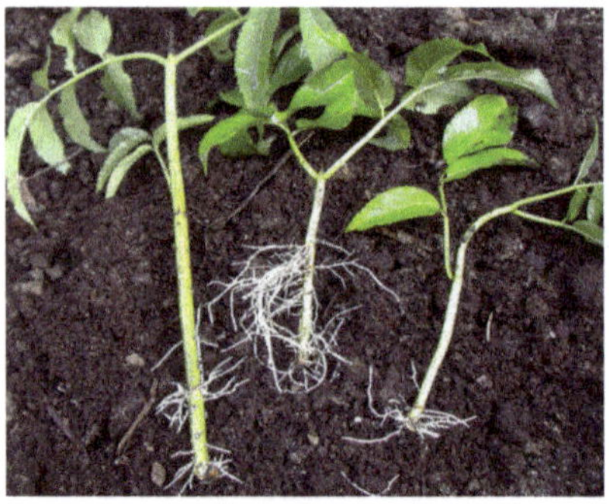

Roots growing on Elderberry stem cuttings

Steps for Stem Cutting Propagation:

❖ Cut a 10-15″ piece of stem from a plant using a knife or clippers. Be sure that the end of the stem contains the leafy tip. Make the cut just below a leaf bud and include at least 3-4 leaf nodes on the stem. Make a sharp, angled cut to allow greater water uptake. Use sharp cutters to make a "clean" slice because this allows water to flow into stem vessels. Be sure to cut side stems rather than the main stem of the plant, which could be very damaging.

❖ Remove any flowers from the top of the cutting and remove leaves from the lower half of the cutting. Leave any buds on the stem because they produce hormones that stimulate the growth of new roots.

❖ Place cuttings in deep pots or a prepared bed in a very moist growing medium, covering the two lower stem nodes with soil. Good growing mediums include combinations of perlite, vermiculite, sand, and potting soil. Some gardeners like to add rooting hormones to the potting mix, but these are often not necessary because many plants produce their own hormones to stimulate root development. Most stem cuttings do best if they are rooted in a very wet potting mix rather than just water.

❖ Keep stem cuttings out of direct sunlight, which can shock the plant and inhibit root growth.

❖ Keep the soil consistently moist but not so wet as to promote fungus and rotting. Adequate air ventilation is helpful. Leaves on the stems can be misted if they get too dry.

❖ Roots will eventually grow out of the stem nodes. This usually takes 2-6 weeks depending on the plant species. When roots are 1-2″ long, the stem cutting can be planted in a permanent bed. Be careful not to tear or damage the delicate roots. Always transplant out of direct sunlight, and apply lots of water and mulch.

Propagation by Layering

Layering is an easy way to start new plants by encouraging roots to sprout on a stem that is still attached to the parent plant. Bend an outer stem of the parent plant down to the ground and bury its mid-section under 1″ of soil, leaving the stem tip exposed to air. Make a tiny cut in the stem portion that is buried to stimulate root formation. Use Y-shaped sticks or garden stakes to hold the stem down and keep it buried. In many plants, roots will eventually develop along the stem buried in the soil. After roots are established, the stem can be cut from the parent plant and either left alone or transplanted to another location. Late spring and early summer are optimal times to propagate by stem layering.

Step Four: Tending Your Garden

After the garden has been prepared and seeds and plants are in the ground, it is important to continue taking good care of the soil and your plants. Mulching, watering, and weeding your garden assures healthy plants and a beautiful garden area. Pruning plants helps them to thrive, and sometimes insect and disease control are required.

Mulch

Mulch is a layer of plant material placed on the soil around plants to conserve moisture, reduce weeds, and ultimately improve soil structure and fertility by breaking down into humus. A thick layer of mulch can practically eliminate the need for weeding. By keeping soil and roots moist, mulch reduces the need to water during dry periods. Protective layers of mulch maintain more consistent soil and root temperatures. It helps insulate roots from extremes of summer heat and parching, and from winter freezing and thawing. Mulch keeps surface dirt from cracking during drought, from erosion by wind and rain, and makes the soil more workable. As mulch slowly breaks down into humus, it provides nutrients for plants, earthworms, and other beneficial soil organisms. Spending time to mulch a garden is a rewarding task, and in the long run it saves hours of labor and allows for healthier crops with bigger yields. And mulch certainly makes gardens look more attractive and manicured. In autumn, mulch that has been applied to annual beds can be tilled in, or turned over with a shovel, to enrich soil. In perennial beds, mulch is left on the ground surface over winter to naturally decompose into humus, and more can be reapplied in spring.

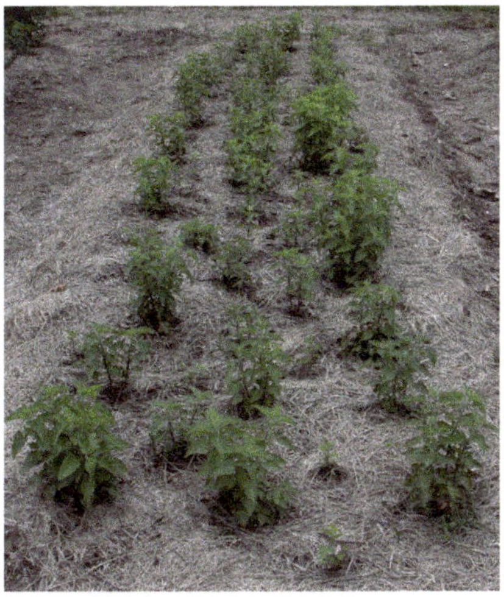

Plants mulched with grass clippings

Grass clippings surpass other kinds of mulch and are a favorite of many gardeners. Lawn grass tends to be a readily available resource. Clippings should always be dry before being applied around plants. Be sure that grass is cut before going to seed to prevent adding grass seeds to your gardens. Grass clippings are rich in nitrogen and plant nutrients that eventually decompose into fertile soil.

Other good mulching materials are straw, leaves, aged sawdust, and ground up wood chips (for faster decomposition). Avoid hay because it contains lots of weed seeds. Some gardeners like using several layers of newspaper placed on the ground and covered with grass clippings or sawdust to hold it down and make it aesthetically pleasing. Use newspaper with black ink instead of colored newspaper. Over 95% of newspapers are printed with soy-based black ink that is acceptable for organic gardening. Plastic is not good mulching material because it deteriorates into small pieces in the sun, scattering everywhere and leaving a big mess to clean up. Be sure all organic mulch is aged before applying it near plants. Fresh manure and freshly cut grass will release heat that may injure or kill plants if applied too closely. Do not allow mulch to touch stems or leaves. Provide good air ventilation between plants to discourage fungus and rotting. Apply a thick layer of mulch material 2-5″ deep. Mulch plants in spring to protect them over summer, and re-mulch perennials in late summer or early autumn to protect them from harsh winter temperatures. All transplants should be protected with mulch.

Old carpets can be laid on top of weeds and grass to kill their roots over time. Many carpets are made from synthetic materials, but as long as they do not deteriorate and get into the soil, they are a great way to create a weed-free garden patch. Another non-organic mulching material is black weed-barrier matting. This matting allows rainwater to permeate into soil, but will not allow weeds to penetrate. It is a fibrous, polyester material that holds up well for several years without deteriorating. It can be purchased in rolls of various widths. The mat is cut to the length of the garden bed, and holes for plants are cut in the mat with scissors or a utility blade. The mat is laid over a prepared bed, staked down, and plants are put in the cut holes. This type of matting material greatly reduces weed growth and can be left in the garden for several years, or pulled up each autumn and reapplied in spring.

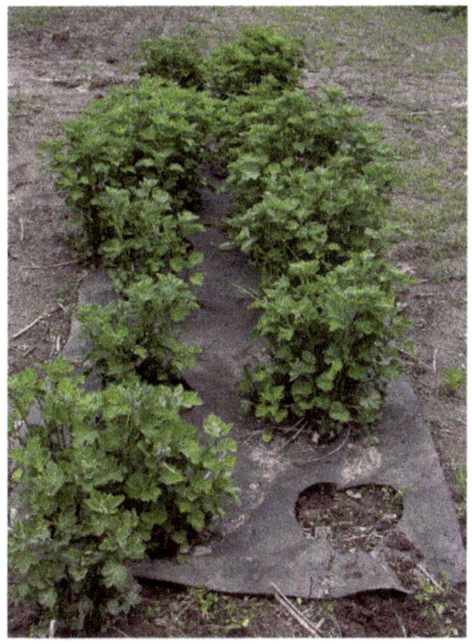

Weed-barrier matting

Organic mulching materials include:

- ❖ Compost
- ❖ Grass clippings are a superior mulch due to availability and high nutrient content. Be sure the grass has not been sprayed with chemical fertilizers or herbicides.
- ❖ Leaves are valuable to build humus, aerate heavy clay soils, and improve sandy soils. Autumn leaves make excellent winter mulch to protect perennial roots.
- ❖ Finely cut wood bark chips and sawdust. Remember that wood chips and sawdust can temporarily rob soil of nitrogen. For best results, mix them with manure or grass clippings.
- ❖ Pine needles (acidic)
- ❖ Straw consists of the stems of grain crops and lacks seeds.
- ❖ Buckwheat hulls and cocoa shells mixed with 50% sawdust are used for small areas due to cost.
- ❖ Newspaper with black ink
- ❖ Old carpets and weed-barrier matting (not organic)

Watering

Plants require water for photosynthesis, growth, respiration, and to carry nutrients through their roots, stems, leaves, and flowers. The water in plants creates turgor (rigidity), which strengthens plant tissue and enables stems to stand upright. Lack of water decreases turgor, causing wilting and drooping. Plants obtain all water through their roots. Leaves typically do not absorb water. However, up to 97% of the water that plants absorb through their roots is lost due to evaporation from leaf and stem surfaces in a process called **transpiration**. Transpiration occurs during the day because pores, or stoma, on the underside of leaves must be open to allow the plant to breath in carbon dioxide, which is necessary for photosynthesis. When leaf pores are open, sunlight and wind pull water out through the pores. On extremely hot, dry days plants can get dehydrated, causing the pores to close, which temporarily inhibits photosynthesis and plant growth.

Use a gentle mist to water delicate seedlings and plants. Water all transplants and root divisions well and mulch around them. Water plants adequately so moisture goes deep into soil to supply root systems. Brief, shallow watering is not recommended because it encourages roots to stay close to the surface for moisture rather than growing deeper. Less frequent but longer watering time allows water to penetrate deeper into soil, encouraging deeper root growth. A few minutes after watering an area, dig into the dirt to determine how far down the water has penetrated. Constantly assess soil to determine if watering is necessary.

It is best to water in the cool of early morning. Watering in midday when the sun is hot can burn the leaves of some plants. If your plants have problems with mold, rust, mildew, and other diseases caused by excess dampness, avoid getting the leaves wet when watering, especially during times of high humidity. Watering in the evening can leave foliage damp overnight when molds and fungi are most active. If molds and fungi are not problems, evening can be a good watering time because roots absorb more water overnight than during the day when the sun dries everything. Mulching definitely decreases the need for watering. Adding plenty of organic matter to the soil improves its ability to both hold water and drain excessive amounts.

Weeding

Gardening involves the selective process of deciding what lives and what dies. Although some people dread weeding, this task can be a peaceful time of reflection and stillness, and an excellent opportunity to weed out our own inner problems and irritations. Weeding helps cultivated plants survive by reducing competition for nutrients, water, light, and growing space. Weed roots help to break up and aerate soil, and when pulled up and left around plants as mulch or thrown into the compost pile, they decompose into fertile organic matter. Weeding presents an opportunity to get to know and enjoy the herbs you are working around, while providing instant gratification by making the garden look more orderly and beautiful! So by all means, please enjoy the practice of weeding!

Pruning

Prune diseased and insect-infected plants, and remove them from the garden to prevent contaminating healthy plants. Harvesting healthy leaves and flowers for medicinal use serves as an effective way to prune herbs. Plants always try to produce flowers and seeds to ensure their survival, and pruning them often encourages new growth and bushier plants. Removing wilted and dead flowers is called **dead-heading**, which also stimulates new growth and flowers. After flowers have gone to seed, dead-heading encourages the energy of the plant to go into root development rather than seed development.

Insect, Animal, and Disease Control

Fortunately, most herbs are not bothered by insects and are less prone to diseases than food crops. The best way to avoid insect and disease damage is to use preventative measures. Growing vigorous plants by providing fertile soil, good drainage, moisture, and mulch provides a natural immunity that helps plants withstand stress. Inspect your garden plants throughout the growing season to keep watch for insect and disease infestation.

Here are tips to help protect your plants from disease, insects, and larger critters:

❖ Plants in nursery beds may need protection from nibbling critters, and can be enclosed with wire screen.
❖ Take all diseased plants out of the garden to prevent contamination and protect healthy plants.
❖ Reduce fungal growth by providing adequate soil drainage and air circulation.
❖ Moles tunnel underground and often eat mild-tasting roots (Ginseng is a favorite) and bulbs. Protect roots by digging a 8-10″ deep bed, lining the bottom and sides with tight-knit screen, and filling the hole with fertile soil. Roots, rhizomes, and bulbs are planted and moles cannot get through the wire screen.
❖ Deer eat many herbs and can be deterred by 7′ high fencing and are sensitive to obnoxious smells.
❖ Aphids are controlled by applying soapy water to plants with a spray bottle. "Safers" soap is organic and can be purchased at garden nurseries. Ivory soap and Castille soap are also effective against aphids.
❖ Cayenne, Feverfew, and Garlic are natural insecticides. Brew a strong tea with one of these, strain out the herb, and add 25% mineral oil to the tea. Put the mix in a spray bottle and shake well before applying it to plants. Mineral oil helps the herbal tea adhere to leaves, but the spray must be reapplied after rain. This method can work well to keep insects, deer, rabbits, raccoons, and other pests away from plants.
❖ Stronger organic pesticides include Neem (from the Neem tree of India), Sabadilla from Sabadilla Lily seeds (*Schoenocaulon officinale)*, and Pyrethrum (from dried flower heads of *Chrysanthemum cinerariifolium* and *C. coccineum*). Rotenone comes from several plants in the Pea (*Fabaceae*) family and is a popular organic pesticide. It is toxic to insects and fish, but safe for people and mammals due to poor absorption through the skin and digestive tract. Once applied to plants, rotenone biodegrades in sunlight within six days.

In Closing

Trust your ability to participate in the exciting and transformative adventure of co-creating with Nature by gardening. If you are a first-time gardener, be sure to start slowly to avoid feeling overwhelmed.

Observing the miracle of life through plants, creating medicines, and eating food from your own garden is a fulfilling and self-reliant way to live on the earth. Plants speak the gentle language of the heart. Be still and listen. They will teach and guide you towards greater peace, contentment, and health. May you be inspired and blessed with abundance from the earth, and be nourished by the joys and gifts of the garden!

Sustainable Harvesting of Medicinal Herbs

Harvesting herbs can be the crowning glory and most fulfilling aspect of cultivation. Medicinal herbs are harvested from gardens or wildcrafted from uncultivated areas in forests, fields, prairies, and other locations. Collecting herbs from your own garden is a satisfying experience, and reaping from the bounty of wild stands can be just as magical. The activity of harvesting herbs is a wonderful blessing and a gift from Mother Earth. When sacrificed for our benefit, plants should always be harvested with an attitude of gratitude and respect, and measures should be taken to preserve them for future generations.

Sustainable harvesting and wildcrafting involve reciprocity, the act of giving and receiving in a mutual exchange. Strive to co-create with Nature by propagating more plants as you harvest them, and try to avoid killing the ones you do collect.

Sustainable harvesting is imperative for the continued survival of medicinal herbs. So many of the earth's plants have been consumed or destroyed without restoration that hundreds of species have become extinct, and the numbers continue to rise at alarming rates. Sustainable harvesting and wildcrafting are all about reciprocity, which is the act of giving something while receiving something else in a mutual exchange. By its very nature, harvesting herbs necessitates a sacrifice from the plants. We either take parts of them or end their lives altogether. Whenever possible, work to co-create with Nature by propagating more plants as you harvest them, and try to avoid killing the ones you do collect.

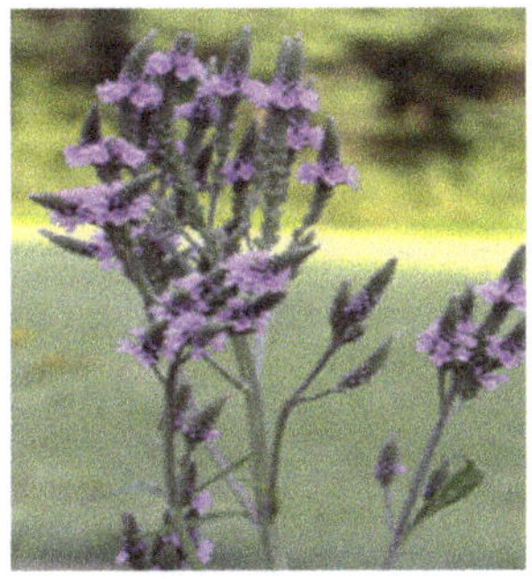

Blue Vervain

Many suggestions for sustainable harvesting are provided in this book. One example can be illustrated by the beautiful Blue Vervain (*Verbena hastata*) plant. This perennial herb is becoming increasingly rare in many parts of the United States, but fortunately it grows quite well in cultivated gardens. The roots, leaves, and flowers all contain phytochemicals traditionally used in healing. When sustainable harvesting is practiced, only the leaves and flowers are taken rather than digging up the roots, which would kill the plant. A portion of the flowers are also left blooming so the plant can reseed itself. Following these methods, Blue Vervain plants can be harvested without being killed, continuing to thrive and reproduce year after year.

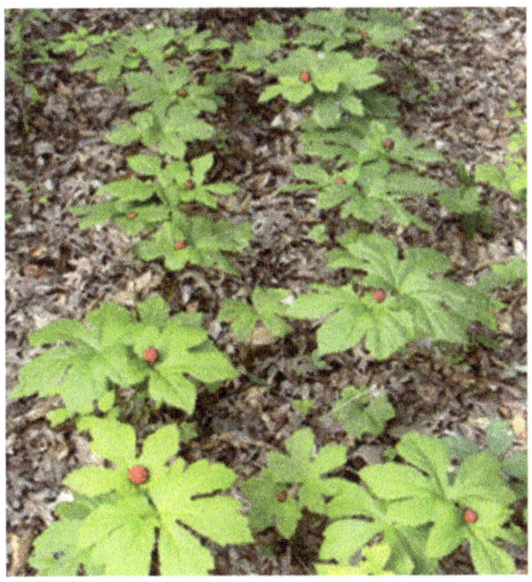

Goldenseal with red berries

Goldenseal (*Hydrastis canadensis*) is a popular but endangered North American woodland herb that provides another example of sustainable harvesting. Wild stands of Goldenseal are so scarce that they should never be harvested by the "clear-cutting" method of taking all the plants in an area. However, wild stands can be "tended" to expand and produce more plants for eventual sustainable harvesting. This can be accomplished on a yearly basis by collecting the ripe, red berries in early summer and planting their black seeds around the parent plant or in separate woodland nursery beds. The seeds must stay hydrated and will germinate readily if they are planted immediately after harvesting. Another way to increase wild stands is to dig up some of the rhizome roots and divide them into ¾-1" pieces. Each root piece is replanted and will grow into a new plant. After several consecutive years of seed planting and root divisions, these cultivation methods will provide enough plants to allow small-scale sustainable harvesting. Woodland beds can also be established quite easily by purchasing roots, then dividing and planting them. The root of Goldenseal is traditionally used for healing and is the most potent part of the plant, but the leaves and stems also contain substantial amounts of medicinal phytochemicals. Leaves and stems can be harvested in summer after the seeds have matured but before the leaves dry up and die away. In this way, plant parts are utilized that would otherwise die. When harvesting Goldenseal roots, always remember never to dig them up until the red berries have matured and fallen off the plant, or have been picked off and planted in woodland nursery beds. Like many perennial rhizomes, Goldenseal roots can be propagated as they are harvested. After digging up a root, chop off a small piece of the root with a bud attached and replant it. A new plant will eventually grow from that one piece, while the remaining root is taken for medicine.

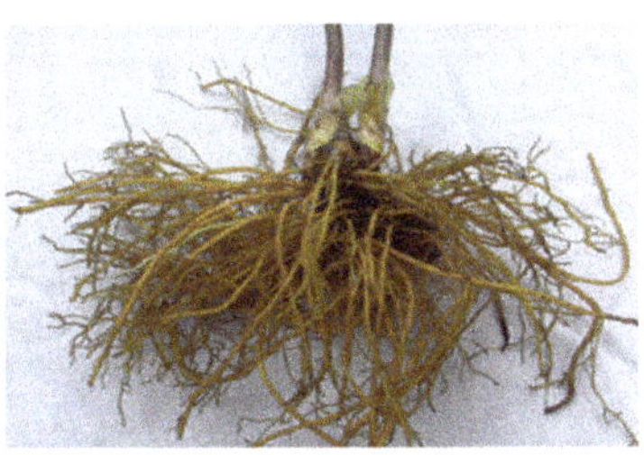

One Goldenseal root

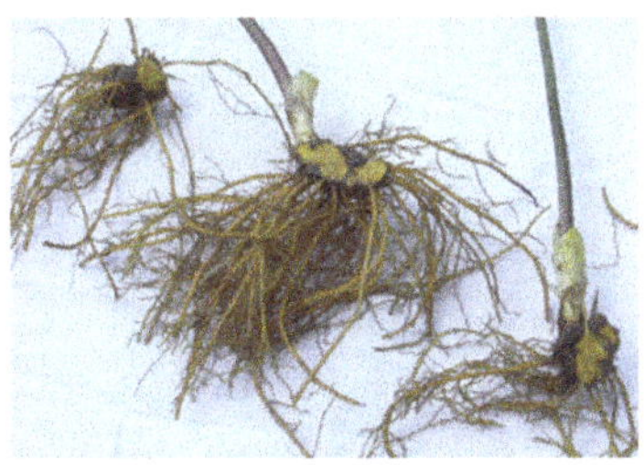

Root divided into 3 pieces

By following these suggestions and applying them to other plants, harvesting becomes a sustainable cultivation practice and we give something back to Nature as we receive her bounty. Through this reciprocity, balance is maintained in our relationship with the earth and the healing plants she offers us. After many years of gardening and wildcrafting to create herbal remedies for my family, friends, and clients in my nursing practice, and after listening to many people's experiences with the herbs, it is my strong belief that plants tended with gratitude and reciprocity provide exceptionally potent healing medicines.

This chapter provides information on the optimal times, situations, and methods of harvesting herbs to obtain the greatest concentration and potency of their healing properties. By following these suggestions, you will reap the greatest benefits from the time and energy you put into harvesting and preparing herbs. More detailed information for harvesting specific herbs is provided in the Materia Medica section.

Differences Between Harvesting Cultivated Herbs and Wildcrafting Naturally Occurring Plants

The issue of harvesting the earth's resources has never been more important than now. In response to the current dilemma of increasing numbers of plant species becoming endangered or extinct, it is vital that we harvest medicinal herbs in ways that do not contribute to this huge loss of life and diversity on our planet. There is currently a massive movement among dedicated herbalists and environmentalists to reduce further loss by encouraging the cultivation of wild medicinal herbs. This is especially urgent for herbs in high demand that are already rare in their naturally occurring stands. In North America alone, there is a long list of endangered herbs, including Goldenseal (*Hydrastis canadensis*), American Ginseng (*Panax quinquefolius*), Black Cohosh (*Cimicifuga racemosa*), and Lady's Slipper (*Cypripedium* spp.). People have wildcrafted these plants from natural habitats until they have nearly disappeared, and now cultivation is necessary to supply market demands. As more growers experiment with cultivating endangered species, they are sharing knowledge and making headway in discovering successful methods of cultivation. This global initiative will help reduce further destruction of remaining native stands. When purchasing endangered herbs, consumers are encouraged to choose organically grown plants rather than wildcrafted ones. For a list of endangered herbs, please refer to the chapter titled "Rare and Endangered Herbs ~ Botanical Sanctuaries to the Rescue."

Although unsustainable wildcrafting of endangered species is now discouraged, many other herbs growing abundantly in the wild can be harvested without reducing their general populations. Commonly occurring medicinal plants such as Dandelion (*Taraxacum officinale*), Burdock (*Arctium* spp.), Chickweed (*Stellaria media*), Yellow Dock (*Rumex crispus*), Yarrow (*Achillea millefolium*), Stinging Nettle (*Urtica dioica*), Red Clover (*Trifolium pratense*), and Goldenrod (*Solidago* spp.) can be freely harvested. Hike around with good herb identification books to discover what grows in your area. As you become more familiar with the plants, you can develop a map-like knowledge of where to go for specific herbs, just as you know which aisle to go down when shopping for specific items in your favorite grocery store.

Growing your own herbs allows the freedom to harvest as much as you grow, and elicits great feelings of abundance and satisfaction. There are plenty of easy ways to continually maintain and even expand your gardens while reaping bountiful harvests and establishing a cycle of sustainability.

Many herbalists and horticulturists believe that herbs growing in their native habitats are superior to those cultivated in gardens. I would certainly agree that herbs living in the wild enjoy the benefits of being in their self-selected environment. However, plants are extremely responsive to human touch and interaction, especially when people have good intentions and work cooperatively with Nature. When plants are lovingly cared for and their needs met, they can grow strong and produce amazingly potent medicine, even in a cultivated garden. In fact, I would venture to say that garden herbs grown in this manner can even surpass those living in the wild in the quality of their healing potential. I have noticed, over many years of gardening herbs and watching those that live in the wild, that plants often grow larger and are more vigorous in gardens compared to plants of the same species growing in the wild.

The Advantages of Harvesting Your Own Herbs

Herbs can be obtained by purchasing them from markets and distributors, or by gathering them yourself. There are several benefits of cultivating and harvesting your own medicinal herbs:

- ❖ It is empowering to harvest your own herbs rather than relying on others to do the job.
- ❖ You are less dependent on commercial manufacturers and vendors for your herbal medicine.
- ❖ It is cost-effective to harvest your own herbs rather than purchasing them.
- ❖ By harvesting herbs from organic gardens or wildcrafting in unpolluted areas, you have more control over the purity of the plants and the herbal preparations made from them.
- ❖ Herbs sold in commercial preparations are sometimes incorrectly identified or adulterated with other plants. You can be certain that the herbs you harvest have been correctly identified.
- ❖ You can gather and process plants at the peak of their potency to obtain freshness and quality.
- ❖ The harvest date of an herb is a marker of its shelf life, which is the period of time in which herbs maintain their potency and biological activity. When purchasing herbs, you can never be sure of the date they were harvested. But as the grower, you know the times of harvest.
- ❖ Harvesting provides opportunities to be outdoors and interact with the elemental forces of nature and the plants, which is healing in itself!

Correct Identification of Medicinal Plants

Accurate identification is imperative when harvesting plants and using them for healing. The best way to develop your identification skills is to take classes with an experienced herbalist or botanist who can walk you through gardens, fields, woodlands, and the surrounding terrain to point out herbs for close observation. Use all of your senses when getting to know a plant. Touch it to feel the texture. Is it smooth or rough, soft or hard, succulent or brittle? Smell it. Look closely at the obvious and more detailed characteristics. Taste the edible parts, but *never* ingest a plant without knowing its exact identification! To become more familiar with the plants you find and to sharpen your memory, it is helpful to photograph them, make a drawing, or gather and dry plant specimens by pressing them in newspapers or a phone book. The photographs, drawings, or dried plant parts can then be placed in notebooks, labeled, and used as reference guides.

Purchasing medicinal herb and plant identification books with good pictures is imperative for correct identification. Owning several different books will provide a helpful assortment of pictures. These might include various angles of the whole plant or close-ups of the leaves or flowers, and occasionally the roots. The more illustrations and written descriptions you have of a plant, the easier it is to determine the correct identification and reduce the possibility of mistakes. It is also very important to become familiar with the Latin botanical names of herbs because it provides greatest accuracy. Always use herb books that list Latin names alongside the common names of plants. If in doubt about the identity of a plant, seek help from a knowledgeable herbalist or botanist. Remember that the best time to accurately identify a plant is during its blooming stage when the color and appearance of the flowers serve as the primary and most reliable guides. Trying to identify an unfamiliar plant only by the leaves and stems can be very difficult, frustrating, and prone to error.

The importance of accurate plant identification cannot be stressed enough! One day many years ago when I was a "budding" herbalist, I hiked through the woodlands surrounding my log cabin home looking for the wonderful women's ally, Black Cohosh (*Cimicifuga racemosa*). I was thrilled when I found several plants whose leaves looked just like Black Cohosh, and I harvested their roots to make a tincture. After returning home, I decided to look through my identification books once more to double-check that I had the right plant before chopping up the roots. To my horror, I discovered that I had picked White Baneberry (*Actaea pachypoda*), whose leaves look nearly identical to Black Cohosh, but the roots and entire plant are actually poisonous! What a great lesson Baneberry provided. After that experience, I never harvested another herb for medicine unless I thoroughly checked my books and was absolutely sure my identification was correct.

When to Harvest Herbs

Time of Season: It is important to understand the energetics of live plants in order to determine the best times for harvesting. Let's use the example of perennial plants that live for several years. Remember that all living things embody an energetic "life force." This life force moves through plants, and during different seasons it is more concentrated in some parts of the plant than in others. During the winter months, the life force lays dormant in perennial roots and the plant appears to be dead. In spring, increased light and warmth activate this life force to move up from the roots for the development of leaves, stems, and flowers. Throughout the warm season, roots absorb nutrients from the soil in order to nourish the whole plant, keep the roots alive during winter, and contribute to new growth each spring. During the spring and summer months, most of the life force in plants is concentrated in their leaves and flowers. The process of photosynthesis within the leaves miraculously transforms sunlight into energy for nourishment and growth. As the flowers eventually fade and develop into seeds, the life force becomes concentrated in the seeds. In fact, the primary biological purpose of all plants is to form seeds or nuts to ensure continual survival of their species. As cold temperatures and diminished light of winter approach, the life force retreats back into the roots, causing seeds to drop and foliage to die. Each spring this cycle repeats itself in perennial plants. In annual plants, this cycle culminates with the dispersal of seeds and is completed within one growing season. In biennials the life cycle takes two years.

When harvesting herbs, always try to obtain the optimal potency of their medicinal constituents by considering where the life force of the plant is concentrated. Reflect on the cyclic movement of energy that moves upward from the roots in early spring to form stems, leaves, flowers and seeds, and then descends down to the earth and into the roots as cold weather approaches.

Time of day: Herbs should be collected on dry, sunny days because their medicinal qualities can be diminished by rain and lack of sunlight. Concentrations of volatile oils in leaves and flowers are greater during dry periods, generally increasing with exposure to the sun. Oils on the surface of plants are washed away during heavy rains. Gather plants in the cool of the morning after all dew has evaporated, or in the afternoon before an excessively hot sun makes leaves dehydrate and wilt. Leaves and flowers can mold and spoil quickly if they are collected damp or wet, and they are more difficult and time-consuming to dry. Roots will be more saturated with water if they are dug up when the ground is very wet.

These are the optimal seasons and times for harvesting herbs to obtain their greatest potential. However, if you have the need and opportunity to collect herbs outside of these guidelines, by all means do so, and do not necessarily be limited by the "ideal" scenario.

Harvesting Leaves and Flowers

As a general rule, leaves and flowers are harvested as the flowers begin to bloom or when the plant has just reached full bloom. This is because the life force, volatile oils, alkaloids, and other chemical constituents in the foliage are typically most concentrated when blooming starts and the leaves and flowers are still very fresh. Select young, healthy looking leaves and flowers that are rich in color. Be sure they are clean and free of dirt. Selectively prune each plant to prevent their damage or death, and do not harvest more than 1/3 to 1/4 of the foliage. If too many leaves are removed the plant will die, because leaves are necessary for photosynthesis and nourishing the roots. Pruning the upper leaves and flowers can sometimes encourage bushier plants with more vigorous and abundant foliage and root growth. The biological goal of plants is always to produce seeds for their reproduction, so when flowers are pruned off, many plants will grow more flowers in an attempt to produce seeds. Always leave some flowers on the plant so they will mature into seeds and contribute to the plant's self-propagation.

Harvesting Roots

Most roots that are used for medicinal purposes come from biennial plants that live for two years or from perennials living for several years. Roots of annual plants are rarely harvested. Biennial roots are typically gathered in late autumn of their first year of growth, or early spring of their second year, when most of the plant's energy is concentrated in the roots. Biennial roots often become woody, pithy, or hollow during their second year of growth, and their energy and vitality become exhausted. Roots of perennial plants are harvested as soon as they reach substantial size, usually in spring or autumn when the life energy of plants is most concentrated in their roots.

During the warm growing season, biennial and perennial roots absorb and store carbohydrates, proteins, vitamins, minerals, and other nutrients that provide nourishment, enabling them to grow and to survive during cold winter months when photosynthesis, occurring in the leaves, comes to a halt. Roots typically weigh more and reach their greatest concentration and potency in late summer and autumn following this growth period. Over winter, these stores become somewhat depleted in order to keep the plant alive. It stands to reason that roots harvested in autumn probably contain optimal quantities of many medicinal constituents. But realize that roots still contain good medicine in spring, and if the need arises, roots can be dug any time for healing. Actually, my favorite time to dig up roots is in early spring because the moist soil allows for easy digging, and after a long winter, some strenuous activity feels good. It is also wondrous to be outdoors in springtime with the musky, earthy smell of the soil and the explosive emergence of all the vibrantly green plants.

There is another, more subtle perspective in understanding the energetics of roots harvested in springtime compared to autumn. In spring, the radiant life force in roots surges upward and outward in a dynamic, expansive movement that stimulates growth of leaves and flowers. In autumn, when this life force moves back down to the earth, leaves and flowers fade away and the energetic quality of the roots is more subdued and sinking. Understanding these energetic differences can be of assistance in using herbs to create balance for healing. The uplifting, stimulating, and energizing quality of roots collected in spring may bring more balance to people who are depressed and lethargic, or be more effective for upper body problems like lung or head imbalances. Roots harvested in autumn can have more of a calming, stabilizing, and grounding effect on people who are hyperactive, overly excitable, or anxious. Autumn roots may be more appropriate for problems in the lower body such as digestive or urinary issues.

Harvesting roots definitely requires more effort than collecting leaves and flowers. Small, short roots are easy to dig up, but large, deep roots require some elbow grease. The upper stems and foliage of the herb may be snipped off at ground level to clear the area. Use a shovel or spade that is large enough to dig up the entire root. Dig a hole around the root that is wide enough and deep enough to avoid breaking off the end of the root or any side-shoots.

Harvesting the roots of endangered species like Goldenseal (*Hydrastis canadensis*), American Ginseng (*Panax quinquefolius*), Blue Cohosh (*Caulophyllum thalictroides*), and Black Cohosh (*Cimicifuga racemosa*) requires special consideration. To help ensure their continuation, it is absolutely imperative that the seeds of all endangered plants are completely mature and planted before taking the roots. Never harvest these plants in the spring or early summer before their seeds mature, and as previously mentioned, never harvest endangered plants unless you are using sustainable methods!

A marvelous attribute of so many plants is their expansive nature and ability to propagate. Remember that when harvesting the roots of some plants, a small piece can be cut off and replanted, and it will sprout leaves and grow into another plant. Many roots grow sprouts at ground level, and when this sprout is cut away with a little bit of root attached to provide nourishment, it will develop into a new plant. This is a perfect solution because the major portion of a root can be harvested to make medicine, while a small part of it can be replanted to perpetuate more plants and provide for future harvests.

Many years ago, the Elecampane plant (*Inula helenium*) taught me this valuable lesson. I dug up a huge Elecampane root containing about 20 round, bulbous sections attached to long tapering roots. The top part of each bulbous section had a sprout and, following my intuition, I decided to separate and replant all 20 sprouts. The results were great! I was able to produce a good volume of tincture from harvesting the long roots, and 20 new Elecampane plants emerged from the bulbous sprouts the following spring. It is the best of both worlds when harvesting becomes sustainable and more plants are propagated in the process.

Harvesting Tree Bark

The inner barks of trees such as Wild Cherry (*Prunus serotina*), White Oak (*Quercus alba*), Sassafras (*Sassafras albidum*), and Slippery Elm (*Ulmus rubra*) are collected in the spring or autumn. The flow of sap, which contains medicinal phytochemicals, is most active in the spring as it moves up the tree when the buds open and again in autumn when sap flows back down into the roots as the leaves fall off.

Harvesting tree bark is a skill that must be performed very carefully to avoid killing the tree. It is less damaging to harvest bark from the branches rather than the main tree trunk. A two-handled draw knife works best for shaving bark, but a sharp knife will also do well. The outer bark is first shaved off in lengthwise strips that are no larger than 4″ long and 2″ wide. This exposes the inner layer that is usually lighter in color and slightly soft and moist. Gently shave off this inner layer in small strips. Only remove bark from 2-4 areas on a tree. When done correctly, the tree wounds will heal up after a few weeks and not weaken or damage the tree. To protect against insect infestation, which would weaken the tree, sealants specific for trees may be applied over the exposed areas. Never girt trees – they will die if the bark is stripped around their entire circumference. The most ecological way to harvest large amounts of tree bark is to find dying trees, those that have been blown down after windy storms, or those that have been devastated by clear-cutting. Since these trees will die anyway, their inner bark can be completely harvested and put to good use. Slippery Elm is now an endangered species due to the epidemic Elm disease, and should only be harvested according to sustainable methods in areas where it is still plentiful.

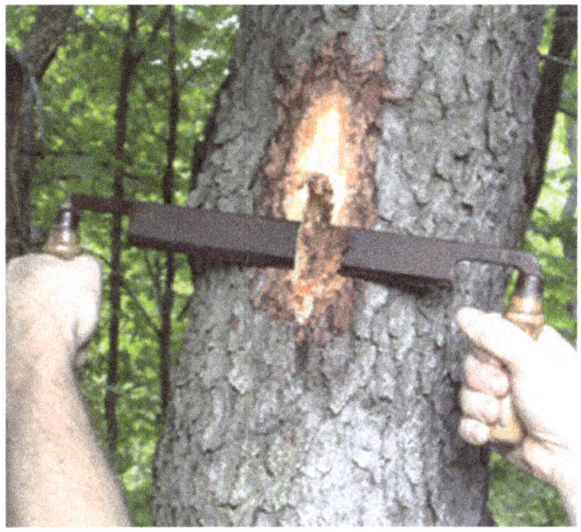

Harvesting tree bark with a two-handled draw knife

Harvesting Seeds and Berries

Many edible berries also possess healing properties and are typically collected when ripe. Elderberries (*Sambucus* spp.) are gathered when they are dark purple, Hawthorn berries (*Crataegus* spp.) are picked when black, and Juniper berries (*Juniperus communis*) should be collected when they are dark blue rather than green. Chaste berries (*Vitex agnus-castus*) are dark shades of purple and emit a strong and pleasant fragrance when they are ready for harvesting. Some seeds are also used medicinally, like those from Burdock (*Arctium* spp.) and Milk Thistle (*Silybum marianum*).

Collect fully mature berries and seeds on a sunny day when they are thoroughly dry. Harvest from the strongest plants to obtain good medicine and good genetic stock for seed planting. Gather clean berries and seedpods so they will not need to be washed. Berries and seeds can be dried or processed immediately while fresh.

When using seeds for medicinal purposes, it is important to separate them from their seedpods and get them as clean and free of debris as possible. An excellent way to separate seeds from their pods is to put the dry seedpods in a paper bag, hold or tie the open end shut, and dislodge the seeds by shaking, pounding, or stomping on the bag. Then turn the bag upside down and open the end that has been closed just enough to allow the seeds to come out without the pods. Once they have been separated from their pods, seeds can go through another cleaning step using screens or wire mesh. Place the seeds on screens that allow them to slip through the spaces without letting larger particles through.

Be sure to utilize seeds not only for making herbal preparations, but also as seed stock for planting. Seeds for planting do not require as much cleaning as those prepared for medicine, but do need be removed from their seedpods. Store seeds in paper bags labeled with the name of the herb and date of collection. Place these in a larger plastic or glass container, which will supply enough air for seed respiration during storage. Keep seeds in a cool, dark, dry area to maintain viable dormancy.

Collecting your own seeds rather than purchasing them saves money and is a great way to increase the size of garden plots. Extra seeds can be given to fellow gardeners or sown in fields and waste areas, making a wonderful contribution to increasing plant populations.

Harvesting Stems

Stems are the transporting structure of plants and generally are not suitable for medicinal use. Most stems are fibrous and lack significant amounts of healing components. It is best to strip the leaves and flowers off the stem in the process called **garbling**. Juicy or succulent stems like those of Chickweed (*Stellaria* spp.) are an exception to this rule and can be used with the rest of the herb for medicine.

Preparation of Plant Parts After Harvesting

Leaves, flowers, bark, and berries should never be washed, so only collect clean samples. Roots will always need to be thoroughly washed with a vegetable scrubber brush or a pressurized water sprayer. When removing dirt, avoid soaking roots for more than a few minutes because they will absorb water, increasing drying time and diluting their medicinal sap and juices. My favorite method is to put the roots on a clean surface outside, or in a large bucket with big drainage holes in the bottom, and use a garden hose with a sprayer to get a forceful stream of water. (Placing roots in a bucket keeps them contained.) This is an efficient method of removing dirt and sand sediments out of even tiny cracks and crevasses in the roots.

The next step after harvesting your medicinal or culinary herbs is deciding whether they will be used fresh as tea, processed into other preparations, or dried and stored for future use. Be sure to either make your medicinal preparations or dry the herbs immediately after harvesting to avoid deterioration and possible mold growth.

Guidelines for Safe and Ethical Harvesting and Wildcrafting

It is more important than ever for people to harvest herbs according to ethical practices of sustainability and promote the continued survival of our medical plants, especially those that are becoming rare and endangered. In a single afternoon, one person can permanently eradicate large areas of very old medicinal plants that have taken Nature many years to establish. Robyn Klein is a researcher who has done excellent work in compiling the age ranges and potential life expectancy of several endangered herbs. Klein discovered that American Ginseng (*Panax quinquefolium*) can live for 50-60 years, Echinacea (*Echinacea angustifolia*) for 17-44 years, Helonias root (*Chamaelirium luteum*) for 30-80 years, Trillium (*Trillium ovatum*) for 70 years, and Yellow Lady's Slipper (*Cypripedium calceolus*) can live between 30-100 years.

If you are fortunate enough to be able to harvest from your own gardens, the issue of eliminating plant species by over-harvesting is not as pressing as in wildcrafting. The following suggestions are specifically intended for wildcrafting, but are also appropriate for harvesting from cultivated gardens:

❖ Use common sense and intuition when harvesting. Conduct research and educate yourself on the current information and uses of the plants you are gathering. Consider the guidance of knowledgeable herbalists, authoritative books, organizations, and other resources. And always be open to following your instincts when interacting with plants. Much is learned by opening *all* of our senses to the subtle aspects of plants – their color, fragrance, texture, and shape – and by experiencing the visions and feelings they elicit from us when we are quiet and paying attention.

❖ Get the owner's permission when wildcrafting on someone else's property.

❖ Harvest or transplant herbs destined for destruction from clear-cutting or land development.

❖ Harvest herbs from areas that are free from pollution and be sure they grow at least 30-40 feet away from roads, railroad tracks, major power lines, and other potentially toxic areas. Avoid farm fields and lawns that have been sprayed with chemicals. If harvesting herbs from your own lawn and gardens, be sure they are organic by avoiding toxic chemicals yourself.

❖ Only harvest plants that grow in abundance. If you find one or two herbs growing alone, without any others of the same species nearby, please leave them so they will be able to reproduce and naturally increase their populations.

❖ Only harvest what you need. No more.

❖ *Never* harvest an entire patch of herbs when wildcrafting. Depending on the size of the patch and scarcity of the plant, take no more than 1/10 to 1/4 of a patch.

❖ When harvesting leaves and flowers, collect no more than 1/4 to 1/3 of the foliage from each plant.

❖ When harvesting roots, propagate the plant by cutting off a piece of the root containing a bud and replanting it.

❖ Be mindful that you are in Nature's garden when wildcrafting or harvesting cultivated herbs. Work with the awareness that you are pruning and thinning the plants to assist in their growth rather than desecrating and ransacking the area. After digging roots, refill the holes and leave the harvested area looking like you found it.

Harvesting in a Conscious Way by Following Native American Traditions

People of all cultures have relied upon the grace and power of the plant kingdom for healing and sustenance of daily life. Our supremely loving and nourishing mother, the Earth, unconditionally and continually provides us with an abundance of medicinal herbs. And so it is especially important to give something back to the Earth when we gather her bounty, whether it is a prayer of gratitude, a silent moment of appreciation, or an offering of Tobacco or cornmeal. Our geographical ancestors, the Native American Indians, understood their close connection and total dependency on the Earth and her plants, and interacted with their environment in a respectful way. Their traditions of gathering and harvesting herbs honored and promoted life, and they serve as sorely needed examples for those who now carelessly take from the earth while leaving pollution and devastation in their wake.

Remember these lessons from our wise ancestors when harvesting and wildcrafting: Plants are like people in that they tend to grow together in communities. Often, one or two plants in a patch will stand out by being taller, larger, or more vibrant than the others. These are considered to be the "grandparents" of the community and, out of respect, these elders should be left undisturbed. Before doing any cutting, select one plant in the patch to stand next to or sit by for a few minutes. Relax. Take a deep breath. Look around at the plants and grasses and trees surrounding you. Feel the Earth under your feet and know she is your ultimate mother. Observe the plant in front of you. Touch it, smell it, get a sense of its presence, feel its essence. Acknowledge the plant as an ally, and speak to it as you would a friend. Greet the plant. Give thanks for its presence and healing gifts, and explain the nature of your needs. Ask the plant to share its wisdom with you. It is good to request its permission to be harvested and ask the plant to provide strong healing medicine for all who will use it. After making your request, be calm. Allow your mind to be quiet. Open your heart to feel into the plant. Then listen and pay attention to what the plant says or to the feelings you receive. I was told the story of a woman who once asked a group of plants for permission to harvest them and they told her "no." Yet she harvested them anyway. As she walked away from the harvest site, she noticed a sign saying that the whole area had been sprayed with chemicals. Then she understood why the plants had refused her request – they were protecting her. A valuable lesson.

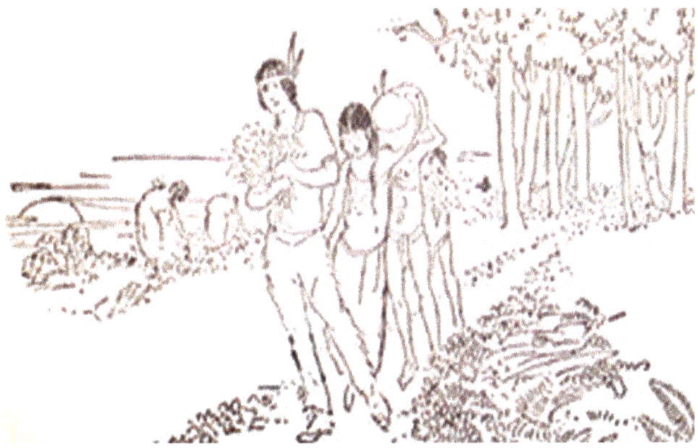

Be open to the possibilities of listening and talking to your plant friends. Over time, your feelings and connection with the plants will develop and deepen, and you can feel their joy in being acknowledged and used in beneficial ways. In the spirit of reciprocity, and to enhance your intentions and awareness of balance, place an offering on the ground next to the plant as a token of gratitude. This can be a pinch of Tobacco, Sage, cornmeal, or any object that has personal value and meaning to you. All this takes a few minutes, and then harvesting can begin.

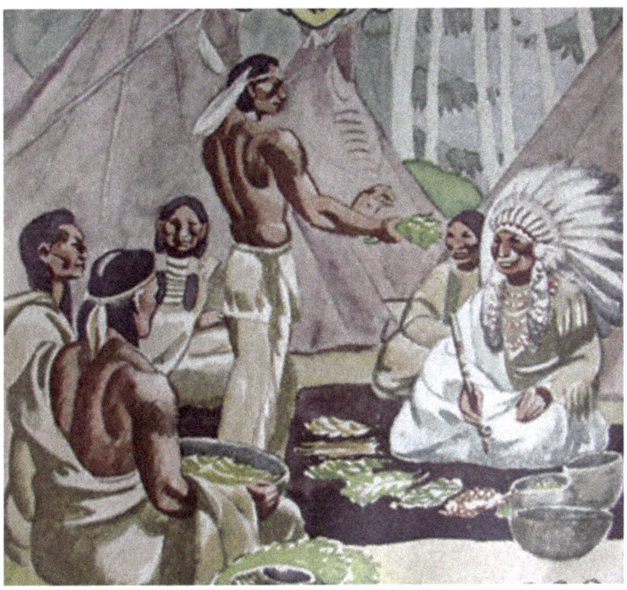

Would you be surprised to know that many long-time gardeners, herbalists, and other plant lovers say that they hear the plants talking to them and teaching them? Do you already hear the voices of the plants? It is not so uncommon. The plants are always delighted when people approach them with good intentions and use their healing gifts. We can be grateful for their amazingly maternal and nurturing presence helping us feel loved, cared for, protected, and healthy. When ingesting herbal medicines that you have harvested and prepared, close your eyes and feel the healing life force of the plant enter your body. Have fun harvesting and wildcrafting the medicinal herbs. Listen to their teachings and use their treasures wisely.

Drying and Storing Medicinal Herbs

Make teas and other medicinal preparations with freshly harvested plants when possible, because they contain peak concentrations of phytochemicals and a vital life force that diminishes during the drying process. If using freshly harvested plants is not feasible, drying is the next best option. Homemade pills and capsules are always made from herbs that have been dried and ground into fine powder.

Before drying or making herbal preparations, freshly harvested plants must go through the **garbling** process, which is the separation of flowers, leaves, or roots from their stems. Garbling is usually done by hand, although large manufacturing operations use machinery to perform this task. Snip flowers off the stems with scissors or pruning shears. Leaves and small flowers can be easily stripped off their stems by grasping the top of the stem with both hands, and with the lower hand, strip away the foliage using a sweeping motion along the entire length of the stem. Wear gloves to save wear and tear on your hands when doing this. Separate roots from stalks with a hatchet, sharp knife or pruning shears, and always clean roots with a strong spray of water and some scrubbing to remove dirt and other extraneous matter. All other plant parts, including the flowers, leaves, seeds, berries and bark, are generally not washed.

General Drying Instructions

Proper drying is crucial to retain the active ingredients of plants for extended periods of time and to avoid the damaging growth of molds. Plants may be dried indoors or outdoors in shady, well-ventilated areas. Attics or sheds with good airflow can be excellent drying locations. Direct sunlight can deteriorate healing substances in herbs and turn their leaves brown or black. Herbs should be dried as quickly as possible to preserve their volatile oils, natural color, aroma, and freshness. Plants will dry out most during daylight hours, but at night they tend to reabsorb moisture, especially when humidity is high. Over time, this constant fluctuation deteriorates herbs, so speedy drying is imperative to preserve the plant's vitality and healing properties. When dried correctly, herbs usually retain their original color and at least some of their fragrance.

The leaves and flowers of most herbs can be dried in 3-4 days. Adequate airflow is essential to speed up the drying process and reduce likelihood of mold growth and deterioration. A fan can be placed in front of herbs to achieve maximum airflow, and works especially well for roots that are more massive and require longer drying time than leaves and flowers. During times of high humidity, fans are particularly helpful in speeding up dehydration, and dehumidifiers may also be placed in drying rooms to remove moisture from the air. People living in arid climates should have no problems drying herbs. Drying plants in humid areas can be more challenging, however, and extra care is needed to ensure enough moisture has been eliminated before storing the finished product. Keep in mind that properly dried leaves and flowers should feel crisp and crumble when they are crushed. Roots should feel hard and snap when broken apart.

Whole plants generally retain 10-20% of their weight as moisture, even after drying. Fresh leaves and flowers typically contain 65-90% water and lose at least ¾ of their weight after drying. Water content of live roots ranges from 45-75%, with about 5%-10% remaining after drying.

There are three basic methods of drying herbs. They may be placed on drying screens, tied and hung in small bundles, or placed inside an oven, dehydrator, or electric heating box.

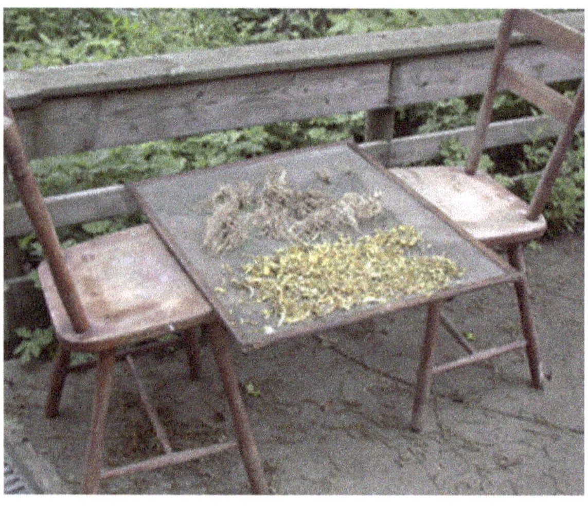

Roots drying on a screen

Drying Screens: Drying herbs on screens is easy and efficient. Old window screens are perfect to use. Metal or fiber mesh screen can also be purchased from hardware stores and made into "screen trays" by stapling or nailing the screen material onto wooden strips to form square or rectangular trays. Ideal sizes for manageable drying trays range from 2-3′ wide by 4-7′ long.

Screens must be placed so air circulates freely through both sides, allowing herbs to receive equal airflow on all their surfaces. Accomplish this by placing screens on the edges of chairs or tables, between sawhorses, or suspended from the ceiling with string attached to their corners. To process large amounts of herbs, make more sophisticated drying racks by assembling multi-layered screens, one above the other, allowing a large quantity of herbs to be dried on a small area of floor space. Spread the plant parts evenly on the screen trays in one layer. Turn the herbs daily to allow uniform drying. Store them as soon as they feel dry.

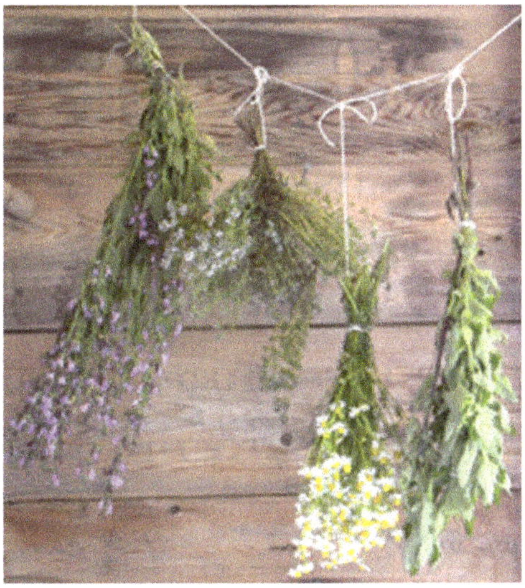

Hanging Bundles: Leaves and flowers can be left on their stalks and tied together with string to make small bundles. Hang the bundles upside down with the flower heads pointing downward and stems pointing up. Be sure not to make the bundles too large or the inner herbs will not dry. After hanging for a few days, bundles may need to be re-arranged for uniform drying. Hang the bundles of herbs from attic rafters and kitchen ceilings, or on a cord that is stretched across a room. The presence of drying herbs hanging from the ceiling is a beautiful and picturesque addition to one's home. Lemon Balm (*Melissa officinalis*), Sage (*Salvia officinalis*), Catnip (*Nepeta cataria*), and Hyssop (*Hyssopus officinalis*) are among the many herbs that hang from my kitchen rafters throughout the spring and summer months. They create a very cozy, earthy feeling as their delightful fragrance and vibrant green colors fill my log cabin.

Artificial Heat: Drying plant parts at a very low temperature in an oven, dehydrator, or electric heating box with interior screen racks works quite well. The temperature must be controlled to stay below 100°F. These appliances are good drying methods because they produce a rapid drying time with minimal heat to preserve the medicinal constituents. The herbs must be watched very closely to prevent over-drying. Excess heat promotes the rapid evaporation of essential oils and induces other detrimental changes in the chemical constituents of the plant. Excessive heat will also dry the outer cellular layers of the plant, causing those cells to harden and seal moisture inside, allowing mold to develop. This can be a particular problem when drying roots, which usually have a thicker mass than leaves. Dehydrating boxes and electric heating boxes often have fans that provide good ventilation and uniform drying.

Drying Tips for Each Part of the Plant

Leaves and flowers are usually removed from their stems to encourage faster drying before they are placed on screens. Large or succulent leaves like Comfrey (*Symphytum officinale*) or Burdock (*Arctium* spp.) and large flowers can be chopped into smaller pieces with a knife to quicken dehydration. Drying leaves and flowers on screens is most efficient in more humid conditions. In dry climates, tying them in bundles with string works well. Large baskets allowing good ventilation are also handy for drying leaves and flowers.

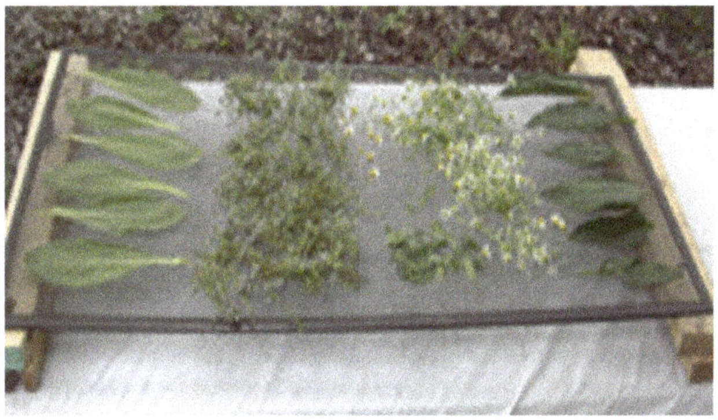

Roots are dried on screens. They can be dried whole or chopped into pieces for increased air contact, reducing drying time and potential for mold growth. Roots may be chopped up with a sharp kitchen knife or a mechanized food processor. Chopping by hand is always the best way to begin, because you can feel the texture of the plant, be more fully immersed in its aroma, and experience greater contact with the plant. Over time, if the quantities of your harvest increase, you may decide to use power tools. Large amounts of roots, leaves, or flowers can be cut into small pieces with an electric garden shredder, which is a great time saver. The quantity of plant parts that would take an hour to chop by hand go through a small shredder in a matter of minutes.

Although chopping whole roots into smaller pieces speeds up drying time, the increased exposure to air also increases the natural process of deterioration. So consider this when deciding how to dry roots. Some roots like Goldenseal (*Hydrastis canadensis*) or American Ginseng (*Panax quinquefolius*) may be dried whole to maintain optimal potency. Using a fan is recommended for drying whole roots because it speeds up the process. Lay the roots on screen trays in one layer and turn them daily for uniform drying. Roots are ready for storage when they feel hard and snap in half when bent.

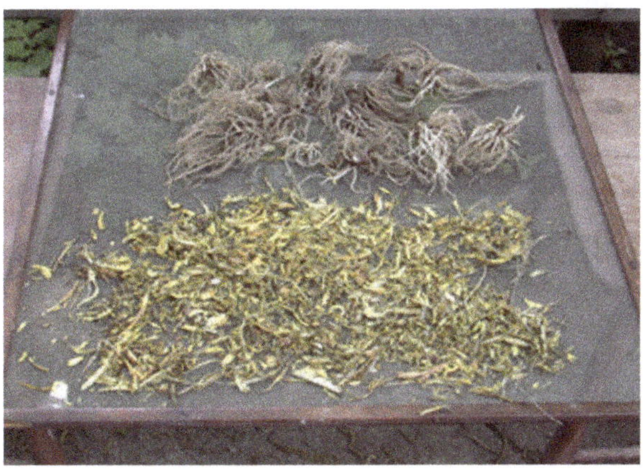

Bulbs may be placed on screens or put in net bags that are hung to dry. Braiding the dried leaves of bulbs is a popular and attractive method of drying and storing Onions and Garlic.

Tree bark is often used fresh but may be cut into small pieces and dried on screen or cardboard. Turn frequently to allow uniform ventilation.

Berries and **seeds** should be dry when they are harvested. To complete the process, place them in an open paper bag or spread them out on newspaper, cardboard or screens, and leave them in a well-ventilated area for a few days.

Always keep a close watch on your herbs during the drying process. Dry them as quickly as possible to retain their freshness and valuable healing properties. Protect them from mice, rats, bats, and other critters that may nibble on them and leave their droppings. If herbs are left out too long to dry, they will collect dust and can reabsorb lots of moisture on humid or rainy days.

Storing Dried Herbs

As soon as herbs are adequately dried, store them in airtight glass or earthenware containers. Be sure to label all containers with the name of the herb and the date it was harvested. Labeling is imperative since herbs can be difficult to identify after they are dry. Remember that exposure to heat, moisture, and air promotes the growth of bacteria and mold, and also stimulates enzyme activity in the plant itself, leading to deterioration. Store herbs away from heat and sunlight in a shaded or dark area that stays relatively cool. Always check the dried herbs 24 and 48 hours after bottling them in their storage containers to be sure the moisture was adequately removed. Dry them again if moisture is detected. If you skip this step, you may open your container at a later time and be disappointed to find a moldy pile of leaves or roots. It is convenient and aesthetically pleasing to have your storage jars of herbs neatly arranged in your medicine chest, cabinet, or closet. But be sure not to hide them away where you may forget about them.

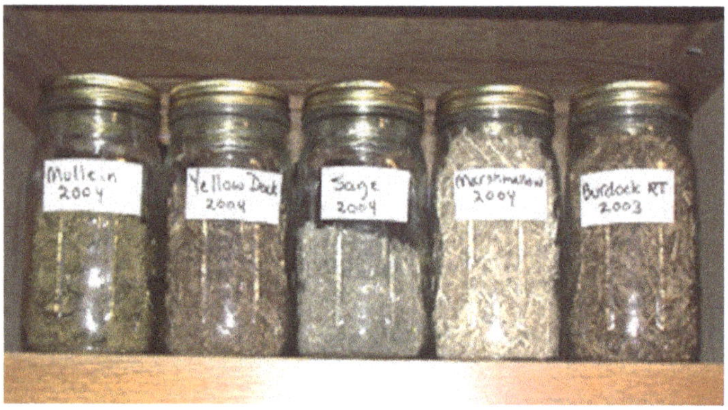

Dried herbs can also be placed in plastic bags and stored in a refrigerator or freezer. Freezing works especially well to retain freshness and extend shelf life.

If seeds are being saved for planting rather than for medicinal purposes, store them in small paper bags or mailing envelopes, and place these inside a larger plastic or glass container to keep out mice and other critters. Put these containers in a cool, dark area for optimal storage.

The Shelf Life of Dried Herbs

Remember that dried herbs slowly begin to deteriorate and lose their potency after being harvested. The amount of time in which they maintain effective biological activity is referred to as their "shelf life." Many herbal preparations on the commercial market provide their shelf life, also known as the expiration date, on their labels. Always check the expiration date when purchasing herbs.

The standard shelf life of dried leaves and flowers is 6 months to 2 years. During that length of time, they start to deteriorate and lose their healing ability. Roots last longer with a shelf life of 2-4 years. To preserve optimal potency, remember that grinding herbs into powder increases damaging oxidation in air and shortens their shelf life, so grind herbs immediately before use. Shelf life is greatly extended when herbs are stored in the freezer after drying.

Drying herbs is an art that is learned and mastered over time with experience. Have fun with this aspect of herbalism, and enjoy making delicious teas and medicinal preparations with your preserved herbs!

Creating Herbal Preparations

Knowing how to create your own medicines from the bounty of Nature is wonderfully gratifying. Imagine the empowering experience as the fruit of your labor culminates in the finished salve, tincture, or cup of tea! A wide variety of herbal preparations can be produced from freshly harvested or dried herbs. This section discusses the most popular preparations and includes teas, tinctures, salves, oils, tablets, capsules, syrups, poultices, liniments, fomentations, compresses, suppositories, douches, enemas, eyewashes, and nasal sprays. Step-by-step instructions describe how to make these herbal remedies in simple ways, allowing you to create your own herbal pharmacy in your kitchen. Most herbalists follow basic principles and recipes in formulating herbal preparations, but there is also opportunity for variation.

The production of quality herbal medicine containing maximum potency and biological activity depends on many variables starting at the level of the grower or wildcrafter. Strong, healthy plants require specific types of soil, good drainage, and adequate amounts of moisture and sunlight. Correct cultivation practices, methods of harvesting, handling, processing, drying, and storing all directly influence the quantity and quality of medicinal phytochemicals in plants. When we grow the herbs ourselves and create our own medicines, we have considerably more control over these variables. All the time, attention, nourishment, and care that we give to plants creates a strong alchemy that further enhances their healing qualities. Almost anyone who has grown and processed his or her own herbal medicines will verify this truth!

Creating our own herbal pharmacy is fun, exciting, and economically worthwhile. It inevitably draws us into a lifestyle that revolves around Nature and the seasons. When medicines come directly from the earth and from our own labor, their value extends beyond the potency of their chemical components or their monetary worth. Perhaps their greatest healing gift is how they help us to connect with, and feel nurtured by, our supreme and unconditional mother, the Earth herself! So enjoy making your herbal remedies and filling your medicine cabinet with Nature's treasures. Friends usually love homemade products, so your herbal preparations also make wonderful and valued gifts.

Choosing Between Fresh or Dried Herbs When Making Preparations

Whenever possible, make herbal preparations with fresh plant material that you gather yourself. Compared to dried and aged herbs purchased from stores, freshly harvested plants still possess their life force and vitality, which produce exceptionally potent medicinal preparations. These are noticeably more effective than those made with dried plants, for several reasons. Firstly, fresh herbs that have been correctly harvested contain the highest concentrations of volatile oils, resins, and other medicinally active phytochemicals. For a short time after being harvested, plants maintain their peak of potency, retaining their vital life force and full flavor and aroma. When herbs dry and begin to age, they naturally deteriorate and their medicinal properties eventually diminish over time.

Another major difference between fresh and dried herbs is their water content. Fresh herbs generally contain about 80% water, while dried herbs contain only 10-20% water. Although phytochemicals in dried herbs are not quite as potent, they are more concentrated by weight because dried herbs contain less water. There are a few ways to compensate for this difference in water volume. When preparing a cup of herbal tea, for example, use 2-3 times as much fresh herb as you would dry. When making tinctures from freshly harvested herbs, add less water and more alcohol to compensate for the water naturally occurring in the plants. Freshly harvested herbs can also be chopped into small pieces and allowed to dry for several hours to reduce their water content before being processed into different preparations. This pre-drying immediately before processing is highly recommended when making tinctures and salves. It will increase the potency of the preparation while the herbs still retain their full vitality, flavor, and aroma.

The vast majority of tinctures, salves, pills, capsules, and other herbal preparations on the market are made from herbs that have been dried and stored for a length of time. This is because most manufacturers typically buy herbs from growers located some distance away. In order to be shipped to the manufacturing companies, plants must be thoroughly dried or they will decompose quickly and be useless. There are a few companies, however, that are owned and operated by people who cultivate, harvest, and immediately process the plants into finished products ready for sale, all in the same location. This is the ideal situation because the maximum concentration of medicinal phytochemicals and vital life force of the plants are retained. When purchasing herbs, always try to buy from reputable companies that handle the herbs from cultivation to processing in order to get the best quality product.

Obviously, cultivating your own herbs and processing them while they are still fresh provides the best opportunity to ensure potent healing. It is fun and enlightening to participate in the entire process from cultivation to packaging, and to experience the magic of using herbal medicines that you and Nature have co-created.

Basic Types of Herbal Preparations

Herbal preparations can be divided into four major categories: those that are dried, water-based, alcohol-based, and oil-based. For the sake of simplification and organization, all the different types of herbal preparations mentioned in this chapter are listed under these four primary categories.

Dried herbs can be stored for extended periods of time and are used in many preparations, including teas, powders, pills, capsules, poultices, salves, and tinctures. Dried leaves and flowers generally last 6 months to 2 years before their potency expires. Roots and bark have a longer shelf life of 2-4 years. Refrigerating or freezing dried herbs helps retain their potency and greatly prolongs shelf life.

Water-based herbal medicines include teas, cough syrups, poultices, compresses, fomentations, baths, eyewashes, suppositories, douches, and enemas. These are made by extracting the healing components from herbs with boiling water. Water-based preparations generally spoil within a few days and must be prepared at, or close to, the time of use. Refrigerating or freezing water-based preparations extends their shelf life.

Teas are digested faster than pills and capsules because they are readily absorbed through the stomach and intestines. Teas are weaker than tinctures, fluid extracts, and the most concentrated preparation, solid extracts. A great benefit of drinking tea is that the herb has direct contact with the tissues in the mouth, throat, stomach, and intestines and can be especially effective in treating problems in these areas. For instance, drinking a cup of Sage tea is more effective in relieving a sore throat than taking a capsule or pill because as the tea is swallowed, it soothes and coats the lining of the throat to ease pain and eliminate bacteria. In the same way, teas are excellent for healing ulcers or inflammation in the stomach and intestines because they have direct contact with these tissues.

Alcohol-based preparations include tinctures, extracts, and liniments. These are processed by soaking or macerating herbs in alcohol to extract their chemical constituents. Processing herbs in alcohol is the best way to preserve their medicinal properties for long periods of time. The alcohol content of tinctures contributes to their long shelf life by preventing the growth of molds and bacteria, and when stored in dark, cool places, tinctures can remain potent indefinitely. Tinctures are very easy to digest and can be fast-acting because alcohol is absorbed directly from the stomach lining.

Oil-based preparations include infused oils and salves. Herbal oils and salves are prepared by baking herbs in oil for several hours to extract their medicinal properties. Oil-based products are used for external healing and, depending on their ingredients, are generally soothing and moisturizing to the skin and mucous membranes. Oils and salves usually maintain freshness for 1-3 years before rancidity starts, which can be detected by its unpleasant, stale odor. Refrigerating or keeping oils and salves in cool areas out of direct light helps maintain freshness and delays rancidity.

Understanding the Process of Herbal Extraction

When creating medicinal preparations, it is important to understand the basic process of extracting chemical constituents from plants in order to obtain optimal potency in the finished products. One plant can contain hundreds of phytochemicals that synergistically exert biological and medicinal effects in the body. Obtaining the maximum quantity and quality of these phytochemicals is always the goal of extraction. The art of extracting, or drawing these chemical components from plant material, follows basic principles.

Herbal extraction occurs by osmosis, the force that pulls phytochemicals from plants into fluid extracts.

Herbal extraction occurs by the process of **osmosis**, which involves the natural tendency for elements to seek balance or equilibrium with each other. Osmosis is the force that draws solvents (particles dissolved in fluids) from areas of greater concentration to areas of lesser concentration until equilibrium has been obtained. For example, imagine that in a gallon container of water divided in half by a permeable filter, two tablespoons of salt are stirred into the water on one side of the filter. Due to osmosis, the salt naturally starts moving through the filter from the side containing high concentrations of salt to the side without any salt. The movement created by this osmotic pull continues until the water on each side of the filter contains one tablespoon of dissolved salt. At this point, the concentration of salt has become equalized on both sides, and osmotic movement is complete and comes to a halt.

When making plant medicines, remember that the process of osmosis is the force that extracts medicinal phytochemicals from herbs. The plant material is called the **marc** and is chopped or ground into small pieces. The marc, containing high concentrations of phytochemicals, is placed in a liquid solvent called the **menstruum**, which contains low concentrations of chemical constituents. The process of osmosis automatically begins to pull the phytochemicals out of the plant material into the liquid. This movement continues until concentrations of phytochemicals in the plant material are equal to their concentration in the liquid menstruum. When this equilibrium has been achieved, herbal extraction is complete.

The color of the liquid solvent changes as osmosis progresses. When making tea, phytochemicals are pulled out of herbs into boiling water, typically turning the water various shades of brown or green. Green leafy herbs, baked to create oils and salves, will turn olive oil from pale yellow to different shades of green. When preparing tinctures, crystal clear grain alcohol and vodka quickly turn dark with the addition of plant material.

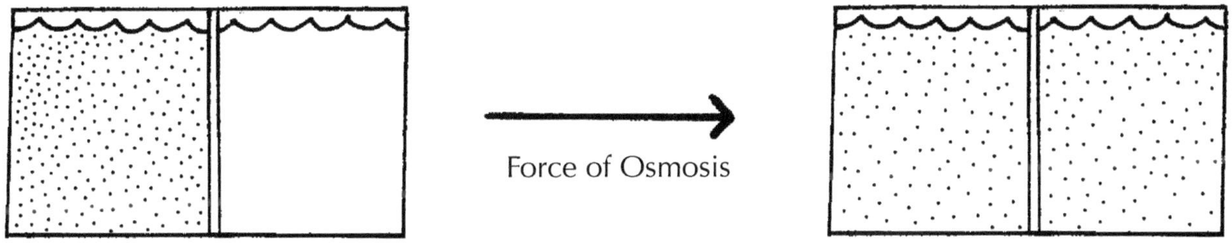

A gallon of water divided by a filter.
The left side contains 2 tablespoons
of salt (represented by dots).
The right side is plain water.

Equilibrium is achieved by the
process of osmosis
when both sides contain
equal amounts of salt

Here are several ways to expedite and maximize the process of osmosis to provide the best extraction of medicinal phytochemicals:

1. It is important to chop or grind herbs into small pieces. This breaks up the cellular structure of plants to allow greater release of their phytochemicals. It also provides the greatest amount of surface area for exposure to the liquid solvents.

2. The liquid solvents must be as pure as possible. Purity means that the solvents contain very few chemical particles. This allows the greatest amount of osmotic pull from an area of dense concentration (the plant material) to an area of sparse concentration (the liquid solvent). For example, distilled water is a much better solvent than tap water or mineral water because it contains fewer particles. 190-proof grain alcohol is a better solvent than 90-proof gin or vodka because grain alcohol is nearly pure alcohol and does not contain many other chemical particles.

3. Heat greatly enhances osmosis when using water or oil as the liquid solvents. Heat increases the movement of molecules in water and oil. This softens and breaks up plant material, forcing a faster flow of phytochemicals out of plant cells into the liquid. When extracting phytochemicals for tea, boiling water is more efficient than simply soaking herbs in cold water. Exceptions to this general rule exist for mucilaginous herbs like Comfrey (*Symphytum officinale*), Slippery Elm (*Ulmus rubra*), Solomon's Seal root (*Polygonatum* spp.), Marshmallow root (*Althaea officinalis*), Plantain (*Plantago* spp.), and Chickweed (*Stellaria* spp.). Their highly water-soluble mucilage dissolves very well in lukewarm water. When making oil preparations, extraction is greater in hot oils than in cold. Keep in mind that heat does denature herbs and excessive amounts should be avoided. Only use as much heat for processing herbs as is needed. One major advantage of preserving herbs with alcohol is that heat is not required for extraction.

4. Allow ample time for complete extraction. Teas made from leaves and flowers typically require 5-30 minutes to steep (soak) in boiled water for extraction. **Sun tea** is made by putting leaves and flowers in a glass jar of warm water and placing it in the sun to heat up for several hours. Roots and bark require more heat to extract phytochemicals from their tough, hard surfaces and must be gently boiled (simmered) for 10-30 minutes. Hot oil will extract medicinal constituents from herbs after baking in a low-heat oven for 2-3 hours. Herbs will also extract into warm oils that are placed in full sun for 7-10 days, although caution must be taken to watch for mold growth. Alcohol tinctures are generally processed for 4-5 weeks to ensure complete extraction, especially when tincturing roots, which are more dense than leaves and flowers.

5. Squeeze or press as much liquid out of the plant material as possible during the decanting process when the plant material (the marc) is separated from the liquid solvents (the menstruum). Remember that osmosis is complete when there is an equal concentration of phytochemicals in the plant material as in the liquid solvent. This means that 50% still remains in the plant material. Good methods of squeezing or pressing the marc are essential for more complete extraction of all the phytochemicals.

Squeezing by hand using a lot of force works fairly well for leaves and flowers, but is not effective for roots. Juicing machines that operate by centrifugal force are wonderful for extracting small volumes, while presses are convenient for larger amounts of plant material.

Dried Herbal Preparations: Powders, Pills, and Capsules

After herbs are dried, they can be stored for future use in preparing many different herbal remedies. Dried herbs store well in airtight containers placed in cool, dark places and have a shelf life of up to 4 years depending on the plant part. Delicate flowers deteriorate faster than thick, dense roots and bark. When freshly harvested herbs are not available, dried herbs can be used to make teas, infused oils, alcohol tinctures, poultices, washes, douches, enemas, and other herbal products. Plant material must always be thoroughly dry in order to be made into powders, capsules, and pills.

Powders

Powders are prepared from herbs that have been dried and ground into fine particles. The powder can then be made into pills, put into gelatin capsules, or used for other preparations like teas, salves, poultices, or tinctures. Very fine powders make wonderful teas because they dissolve into the water and are completely consumed without any waste.

Small coffee bean grinders do an excellent job of making fine powders from dried plant parts, including hard roots and seeds. Small grinders are inexpensive and available at discount stores. Larger commercial coffee bean grinders can be helpful for processing greater quantities of herbs. Keep in mind that powders deteriorate and lose their potency faster than whole plants because the tiny, ground-up particles have much greater exposure to air, which causes them to oxidize (combine with oxygen). For this reason, it is best to grind herbs into powder just before using them. The shelf life of herbal powders is 3-12 months. To maintain maximum freshness, they should be stored in airtight glass containers in a dark, cool location. Refrigerating or freezing powders will extend their shelf life considerably. In this case, place the freshly ground powder into a small plastic bag, remove the air from the bag, and seal it securely to reduce oxidation.

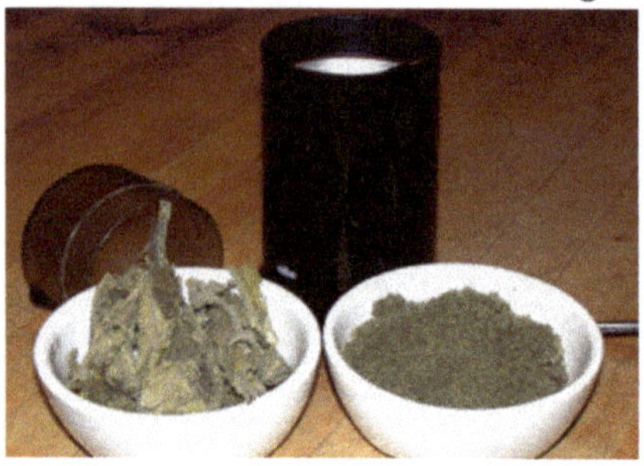

Grinding herbs into powder

Capsules

Herb powders can be inserted into gelatin capsules and conveniently swallowed. One major advantage of both pills and capsules is their ability to make bitter and not-so-pleasant-tasting herbs much easier to take. Goldenseal (*Hydrastis canadensis*) is an example of a bitter herb that most people prefer to consume in capsules rather than drinking as a cup of bitter tea. Pills and capsules are also convenient to use when traveling. Capsules are usually easy to digest because the powder is released for fast absorption as soon as the capsule dissolves in the stomach. Capsules and pills should always be taken with water or tea. Do not take herbs with alcohol, soda, coffee, or citrus juices because the pH balance and chemistry of the herbs can be altered. It is best to ingest herbal capsules and pills on a fairly empty stomach for better absorption.

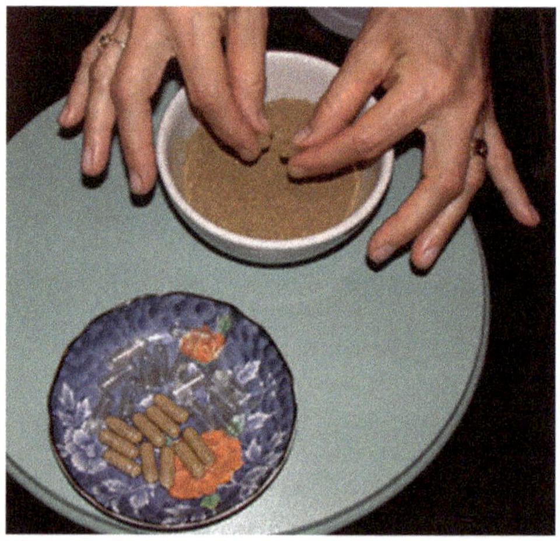

Making herbal capsules at home is easy and less time consuming than making pills. Gelatin capsules (regular or vegetarian) can be purchased from most health food stores. There are a variety of capsule sizes, but the most common are the small "0" size for children or adults who have a difficult time swallowing pills, and the larger "00" size for regular adult use. A well-packed "00" size capsule holds about ½ teaspoon of powdered herb.

Place the pulverized herb in a shallow bowl and pack it into the capsule by hand. Simply separate the two parts of the capsule, holding one part in each hand, and push them through the powdered herb toward each other to compress the powder, forcing the capsules to fill. When you have packed them as full as possible, fit the two halves of the capsule together tightly to close it. Handy plastic trays used for this purpose are available in many health food stores. Store your capsules filled with powdered herb in an airtight glass jar in a dark, cool place. Or put them in a plastic bag and store them in a refrigerator or freezer to extend their freshness and potency. Always label the storage container with the date and name of the herb. Pills and capsules have a shelf life of 1-3 years, so keep this in mind when making your own preparations. And when purchasing dried herbs, always remember to look at the label for expiration dates.

Pills

Herbal pills and tablets are convenient to use and are made in a variety of ways. Basically, pills are powdered herbs pressed into a compact form. They can be made by hand or produced commercially with machinery and more advanced technology. One commercial production method is to boil the herb in water until it is reduced to a pasty gruel. This paste is scraped off the bottom of the pan, combined with several additives, rolled into balls, and dried. Binding agents like natural acacia gum keep the herbs compacted into pill form and prevent crumbling. Flowing agents are added to prevent stickiness, which allows the pills to flow through the machinery smoothly without getting stuck. Disintegrating agents are added to ensure fast digestion. And filling agents are used to make the pill a uniform shape and size. Finally, the pill is often glazed with clear vegetable shellac or, unfortunately, some manufacturers use colorful chemical dyes or sugar to coat the outer surface.

Making herbal pills by hand is fun and easy! Additives used for the commercial production of pills are unnecessary when making your own. Pills can be made with flowers, leaves, or roots. A wide variety of herbs can be used alone or combined to make pills for various healing purposes. After deciding which herbs to use, chop them into small pieces that are then dried and ground into a fine powder. Cook the powder in water for a couple minutes to break down the cellular fibers, making them easier to digest. Cooking also kills any bacteria and mold on the plants.

Instructions for Making Herbal Pills

Put powdered herbs in a stainless steel cooking pan. Cover them with a little water and simmer very gently until they are reduced to a thick, pulpy mash. Cover with water slowly – an excess will have to be boiled off, and the herbs should not cook for more than 4-5 minutes. At the same time, be sure there is enough water to prevent burning. When cooking is complete, allow the pulpy mash to cool. If you are making cough drops or throat lozenges, add honey or maple syrup to make bitter herbs more palatable, especially for children. One drop of essential oil such as Peppermint (*Mentha x piperita*) or Wintergreen (*Gaultheria procumbens*) can be added for flavoring, but do not exceed this amount since essential oils are extremely strong. Very finely powdered Marshmallow root (*Althaea officinalis*) and psyllium powder (*Plantago ovata*) are excellent thickeners and sticky binders for hand-made pills, and small amounts of either herb can be slowly added to your mix as it cools and thickens. The mucilaginous qualities of Marshmallow root and Psyllium are ideal for soothing and coating inflamed sore throats, stomachs and intestinal tracts, so they are a welcome addition to any pill.

Next, form pills by rolling a pinch of the pasty mash between the palms of your hands. Roll it into tightly compacted little balls small enough for easy swallowing and fast drying. In the same way bakers use flour to make bread dough more manageable and prevent sticking, you can dust your palms with powdered Marshmallow root or Psyllium to make rolling the pills easier.

Place the herb balls on a flat surface or cookie sheet to dry. They can be dried in an oven with very low heat (100-120°F) or placed in a shady, well-ventilated area. Drying pills close to a radiator or wood stove works well. Some herbalists dry pills in the sun, although this can have a deteriorating effect. Experiment to decide which method works best for you.

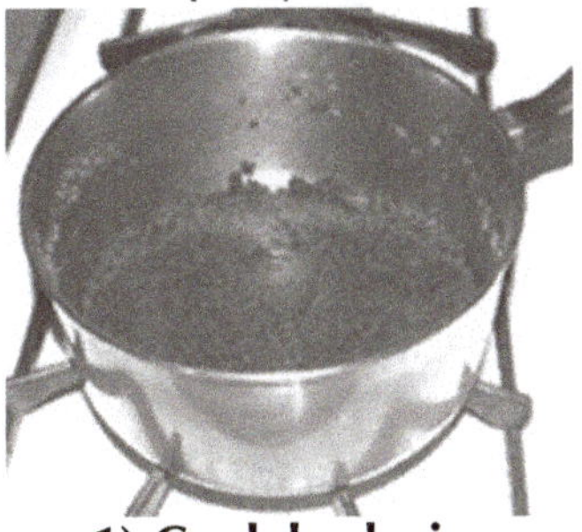

1) Cook herbs in pan to make mash

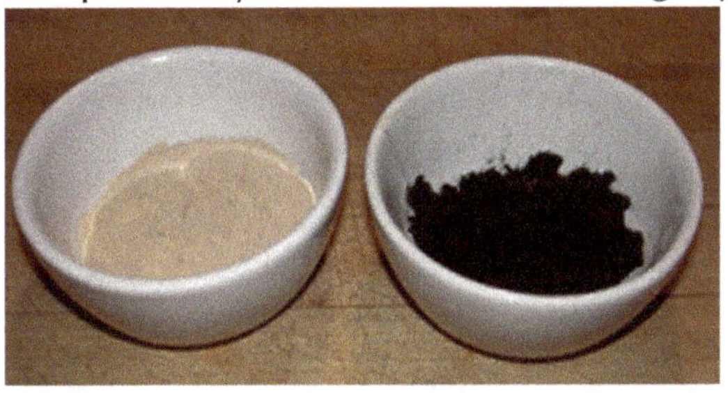

2) White powdered Marshmallow root and dark herbal mash

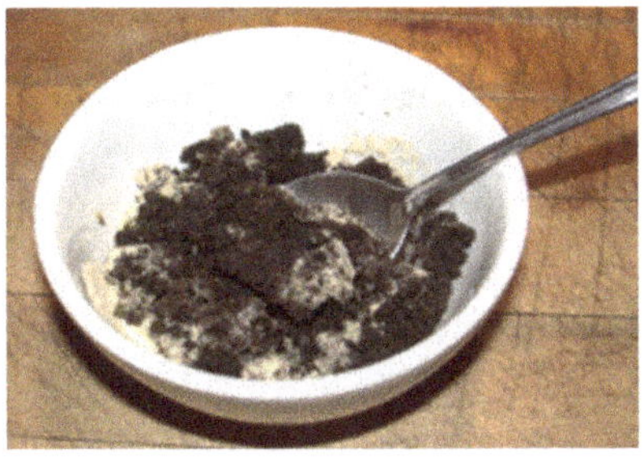

3) Mix mash and Marshmallow root

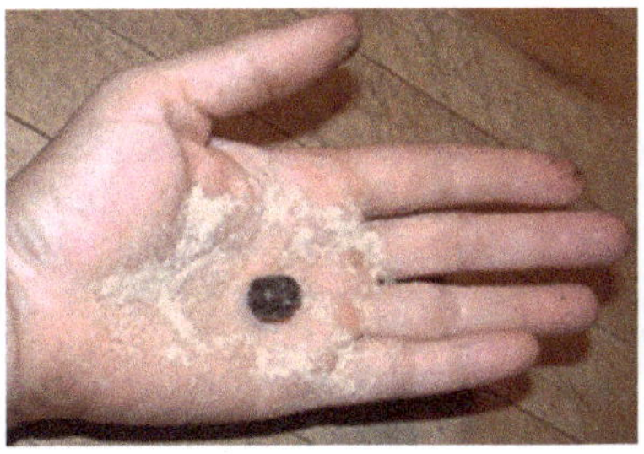

4) Roll mixture into balls

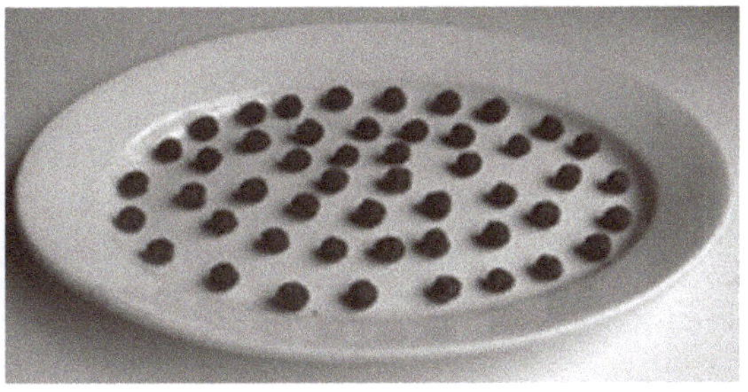

5) Finished pills ready to dry

When thoroughly dry, place the pills in an airtight glass jar labeled with the name of the herbs and date, and store them in a cool, dark place. It is a good idea to recheck the pills after the first 24-48 hours to be sure that all the moisture was removed. Break a few of the largest pills in half to be sure that they are completely dry. Mold will grow on moist pills. If any mold or moisture is present, immediately re-dry your pills in a low-heated oven. If caught in time, you will probably be able to save your herb pills. Pills may be stored in the freezer, which extends shelf-life and eliminates moisture or mold concerns.

An Alternate Method for Making Herbal Pills

This method is identical to the previous one except that the cooking step to eliminate potential bacteria or mold is skipped. Put the powdered herbs in a bowl and add enough water, honey, or maple syrup to make a very thick, sticky paste. Mix and knead the herbal brew to thoroughly combine the ingredients. Add enough powdered Marshmallow root or Psyllium powder to obtain the desired thickness. Roll the paste into pills and dry them.

Water-based herb pills dry much faster than honey or syrup-based pills, usually within 1-2 days if the weather is dry. Pills made with honey, maple syrup, or glycerin can take a couple of days to dry around a wood stove or in a drying box, or up to 5-7 days to dry in the shade.

Water-Based Preparations:
Tea, Syrup, Poultice, Fomentation, Compress, Wash, Flower Essence, Eyewash, Nasal Spray, Douche, Enema, and Suppository

Tea

For thousands of years, people around the globe have been enjoying the delicious flavors and superb healing qualities of herbal teas. A warm, soothing cup of tasty tea offers a great way to start and end each day. Drinking herbal tea contributes to a healthy diet and lifestyle. Teas contain minerals, vitamins, and many phytochemicals that are nourishing as well as healing. Pleasant-tasting herbal teas provide smart alternatives to soda pop and coffee, which leach calcium and other minerals out of the body due to their acidic chemistry. Mothers are encouraged to give their children mild herbal teas that taste good like Peppermint (*Mentha x piperita*), Catnip (*Nepeta cataria*), Chamomile (*Matricaria recutita*), or Lemon Balm (*Melissa officinalis*) instead of soda pop and sugary fruit juices that promote tooth decay, sugar craving, and blood sugar imbalances.

Teas can be created from either freshly harvested or dried herbs. If you are fortunate enough to have herbs growing nearby, take advantage of harvesting this fresh bounty. Most herbs in North America, with some exceptions, are fine to use fresh for teas and have a stronger potency and flavor than dried herbs. Use twice as much fresh herb as dried when making tea. **Mucilaginous herbs** like Slippery Elm, Marshmallow root, and Chickweed have a moist and slippery texture and are most effective when prepared as tea because water dissolves and holds their medicinal mucilage better than alcohol extracts.

Infusions and decoctions are the two basic types of teas. Both are made with boiling water, which is the menstruum that extracts the active ingredients from the plant. Dried plants are powdered or crumbled into small pieces to allow for optimal extraction. Fresh herbs are chopped into small pieces. Allow your taste buds and knowledge about each herb guide you when deciding the proportions of herbs to use in your teas. When making infusion teas from pre-packaged tea bags, it is easy to make one cup at a time. But when using bulk herbs to brew your tea, it is more efficient to make a large batch to drink over a few days. Large amounts of infusion and decoction teas can be prepared in a big pot and kept in the refrigerator for no longer than 3-4 days. Teas can also be poured into plastic bags or containers and stored in the freezer to last several months.

Infusion teas are prepared by steeping (soaking) leaves and flowers in boiling hot water. **Tisane** is another name for infusion teas used as tasty beverages or medicinal remedies. The standard method of making infusions is to steep 1-2 teaspoons of dried leaves or flowers in 1 cup of boiled water. For freshly harvested herbs still containing moisture, use 2-4 teaspoons in 1 cup of water. More potent medicinal infusions are made using greater amounts of herbs, often up to ½-1 ounce of leaves or flowers to a pint of water. Teas may be prepared using only one herb or a blend of several.

Begin by chopping the herb or herbs into small pieces. Put the desired amount of water in a stainless steel pan and bring it to a boil. Turn off the heat, add the herb, stir, and let it steep for 5-30 minutes depending on the herb. Cover the pan with a lid while the herbs steep to prevent loss of volatile oils. When steeping is complete, pour the tea into a cup while straining off the leaves and flowers. Be sure to squeeze the remaining water out of the plant material for more complete extraction of phytochemicals. A little sweetener and milk may be added to the tea to enhance its flavors.

One-quart glass canning jars are convenient for making larger amounts of infusion. Put the desired amount of herbs in the quart jar, pour boiling hot water over them, cover with a lid, and allow the brew to steep. Canning jars will not crack or break when boiling water is poured into them.

The length of steeping time for infusions depends on the herbs being prepared. Some herbs like Stinging Nettle (*Urtica dioica*) and Alfalfa (*Medicago sativa*) need more time for full extraction of their healing properties, and can be steeped for a few hours or overnight. Other teas like Fenugreek (*Trigonella foenum-graecum*) taste delicious after only 3-4 minutes of steeping, but become increasingly bitter if steeped for longer periods. Green and Black teas (*Camellia sinensis*) containing tannins become bitter and astringent with longer steeping times.

Cold water infusions are made by adding leaves and flowers to cold water and letting them soak for at least 1 hour or as long as 12 hours. This is not the best method for most herbs since it extracts only small amounts of minerals, alkaloids, and other important healing components. Cold-water infusions are primarily used for herbs with delicate volatile oils like the Mints and Lemon Grass. **Mucilaginous herbs** also extract better in lukewarm water. **Sun tea** is a form of cold-water infusion in which herbs are placed in a glass jar, covered with water, and placed in the sun to brew for several hours.

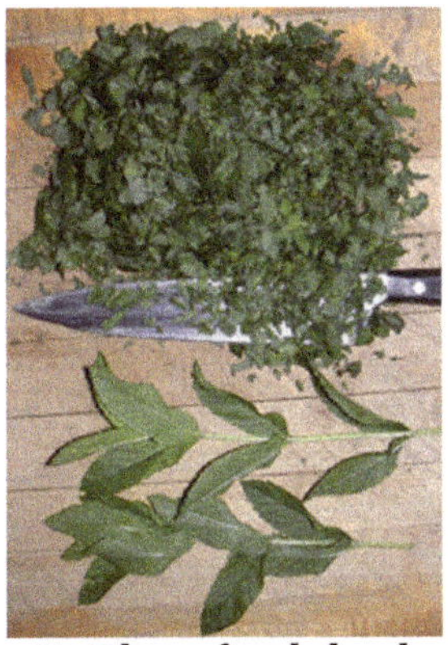

1) Chop fresh herb into small pieces

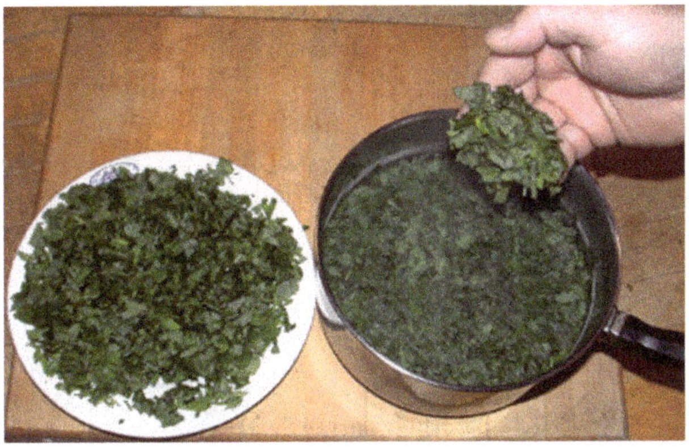

2) Add chopped herb to boiling hot water, cover with a lid, and steep

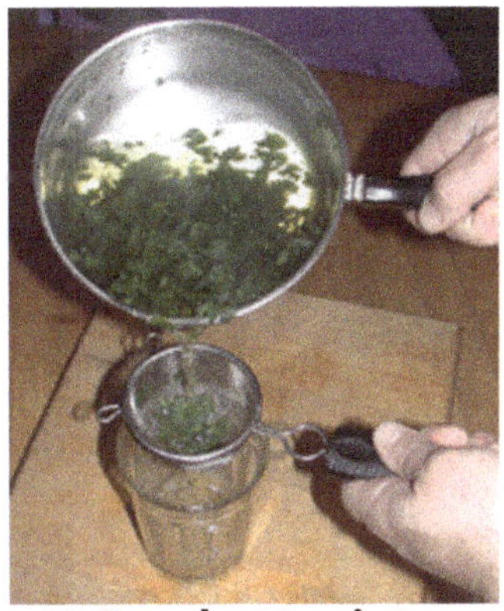

3) Pour hot tea into a cup through a strainer

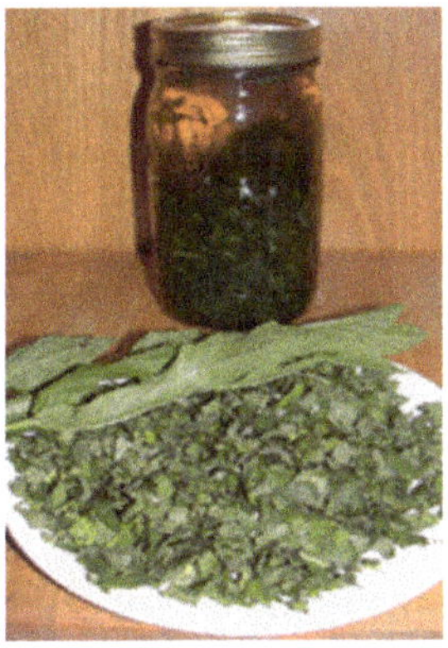

4) Quart jar of herbs steeping in boiled water

Decoction teas are prepared by chopping or pounding fresh bark, roots, twigs, seeds, or nuts into small pieces and gently boiling them in water. Dried parts can be ground into powder and boiled. Compared to softer leaves and flowers, these dense and tough plant parts require more heat and longer boiling time to extract their medicinal properties. They should be very gently boiled at no more than a simmer to allow for extraction of their medicinal components, but not enough to denature or damage them. Use your intuition and experiment in deciding how long to simmer tough plant parts. Some roots like Goldenseal (*Hydrastis canadensis*), Burdock (*Arctium* spp.), and Valerian (*Valeriana officinalis*) contain delicate essential oils that are destroyed by excessive heat. Slippery Elm bark (*Ulmus rubra*), Comfrey (*Symphytum officinale*), and Marshmallow (*Althaea officinalis*) roots contain soothing and healing mucilage that is destroyed by high temperatures, and should be steeped for several hours or overnight in warm water rather than simmered. Many roots like Sassafras, Astragalus, Dandelion, Echinacea, Ginger, Ginseng, and Licorice can be simmered for 20-40 minutes for extraction. Whole roots or large pieces of bark need longer simmering time, from 1-2 hours. Soaking dense plant material in water for up to 12 hours helps soften them before any cooking actually begins and is recommended. Chopping herbs into very small pieces or grinding them into powder greatly enhances extraction capacity and reduces the required length of boiling time.

Weak decoction teas are made by simmering 1-2 teaspoons of the herb in 1 cup of water. Strong decoctions can contain as much as an ounce of herb in 1 pint of water. Boil the herbs at a gentle simmer for the appropriate time in a stainless steel pot covered with a lid to prevent the loss of valuable oils and resins. The longer the decoction simmers, the stronger and more concentrated it becomes. Longer cooking times for decoctions typically reduce the final amount of water to ¼-½ of its original volume. Cool the tea for 20-30 minutes, strain, and drink. For a more potent tea, allow the decoction to steep for several hours or overnight before straining and drinking.

Extra Suggestions for Preparing Herbal Teas

Herbs for preparing teas can be harvested and used fresh or dried. When purchased from stores, bulk herbs are always less expensive than pre-packaged.

Different herbs blend well to make tasty teas. Explore different flavored herbs and decide which combinations you enjoy. There are also many excellent herbal combinations packaged in tea bags that are sold commercially.

If you want to make tea with a combination of roots, leaves and flowers, start by simmering the roots. Then turn the heat off and add the leaves or flowers to steep. In this way, several herbs may be prepared together in one pot.

A small amount of honey, maple syrup, or other natural sweetener can be added to bitter or less-than-pleasant-tasting teas to entice children and adults with sensitive palates. Soy milk, almond milk, coconut milk, rice milk, or dairy milk can also enhance flavor and add creaminess to the tea.

Herbs should be prepared in glass, enamel, or stainless steel containers. Do not use aluminum or iron cookware due to aluminum toxicity and questionable chemical interactions between metals and herbs.

Always cover pans with a lid when making teas to prevent the escape of essential oils and steam.

Do not use microwave ovens when preparing herbs. Research is still pending on the questionable safety of microwaves and their damaging effects on nutrients and other phytochemicals.

Syrups

Syrups are created by combining a strong brew of herbal tea with large amounts of sugar. Sugars improve the flavor of bitter herbs. Since syrups tend to be tasty, they can be valuable herbal preparations for children. Depending on the herbs they contain, syrups can be soothing and healing for inflamed and irritated tissues, sore throats, coughs, and gastrointestinal problems. Refer to **"Index of Health Issues and Herbal Recommendations"** in Section Three for listings of appropriate herbs to make syrups to address your needs.

Sugar is also a preservative, and syrups must contain at least 65% sugar to avoid spoiling when they are stored at room temperature. Refined sugar is the sweetener most commonly used in syrups. Glycerin is sometimes used and is available in drug stores and some health food stores. The best alternatives to these refined sugars are honey and maple syrup because they are naturally occurring sugars. For children younger than 3 years old, do not use honey unless it is thoroughly cooked due to the possibility of botulism.

The main drawback of syrup, however, is the large amount of sweetener it contains. Whether natural or refined, excessive amounts of sugars can cause health problems such as diabetes or hypoglycemia (low blood sugar), Candida yeast infections, weakened immune response, and hyperactivity. When we are sick, our immune system needs to be strong and responsive, so ingesting large amounts of sugary syrups for medicine can be counterproductive. Most syrup recipes traditionally contain huge amounts of sugar, but I have experimented with using smaller portions and have discovered that one-fourth the traditional amount of sugar makes excellent syrup if it is refrigerated. The large reduction of sugar preservative shortens shelf life, but the syrup will keep for over 6 months in a refrigerator and indefinitely in a freezer.

Over time, the high sugar content in syrups may cause crystallization. Sugar crystals will melt back into liquid form when the container of syrup is placed in very hot water for a short time. Syrups containing less

Syrup Recipes

The basic method of preparing herbal syrups is to make a strong, concentrated tea that is preserved with substantial amounts of sweetener. Traditional ratios of sweeteners to a strong infusion or decoction tea include the following:

- ❖ Sugar syrup is made by combining 2 parts sugar (by weight) with 1 part tea (by volume). For example, 500 grams (gm) of sugar (equaling 1 pound and 2 ounces) is combined with 250 milliliters (mL) of tea (equaling 1 cup).
- ❖ Glycerin syrup is made by adding 3 parts glycerin to 2 parts tea.
- ❖ Honey and maple syrup are made by adding 3 parts syrup (by volume) to 1 part tea (by volume).

For a reduced-sugar syrup, try using these ratios:

1/8 pound (56 gm) to 1/4 pound (112.5 gm) of sugar combined with 1 cup (250 mL) of concentrated tea or

1/2 pound (225 gm) to 1 pound (450 gm) of sugar combined with 1 quart (1,000 mL) of concentrated tea

Add 1-2 parts honey or maple syrup (by volume) to 1 part tea (by volume). For example, 1-2 cups of honey are added to 1 cup of tea.

Begin making syrup by preparing a strong tea with the herbs of your choice, either dried or freshly harvested (the best option). Make tea the standard way, except use large amounts of herb to make it very concentrated. A good ratio of herbs-to-water is 2-3 cups of dried herb per 1 quart of water, or 4-6 cups of freshly harvested herbs per 1 quart of water.

Chop or crumble the plant material into small pieces for maximum extraction and put it in a stainless steel cooking pot. Cover with the appropriate amount of water. When making teas with both hard and soft plant parts, the roots or bark should be cooked first by gently simmering for 15-30 minutes. Then turn off the heat, add leaves and flowers to the root brew, and allow the herbs to steep for 60 minutes.

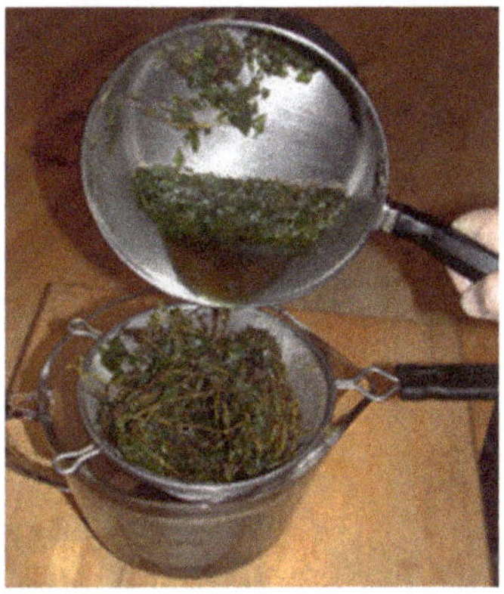

1) Strain and measure tea

Keep a lid on the pot during the entire tea-making phase to avoid losing essential oils through steam. Strain off the plant material and squeeze out as much water as possible from the herbs for maximum extraction of their healing properties. Measure the amount of finished tea to determine the correct amount of sweetener to be added. The sugar, honey, maple syrup, or other natural sweetener may be added directly to the concentrated tea. Heat the tea and sugar mixture while stirring constantly to help the sugar dissolve quickly. Do not boil this mixture. As the sugar dissolves, the tea turns into thick syrup. A few tablespoons of brandy or vodka, or 1-2 drops of an essential oil like Peppermint (*Mentha x piperita*), may be added to the syrup. The alcohol helps stabilize and preserve syrup, adding another dimension to its flavor.

Pour the hot syrup into sterilized glass jars, cool, and refrigerate. If the syrup is to be frozen for longer storage, allow it to cool and pour it into plastic bags or containers. Be sure to label your containers with the date and names of the herbs in your syrup.

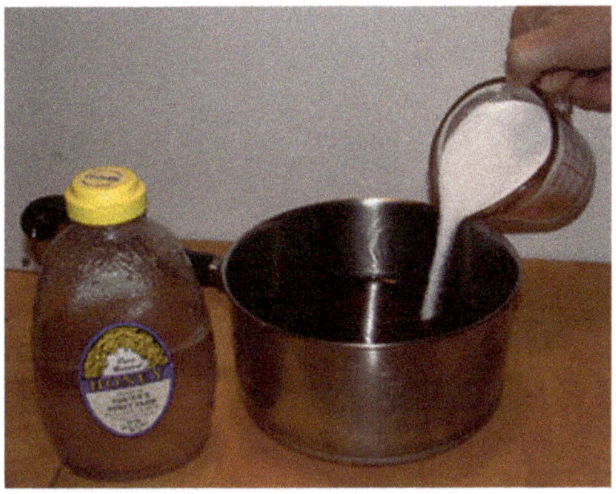

2) Add sugar, honey, or other sweetener to strained tea

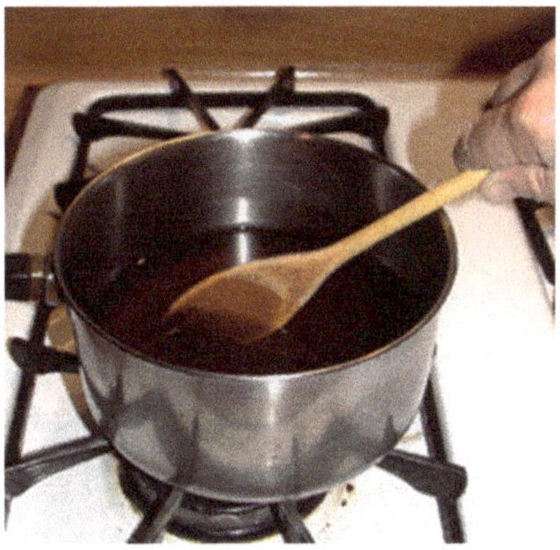

3) Heat tea and sweetener to form a thick syrup

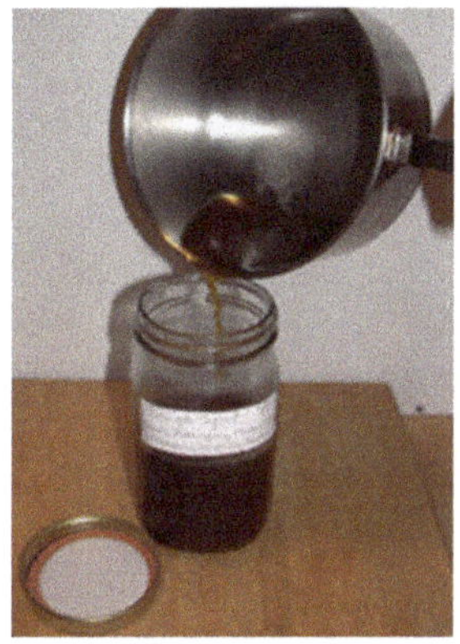

4) Pour syrup into a sterile jar

than 65% sugar will go bad eventually, even in the refrigerator. Discard the syrup if mold is present.

A **cordial** is a tincture sweetened with syrup. Cordials are made by combining 1 part tincture to 2-4 parts syrup made from water and sweetener.

Poultice

A poultice is a moist, pasty mash made from roots, leaves, or flowers that is applied externally on skin for the treatment of irritations, wounds, and injuries. A **cataplasm** is an older name for a poultice that is applied hot. Herbs may be used fresh or dried for poulticing, and are first chopped, crushed, pounded, grated, or ground. This can be accomplished with a knife, hammer, grater, grinder, or mortar and pestle.

Gently simmer the plant material in a small amount of water for a few minutes to make a thick paste. If dry herbs are used, more water is required for the desired paste consistency. Roots like Goldenseal or Yellow Dock (*Rumex crispus*) work best when they are dried, ground into powder, and mixed with a little water. Fresh succulent herbs like Chickweed (*Stellaria* spp.) contain enough water that cooking is not required. Fresh mucilaginous roots like Comfrey (*Symphytum officinale*) and Marshmallow (*Althaea officinalis*) also fall into this category, and can be chopped into a moist, pulpy mash without being cooked. The large leaves of Comfrey, Burdock (*Arctium* spp.), Yellow Dock, and Plantain (*Plantago* spp.) are wonderful poulticing herbs that can be chopped or ground into a paste. Whole fresh leaves can be placed on the skin if several slices are made through them, allowing their healing juices to flow out. Some leaves, like Comfrey, are covered with fine hairs that can be irritating, but simmering hairy leaves in a small amount of water eliminates this problem and provides soothing poultice material.

When preparation is complete, the herbal mash is applied over the desired area and covered with a cloth. Use an ace wrap or other bandage material to hold everything in place. Poultices are applied for 30 minutes to several hours, depending on the condition being treated and herbs that are chosen. Poultices may be applied hot, cold, or at room temperature. When hot poultices are applied, their heat opens skin pores, allowing healing components in the herbs much greater penetration into deeper tissue layers. Heat also increases blood and lymphatic circulation in the surrounding areas to promote healing. Cold poultices are best for bleeding wounds, acute inflammation, and burns. Poultices should always be kept moist and can be sprinkled with water during application if they become dry.

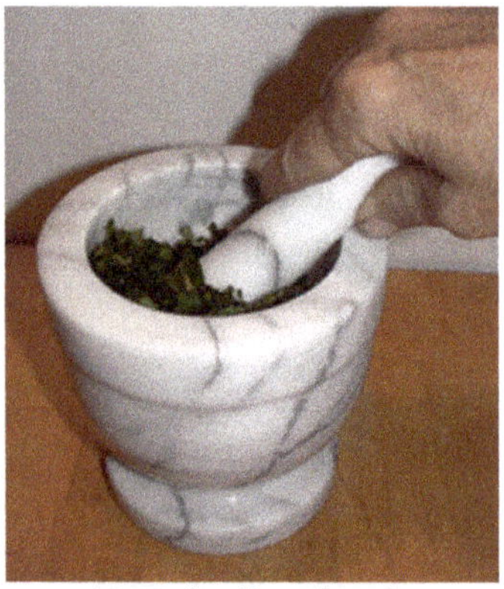

1) Grinding herbs into mash with a mortar and pestle

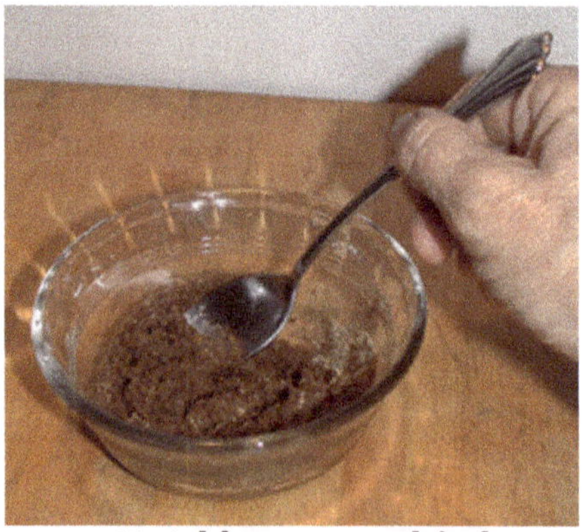

2) Add water to dried, powdered herbs to make a pasty mash

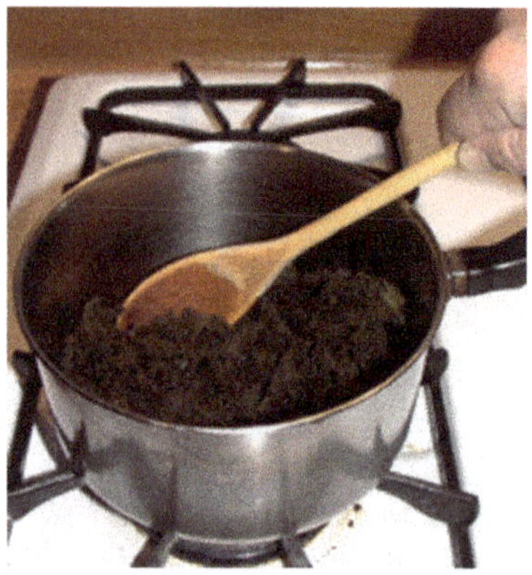

3) Or simmer either dry or fresh herbs in water to make a mash

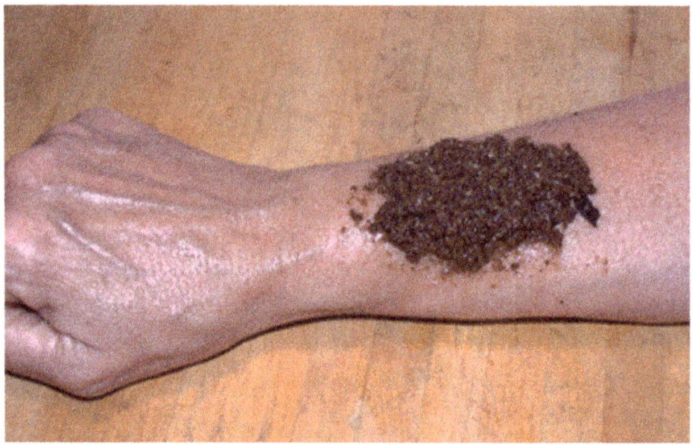

4) Apply a thick layer of moist herbal mash on affected skin

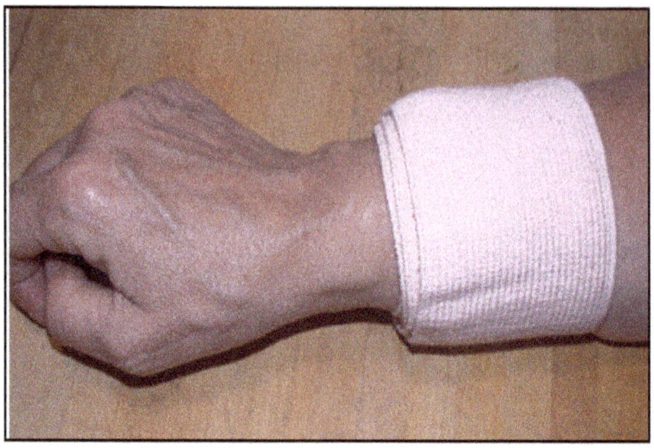

5) Cover and wrap herbal mash to keep it in place

Various herbs are prepared as poultices for their soothing and healing properties, ability to relieve pain, and to draw out infections, toxins, and other irritants such as splinters. Poultices are used for cuts, wounds, burns, sprains, muscle aches, joint inflammation, fractures, dermatitis, boils, abscesses, hives and other skin eruptions, plant toxins like poison ivy, and animal toxins such as bee stings and snake or insect bites. Since healing chemical constituents in herbs penetrate the pores of the skin, poultices are also used to heal injured or diseased organs deeper in the body. When making poultices, refer to the **"Index of Health Issues and Herbal Recommendations"** in Section Three to find appropriate herbs that address your specific concerns.

Fomentation, Compress, and Wash

A fomentation or compress is an application of moist, warm herbs for external healing. They are used for the same conditions as poultices. A fomentation or compress can be either a liquid or solid preparation.

To make a liquid preparation (also called a wash), prepare a stronger, more concentrated tea. Soak a cloth in the tea and place the cloth over the affected area. Hot fomentations are applied as hot as can be tolerated. Cover the cloth with a dry towel, and if more heat is desired, put a heating pad or hot water bottle on top of the towel. This can be left on for an hour or overnight. Be sure not to burn yourself if using a heating pad. If the hands, arms, legs, or feet are being treated, soak them in a pot or bathtub of tea.

Fomentations or compresses can also be made using herbal oils or liniments. The oil or liniment is heated and a cloth is dipped into it, wrung out, and applied over the affected area. Castor bean (*Ricinus communis*) oil compresses are commonly used for softening tissues, drawing out toxins, and treating fibroids.

A solid fomentation or compress is made by mixing or steeping macerated herbs in hot water to form a mash. This is wrapped in muslin or cotton cloth and applied to the afflicted area. The cloth is then covered with a dry towel or plastic wrap to stay warm and moist. This type of solid fomentation or compress is similar to a poultice, except the herbs are contained in a cloth when applied to the skin.

Flower Essences

These are vibrational remedies prepared from flower petals, whose life force and healing patterns are transferred into pure water. When ingested, flower essences restore the human energy field to heal emotional and spiritual imbalances. On a sunny day, fill a clean glass bowl with spring or rainwater (not tap water) and cover the water surface with fresh, whole flowers. All equipment must be sterile and tweezers are used to handle flowers rather than fingers. Leave the bowl in sunlight for 3 hours. Remove the flowers and filter the water into another container. Add 50% brandy to preserve the water, which is called the mother essence. From this, 2-7 drops are added to a 1-ounce dosage bottle in a 50/50 mix of brandy and pure water. Shake the final product to potentize (activate) it and put 2-4 drops under the tongue or on the wrists as needed.

Herbal Eyewash

Eyewashes are made from herbal teas that are strained through coffee filter paper to remove all plant sediment. Place drops of the warm filtered tea in the eyes with a sterilized dropper or eyewash cup purchased from drugstores. Store the tea in sterile glass bottles and refrigerate it for no longer than 5 days. After this length of time, a new batch must be brewed to assure freshness. Goldenseal, Echinacea, Marshmallow, and Chickweed teas are excellent eyewashes to treat infections like conjunctivitis and allergy or hay fever symptoms of itching, irritation, swelling, and redness.

Herbal Nasal Spray

Nasal sprays are wonderful for reducing sinus inflammation, infection, drainage or congestion, and for treating the common cold, sinus allergies, and chronic sinusitis. Herbal extracts that directly contact the tissues of the sinus cavities can work wonders in soothing delicate membranes, opening up the nasal passages, and eliminating bacterial and fungal infections that often accompany colds, especially chronic sinusitis. Nasal sprays are easy to prepare and can be made from herbal teas. These nasal sprays can last for 5 days without refrigeration or as long as 1-2 weeks in the refrigerator.

Goldenseal is my favorite herb for all sinus problems. It can be used alone or with other herbs, including Echinacea, Hyssop (*Hyssopus officinalis*), Sage (*Salvia officinalis*), Yarrow (*Achillea millefolium*), Yerba Mansa (*Anemopsis californica*), Myrrh (*Commiphora myrrha*), Calendula (*Calendula officinalis*), Isatis (*Isatis tinctoria*), and Lavender. Refer to the **"Index of Health Issues and Herbal Recommendations"** in Section Three and look at the herbs under the listing "Sinus Problems, Allergies, and Sinusitis" for other options.

To prepare nasal spray, put 1 cup of water in a pan. Add 1/16 teaspoon of Goldenseal root powder and small amounts of other herbs of your choice. Cover with a lid and gently simmer for 2-3 minutes. Turn off the heat and allow it to cool. Strain the tea through coffee filter paper, making sure all sediment is removed.

After preparing the herbal tea, pour it into a neti pot or plastic nasal spray container. Spray containers of saline water can be purchased at drugstores. Dump out the water and replace it with the herbal formula. Sniff deeply while squirting the formula into the nose several times a day for best results.

Herbal Douches

Herbal douches are teas used for vaginal infections caused by Candida yeast, bacteria or viruses, abnormal pap smears and growths, and for cleansing. Douching as a daily practice is not recommended because the balance of naturally occurring vaginal bacteria becomes disrupted. Only douche for specific reasons. To prepare an herbal douche, make a strong herbal tea, let it cool to a warm temperature, and pour it into a douche bag. Gently insert the application end of the douche bag high into the vagina while in the bathtub or shower and allow the tea to flow. Pregnant women should not douche unless they are under the supervision of a health care professional. Refer to the **"Index of Health Issues and Herbal Recommendations"** in Section Three and look under "Vaginal Infections" for a listing of appropriate herbs to use for douches.

Herbal Enemas

Herbal enemas are made with teas and are used for treating hemorrhoids, constipation, polyps, tumors, pain, and toxicity. Many enemas contain herbs that have laxative or peristaltic action on the bowels. Enemas also provide a means to increase fluids to treat dehydration and to cool the interior in cases of high fevers. This can be especially valuable for small children who are dehydrated from high fevers and cannot be persuaded to drink fluids. Coffee enemas are an old remedy to detoxify the bowels and body. Refer to the **"Index of Health Issues and Herbal Recommendations"** in Section Three to find herbs to use for enemas.

To make an herbal enema, prepare a strong tea with the desired herbs, cool it to lukewarm, and pour it into an enema bag purchased from drugstores. Lie on the bathroom floor or in the bathtub and insert the application tip of the enema bag into the rectum. Retain the herbal tea in the colon for 10-15 minutes or as long as possible. To help the fluid move through as much of the large intestine as possible, insert the application tip while lying on your left side, turn over on your hands and knees or lie on your stomach for 1-2 minutes, and then lie on your right side. If this specific sequence is followed, the tea will move up through the descending colon on the left side of the abdomen, into the transverse colon crossing the abdomen, and down the ascending colon on the right side.

Herbal Suppositories

Suppositories are used vaginally to treat infections, inflammation, irritations, and abnormal growth of cells, tumors, or cysts. A vaginal suppository is called a **pessary**. Suppositories administered rectally for hemorrhoids, cysts, and polyps are known as a **bolus**. Herbal suppositories can draw toxins and infectious material out of tissues, and they contain healing compounds that disperse into tissues. Suppositories are simple to make and effective for healing. They are prepared with water or cocoa butter purchased from drug stores or health food stores. Cocoa butter is solid at room temperature and melts into liquid when heated.

To make suppositories with cocoa butter, melt it into a liquid over hot water (using a double-boiler) or use very low heat because cocoa butter can burn quickly. Choose the appropriate herbs (refer to the **"Index of Health Issues and Herbal Recommendations"** in Section Three) and pulverize them into a fine powder with a small coffee bean grinder. Slowly stir the liquid cocoa butter into the powdered herbs until the mix has the consistency of thick peanut butter. After allowing the mixture to cool a little, roll the thick paste into strips about the size of your little finger, place them on a flat surface, and refrigerate them to harden.

Suppositories can also be made with water. Add enough water to the powdered herbs to create a thick paste, roll it into little round strips, and allow them to dry. Finely powdered Psyllium or Marshmallow root are good plant-based binders to add to suppositories made with water because their gluey and slippery mucilage holds the herbal mix together, and allows smooth sliding through body orifices. Dry the finished products in the sun for a few hours and periodically turn them to allow uniform drying, or put them in an oven set at 100-120°F until they are dry. Water and oil-based suppositories can be stored in a glass container or plastic bag in the refrigerator for several weeks, or put in a freezer where they will last indefinitely. If refrigeration is not possible, suppositories will last for several months in an airtight glass jar if they are thoroughly dry and kept in a cool, dark place.

It is best to insert suppositories at bedtime since they will slowly melt at body temperature. In the morning, place a pad of tissue inside underwear because whatever has not dissolved in the suppository will slide out. Herbal suppositories can be used every night at bedtime until the problem resolves. After several nights of using vaginal suppositories, douching with herbal tea will thoroughly clean the vaginal area.

Hydrotherapy ~ the Herb Bath and Sitz Bath

Hydrotherapy uses water as therapy for illness, anxiety, and to restore balance to the body. To prepare an herbal bath, pour a large pot of very strong tea into hot bath water. Lavender, Chamomile, and the Mints create a wonderfully soothing, aromatic bath. In a sitz bath, a person sits in water up to their hips to relieve pain, heal hemorrhoids, anal fissures, episiotomies, ease uterine cramps, and heal tissues after rectal surgery. To prepare a sitz bath, pour hot, strong tea into a basin or bathtub and sit in it for 15-30 minutes. Refer to the "Index of Herbs for Specific Health Issues" in Section Three to find herbs to use for different conditions.

Alcohol-Based Preparations: Herbal Tinctures and Liniments

Tinctures

Tinctures are liquid extracts of herbs. Most are made with alcohol and varying amounts of water, although some tinctures are made from vinegar or glycerin. Alcohol tinctures are significantly more potent than dried herbal preparations because alcohol is the best extractor of phytochemicals.

Tincturing is the process of soaking shredded plant material in a liquid solvent to infuse the liquid with active components of the herb. The liquid solvents that extract phytochemicals out of herbs are called the **menstruum**. The herb material being tinctured, or macerated, is called the **marc**. The process of extracting the marc into the liquid menstruum is called **maceration**. Remember that extraction occurs by the process of **osmosis** in which the chemical substances held within the plant are drawn out into liquid solvents by the natural tendency for particles in high density concentration (within the herb) to move to lower density areas (in fluids) in order to achieve equilibrium. **Maceration, the tincturing process**, is complete when there is an equal amount of chemical components left in the marc as in the liquid menstruum. The tincture is then **decanted**, meaning that the menstruum is separated and squeezed from the marc. At this point, the marc should be nearly dry and can be added to the compost bin. The remaining liquid is the finished tincture. Filter the tincture to remove all sediment, pour it into bottles, and store these in a cool, dark place.

Benefits of Herbal Tinctures

❖ Herbal tinctures are quick and easy to use. Taking a tincture in a small amount of water is much easier than drinking a whole cup of bitter or unpleasant-tasting tea. Even children can be encouraged to drink a little tincture in water or juice. Tinctures are perfect for emergency and first-aid situations, and are handy for use away from home at school, work, or when traveling.

❖ The body digests tinctures easily and rapidly. The tincturing or maceration process "pre-digests" the herbs by drawing their medicinal constituents out of the cellular plant material into a liquid solution. Once these constituents dissolve in the liquid tincture and are ingested, they are readily absorbed through the lining of the stomach and small intestines, passing quickly into the bloodstream.

❖ Alcohol tinctures retain their medicinal properties far longer than other herbal preparations, with a shelf life that can extend for many years. Vinegar and glycerin tinctures do not last as long.

❖ The alcohol content in tinctures provides a sterile environment where no bacteria, mold, or other microbes can grow. This contributes to a long shelf life.

❖ The tincturing process does not require heat and eliminates heat-induced deterioration of herbs.

❖ Alcohol can extract substances from medicinal plants that are not completely soluble (meaning that they will not dissolve) in plain water, such as essential oils, resins, and alkaloids.

How to Use Tinctures for Medicine

❖ Always dilute tinctures by putting them in ¼-½ cup of water. Although some herbalists and product labels advise putting tinctures directly into the mouth, it is best to add them to water. High quality tinctures are very strong, concentrated herbal preparations that are safer to use when diluted. Dilution decreases possibilities of unwanted reactions in people with sensitive systems.
❖ Although water is preferable, tinctures can be added to a little tea or juice, especially when the herbs taste strong or bitter and their flavor needs to be masked. Never take tinctures or other herbal preparations with coffee, soda pop, or citrus juices because their acidic chemistry can reduce the beneficial effects of the herbs.
❖ Herbs should be taken on an empty stomach for the best and fastest absorption through the stomach and intestinal. Exceptions include Cayenne and other strong herbs that may be irritating to the stomach.
❖ Different herbal tinctures may be combined and added to the same glass of water.
❖ Pregnant women, recovering alcoholics, and people with liver or kidney problems should not use alcohol in any form. Most of the alcohol in tinctures will evaporate if the tincture is put in a cup of boiling hot water for 10-15 minutes and stirred occasionally.

Different Types of Liquid Solvents (Menstruums) Used for Making Tinctures

The menstruums (liquid solvents) used in tincturing are **alcohol, glycerin**, or **vinegar**. Alcohol is the best solvent and the one most commonly used by herbalists and manufacturers. Distilled water is often added to alcohol, glycerin, and vinegar menstruums.

Alcohol is the most potent and effective solvent to extract water-soluble and fat-soluble phytochemicals from herbs. It specifically extracts fats, resins, volatile oils, waxes, and alkaloids from plants and dissolves them into a liquid solution. Because alcohol eliminates all potential for bacterial or fungal growth in tincture preparations, it is the best preservative to hold and stabilize the medicinal properties and potency of herbs for many years.

Herbalists use many different kinds of liquor to make tinctures, from 80-proof to 190-proof alcohol. "Proof" indicates the ratio of alcohol and water in liquor, and represents twice the percentage of alcohol. For instance, 80-proof liquor means that it contains 40% alcohol and the remaining 60% is water. Many herbalists use straight gin, vodka, or brandy (without additional water for tincturing) because they are usually 90- to 95-proof, meaning that they contain about 45-50% alcohol and 50-55% water. Pure grain alcohol is 190-proof and is almost 100% pure alcohol. It may be used alone but is often combined with distilled water when preparing tinctures. Grain alcohol is available in liquor stores in some states under brand names such as "Clear Spring" and "Everclear."

When deciding which type of alcohol to use as a menstruum, several factors should be considered. Different liquors affect the taste of tinctures. Brandy is a favorite used for the creation of pleasant-tasting preparations. Tincturing aromatic and tasty roots like Licorice (*Glycyrrhiza glabra*), Anise (*Pimpinella anisum*), or Sarsaparilla (*Smilax* spp.) with good brandy makes a delicious **cordial**. However, when the primary objective of tincturing is to obtain maximum quantities of phytochemicals for medicinal use, crystal clear 190-proof grain alcohol, which is the purest form of liquor, is the best solvent for extraction. When plant material is soaked in grain alcohol, which contains very few solutes (chemicals held in liquid solution), a strong osmotic pull naturally draws their phytochemicals into the alcohol until there is an equal amount of constituents in the plant material as there is in the liquid. But when herbs are tinctured in liquors like brandy and vodka, or in wines that contain many more solutes, the osmotic pull is not nearly as great and less extraction occurs. For these reasons, I generally recommend using 190-proof grain alcohol for the production of medicinal tinctures. Depending on the herb being processed, tinctures are made with 100% grain alcohol or with a ratio of alcohol and water. Likewise, distilled water works better than tap water or mineral water because distilled water contains fewer minerals and chemical additives, exerting a stronger osmotic pull.

Most herbs contain medicinal phytochemicals that are both water-soluble (requiring only water to dissolve) and fat-soluble (requiring alcohol to dissolve). Thus, a combination of alcohol and water extracts most completely. I observed this many years ago when I worked as a lab technician for Hulda Clark, Ph.D., the well-known orthomolecular nutritionist and author. She requested that I create different homeopathic substances starting with basic plant tinctures. To prepare each tincture, I divided the plant material and put half in a container of distilled water and the other half in a container of 190-proof grain alcohol. The quantity of liquid was the same in each container. After several days of maceration, the color of the water and alcohol solutions were always different, demonstrating that water and alcohol extract different chemical constituents out of the same plant. For this reason, I usually like to combine 190-proof grain alcohol with distilled water when making tinctures in order to extract the full spectrum of healing components from herbs.

When preparing the menstruum for tinctures, deciding on the best ratio of grain alcohol to distilled water depends on several variables that include the water content of the plant material, the part of the plant being processed, and the solubility factors of specific plant constituents.

1) Water content of the plant:
The amount of alcohol necessary to tincture dry herbs must be at least 45-proof (22% alcohol).
The amount of alcohol to preserve fresh herbs holding moisture must be at least 80-proof (40% alcohol).
2) Part of plant being processed:
The menstruum must contain at least 35-45% alcohol to extract medicinal constituents from leaves and flowers and to prevent mold and bacterial growth in tinctures.
Soft seeds, fruits, and moist roots generally need a menstruum of at least 45-60% alcohol for extraction.
Hard seeds, dry roots, and bark require a menstruum containing 60-90% alcohol.
3) Solubility factors of specific plant constituents:
Plants containing large amounts of resins, essential oils, and gums that are alcohol-soluble, but not water-soluble, need a menstruum containing 75-95% alcohol for maximum extraction. 190-proof grain alcohol works best for these substances.
Herbs containing polysaccharides and mucilage (Chickweed, Slippery Elm, and Marshmallow) are water-soluble and require only 22-25% alcohol, which is the least amount necessary for preservation.
Plant material containing saponins, sterols, and alkaloids needs a menstruum containing at least 45% alcohol for extraction.

Vinegar tinctures substitute vinegar as the main solvent rather than alcohol. When acidic vinegar is used to tincture alkaline herbs, chemical reactions dissolve the alkaline components and suspend them in the vinegar solution. Although vinegar successfully extracts plant minerals and alkaloids, it extracts other phytochemicals very poorly. This is one reason why vinegar-based tinctures are often not as potent as alcohol tinctures. Vinegar tinctures also have a shorter shelf life than alcohol tinctures. For this reason, alcohol is sometimes added to vinegar menstruums to enhance extraction and preservation. Tinctures made with 100% vinegar are called **aceta**, and tinctures processed with a combination of vinegar and alcohol are called **acetous**.

Vinegar-based tinctures are typically prepared to extract specific alkaline constituents from various herbs. Western herbalists often make a vinegar tincture of Lobelia (*Lobelia inflata*) since the primary active ingredient is an alkaloid. A medicinal vinegar tincture is made in the same way as an alcohol tincture, and unless alcohol is added, the menstruum is 100% vinegar. Many herbalists prefer apple cider vinegar. Remember that the acids in vinegar rust metal, so do not use metal lids on your containers unless a piece of Saran wrap or wax paper is placed between the jar and the lid.

For a tasty culinary treat, try making **herbal vinegars** by soaking garden herbs such as Basil, Thyme, Rosemary, Tarragon, Oregano, Chives, Sage, and Marjoram in apple cider vinegar for 2-6 weeks. Herbal vinegars taste wonderful in salad dressings, marinades, and other seasonings.

Glycerin is a sweet, thick, mucilaginous liquid that naturally occurs in animal fats and plant oils, and is obtained as a by-product from the manufacture of fatty acids and soaps. Only vegetable glycerin is used for herbal preparations, and it can be purchased from health food stores and drug stores.

Glycerin herbal preparations are non-alcoholic and are made in various ways. Some preparations are processed using glycerin as the sole medium for extraction. Many manufacturers first extract plant material in a water and alcohol menstruum. When the tincturing process is complete, this mixture is heated to promote evaporation of the water and alcohol, leaving a thick glob of concentrated plant material. Glycerin is added to this to make the final product. Other companies extract herbs in chemical solvents such as acetone, hexane or dichloromethane, which are then distilled into concentrated substances and added to glycerin. Both types of preparations require exposure to long periods of heat, which denatures medicinal properties, and trace amounts of chemical residues can remain in the finished product.

Glycerin preparations can be milder and more soothing to the digestive system than alcohol tinctures, although an excess of glycerin may be irritating to the stomach and intestines. Glycerin remedies offer an alternative for children (who like the sweet taste), pregnant women, and others who should not or do not want to ingest alcohol.

There are several disadvantages to glycerin preparations, however. Glycerin is not as effective at extraction as alcohol. While it will extract vitamins, minerals and mucilage, it does not extract resins, oils, alkaloids, and other important phytochemicals. At best, glycerin preparations contain only half the potency of alcohol tinctures. Many important herbs contain bitter-tasting constituents with medicinal activity that is diminished in the presence of sweet glycerin. Bitters such as Dandelion (*Taraxacum officinale*), Yellow Dock (*Rumex crispus*), Gentian (*Gentiana lutea*), and American Centaury (*Sabatia angularis*) lose potency in glycerin extracts. Another disadvantage is the excessive sweetness that may contribute to sugar cravings and weight gain. Research shows that ingesting sugar weakens immunity for a period of several hours, so its use as a base in medicinal preparations can be counterproductive to healing. Glycerin is not as sterile a medium as alcohol, so extra care must be taken to maintain cleanliness when making glycerin extracts. All utensils and containers must be sterile, and herbs should be thoroughly dried prior to the tincturing process to avoid introducing fungus or bacteria. It may be necessary to add preservatives like vitamin E or benzoin. Glycerin preparations last longer when stored in a cool, dark place, but have the longest shelf life when refrigerated.

Despite these drawbacks, if you want to make a glycerin extract, here are two easy methods:
Method One: Mix glycerin with warm water. Different ratios are used, from 1:1 (1 part glycerin to 1 part water) to 1:4 (1 part glycerin to 4 parts water). Experiment to decide which ratio you prefer. Put the powdered or chopped herb into a glass jar and cover it with the glycerin menstruum. Screw the lid on tightly and label the jar with the name of the herb, the ratio of water and glycerin used in the menstruum, and the date. Let it sit and percolate for 4 weeks, shaking it every day. Then strain and separate the herb from the glycerin. Store the glycerin preparation in sterile glass containers that are labeled and dated.
Method Two: Make a strong herbal tincture using grain alcohol and water for the menstruum. Pour the finished tincture into a cooking pan and heat it below the boiling point until most of the liquid has evaporated and the remaining product is a wet mass. Add glycerin to this, mix well, and bottle in sterile containers.

Creating Alcohol Tinctures

Making alcohol tinctures is easy, fun, and extremely rewarding. It does not require fancy equipment, especially for small batches, and can be accomplished in your own kitchen. There are many ways to make tinctures, and the more herb books you read, the more you will discover variations among herbalists. One method that may appeal to scientifically oriented people requires making mathematical calculations and measurements, weighing with scales, determining variables between tincturing dry and fresh herbs, and figuring out desired ratios of herbs and liquid solvents. The older and more traditional **simpler's method** is much less complicated and exacting, with the end product being nearly identical to the more complex version. Several years ago when I was teaching an herb class about these two methods of tincturing, one of my apprentices came up with the term **"complexer's method"** to describe the more complex process involving mathematical calculations and measurements. This is a perfect description that I have adopted into my herbal vocabulary. Try both methods of making tinctures and decide which works best for you. You may want to begin with the less demanding simpler's method.

Making Tinctures by the Simpler's Method

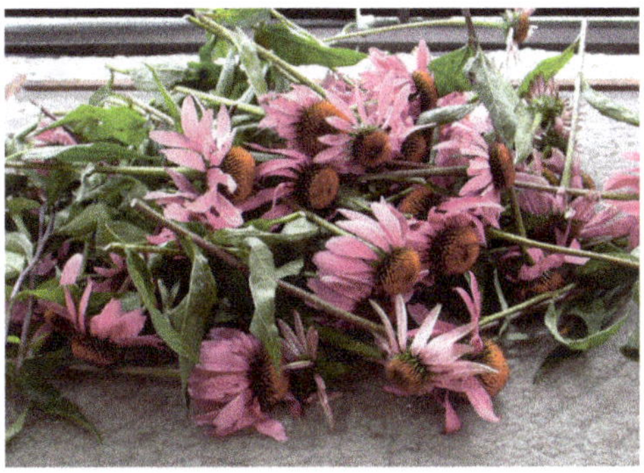

1) Freshly harvested Echinacea

❖ Gather the herbs you want to tincture from your gardens, by wildcrafting, or by purchasing dried herbs from health food stores. Most tinctures on the market are made with herbs that have been pre-dried and stored for questionable periods of time. If you have the opportunity to use freshly harvested herbs, take advantage of it because they always produce more potent tinctures than dried, aged plants.

❖ If herbs have been freshly harvested, they can be dried for several hours to remove at least some of their water content. Roots that have been washed should be allowed to dry for a few hours.

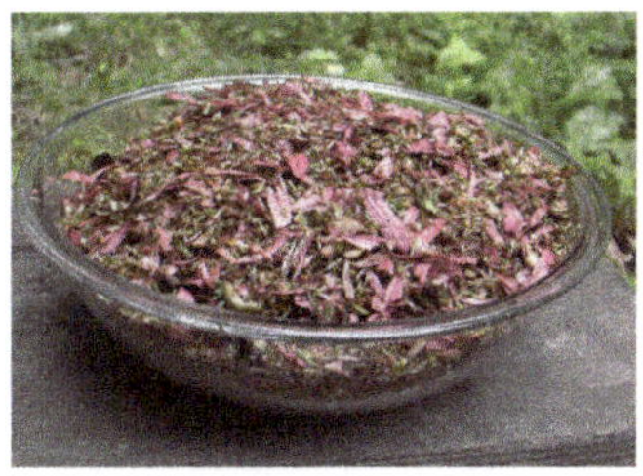

2) Chopped herbs

❖ Chop fresh flowers, leaves, or roots into small pieces, or crumble dried herbs into tiny particles. This increases their surface area, allowing for better extraction. Remember that breaking up the fibrous cells of plants allows their chemical constituents to be released into liquid solvents more efficiently than if they are left whole.

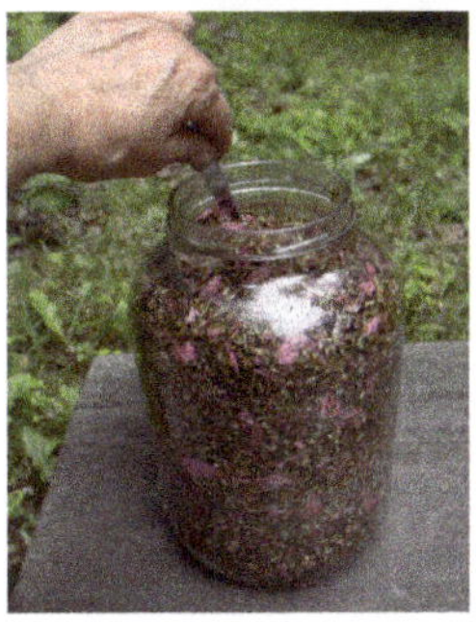

3) Pack herbs in glass jar

❖ Put the plant material into a clean glass jar and pack it tightly so the jar is completely full. The size of the jar is determined by the amount of herb material you have. Quart and half-gallon canning jars work well. Glass gallon jars are great for larger amounts of plant material.

❖ Prepare the liquid menstruum by combining the desired ratio of 190-proof grain alcohol with distilled water in a measuring cup. A **standard menstruum ratio for <u>moist</u>, <u>freshly harvested</u> plants that hold a lot of water is typically 75% grain alcohol mixed with 25% distilled water, which is abbreviated as (75A:25W). Fresh plant material that has been <u>partially pre-dried</u> for a short time can be prepared with 65% grain alcohol and 35% distilled water (65A:35W). The menstruum ratio for <u>dry</u> herbs is usually 50% grain alcohol to 50% distilled water (50A:50W).** If the menstruum is 90- to 95-proof liquor like brandy, vodka or gin, no water is added.

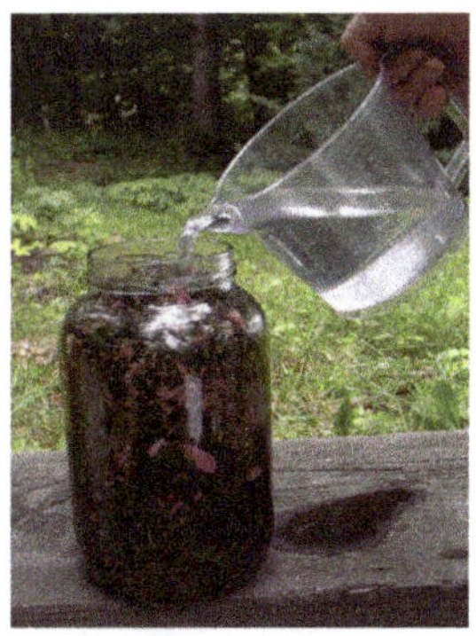

4) Cover herbs with alcohol and water menstruum

❖ When the menstruum is prepared, pour it into the glass jar and completely cover the plant material.

❖ Eliminate air in the jar by using an implement, like a long knife or poker, to stir the marc and menstruum so air bubbles rise to the surface. This usually creates extra space at the top of the jar, so add more liquid menstruum to completely cover the

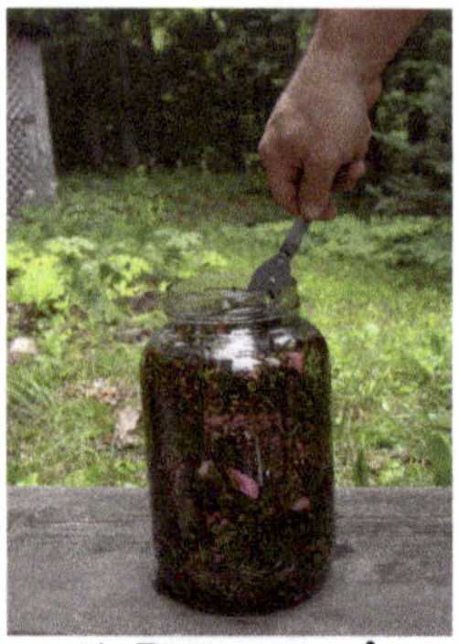

5) Remove air bubbles

herbs. If air space remains, exposed plant material typically oxidizes and turns black.

❖ Screw the lid tightly onto the jar. Be sure that no liquid dribbles out when the jar is vigorously shaken and turned upside down. If there is leakage, fold a piece of plastic wrap 3-4 times and place it between the lip of the jar and the lid to create a tight seal.

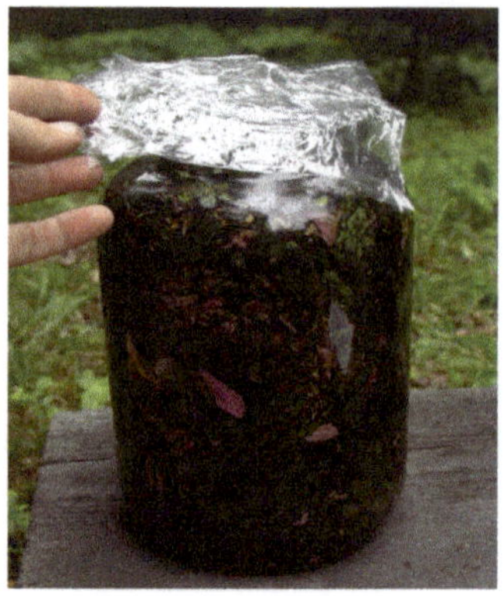

6) Cover jar with plastic wrap

❖ Label the jar with the name of the herb, ratio of alcohol to water used in the mix, and the date.

❖ Place the jar out of direct sunlight and shake it on a daily basis to encourage the osmosis process. Keep your tincturing jars in plain view as a reminder to tend them daily. As more constituents are drawn out of the herb, the color of the menstruum usually darkens.

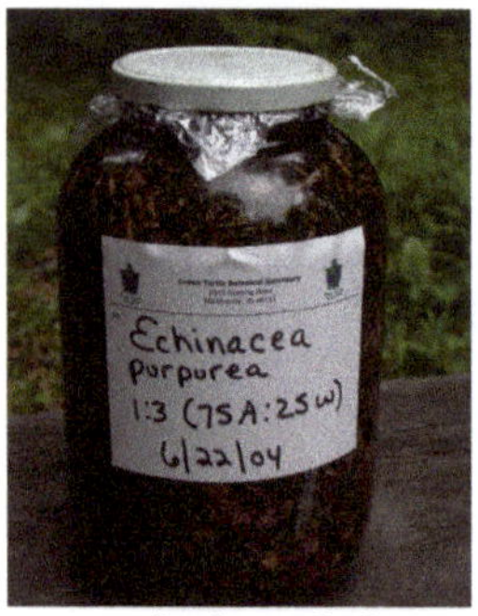

7) Label and date the jar

❖ Allow the tincture to sit for 4-6 weeks for maximum extraction.

❖ After 4-6 weeks the tincture is ready to **decant**, which is the separation of the liquid menstruum from the herbal marc. It is fine if it takes you longer than 4-6 weeks to get to this decanting process, because the tincture will not deteriorate over time.

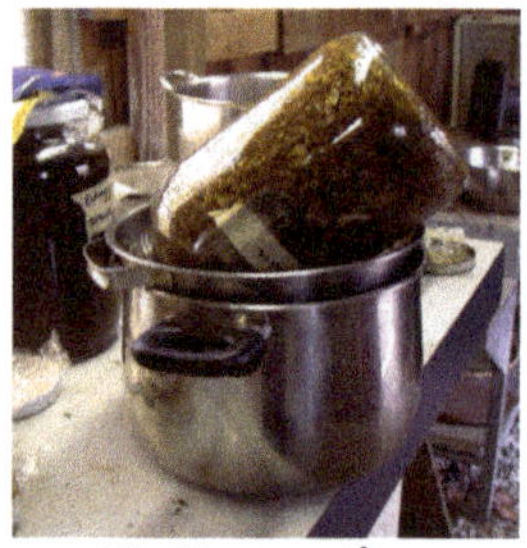

8) Decanting

❖ To decant, line the inside of a strainer or colander with several layers of cheesecloth. Place the strainer over a large bowl, then dump the contents of the jar into the strainer. The liquid will empty into the bowl while the cheesecloth captures the plant material.

❖ Next, squeeze as much of the menstruum as possible out of the remaining marc. This is important because the marc still contains substantial amounts of chemical constituents that should not be wasted. Plant material remaining in the cheesecloth can be squeezed by hand. If you are tincturing large amounts of herbs, you may want to use a juicing machine or press. Juicing machines that operate by centrifugal force are excellent for small amounts. Put the remaining marc into the juicer (without the slicing bade), turn it on, and let it spin around. More liquid will be spun out, leaving the marc almost dry. Investing in a juicer is also a great opportunity to make delicious fruit and vegetable juices at home. Juicing machines are available at department stores and in some health food and kitchen specialty stores. Presses made specifically for processing herbs can be purchased from herbal equipment suppliers. With a few modifications, apple cider presses can be converted into tincture presses. They work well and save a lot of time, especially when processing large amounts of herbs.

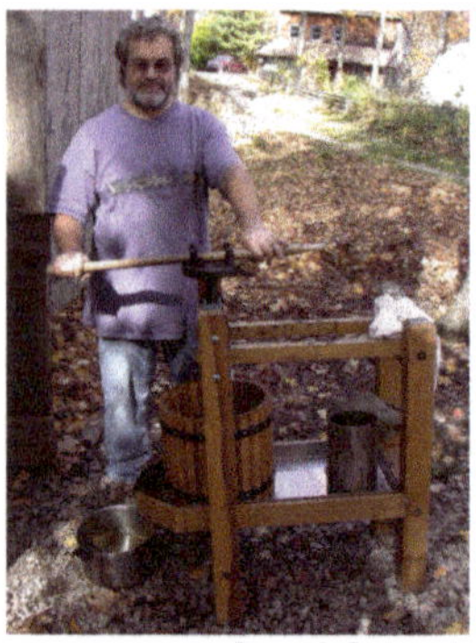

9) Apple cider press for decanting

❖ Put the discarded herbs in a compost bin or back on the earth as compost.

❖ Next, filter the menstruum to remove all sediment. Knee-high nylon stockings are the fastest filters I've found, while coffee filter paper is a slower but more complete filtration. Put the foot section of a clean stocking in a glass jar and pour the liquid into it. Or coffee filter paper can be placed in a large funnel or colander, and the menstruum is poured through this. As it passes through these filters, extraneous plant material and sediment are captured. The filtered liquid is the finished tincture.

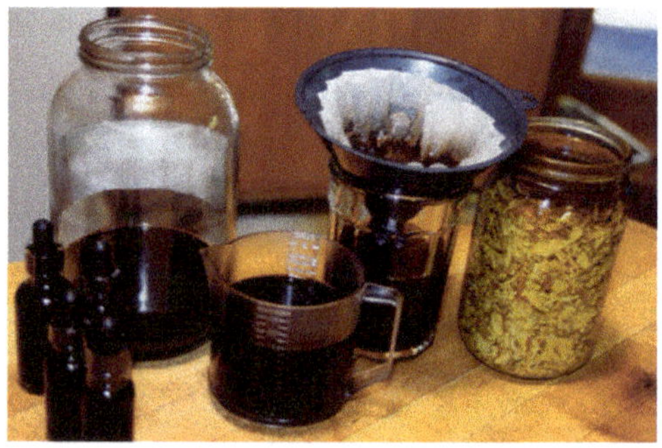

10) Final cleaning with filter paper

❖ The last step is to pour the finished product into glass jars. Tinctures can be stored in empty alcohol bottles, glass gallon or quart jars, or smaller glass bottles. One- and two-ounce dark glass bottles with droppers, called Boston amber round bottles, are perfect for administering doses of tinctures and can be purchased from many pharmacies or in bulk from glass manufacturers. Never store herbs in plastic containers due to questionable chemicals in plastics.

❖ Label your jars and bottles with the name of the herb, the alcohol-to-water ratio, and the date.

❖ Store the finished tincture in a cool, dark location.

A Few More Tincturing Tips

Fresh plant tinctures: For exceptionally potent tinctures, gather your own fresh plant material. Prepare herbs for tincturing immediately after harvesting to maintain their freshness and maximum quality.

Drying: The vast majority of herbs can be tinctured fresh while they still contain moisture. However, chopping the plant material and allowing several hours of drying time prior to maceration reduces much of the moisture, which is helpful for plants with a high water content. Some herbs must be dried prior to tincturing because of their unique chemistry. Cascara Sagrada (*Rhamnus purshiana*) and Buckthorn (*Rhamnus cathartica*) bark can cause intestinal spasms unless they are dried for at least one year before being processed into tinctures.

Electric blenders: Mixing the herbal marc with the liquid menstruum in an electric blender works well. This makes a thick slurry or paste that is more difficult to decant without a centrifugal juicer or press. Blenders are a great way to chop the herb into very small pieces.

Precipitation: Tinctures are solutions of plant constituents dissolved in liquid solvents. Over time, particles in tinctures may clump together and precipitate to form sediment that settles on the bottom of the storage bottle. Precipitation can result from poor filtering techniques, exposure to excess light during storage, temperature changes, or chemical reactions within the tincture itself. Alcohol can precipitate or draw proteins, tannins, and high molecular weight polysaccharides out of liquid solution. Precipitate particles are easily removed by filtering the tincture through coffee filter paper or nylon stockings.

Mucilaginous herbs: Do not make tinctures with plants that are high in mucilage. These include Marshmallow (*Althaea officinalis*), Comfrey (*Symphytum officinalis*), Slippery Elm (*Ulmus rubra*), Fenugreek seeds (*Trigonella foenum-graecum*), Chickweed (*Stellaria* spp.), and Psyllium (*Plantago* spp.). Prepare these as teas using water because alcohol "cuts" through and destroys the healing properties of the mucilage. If mucilaginous herbs are prepared as tinctures, only a small amount of alcohol (25%) is used for preservation.

Tincture one herb species per jar: It is generally best to tincture only one species of herb per glass jar rather than mixing several together. After each species has been processed, filtered, and poured into their storage jars, they can be mixed together to create combinations for different formulas.

Lunar influences on preparing tinctures: Herbalists usually let herbs macerate or soak in liquid solvents for 2-4 weeks, although some use less time. In Europe during the Middle Ages, astrologer-herbalists like Nicholas Culpeper, who were aware of the astrological influences of the moon and other heavenly bodies, recommended that herbs be harvested at the time of the new or full moon, macerated for 2-4 weeks, and decanted during the time of the full moon. Just as the energies of the new moon and full moon influence the ocean tides, they also affect the flow of fluids in the earth and in plants. The waxing of the moon as it becomes full allows phytochemicals in plant material to be drawn out more easily into liquid solvents. If you have the time and opportunity to work in correlation with the moon cycles, it is interesting and worth the experience. However, since many people have busy and hectic lifestyles, it may be more realistic to harvest herbs whenever the opportunity arises rather than being limited to specific times of the moon cycle. It is much easier to let herbs macerate for 4-6 weeks so the moon travels through its entire cycle, especially the time of the full moon, to take advantage of its beneficial drawing effects. Creating potent remedies by working cooperatively with the powerful forces of the cosmos is fun and quite an education in itself!

How to remove alcohol from tinctures: Remove alcohol for children, pregnant women, people with liver or kidney problems, and others not wanting to ingest alcohol. Just add the dose of tincture to a cup of boiling water, stir, and let it cool. Most of the alcohol evaporates off.

Making Tinctures by the Complexer's Method

The complexer's method involves exactly the same tincturing or macerating process as the simpler's method. The only difference is the use of standardized formulas and mathematical calculations for weights, volumes, and ratios of plant material (the marc) and liquid solvents (the menstruum). Rather than simply covering the herbs with the menstruum, exact amounts are weighed and calculated. Creating tinctures according to standard formulas provides more consistent, uniform batches and appeals to those who enjoy more precise mathematical methods. It is fun to experiment with both methods for a broader understanding of the tincturing process!

The metric system measuring weight and volume is used for these mathematical calculations.
Grams are units that measure the weight of solid mass.
Liters are units measuring the volume of liquid.
According to the metric system:
1 pound = 16 ounces = 450 grams (gm) = 450 milliliters (mL)
28 gm = 1 ounce   1000 mL = 1 liter

There are two ratios to consider and calculate when making tinctures by the complexer's method:

The **marc to menstruum ratio** expresses the weight of the herb (marc) measured in grams (gm) to the volume of liquid (menstruum) measured in milliliters (mL). A ratio of 1:3 means that 1 part herb measured in grams is combined with 3 parts menstruum measured in milliliters. A stronger extract with a 1:1 strength means that 1 part herb measured in grams is combined with 1 part liquid measured in milliliters.

The **alcohol to water ratio** describes the proportions of alcohol, water, vinegar, or glycerin that are combined to make the menstruum. A formula expressed as (50A:50W) means that 50% grain alcohol is combined with 50% water. The formula for a vinegar tincture may be written as (60V:40A), meaning that 60% vinegar is mixed with 40% grain alcohol. A glycerin tincture may read (50G:40A:10W), which translates as 50% glycerin mixed with 40% grain alcohol and 10% water to make the menstruum. A tincture containing only alcohol is expressed as (100A).

Three Basic Formulas for Tincturing Herbs

Dried herbs: 1:5 (50A:50W). 1 part dried herb (marc) measured in grams is mixed with 5 parts liquid (menstruum) measured in milliliters. The menstruum is 50% grain alcohol and 50% water.

Freshly harvested herbs containing large amounts of water: 1:2 (75A:25W). 1 part marc measured in grams is combined with 2 parts menstruum measured in milliliters, which is a combination of 75% grain alcohol and 25% water. Fresh herbs can also be tinctured using a **1:3 (75A:25W)** formula. Since fresh plants contain between 40-90% water in their tissues, their preparation requires one more step to determine their water content and figuring that amount into the calculations.

Freshly harvested herbs that are pre-dried for several hours: 1:3 (65A:35W). 1 part marc is covered with 3 parts liquid menstruum. The ratio of alcohol to water in the menstruum is adjusted according to loss of moisture from drying. I believe that this formula may be the best one to use in producing a tincture with the strongest potency and vital force because the herbs are freshly harvested and only partially dried, and this is the one I most often use.

Step-by-step instructions for making tincture with <u>dry herbs using the standard formula 1:5 (50A:50W)</u>, which means 1 part plant material to 5 parts menstruum (made with 50% alcohol and 50% water):

1. Weigh the dried plant material using a scale that weighs in ounces and grams.
2. Calculate the amount of liquid menstruum needed (5 times the weight of the plant material).
3. Prepare the menstruum by combining 50% grain alcohol with 50% distilled water.
4. Combine the calculated proportions of menstruum and marc in a glass jar.
5. From this point, complete the process as described for the simpler's method.

Look at an example. You have a batch of dried leaves that needs to be tinctured and you want to use the standard formula for dried herbs, which is 1:5 (50A:50W).

1. Weigh the herb. The leaves weigh 2.5 pounds, which is equal to 1,125 gm.
   Use the metric formula to convert pounds into grams.
   1 pound = 450 gm, so 2.5 pounds x 450 gm = 1,125 gm of leaves.
2. Calculate the amount of menstruum needed for 1,125 gm of leaves (the marc).
   Using a 1:5 ratio means that 1 part herb is combined with 5 parts liquid.
   5 x 1,125 gm of marc = 5,625 mL of menstruum needed
3. Calculate and measure the amount of grain alcohol and distilled water needed for the menstruum.
   Using a (50A:50W) ratio for 5,625 mL means that 50% grain alcohol and 50% water are used, so:
   5,625 mL x .50 (50%) = 2,812.5 mL of grain alcohol are added to
   5,625 mL x .50 (50%) = 2,812.5 mL of distilled water.

So, for 2.5 pounds of dried leaves, the formula <u>1:5 (50A:50W)</u> translates as:
<u>1,125 gm leaf:5,625 mL menstruum (2,812.5 mL grain alcohol:2,812.5 mL distilled water)</u>

Step-by-step instructions for making tincture with <u>fresh herbs using the standard formula 1:2 (75A:25W)</u>, or 1 part plant material to 2 parts menstruum (made with 75% alcohol and 25% water):

Since fresh plants contain so much water, this variable is figured into the alcohol and water ratio to ensure enough alcohol is added to the tincture to provide adequate extraction and preservation.

A Formula to Determine Water Content of Fresh Herbs:

$$\frac{\text{weight of dry herb}}{\text{weight of fresh herb}} = \text{\% of dry weight}$$

100 minus the % of dry weight = weight of water content

The specific gravity of water is 1, and **1 gm of water conveniently equals 1 mL of water, which makes the weight of water equal to the amount of water.**

These are the steps to determine exactly how much water a fresh plant contains:

1) Weigh a sample of fresh herb. A sample weighing 50 or 100 gm makes for easy figuring.
2) Let the sample dry completely so that it snaps or crinkles when crushed. It may be dried quickly in an oven using very low heat, but do not let it burn.
3) Weigh the dried sample.
4) The difference in weights is equal to the amount of water in the fresh sample.

For example: A sample of 100 gm of fresh Thyme is dried and reduced to a weight of 30 gm.

This is expressed as $\frac{\text{30 gm dry herb}}{\text{100 gm fresh herb}}$ = 0.3 (30% dry weight)

100% - 30% dry weight = 70% water in the fresh plant

So, 100 gm of fresh Thyme contain 70% water. Since **1 gm of water equals 1 mL of water**, 100 gm of fresh Thyme already contains 70 mL of water. This amount of water is then figured into the equation when calculating the amount of grain alcohol and distilled water in the menstruum.

Another example: A sample of 51 gm of fresh Black Cohosh root is dried and reduced to 18 gm.

This is expressed as $\frac{\text{18 gm dry root}}{\text{51 gm fresh root}}$ = 0.35 (35% dry weight)

100% - 35% dry weight = 65% water in the fresh roots

Remember that various species of herbs absorb liquids differently. If you prepare tinctures according to these standard formulas and discover that there is not enough liquid menstruum to completely cover the herbal marc, measure and add enough to accomplish this, and then recalculate to determine the actual ratio of marc to menstruum that you used. For example, I once tinctured 500 gm of freshly harvested Passion Flower leaves using a standard formula for fresh herbs, which is 1:2 (75A:25W). According to this formula, 500 gm of herb should be covered with 1,000 mL of liquid menstruum (2 x 500 gm = 1,000 mL). However, 1,500 mL were needed to completely cover the marc, so the ratio of marc to menstruum turned out to be 1:3 (3 x 500 gm = 1,500 mL).

Let's look at some examples and go through the calculations for making fresh plant tinctures.

Example 1: You have harvested fresh Sage leaves to make a tincture.

1. Decide the strength of the tincture. Use a standard formula for fresh herbs, which is **1:2 (75A:25W).**

2. Weigh the herb. The leaves weigh 4 pounds, which equals 1,800 gm.
   To calculate: 1 pound = 450 gm
   4 pounds x 450 gm = 1,800 gm

3. Calculate the amount of menstruum needed to cover 1,800 gm of leaves.
   Using a 1:2 ratio means that there is twice as much liquid as plant material, so:
   2 x 1,800 gm of leaf = 3,600 mL of liquid menstruum needed

4. Calculate the percentage of water in a sample of the fresh herb:
   The weight of a fresh sample is 30 gm and is reduced to 16 gm when dried:
   $\frac{\text{16 gm of dry leaves}}{\text{30 gm fresh leaves}}$ = 0.53 (53%) of dry weight

   100% - 53% = 47% water in the fresh plant

5. Calculate how much water is in the total amount of fresh leaves by multiplying the weight of the fresh plant material (1,800 gm) by the percent of water in the plant (47%):

   1,800 x .47 = 846 mL of water in 1,800 gm of leaves

6. Calculate the total amount of liquid:
   3,600 mL of menstruum + 846 mL of water in leaves = 4,446 mL of liquid

7. For a (75A:25W) menstruum ratio, calculate 75% alcohol and 25% water from 4,446 mL:

    4,446 mL x .75 = 3,334.5 mL of alcohol
    4,446 mL x .25 = 1,111.5 mL of water

8. Compensate for water in the herb to determine the amount of alcohol and water in the final menstruum.

    The leaves already contain 846 mL of water.
    This amount is subtracted from 25% of the total water (1,111.5 mL):
    1,111.5 – 846 = 265.5 mL.

   The menstruum will contain 3,334.5 mL of grain alcohol and 265.5 mL of distilled water.

9. Add this amount of menstruum to the marc and complete the process as described in the simpler's method.

Example 2: You just harvested 3 pounds of Yellow Dock roots and want to make a tincture.

1. Use the other standard formula for fresh herbs, which is **1:3 (75A:25W).**

2. Weigh the herb. Use the metric formula to convert pounds into grams:
    1 pound = 450 gm
    3 pounds x 450 gm = 1,350 gm of roots

3. Calculate and measure the amount of menstruum needed for 1,350 gm of roots.
    Using a 1:3 ratio means that 3 times as much liquid is needed for the roots, so:
    3 x 1,350 gm of root = 4,050 mL of menstruum needed

4. Calculate the percentage of water in a sample of the fresh root:
    The weight of a fresh sample is 100 gm and is reduced to 50 gm when dried:

    $$\frac{\text{50 gm of dry root}}{\text{100 gm fresh root}} = \text{0.5 (50\%) of dry weight}$$

    100% - 50% = 50% water in the fresh plant

5. Calculate how much water is in the total amount of fresh roots by multiplying their weight (1,350 gm) by the percent of water in the plant (50%):

    1,350 x .50 = 675 mL of water in 1,350 gm of roots

6. Calculate the total amount of liquid:
    4,050 mL of menstruum + 675 mL of water in roots = 4,725 mL of liquid

7. For a (75A:25W) menstruum ratio, calculate 75% alcohol and 25% water from 4,725 mL:

    4,725 mL x .75 = 3,543.75 mL of alcohol
    4,725 mL x .25 = 1,181.25 mL of water

8. Compensate for water in the roots to determine the amount of alcohol and water in the final menstruum.

    Roots already contain 675 mL of water.
    This amount is subtracted from 25% of the total water (1,181.25 mL):
    1,181.25 – 675 = 506.25 mL of water.

   The menstruum will contain 3,543.75 mL of grain alcohol and 506.25 mL of distilled water.

9. Add this amount of menstruum to the marc and complete the process as described in the simpler's method.

As you can see, the complexer's method is much more technical and it takes a while to go through all the formulas and calculations. It will become easier with practice. If you find the complexer's method too technical or difficult, use the simpler's method to create very potent tinctures and have lots of fun with the herbs.

Elixirs

Elixers are drinks containing herbal tea, a sweetener like honey or glycerin, and small amounts of alcohol. Brandy is a good alcohol to use because it makes elixirs with the best flavor. Elixirs are generally tastier than tinctures, but larger doses are usually necessary to get the same physiological effects.

Liniments

Liniments are alcohol- or oil-based preparations used externally for massage and to rub into the skin to treat sprains, inflammation, and achy arthritic pain in the muscles and joints. Liniments are usually alcohol-based herbal extracts made in exactly the same way as tinctures. Since liniments are only used externally, less expensive isopropyl alcohol (rubbing alcohol) may be used to make them. Always label your bottle "for external use only" when using rubbing alcohol. Tinctures made with grain alcohol can be diluted with a little rubbing alcohol or water to be used for external problems. Infused oils, which are oil-based preparations, may also be applied as liniments.

Extracts

More concentrated and potent than tinctures, extracts are liquid or solid preparations made with alcohol and water. Extracts are usually produced by commercial manufacturers using technological equipment capable of further concentrating tinctures by evaporating most of the water and alcohol. The potency or strength of extracts is expressed in two ways. If the active chemicals are known, their strength can be expressed in terms of their amount. For example, Milk Thistle (*Silybum marianum*) extract is often standardized to contain 80% silymarin, one of its primary phytochemicals. Extracts are also measured by the "extract ratio," which is the ratio of the raw plant material to the finished product. When extracts are more concentrated than the amount of raw material, the final product is expressed as "1" and is the second number in the ratio. For example, a 9:1 solid extract means that 9 parts dried herb (measured in grams) is used to produce 1 part solid extract (also measured in grams). A 1:5 liquid extract means that 1 part dried herb (measured in grams) is used to produce 5 parts liquid extract (measured in milliliters). Many tinctures sold in North America are typically made in a 1:5 concentration.

Fluid extracts are usually a 1:1 concentration, meaning that they contain 1 part herb material to 1 part liquid solvent. An easy way to make a fluid extract at home is to boil off almost all the alcohol in the tincture until very little remains, leaving a more concentrated product. The heating will alter the preparation in some ways, so use a low heat.

Solid extracts are produced by further concentrating liquid extracts. The liquid (alcohol and water) is completely removed through different methods of evaporation, leaving a soft solid or dry residue that is usually a powder. Freeze-drying, called sublimation, is one common method of removing moisture from herbs. Solid extracts are the most concentrated and potent of all herbal products, and are typically produced in 2:1 to 8:1 concentrations. Solid extracts can be diluted with alcohol and water to make a fluid extract or tincture.

Oil-Based Preparations: Oils and Salves

Infused Oils

Infused oils are also called **fixed oils**. They are easy to make and can be processed in the comfort of your own kitchen. The selected herbs are chopped, covered with oil, and the mix is heated. The heated oil acts as the solvent (menstruum) to infuse or extract the medicinal components out of herbs (the marc). Any kind of vegetable oil can be used to infuse herbs, as long as it remains liquid in cooler temperatures. I prefer olive oil because it readily absorbs into the skin and resists rancidity longer than most other oils. When beeswax is melted into the hot oil, the mixture hardens and thickens into a **salve** or **ointment**. The olive oil does not have to be "extra virgin" or "cold pressed" since it is heated during the infusion process.

Infused oils are delightful to apply to the skin for healing and soothing purposes. They may be preferred over herbal salves made with beeswax because oils do not cause a waxy buildup on skin or hair, and can be applied on a daily basis for softening and healing the skin, treating chronic skin problems, and even caring for pets. Oil infusions make wonderful massage oils and moisturizing body lotions. Combining infused oils with commercially purchased body lotions in a 40% oil to 60% lotion ratio makes a wonderful body moisturizer.

I have been making infused oils for many years and use them on a daily basis combined with body lotion or prepared as salve. When you have infused your own oils, it is a wonderful feeling to envision all the colorful and fragrant herbs intermingling in your creation as you rub it on your skin. Have fun creating oils and add them to your herbal pharmacy. Enjoy the luxury of using their healing essence to heal and soothe your skin!

For listings of appropriate herbs to use in creating infused oils and salves, refer to the **"Index of Health Issues and Herbal Recommendations"** in Section Three and look under the heading "Skin."

Recipe for Infused Oils

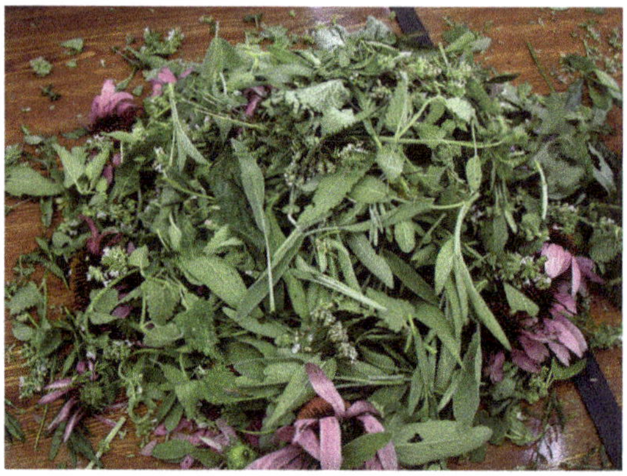

1) Freshly harvested herbs

❖ First, gather the herbs of your choice. Using freshly harvested herbs to make oils and salves ensures a vitally potent end product, but if this is not possible, dried herbs will do.

❖ Chop the herb material into small pieces with a knife. For large quantities, food processors or leaf shredders are helpful. Be sure that freshly harvested herbs are free of excess moisture to discourage the formation of mold. After chopping the herb into small pieces, they may be allowed to dry for 3-6 hours.

❖ Place the chopped herbs in a glass, enamel, or stainless steel pan. Do not use aluminum or cast iron.

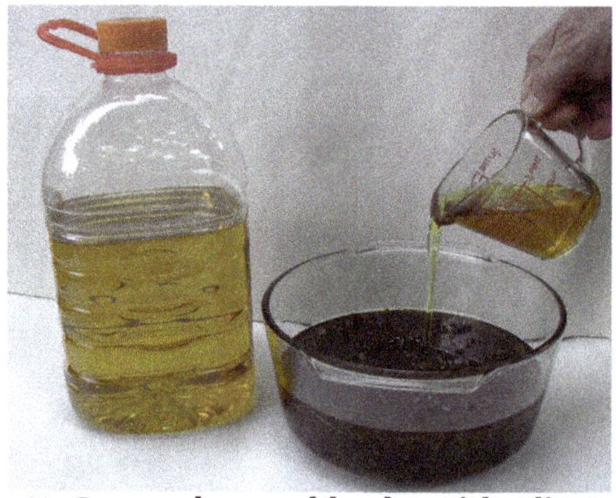

2) Cover chopped herbs with olive oil and bake them in an oven

❖ Pour olive oil into the bowl and completely cover the herbs.

❖ Put the pan of herbs and olive oil in an oven and bake for 3-4 hours at a very low temperature of 180-200°F. Stir occasionally to prevent the plant material on top from drying and turning crispy. Do not overheat the oil or let it boil!

❖ Keep the pan uncovered when baking the herbal oil. Some herbs like Yellow Dock, Comfrey, and Chickweed release gas as they infuse, so if you see bubbles in your oil, do not be alarmed. Any water left in the oil will sink to the bottom.

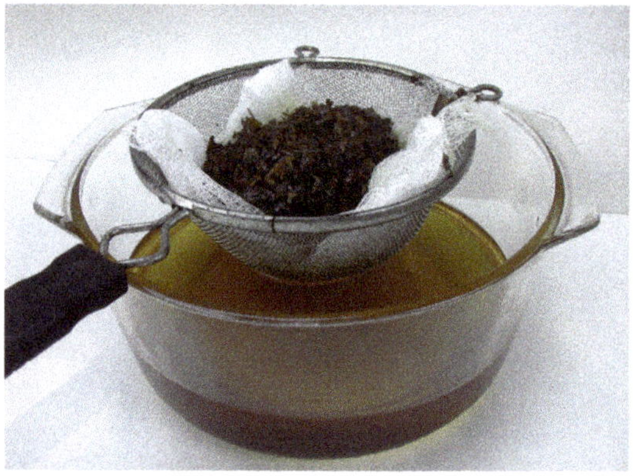

3) Baked herbs and oil being strained through cheese cloth

❖ When the baking is complete allow the oil to cool until it is warm.

❖ The warm oil is then separated (decanted) from the herb material. This is done in two steps:

❖ First, prepare a wire strainer or colander by lining it with several overlapping layers of cheesecloth and place this over a large bowl.

❖ Pour or scoop the mixture of herbs and oil into the strainer, which will collect the bulk of the plant material and allow the oil to pass through into the bowl underneath. Squeeze and wring out as much of the remaining oil from the plant material as possible. You can use latex gloves for this or simply enjoy the delightfully warm oil.

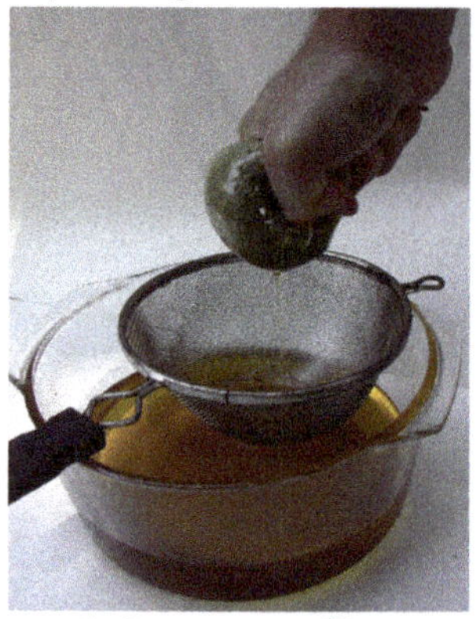

4) Squeeze oil out of the herbs

❖ Next, use the "nylon stocking method" to remove the final remnants of plant particles from the oil. Put a clean knee-high nylon stocking in a container, placing the toe end at the bottom of the container. Lip the open end of the stocking over and around the mouth of the container, and use a rubber band to hold it in place.

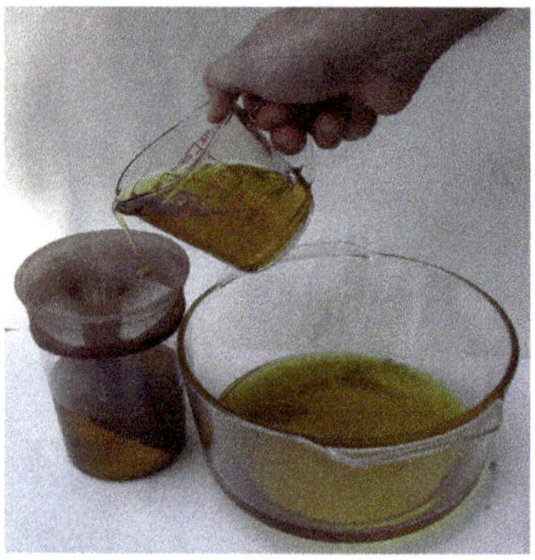

5) Pour oil into nylon stocking to remove all plant particles

❖ Carefully pour the strained oil into the nylon, which will hold the remaining plant material while allowing the clean oil to filter through. Be sure the oil is not too hot, or it will scald the nylon.

❖ Some people like to add fragrances to their infused oils. Aromatic essential oils are added after baking is complete, immediately before pouring the finished oil into jars.

❖ Finally, pour the herbal oil into clean jars or bottles. Fill jars to the very top to reduce as much air space as possible. This discourages growth of mold.

❖ Label the jars with the names of the herbs they contain and the date. Store them in a cool, dark place. Refrigerating the oil will increase its shelf life. Refrigeration makes olive oil solidify, but it quickly returns to liquid at room temperature.

❖ Oils and salves typically stay fresh for 6-9 months after a jar has been opened and for 2 or 3 years in unopened jars. Exposing oils and salves to warm air accelerates the rancidity process. You can tell when oils go rancid by their stale odor.

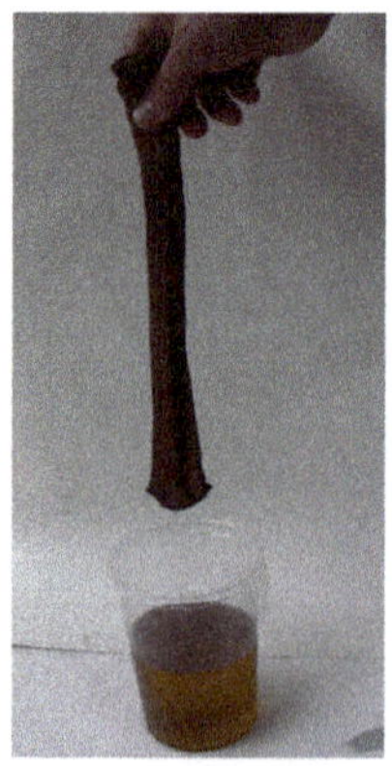

6) Drain oil from stocking

Tips for Making Infused Oil with Herbs Harvested During Different Times of the Year

The herbal oil that I have been making for many years is a blend of roots, leaves, and flowers from about 20 different herbs. Some of these herbs are harvested in spring while others are gathered throughout summer and into autumn. Therefore, harvesting is a process that takes the whole growing season to complete. If you make oil with several herbs that must be harvested at different times, there are two ways of accomplishing this. With the first method, each herb is gathered at its peak time of freshness, cleaned, and chopped into small pieces. Allow the chopped herb to dry for several hours to reduce moisture. Then put each prepared herb in a plastic bag, squeeze the air out of the bag, label it with the name of the herb and date of harvest, and store it in the freezer. At the end of the growing season when all the herbs have been collected, they are processed into oil. Put all the frozen herbs in a large pan to thaw and dry out. Cover them with oil and bake according to the recipe above for infused oils.

The second method eliminates the need to freeze herbs, and is the one I use and prefer. Rather than being frozen, each batch of herbs collected throughout the growing season is baked in olive oil. The oil is then strained from the plant material, stored in jars, and labeled. At the end of the growing season when all the plants have been harvested and processed into oil, all the batches of oil are thoroughly mixed together in one large container. The oil is then poured into bottles and labeled, or further processed into salve. These methods work well and allow you to use a wide variety of herbs that have to be harvested during different times, while maintaining very fresh quality.

Herbal Salves

Salves are also called **ointments**. Most salves are now made by adding beeswax to infused oils to thicken and harden the liquid oil into a solid paste. Prior to the industrialized production of olive and other vegetable oils, salves and ointments were made with lard and other fats rendered from animals. My friend, Dark Rain Thom of the Shawnee Nation, still follows the old traditions of her Native American ancestors and sometimes melts bear fat to thicken her herbal salves. Salves and ointments are used to heal, soothe, and disinfect external wounds, sprains and fractures, skin irritations, rashes, bites, and stings. The thick consistency of salve allows it to stick on the skin and stay in place. Salves are often easier to manage than oils and are not as messy. They can be applied in a thin layer or a thick glob, and covered with a non-absorbent dressing to stay in place for several hours and have long-lasting effects.

The oils in salves naturally soothe and moisturize all tissues they directly contact. This relaxes and opens skin pores, allowing the herbal components to be absorbed and penetrate into the deeper tissues. For this reason, salves and ointments can assist in healing and soothing muscles, joints, and deeper organs. Depending on the herbs they contain, salves can reduce pain and inflammation, and exert an excellent drawing effect to pull out toxins from bites, stings, and deeper toxins and pus released through pimples, abscesses, or hive-like rashes.

Have fun making salve! I have been making salve since the early 1980s and use it every day to soothe and heal dry skin, chapped lips, cuts, bruises, burns, bug bites, and occasionally for more serious injuries or problems. I cannot imagine life without my salve and am constantly grateful to the plants for their beautiful presence and remarkable healing gifts.

Instructions for Making Herbal Salve

Salve production begins with the creation of infused oil that is then combined with beeswax to produce a thicker, more solidified consistency.

❖Follow the directions for making infused oils provided in the section above. Herbs are chopped, baked in olive oil, and the oil is separated from the plant material. At this point, the herbal oil should be warm and clean. It is then ready for the beeswax to be added.

❖The amount of beeswax will determine the thickness and solidity of the salve. People's preferences vary, so experiment with different amounts to find what works best for you.

Commonly used ratios of beeswax to infused oil:

2:8 means that 2 ounces of beeswax are added to 8 ounces of oil
(this makes a very thick, solid salve)

1:8 means that 1 ounce of beeswax is added to 8 ounces of oil
(1:8 is the ratio I use and recommend for medium thickness)

1/2:8 means that ½ ounce of beeswax is added to 8 ounces of oil
(this makes a thinner, softer, less solid salve)

When measuring remember:
8 ounces = 1 cup

❖Beeswax usually comes in blocks that have to be cut into pieces to be measured and added to the oil. Beeswax can be cut by heating a long knife blade over a gas burner until it gets hot enough to slowly cut through the wax, or by using a hammer and large screw driver to break the block into small pieces.

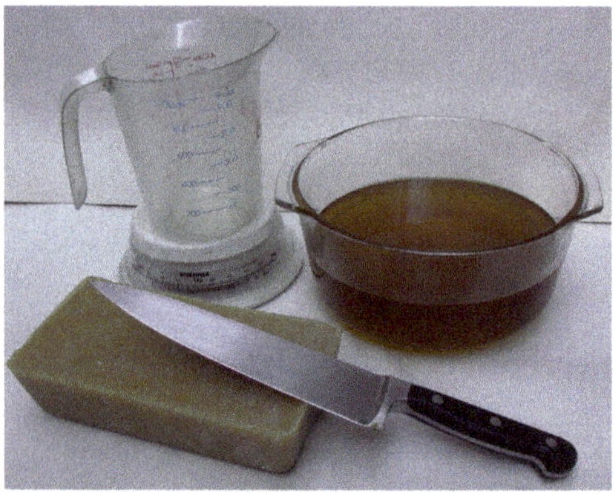

1) Infused oil and beeswax

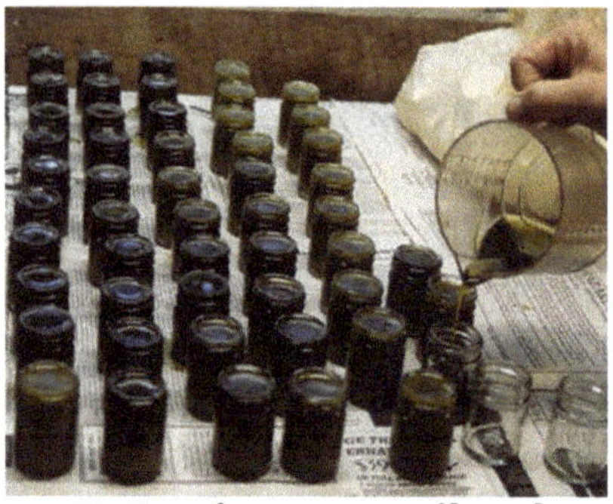

3) Pouring warm oil and wax mixture into jars

❖ After adding beeswax to the pan of oil, place it on the stove top and very slowly reheat the oil until the wax is completely melted. Constantly stir the mixture and do not let it overheat. The oil should be warm enough to melt the wax but not allowed to get too hot.

❖ When the wax has melted and disappeared, it is always wise to check the consistency of the salve before pouring it into your containers. To do this, create a test sample by placing 1-2 tablespoons of the warm oil and melted beeswax into a jar and allow it to stand at room temperature until it cools and solidifies. Placing it in the refrigerator for a few minutes speeds up this process. Then check to make sure it is the consistency you want. If it is too soft, add more beeswax to your pan of oil and let it melt down into the brew. Then retest.

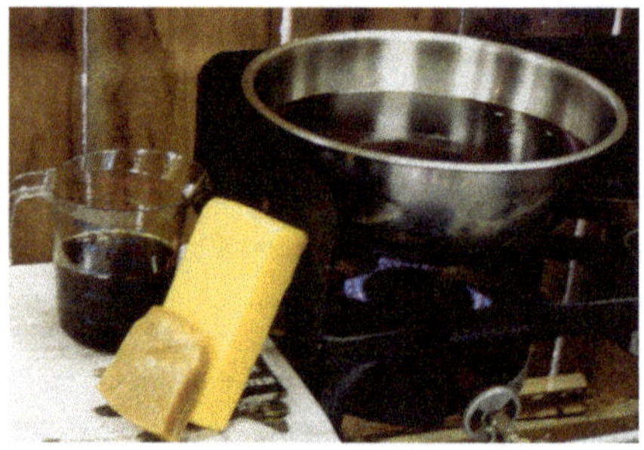

2) Melting beeswax in hot oil

❖ When you are satisfied with your test results, pour the warm oil and wax mixture into clean glass jars, carefully filling them to the top. A large air space in the jar increases the possibility of mold and bacterial growth. As the mixture cools it will solidify into a wonderful salve.

❖ Screw the lids tightly onto the jars.

❖ Label the jars and store them in a cool place out of direct sunlight. If you have room in your refrigerator, cool conditions retard the tendency for oils to go rancid and extend shelf life. Keep your oils and salves away from heat and the sun, which eventually deteriorates oils and the healing qualities of herbs.

Beeswax

Beeswax is a golden-yellow substance made by bees when they are inside their hives. They secrete and deposit the wax to form cup-like containers that hold honey. When honey is extracted from hives, beeswax is a natural by-product. It can be melted and made into beautiful, heavenly-smelling candles, and is also used as the hardening agent in salves. Beeswax contains natural antibiotics that help keep bee hives clean and sterile, and it also contributes to the healing properties of herbal salves.

When beeswax is taken directly from hives, it is full of debris and must be cleaned and filtered. Do this by melting the wax in a stainless steel pan over low heat until it liquefies. Turn off the heat and, when the wax has cooled to a warm temperature, use a knee-high nylon stocking to strain out the debris. If the wax is too hot, it will singe the nylon. Have someone help you by carefully holding the end of the stocking wide open so you can pour the melted wax through the nylon. The debris will be neatly contained in the foot of the stocking, which can be discarded. Place a container under the stocking to hold the beeswax. For this purpose, you can use plastic food containers, small boxes, or bread pans lined with waxed paper. After the clean beeswax is poured into a container and has cooled, the wax paper holding the solid block of wax can be easily lifted out of the pan. Then you have a block of clean beeswax that looks beautiful and smells great! At this point, it is ready to be cut, measured, and added to your salve. Clean your utensils by pouring boiling water over them to melt the beeswax.

Many health food stores sell blocks of beeswax that are clean and ready to use. You can also check labels in the honey section of health food stores to find local beekeepers. They often have extra beeswax and are happy to sell it.

Solar Infused Oils

Solar infusion is an old method of preparing herbal oils using the heat of the sun. Herbs are chopped into small pieces, placed in a glass jar, covered with olive oil, and a lid is securely screwed onto the jar. Put the jar in a warm, sunny location for 1-2 weeks. It is important to fill the jar to the top without leaving any air space in order to reduce oxidation and the potential for mold growth.

Essential (Volatile) Oils

Essential oils, also known as volatile oils, are extremely concentrated plant oils obtained by distillation. Hundreds of pounds of fresh herbs may produce only a few ounces of essential oil. Their production requires expensive, sophisticated equipment and is more challenging for the "kitchen" herbalist to make at home.

Essential oils are used both externally and internally, exerting a wide range of healing properties determined by their chemical constituents. They are very potent and must be used with caution and respect. Be aware that everything applied to the skin permeates through the porous tissues and can get into the bloodstream where it is transported throughout the body. This includes herbal oils, salves, poultices, hair spray and chemical coloring agents, deodorants, insect repellents, hand lotion, and much more. Pennyroyal oil applied to the mid-forehead has been known to stimulate uterine contractions in women. Always think twice about what you put on your skin!

Avoid skin irritation when applying essential oils to the skin by diluting them in a base of olive oil or other vegetable oil. The amount of dilution can range from 1-5%, which amounts to 6-30 drops of essential oil to 1 ounce of vegetable oil. A 2.5% preparation equates to 15 drops of essential oil to 1 ounce of vegetable oil. Essential oils can be used for aromatherapy or applied to the skin to repel insects, increase blood and lymphatic circulation, relieve spasms, inflammation and pain, treat skin eruptions and dermatitis, prevent and reduce infection, and heal injuries.

Be *extremely* careful when using essential oils internally! They are very strong and should always be diluted in tea or water. Some should never be ingested, so always check labels. No more than 1 or 2 drops of essential oil should be ingested, and even this may be too much for children and more sensitive adults. Always keep essential oils out of the reach of small children because ingesting large amounts can be damaging or even fatal.

Standardized Herbal Products

A **standardized extract** is an herbal extract produced according to specific criteria. There are different types of standardized extracts and some may be very simple, such as the ratio of crude plant material to the finished product. A standardized extract of 3:1 means that 3 kilograms of raw herb material is processed to yield 1 kilogram of finished product. A **galenical extrac**t is made by the ancient method of extracting herbs in an alcohol and water combination, and is named after Galen, the Greek herbalist and physician who lived around A.D. 150. Galenical preparations are standardized according to their ratios of herb to alcohol and alcohol to water. In the past, all galenical preparations were fluid extracts or tinctures, but with the advent of technology, liquid extracts are often dried to solid residues and produced as pills or capsules. Herbalists generally view galenicals as "whole herb" extracts because they contain the full spectrum of phytochemicals in plants rather than focusing on only one or two constituents.

In the herbal manufacturing industry, standardization implies that an extract has been produced to contain a specific and consistent amount of one or more phytochemicals. Plants of the same species typically contain different concentrations of chemical constituents due to variables that include the type of soil they are grown in, amount of rain and sunlight, the health and age of individual plants, time of harvest, and methods of preparation. The process of standardization is an attempt to ensure that an herbal preparation contains measurable amounts of specific phytomedicines to provide reliable and consistent activity from batch to batch. Manufacturers producing standardized extracts guarantee customers that every dose contains a "standardized" or precise amount of one or more chemical constituents.

The herb industry has three basic classifications of standardized herbs: guaranteed potency herbs, fortified herbs, and phytopharmaceuticals. **Guaranteed potency** products have been tested for the chemical components listed on the label. These herbs have not been altered and are considered to be "whole herb" products. **Fortified herbal preparations** have one or more chemical constituents added to them. This practice is acceptable if the added constituents are combined with whole, potent herbs. But sometimes manufacturers add constituents to a poor quality and inferior herbal base, similar to fortifying white processed bread with vitamins and minerals to make it nutritious. When extracts are produced from potent herbs grown and processed under optimal conditions, there is no need to fortify them. **Phytopharmaceutical products** only contain one or more isolated chemical constituents in a filler base. They do not contain the whole herb and are more like pharmaceutical drugs that typically contain only one active ingredient.

In July 2003, the American Herbal Products Association (AHPA) published *Standardization of Botanical Products*, a 33-page document providing an authoritative reference that discusses and defines standardization of herbal products. In it, the AHPA defines standardization as "the complete body of information and controls to optimize the batch-to-batch consistency of botanical products. Standardization is achieved by reducing the inherent variation of natural product composition through quality assurance practices applied to agricultural and manufacturing processes." It is a complex and confusing subject because "herbal standardization" means different things to different people. In its broadest scope, standardization involves consistent agricultural and manufacturing methods.

The practice of standardizing is an attempt to enhance the consistency of an herb's safety and efficacy. Standardized herbal preparations are produced to contain defined amounts of specific phytochemicals or active constituents called "marker compounds." When specified amounts of marker compounds are present in raw herb material, it is an indication that other important constituents are also present in relative amounts. In this way, marker compounds make it possible to reproduce multiple batches of an herbal product with consistent biological activity, which is a primary aim of the standardization process.

A major advantage of standardized herbs is their ability to supply an accurate dose of the desired phytochemicals. Physicians and pharmacists prefer standardized botanicals because they provide a level of reliability and consistency, and are a step closer to pharmaceutical drugs that can be measured, prescribed, and dispensed in specific amounts. Standardization can promote consistent guidelines and better regulation during the manufacturing process. Standardized preparations provide more scientifically measurable and reliable outcomes in research and clinical trials, and most of the herbal research in Europe and the United States has been done using standardized extracts.

However, standardized extracts are controversial among some herbalists for several reasons. Although researchers can prove the biological and medicinal efficacy of standardized herbs, this does not necessarily establish that these herbal preparations are the best to take for medicinal purposes. Some people feel that these artificially manipulated preparations, achieved with sophisticated technology, are moving away from the time-honored traditional roots of herbalism grounded in the perspective of holism and "whole plant" remedies. Plants contain complex mixtures of hundreds or even thousands of chemical compounds responsible for their unique properties and biological actions. Every plant is a perfect balance of phytochemicals that nature has engineered and evolved over eons of time. The more that people alter and tamper with the structure and chemical balance of plants, the further we move away from this perfect balance and holistic perspective that has always been at the heart of herbalism. It is important to realize that the medicinal effects of herbs always result from the synergistic combination of *all* chemical substances in the plant, and are never limited to the activity of only a few. The process of standardization often focuses on only one or two chemical "marker compounds," presuming that these, rather than the combination of all phytochemicals, produce the important benefits. This tends to follow the reductionistic model of pharmaceutical medicines consisting of only one isolated chemical. Using herbal products containing the whole herb is like eating whole foods that provide complete and optimal nutrition.

Another potential problem with standardization is deciding upon suitable markers to measure as standard criteria. The industry determines which constituents are chosen to be the marker compounds based on constantly expanding research. Often the marker chemicals are not the active constituents in herbs. For example, *Ginkgo biloba* leaf standardized extract (GBE) was initially manufactured to contain 24% ginkgo flavonol glycosides, but later research indicated that a different group of terpenes was more important, and now GBE is also standardized for these. It is important to remember that marker compounds are not necessarily the only active constituents in herbs and do not reflect the totality of herbal activity.

There are definitely some benefits to standardizing herbal products. But it does not necessarily guarantee quality, as is usually assumed. Choosing the right raw materials, marker compounds, analytical methods, and processing techniques is necessary for optimal quality and potency of standardized herbal products. Standardized preparations do not contain the benefits of the whole plant unless the extracted chemical compounds are added to a base of whole herb extract.

Pharmaceutical companies have been the primary force promoting and establishing the production of standardized herbal preparations, which can legally be patented and provide much greater monetary profits compared to non-standardized products. But there are many flaws in the system, and several analytical studies have found that potency claims on many labels of herbal preparations are not accurate. On August 31, 1998, the *Los Angeles Times* reported about false potency claims on the labels of 10 different standardized St. John's Wort products purchased from health food stores. An independent lab tested their content of hypericin, a primary constituent used for standardizing, and discovered that 8 out of 10 products had less than 90% of the hypericin claimed on the label. The two lowest-potency products only contained 20% and 22% of the amount claimed on the label.

Standardized extracts are sold in the form of liquids, tablets, and capsules in pharmacy, grocery, and discount stores in the United States and Europe. They are becoming more popular among the general population due, in part, to mass media and advertising. Following the scientific method and an analytical, reductionistic approach to medicine and healing, the pharmaceutical companies, scientific research community, and medical profession continue to move in the direction of herbal standardization. Standardized herbal preparations certainly serve important functions and are important for valid research and the advancement of herbalism in the modern medical system. However, always remember that whole herb extracts processed from plants that have been properly grown, harvested, handled, and prepared are vital and potent remedies that provide adequate biological activity on their own. Fortifying or standardizing them does not necessarily improve the quality or efficacy that is provided by the master chemist, Mother Nature.

In Closing

For many years, I have relied on herbal allies for their trusted assistance in keeping me well and helping my family, friends, and clients stay healthy. I am always grateful to be able to go to the herbal medicine cabinet and pull out one of my homemade preparations to ward off an impending cold, relieve a painful injury, or deal with other problems that arise. These guidelines and instructions will hopefully provide you with the information and inspiration to create your own herbal pharmacy, and to receive the healing gifts that the plants have to offer. Learning the art and science of plant alchemy to transform live plants into potent healing medicines is an empowering, exciting way to interact and co-create with Nature and the elements. Making your own herbal medicines, especially from plants you grow and harvest, is a blessing that brightens your life and calms the heart and mind. Learn from all your successes and failures as you create your medicines, and be sure to experiment and follow your intuition in a spirit of adventure!

Creating Herbal Formulas

After researching and learning about an assortment of individual herbs by reading, classes, growing, and gaining the practical experience of using them in your own health care, you may want to consider combining them into formulas for specific health purposes. A fundamental knowledge of human anatomy, physiology, and disease processes is vital when choosing the herbs that will work best to promote and maintain health and heal illness. It is helpful to understand the biological activities and healing qualities of each herb in terms of how they interact with each other in a formula, and how they will affect the individual taking them. A person's constitution should be considered, along with the nature of the health problem. Herbs should be chosen to heal underlying causes of the imbalance and improve symptoms. The skill of creating herbal formulas is acquired over time with study and experience. The science and art of herbal formulation can be rather complicated and challenging, but the results are worth the effort!

Differences Between Polypharmacy and Simpling

Polypharmacy is the ancient practice of combining several herbs to create a formula. Many herbalists prefer using these more complex formulas when treating a specific problem rather than relying on only one or two herbs, which is called **simpling**. Over the centuries, many sophisticated plant-based healing systems around the world have developed extensive formulations of remedies that continue to be popular in modern times. In Traditional Chinese Medicine and the Indian tradition of Ayurvedic medicine, the majority of practitioners prescribe herbal formulas containing anywhere from five to twenty different herbs. In my personal life and nursing practice, I have found that the practice of polypharmacy is usually superior to simpling for a few reasons.

Polypharmacy is the art of combining several herbs into one formula to treat a specific problem.

Simpling is the other ancient practice of using only one or two herbs to address a health problem.

First, the healing potential of the whole formula is greater than that of the individual herbs. Combining several herbs to treat a health problem provides a greater broad-spectrum effect that allows a variety of symptoms to be treated with one formula. For example, if a person is suffering from a bacterial bladder infection and complaining of pelvic pain, burning urination and bloody urine, an herbal formula is needed to address all these problems. One herb would probably not be up to the task, but several herbs combined in a formula would be able to address these various problems and provide greater healing potential. Such a formula may include three or four antibiotic herbs such as Goldenseal (*Hydrastis canadensis*), Yarrow (*Achillea millefolium*), Sage (*Salvia officinalis*), or Pau D'arco (*Tabebuia* spp.) to fight the infection. Goldenseal and Yarrow are also anti-inflammatory to reduce tissue irritation, as is Stinging Nettle (*Urtica dioica*). Soothing herbs like Marshmallow (*Althaea officinalis*), Corn Silk (*Zea mays*), or Oatstraw (*Avena sativa*) help ease pain, and cool and heal irritated, inflamed tissues. Astringent herbs such as Cranesbill (*Geranium maculatum*), Cinquefoil (*Potentilla* spp.), Sage, or Yarrow can be included to tone and contract tissues to stop bleeding. This type of formulation would be much more effective than using only one herb.

Secondly, when treating acute or chronic problems, herbal formulas usually provide much faster results and reduce more symptoms than taking only one herb. Combining several herbs is often more effective than the simpling method because of the synergistic relationship of plants in which they harmoniously blend together to activate and balance each other. For example, when herbs in a formula are strong or bitter, sweet-tasting herbs like Licorice (*Glycyrrhiza glabra*), Anise (*Pimpinella anisum*), or Fennel (*Foeniculum vulgare*) can be added to improve the flavor. Excessively warming herbs in a formula can be neutralized with cooling herbs like Dandelion (*Taraxacum officinale*), Burdock (*Arctium* spp.), or Isatis (*Isatis tinctoria*). Combining three or four antibacterial herbs to fight an infection is more effective than using only one, because each herb acts in its own way on specific bacteria, and their combined qualities provide greater strength and broad-spectrum effect.

Combining herbs is usually superior to simpling because synergistic actions of several herbs provide greater broad-spectrum effect than one herb alone.

It is also important to remember that herbs have primary actions providing the strongest healing activity as well as secondary actions. For instance, Wormwood (*Artemisia absinthium*) is used to kill parasites as its primary action, but it also has secondary qualities as a stomach bitter to promote better digestion. St. John's Wort (*Hypericum perforatum*), known to help with mild to moderate depression, is also an analgesic for pain and a powerful antiviral with special affinity for the nervous system and treating the herpes virus.

Creating Formulas According to the "Three Cornerstones" Model

There are three fundamental guidelines or cornerstones to follow when preparing potent and balanced herbal formulas. View these three guidelines as a triangle.

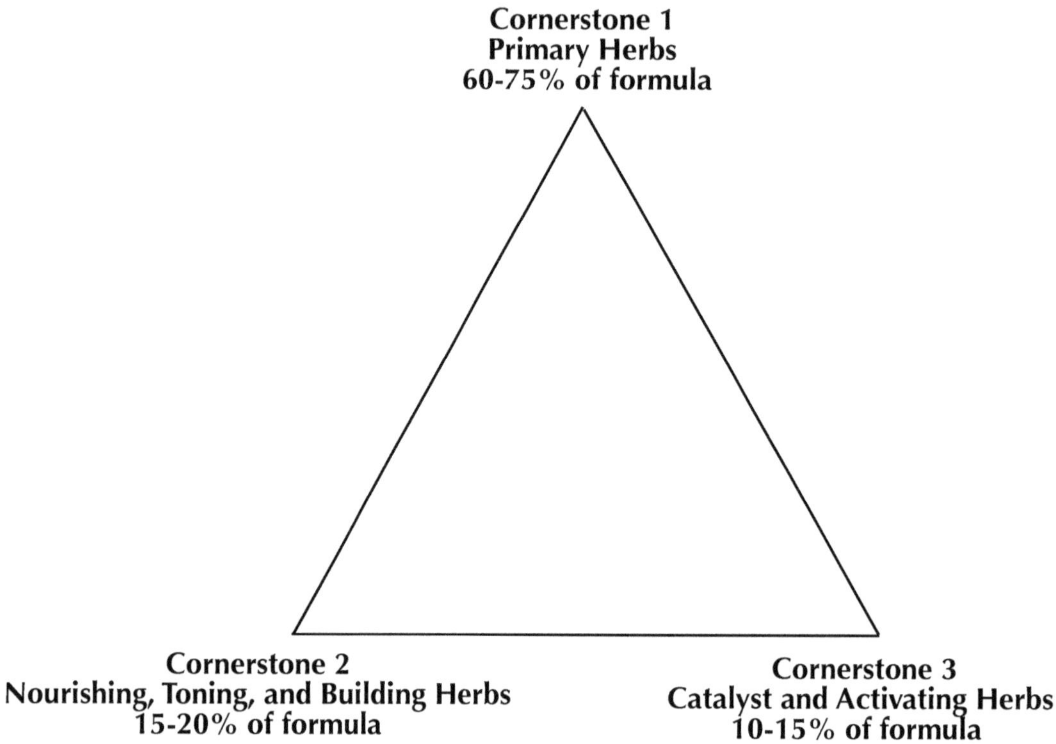

The **first cornerstone** consists of several primary herbs that target specific ailments or imbalances. Primary herbs are the most potent and exert the major activity. They usually comprise 60-75% of the formula. Other herbs in the formula should support and balance activities of these primary herbs.

The **second cornerstone** consists of herbs that support and nourish the body. They tend to be nutritive tonics containing significant amounts of vitamins, minerals, and other substances that build, tone, and fortify the specific body systems being targeted. Secondary herbs are milder and often contain mucilaginous or demulcent materials that are soothing and can buffer the powerful nature of some primary herbs. They may also be pleasant-tasting or fragrant, and are added to improve the flavor and aroma of the formula. Secondary herbs comprise about 15-20% of the formula, and strengthen the properties and support the actions of the primary herbs.

The **third cornerstone** is composed of the "movers and shakers." These are the herbs that activate and catalyze both the formula and the body systems. They increase blood and lymphatic circulation, stimulate energy and movement throughout the body, and promote elimination. They perk up the system, break up congestion, contribute warmth, and help move the primary herbs throughout the body. Third cornerstone herbs are typically diuretics, stimulants, laxatives, diaphoretics, and adjuvants that promote circulation and carry other herbs to their target sites in the body. These herbs usually make up 10-15% of the formula.

General Guidelines for Making Formulas

1. Familiarize yourself with each herb you put in your formula through study and personal experience. Be aware of its taste, medicinal properties, and how it will function in the formula and in the human body. Think through your choices so you produce a balanced formula for the person and conditions being treated.

2. An herbal combination can include as few as three or four herbs or as many as twenty. Choose your herbs wisely for their specific qualities to promote balance. Choices for ingredients in your formulas are also determined by the plant species that are available in your area.

3. When preparing formulas for tea, roots and bark are thick and dense so they must be simmered first. When this simmering is complete, turn off the heat and add the more delicate leaves and flowers to be steeped.

4. You can base your formulas on older traditional ones that have been successfully used and handed down over time. But also be willing to trust your instincts and rely on your "hunches" when creating new formulas or altering older ones. It is fun and exciting to experiment with some of your own ideas.

5. Always pay attention to the condition of the digestive, nervous, and endocrine systems. The digestive organs (stomach, pancreas, liver, gallbladder, and intestines) must function properly to provide nutrients essential for the healing process. The nervous and endocrine systems must be in balance to facilitate the regulation of all body functions.

6. When creating a formula for a person with a specific problem, consider the individual's case history. Work with the intention of bringing his or her system into dynamic balance by treating the underlying causes and resulting symptoms. This is a precise and refined skill requiring knowledge of human anatomy, physiology, and disease processes. The ability to understand energetic qualities of herbs and disease processes, and to choose herbs according to their energetics, involves a complex study of the dynamic energies of the human body and medicinal plants. Knowledgeable practitioners of Traditional Chinese and Ayurvedic Medicine have highly refined this art of balance, basing their herbal remedies on the system of energetic dynamics. Hippocrates and other early European physicians understood these energetic forces and implemented them in their medical system as the "four humors." Further study of these traditions is highly recommended and extremely enlightening for greater appreciation of the life forces.

The basic energetics of balance include the elements of damp/dry, cold/hot, deficiency/excess, and internal/external. The qualities of a person's illness are matched with the energetics of medicinal herbs to restore health. For example, conditions caused by too much dampness such as edema (water retention) are treated with drying and diuretic herbs. Conditions of excess heat that are drying to tissues are treated with cooling and moisturizing herbs like Chickweed (*Stellaria* spp.), Marshmallow, Burdock, or Plantain (*Plantago* spp.). Cold-natured people with poor circulation and sluggish digestion can benefit from stimulating, warming herbs. On the other hand, hyperactive and hot-tempered people benefit from sedating, calming, and cooling herbs. For problems caused by deficiency such as anemia or osteoporosis, use nutritive herbs like Dandelion, Burdock, and Stinging Nettle that contain iron, calcium, and other minerals. For conditions of excess, such as constant sinus drainage or constipation, use detoxifying and decongesting herbs.

7. To create a formula, write the symptoms you want to address in the order of highest priority. Assign several appropriate primary herbs to address these major problems and symptoms. If infection is the primary issue, use several antibiotic herbs such as Yarrow, Boneset (*Eupatorium perfoliatum*), Echinacea, or Goldenseal. If the infection is viral, include antiviral herbs like Licorice, St. John's Wort, Thyme (*Thymus vulgaris*), Hyssop (*Hyssopus officinalis*), or Isatis. For wound healing, add vulnerary herbs such as Calendula (*Calendula officinalis*) and Comfrey (*Symphytum officinale*) to promote tissue repair and growth.

8. Next, decide which botanicals are appropriate to use as secondary herbs. If nutrition is poor and the person needs strengthening, select nutritious herbs such as Stinging Nettle, Chickweed, Astragalus (*Astragalus membranaceus*), Burdock, or Alfalfa (*Medicago sativa*). If there is a problem with poor digestion, include Peppermint (*Mentha x piperita*), Horehound (*Marrubium vulgare*), Ginger (*Zingiber officinale*), or Dandelion to promote digestion and assimilation of the primary herbs. For inflammation and irritated tissues, add mucilaginous demulcents such as Marshmallow root or Chickweed. If the primary herbs are bitter, include Stevia (*Stevia rebaudiana*), Licorice, Fennel, or Anise to sweeten and modify the flavor.

9. Choose which tertiary (third level) herbs to employ for promoting activity and energy in the body. When circulation is slow, warming stimulants such as Cayenne (*Capsicum annuum*), Ginger, Garlic, or Peppermint may be added. Cayenne and Ginger are often used because they stimulate circulation and assist the other herbs in the formula in traveling through the body. For lymphatic congestion, select Echinacea or Poke root (*Phytolacca decandra*), which is only taken in small doses. Laxative herbs such as Senna (*Senna* spp.), Cascara Sagrada (*Rhamnus purshiana*), or Buckthorn (*Rhamnus cathartica)* are appropriate for constipation problems. If detoxification is indicated, use blood-cleansing herbs such as Calendula, Hyssop, and Milk Thistle (*Silybum marianum*), or the roots of Dandelion, Yellow Dock (*Rumex crispus),* and Burdock.

10. Mix all primary, secondary, and tertiary herbs together and try your formula. Notice its taste, aroma, and effect after using it. With time and experience, you may decide to change ingredients or alter measurements to improve the formula. Record all the formulas you prepare and their effects.

For your assistance when preparing formulas, the chapter **"Healing Qualities of Herbs"** in Section One explains the biological effects various plants produce in people. The **"Index of Health Issues and Herbal Recommendations"** in Section Three is helpful in choosing appropriate herbs. The energetic qualities of each of the 50 herbs in the Materia Medica section are also provided.

Over the years, I have created and improved many formulas as I learn more about individual herbs, discover new plants growing in the wild, and grow additional herbs in my gardens. My salve formula was created over a period of eight to ten years, as I discovered two or three new vulnerary (wound-healing) herbs that I added to the original formula each year. Devising herbal formulas can be a very creative and expansive experience that has no end or limitations. Experiment and enjoy making your own herbal formulas!

How to Calculate Dosages

Calculating dosages for children and the elderly is always necessary, especially when using tinctures, pills, or capsules. Knowing the appropriate dosage is vital to ensure safety and the desired outcome when using herbal preparations. Commercially available herbal products like pills, capsules, tinctures, and cough syrups always specify recommended dosages on their labels. Standardized botanical extracts provide specific amounts of guaranteed active ingredients measured in units to make dosages more accurate for these compounds. If you make your own herbal medicine or acquire a preparation that does not provide a recommended dosage, you will need to do some research. Specific dosages are provided for each herb listed in the Materia Medica section of this book.

Methods Used to Calculate Dosages for Medicinal Herb Preparations

There are several ways to calculate dosages. The King's American Dispensatory, Fried's Rule, and Young's Rule determine dosage by age. **Clark's Rule is the most accurate and reliable method because it measures according to weight, which can vary greatly within the same age group.** Clark's Rule can be used to calculate dosages for children, the elderly, and other adults who are smaller or larger than average. **Most dosages appearing in literature and on labels are recommended for people who weigh about 150 pounds.** A person who weighs at least 20-30 pounds less or more than that should adjust the dose for best results.

Clark's Rule for Dosages
(the safest and most reliable method)

$$\text{Child's dose} = \frac{\text{Child's weight in pounds}}{\text{150 pounds (average adult weight)}} \times \text{adult dose}$$

Young's Rule for Dosages

$$\text{Child's dose} = \frac{\text{child's age (in years)}}{\text{child's age (in years)} + 12} \times \text{adult dose}$$

Fried's Rule for Dosages

This is calculated by months and is used for infants 2 years of age and younger.

$$\text{Child's dose} = \frac{\text{child's age in months}}{\text{150 months}} \times \text{adult dose}$$

King's American Dispensatory Rules for Dosages

For the **Elderly** over 63 years . . . . 5/6 (of a full adult dose)
over 77 years 2/3
For **Children** under 1/2 year . . . . . . 1/15 (of a full adult dose)
under 1 year 1/12
under 2 years 1/8
under 3 years 1/6
under 4 years 1/5
under 5 years 1/4
under 7 years 1/3
under 14 years 1/2

For example, you need to give a tincture to a 5-year-old child weighing 40 pounds. The bottle of tincture recommends an adult dose of 60 drops every 4 hours. Figure the correct dosage for the child using Clark's or Young's rules. Use Fried's rule to calculate dosages for infants.

Using **Clark's Rule**: the child's dose = $\frac{\text{40 lbs (child's weight)}}{\text{150 lbs}}$ x 60 drops (adult dose) =

$$\frac{40}{150} \times \frac{60}{1} = \frac{2400}{150} = 16 \text{ drops is the child's dose}$$

Using **Young's Rule**: child's dose = $\frac{\text{5 (child's age)}}{5 + 12}$ x 60 drops (adult dose) =

$$\frac{5}{17} \times \frac{60}{1} = \frac{300}{17} = 17.6 \text{ drops is the child's dose}$$

Using **Fried's Rule** for a 20-month-old infant:

the child's dose = $\frac{\text{20 months}}{\text{150 months}}$ x 60 drops (adult dose) =

$$\frac{20}{150} \times \frac{60}{1} = \frac{1200}{150} = 8 \text{ drops is the infant's dose}$$

Factors Determining the Quality and Potency of Herbal Preparations

The strength and concentration of an herb are important to consider when calculating dosages correctly. Herbal preparations with strong potency and fast absorption rates require smaller doses. Several factors determining the quality and potency of herbs should be considered and include the following:

1. The basic quality of an herb plant is affected by growing conditions, fertility and type of soil, amount of rainfall and sunlight, time and process of harvesting, drying techniques, and methods of product preparation. Herbal products that have been carefully grown and processed have a higher quality and stronger potency. Products prepared from freshly harvested rather than aged plants retain more of their vital life force.

2. The type of herbal preparation determines the availability and potency of its chemical constituents. Teas are easily digested and absorb well, but are relatively weaker than tinctures and fluid or solid extracts. A great benefit of drinking tea is that the herb has direct contact with the tissues in the mouth, throat, stomach and intestines, and can be especially effective when treating problems in these areas. Capsules tend to be fairly easy to digest because the finely ground powder is released as soon as the gelatin capsule dissolves. Pills can take longer to digest depending on the coating and binding materials used in their production. Alcohol preparations (tinctures) are probably the easiest to digest because the alcohol has extracted the chemical constituents out of the plant material so well that absorption in the digestive system is fast and complete. Since water and alcohol are easily absorbed through the stomach and intestinal walls, tinctures quickly find their way into the bloodstream and are excellent for emergency situations.

3. The age of the person using the herb is important and involves several variables. Children are much more sensitive to herbs than adults and should always be given smaller doses depending on their weight. Calculate children's dosages according to Clark's Rule. The elderly are also more sensitive and may require smaller doses. Some elderly people experience digestive problems due to insufficient stomach, liver or pancreatic enzymes, which decrease their ability to digest and assimilate foods, herbs, and pharmaceutical drugs. In this case, slightly higher doses are appropriate. On the other hand, as the liver and kidneys age, they lose their ability to process and excrete drugs and herbs, resulting in an overall increase in effects. For these reasons, it is usually wise to start with smaller doses determined by Clark's Rule and gradually increase the dosage over time to get the desired effects.

4. The weight of the person must be figured into the equation. Since doses for herbal preparations are typically based on the needs of a 150-pound person, they should be adjusted if the person weighs significantly more or less than 150 pounds. Weight-dependent doses should be calculated for children, the elderly, and for people who weigh less than 130 pounds. Use Clark's Rule to determine dosages according to weight rather than age.

5. Individual sensitivities. People have different levels of sensitivity and allergy thresholds, and some require smaller or larger doses regardless of their age or body weight. This is another reason to start with small doses to determine tolerance of the herbal preparation and gradually increase the dosage as needed.

Suggestions for Deciding Dosages of Herbal Preparations

1. Follow directions on herbal preparations that are purchased, or follow directions from your health care practitioner.
2. Always begin with small amounts and gradually build up to the recommended dose when starting a new herb or any type of supplement. This decreases possibilities of side effects or reactions in people with more sensitive systems.
3. Be familiar with the herbs you are using. Mild herbal teas like the Mints, Stinging Nettle (*Urtica dioica*), Chamomile (*Matricaria recutita*), Raspberry leaf (*Rubus idaeus*), and Green tea (*Camellia sinensis*) can usually be enjoyed on a daily basis without concern about excessive amounts causing side effects. Most commercially available herbal tinctures, pills, and capsules are safe when taken according to directions on labels, and troublesome reactions are much less problematic than reactions to pharmaceutical drugs. Other herbs like Poke (*Phytolacca decandra*), Bloodroot (*Sanguinaria canadensis*), or Wild Indigo (*Baptisia tinctoria*) can cause strong reactions and toxicity in excessive amounts, and must be taken in small, very specific doses.
4. The typical dosage for herbal tinctures is 25-100 drops (1-4 mL). However, this can vary greatly according to specific herbs and different concentrations of liquid extracts.
5. Essential oils are *extremely* potent and only 1-2 drops are taken internally. They should always be diluted in a cup of water or tea, and caution is emphasized regarding their potential toxicity.
6. For acute problems such as the common cold, flu, fever and infections, stronger herbs are indicated in larger doses, and are taken 4-6 times throughout the day for a short period of time.
7. For chronic problems like asthma, hypertension, poor circulation or diabetes, small to moderate doses are used on a daily basis over an extended period of time to elicit gradual improvement.
8. Herbs can exert different actions depending upon the amount taken. As a general rule, low doses tend to have a restoring, nourishing effect, moderate doses are more stimulating, while high doses promote the most activity with moving or draining actions. For example, when *Lobelia inflata* tincture is taken in small doses of 3-6 drops, it is stimulating and helpful for bouts of low blood pressure or reviving consciousness after fainting. In medium doses, it relaxes smooth muscles and relieves cramps and spasms. In large doses of 60-100 drops, it can act as an emetic to induce nausea and vomiting. Many aromatic herbs with large concentrations of essential oils, such as Thyme (*Thymus vulgaris*), Rosemary (*Rosmarinus officinalis*), Peppermint (*Mentha x piperita*), Ginger (*Zingiber officinale*), Hyssop (*Hyssopus officinalis*), Lavender (*Lavandula* spp.), Lemon Balm (*Melissa officinalis*) and Sage (*Salvia officinalis*), typically act as digestive stimulants and carminatives (relieve gas and indigestion) in small doses. In moderate doses, they stimulate increased circulation and movement in the system. And in larger amounts, they act as diaphoretics to promote perspiration, which reduces fevers and expels toxins.

Helpful Hints on Drop Dosages When Using Tinctures (Liquid Extracts)

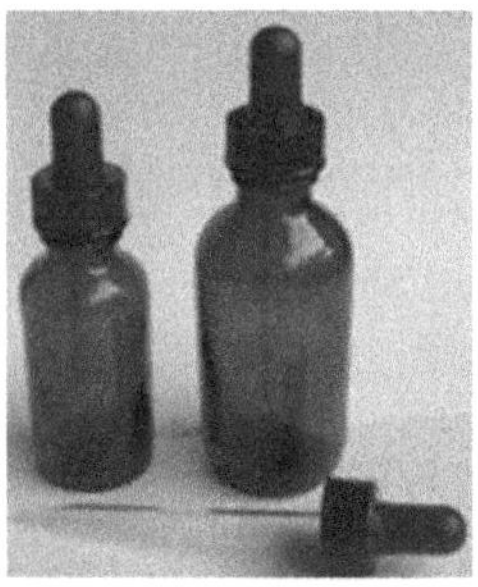
1- and 2-ounce Boston amber round bottles

Doses for tinctures are measured by the drop, milliliter, or teaspoon. Tinctures are usually bottled and dispensed in one- and two-ounce Boston amber round bottles, which are glass bottles with glass droppers attached to rubber-capped lids. Glass droppers allow for easy administration of the liquid, especially for doses according to drops. The drop method of dosing can be a little confusing because the size of the drop depends on the size and edge of the dropper. A large dropper will release a larger water droplet than a very tiny dropper. The size of the drop also depends on the viscosity (ability of fluids to adhere or stick together) of the fluid being measured. For example, when using the same dropper, one drop of water is larger than one drop of alcohol. One teaspoon of water contains about 70 drops, a teaspoon of grain alcohol contains about 184 drops, and a teaspoon of olive oil contains approximately 142 drops. The viscosity of water is much greater than alcohol and olive oil, and it forms a larger drop. Viscosity is also affected by any materials contained in liquids. A drop of Fenugreek tea is much thicker and more viscous than a drop of distilled water because the tea contains more solutes (dissolved substances).

When instructions call for a **dropperful** of tincture, this does not mean that the entire dropper is full of liquid. To measure a dropperful of tincture, completely squeeze the rubber cap holding the glass dropper to push all liquid out. While holding the cap closed between your fingers, place the dropper in the liquid extract and release the cap. The amount of fluid that is drawn into the dropper is measured as a "dropperful." A dropperful of tincture contained in a dropper for a one-ounce bottle contains the same amount as a dropper for a two-ounce bottle.

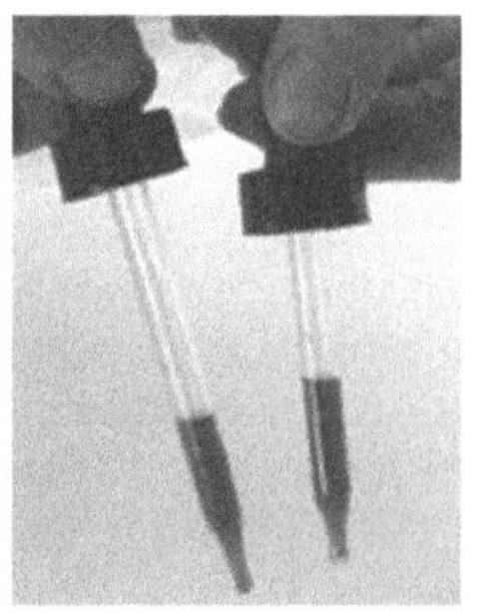
A "dropperful" using a 1- and 2-ounce dropper

Examples of differences in the number of drops of liquid solvents used in herbal preparations:

Substance	Number of drops in 1 dropperful (1 dropperful = approximately 0.7 mL)	Number of drops in 1 mL
Distilled water	15	22
Glycerin	15	22
Olive oil	28	40
St. John's Wort tincture	30	43
Echinacea tincture	31	44
190-proof grain alcohol	34	49

According to the figures above, 190-proof grain alcohol is less viscous (thick) and makes smaller droplets than the other solvents. When plant material is added to a combination of grain alcohol and distilled water, the viscosity of the remaining tincture is greater than plain alcohol, so drops of tincture are larger than drops of grain alcohol. Glycerin is equal to tap water, and olive oil is in the middle range of viscosity.

Calculating How Long a Bottle of Tincture Will Last When Taking a Specific Dose

Sometimes it is helpful to know how long a one- or two-ounce bottle of tincture will last. Here are a few points to remember in your calculations according to the metric system:

1 ounce of tincture = 30 mL (milliliters)
1 mL ≅ (equals approximately) 40 drops of tincture

1 ounce ≅ 1,200 drops of tincture (30 mL x 40 drops ≅ 1,200 drops)
2 ounces ≅ 2,400 drops of tincture

Example 1: If you take 60 drops of tincture twice daily, how many days will a one-ounce bottle last?

1 oz bottle ≅ 1,200 drops
60 drops x 2 = 120 drops a day
1,200 drops in 1 oz ÷ 120 drops = 10 days

Example 2: If you take 50 drops of tincture three times a day, how many days will a two-ounce bottle last?

2 oz bottle ≅ 2,400 drops
50 drops x 3 = 150 drops daily
2,400 drops in 2 oz ÷ 150 drops = 16 days

Weights and Measurements for the Herbalist

The science of weights and measures provides a universal system and language that defines and describes matter by its weight, volume, and other measurements. A few different systems have developed over time including the avoirdupois, apothecaries' and metric systems, which are discussed in this section. Depending on how deeply you immerse yourself in herbology and which books you read, you will probably need reliable references to understand how to weigh and measure herbs.

Weight is a measurement of heaviness and the degree to which material is drawn towards the earth by gravity. **Capacity** is a measurement of the amount of space or volume that a substance fills.

Avoirdupois weight is the system of measurement commonly used in the United States and many other English-speaking countries for all commodities except pharmaceutical drugs, precious stones, and precious metals. Avoirdupois units of measurement are the grain, dram, ounce, and pound.

Avoirdupois Weight

Pounds (lb)	*Ounces (oz)*	*Drams (dr)*	*Grains (gr)*	*Metric Equivalent in Grams (gm)*
1	16	256	7000	453.59
	1	16	437.5	28.35
		1	27.34	1.77
			1	0.0648 (64.8 mg)

Apothecaries' weight is used for weighing and measuring pharmaceutical drugs. This system was brought to the United States from England during the colonial period and is gradually being replaced by the metric system. In the apothecaries' system, the basic unit of measurement is the grain followed by the scruple, dram, ounce, and pound. The main difference in this system is that a pound contains 12 ounces.

Apothecaries' Weight

Pounds	*Ounces*	*Drams*	*Scruples*	*Grains*	*Metric Equivalent in Grams (approximate)*
1	12	96	288	5760	373.24
	1	8	24	480	31.1
		1	3	60	3.89
			1	20	1.33
				1	0.065 (64.8 mg)

Apothecaries' measure of capacity or volume is a system of graduated liquid volumes. The basic unit is the minim, which is equal to one drop, and is now standardized to equal 0.06 milliliters (ml). The unit of minim is followed by the scruple, dram, ounce, pint, quart, and gallon.

Apothecaries' Measure of Fluid Capacity or Volume

Gallon	*Quart*	*Pint*	*Ounce*	*Dram (=1 tsp)*	*Scruple*	*Minim (=1 drop)*	*Metric Equivalents in Milliliters (mL) (approximate)*
1	4	8	128	1,024	3,072	61,440	3,785
	1	2	32	256	768	15,360	946
		1	16	128	384	7,680	473
			4	32	96	1,920	118
			1	8	24	480	30
				1	3	60	3.7
					1	20	1.3
						1	0.06

Metric measures of weight, volume, and length are established on a decimal system. The system is based on units of the gram (measuring weight of mass), liter (measuring capacity or volume), and meter (measuring length). New units of measurement are formed by adding prefixes denoting the power of ten. For example, 1,000 milligrams equals one gram, 1,000 grams equals one kilogram, and 1,000 milliliters equals one liter.

Metric Measure for Weight

Microgram (mcg)	*Milligram (mg)*	*Gram (gm)*	*Kilogram (kg)*	*Apothecaries' Equivalents: (approximate)*
1,000	1	0.001		0.015 grain (1/65 grain)
6,000	6	0.006		0.09 grain (1/10 grain)
10,000	10	0.01		0.15 grain (1/6 grain)
12,000	12	0.012		0.185 grain (1/5 grain)
20,000	20	0.02		0.3 grain (1/3 grain)
65,000	65	0.065		1 grain
75,000	75	0.075		1.16 grains
100,000	100	0.1		1.5 grains
600,000	600	0.6		9.3 grains
1,000,000	1,000	1		15.4 grains
10,000,000	10,000	10		5.6 drams (154 grains)
		15		8.5 drams (231 grains)
		28.3		1 ounce
		100		3.5 ounces
		500		17.6 ounces
		1,000	1	2.2 pounds

Metric Measure for Volume or Capacity of Fluids

Milliliter (mL)	*Liter*	*Apothecaries' Equivalents (approximate)*
1	...	15 minims (15 drops)
4	...	1 fluid dram (1 teaspoon)
10	...	2.5 fluid drams
30	...	1 fluid ounce
100	...	3.5 fluid ounces
500	...	1 pint
1,000	1	2.11 pints = 1.06 quarts
10,000	10	2.64 gallons

Weight and Volume Equivalents (approximate)

1 milligram (mg) = 0.001 grams = 0.015 grains
1 grain = 0.065 gram = 65 milligrams
1 gram = 1,000 mg = 15.4 grains
1 kilogram (kg) = 1,000 grams = 2.2 pounds
1 pound = 16 ounces (oz) = 454 grams
1 ounce (oz) = 28 grams
1 drop = 1 minim = 0.06 mL
1 milliliter (mL) = 16 minims (16 drops)
1 teaspoon (tsp) = 3.7 mL
1 tablespoon (Tbs) = 3 tsp = 11 mL = 0.5 fluid oz
1 fluid oz = 6 tsp = 30 mL = 8 drams
1 cup (C) = 8 oz = 16 Tbs = 237 mL
1 pint (pt) = 16 oz = 2 cups = 473.2 mL
1 quart (qt) = 2 pt = 4 cups = 32 oz = 946.4 mL

Converting Measurements to Calculate Equivalent Values

When working with herbs and reading herbal books, sometimes it is necessary to convert one measurement to another. One way to solve these math problems is to calculate by ratio and proportion.

A **ratio** is composed of two related numbers separated by a colon. For example, "16 ounces is equal to 1 pound" is written as 16:1, and "2 grains is equal to 130 mg" is written as 2:130.

A **proportion** consists of two ratios separated by an equal (=) sign indicating that the two ratios on both sides of the equal sign are equal in proportion to each other.
For example, "16 ounces (oz) = 1 pint (pt) and 40 oz = 2.5 pt" is written as 16 oz : 1 pt = 40 oz : 2.5 pt.

The numbers on the ends of the proportion are the **extremes** (16 oz and 2.5 pts).
The numbers in the middle by the = sign are the **means** (1 pt and 40 oz).
In a proportion, the product of the extremes equals the product of the means.

If 16 oz : 1 pint = 40 oz : 2.5 pints
Then 16 x 2.5 (the extremes) = 1 x 40 (the means)
40 = 40

This mathematically proves that the ratios are equal. This equation can be used to calculate any conversion problem.

Example 1: How many Apothecaries' grains are in 2.3 grams (gm)? Set up the problem using the ratio/proportion formula. By looking at the Apothecaries' Weight chart, you find that:

1 grain (gr) = 0.065 gm

1 gr : 0.065 gm = N (unknown) gr : 2.3 gm

1 gr x 2.3 gm = 0.065 gm x N gr

2.3 = 0.065 x N

$$\frac{2.3}{0.065} = N$$

35.38 gr = N

1 gm : 0.065 gm = 35.38 gr : 2.3 gm
There are 35.38 Apothecaries' grains in 2.3 grams.

Example 2: How many drams are in 10 ounces according to Apothecaries' Weight? The equation is set up like this:

1 dram = 0.125 oz (8 drams = 1 oz, so 1 ÷ by 8 = 0.125)

1 dram : 0.125 oz = N (unknown) drams : 10 oz

1 x 10 = 0.125 x N drams

10 = 0.125 x N drams

$$\frac{10}{0.125} = N$$

80 = N

1 dram : 0.125 oz = 80 drams : 10 oz
There are 80 drams in 10 ounces.

The Safety of Medicinal Herbs

The renaissance of medicinal herbalism currently interfacing with the modern medical system and pharmaceutical industry has made the questions of herbal safety, contraindications, and adverse drug interactions important and sometimes controversial issues. Many herbs used for medicinal purposes are very safe, especially those that are consumed as culinary herbs and spices. However, some herbs contain toxic alkaloids and other powerful phytochemicals that can cause undesirable and potentially dangerous side effects when ingested. Just as certain foods can cause adverse reactions in some people, even mild herbs can elicit side effects in sensitive individuals. All plants contain hundreds of different chemical constituents, including vitamins, minerals, proteins, oils, oxidants and antioxidants, carcinogens and anticarcinogens, toxins and antitoxins, and many other biologically active compounds. Most plants, even those that are considered very safe like apples or wheat, contain chemicals that can be toxic if they are isolated and ingested in large amounts over an extended period of time, resulting in inflammation, allergies, tumors, and other symptoms. For example, anaphylactic shock from eating peanuts kills at least two Americans each year (Duke, 2000). Other common foods like dairy milk, gluten breads and grains, corn, shellfish, mangoes, and members of the Nightshade family (tomato, potato, eggplant) cause inflammation and allergic reactions in some people. Sassafras and Cinnamon oils contain safrole, which induces cancer when isolated and injected into lab animals. Interestingly, Sassafras is deemed toxic by the Food and Drug Administration (FDA), although Cinnamon is not. Always remember that most chemicals from plants or medicine, whether natural or synthetic, can be toxic in overdoses. The concept of safety is relative and there are many factors to consider.

The premise that all herbs are safe because they occur in nature is a false and potentially dangerous assumption.

The Primary Causes of Herbal Side Effects and Toxicity

There are many causes of side effects and toxic reactions induced by certain herbs. Many plants contain phytochemicals with strong biological activity and potential toxicity. These should be avoided or used cautiously in very small and specific dosages according to traditional models, and ideally under the supervision of an experienced herbal practitioner. Side effects can occur after ingesting an herb because of individual sensitivities and chemistry. People may have allergic responses and idiosyncratic reactions to substances that do not bother other people. Many plants can cause contact dermatitis when sensitive individuals handle or brush against live plants. This type of dermatitis is short-lived and can be eliminated by dousing the affected area with rubbing alcohol two or three times. Overdosing and the excessive use of an herb over an extended period of time can obviously create many problems. Actions of herbs can also interact with pharmaceutical drugs in beneficial or adverse ways.

Toxic reactions from herbs are caused by:
- *Powerful phytochemicals in some plants*
- *Allergic and idiosyncratic reactions*
- *Overdose and/or extended use*
- *Interaction with pharmaceutical drugs*
- *Incorrect identification of an herb*
- *Mislabeling or omission of ingredients*
- *Presence of heavy metals, pesticides, herbicides, bacteria, viruses, fungi, or mold*

Most serious adverse effects of herbs result from the incorrect identification of plants. For example, Foxglove (*Digitalis purpurea*) is a lethally toxic plant that contains digitalis, a chemical that exerts major effects on the heart, and its leaves look similar to those of Comfrey (*Symphytum officinale*). An elderly Englishman once mistakenly harvested and ingested Foxglove, thinking it was Comfrey, and required hospitalization for life-threatening digitalis poisoning. Germander (*Teucrium canadense*), a plant that can cause liver toxicity when taken in large doses over time, is somewhat similar in appearance to Scullcap (*Scutellaria lateriflora*), a harmless herb. Germander has occasionally been mistakenly harvested and marketed as Scullcap, and the toxic effects have sometimes been inappropriately blamed on Scullcap.

According to the Centers for Disease Control and Prevention, about six people die in the United States each year after ingesting a poisonous plant that was misidentified as an edible herb. Plant adulteration, which is mistaking and misplacing a toxic plant for a medicinal herb, is one of the most common causes of herbal side effects and toxicity. Other causes are due to the intentional addition of pharmaceutical drugs and unintentional contamination from herbicides, pesticides, or other environmental poisons. There are many reports of imported Chinese and Ayurvedic herbal formulas that have been analyzed and found to contain steroids and other pharmaceutical drugs not listed on the label, as well as heavy metals, including lead, mercury, gold, cadmium, and arsenic. The presence of heavy metals may be due to processing with metal containers and utensils. Other sources of toxicity can include contamination of the crude or unprocessed plant material by bacteria, yeast, mold, fungi, and animal feces containing *E. coli* and *Salmonella* toxins.

Avoid many of these potential problems by purchasing herbal products from reliable companies that maintain high standards of quality and production. However, thorough research and cultivating, harvesting, and processing your own herbal medicines is the best way to ensure the correct identification and purity of herbal products.

Factors in Determining the Safety of Herbs

The safety of most commercially available herbs is supported by more evidence than most people realize. Current research studies, statistics, and published reports show that severe adverse reactions to correctly prepared and administered herbs are rare, especially when compared with reactions to pharmaceutical drugs. However, some people are prone to allergic reactions from herbal plants as well as foods. When evaluating the safety of herbs, be sure to consider these four primary factors:

1) Their historic use in well-established and traditional medical systems such as European herbalism, Traditional Chinese Medicine, India's Ayurvedic system, Islamic Unani medicine, Native American Indian herbalism, and early American Eclectic medicine;
2) Laboratory research and chemical analysis for identification of chemical constituents, their biological actions, and toxicity;
3) Reports and data of side effects, illness or fatalities observed in clinical practice, research trials, and individual cases of people using specific herbs; and
4) The relative lack of side effects or toxicity reported after decades of herbal use among large populations of people throughout the world.

Rules of Safety When Using Medicinal Herbs

Many herbs that have been enjoyed by millions of people over the decades are regularly ingested as popular culinary spices and flavorings, and prepared as teas. These herbs have withstood the tests of time and are generally regarded as safe to consume in the usual amounts. This category of herbs typically includes milder-tasting and more nutritive plants that do not contain as many of the more potent, medicinal secondary metabolites. Herbs containing greater concentrations of powerful, bioactive phytochemicals are traditionally employed for medicinal purposes in treating various health conditions and disease states. These herbs do require more caution and specific directions for their use. Their stronger actions are more likely to cause side effects or interact with pharmaceutical drugs. When using herbs for medicinal purposes, always follow these basic safety guidelines!

❖ Be wise in your choice of health care practitioners and healing tools. The best health care system embraces a wide range of modalities rather than depending on only one model. Try to find a holistically oriented medical doctor who is willing to be a cooperative member of your health care team, and is open to working with people who use herbs and other supplements. Also seek out a holistic practitioner such as a holistic nurse practitioner or naturopath who has graduated from a four-year college-accredited program. Acupuncturists often have clinical knowledge of medicinal herbs. Always tell your health care provider about the pharmaceutical drugs, herbs, and other supplements that you may be taking.

❖ Do not rely exclusively on herbs for the treatment of serious or life-threatening conditions! And do not exclude pharmaceutical drugs and treatment by medical physicians when they are necessary.

❖ Research herbs before using them. Be sure they match your health needs and investigate how they have been historically used in traditional healing systems. Learn whether an herb is considered generally safe or if there is potential for strong effects and toxicity. Take advantage of the wealth of resources, including books and journals, libraries (university libraries are excellent), the Internet, herbalists who teach, and health professionals knowledgeable about herbal medicines. The most accurate and reliable books are those written by health professionals who use herbs in their personal lives and clinical practice. They tend to have the greatest amount of practical experience and usually try to keep up with current scientific research.

❖ Take high-quality herbs that have been correctly identified and not adulterated with other plants. When purchasing medicinal herbs, buy products from a trustworthy company, health professional, or health food store. Avoid cheaper products containing fillers and artificial ingredients. ***Do not purchase herbs or supplements over the Internet*** because many cases of tampering, adulteration, and substitution have been reported. (This happened to one of my clients, and the product made her and her child sick.)

❖ Dosage and correct administration are important. Use herbs according to their recommended doses and do not exceed these! Follow the directions on product labels or recommended by a health professional.

❖ Be cautious when starting an herb or other type of supplement for the first time. Always start with a low dose and gradually work up to the recommended dose to reduce or eliminate any possible reactions. Pay attention to how your body feels and adjust dosages accordingly.

❖ If you experience a reaction to an herb, stop taking it immediately and inform your health care practitioner. One of the most serious allergic reactions is anaphylactic shock. Although this is a very rare reaction to herbs, it is wise to be aware of all possibilities and know how to respond. Symptoms include tissue swelling, irritation, itching, difficulty breathing, rash or hives, edema, dizziness, heart palpitations, or eventual loss of consciousness. The medical treatment consists of antihistamines for mild reactions, and epinephrine and steroids for more serious cases. If you experience any of these symptoms after ingesting an herb, immediately treat yourself by taking detoxifying herbs and/or get medical assistance. Large doses (2-3 teaspoons) of tincture containing Dandelion (*Taraxacum officinale*), Burdock (*Arctium* spp.), Yellow Dock (*Rumex crispus*), and St. John's Wort (*Hypericum perforatum*) taken every 5-10 minutes in a cup of water can often eliminate symptoms of anaphylactic shock. Milk Thistle (*Silybum marianum*) is also excellent to detoxify ingested poisons. If these fail to help, get medical attention!

❖ Pregnant and nursing women must take particular caution when using herbs. Many botanical medicines are questionable or potentially not safe for infant development, and should be avoided. Refer to **"Herbs for Pregnancy, Childbirth and Lactation"** in Section Three for basic guidelines.

❖ People who take prescription medicines, over-the-counter drugs, or have serious medical problems need to be informed and cautious when using herbs for medicinal purposes. In these cases, it is best to have the assistance of a health professional with herbal knowledge. To decrease the possibility of herb-drug interactions, always take herbs 1½-2 hours before or after taking pharmaceutical drugs.

❖ Children and the elderly should use herbs with care. Both age groups tend to have more sensitivity and should be given lower doses according to individual body size and weight. Children younger than two years of age should not be given herbal medicines unless there is a specific need for gentle herbs like Catnip (*Nepeta cataria*), Fennel (*Foeniculum vulgare*), or Marshmallow (*Althaea officinalis*). Refer to the chapter **"How to Calculate Dosages"** in Section One for specific methods for calculating dosages by body weight.

Comparing the Safety and Toxicity of Herbal Medicines and Pharmaceutical Drugs

It is unfortunate that many herbs have received such harsh criticism concerning their overall safety. Hypothetical statements, media misinformation, and bias against herbs have exaggerated the issue of herbal safety and made herb-drug interactions a controversial topic. When a potentially harmful phytochemical is detected in a plant, or a few people experience side effects, the herb in question is often regarded as dangerous. Sometimes it is banned from the commercial market even though it has been used by large populations for hundreds of years. Reports of hypothetical or potential problems caused by herbs are often accompanied by excessive negativity and biased comments that question the validity and safety of using any herb. The news media tend to conceal and downplay the dangers of pharmaceutical medicines, which pose a much greater potential for harm. When looking at the issue of safety, it is important to acknowledge the tremendous discrepancy and bias against herbal medicines, which are scrutinized much more rigidly than pharmaceutical drugs. A survey of the historical evidence, clinical references, research, documentation, and statistics unequivocally validates the fact that herbs are generally much safer than pharmaceutical drugs. Many more people suffer from side effects and deaths caused by pharmaceutical drugs and iatrogenic (physician-induced) incidents than from herbal medicines. Although pharmaceuticals have more potential side effects than herbs, many drugs are extremely beneficial and are an important contribution of the health care system. Nevertheless, safety issues need to be determined from a realistic perspective.

Pharmaceutical drugs are "new age" compared to herbal medicines.

When considering the general safety of herbs in relation to modern medicines, it is important to realize that pharmaceutical drugs were introduced only 100-150 years ago. Many drugs have been around for just 10-20 years, and new ones appear on the market all the time. These drugs are "new age" compared to herbs, which people have been ingesting since the beginning of human life on this planet. Over eons of time, the human body has developed the ability to digest and assimilate naturally occurring plant foods and medicines. One of the many benefits of using whole plant herbal preparations is the inclusion of all their phytochemicals that act synergistically not only to heal, but to reduce or eliminate potential for side effects and toxicity. In contrast, pharmaceutical drugs are usually composed of one chemical isolated from a plant or synthetically produced in the laboratory into new forms that our bodies do not necessarily know how to process. This is one reason why all pharmaceutical drugs have potential side effects, and many reports have documented their damaging or toxic effects.

Herbs and pharmaceutical drugs are judged by different safety standards.

Double standards exist in judging the safety of herbal medicines compared to pharmaceutical drugs. The medical community demonstrates much more tolerance for adverse reactions caused by pharmaceutical drugs than it has for herbal side effects. For example, excessive ingestion of Comfrey (*Symphytum officinale*) over extended periods of time caused several cases of a serious and potentially fatal veno-occlusive liver disease between 1980 and 1990. Consequently, the internal use of Comfrey was banned from the commercial market despite its long history of safe use throughout Europe and North America. In contrast, according to the American Association of Poison Control Centers, overdose of acetaminophen (found in Tylenol, Darvocet, Lortab, Percocet, and Vicodin) is the most common cause of liver failure. Acetaminophen can cause liver toxicity when daily dosage exceeds 3,000 mg, which many people with intractable pain take for months or years. In 1997, regional Poison Control Centers treated more than 10,000 cases of acetaminophen overdose. A 1998 study of 47 children suffering from acetaminophen overdose reported 23 deaths. Another study involving more than 600 patients from 22 American care centers discovered that acetaminophen-related liver damage is the primary cause of acute liver failure in the country. About half of these cases resulted from unintentional overdoses (Larson, 2005). Despite mounting evidence of problems, a multitude of acetaminophen products remain on the market, and Tylenol is an over-the-counter drug that does not require a prescription.

In another example of double standards, the American Association of Poison Control Centers documented that non-steroidal, anti-inflammatory drugs (NSAIDs) caused approximately 100,000 toxic reactions resulting in hospitalization and 10,000 deaths in 1997. A study published in the *New England Journal of Medicine* estimated that about 16,500 Americans died from gastrointestinal toxicity from NSAIDs in 1997 (Wolfe, 1999). There were 52,751 reports of toxic reactions caused by ibuprofen and 4 reported deaths (TESS Annual Report, 1999). Statin drugs are routinely prescribed for high cholesterol levels despite the well-known fact that they can cause liver and muscular damage, and evidence published in the *New England Journal of Medicine* showed that almost 50 percent of the children born to women who took statins during their first trimester of pregnancy were born with birth defects or malformations (Edison, 2004). Synthetic estrogens in hormone replacement therapy and birth control pills are proven to cause reproductive cancers, blood clotting, and heart attacks in some women, and many studies substantiating this fact have been widely publicized in medical journals. And yet the Food and Drug Administration (FDA) allows physicians to continue prescribing synthetic estrogens even though safe, bio-identical hormones are available. Since bio-identical hormones have the same molecular structure as the hormones our bodies produce (making them safe for women), they cannot be patented, so drug companies cannot profit by producing them. Although many drugs cause toxic reactions, birth defects, cancers and deaths, even when taken as prescribed, they remain on the market because the FDA has determined that their benefits override the risks. Yet herbs are quickly banned when side effects occur, even when the problems are caused by incorrect or excessive use and the herb in question has a long history of safety in large populations. Considering the evidence, it is obvious that herbs and pharmaceutical medicines are scrutinized and regulated very differently.

Are FDA-approved pharmaceutical drugs really safe?

In the United States, all new pharmaceutical drugs must meet specific standards before the FDA approves them to be put on the market. The research, development, and approval process for each drug can cost millions of dollars and last 8-12 years. Drug companies are responsible for research studies on the safety and efficacy of the drugs they produce, which are sent to the FDA for final approval.

Herbs are categorized as dietary supplements rather than drugs and do not require FDA approval. For this reason, medicinal herbs receive harsh criticism by some members of the medical establishment, pharmaceutical industry, media, and regulatory agencies for being "unproven" and "unregulated." There is concern that public safety is at risk because herbs are not tested and approved by the same standards as pharmaceutical drugs. Unfortunately, many people falsely belief that FDA approval guarantees that a drug is safe for consumer use. But in reality, hundreds of FDA-approved drugs have been recalled and taken off the market due to dangerous side effects and deaths. Although scientists and manufacturers conduct rigidly controlled tests on synthetic drugs, every pharmaceutical drug carries potential side effects that are listed in fine print on information papers accompanying all prescriptions and they continue to cause thousands of deaths each year. As an example, prior to its removal from the market in 2004, the anti-inflammatory arthritis drug, Vioxx, had been implicated in about 160,000 cases of heart attacks and strokes in the United States between 1999 and 2004, and about 100,000 unnecessary deaths (Topol, 2004). Although very few herbs have been thoroughly researched in the United States to determine their safety or effectiveness, research shows that they are responsible for very few deaths each year.

Statistics comparing the safety and toxicity of botanicals with pharmaceutical drugs:

❖ The incidence of adverse, drug-related fatalities in American hospitals between 1966 and 1996 was studied in a meta-analysis conducted by researchers at the University of Toronto. The results, published in the prestigious *Journal of the American Medical Association* (*JAMA*), reported that properly prescribed FDA-approved drugs that were used as directed killed over 106,000 hospital patients in 1994 due to toxic reactions, and injured over two million more. Researchers were surprised by these large numbers of fatal adverse drug reactions, estimated to be the fourth to sixth leading cause of death that year (Lazarou, 1998).

Other studies show that hospital costs directly attributable to adverse drug reactions can total an additional $1.56 billion to $4 billion per year in the United States (Classen, 1997; Bates, 1997).

❖ In 1990, the General Accounting Office (GAO), an agency of the United States government, conducted a study on 198 drugs approved by the FDA between 1976–1985. The GAO reported that over half of these (102 drugs) caused serious safety problems, including anaphylactic shock, failure of the heart, liver and kidneys, respiratory depression and arrest, seizures, severe blood disorders, toxicity, birth defects, cancers, and blindness (GAO, 1990).

❖ In 1988, there were 1.2 million reports of exposure to poisons in the United States. Of these cases, 7% (84,400) involved plant poisoning from common household plants, while Poke (*Phytolacca decandra*) was the only medicinal herb implicated (*U.S. News and World Report*, 1988).

❖ From 1989–1992, when an increased number of Americans were using herbs, the American Association of Poison Control Centers recorded a total of 4 deaths attributed to ingestion of poisonous plants. In Germany, where an estimated 65% of the population uses herbs, such deaths are equally as rare.

❖ The American Association of Poison Control Centers reported that during 1995, only 5.2% (104,187 cases) out of about two million reported poisonings were caused by plants. Only three of these cases resulted in death (Litovitz, 1996). The Center reported no deaths from herbs or dietary supplements during 2007–2009 (Lindstrom, 2011).

❖ The 1997 annual report of the American Association of Poison Control Centers stated that synthetic drugs are the leading cause of fatal poisonings (Litovitz, 1998).

❖ Less than 10 people die yearly from ingesting herbs.
About 6,000 people die yearly from intentional consumption of narcotics.
Alcohol-related deaths number around 100,000 each year.
Approximately 300,000 people die every year from Tobacco smoke (Foster, 2000).

The impact of pharmaceutical drugs on the environment is devastating!

Botanical medicines are biodegradable and do not harm the environment, although some herbal products are manufactured using questionable chemicals. Most pharmaceutical drugs are not biodegradable. After being consumed and excreted, many of these drugs and their metabolites are dumped into the ecosystem, mainly through waste treatment plants. Extensive evidence documents that measurable quantities of drugs are ending up in soil over vast land areas and in most bodies of water. Dangerous concentrations of pharmaceuticals are being discovered in animal, human and fetal tissues, causing metabolic abnormalities, birth defects and deformities, cancers, and other diseases. Antibiotics, synthetic estrogens, steroids, statin drugs, serotonin-enhancing drugs like Prozac, Paxil and Zoloft, chemotherapy drugs, and radioactive materials are just a few examples of drugs that remain in the environment, disrupting the natural order of life for unknown lengths of time (Buhner, 2002). Considering the huge amounts of pharmaceutical drugs manufactured and ingested worldwide, the harmful impact on our bodies and ecosystem is alarming!

Research on Herbal Safety

Research on whole herbs and isolated compounds in plants is necessary to expand our knowledge about botanical safety and potential risks. These studies potentially provide good information, but unfortunately they are sometimes flawed and become the source of exaggerations and incorrect conclusions about the dangers or ineffectiveness of herbal medicines. This misinformation can then become widely publicized, and herbs that have been utilized as medicines for hundreds of years are suddenly under attack.

> *Research studies must be designed to investigate herbs according to their typical dosages and routes of administration. Outcomes must be carefully scrutinized and evaluated.*

Before blindly accepting the results of one or two tests, it is wise to consider all the factors involved, including the testing methods, who funded the research, and the actual incentive for the research. Toxicity studies are often designed to give laboratory animals huge doses of an isolated phytochemical orally or in an injected form, which does not reflect the normal action of the entire herb when ingested in standard doses. Laboratory *in vitro* (in test tubes or petri dishes) and *in vivo* (in animals and humans) tests only suggest possible biological activity of herbs and their chemical constituents. While acknowledging the sacrifice of animals used for experimental testing, it should be pointed out that animal testing does not necessarily provide accurate information on how herbs interact in humans. Thalidomide is a drug that was nontoxic to animals but caused severe birth defects in humans before it was recalled from the market in 1961. Since rodents do not menstruate, it is ludicrous to use them for testing estrogenic or emmenagogue (promoting menstruation) effects of herbs. Some herbs affect animals very differently than they do people. Catnip (*Nepeta cataria*), for example, is relaxing to people but has obvious and perhaps hallucinogenic effects on many cats, who get very excited and exhibit bizarre behavior after chewing on the leaves. Human studies involving clinical trials and individual case reports are the most accurate and realistic sources of information to determine herbal safety. Equally as important is the long term historic use of the herb among the general populace and by practitioners in respected health care traditions.

Potentially Toxic Herbs

Names of plants can provide clues about their safety. Plants with "bane" in their names indicate potential toxicity and should not be ingested. Examples include Wolfbane, Fleabane, Henbane, and Baneberry. The old Anglo-Saxon term "wort" means "having medicinal value" and has been included in names of herbs with long histories of medicinal use such as Motherwort, St. John's Wort, Mugwort, and Lungwort. Plants with species names of *officinalis* or *officinale* indicate that they were safely used as officially medicinal drugs. Examples include *Salvia officinalis* (Sage), *Althaea officinalis* (Marshmallow), *Borago officinalis* (Borage), *Hyssopus officinalis* (Hyssop), *Calendula officinalis* (Calendula), and *Jasminum officinale* (Jasmine).

Most commonly used herbs available in the commercial market are very safe when taken according to the correct indications, dosages, and administration. But many plants contain strong chemical constituents that cause toxicity with only one or two large doses, or following long-term ingestion. Some of these should not be used at all, and others, when used wisely in specified doses and time frames, are very effective and less dangerous than many pharmaceutical drugs. Many medical doctors in Europe, especially in Germany, prescribe some of these potentially toxic herbs that practitioners in North America generally avoid.

The question of toxicity can be confusing because the presence of a toxin in a plant does not necessarily pose a threat to health. According to J. Kingsbury, a recognized authority on plant toxicology:

> In order for a plant to be functionally poisonous, it must not only contain a toxic secondary compound, but must also possess effective means of presenting that compound to an animal in sufficient concentrations, and the compound must be capable of overcoming whatever physical or biological defenses the animal may possess against it. Thus the presence of a known poisonous principle, even in toxicologically significant amounts, in a plant does not automatically mean that either man or a given species of animal will ever be effectively poisoned by the plant. (Upton, 2004)

Many warnings of plant toxicity that appear in popular and professional references are derived from *in vitro* studies and case reports of individual reactions to ingesting an herb. However, these sources provide suggestive evidence at best. *In vitro* studies of an isolated phytochemical do not indicate how the whole herb containing the chemical will react in an animal or human. Herbal remedies have traditionally been prepared from whole plant parts containing hundreds of substances that interact with each other, often neutralizing toxic effects of other chemicals in the same plant. When ingested, plants are broken down by multiple enzymes in the digestive system, and many potential toxins are neutralized or destroyed. Another toxicology authority and editor of *Botanical Safety Handbook*, Roy Upton, believes that individual case reports of alleged toxic reactions to ingesting herbs are frequently unreliable due to three primary factors:

1) A reaction may have been coincidental to ingesting the herb;
2) Other toxic compounds or pharmaceutical drugs may have been ingested with the herb; and
3) The reaction may be due to adulteration of the herbal product with a toxic botanical or contamination due to the presence of heavy metals, bacteria, fungi and other microbial substances (Upton, 2004).

For these reasons, warnings and hypothetical statements about potential toxic effects of an herb should be carefully scrutinized when they originate from laboratory tests and individual human cases. This is especially true when the herb in question has been safely used over many centuries by large groups of people.

Classes of Potentially Toxic Phytochemicals

Modern scientific research has identified many phytochemicals with potential toxicity. The following are examples of some toxic phytochemicals that have historically been employed in medicine. Some plants containing these phytochemicals should be completely avoided, some may be safely administered in small doses with the aid of a health professional, while others are safe for use by the general public.

Aristolochic acid primarily occurs in members of the *Aristolochiaceae* family, including *Aristolochia clematitis* (Birthwort), *A. serpentaria* (Virginia snakeroot), *A. reticulata* (Texas Snakeroot), and also in *Asarum canadense* (Wild Ginger/Canadian Snakeroot). Plants containing aristolochic acid have been used medicinally for more than 2,500 years. However, carcinogenic and nephrotoxic (kidney toxin) effects have been established, and plants containing this phytochemical should be used short-term in small amounts.

Atropine and **hyoscyamine** are alkaloids with high potential for toxicity. These occur in several members of the *Solanaceae* (Nightshade) family, including *Atropa belladonna* (Deadly Nightshade), *Hyoscyamus niger* (Henbane), *Mandragora officinarum* (Mandrake), and *Datura stramonium* (Jimson Weed). Atropine blocks the parasympathetic nervous system, resulting in mental confusion, hallucinations, memory loss, dry mouth and mucous membranes, constipation, difficult urination, nervousness, and reduced heart rate. Although atropine and hyoscyamine are prescribed by physicians, plant sources should *never* be taken internally.

Cardiac glycosides affect the rhythm and function of the heart. *Digitalis* (Foxglove), *Convallaria majalis* (Lily-of-the-Valley), and *Urginea maritima* (Squill) contain cardiac glycosides used for many years in Europe to treat heart conditions. They are potentially toxic in large doses and should be ingested very carefully, if at all. American herbalists tend to avoid using or recommending these herbs.

Pyrrolizidine alkaloids (PAs) are a large class of over 200 compounds having a wide range of toxicity. More than 60 plants that are used medicinally contain PAs, including *Symphytum* spp. (Comfrey), *Tussilago farfara* (Coltsfoot), *Borago officinale* (Borage), *Petasites hybridus* (Butterbur), *Senecio aureus,* spp. (Ragwort), and several species of *Eupatorium*. Borage seed oil contains such small traces of these compounds that it is considered safe. Laboratory animals that were fed large amounts of pure PAs experienced liver damage, toxicity, and eventual death. Large doses of toxic PAs ingested over extended periods of time have been associated with liver disease and a few cases of death in humans and livestock. Toxic PAs can cause liver veno-occlusive disease (blockage of blood vessels) and liver failure. PA metabolites impair cell division in the liver and cause cellular necrosis (death). Plants containing PAs should only be ingested in small doses over short periods of time.

Thujone is found in many volatile oils. When ingested in large doses over a long period of time, it is a neurotoxin (toxic to the nervous system) that can cause restlessness, vomiting, vertigo, tremors, kidney damage, convulsions, and hallucinations. Many herbs containing thujone are safe to use in standard doses, and these include *Achillea millefolium* (Yarrow), *Artemisia absinthium* (Wormwood), *Salvia officinalis* (Sage), and *Tanacetum vulgare* (Tansy).

Herbs Containing Potentially Toxic Phytochemicals

Arnica *(Arnica montana)* is only used externally for bruises and injuries where the skin is not broken. Ingestion can cause serious toxic side effects, including stomach and intestinal problems, nervous disorders, and muscle weakness.

Bloodroot *(Sanguinaria canadensis)* contains sanguinarine and chelerythrine, which are skin irritants, plus proteolytic enzymes that dissolve proteins. These chemicals slowly dissolve and destroy tissue, making external applications of Bloodroot useful for removing warts, moles, and some cancers. People ingesting Bloodroot have various responses ranging from none at all to severe and unpleasant side effects. These can include nervous system depression causing a reduction in blood pressure, heart rate and respirations; nervous system stimulation causing pounding heart beat and elevated blood pressure; digestive disturbances of nausea, vomiting and diarrhea; visual disturbances and dizziness; and changes in thought processes and mental acuity. This herb can be a valuable remedy, but should always be used very cautiously in small amounts under the guidance of an experienced herbalist.

Chaparral *(Larrea tridentata)* has been used for the treatment of cancer because it contains a strong antioxidant and anti-cancer substance called nordihydroguaiatetic acid (NDGA). Two or three cups of the tea and isolated NDGA have been given to cancer patients on a daily basis, and the only side effects were occasional nausea or diarrhea. Very large doses reduced blood pressure. According to surveys published by the herb industry, over 200 tons of Chaparral were sold in the United States between 1970 and 1990. There were no complaints of side effects from using the herb during this 20-year period. In 1989, the National Cancer Institute declared that incidence of NDGA toxicity is minimal.

Since then, several cases of liver toxicity linked to Chaparral have been reported in the United States. One woman developed hepatitis after taking 15 tablets a day for three months to treat breast lumps. This incident did not attract attention until 1992, when three people who were taking 2-3 tablets daily developed liver problems that did not improve until they stopped ingesting the herb. As a result of these cases, the FDA issued a public warning that Chaparral can cause liver problems. However, a doctor review funded by the American Herbal Products Association found insufficient evidence that Chaparral actually caused the alleged incidents of liver toxicity (McCaleb, 2000). If Chaparral is used medicinally, it should only be ingested in small amounts that are taken intermittently, and liver enzymes and function should be monitored.

Coltsfoot *(Tussilago farfara)* has been used as a cough remedy since ancient times. Like Comfrey, it contains pyrrolizidine alkaloids (PAs) linked to liver damage, and many people caution against using it. Case reports suggest it causes liver toxicity, but in at least one case the person was also taking pharmaceutical drugs known to cause liver toxicity. Other cases involved patients with previously diagnosed liver disease, so the role of Coltsfoot was questionable. The German Commission E, a recognized authority on herbal standards, has documented that Coltsfoot is safe when the dosage is limited to 4.5–6 grams taken only for 4-6 weeks per year for acute illness.

Comfrey ***(Symphytum officinale)*** has been a favorite healing plant throughout the world for thousands of years, but it has developed a bad reputation in the scientific community due to the presence of pyrrolizidine alkaloids (PAs). Although there are only a few documented cases of liver damage caused by excessive doses of Comfrey taken over extended periods of time, the FDA ordered that it be removed from the market. According to the findings of biochemist Bruce Ames, PhD, of the University of California in Berkeley, who specializes in estimating the cancer-causing potential of food, a cup of Comfrey tea is about 1/100 as carcinogenic as a can of beer (Ames, 1987).

False Hellebore ***(Veratrum viride)*** should be avoided because its sedating action reduces heart rate and respirations, and it can damage the nervous system.

Foxglove ***(Digitalis purpurea)*** is the source of the popular drug digoxin/lanoxin. The herb exerts a significant effect on the heart, and excessive doses cause arrhythmias and cardiac arrest. Foxglove should never be used unless under the direction of an experienced practitioner who works with this herb.

Gelsemium/Yellow Jasmine ***(Gelsemium sempervirens)*** toxicity can cause double vision, dizziness, depression, impaired breathing and heart function, and paralysis.

Germander ***(Teucrium chamaedrys, T. canadense)*** has been used over many centuries for menstrual problems in Argentina, as an anti-inflammatory in Italy, and as an emmenagogue in Arabic countries. Seven people from France experienced acute hepatitis after taking capsules or tea of Germander to lose weight. All seven recovered after discontinuing the herb, but three of them developed signs of liver problems as soon as they started taking it again. Consequently, French manufacturers voluntarily stopped marketing Germander and the government banned its use in 1982. Germander has also been implicated as a cause of liver problems when it has been adulterated and marketed as Scullcap *(Scutellaria lateriflora)*, a safe herb.

Hemlock, Poison ***(Conium maculatum)*** is very toxic and deadly. It can cause birth defects. There are many historical accounts of Hemlock used as a poison.

Henbane ***(Hyoscyamus*** **spp.*)*** contains the dangerous alkaloids scopalamine, atropine, and hyoscyamine. It causes marked depression of the nervous and respiratory systems, and should never be ingested.

Jimson Weed ***(Datura stramonium)*** also contains scopalamine, atropine and hyoscyamine, which can cause hallucinations, vomiting, rapid weak pulse, and eventual convulsions. A beautiful plant, but do not ingest it!

Kava Kava ***(Piper methysticum)*** has been a traditional recreational drink enjoyed by people in South Pacific countries and Polynesia for hundreds of years. Until its international ban in 2002 due to potential liver toxicity, it was widely used in Europe and America as a treatment for anxiety and premenstrual syndrome (PMS) and as a muscle relaxant, mood enhancer, and sedative to induce sleep. There have been at least 25 reports of serious liver toxicity in Germany and Switzerland, including cases of cirrhosis, hepatitis, and liver failure. There was also a case in the United States of a previously healthy young woman who required a liver transplant after using a supplement containing Kava. Out of 56 reports about Kava's potential to cause hepatotoxicity, only four reports of liver toxicity could be directly related to the consumption of Kava (Upton, 2004). Toxic effects may be due to use of excessive amounts of the herb or ingestion of the stem rather than root, which is the plant part traditionally used by Polynesians.

Lily-of-the-Valley ***(Convallaria majalis)*** contains convallarin and convallamarin, which are potent cardiac glycosides exerting strong actions on the heart. An overdose can cause dangerous heart arrhythmias. This herb should only be used under the guidance of an experienced herbalist.

Mayapple ***(Podophyllum peltatum)*** root, young shoots, and unripe fruit are all toxic. The root has a strong cathartic effect causing severe stomach and intestinal irritation and pain, nausea, vomiting, and diarrhea. The ripe yellow fruit has a citrus flavor and is edible, but you have to beat the deer to harvest the fruit because they love to eat it.

Mistletoe ***(Viscum album)*** has been used by European physicians for many years to treat cancers, tumors, hypertension, arteriosclerosis, and tachycardia (rapid heart rate). Overdose can cause gastrointestinal bleeding and central nervous system depression, including low blood pressure and slow heart rate.

Monkshood/Aconite ***(Aconitum*** **spp.*)*** should be avoided because it lowers blood pressure and is very toxic to the heart and nervous system.

Mormon Tea ***(Ephedra nevadense)*** and **Ma Huang** ***(Ephedra sinica)*** contain the alkaloids ephedrine and pseudoephedrine, which are central nervous system stimulants. Ma Huang has been safely used in Traditional

Chinese Medicine for centuries to treat allergic reactions, nasal congestion, asthma, and other respiratory problems. This is an herb with powerful medicinal properties that should be used for the correct reasons in reasonable dosages. Excessive amounts can cause insomnia, anxiety, restlessness, and increased heart rate and blood pressure. More recently, American food and supplement industries included Ephedra in products for weight loss and improving athletic stamina. This trend, which was not supported by historical use of the herb, caused many cases of Ephedra overdose and some severe side effects. Consequently, rather than banning the inappropriate use of Ephedra in diet and athletic endurance products, the FDA has banned its complete use. This is very unfortunate because, when applied in normal doses for respiratory distress and allergic reactions, it is a remarkably safe and effective herbal medicine.

American Pennyroyal *(Hedeoma pulegioides)* and **European Pennyroyal *(Mentha pulegium)*** are used to induce menstruation and abortion because they irritate the uterus and cause contractions. Pennyroyal has also been used for treating colds, flu and fever, cramps, colic, and as an insect repellent. Excessive amounts cause toxic effects when ingested, and even the external application of Pennyroyal oil can cause uterine contractions or toxicity in some people.

Poke root *(Phytolacca decandra)* is a popular and potent lymphatic cleanser and anti-inflammatory. It is ingested in small amounts of 4-8 drops of the tincture 1-3 times a day. An excess can cause respiratory depression and digestive problems, including vomiting and bloody diarrhea.

Ragwort *(Senecio aureus,* spp.*)* contains pyrrolizidine alkaloids that can cause liver disease and toxicity when ingested over time. Do not use Ragwort internally.

Rauwolfia *(Rauwolfia serpentina)* is used in India's Ayurvedic medical system and is prescribed in low doses for hypertension. It can easily cause side effects of headaches, constriction of the pupils, diarrhea, and can induce or aggravate depression. It should only be used for short periods of time under the supervision of a qualified medical herbalist.

Tansy *(Tanacetum vulgare)* leaves and flowers contain tanacetin, which is poisonous to humans and animals when ingested in sufficient amounts. The plant also has the potential to induce abortions. It can be safely used as an external wash to kill scabies and lice.

Herbs Incorrectly Accused of Being Toxic

For a variety of reasons, many herbs have been judged incorrectly of being toxic and unsafe to use. The following are a few examples:

Burdock *(Arctium* spp.*)* is a common and relatively mild herb that has been safely ingested as a medicinal remedy for many centuries throughout Europe, Asia, and North America. The root is eaten as a vegetable in Japan. Erroneous reports of toxicity originated from one incident, in which a batch of Burdock was contaminated with Belladonna root containing toxic atropine.

German Chamomile *(Matricaria recutita)* and **Roman or English Chamomile (*Chamaemelum nobile)*** have historically been used as a beverage tea and calming, anti-inflammatory medicinal. Although allergic reactions have only been reported by a few people, the American medical profession considers it a potentially toxic plant. Most plants in the *Compositae* (Daisy) family contain sesquiterpene lactones, a class of allergenic substances. Although allergic reactions tend to be rare, many modern references recommend that those with allergies to Ragweed and plants in this family should avoid using any of its members for medicine. This is a notorious misconception and most herbalists consider Chamomile to be a very safe and beneficial herb.

Asian Ginseng *(Panax ginseng)* and **American Ginseng *(Panax quinquefolius)*** have long histories of safe use. In 1979, the *Journal of the American Medical Association* (*JAMA*) published an article describing a study in which 10% of the participants experienced symptoms of nervousness, insomnia, and diarrhea that were labeled the "Ginseng abuse syndrome." The study was flawed because the 10% experiencing symptoms were drinking large amounts of coffee with the Ginseng. *JAMA* and the press spread the erroneous message about Ginseng but never mentioned that coffee could have been the precipitating factor.

Lobelia *(Lobelia inflata)* is often listed as a toxic herb, but this is incorrect. This misconception originated in the early 1800s when American herbalist Samuel Thomson was taken to court after being accused of killing his patient with Lobelia. All charges were dropped due to lack of evidence, and there have been no reports of death since that time. Unfortunately, many references continue to label Lobelia as toxic.

Sassafras *(Sassafras albidum)* is a popular herb with a long history of safe use. The root bark of Sassafras contains the compound safrole, which has caused cancer in lab mice and rats fed and injected with large doses over extended periods of time. Although there are no reported incidences of Sassafras causing cancer in humans, the FDA instituted a ban on putting the herb in foods or drinks. This ban lasted from 1960 until the passage of the Dietary Supplement Health and Education Act (DSHEA) in 1994. Sassafras root extracts that do not contain safrole, or from which the safrole has been removed, are now permissible and used commercially in teas and root beers. Small amounts of safrole are also found in Black Pepper, Cinnamon and Sage, but these herbs have never come under fire.

Contraindications

A contraindication typically refers to the limitation or avoidance of an herb due to the possibility that it may worsen or aggravate a pre-existing condition, disease, or imbalance. The range of contraindications can include restrictions due to allergic reactions, pregnancy and lactation, the young age and sensitivity of infants and children, and medical conditions like diabetes, cardiovascular disease, or hypertension.

Many contraindications listed in current books are theoretical considerations based on the activity of one or two isolated constituents in a plant, which does not necessarily reflect the actual effect of the whole plant. Many theoretical considerations are not based upon or proven by case studies or clinical experience. The following list provides examples of several herbs that are contraindicated for specific conditions:

Common name	**Botanical name**	**Do not use in cases of:**
Buckthorn	*Rhamnus cathartica*	Diarrhea, ulcerative colitis, Crohn's, appendicitis
Cascara Sagrada	*Rhamnus purshiana*	Diarrhea, ulcerative colitis, Crohn's, appendicitis
Comfrey	*Symphytum officinale*	Liver disease
Dandelion	*Taraxacum officinale*	Bile duct obstruction
Echinacea	*Echinacea* spp.	AIDS, multiple sclerosis, other autoimmune diseases
Ephedra	*Ephedra* spp.	Anxiety, hypertension, rapid heart beat, insomnia
Juniper berry	*Junipurus communis*	Kidney inflammation
Kava Kava	*Piper methysticum*	Depression
Licorice	*Glycyrrhiza glabra*	Hypertension, water retention, liver cirrhosis
Milk Thistle	*Silybum marianum*	Diarrhea
Peppermint	*Mentha x piperita*	Gastric reflux, heartburn, bile duct obstruction
Senna	*Senna marilandica*	Diarrhea, ulcerative colitis, Crohn's, appendicitis
Turmeric	*Curcuma longa*	Bile duct obstruction

Herb-Drug Interactions

Herb-drug interactions refer to the effects that occur when herbs are taken with pharmaceutical drugs. This is a relatively new field of research, often providing limited amounts of information and inadequate clinical observation to make reliable conclusions. Physician and nursing herbal reference books are the most notorious for listing hypothetical herb-drug interactions, side effects, and toxic reactions that are not backed by human experience or clinical trials. It is difficult to substantiate herb-drug interactions without thorough knowledge of chemical properties and biological actions of the herb. Whole-plant herbs contain so many chemical constituents that analysis is very complicated. However, researchers are making attempts to identify herbal ingredients with the potential to interfere with specific types of pharmaceutical drugs based on the known chemical constituents and actions of the herb, and on clinically observed side effects.

> *Several herb-drug interactions are well documented, but many interactions appearing in the literature are based on laboratory findings or theory, and are not determined by actual clinical proof or case studies.*

It is interesting to note the double standard evidenced by the extreme degree of scrutiny and critical bias focused on herb-drug interactions when there is very little interest in or research on drug-drug interactions, which have significantly greater potential for harm. The biological activity of pharmaceutical drugs is typically much greater than that of herbal remedies. Considering the vast number of people who use both herbs and pharmaceutical medicines, relatively few herb-drug interactions have been reported in the literature. These are uncommon compared with drug-drug interactions, which tend to be much more serious. Herb-herb interactions are very rare, which is why many herbal traditions employ polypharmacy, the practice of combing several herbs into one formula.

Interactions occur when one substance reacts with another to increase or decrease their effects. Herb-drug interactions can be pharmacokinetic or pharmacodynamic. Herbs create pharmacokinetic interactions by changing the absorption, distribution, metabolism or excretion of a drug, which alters its dosage level and duration of availability at the site of action. Herbs elicit pharmacodynamic effects by increasing or decreasing the effects of drugs.

Herb-drug interactions fall into four basic categories:
1) Synergistic, complimentary, or agonist effects
2) Opposite or antagonistic effects
3) Drug absorption
4) Drug metabolism

Synergistic or agonist effects occur when herbs with similar properties as a pharmaceutical drug compliment and increase the actions of the drug. This interaction can be dangerous when the herb and drug are used together and excessive amounts accumulate to cause imbalance or toxicity. But synergistic effects can be a beneficial tool used to reduce or discontinue pharmaceutical drugs that may have potentially dangerous side effects. People can often safely wean themselves off drugs by gradually replacing them with herbal remedies. The herb is taken while gradually reducing the dosage of the pharmaceutical drug, and eventually the drug can be discontinued. During this period of replacement, drug doses may need to be monitored and adjusted accordingly. This process should be guided by a qualified health professional.

The following are several examples of synergistic or agonist herb-drug interactions:
❖ Combining stimulating herbs like Guarana, Ephedra, Ginseng, and Kola Nut with caffeine or amphetamines will increase their stimulating effects, possibly to the point of dangerous excess causing increased heart rate and blood pressure, or damage to the nervous system in extreme cases.
❖ Combining sedating herbs such as Kava Kava, Valerian, Scullcap, and Hops with sedative drugs, anti-anxiety medication, sleeping pills, or psychiatric drugs may cause excessive sedation that can reduce heart rate and blood pressure.
❖ Taking an anti-depressant herb like St. John's Wort can increase or complement the action of pharmaceutical anti-depressants. If individuals want to reduce or discontinue prescription anti-depressants, this synergistic effect can be beneficial. Although some sources caution against using St. John's Wort with anti-depressants, I have seen many people use both, and the herb allows them to decrease and eventually go off the drugs, which have much greater risk of side effects.
❖ There are many concerns about suspected interactions caused by combining blood-thinning herbs with aspirin and anticoagulant drugs. Blood-thinning botanicals like Bilberry, Dong Quai, Gingko, Garlic, and Ginger reduce blood platelet aggregation and can increase the effects of anticoagulant, antiplatelet drugs (like warfarin/coumadin) and increase possibilities of hemorrhaging. If the patient is monitored, however, these herbs can be used advantageously by enabling people to decrease the dosage of their prescription drug. All blood-thinning herbs should be avoided before surgery to reduce risk of hemorrhage.
❖ The antibiotic and immune-stimulating properties of Goldenseal and Echinacea can beneficially augment the action of prescription antibiotic drugs.
❖ Herbs like Hawthorn and Aloe Vera contain cardiac glycosides that should not be taken with pharmaceutical cardiac glycosides and beta-blockers because excessive doses can be dangerous to the heart.
❖ Herbal diuretics like Dandelion and Aloe Vera can increase the action of pharmaceutical diuretics and can be used to replace them.
❖ Stinging Nettle is an anti-inflammatory herb that can increase the therapeutic effects of nonsteroidal anti-inflammatory drugs (NSAIDs).
❖ Valerian increases the effects of GABA (gamma-aminobutyric acid), which is a brain neurotransmitter that reduces anxiety.
❖ Immune-enhancing herbs like Astragalus and Echinacea can increase the action of immune-stimulating drugs such as interleukin-2 and acyclovir, and can be taken together for greater effects.

Opposite or antagonistic effects occur when herbs and drugs have opposite biological effects, and the herb reduces or cancels out actions of the drug. In most cases, these effects should be avoided.
❖ Stimulating herbs should not be taken in conjunction with calming medications like anti-anxiety or insomnia drugs.
❖ Since Astragalus and Echinacea stimulate immunity, they should not be taken with drugs that suppress the immune system.
❖ Laxative herbs like Senna, Cascara Sagrada, and Yellow Dock should not be taken with anti-diarrhea drugs like Lomotil or Imodium.
❖ Milk Thistle can be taken with drugs that are toxic to the liver and following conventional cancer treatments to reduce liver damage.

Drug absorption can be reduced or increased by different herbs.
❖ Stimulating herbal laxatives can speed the transit time of drugs moving through the intestinal tract to reduce their absorption and biological effects.
❖ Mucilaginous and fibrous herbs like Marshmallow root, Slippery Elm, and psyllium seeds can absorb drugs and reduce their effects. This can be avoided by ingesting these herbs at different times than the drug.
❖ Cayenne and Ginger stimulate blood circulation, which can promote increased drug absorption and speed up the peak time of drug effects.

Drug metabolism can be affected by herbs and foods.

- ❖ St. John's Wort can interfere with enzyme systems and has been shown to interact with some drugs, such as cyclosporine and protease inhibitors.
- ❖ Grapefruit juice has been clinically proven to interact with dozens of drugs.

Although many herbs are assumed to create potential drug interactions, actual clinical experience often contradicts these assumptions. Ginkgo, for example, is one of the most widely utilized herbs in the world, and many references caution against using it with blood-thinning and anticoagulant pharmaceuticals. Based on the marketing data of Dr. Willmar Schwabe, the world's leading producer and marketer of Ginkgo extract, over two billion daily doses of Ginkgo extract were distributed worldwide from 1979 to 1997. From 1997 to 2002, 1.3 billion daily doses of Ginkgo were administered in Germany alone. Until 2003, only four case reports of potential interactions between Ginkgo and conventional drugs had been published. Over 40 clinical trials involving several thousand people have been conducted with Ginkgo, and there have been no reports of increased bleeding (Upton, 2004). This shows that although this is commonly listed as a problem interaction, there is little or no clinical evidence to support the hypothesis. Nevertheless, caution and common sense are always advised.

Final Analysis of Herbal Safety

To put the issue of herbal safety into realistic perspective, understand that as a general rule, herbal medicines are much safer than conventional drugs and cause significantly fewer side effects when they are used correctly according to their normal dosages. The World Health Organization has developed guidelines to integrate medicinal herbs into modern health care systems, and recommends that herbal medicines should be considered safe if they have been widely used by large populations over long periods of time without causing side effects or toxicity, unless proven otherwise (WHO, 1992). The statistics definitely favor herbs over pharmaceutical medicines when it comes to safety. World-renowned herbal authority Norman Farnsworth, Research Professor of Pharmacognosy and Senior University Scholar at University of Illinois in Chicago, affirmed:

Herbal medicines do not present a major problem with regard to toxicity based on a survey of the scientific literature. In fact, of all classes of substances reported to cause toxicities of sufficient magnitude to be reported in the United States, plants are the least problematic. However, this does not minimize the need to have quality assurance procedures in place for products being offered to the public that are intended to have a palliative or curative effect on selected disease states. (Farnsworth, 1993)

> *For people, herbal medicines are safer than conventional drugs and cause significantly fewer side effects when correctly used in normal dosages.*
>
> *For our planet and local ecosystems, herbs are also safe, unlike pharmaceutical drugs that do not breakdown but remain in the soil and water to find their way into animal and human tissues.*

In the holistic perspective, Mother Nature is the supreme master chemist. Life exists within a delicate balance of thousands of complex chemical combinations and interactions. When left undisturbed by humans, life maintains a dynamic balance and flow. When we look at the self-destructive tendencies and effects humanity has on the planet resulting in air and water pollution, toxins in our foods, the destructive effects of global warming, and the extinction of many animals and plants, one wonders why people assume that we are so intelligent as to improve upon Nature. When it comes to our medicines, why is there such trust in synthetic drugs while excluding Nature's offerings of herbal medicines? There is a tendency to be so immersed in our sophisticated technology that it can be easy to lose sight of common sense and living in more natural ways.

Pharmaceutical drugs definitely play an important role in modern health care, and although they are laden with potential side effects, many are important and appropriate for certain conditions. However, when comparing the safety of herbs to pharmaceutical drugs, it is wise to exclude biases and to be realistic in judging differences. When deciding between the safety of an herb that has been used by large populations for hundreds of years compared to a pharmaceutical drug that has been on the market less than 10 years, I am much more comfortable using the herb.

Do not allow unsubstantiated fears of toxicity, side effects, or herb-drug interactions to prohibit you from incorporating herbs into your life and using plants as part of your health care. Have a healthy respect for the powerful chemicals in plants and thoroughly research any herb you decide to ingest. Enlist the guidance of a qualified medical herbalist. Use common sense, take herbs according to their traditional uses and dosages, and benefit from their healing gifts!

Chemical Constituents in Plants

Thousands of different chemical constituents are found within the plant kingdom, and hundreds can occur in one individual plant. Plants are living, breathing, chemical factories that have been evolving over a span of more than 400 million years. In their process of evolution, plants have developed **phytochemicals (plant chemicals)** that are vital for their biochemistry and survival, and many are responsible for their characteristic odors and flavors. Phytochemicals also exert their biological influence on animals and people. Many plant constituents have medicinal properties that promote health and healing, while others can be toxic and dangerous when ingested. Becoming acquainted with some of the common chemical constituents in medicinal herbs is helpful in unraveling their diverse "personalities" and understanding their effects on animal and human physiology.

All forms of life are composed of chemical compounds. Plants, animals, and humans exist by the processes of metabolism involving complex chemical reactions mediated by enzymes. The metabolic process either breaks down living matter (catabolism) or creates new life forms (anabolism). The metabolic pathways for catabolism or anabolism in all organisms are similar and require many of the same nutrients, enzymes, and chemical constituents. **Primary metabolites** are nutritional substances essential for the life and physical structure of the organism, and generally occur in plants in substantial amounts. They are the building blocks necessary for the production of **secondary metabolites** that usually occur in much smaller concentrations. Secondary metabolites are substances that have specific functions in the biochemistry of plants.

Primary metabolites are proteins, fats, and sugars. Plants depend on these for nutrients and to provide their form and structure. Herbs containing large amounts of these primary substances are generally used as nourishing tonics to support growth, maintenance, repair, and optimal health in the human body. Smaller amounts of secondary metabolites in plants have naturally evolved to help them survive in nature. Secondary metabolites, which are paramount to the life of plants, also benefit people because they often possess biological and medicinal properties, and are the active components in many herbal remedies and pharmaceutical drugs.

These specialized secondary metabolites reveal the ability of plants to adapt to their environment and defend themselves against predators. Some of these phytochemicals regulate sprouting, budding, and growth of plants. Others are involved in pollination and seed dispersal by attracting birds and insects with

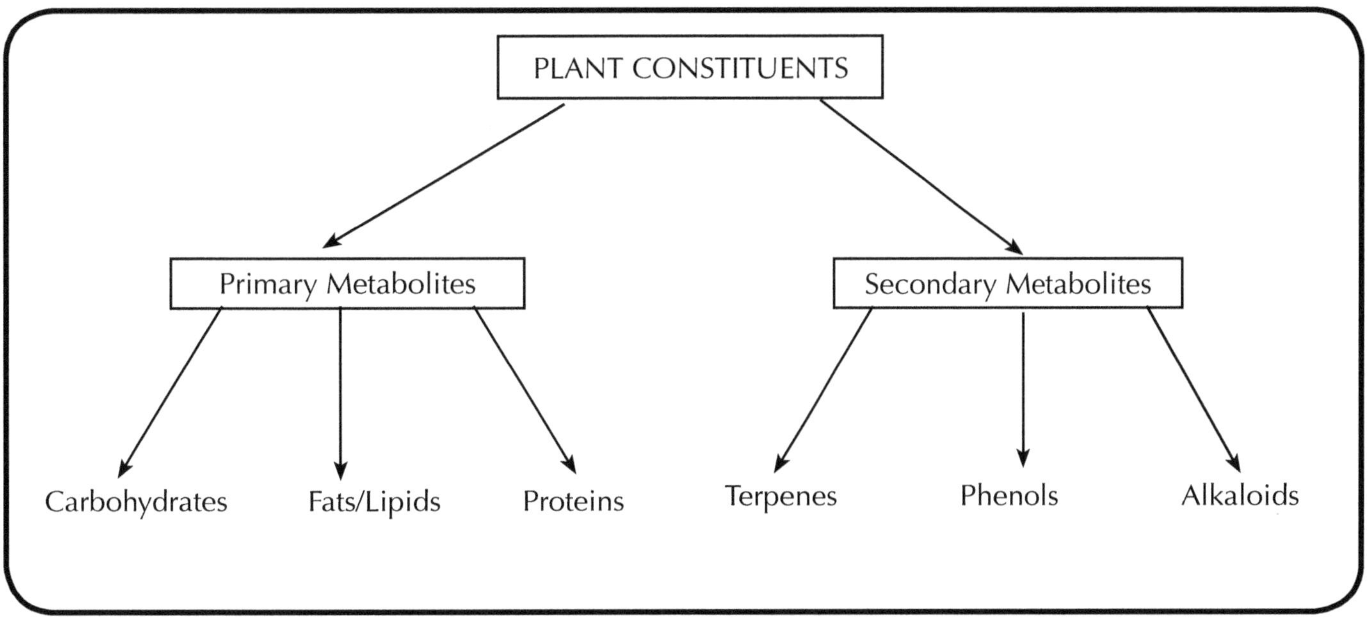

alluring fragrances and colors. Antimicrobial phytochemicals that protect plants against bacteria, viruses, fungi, and mold infections also benefit people. Tannins are chemical constituents occurring in many leaves, unripe fruit, bark, and roots. They have an astringent effect and act as strong deterrents to insects and other herbivores, as well as inhibiting fungal and bacterial growth in plants and humans. Alkaloids are nitrogen compounds with bitter flavors that serve as self-protective mechanisms deterring animals and insects from eating plants. Some insects have adapted this plant defense to their own benefit. For example, the monarch butterfly in its caterpillar stage is able to eat the leaves of Rue *(Ruta graveolens)*, an extremely bitter plant, and the bitter phytochemicals stay in the butterfly's body to protect it from being eaten by birds. Gums and resins provide a thick, sticky, protective layer on plants to shield them from intense heat, weather, and nibbling animals. The complex quality and concentration of active plant constituents depend on many factors, including plant genetics, environmental conditions like temperature, rainfall, altitude, soil type and fertility, amount of daylight and sunlight, and the methods of harvest and preparation of medicinal products. The age and general health of plants at the time of harvest are also major factors.

Joel Swerdlow provides fascinating information in his book, *Nature's Medicines*, when he explains:

> A plant's chemical-based defense system, recent research has documented, can be as complex as the human immune system. Plant defenses even have chemical memory. After combating a particular disease-causing virus, a plant can retain a resistance to that virus and related microbes. Among other components of plant defenses is the capacity to order cells near an invader to die, exuding poisonous and acidic chemicals. Some cells stiffen to exude and wall off invaders, while still others produce the equivalent of antibiotics.
>
> Sophisticated plant defense mechanisms include those that time the greening of leaves to the absence of herbivores and the production of chemicals that protect plants during constant exposure to sunlight. The chemicals responsible for such defensive actions may have beneficial effects on humans, as could plant capabilities that go far beyond defensive functions. Many plants generate an amino acid called glutamate that they use for internal communications. Humans also produce glutamate, which serves as a chemical messenger in the brain. Other instances of commonality are evident in the apparently countless ways that plant-generated chemicals bind to human receptors. Licorice, to cite one example, produces glycyrrhizic acid, a compound that binds to human kidney cells – which respond as if it is aldosterone, a chemical that the adrenal glands release to combat low blood pressure. These links between plants and animals may be coincidences, but growing genetic evidence indicates that they are vestiges of the time billions of years ago before plants and animals evolved in different directions. (Swerdlow, 2000)

All drugs, whether they are derived from crude plant material or refined and synthesized in the laboratory, must go through the same biochemical pathways and metabolic processes in the body. The **cell receptor model**, which explains the mechanism allowing chemicals to affect the human body, has become the basis of modern drug research. According to this model, the outer surface of human and animal cells contains receptors that are specific areas of reactive chemical groupings. When chemical constituents from herbs or drugs make contact with these receptors, they set off a chemical reaction known as the therapeutic effect. However, receptors will only react if a constituent can structurally fit into the site, like a key fitting into a lock. This reaction occurs whether the chemical constituent comes from a plant or is synthetically produced in a laboratory.

> *Plants are complex and dynamic forms of life.*
>
> *The medicinal properties of herbs come from the synergistic activity of all chemical constituents within each plant, and are not determined by the activity of only a few phytochemicals.*

One way to collect information about the properties of herbs and their effects on the human body is by experimentation and observation, which is documented and tried by the test of time. This is the ancient and traditional method of herbalists, whose perspective is innately holistic by focusing on the whole organism and by understanding the interconnection and interactions of all life. This tradition is the foundation of our modern knowledge and application of medicinal herbs. Another valuable method to analyze the therapeutic potential of herbs is the scientific approach, which uses various laboratory techniques to identify and isolate specific chemical compounds in plant material. The scientific method, embraced by the pharmaceutical and medical industries, is based on the reductionist model that attempts to reduce the whole plant to its primary active constituents in order to use them as individualized substances in many pharmaceutical drugs.

Plant chemistry became an established science and discipline included in university curriculums by the end of the 1800s. The science of **pharmacognosy** deals with the biological, chemical, and economic aspects of natural and synthetic drugs and their applications in medicine. It involves the study of crude plant and animal drugs, and their natural chemical derivatives that are isolated and purified. **Pharmacology** is the study of drug preparations and applications and their effects on living organisms. Both employ a multitude of laboratory tests to research and analyze herbs. The goal of scientific analysis is to identify and isolate plant chemicals that possess potential healing activities. These chemicals are then tested in the laboratory to determine their physiological effects and potential as medicinal agents.

Knowing the chemical constituents in plants is beneficial for several reasons. Discovering the identities and activities of herbal constituents often validates their historic uses and increases the credibility of traditional herbalism. The scientific approach expands our herbal knowledge and understanding of the medicinal and therapeutic actions of herbs in the body. Greater awareness of the specific chemical properties and actions of plants helps guide us to tap into their full healing potential. Knowing the primary chemical constituents of an herb is also helpful when deciding the best method of preparation and menstruum (liquid solvent) to use for their extraction. For example, herbs like Marshmallow (*Althaea officinalis*) and Comfrey (*Symphytum officinale*), which contain mucilage as their active constituents, are best extracted in cool or warm water and ingested as a tea. On the other hand, plants containing alkaloids and essential oils need alcohol for best extraction. Many herbs contain active constituents that are soluble in both water and alcohol, so the menstruum should contain a combination of water and alcohol for optimal extraction.

It is important that scientific research on medicinal plants and identification of their phytochemical content continues to evolve. And it is equally vital that our understanding of herbal medicine not be reduced to the inherently limited application of a few isolated chemical constituents labeled as "active ingredients." Plants are complex and dynamic forms of life, and their biological effects cannot be reduced to the activities of only one or two chemical constituents. Researchers can identify and analyze plant chemicals and make scientifically based statements about their properties and actions, but the biological effects of isolated chemicals do not necessarily reflect how the whole plant interacts within the human body. The physiologic effects of herbs result from the complex and synergistic activity of all the chemical constituents blended together within each plant, and do not depend on the activity of a few phytochemicals.

The long-standing historic use of an herb within respected medical traditions provides realistic assurance of its safety and should be considered along with scientific research.

Another limitation of defining and applying herbs solely based on scientific analysis is that the testing methods themselves can be biased and incongruent with traditional uses of herbs. After a specific chemical with suspected biological activity is identified and isolated by the pharmaceutical industry, it is typically tested on laboratory animals. The animals are often fed or injected with abnormally large amounts of a chemical, and the resulting test conclusions do not necessarily reflect normal human dosages or the normal route of administration. These tests can be inherently biased because isolating one chemical from a plant and studying the effects of unreasonably large doses is not an equal comparison to the biological effects of the entire root, leaf, or flower normally used as medicine.

A common problem with modern research and scientific data analysis occurs when researchers postulate theories about possible adverse reactions and interactions of many herbs, even though these effects have never been proven or seen in actual clinical practice, and thousands of people have safely used the herbs for centuries within respected herbal traditions. When these theories appear in herbal publications and the media, herbs are branded with negative publicity and misinformation about their safety. These distorted perspectives about medicinal herbs can be confusing and misleading to health professionals and laypersons.

A complete understanding of the therapeutic actions of herbs is not possible through biochemical analysis alone. Greater accuracy and reliability are obtained when scientific research and outcomes are measured alongside the long historic use of herbs and a broader, more holistic perspective is considered. Medicinal herbalism has been practiced for thousands of years among common people and within respected medical traditions in countries around the world. This long-standing history and years of anecdotal evidence definitely provides realistic assurance of the effectiveness and safety of many plants, and should be taken into account along with the scientific research.

Chemical Pathways of Phytochemical Synthesis

Scientists have isolated and classified several thousand chemical constituents from different plant groups. The groups are determined by their chemical structure rather than their function, which relates to the healing properties of phytochemicals. Despite their numerous and varied structures, all phytochemicals are synthesized by only a few pathways (a series of chemical reactions), including the **pentose phosphate pathway**, **shikimate pathway**, **acetate-malonate pathway**, and **mevalonic acid pathway**. As mentioned earlier, phytochemicals are broadly classified as primary and secondary metabolites. **Primary metabolites** are nutritional substances essential to the life and physical structure of the organism as well as necessary building blocks for the production of secondary metabolites that occur in much smaller concentrations. **Secondary metabolites,** generally divided into three large groupings determined by their metabolic pathway of biosynthesis, include terpenes, phenols, and alkaloids. **Terpenes** are lipids (fats) synthesized from acetyl coenzyme A via the mevalonate pathway. **Phenols** are aromatic substances formed in various ways via the shikimate and malonate pathways. Nitrogen-containing **alkaloids** are made from amino acids via the shikimate pathway. Since scientists first recognized and began studying secondary plant metabolites at the end of the 1800s, over 200,000 have been identified.

Modern analytical research using techniques such as chromatography, electrophoresis, isotopes, and enzymology have provided much information about the structural formulation and the most important biosynthetic pathways of many secondary plant metabolites. References to many of these chemical constituents are found throughout herbal literature, and knowing a bit about them will contribute to better understanding and application of medicinal herbs. The science of plant constituents is immense and continually expanding. The following is a brief description and discussion of some of the most common groups of constituents comprising primary and secondary metabolites, and is by no means meant to be a complete presentation of this very intricate topic.

Pathways of Primary and Secondary Plant Metabolites

CO_2 (carbon dioxide) + H_2O (water) + Sunlight = CH_2O (carbohydrates) + O_2 (oxygen) via Photosynthesis

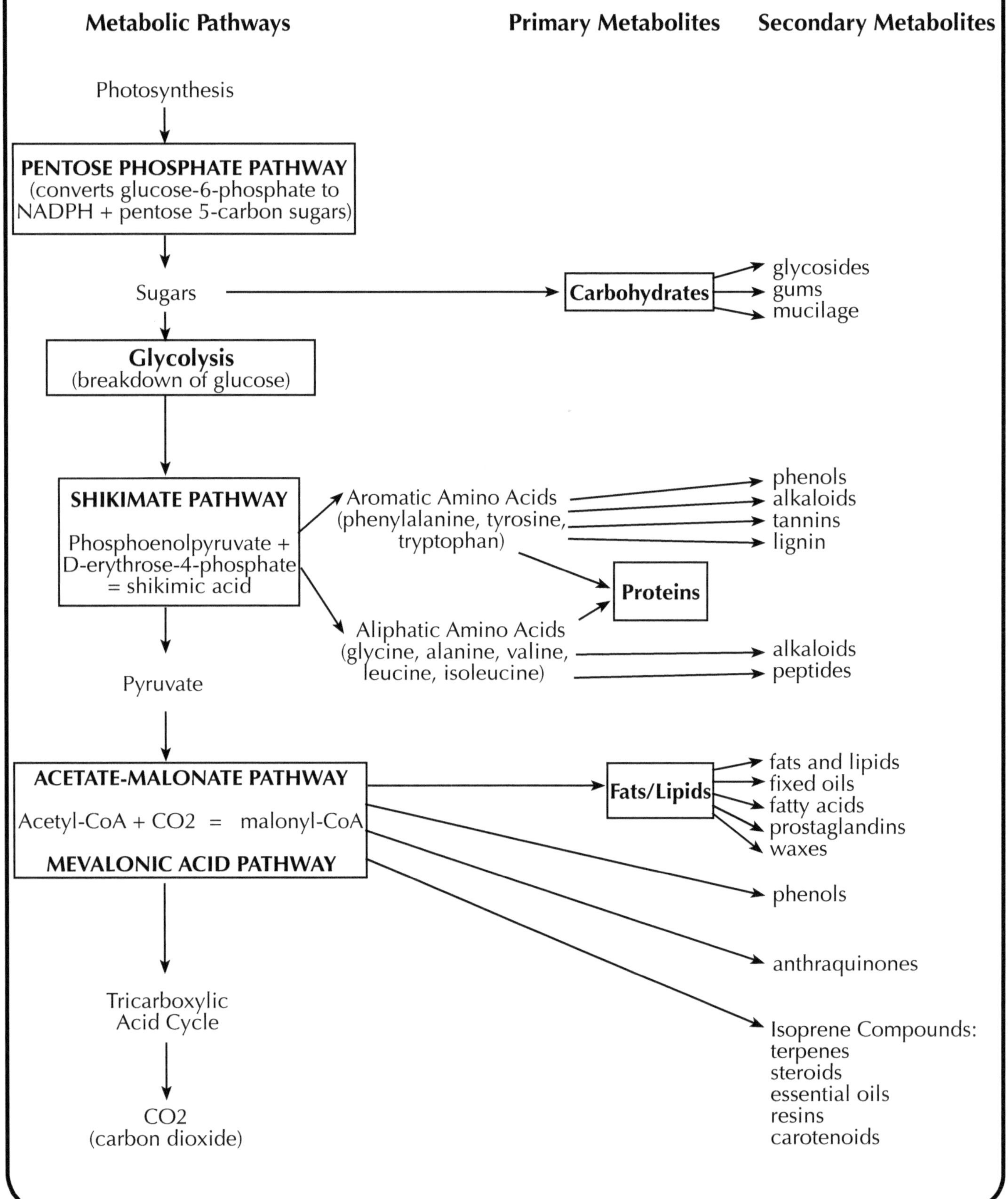

Carbohydrates

Carbohydrates are primary metabolites composed of sugar molecules. They occur in plants and animals as a primary food source. Sugars provide energy needed for plant growth, mineral transport, and water uptake. They are formed by photosynthesis, the mechanism that transforms solar energy into plant material. Without this incredible process of photosynthesis and the formation of carbohydrates, no life would exist on earth. Many secondary plant metabolites are glycosylated, meaning that they contain sugar molecules that increase their solubility in water.

Carbohydrates are divided into simple and complex sugars. There are three types of simple sugars, or saccharides. **Monosaccharides** contain one sugar and include glucose and fructose. **Disaccharides** are a subcategory of oligosaccharides and contain two sugars bonded together. Disaccharides include sucrose (common table sugar formed by the combination of glucose and fructose), maltose (malt sugar), and lactose (milk sugar formed from glucose and galactose). **Oligosaccharides** have 2-10 sugars on a chain and include mannose and galactose (derived from milk sugar). Complex carbohydrates consisting of many sugar chains are called **polysaccharides**, which form starch, cellulose, gums, mucilage, inulin, and pectin. Plants use starch as a primary source of stored energy. Cellulose is the fibrous substance surrounding the cells of almost all plants, and is the basic structural component of plants and wood. Glycosides are a large group of polysaccharides that are secondary plant metabolites.

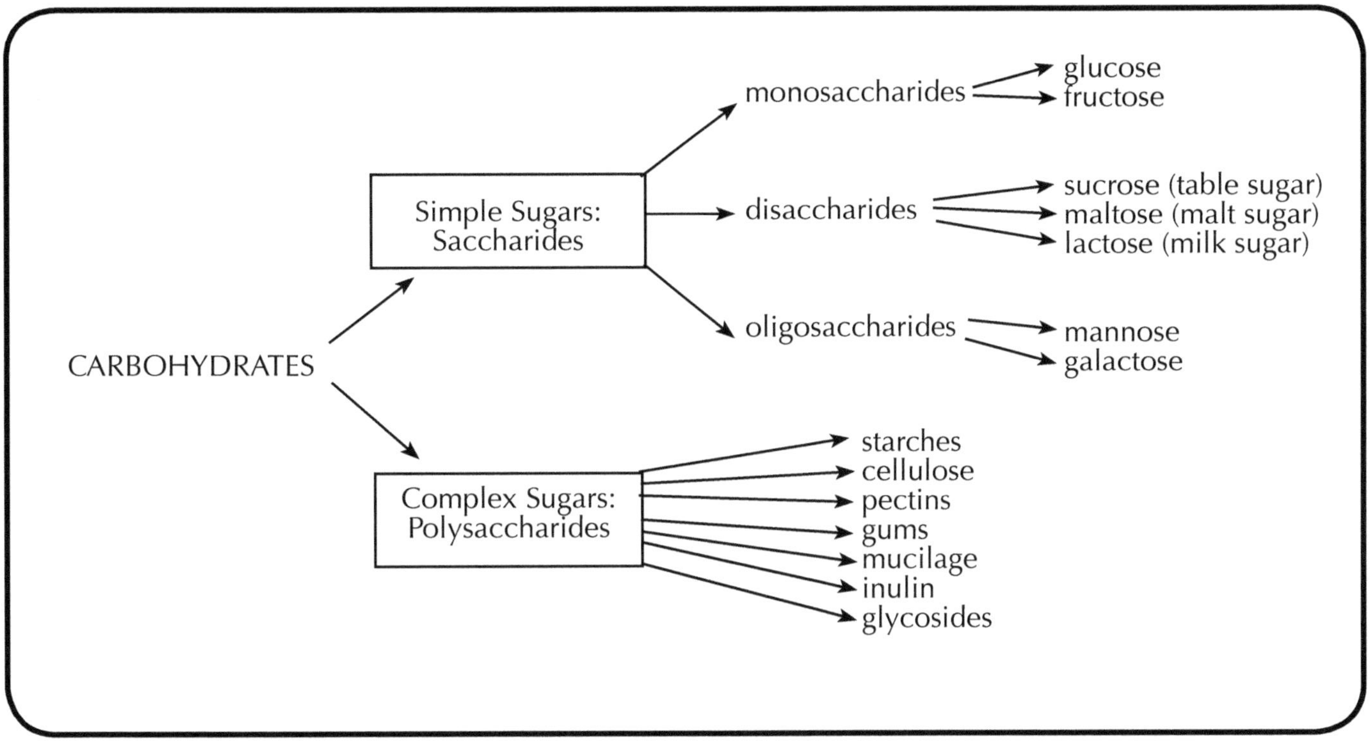

Plants with high contents of carbohydrates such as carrots, beets, potatoes, beans, and grains are nutritious and often used as food sources. Simple sugars do not play a medicinal role, but polysaccharide sugars are key components in the biochemistry of green plants and are used in medicine. They are the precursors (original ingredients) for the synthesis of many other compounds. An important property of some polysaccharides is their ability to stimulate the immune system. Tests have shown that herbs with high concentrations of polysaccharides, such as Astragalus, Cordyceps, Echinacea, Eleuthero (Siberian Ginseng), Ginseng, and Reishi and Shiitake mushrooms, can assist in treating tumors, AIDS, and chronic fatigue syndrome. Examples of other plants containing high amounts of polysaccharides include Alfalfa, Boneset, Burdock, Codonopsis, Comfrey, Dandelion, Irish Moss, Marshmallow, Oatstraw, Plantain, Raspberry leaf, Red Clover, Slippery Elm, and Solomon's Seal root,.

Carbohydrates, starches, and polysaccharides are generally soluble in water and only partially in alcohol. Polysaccharides can be precipitated out of solution by alcohol.

Mucilage is a thick, slimy, slippery, lubricating substance composed of polysaccharides. It is formed in plants by specialized organs, and plants containing large amounts of mucilage feel rather slick and slimy. Mucilage has a mild flavor, absorbs moisture, and expands in the presence of water. Mucilaginous herbs provide wonderful healing properties. They are used medicinally both internally and externally to provide a cool, soothing, protective, moisturizing, and lubricating coating to injured, irritated, and inflamed tissues. Mucilage is excellent for burns, toxin-induced rashes, and itchy, irritated dermatitis. For internal use, mucilage herbs work best when taken as a tea instead of tincture. As a tea, the healing constituents maintain physical contact with the tissues as they move through the digestive system. Mucilage herbs are used internally to sooth and heal sore throats, stomach and intestinal ulcers, spasms, inflammation, and lung problems such as coughs (especially dry, unproductive coughs). Their soothing quality and ability to absorb and hold water make them excellent bulk laxatives. Mucilage also absorbs toxins from the intestines, helps lower cholesterol levels, and can reduce elevated blood sugar levels.

Mucilage herbs provide the best healing activity when they are prepared with water that is warm rather than boiling hot. Alcohol negates the beneficial effects of mucilage and causes it to precipitate out of solution. If tinctures are made from mucilaginous herbs, only 24% alcohol should be used, which is the minimum amount to ensure preservation of the tincture.

Mucilage herbs include Aloe Vera, Astragalus, Borage, Coltsfoot, Comfrey, Dandelion, Flaxseed, Fenugreek, Marshmallow, Mullein, Plantain, Psyllium seed from *Plantago ovata*, Purslane, Slippery Elm bark, and Solomon's Seal root.

Gums are a complex mixture of colorless, tasteless polysaccharides and glycoproteins that are edible. They are similar to mucilage but are generally thicker, denser, and stickier. When gums absorb water, they swell up in size and form a gelatinous glue consistency. Like mucilaginous herbs, gums are demulcents that cleanse and soothe inflamed and irritated tissues or mucous membranes, and are used as bulk laxatives. They are commonly used as stabilizers and adhesives in the food, cosmetic, and pharmaceutical industries because their sticky consistency prevents mixtures from separating. As emulsifiers, gums are added as a thickener to prevent ingredients from separating and to extend shelf life. Gums are also used by manufacturing companies to coat and bind pills.

Gums are secreted at the surface of plants where they act as protective sealants against mechanical injury. Gum arabic, also called acacia gum, comes from the Acacia tree (*Acacia senegal*). Guar gum is extracted from the seeds of the Guar bean (*Cyamopsis tetragonoloba*), agar is derived from red algae sodium alginate or algin is extracted from all species of brown seaweeds, and carrageenan comes from red edible seaweeds like Irish Moss (*Chondrus crispus*). Gums are very soluble in water but not in alcohol. They can be precipitated from liquid solutions by alcohol.

Inulin is a commonly occurring polysaccharide that plants store and use as food. It has a mildly sweet taste but is not absorbed well through the digestive system. It feeds beneficial lactobacilli in the intestinal tract to improve intestinal health, and helps protect against colon cancers. Inulin can be beneficial to reduce high cholesterol and blood sugar levels, kill microbial infections, and prevent osteoporosis by improving mineral absorption through the small intestines. Despite similarity in names, inulin has no relationship with insulin. Inulin is soluble in hot water and less soluble in cold water and alcohol. In tincture preparations, inulin precipitates into a white substance that sinks to the bottom of the container.

Inulin is present in the roots of many members of the *Compositae* family, including Burdock, Chicory, Codonopsis, Dandelion, Echinacea, Elecampane, and Jerusalem artichoke. These herbs are traditionally prepared as hot decoction teas.

Glycosides are an important class of polysaccharides consisting of organic sugar compounds called glycons and a non-sugar, or aglycone, component. Glycosides are typically divided into 11 groups, each named according to the chemical composition of its non-sugar aglycone component. This non-sugar compound is chemically variable and often has biological activity. Plants produce glycosides to regulate their chemical processes and provide protection. In humans, glycosides exert many different medicinal properties affecting all systems of the body. Some glycosides are toxic. Most glycosides are soluble in water and alcohol, but not in oils.

❖ **Cardiac Glycosides** exert a characteristic action on the contractile force of the heart. They help strengthen and restore normal heart function, regulating normal rhythm without increasing the amount of oxygen needed by cardiac muscles. Due to their ability to increase heart function, they also have a diuretic effect that removes excess fluids from the body. Cardiac glycosides are terpene sterol derivatives closely related to saponins, which also have a beneficial effect on the heart. Herbs containing cardiac glycosides must be used very cautiously, if at all, because the therapeutic dose tends to be close to the toxic dose and must be carefully monitored. These herbs include Foxglove (*Digitalis*), the source of the popular heart drug digitalis, Lily-of-the-Valley, Squill (*Urginea maritima*), and the Milkweed (*Asclepias*) and Dogbane (*Apocynales*) families. Foxglove is rarely used due to its high potential for toxicity, but small amounts of Lily-of-the-Valley can be quite beneficial for the heart. These plants developed cardiac glycosides to deter plant-eaters, but the larvae of monarch butterflies have adapted the ability to eat large amounts of milkweed without being affected. The caterpillars concentrate large amounts of these compounds in their bodies to deter birds from eating them.

❖ **Anthraquinone glycosides** are bitter-tasting compounds that stimulate laxative action by encouraging peristaltic movement of the colon to promote bowel movements about 8-12 hours after ingestion. Herbal laxatives and cathartics contain anthraquinone glycosides and include Aloe, Buckthorn, Cascara Sagrada, Pau

D'arco, Rhubarb, Senna, and Yellow Dock root. The botanical families richest in anthraquinone glycosides are *Rubiaceae* (Madder Family), *Rhamnaceae* (Buckthorn Family), and *Polygonaceae* (Buckwheat Family). Anthraquinones are also used as plant dyes.

❖ **Saponins** are a group of glycosides with sugars attached to either a steroid or triterpene. Saponin glycosides, or steroidal glycosides, have a soapy, frothy detergent quality and foam up when crushed leaves and roots are shaken in water. The name "saponin" is derived from the Latin word *sapo*, meaning "soap." They are effective in removing dirt but not oils. Saponins occur in many plants in a wide variety of forms with different potencies. Plants produce antibiotic and antifungal saponins to protect their roots and leaves from soil bacteria and fungi. Saponins have soothing and healing demulcent properties, and exert anti-inflammatory, expectorant, and diuretic activity. They are chemically similar to cardiac glycosides and can have a beneficial effect on the heart. They enhance digestion and promote assimilation of nutrients. Others stimulate immunity, inhibit the growth of cancers, and have potential as chemotherapeutic drugs. Herbs such as Chickweed, Soapwort (*Saponaria officinalis*), and Yucca contain substantial amounts of saponins and have a cleansing and dissolving action on tissues and some tumors. Steroidal glycosides affect insect and animal reproduction, and chemists use these for the synthesis of sex hormones and cortisone (a powerful anti-inflammatory drug). Alfalfa, Black Cohosh, Blue Cohosh, Fenugreek, Licorice, Sarsaparilla, and Wild Yam root contain steroidal saponins that the body can use as raw materials or chemical precursors for the production of steroids and hormones. When ingested in appropriate quantities, these herbs can exert mild hormone-like actions. The other type of saponin has a terpene structure and can also exert hormone-like activity in people. Devil's Claw, Ginseng, Horse Chestnut, Mullein, Primrose, Sassafras, and Schisandra contain saponins. <u>All saponins are soluble in water and oil.</u>

❖ **Cyanophose glycosides** are the largest group of organic cyanides. They are used as flavoring agents, anti-anxiety remedies, and as anticancer herbs. Amygdalin and mandelonitrile are two of the most common cyanophose glycosides. Amygdalin has anticarcinogenic properties and occurs in sizable amounts in almonds and the kernels of apricots, cherries, peaches, plums, and many other seeds. Laetrile from apricot kernels contains amygdalin. Several people have reportedly died while taking laetrile, while others have experienced a remission of their cancer. Prunasin, a cyanophose glycoside found in many Prunus species of pitted fruits, including Wild Cherry bark, is used to treat coughs.

❖ **Isothiocyanate glycosides,** also called glucosinolates, consist of nitrogen-sulfur compounds attached to glucose. Many cruciferous plants (Bok Choy, Broccoli, Cabbage, Cauliflower, Kale, and Mustards) contain this type of glycoside, which is believed to protect plants against parasites and to possess antibiotic activity. Research indicates that a regular diet of the cruciferous family helps prevent colon cancer. Different types of isothiocyanate glycosides include sinigrin extracted from Black Mustard, sinalbin derived from White Mustard, and gluconapin from Rapeseed. Horseradish root also contains isothiocyanate glycosides. Some, like those in Mustard, can be irritating when applied to the skin.

❖ **Anthocyanin glycosides** are pigments responsible for most of the blue, purple, and red colors found in plant buds, leaves, fruits, and berries. They are similar to flavonoid glycosides in their structure and most of their properties. They are extremely valuable, health-promoting anti-oxidants and are <u>soluble in water</u>.

❖ **Coumarins** are also called coumarin glycosides and are blood thinners and anticoagulants (prevent blood clotting). Plant coumarins are the basis for the commonly used anticlotting drug known as warfarin. They generally have anti-inflammatory and antibacterial properties, and some have antitumor activity. There are more than 100 types of coumarins, many having the sweet, characteristic smell of recently mown grass. Alfalfa, Angelica, Cleavers, Red Clover, Sweet Clover, Mullein, and Sweet Woodruff contain coumarins.

❖ **Flavonoids**, also known as flavonoid glycosides, are the largest group of phenols that are commonly found in many plants worldwide. They are especially abundant as colorful pigments in fruits, vegetables, and dark berries. Many flavonoids have been identified and divided into several classes, including anthocyanins, proanthocyanidins, flavones, flavonols, and isoflavones. They are safe for human and animal consumption, but can be toxic to microorganisms. Botanists believe that plants produce flavonoids as protection against infectious diseases. The most common flavonoids are bioflavonoids, which include rutin, hesperidin, and quercetin. Flavonoids have yellow or white pigmentation, and exert a variety of actions having many medicinal applications. One of the most important actions affects the vascular (blood vessel) system. Flavonoids decrease capillary fragility and permeability, and are helpful for peripheral circulation, varicose veins, and hypertension. They can also decrease inflammation, cramps and spasms, water retention, and are antiseptic, antiviral, and anticarcinogenic. They are strong antioxidants that protect cells from damage and reduce allergic reactions. <u>Flavonoids are water-soluble.</u> Plants containing flavonoids include citrus fruits, Blueberries, Buckwheat, Elder berries, Ginkgo, Hawthorn berries, Milk Thistle, Peppers, Rue, Rose hips, and Yarrow.

Lipids

Fixed oils and fats (lipids) are primary metabolites occurring in many forms throughout the plant kingdom. They include fatty acids, phospholipids, waxes, steroids, vitamins A, D, E and K, and the familiar vegetable oils and fats used in cooking. Lipids often bond with carbohydrates or proteins to form lipopolysaccharides or lipoproteins. There are many types of saturated fatty acids, including arachidic, butyric, capric, caproic, caprylic, isovaleric, lauric, myristic, palmitic, and stearic acids. Unsaturated fatty acids include omega-3 fatty acids (alpha-linoleic acid or ALA, eicosapentaenoic acid or EPA, and docosahexaenoic acid or DHA) and omega-6 fatty acids (linoleic acid or LA and gamma-linolenic acid or GLA). ALA is found in edible seeds, Flaxseeds and Walnuts, while EPA and DHA fatty acids occur in fish oils and eggs. GLA is found in Black Currants and the seeds of Borage, Evening Primrose, and *Cannabis sativa* (Hemp and Marijuana). Omega-3 and omega-6 fatty acids tend to be anti-inflammatory and are beneficial for dry skin, different types of dermatitis, and the cardiovascular, nervous, and reproductive systems. Prostaglandins are important chemicals for the regulation of many body processes and are synthesized from fatty acids. Waxes are combinations of fatty acids and alcohols that protect leaves and other plant parts with a waxy coating.

Fixed oils are liquid at room temperature, and fats are partially or completely solid at room temperature. Fixed oils and fats have similar chemical structures consisting of three fatty acid molecules bonded to one glycerol (sugar) molecule. They occur in all parts of plant and animal tissue, forming a protective membrane surrounding cells. Fats in seeds and other parts of plants provide stored energy reserves. Herbalists use oils for their rich, moisturizing, soothing effect on the skin, and as menstruums when extracting herbs for salves and ointments. Fixed oils and fats are soluble in alcohol and other oils, but not in water. Castor Bean oil (*Ricinus communis*) is applied externally for its stimulating activity. Flaxseed oil (*Linum usitatissimum*) is ingested for its high concentrations of essential fatty acids.

Essential oils are also called volatile oils and occur in a wide range of plant species, including herbaceous plants, deciduous trees and shrubs, and evergreens. They have a different chemical structure than fixed oils. Essential oils are chemically complex, fragile, and unstable oils that easily oxidize, separate from plant material, and evaporate when exposed to air. They give some plants their characteristic fragrance and flavors, and herbs containing large amounts of essential oils are called "aromatic." Plants have developed essential oils to attract pollinators, to cover and heal wounds, to protect against microbial infection, herbivores, and intense weather conditions, and to act as hormones and catalysts in biochemical processes. Essential oils are usually secreted from specialized secretory structures on the surface of plants or inside their tissues. Essential oils are generally composed of simple isoprene molecules that can combine in a variety of ways to form terpenes, which are secondary plant metabolites.

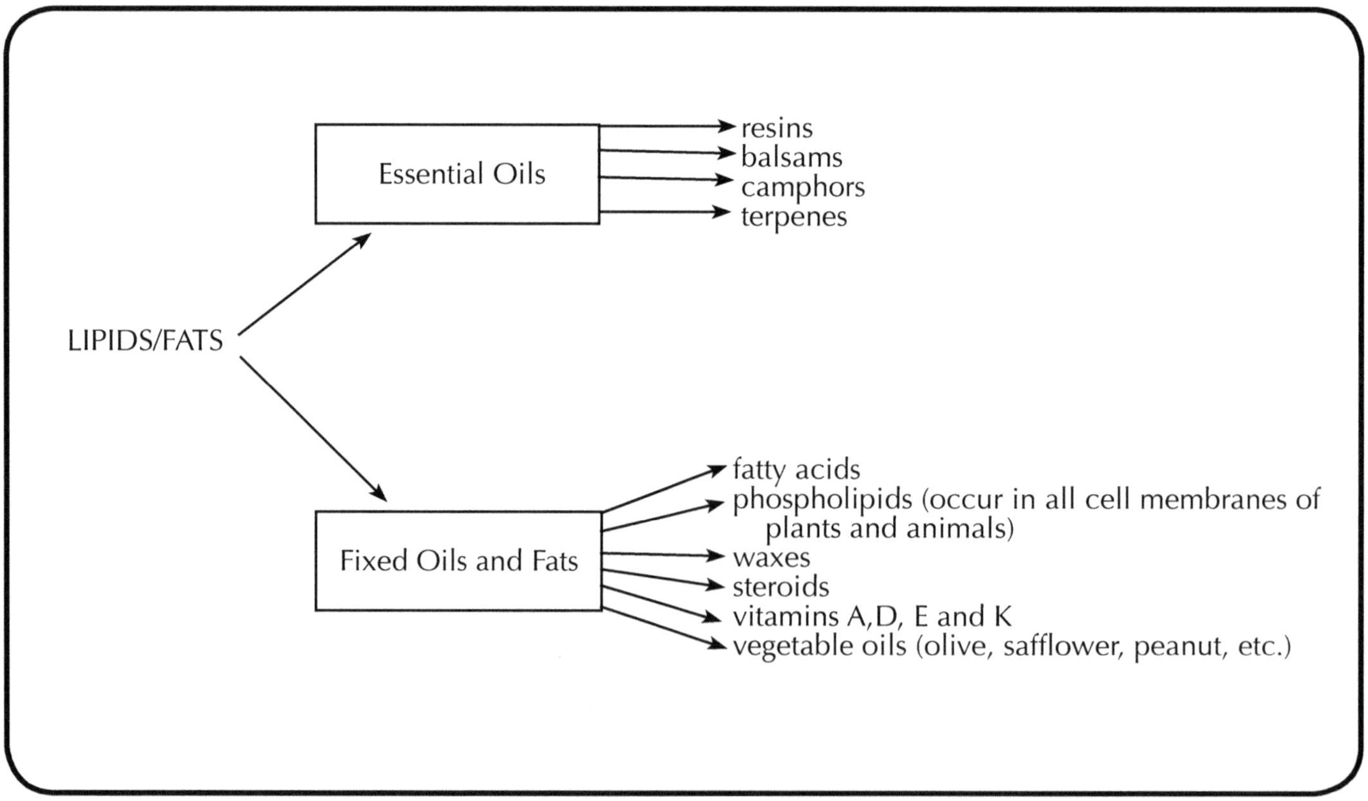

Since ancient times, the pronounced aroma of herbs containing essential oils has drawn people to use them for spices and medicines. Essential oils permeate through tissue extremely well, and many people experience tasting or sweating a strong odor of herbs shortly after they have been applied externally or taken internally. Essential oils circulate in blood through the placenta into the fetus and into mother's milk. They have many healing applications that can have a strong impact on the body, and they affect the nervous system in a variety of ways. The essential oils in some herbs like Chamomile, St. John's Wort, and Valerian are calming and sedating to ease tension and promote sleep. Essential oils in Cayenne, Ginger, and Peppermint stimulate the nervous system and digestive organs. Many oils are analgesic, anti-inflammatory, and soothing for muscle cramps and spasms. They are usually antiseptic, anti-fungal, and enhance immunity by increasing the production of white blood cells. The stimulating and warming properties of many essential oils promote better blood circulation and open sweat pores to increase perspiration. This diaphoretic property is used to reduce fevers and eliminate toxins from the body. Essential oils act as helpful decongestants for coughs and dispel gas from the intestines. Aromatic oils are also used for perfumes and aromatherapy.

The amount of essential oils in plants is minute. Oils are primarily extracted from plants by the distillation process requiring huge amounts of herb material. For example, it takes 50 pounds of Eucalyptus, 150 pounds of Lavender, and 500 pounds of Sage, Thyme, or Rosemary leaves to obtain one pound of essential oil from each of these herbs. Most essential oils are lighter than water. Essential oils are insoluble in water and are very soluble in alcohol and in fixed oils such as olive oil. Medicinal plants containing large amounts of essential oils have a short shelf life, and are best preserved as alcohol-based tinctures. Heat applied during the process of cooking, drying, and extraction results in loss of essential oils and medicinal efficacy.

Substantial amounts of essential oils occur in Bergamot, Cedar, Cinnamon, Cloves, Eucalyptus, Garlic, Hyssop, Juniper, Lavender, Lemon Balm, Rose, Rosemary, Sage, Sassafras, Thyme, Wild Ginger, Wintergreen, and many members of the Mint family. In some herbs, like Peppermint and Thyme, up to 50 or more different essential oils in each plant combine to produce its unique fragrance.

Resins are thick, sticky substances produced by plants and trees for self-protection against injury, fungal or bacterial infections, and as deterrents to nibbling animals. Sap from Pine trees is an example. Resins form when essential oils mix with air and are oxidized, becoming solid at room temperature. Resins have warming, stimulating, and diaphoretic properties that are used medicinally. They are strong antimicrobials against a wide range of bacteria, viruses, yeast and fungi, and can stimulate the immune system to increase production of white blood cells. Resins are effective expectorants for the lungs, promoting easier breathing and mucous discharge. They tend to be hard and are heavier than water. Resins are soluble in alcohol and hot oils, but do not dissolve in water. They occur in nature with essential oils, which give them their characteristic odors. *Cannabis sativa* (Hemp and Marijuana), Cayenne, Ginger, Kava Kava, Myrrh, Pine and Rosemary contain large amounts of resins.

Balsams are gummy resins from various trees and shrubs that contain large amounts of cinnamic or benzoic acids. They occur as liquids or solids. Like other oil-based constituents, balsams are only soluble in alcohol and hot oils, and are insoluble in water. Examples include Balsam of Tolu (*Myroxylon balsamum*) and Benzoin (*Styrax benzoin*).

Camphors are closely related to essential oils in their chemical and physical structure. They are solid at room temperature but melt easily when heated. Camphors occur in many essential oils. Menthol is a camphor in Peppermint oil. Camphors are soluble in alcohol and hot oils, and insoluble in water. Plants containing large amounts of camphors include Anise, Camphor (*Cinnamomum camphora*), Mugwort, Peppermint, Rosemary, and Spearmint.

Proteins

Amino acids are nitrogen compounds that combine to form proteins, which are primary metabolites. Proteins provide nutrients and enzymes to build plant tissue and maintain life. They provide building blocks for animal and human muscle, neurotransmitters regulating nerve and brain chemistry, and immunoglobulins for strong immunity. The largest concentration of proteins in plants is often found in their seeds. Alfalfa, Chickweed, Fenugreek, Feverfew, Ginseng, Parsley, Peppermint, Soybeans, Stinging Nettle, Yellow Dock, and Spirulina and Chlorella (types of fresh water algae) contain relatively large amounts of amino acids.

Terpenes

Terpenes, also called terpenoids or isoprenoids, occur in most plants as the largest and most varied class of secondary plant metabolites. Over 22,000 terpenoid compounds have been identified, and all of them originate via the mevalonate pathway that transforms them into a phosphorylated isoprene. Terpenoids are composed of isoprene units arranged in a multitude of chemical variations. All terpenes are classified according to the number of isoprene units they contain. Isoprene is emitted from the leaves of many plant species during daylight, and is responsible for the bluish haze that hovers over wooded hills and mountains in summer. Camphor and essential oils are monoterpenes (monoterpenoids) consisting of two isoprene units. Monoterpenes are responsible for the fragrances of many plants and are used for aromatherapy and producing perfumes. They often produce significant responses in people, and this biological activity forms the basis for many herbal remedies. Examples of monoterpenes include 1) limonene, a primary constituent of essential oils in citrus fruits, Caraway, Dill, and the Mints; 2) pinene, occurring in essential oils from Pine trees and the Mint family; 3) borneol, found in Lavender, Rosemary, and Nutmeg oils; 4) geraniol, a main constituent in the oils of Lemongrass *(Cymbopogon citratus)* and Roses; 5) menthol, found in Peppermint and other Mints; 6) citronellal, occurring in Lemon Balm and Lemongrass; and 7) linalool, in Cinnamon, Citrus fruits, and many of the Mints.

Sesquiterpenes (sesquiterpenoids) have three isoprene units and occur in highly aromatic plants and essential oils. They tend to stimulate liver and glandular activity, and have antispasmodic and anti-inflammatory properties. Diterpenes (diterpenoids) have four isoprene units and include resins, saponins, gums, vitamin A, and taxol from Yew trees (*Taxus* spp.). Triterpenes (triterpenoids) also include resins, saponins, cardiac glycosides, and phytosterols. Phytosterols are widely distributed in the plant kingdom and include sitosterol, stigmasterol, diosgenin, and campesterol. Sterols are important components in the cell membranes of almost all plants. Cholesterol is the most widely occurring sterol. Ergosterol is the principle sterol in fungi, and sitosterol is the principle sterol in green plants and algae. Other sterols are similar in structure to cholesterol, but many sterols have unique health benefits such as lowering cholesterol, improving immune function and reproductive health, and reducing prostate problems and menopausal hot flashes. Sterols may also function as hormones. Sterols occur in Black Cohosh, Chaparral, Red Clover, Coltsfoot, Hops, Hyssop, Sarsaparilla, Soybeans, and Yam. Tetraterpenes include carotenoid pigments that are found in all plants and give flowers and fruits their colors. Carotene and lycopene are two examples of carotenoids.

TERPENES
The 5 primary chemical classes of terpenes

Number of isoprene units	
2	Monoterpenes
3	Sesquiterpenes
4	Diterpenes
6	Triterpenes
8	Tetraterpenes

Individual plants can synthesize many different terpenes in their roots, leaves, or flowers. Plants produce terpenes for a variety of reasons necessary for their survival. Many are toxins that act as feeding deterrents to herbivores. Some plants release terpenes from their leaves or roots into the soil, where they act as toxins prohibiting other plants from growing close by. In this way, plants can establish and defend territory for their own growth and expansion. For example, Black Walnut trees (*Juglans nigra*) release juglone from their roots to inhibit growth of herbaceous and woody plants around them. Wormwood (*Artemisia absinthium*) also releases substances that can be toxic to other plants. Terpenes in essential oils and resins provide protection against insect damage by forming a protective barrier on plants against bacterial and fungal diseases, and their pleasant and unique fragrances attract pollinators.

Terpenes are responsible for the fragrance of Pine trees and citrus fruits, and their name is derived from "turp" in turpentine. Triterpenes and saponin glycosides are chemically related to steroid hormones, so they can strengthen, normalize and regulate the endocrine organs, and they tend to exert strong actions throughout the body. Many herbs containing significant amounts of triterpenes are known as "adaptogens," which help the body respond and adapt to stress. Adaptogen herbs include Ashwagandha, Astragalus, Eleuthero (Siberian Ginseng), American and Asian Ginseng, Gotu Kola, Holy Basil (Tulsi), Licorice, and Reishi mushrooms.

Phenols

Phenols comprise a huge class of secondary plant metabolites that are almost universally present in all plant parts and contribute to the colors and flavors of plants. Plant tissues can contain as much as several grams of phenolic compounds per kilogram. Plants synthesize phenols via the shikimate and malonate pathways in response to microbial infections, chemical stressors, and ultraviolet radiation. About 8,000 phenols have been identified. Phenols are chemically distinct from terpenes, although, like terpenes, many phenolic compounds are attached to sugar molecules and are called glycosides. Phenols are basic building blocks and major components of a large portion of plant constituents, including coumarins, anthroquinones, flavonoids, saponins, tannins, lignans, cardiac glycosides, and some alkaloids and terpenes. Vitamins C and E are phenolic substances. The structure of phenolic compounds varies from simple to very complex chemical combinations having many different medicinal applications. Salicylic acid is an example of a simple phenol glycoside that exerts analgesic and anti-inflammatory properties, and is found in Cramp Bark,

PHENOLIC COMPOUNDS
and some of their derivatives

Antioxidants
- occurring in fruits and berries
- vegetables
- grains

Flavonoids
- flavones: apigenin, luteolin, scutellarein
- flavonols: quercetin, rutin, kaempferol
- isoflavones: exhibit estrogen activity and include genistein and daidzein found in Soy, Alfalfa, and Yams
- dihydroflavones: catechins found in Green and Black Tea, silybin in Milk Thistle
- anthrocyanins: color pigments in fruits and vegetables

Phenolic Acids
- salicylic acid: occurs in Willow bark, Meadowsweet, and aspirin
- vanillin: in Vanilla Beans, Cloves, Asparagus, and Rue
- arbutin: in Uva-ursi, Bilberry, and Marjoram
- gallic acid: in Nettles, Hops, Raspberry, Black Walnut
- ellagic acid: Grapes, Raspberries, Cranberries, Oak bark
- tannic acid: Green and Black Tea, Cranesbill, Cinquefoil

Hydroxycinnamic Acid derivatives
- caffeic acid: in fruits, vegetables, Poppies, Yarrow, Coffee, Foxglove, Dandelion
- ferulic acid: occurs in fruits and vegetables
- curcumin: in Turmeric and Mustard
- coumarins: in Citrus, Sweet Clover, Khella, Horse Chestnut, and Rue
- myristicin: in Nutmeg, Parsley, and Cinnamon
- cimicifugin: in Black Cohosh
- umbelliferone: occurring in many members of the Carrot/ Parsley family

Lignans
- Exhibit estrogen activity
- found in Flaxseeds
- Bran in grains
- in Milk Thistle

Quinones
- naphthoquinones: in Walnut and Butternut trees
- juglone: in Black Walnut
- anthraquinones: occur in Yellow Dock, Rhubarb, Senna, and Buckthorn

Meadowsweet, Willow, and Wintergreen. Eugenol oil in Cloves is an analgesic phenol. Thyme contains thymol oil, another phenol that shares similar healing properties with salicylic acid. Other examples of phenols include arbutin found in Bilberry, Marjoram, and Uva-ursi; hesperidin occurring in citrus fruits; baptisin from Wild Indigo; and iridin from Iris plants. Phenols have antimicrobial activity.

Phytoestrogens are phenolic compounds with a chemical structure similar to estradiol, the most potent form of estrogen produced by the human body. Due to this similarity, phytoestrogens elicit estrogenic effects that usually mimic estradiol, but can also act as antagonists to estradiol. The three classes of phytoestrogens are isoflavones (including diadzein, formononetin, genistein, and biochanin A), lignans (found in Flaxseed,

Sesame seeds, Brassica vegetables, and bran in grains), and coumestans (occurring in Alfalfa, Clover, Pinto and Lima beans, and split peas). Isoflavones are found in Alfalfa, Beans, Red Clover, and Soybeans.

Evidence verifies the ability of these phytoestrogens to protect against many menopausal problems, osteoporosis, cardiovascular issues, and cancers of the intestines, prostate, and breast. The National Institute of Health (NIH) published the outcome of the Woman's Health Initiative Study in 2002, which clearly implicates synthetic hormones commonly prescribed in hormone replacement therapy (HRT) in promoting breast cancer, heart attacks, and strokes in menopausal women. In light of this research, the use of phytoestrogens offers a safe and effective alternative for normalizing hormone levels.

Tannins

Tannins occur in many plants and are especially concentrated in bark, leaves, and unripe fruit. About one-third of all flowering plant families contain tannins. These antiseptic phytochemicals stored in plant cells have evolved over time to deter insects and animals from eating them, and to protect against fungal and bacterial infections.

Tannins are derived from phenolic acid and are complex polyphenols that combine with proteins. They inhibit and reduce enzyme activity, especially in the mouth and gastrointestinal tract. For this reason, tannins can reduce nutrient availability if taken in excessive amounts over time. They are somewhat bitter and have strong astringent properties that constrict, tighten, tone, and strengthen tissues and blood vessels. When taken as a tea or tincture, herbs containing tannins taste astringent, making the tissues in the mouth pucker and feel dry. Tannins affect the permeability (the ability of fluids to pass through membranes) of tissues, and their tightening and constricting qualities tend to dry up secretions and discharges. When applied on the skin, tannins constrict protein molecules in tissues to form a protective layer on the skin and mucous membranes. Research shows that tannins are antioxidants that inhibit harmful free radicals responsible for cellular damage and aging. Tannins also inhibit the growth of many bacteria, fungi, and viruses in laboratory settings. Herbs with high concentrations of tannins have historically been externally applied for treating burns and infections, sealing wounds, and reducing inflammation. They are taken internally for the treatment of abnormal or excessive bleeding, diarrhea, hemorrhoids, varicose veins, vaginal infections, and sore throats.

Tannins are soluble in water, alcohol, vinegar, and glycerin. They change the structure of protein molecules and precipitate alkaloids, proteins, starch, and gelatin by drawing them out of liquid solution and making them clump together into small particles. When preparing formulas containing herbs with tannins and alkaloids, 10% glycerin can be added if precipitation is a problem. Tannins can be used to treat alkaloid poisoning because they are able to precipitate alkaloids. Types of tannins include catechol, pyrogallotannins, gallic acids, catechins, chlorogenic acid, and ipecacuanhic acid. Agrimony, Bayberry, Bistort, Cinquefoil, Cranesbill, Goldenrod, Horse Chestnut leaves, Lady's Mantle, Meadowsweet, Mullein, Plantain, Raspberry leaf, Rosemary, Sage, Shepherd's Purse, Uva-ursi, White Oak bark, Witch Hazel, Yarrow, and Black and Green Tea contain substantial amounts of tannins.

Alkaloids

Alkaloids are secondary metabolites comprising a large and chemically complex group of alkaline substances with a nitrogen base. Only a few alkaloids are derived from purines (caffeine is an example) or pyrimidines, while the vast majority are produced from amino acids. They are organic compounds (containing carbon) constructed around rings of nitrogen atoms. Although about 60% of all plant families do not contain alkaloids, many families contain dozens or hundreds of them. About 10,000 alkaloids have been identified, each one having specific activities. They are highly reactive and exert biological activity in small doses. Alkaloids are diverse in structure and are chemically divided into 14 groups. They are very important compounds in medicine because of their powerful physiologic activity on the nervous system, brain and cognitive processes, and many other body functions.

Alkaloids tend to taste extremely bitter and some are poisonous, which are protective mechanisms plants have developed to repel nibbling insects and other destructive animals. Many alkaloids inhibit and kill pathogens, including bacteria, viruses, fungi and yeasts, providing more protective devices for plants and sources of potent medicines for people. They exert many properties such as analgesic, anticancer, anti-inflammatory, emmenagogue, expectorant, antispasmodic, sedative, stimulant, and nervine actions. Some are very potent, hallucinogenic, and potentially toxic.

Alkaloids in plants typically remain active after the drying process. In their pure form, alkaloids are not very soluble. However, when they occur in plants, their crystalline structures bind to organic acids forming alkaloid salts, which are safer and more soluble forms of alkaloids. Plant alkaloids are very soluble in alcohol and only partially water-soluble. Vinegar is sometimes used in extracting alkaloids from specific plants because its acidic nature breaks them down, as alkaloids are alkaline.

Alkaloids are given names ending with the suffix "–ine." Some examples of plant-derived alkaloids include hydrastine and berberine from Goldenseal (*Hydrastis canadensis*), lobeline from Lobelia, morphine from the Opium Poppy (*Papaver somniferum*), cocaine from leaves of the Coca plant (*Erythroxylum coca*), quinine from the Cinchona plant native to the Andes Mountains in South America, nicotine from Tobacco (*Nicotiana tabacum*), strychnine from Peyote, curarine from the Strychnos plant native to the Amazon region, as well as caffeine derived from the Coffee bean, Green and Black tea (*Camellia sinensis*), and Cocoa (*Theobroma cacao)*. The nightshade (*Solanaceae*) family contains atropine, scopalomine, and hyoscyamine. Pyrrolizidine alkaloids in Comfrey and Coltsfoot have a detrimental effect on the liver if taken in large amounts over long periods of time. Other plants containing medicinal alkaloids include Barberry, Bloodroot, Cayenne, Ephedra, Marijuana and Hemp (*Cannabis sativa*), Motherwort, Oregon Grape Root, Pau D'arco, and Valerian.

Enzymes

Enzymes are large, complex proteins that catalyze, regulate, and control the biochemical reactions vital to all life forms. Hundreds of different enzymes in plants and animals direct and accelerate chemical reactions in cells. Each type of enzyme is very specific in its biological activity and catalyzes only one, or a few, chemical reactions. To produce chemical reactions, enzymes must have the exact chemical structure to attach to special areas on cellular membranes, called cell receptors sites. This selective lock-and-key situation limits enzyme activity to specific cells. Herbs containing enzymes are used medicinally to improve digestion and reduce inflammation. Large concentrations of enzymes occur in Alfalfa, Hawthorn berries, Papaya fruit, and Pineapple.

Acids

Many different types of organic acids are widely distributed throughout the plant kingdom. Some acids are weak and some, like formic acid found in Stinging Nettle and bee venom, are very strong. Organic acids possess a variety of medicinal properties depending on their chemical structure. They affect the activity of enzymes in the body, play a vital role in many biological processes, and are necessary for normal function of cells and tissues. Acids generally exert antibiotic activity, and are nourishing and cooling to the body. They tend to have a sour taste that makes the mouth pucker. Citrus fruits contain citric acid, Valerian and Hops contain valeric acid, isocitric acid occurs in Blueberries, and malic acid is in Apples. Oxalic acid is found in Rhubarb and in the Buckwheat and Wood Sorrel families. Rosmarinic acid occurs in Basil, Rosemary, Sage, and the Mints. Aromatic acids, like benzoic acid, are highly complex chemical structures found in many plant resins and balsams. The strong properties of many organic acids often give plants their characteristic fragrance and flavor. <u>Acids are soluble in water, alcohol, and vinegar</u>.

Minerals

Minerals and mineral salts naturally occur in almost all plants. Their mineral content is affected by the mineral content of the soil in which they grow. Plants are able to transform inorganic minerals from the soil into organic plant tissue. Organic minerals in plants are much easier for people and animals to digest and assimilate than elemental minerals from rock sources. Minerals are necessary for normal growth and maintenance, strong bones, and iron-rich blood. Minerals regulate electrolyte balance and reduce acidity in the body. Alfalfa, Catnip, Chamomile, Chickweed, Comfrey, Fennel, Horsetail, Oatstraw, Peppermint, Red Clover, Red Raspberry leaf, Scullcap, Stinging Nettle, and the roots of Burdock, Dandelion, Licorice, Marshmallow, and Yellow Dock contain substantial concentrations of minerals. <u>Significant mineral extraction requires long cooking on low heat when preparing tea.</u>

Plants sense what is happening in their environment and respond by producing specific phytochemicals in the required amounts.

Plants display profound intelligence in their ability to develop nutrients for their growth and secondary metabolites to protect themselves from disease and animal predators, attract pollinators, and fulfill requirements necessary for their survival.

Because of the fundamental physiological similarities between plant and human bodies, many of the same chemical constituents that serve plants are used by people for food and medicine.

Healing Qualities of Herbs

Medicinal plants contain hundreds of chemical constituents with healing properties that affect the human body in a multitude of ways. **"Healing qualities" are terms that define and describe the properties, functions, and biological activities of medicinal herbs.** Throughout the ages, herbalists have classified plants according to specific healing qualities that describe their primary or secondary actions on target tissues and organs. For example, all herbs that are generally beneficial to the liver are called "hepatics." Herbs that promote menstruation are "emmenagogues." Some terms like "diuretic" and "analgesic" are commonly used today. Other terms like "aperient" (a mild bowel stimulant) or "anthelmintic" (an herb that kills parasites) are antiquated and less familiar. Most terms describing the healing qualities of herbs date back to early European times, when they were used to describe both herbal and early pharmaceutical medicines.

Although it takes a little study, knowing the most commonly used terms for healing qualities of plants provides an instant understanding of the nature and appropriate use of each herb, and is an important aspect in the language of herbalism. Just as "one picture is worth a thousand words," each healing quality describes a complete picture of herbal and biological activity. For instance, demulcent herbs are soothing, cooling, anti-inflammatory, and nourishing to tissues, and are excellent for wound healing. If you read that Marshmallow root is a demulcent, it would be safe to assume that this herb would be helpful for healing stomach ulcers or an irritated bladder during an infection because the demulcent properties would soothe these inflamed tissues. Knowing that emmenagogue herbs stimulate the onset of menstruation, you would know never to give this class of herb to pregnant women due to threat of miscarriage. Herbs with astringent qualities constrict tissues and blood vessels, and are employed to stop abnormal bleeding or diarrhea and relieve sore throats. If you learn that Sage, Shepherd's Purse, Cranesbill, and Yarrow are astringents, you automatically know one of their primary properties and how to use them in healing.

Many herb books and herbalists commonly refer to the terms for healing qualities that are listed below. Familiarity with them will be helpful in your understanding and wise use of medicinal herbs. Be patient and over time they will become part of your herbal vocabulary.

Use this chapter and the **"Index of Health Issues and Herbal Recommendations"** in Section Three when deciding which herbs are appropriate for treating specific health conditions. The Latin names of herbs listed below and throughout the book are found in the Appendix under **"Cross-Reference of Common and Botanical Plant Names."**

Abortifacient herbs have very stimulating and often irritating activity on the uterus, which can cause expulsion of the fetus when taken in large amounts. Women must be sure they are not pregnant when using these herbs because they can stimulate a miscarriage, especially when taken over a period of time. Women who choose to use a combination of abortifacient herbs to induce abortion must be warned that when taken in the large amounts necessary, these herbs are toxic to the fetus and possibly to the woman. Sometimes they work to terminate a pregnancy, and sometimes they do not. But they can damage the fetus if the abortion attempt fails. Abortifacients include Black Cohosh, Blue Cohosh, Feverfew, Mugwort, Pennyroyal, Rue, and Tansy.

Adaptogens increase the body's resistance to illness and ability to handle stress. They have a strengthening and normalizing effect on the immune, endocrine, nervous, and cardiovascular systems, and are helpful for adrenal exhaustion and all stress-related conditions. Adaptogens are safe, well-tolerated herbs that usually have antioxidant activity, protect the liver and adrenals, reduce elevated cortisol levels, help stabilize blood sugar levels and glucose metabolism, and increase stamina and endurance. Examples are Asian and American Ginseng, Ashwagandha, Astragalus, Dang Shen (*Codonopsis pilosula*), Eleuthero (Siberian Ginseng), Gotu Kola, Holy Basil (Tulsi), Licorice, Reishi mushroom, Rhodiola (*Rhodiola rosea*) and Schisandra.

Adjuvant herbs are added to formulas to increase their effectiveness. Cayenne and Ginger are common adjuvants because they increase circulation and assist in transporting other herbs through the bloodstream to their target tissues and organs. Lobelia is an adjuvant for the respiratory system.

Agonist substances increase or prolong actions of other herbs, medicines, or endogenous chemicals.

Alteratives are blood, lymphatic, liver, and bowel cleansers that help the digestive system absorb nutrients and eliminate waste products. They are tonics used over a period of time to gradually repair and restore normal function to the body, and promote general health and vitality. Alteratives work by gently stimulating and supporting metabolic processes involved in many body functions, and are excellent for improving chronic health problems. Alteratives are used to treat toxicity, skin eruptions, infections, cancer, arthritis, and many chronic and degenerative diseases. Astragalus is an alterative that tones and strengthens the liver, kidneys and spleen, and boosts immunity. Other alteratives include Chlorella, Elder berries, Milk Thistle, St. John's Wort, and the roots of Burdock, Dandelion and Yellow Dock, which are excellent blood and liver cleansers, cooling, and full of minerals that fortify the blood. Calendula, Echinacea, Hyssop, Red Clover,

Stinging Nettle, and Poke root neutralize excess acids in blood and lymphatic tissues, acting as cleansing detoxifiers to the blood and lymphatic fluids. Poke root tincture is specific for the lymphatic system, but it is only used in small doses. Black Cohosh, Chasteberry, and Dong Quai are alteratives for the female reproductive system. Garlic, Hawthorn, and Peppermint are alteratives for the cardiovascular system. Wood Betony, Scullcap, and Holy Basil (Tulsi) are alteratives for the nervous system. Other alteratives include Alfalfa, American and Asian Ginseng, Blue Vervain, Cayenne, Chickweed, Elderberry flowers, Marshmallow, Sarsaparilla, and Sassafras.

Analeptic substances stimulate the central nervous system. See **stimulants.**

Analgesics relieve pain and can be taken internally or applied externally. Analgesic herbs include Black Cohosh, Catnip, Cayenne, Chamomile, Cloves, Hemp, Marijuana, Hops, Jamaican Dogwood, Kava Kava, Lavender, Lobelia, Meadowsweet, Sweet Melilot (Yellow Clover), Mullein, Opium Poppy, Passion Flower, Peppermint, St. John's Wort, Scullcap, Valerian, Wild Lettuce, Willow, Wintergreen, and Wood Betony.

Anodyne is another term for analgesic, pain-relieving herbs and medicines. See **analgesic.**

Antacids are generally alkaline or soothing herbs that neutralize excess acids in the stomach, intestines, and blood stream. These include Agrimony, Angelica, Astragalus, Bladderwrack, Burdock, Caraway, Catnip, Chickweed, Dandelion, Hops, Irish Moss, Parsley, Peppermint, Stinging Nettle, Wood Betony, and Yucca. Some antacid herbs such as Fennel, Slippery Elm, and Marshmallow root contain mucilage which has soothing properties that protect the stomach and intestinal lining from the damaging effects of excess acids.

Antagonist herbs oppose the actions of other herbs or pharmaceutical drugs.

Anthelmintic herbs kill and expel worms and parasites. **Vermicide, vermifuge, parasiticide** and **antiparasitic** are other terms for anthelmintic herbs. See **antiparasitic**.

Antibiotic or **antibacterial** herbs inhibit or destroy the growth of bacteria and often stimulate the immune system. These include Andrographis (*Andrographis paniculata*), Astragalus, Black Walnut, Bloodroot, Blue Vervain, Boneset, Calendula, Cayenne, Chamomile, Chaparral, Clary Sage, Cloves, Coptis (*Coptis chinensis*), Echinacea, Elderberry flowers, Elecampane, Eucalyptus, Garlic, Goldenseal, Holy Basil (Tulsi), Horehound, Horseradish, Hyssop, Isatis, Lavender, Lungwort, Motherwort, Mugwort, Myrrh, Oregano, Oregon Grape Root, Pau D'arco, Peppermint, Rosemary, Sage, Tea Tree oil (*Melaleuca*), Thyme, Wild Indigo, and Yarrow.

Anticarcinogenic herbs help prevent and inhibit the growth of cancer and tumor cells. Due to the serious nature of cancer, herbs should be part of a comprehensive care plan and not be relied upon as the only treatment. Anticarcinogenic herbs include Astragalus, Burdock, Calendula, Cat's Claw, Cayenne, Chlorella, Dandelion, Echinacea, Elder berries, Goldenseal, Holy Basil (Tulsi), Hops, Motherwort, St. John's Wort, and Maitake, Reishi, and Shiitake mushrooms.

Anti-catarrhal herbs decrease the production and secretion of mucous from the sinus cavities, lungs, and other mucous membranes throughout the body. **Catarrh** is an old term for mucous. Mucous is a natural secretion of moist membranes and serves many important functions, so attempts to completely eliminate it are not wise. Anti-catarrhal herbs are only used for excessive amounts of mucous caused by acute or chronic problems. It is important to address the causes of chronically excessive mucous production, which are often related to diet and overconsumption of dairy foods, sugar, or white flour and gluten products. Remember that during an acute illness like a cold, respiratory infection, or flu when the body produces more mucous as part of the immune response, it is better to thin the mucous rather than stop its secretion. In this way, herbs assist the body in its natural healing process. Several types of phytochemicals exert anti-catarrhal actions. **Tannins** are astringents that contract mucous membranes to reduce secretions. Volatile oils reduce excessive mucous by their anti-inflammatory and antimicrobial properties. Stinging Nettle reduces mucous due to antihistamine effects.

Anti-catarrhal herbs include Anise, Balloon Flower, Barberry, Bladderwrack, Bloodroot, Blue Vervain, Boneset, Burdock root, Cayenne, Chamomile, Cinnamon, Cinquefoil, Cranesbill, Echinacea, Elder flowers, Elecampane, Ephedra (*Ephedra sinica)*, Eyebright, Feverfew, Garlic, Ginger, Goldenrod, Goldenseal, Gotu Kola, Holy Basil (Tulsi), Horehound, Horseradish, Hyssop, Iceland Moss, Lemon Balm, Lemons and other citrus fruits, Linden, Marshmallow, Motherwort, Mullein, Oregon Grape Root, Pau D'arco, Peppermint, Sage, Stinging Nettle, Thyme, Uva-ursi, Wild Cherry bark, Wild Indigo, and Yarrow.

Anti-emetic herbs prevent and relieve nausea and vomiting. These include Anise, Catnip, Cayenne, Chamomile, Cinnamon, Cloves, Dill, Fennel, Ginger, Lavender, Lemon Balm, Peppermint, and Spearmint.

Antifungal herbs destroy and suppress the growth of **fungus** and **yeast** (a type of fungus). Herbs include

Black Walnut hulls, Bloodroot, Boneset, Burdock, Calendula, Cayenne, Chamomile, Cinquefoil, Clary Sage, Cloves, Coptis, Cranesbill, Dandelion, Echinacea, Elecampane, Garlic, Goldenrod, Goldenseal, Holy Basil (Tulsi), Hops, Hyssop, Isatis, Lavender, Lemon Balm, Mugwort, Oregano, Oregon Grape Root, Pau D'arco, Sage, Tea Tree oil, Thyme, Wormwood, and Yarrow. Another term for antifungal agents is **antimycotic**.

Antihistamine herbs reduce the release of histamine, a protein causing allergic reactions and inflammation. Herbs include Black Walnut, Cayenne, Lemon Balm, and Stinging Nettle.

Antihydrotic herbs eliminate excess body fluids and prevent or reduce excessive perspiration. These include Agrimony, Astragalus, Bladderwrack, Blessed Thistle, Buchu, Buckthorn, Cinquefoil, Cleavers, Cranesbill, Lobelia, and Sage. Many diuretic herbs are antihydrotic. Another term for this type of herb is **anhydrotic**.

Anti-inflammatory herbs reduce inflammation throughout the body through the actions of volatile oils, salicylates, steroids, and antioxidants. Inflammation is a natural response to infection, tissue irritation, physical trauma and injury, and excess heat. Modern medicine often attempts to suppress inflammation, but underlying causes need to be addressed for true healing to occur. Many herbs have anti-inflammatory activities that work with the body's natural healing and restorative processes rather than suppressing them.

Anti-inflammatory herbs high in volatile oils include Bergamot, Calendula, Chamomile, Holy Basil (Tulsi), Hyssop, Lavender, most of the Mints, Oregano, Peppermint, Rosemary, Sage, and St. John's Wort. Herbs deriving anti-inflammatory actions from salicylates include Cramp Bark (*Viburnum opulus*), Meadowsweet, Willow, and Wintergreen. Other anti-inflammatory herbs include Andrographis, Angelica, Astragalus, Black Cohosh, Blue Vervain, Boneset, Boswellia, Bupleurum, Burdock, Cat's Claw, Cayenne, Cleavers, Comfrey, Dandelion, Devil's Claw, Echinacea, Elder berries and flowers, Elecampane, Fenugreek, Feverfew, Ginger, Ginkgo, Goldenrod, Goldenseal, Horse Chestnut, Hops, Isatis, Licorice, Linden, Lobelia, Marshmallow, Mullein, Pau D'arco, Plantain, Solomon's Seal root, Stinging Nettle, Thyme, Turmeric, Wild Yam, Witch Hazel, Wood Betony, Yarrow, and Yucca. Many demulcent, mucilaginous, emollient, and vulnerary herbs also have anti-inflammatory properties due to their ability to soothe and cool mucous membranes and the skin. **Antiphlogistic** is another term meaning anti-inflammatory.

Antilithic herbs prevent and treat kidney, bladder, and gallbladder stones. See **lithotropic/lithotryptic**.

Antimicrobial herbs support immunity and kill microbial pathogens (bacteria, viruses, fungi, yeast, and parasites) or inhibit their growth. See **antibiotic, antiviral, antifungal**, and **antiparasitic**.

Antimycotic herbs reduce fungal and yeast growth. See **antifungal**.

Antioxidants protect the body from cellular damage caused by oxidative stress and free radical damage from toxins and radiation. They can be used on a daily basis to promote optimum wellness and treat chronic illness. Herbal sources of antioxidants include Andrographis, Ashwagandha, Astragalus, Bacopa, Bilberry, Calendula, Catnip, Cat's Claw, Cayenne, Elder berries, Garlic, Ginger, Ginkgo, American and Asian Ginseng, Green Tea, Hawthorn berries, Holy Basil (Tulsi), Lemon Balm, Linden, Marjoram, Milk Thistle, Oregano, Peppermint, Rose hips, Rosemary, Sage, St. John's Wort, Schisandra, Thyme, Turmeric, and Yarrow.

Antiparasitic plants destroy worms and parasites, and often help with their elimination. They should be used for short periods of time through several cycles to kill parasites and their eggs. Since parasites are most active around the full moon, take antiparasitic herbs for one week before and one week after the full moon. Then stop for two weeks, and continue this regime for two to three months. Some antiparasitic herbs are very strong and tend to become toxic to people if they are used in excess for an extended time.

Antiparasitic herbs include Black Walnut hulls, Blue Vervain, Buckthorn, Butternut, Cascara Sagrada, Cayenne, Cloves, Coptis, Elecampane, Feverfew, Garlic, Gentian, Holy Basil (Tulsi), Hops, Horehound, Hyssop, Isatis, Lavender, Motherwort, Mugwort, Rue, Senna, Sweet Annie, Tansy, Thyme, Turkey Rhubarb, and Wormwood. Food grade diatomaceous earth consisting of silica crystals that slice and destroy the bodies of parasites is highly recommended! Safe and non-toxic for human (including young children) and pet consumption, diatomaceous earth is excellent when used in conjunction with a blend of antiparasitic herbs. **Anthelmintic, vermicide, vermifuge,** and **parasiticide** are other terms for herbs that kill parasites.

Antiperiodic herbs relieve alternating fevers and chills typically seen in malaria. These include American Centaury, Blue Vervain, Boneset, Goldenseal, Sweet Annie, and quinine produced from Peruvian Cinchona tree bark.

Antipyretic herbs reduce fevers. See **diaphoretic.**

Antirheumatic herbs decrease pain and inflammation in arthritic joints and reduce excess acids in the blood and tissues that contribute to inflammation. They include Angelica, Black Cohosh, Boneset, Boswellia,

Burdock, Cat's Claw, Cayenne, Devil's Claw, Elder berries and flowers, Feverfew, Ginger, Holy Basil (Tulsi), Juniper, Meadowsweet, Mugwort, Oregon Grape Root, Peppermint, Prickly Ash, Rosemary, Sage, Sarsaparilla, Stinging Nettle, Wild Yam, Willow, Wintergreen, Wood Betony, Yarrow, and Yellow Dock.

Antiscorbutic plants contain ascorbic acid (vitamin C) and help prevent scurvy, a disease caused by severe vitamin C deficiency. Alfalfa, Cayenne, Chickweed, Citrus fruits, Dandelion, Elder berries, Red Sumac berries, Rose hips, Shepherd's Purse, Stinging Nettle, Wood Betony, Violets, and Yellow Dock contain vitamin C.

Antiseptics are applied to the skin to prevent and kill bacterial growth. Herbal antiseptics include Black Walnut hulls and leaves, Calendula, Catnip, Cayenne, Chamomile, Echinacea, Elecampane, Feverfew, Garlic, Goldenrod, Gotu Kola, Goldenseal, Holy Basil (Tulsi), Lavender, Lemon Balm, Myrrh, Oregano, Peppermint, Rue, Sage, St. John's Wort, Tea Tree oil, Thyme, Wild Indigo, Wood Betony, and Yarrow.

Antispasmodic herbs relax nerves and muscles to relieve cramps and spasms. They relax the autonomic nervous system but do not necessarily have a sedating effect. There are many antispasmodic herbs, such as American Ginseng, Angelica, Anise, Black Cohosh, Black Haw, Blue Cohosh, Blue Vervain, Boneset, Bugleweed, Calendula, California Poppy, Caraway, Cardamom, Catnip, Cayenne, Chamomile, Clary Sage, Coriander, Cramp Bark, Damiana, Dong Quai, Elderberry flowers, Elecampane, Eucalyptus, Fennel, Fenugreek, Feverfew, Ginger, Goldenrod, Holy Basil (Tulsi), Hops, Horehound, Hyssop, Jamaican Dogwood, Kava Kava, Khella, Lavender, Lemon Balm, Licorice, Linden leaf and flower, Lobelia, Marjoram, Motherwort, Mugwort, Mullein, Parsley, Passion Flower, Pennyroyal, Peppermint, Raspberry leaf, Rosemary, Sage, St. John's Wort, Scullcap, Stinging Nettle, Thyme, Valerian, Wild Yam, and Yarrow. **Spasmolytic** is another term for antispasmodic.

Antitumor herbs inhibit and reduce tumor growth without suppressing the immune system. Some anti-tumor herbs contain very powerful constituents that can destroy tissue, thus providing the anti-tumor quality. Bloodroot and Poke are potentially toxic and must be used carefully with specific doses. Milder herbs without potential harm include Astragalus, Burdock, Calendula, Echinacea, Garlic, Ginseng, Goldenseal, Hops, Licorice, Red Clover, Sorrel, Turkey Rhubarb, and Maitake, Reishi, and Shiitake mushrooms.

Anti-uric herbs prevent and reduce excess acid in urine. They include Burdock, Dandelion, Hops and Stinging Nettle. Another name for anti-uric herbs is **anti-uricaemic.**

Antiviral herbs inhibit or destroy viruses, and some stimulate immunity. These include Andrographis, Astragalus, Bloodroot, Blue Vervain, Boneset, Calendula, Cat's Claw, Clary Sage, Echinacea, Elder berries and flowers, Elecampane, Garlic, Holy Basil (Tulsi), Horehound, Hyssop, Isatis, Lemon Balm, Licorice, Lomatium, Oregano, Sage, St. John's Wort, Thyme, Wild Indigo, and Maitake, Reishi, and Shiitake mushrooms.

Antiyeast or **candidicide** herbs kill yeast, which is a type of fungus. See **antifungal**.

Aperient herbs are mild laxatives that enhance the production and secretion of digestive enzymes. They include American Centaury, Blue Vervain, Boneset, Catnip, Cayenne, Dandelion, Goldenseal, Hops, Horehound, and Peppermint. Also see **laxative**.

Aphrodisiac herbs stimulate sexual desire and vitality. They include Damiana, Ginseng, Muira Puama (*Ptychopetalum olacoides*), and Yohimbe (*Pausinystalia yohimbe*).

Aromatic herbs contain strong volatile oils that are fragrant and often pleasant. Aromatics have many properties, including antispasmodic, carminative, and antimicrobial activities. They are also used in aromatherapy and for the production of essential oils and perfumes. Examples include Anise, Basil, Cardamom, Catnip, Cinnamon, Cloves, Dill, Eucalyptus, Fennel, Ginger, Holy Basil (Tulsi), Hyssop, Lavender, Lemon Balm, Nutmeg, Oregano, Pennyroyal, Peppermint, Rosemary, Sage, Spearmint, Tea Tree oil, and Thyme.

Astringents have constricting, tightening, firming and binding effects on tissues, mucous membranes, and blood vessels. Most herbal astringents contain **tannins**, which are bitter substances found in tree barks and many plants. When plant tannins contact human flesh, they make proteins coagulate, or clump together, causing the tissues to contract and reduce their secretions. Astringents form a protective coating over injured skin, and the tightening effect tones weak, boggy tissues. When put in the mouth, astringent teas and tinctures create a dry sensation that make the tongue and cheeks contract and pucker. Astringents have a toning effect on the tissues and are traditionally used for diarrhea, excessive and abnormal bleeding, and sore, swollen throats. They improve sluggish blood circulation and are used in the treatment of hemorrhoids and varicose veins. Blood loss from wounds is reduced with astringent herbs and tissue healing is accelerated. Some of the more potent astringents include Agrimony, Bayberry bark, Bistort, Black Tea (*Camellia sinensis*), Calamus, Cinnamon, Cinquefoil, Cranesbill, Eyebright, Goldenrod, Ground Ivy (*Glechoma hederacea*),

Horse Chestnut, Lady's Mantle, Mullein, Plantain, Purple Loosestrife, Raspberry leaf, Rosemary, Sage, St. John's Wort, Shepherd's Purse, Stinging Nettle, Thyme, Uva-ursi, White Oak bark, Witch Hazel, Wood Betony, Yarrow, and Yellow Dock. **Styptic** and **hemostatic** herbs have astringent properties that stop bleeding.

Bitters are highly respected by herbalists because they work so well to stimulate and regulate digestion, absorption, and elimination of food. Many herbs contain bitter-tasting constituents with these beneficial and normalizing actions. Their bitter flavor on the taste buds of the tongue initiates a reflex reaction that stimulates the production and secretion of digestive enzymes in the stomach, pancreas, liver, and gallbladder. Bitters have a wonderful regulatory effect on the liver and gallbladder, and they are used to treat and prevent the formation of gallstones and elevated cholesterol levels. Their ability to increase bile flow makes them reliable laxatives, and they assist in removing toxins and waste products from the body. The stimulating effects of bitters also activate glandular functions and secretions. Research demonstrates that many bitters have antibiotic, antifungal, and even antitumor activity. They are indicated for many types of indigestion, gas and bloating after eating, poor appetite, chronic constipation, and for elderly people who often produce less digestive enzymes as they age. Strong bitters are generally contraindicated for gallbladder disease, kidney stones, pregnancy, acid reflux disease, hiatal hernia, stomach ulcers, and gastritis. Bitter herbs include American Centaury, Artichoke leaves, Barberry, Blue Vervain, Bogbean, Boneset, Catnip, Chicory, Dandelion, Elecampane, Feverfew, Gentian, Goldenseal, Hops, Horehound, Hyssop, Motherwort, Mugwort, Oregon Grape Root, Rue, Turmeric, Uva-ursi, Valerian, Wormwood, Yarrow, and Yellow Dock.

Bronchodilators relax and dilate constricted bronchial passages to improve breathing. They are taken to relieve coughs, lung congestion, shortness of breath, asthma, and emphysema. Anise, Balloon Flower, Cramp Bark, Dong Quai, Elecampane, Ephedra, Lobelia, Peppermint, Thyme, Wild Yam, and Yarrow are bronchodilators.

Cardiac herbs exert beneficial and restorative actions on the heart. **Cardioactive** herbs contain powerful phytochemicals called cardiac glycosides that have strong effects. These should only be used by qualified experts or not at all, and include Foxglove and Lily-of-the-Valley. **Cardiotonics** do not contain cardiac glycosides and exert much gentler and safer actions. These include Astragalus, Bugleweed, Calendula, Cayenne, Elder berries, Figwort, Garlic, Ginger, Ginkgo, Hawthorn, Hops, Horse Chestnut, Lavender, Lemon Balm, Linden leaf and flower, Motherwort, Peppermint, Prickly Ash, and Rosemary.

Carminative herbs reduce gas. They are typically rich in volatile oils that relax muscles and tone and normalize the digestive system, especially the stomach. They help normalize hydrochloric acid production in the stomach, and relieve stomach and intestinal gas, inflammation, pain, and spasms. They promote peristalsis, the rhythmic contractions of muscles lining the intestines that provide the mobility necessary for bowel movements. Carminatives include American Centaury, Angelica, Anise, Balloon Flower, Basil, Bergamot, Blue Vervain, Boneset, Caraway, Cardamom, Catnip, Cayenne, Celery seed, Chamomile, Cinnamon, Clary Sage, Cloves, Coriander, Cumin, Dandelion, Dill, Elecampane, Eucalyptus, Fennel, Garlic, Ginger, Goldenrod, Ground Ivy, Holy Basil (Tulsi), Hops, Horehound, Hyssop, Lavender, Lemon Balm, Licorice, Marjoram, Motherwort, Mustard, Nutmeg, Oregano, Parsley, Peppermint, Rosemary, Sage, Spearmint, Thyme, Valerian, Wild Yam, Wintergreen, Wood Betony, Wormwood, and Yarrow. Carminatives have similar properties as **stomachic** herbs.

Cathartic herbs are powerful laxatives causing rapid evacuation. Laxatives are gentle compared to cathartics and **purgatives**, which have much stronger and more irritating actions on the bowels. See **laxative**.

Caustic herbs have strong, corrosive actions capable of burning or dissolving tissue. They can create blisters and cause tissues to slough off. Bloodroot, Poison Ivy, and Poison Oak are strong caustics. Caustic herbs are also called **epispastic, escharotic,** and **vesicant**.

Cholagogue or **choleretic** herbs act on the liver and gallbladder to promote the production and flow of bile. They help normalize all liver and gallbladder functions, and stimulate normal contractions of the gallbladder and bile ducts to deliver bile into the small intestine. Bile is necessary for digestion of fats and stimulation of bowel movements. Cholagogues help reduce stagnation and blockage in the liver and gallbladder, the cause of many problems, including high cholesterol levels, inflammation and pain, gallstones, constipation, flatulence, and other symptoms of indigestion and malabsorption. This common condition is called "Liver Qi Stagnation" in Traditional Chinese Medicine. Cholagogues should be avoided in cases of painful gallstones because their ability to stimulate contractions can constrict bile ducts and cause more pain. They are also contraindicated for any type of liver, gallbladder, and bile duct obstruction or acute inflammation.

Many cholagogues are bitter herbs and include American Centaury, Artichoke, Balmony, Barberry, Black Walnut hulls, Blessed Thistle, Blue Flag, Blue Vervain, Boneset, Burdock, Butternut, Cascara Sagrada, Cayenne, Coptis, Culver's root, Dandelion, Devil's Claw, Dodder, Elecampane, Fringe Tree, Fumitory, Gentian, Ginger, Goldenseal, Hops, Horehound, Hyssop, Lemon Balm, Licorice, Mugwort, Oregon Grape

Root, Peppermint, Rosemary, Sage, Turmeric, Turkey Rhubarb, Wild Indigo, Wild Yam, Yarrow, and Yellow Dock root.

Demulcent herbs contain mucilage and/or oils that soothe, heal, and protect tissues and mucous membranes lining the gastrointestinal, urinary, and respiratory tracts. They are moisturizing and reduce heat, inflammation, and irritation. Demulcent herbs are commonly used for conditions of excess dryness, skin injuries and inflammation, burns, dermatitis, sore throats, and stomach, intestinal, and skin ulcers. They are excellent for treating digestive problems like excess stomach acid, diarrhea, irritable bowel syndrome, ulcerative colitis, spasms, colic, and painful urinary tract infections. Demulcents also soothe bronchial inflammation and irritation and ease dry coughs.

Mucilage is a carbohydrate consisting of complex polysaccharides that become slimy and viscous when they come into contact with water. Demulcent and mucilaginous herbs are usually bland-tasting and are best taken as tea to obtain optimal healing activity. Warm water, rather than boiling water, works best to extract mucilage. Tincturing demulcents with alcohol is not recommended because it reduces the mucilage and healing potential.

Demulcent herbs include Aloe Vera, Borage, Burdock root, Calendula, Chickweed, Comfrey, Corn Silk, Couch Grass, Fenugreek seed, Flaxseed, Guar Gum, Hollyhock, Iceland Moss, Irish Moss, Licorice, Marshmallow, Mullein, Oats, Plantain, Psyllium, and Slippery Elm bark. See **mucilaginous** and **emollient**.

Deobstruents remove obstructions in the body, specifically from the gastrointestinal tract. These include Asparagus, Barberry, Blue Vervain, Goldenseal, Horehound, Lobelia, Plantain, Poke, and Turkey Rhubarb.

Depurant or **depurative** herbs remove waste products and toxins from blood by promoting elimination by the liver, kidneys, and intestines. These include laxatives and American Centaury, Black Walnut, Burdock, Calendula, Cayenne, Dandelion, Echinacea, Elecampane, Hyssop, Stinging Nettle, and Yellow Dock.

Detergent herbs are cleansing to the skin, boils, ulcers, wounds, and sores. They can be used internally and externally, and include Black Walnut, Calendula, Comfrey, Cranesbill, Echinacea, Goldenseal, Hyssop, Plantain, and Yellow Dock.

Diaphoretic plants stimulate increased blood flow to the surface of the body and induce sweating. They are used to reduce fevers and eliminate toxins through the skin. Tinctures and teas of diaphoretic herbs should be taken hot to induce sweating, and cold for diuretic action. Examples include Angelica, Blue Vervain, Boneset, Catnip, Cayenne, Chamomile, Cinnamon, Cloves, Elder berries and flowers, Elecampane, Fennel seed, Feverfew, Garlic, Ginger, Goldenrod, Holy Basil (Tulsi), Horehound, Hyssop, Lavender, Lemon Balm, Linden leaf and flower, Motherwort, Peppermint, Pleurisy Root, Prickly Ash, Sage, Spearmint, Thyme, and Yarrow. Very strong diaphoretic herbs are called **sudorific**. See **sudorific.**

Discutient herbs reduce swellings and dissolve and remove tumors, polyps, and other abnormal growths. They are also called **resolvents**. See **resolvents**.

Diuretics reduce excess body fluids by acting on the kidneys to stimulate urine production and output. They are used for edema (water retention), swollen lymph glands, congestive heart failure, and cases of high blood pressure involving water retention. Diuretics support inner cleansing by removing waste products.

Diuretic herbs include Agrimony, Blue Vervain, Boneset, Buchu, Burdock root, Celery seeds, Cleavers, Corn Silk, Couch Grass, Dandelion, Elder berries and flowers, Elecampane, Goldenrod, Gravel Root, Green and Black Tea, Hawthorn berries, Holy Basil (Tulsi), Horsetail, Hydrangea, Juniper berries, Linden leaf and flower, Marshmallow, Motherwort, Parsley, Plantain, Saw Palmetto, Shepherd's Purse, Stinging Nettle, Stone Root, Uva-ursi, Wood Betony, and Yarrow.

Emetics are herbs that induce nausea and vomiting when taken in large amounts. They are taken after the ingestion of poisons to expel toxins from the stomach. Historically, emetics were often employed for purging and purifying the body. Some emetics like Bloodroot are toxic when taken in large amounts. Lobelia is not toxic (a common misconception), but it will cause nausea in large doses. Boneset and Catnip are only emetic in very large doses. Ipecacuanha (*Cephaelis ipecacuanha*) is another strong emetic and the syrup, known as Ipecac, is used in modern medicine to induce vomiting in cases of poisoning, although large amounts are toxic. Emetics are also called **nauseant** herbs.

Emmenagogues stimulate menstruation and help regulate the menstrual cycle. Some can induce abortions when taken in large amounts and are contraindicated during pregnancy. Emmenagogues include Bergamot, Black Cohosh, Black Haw, Blessed Thistle, Blue Cohosh, Blue Vervain, Calendula, Catnip, Chamomile, Chasteberry, Clary Sage, Cramp Bark, Elecampane, Fenugreek, Feverfew, Gentian, Ginger, Goldenseal, Hops, Horehound, Hyssop, Lavender, Linden leaf and flower, Motherwort, Mugwort, Partridge Berry, Pennyroyal, Rosemary, Rue, Sage, Shepherd's Purse, Southernwood, Tansy, Thyme, Valerian, Wormwood, and Yarrow.

Emollient herbs are mucilaginous or oily substances applied topically on the skin to soothe, moisturize, and heal tissues. They soften and protect skin, relieving inflammation and irritation. The oils of almonds, wheat germ, olives, Sesame seeds, and Flaxseeds have emollient properties. Emollient herbs include Borage, Chickweed, Comfrey, Elderberry flowers, Elecampane, Fenugreek seeds, Hollyhock, Licorice, Marshmallow, Mullein, Plantain, Psyllium seed, and Slippery Elm bark. Emollients are similar to **mucilagens** and **demulcents**.

Epispastic and **escharotic** herbs burn or eat away tissue, and can cause blisters. They are also called **caustic** and **vesicant**. See **caustic**.

Exanthematous herbs are taken internally or applied externally to treat skin diseases and eruptions. They include American Centaury, Balloon Flower, Black Walnut leaves and hulls, Bloodroot, Burdock, Calendula, Catnip, Dandelion, Echinacea, Elecampane, Goldenseal, Hyssop, Sassafras, Stinging Nettle, and Yellow Dock. Exanthematous herbs have **vulnerary** (wound healing) properties.

Expectorants expel mucous from the lungs and bronchi. They relax bronchial muscles, reduce inflammation and spasms, thin and loosen mucous secretions, and stimulate the cough reflex. Expectorant herbs usually contain volatile oils. **Relaxing expectorants** include Anise, Balloon Flower, Blue Vervain, Chickweed, Comfrey, Goldenseal, Grindelia, Holy Basil (Tulsi), Hyssop, Iceland Moss, Irish Moss, Licorice, Linden, Lobelia, Lungwort, Marshmallow, Peppermint, Plantain, Pleurisy Root, Slippery Elm, Thyme, and Wild Cherry bark. Other expectorants are more stimulating and typically contain alkaloids and saponins that promote the cough reflex to remove excess phlegm. **Stimulating expectorants** include Bergamot, Bloodroot, Boneset, Catnip, Cayenne, Elder berries and flowers, Elecampane, Ephedra, Garlic, Ginger, Ground Ivy, Horehound, Mormon Tea, Mullein, Oregano, Sage, Spikenard, Stinging Nettle, and Wild Indigo. The Poppy (*Papaver somniferum*) is one of the few herbs that affects the brain center controlling respiration and coughing. **Antitussive** herbs suppress coughs.

Febrifuge herbs are cooling and remove heat from the body. They are used to reduce fevers and conditions of excess heat. Examples include Alfalfa, Aloe Vera, Angelica, Basil, Blue Vervain, Boneset, Borage, Burdock, Calendula, Catnip, Chamomile, Chickweed, Echinacea, Elder flowers and berries, Feverfew, Goldenseal, Gotu Kola, Holy Basil (Tulsi), Hyssop, Isatis, Lemon Balm, Peppermint, Thyme, and Yarrow. Febrifuge herbs are also called **antipyretic** and **refrigerant**.

Galactogogues promote the production and flow of breast milk in nursing mothers. These herbs tend to contain many nutrients contributing to rich milk. They include Alfalfa, Anise, Blessed Thistle, Blue Vervain, Borage, Catnip, Chasteberry, Dandelion, Dill seeds, Fennel, Fenugreek seeds, Goat's Rue, Hops, Marshmallow, Raspberry leaf, Slippery Elm, and Stinging Nettle. Galactogogues are also called **lactagogues**.

Hemostatics stop abnormal bleeding. They have similar properties as **astringents** and **styptics**. See **astringent.**

Hepatics tone, strengthen, and promote normal liver function. They stimulate and increase bile flow and benefit the gallbladder. See **bitters** and **cholagogues**, which act as hepatics. **Hepatoprotective** herbs protect the liver from chemical and environmental toxins, and are included in the hepatic category.

Examples of hepatic herbs include Agrimony, Aloe Vera, American Centaury, Andrographis, Artichoke, Astragalus, Balmony, Barberry, Blue Vervain, Bogbean, Boneset, Buckthorn, Bupleurum, Burdock root, Calendula, Cascara Sagrada, Celandine, Celery seed, Chlorella, Cleavers, Culver's Root, Dandelion, Eclipta, Elecampane, Fennel, Fumitory, Fringe Tree, Gentian, Goldenseal, Hops, Horehound, Hyssop, Lemon Balm, Licorice, Milk Thistle, Motherwort, Mugwort, Oregon Grape Root, Prickly Ash, St. John's Wort, Schisandra, Turmeric, Wild Indigo, Wild Yam, Wormwood, Yarrow, and Yellow Dock root.

Hypnotic herbs are strong sedatives that induce deep sleep when taken in adequate amounts. Those containing volatile oils exert a milder, relaxing action, while others that contain powerful alkaloids have greater ability to sedate the central nervous system. Hypnotic herbs are also called **soporific** and **somnifacient**. They include California and Opium Poppy, Chamomile, Hops, Jamaican Dogwood, Kava Kava, Marijuana, Passion Flower, Scullcap, Valerian, and Wood Betony.

Hypotensive herbs help reduce high blood pressure and include American Ginseng, Astragalus, Black Cohosh, Blue Vervain, Cayenne, Eleuthero (Siberian Ginseng), Evening Primrose oil, Fenugreek, Garlic, Hawthorn berries, Holy Basil (Tulsi), Lemon Balm, Linden leaf and flower, Motherwort, Parsley, Passion Flower, Scullcap, Stinging Nettle, Valerian, and Yarrow.

Immunomodulators strengthen and regulate the immune system to fight bacteria, viruses, fungi, parasites, tumors, and cancers. They are used to treat HIV infection, chronic fatigue and weakness, hepatitis, lupus, chronic immune deficiency, and degenerative and malignant diseases. Examples include Ashwagandha,

Astragalus, Boneset, Bupleurum, Burdock, Calendula, Cat's Claw, Chamomile, Chlorella, Codonopsis, Echinacea, Elder berries, Elecampane, Garlic, Ginger, Gotu Kola, Goldenseal, Holy Basil (Tulsi), Oregon Grape Root, Pau D'arco, Prickly Ash, Schisandra, Wild Indigo, and Maitake, Reishi, and Shiitake mushrooms.

Immunostimulant herbs strengthen the immune system by stimulating it to produce and activate necessary compounds to fight active infections, cancers, and immune deficiency diseases like AIDS. They include Andrographis, Astragalus, Boneset, Calendula, Cat's Claw, Echinacea, Elder berries and flowers, Elecampane, Eleuthero, Garlic, Goldenseal, Licorice , Oregon Grape Root, Wild Indigo, and Maitake, Reishi, and Shiitake mushrooms. Immunostimulants are contraindicated for autoimmune diseases, organ transplants, and hypersensitivity reactions because they may worsen the condition.

Lactagogue: see **galactogogue.**

Lactifuge herbs stop or decrease production and flow of breast milk. Astringent herbs can exert a lacifuge effect. These herbs should be avoided by nursing mothers, but work well when taken to wean young children. Agrimony, Cinquefoil, Cranesbill, Parsley, Sage, and Yarrow are well-known lactifuges.

Laxatives promote bowel movements and are used to treat constipation. The most popular and strongest are Barberry, Black Walnut hulls, Buckthorn, Cascara Sagrada, Rhubarb, and Senna. Milder laxatives include Boneset, Chickweed, Dandelion, Elder berries and flowers, Feverfew, Goldenseal, Mugwort, Oregon Grape Root, and Yellow Dock. Bulk forming herbs can reduce constipation and these include Aloe Vera, Fenugreek seeds, Flaxseeds, Guar Gum, Marshmallow root, Oat seed and Oat bran, Psyllium seed or husk, and Slippery Elm bark. *Always* drink plenty of water when taking laxative herbs and eat lots of fresh fruits, vegetables, and whole, non-gluten grains. **Aperient** is an older term for gentle-acting laxatives. **Purgative** and **cathartic** herbs are very strong laxatives that produce vigorous emptying of bowels, often causing a watery evacuation.

Lithotropic or **lithotryptic** herbs help prevent the formation of kidney, bladder, and gallbladder stones. They dissolve and eliminate existing stones and mineral deposits in joints. Examples are American Centaury, Blue Vervain, Buchu, Burdock, Cascara Sagrada, Cleavers, Corn Silk, Couch Grass, Dandelion, Elecampane, Goldenrod, Goldenseal, Gravel Root, Hops, Horsetail, Hydrangea, Oregon Grape Root, Pellitory-of-the-Wall, Parsley, Stinging Nettle, Stone Root, Uva-ursi, and Yucca. These are also called **antilithic** herbs.

Lymphagogues act on the entire lymphatic system to detoxify lymphatic fluids and fight infections in the lymph nodes. They are used for sore, swollen lymph nodes, lymphatic congestion causing toxic problems like skin rashes and dermatitis, and lymphatic cancers. The lymphatic system is an important part of immunity. Lymph nodes are fibrous capsules containing lymphocytes (white blood cells) equipped to fight pathogens. Lymph fluids permeate through all tissues of the body like a vast ocean. Lymph vessels, especially numerous in the groin, chest and neck areas, collect lymph fluids circulating through tissues into the lymphatic circulatory vessels, where lymph is drained into the bloodstream. Lymph nodes are scattered along the vessels. During an infection, when greater numbers of pathogens are present, some nodes get sore and swollen, and sometimes they become hard for an extended time. Lymphagogue herbs are excellent for these conditions.

Poke root (3 drops of tincture) combined with Echinacea (1 teaspoon of tincture) is excellent for all lymphatic problems when taken 2-3 times a day. Other lymphagogues include Black Walnut leaf, Burdock, Calendula, Chickweed, Chlorella, Cleavers, Dandelion, Echinacea, Goldenseal, Mullein, Pau D'arco, Plantain, Prickly Ash, Red Clover, Violet leaf, Wild Indigo, Woundwort (*Prunella vulgaris*), and Yellow Dock.

Mucilage or Mucilaginous herbs have a gummy, gelatinous consistency that feels somewhat slimy and slippery when made into a tea. This mucilage is exceptionally cooling, soothing, softening and moisturizing to hot, dry, inflamed, and injured tissues. It is especially beneficial and protective to the mucous membranes lining the throat, stomach, intestines, lungs, bladder, kidneys, and uterus. All mucilaginous herbs work well when taken as tea to obtain optimal healing activity. Warm water, rather than boiling water, works best to extract mucilage properties. Tincturing with alcohol is not recommended, as alcohol greatly reduces the mucilage. Mucilaginous herbs include Aloe Vera, Burdock root, Chickweed, Comfrey, Corn Silk, Fenugreek seeds, Flaxseed, Hollyhock, Iceland Moss, Irish Moss, Licorice, Marshmallow, Mullein, Oats, Plantain, Psyllium seeds, Sassafras leaves, Slippery Elm bark, and Solomon's Seal root. Many **demulcent** and **emollient** herbs are mucilaginous. Also see **demulcent**.

Nauseant herbs stimulate vomiting and are used to expel poisons from the stomach. See **emetic**.

Nephritic herbs help the kidneys produce urine and are taken to eliminate waste products and toxins from the body. Nephritic herbs include American Centaury, Astragalus, Blue Vervain, Burdock, Chicory, Corn Silk, Couch Grass, Dandelion, Eclipta, Elder flowers, Goldenrod, Goldenseal, Gravel Root, Hops, Juniper berries, Mullein, Parsley, Stinging Nettle, Uva-ursi, and Yarrow.

Nervines are restorative herbs that tone, strengthen, and nourish the nervous system. Some exert energizing and revitalizing activity, while others act as calming, subduing relaxants. Some herbs have both nervine and sedative actions. Nervines are used for all types of anxiety and nervousness, stress headaches, insomnia, tremors, and nerve injuries, pain, and deterioration. They are beneficial for treating diseases of the nervous system such as multiple sclerosis, Parkinson's disease, and trigeminal neuralgia. Many nervines also have anti-inflammatory or analgesic actions. Nervines include American and Asian Ginseng, Black Cohosh, Blue Vervain, Borage, Catnip, Chamomile, Damiana, Elder berries and flowers, Hawthorn berries, Holy Basil (Tulsi), Hops, Hyssop, Jamaican Dogwood, Kava Kava, Lavender, Lemon Balm, Linden leaf and flower, Lobelia, Marshmallow, Motherwort, Mugwort, fresh milky Oats, Passion Flower, Peppermint, Rosemary, Sage, St. John's Wort, Scullcap, Thyme, Valerian, Wood Betony, and Yarrow.

Nutritives contain substantial amounts of nutrients that sustain life and nourish the body, and nutritive plants promote food digestion and assimilation. Examples are Alfalfa, Astragalus, Bladderwrack, Burdock root, Cayenne, Chickweed, Chlorella, Comfrey, Dandelion, Elder berries, Holy Basil (Tulsi), Marshmallow, Oats, Plantain, Raspberry leaf, Shepherd's Purse, Spirulina, and Stinging Nettle.

Opthalmicum herbs are specific for eye problems, including dryness, irritation, itching, inflammation, styes, and infections. Goldenseal is one of the best remedies for styes and infections like conjunctivitis (pink eye). Other opthalmicum herbs are Calendula, Catnip, Chickweed, Clary Sage, Comfrey, Echinacea, Eyebright, and Marshmallow. Prepare the desired herbs as a tea, filter it well to remove all sediment, and apply it as eye drops or eyewash.

Oxytocic herbs stimulate the production and release of the hormone oxytocin, which increases uterine contractions during childbirth and breast milk production during lactation. Oxytocics include Black Cohosh, Blue Cohosh, Cramp Bark, Partridge Berry, and Trillium. Oxytocic herbs are also known as **parturients.**

Parasiticide herbs kill and expel worms and parasites. **Antiparasitic, anthelmintic, vermicide**, and **vermifuge** are other terms for parasiticide herbs. See **antiparasitic.**

Parturient: see **oxytocic**.

Pectorals have a general strengthening and healing effect on the lungs and respiratory system. They include Angelica, Astragalus, Balloon Flower, Blue Vervain, Boneset, Catnip, Cayenne, Elder berries and flowers, Elecampane, Fenugreek seeds, Garlic, Goldenseal, Horehound, Hyssop, Irish Moss, Licorice, Linden, Lobelia, Lungwort, Marshmallow, Mullein, Pleurisy Root, Stinging Nettle, and Thyme.

Purgative herbs are very strong laxatives that stimulate vigorous emptying of the bowels and can cause a watery evacuation. Purgatives and **cathartics** are both very strong laxatives. See **laxative.**

Refrigerant herbs have a cooling effect to reduce body temperature and are used for fevers, inflammation, and conditions of excess heat. They are also called **febrifuge** and **antipyretic**. See **febrifuge**.

Resolvent herbs reduce swellings and help dissolve and remove tumors, polyps, and other abnormal growths. They include Bayberry, Black Walnut hulls, Bladderwrack, Bloodroot, Blue Violet, Burdock root, Chickweed, Garlic, Goldenseal, Mugwort, Plantain, Red Clover, White Oak bark, and White Pond Lily. Resolvent herbs are also called **discutient**.

Restoratives act over time to nourish and balance the body, restoring normal function and vitality. Examples are Astragalus, Burdock, Cayenne, Chlorella, Dandelion, Elder berries, Ginkgo, Lemon Balm, Lobelia, Motherwort, St. John's Wort, Solomon's Seal, and Stinging Nettle.

Rubefacients are applied topically to increase circulation. They can cause mild local irritation and redness due to dilation of the capillaries (vasodilation). This increases blood flow to the skin, relieving congestion in the deeper tissues and organs. Rubefacients include Black Pepper, Bloodroot, Cayenne, Cloves, Garlic, Ginger, Horseradish, Lavender, Mustard, Pennyroyal oil, Peppermint oil, Rosemary oil, Rue, Stinging Nettle (the fresh nettles), and Thyme.

Sedatives calm and sedate the nervous system to reduce stress and tension throughout the body. They are beneficial for all conditions involving anxiety, restlessness, and hyperactivity. These include nervous headaches, migraines, high blood pressure, rapid heart rate, insomnia, muscle tension, spasms, and panic attacks. Sedative herbs include Black Cohosh, Blue Vervain, California Poppy, Catnip, Chamomile, Hops, Jamaican Dogwood, Kava Kava, Lavender, Lemon Balm, Linden leaf and flower, Motherwort, Passion Flower, St. John's Wort, Scullcap, Valerian, Wood Betony, and Yarrow.

Sialagogue herbs stimulate secretion of saliva from the salivary glands in the mouth. They are used to promote appetite and improve digestion. They include American Centaury, Cayenne, Dandelion, Gentian, Ginger, Lobelia, and Prickly Ash.

Somnifacient: see **hypnotic**.

Soporific herbs have strong sedative properties that induce relaxation and sleep. They are also called **hypnotic** and **somnifacient**. See **hypnotic**.

Stimulants increase nerve stimulation to tissues and organs. They promote energy, invigorate blood and lymphatic circulation, break up congestion and obstructions, and warm the body. Stimulants include Angelica, Black and Green Tea, Caraway, Cardamom, Catnip, Cayenne, Cinnamon, Cloves, Cocoa (*Theobroma cacao*), Coffee, Garlic, Ginger, Ginseng (Asian Ginseng is warmer and more stimulating than American Ginseng), Goldenrod, Guarana, Horseradish, Hyssop, Kola nuts, Lavender, Lobelia, Nutmeg, Black Pepper, Peppermint, Rosemary, Sage, Sarsaparilla, Thyme, and Yarrow. Stimulating herbs are also called **analeptic.**

Stomachic herbs strengthen, stimulate, tone, and heal the stomach. See **carminative.**

Styptic herbs are astringent and stop bleeding and diarrhea by contracting tissues and blood vessels. Styptics that stop bleeding are also called **hemostatic**. See **astringent**.

Sudorific herbs stimulate the sudoriferous (sweat) glands on the skin to increase their activity and secretions. Sudorifics have stronger properties than diaphoretic herbs. They induce profuse sweating when taken hot, and act as tonics when taken cold. They are used for fevers and detoxification. Sudorific herbs include Boneset, Cayenne, Ginger, and Yarrow. Also see **diaphoretic.**

Tonic herbs tone, balance, and strengthen the whole body or target specific organs and tissues. Tonics are generally taken over a period of time, and many herbs have tonic effects. **General tonics** include Angelica, Astragalus, Cayenne, Chlorella, Elder berries, Ginger, Ginseng, Holy Basil (Tulsi), Hyssop, and Stinging Nettle. **Heart tonics** include Hawthorn berries, Motherwort, and Peppermint. **Liver tonics** include Burdock, Dandelion, Hepatica, Milk Thistle, Turmeric, and Yellow Dock. **Uterine tonics** include Black Cohosh, Raspberry leaf, and Wild Yam. **Nerve tonics** include Eleuthero (Siberian Ginseng), American and Asian Ginseng, Gotu Kola, Lemon Balm, Scullcap, Valerian, and Wood Betony. **Tonic** and **alterative** herbs are similar in that they are both used for several weeks to strengthen and tone the body.

Vascular tonics nourish and support the normal function of blood vessels. Calendula, Cayenne, Elder berries, Ginger, Ginkgo, Gotu Kola, Hawthorn berries, Linden leaf and flower, and Motherwort are examples.

Vasoconstrictors are astringent herbs that tighten blood vessels and are taken to stop hemorrhaging. See **astringents.**

Vasodilators cause dilation (relaxation and expansion) of peripheral blood vessels. They improve circulation and can reduce elevated blood pressure. They include Astragalus, Balloon Flower, Black Cohosh, Calendula, Catnip, Cayenne, Echinacea, Evening Primrose oil, Feverfew, Garlic, Ginger, Ginkgo, Holy Basil (Tulsi), Horehound, Lavender, Lemon Balm, Linden, Lobelia, Motherwort, Passion Flower, Peppermint, Prickly Ash bark, Thyme, and Yarrow.

Vermicide and **vermifuge** herbs kill and expel worms and parasites. They are also called **anthelmintic, antiparasitic**, and **parasiticide** herbs. See **antiparasitic.**

Vesicant plants produce blisters upon contact. Poison ivy and poison oak are vesicants. Vesicants are also called **caustic, epispastic,** and **escharotic**. See **caustic**.

Vulnerary herbs are applied externally to heal injuries to the skin and underlying tissues and muscles, eliminate external infection, and to promote cell growth and repair. Examples are Aloe Vera, Arnica, Blue Vervain, Burdock leaf, Calendula, Chamomile, Chickweed, Clove, Comfrey, Echinacea, Elderberry flowers, Goldenrod, Goldenseal, Holy Basil (Tulsi), Horsetail, Hyssop, Lavender, Lemon Balm, Marshmallow, Mugwort, Mullein, Oregano, Plantain, Sage, St. John's Wort, Slippery Elm, Solomon's Seal, Thyme, Witch Hazel, Wood Betony, Woundwort, Yarrow, and Yellow Dock.

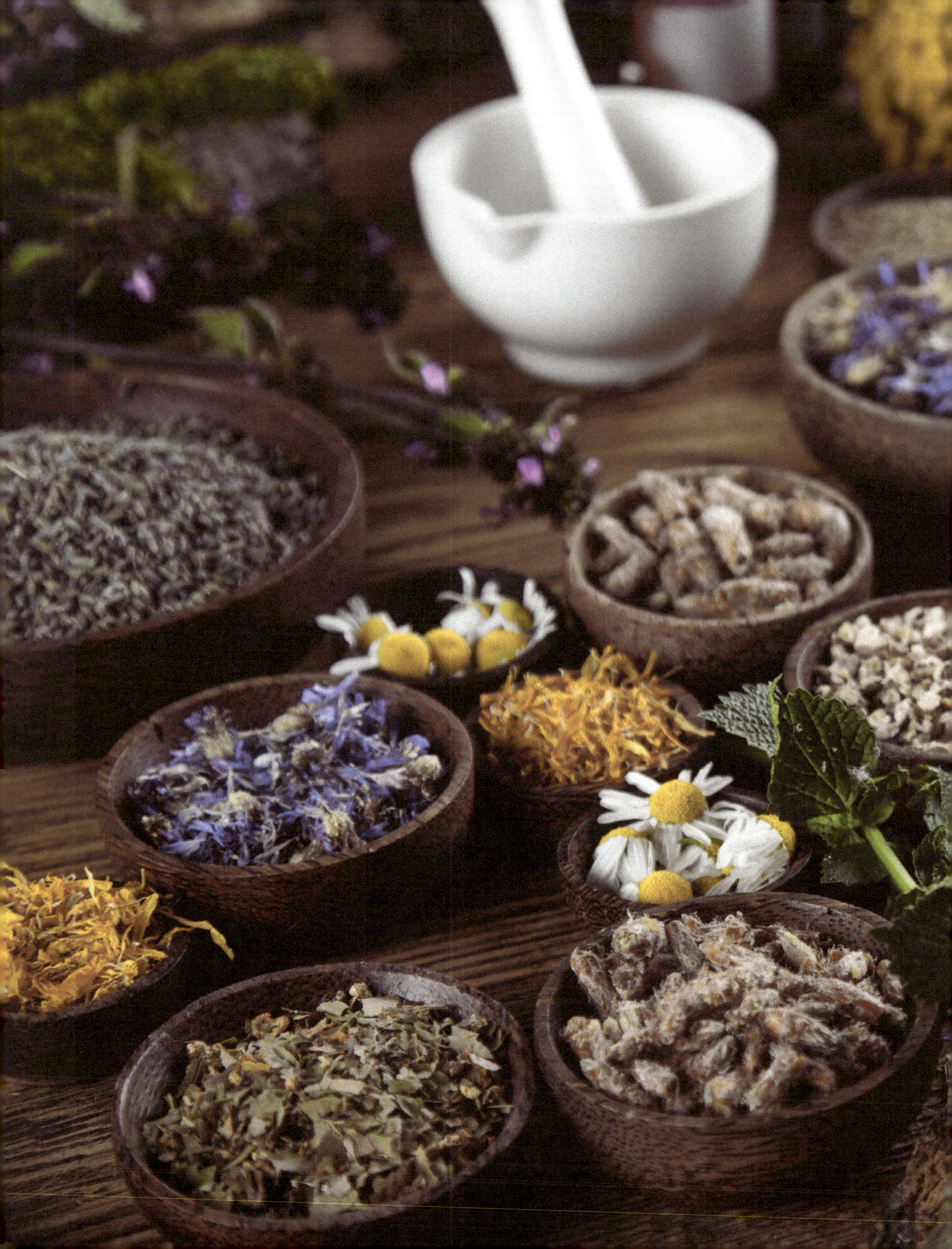

SECTION TWO

The Materia Medica

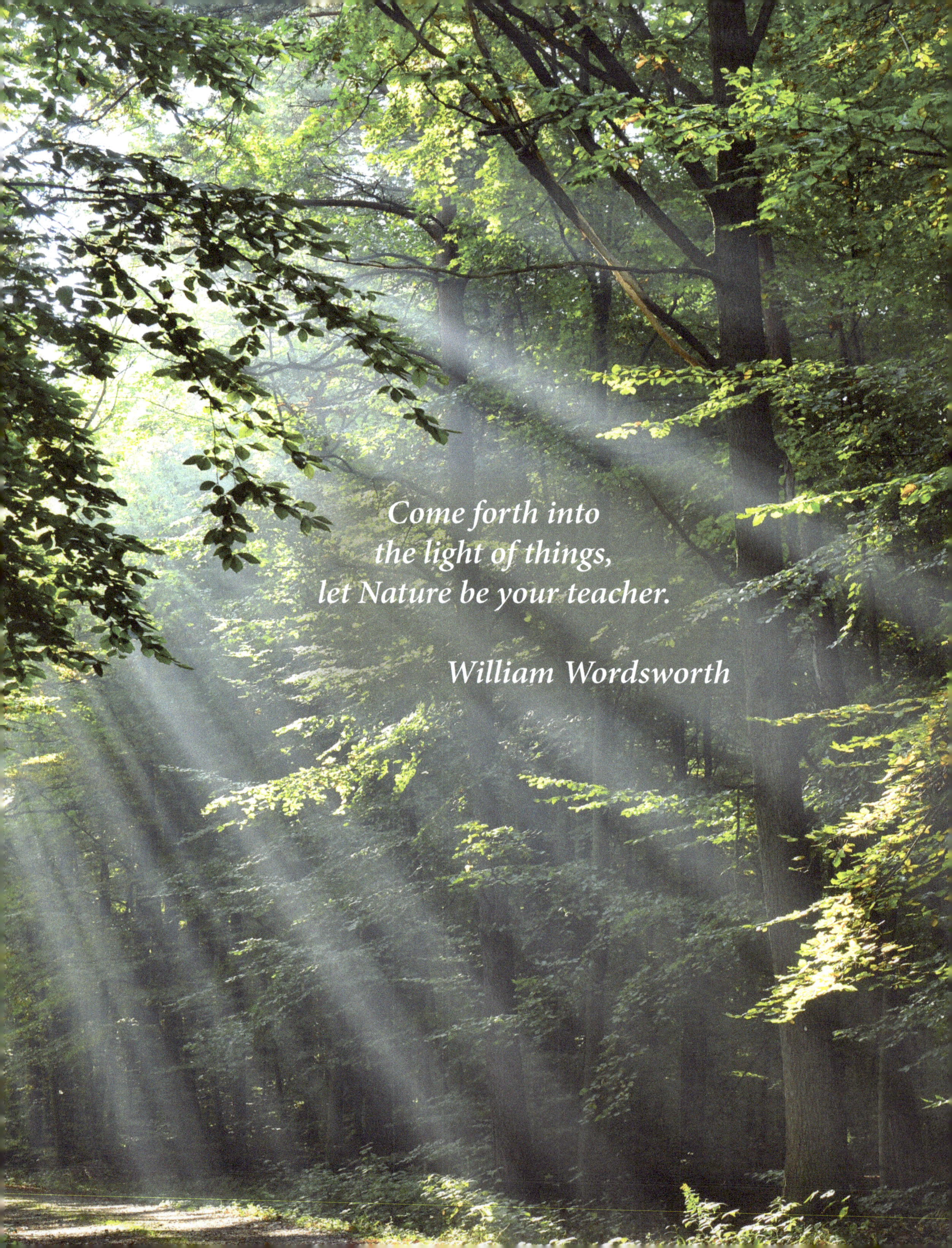
Come forth into
the light of things,
let Nature be your teacher.
William Wordsworth

How to Use the Materia Medica

The Materia Medica, which literally means "medical material," is a compilation of information on 50 medicinal plants. I have selected these after coming to know them over many years. These are the plants I cultivate in my gardens or sustainably wildcraft from the surrounding countryside, providing material for the creation of an "herbal pharmacy" that continues to benefit family, friends, clients, and myself.

In an attempt to present as complete a picture as possible for each herb, a broad spectrum of information is provided. This is drawn from the expertise of numerous herbalists and clinical practitioners, modern scientific research, and from my own personal experience derived over many years as an herbalist and holistic nurse practitioner engaged in private practice.

Over time, my relationship with the plants has become more focused on cultivating a wide variety of healing herbs and encouraging other people to do the same. Without cultivation, many of our most popular and beneficial herbs are becoming endangered, so I consider the information on cultivation to be especially important and a feature offered too rarely in other herbals.

In order to make this a user-friendly manual for quick and easy reference, information on each herb is arranged in a specific sequence of topic headings that are explained below. The explanations will help the reader obtain optimal benefit from the Materia Medica.

The index in Section Three titled **"Index of Health Issues and Herbal Recommendation"** is a helpful guide to choosing appropriate herbs for promoting wellness and dealing with health problems. The chapter titled **"Healing Qualities of Herbs"** in Section One also lists herbs for specific health care issues.

Botanical Name and Family

The botanical name and family are given for each herb in the Materia Medica. Just like people, all plants are members of families evolved from a distant ancestry. Based upon their structure and other characteristics, plants are divided into large groups called **families** that are separated into classes called **genus** and further subdivided into **species**.

The Appendix contains an alphabetically arranged cross-reference of common and botanical names of many herbs. For more information about botanical names, refer to the "Nomenclature and Classification of Plants" chapter in Section One.

Common Names

Although all medicinal herbs have been assigned Latin names, most plants have acquired several common names derived from their medicinal uses, appearance, taste, or other qualities. Many common names describe herbs in interesting ways and shed light on their characteristics. For instance, a common name for Comfrey (*Symphytum officinale*) is "knitbone," indicating its historic use in mending broken bones. Another common name is "slippery root," describing the slimy texture of the medicinal mucilage in the root. Bloodroot (*Sanguinaria canadensis*) is named for the bright blood-red juice contained within the roots. The Latin genus name *Sanguinaria* translates as "bloody."

Common names of a plant may differ depending on locality or language, and can be a source of confusion when the Latin botanical name is excluded. For example, I once attended a class in which the speaker talked about an herb she called Klamath. I didn't realize that she was talking about the plant I know as St. John's Wort until she eventually referred to it as *Hypericum perforatum*, its universally accepted Latin name.

Medicinal Parts of the Plant

It is imperative to know which parts of the plant to use for medicinal purposes so that no mistakes are made when creating and administering herbal preparations. With many plants like Blue Vervain (*Verbena hastata*) and Dandelion (*Taraxacum officinale*), the whole plant is safe to use, including the roots, leaves, and flowers. Do not generally assume, however, that all parts of medicinal plants are safe to consume. Herbs like Blue Cohosh (*Caulophyllum thalictroides*) and Solomon's Seal (*Polygonatum* spp.) bear poisonous berries, while the roots are used medicinally. Rhubarb leaves are considered to be toxic due to high levels of oxalic acid, but the stalks are edible. Although the entire Burdock (*Arctium* spp.) plant is safe to consume, the mild-tasting roots are a far cry from the extremely bitter leaves.

Range and Habitat

The range or geographical distribution of each herb is provided, including the regions where it is indigenous or naturally occurring. Habitat is the type of environment where plants grow, such as a sunny meadow, a dry sandy desert, a boggy marshland, or shaded woodland of rich, loamy soil. Remember that although plants are stationary life forms with their roots anchored in the ground, many are travelers, whose seeds can be broadcast over many miles, spreading out to populate distant areas. Plants travel and set their roots according to the climate, temperature, elevation, moisture, light requirements, and type of soil specific to each of their needs, without being restricted to man-made boundaries drawn on maps. When cultivating medicinal herbs, it is most productive to grow plants that will do well in your specific range and habitat.

Description of the Plant

In this section, the appearance and physical characteristics of each herb are described in botanical terms. Information is included on whether herbs are annual and live for only one year, biennial with a two-year life cycle, or perennial living for several years. A clear and concise description is imperative to ensure correct identification of herbs. To fully understand the botanical language of plant descriptions, please refer to "Botany for Herbalists" in Section One.

Enjoy bringing plant botany to life by spending time outdoors and studying the plants according to this reference. To observe a typically unnoticed dimension of our amazing world, use a 16X loupe magnifying glass (available at camera shops) to view the plants. Tiny hairs, oil glands, sparkling drops of oil and water, intricate parts of the flower, and even insects are visually enhanced to reveal inspiring aspects of life on our beautiful planet!

Cultivating Medicinal Herbs

I am passionately dedicated to ensuring the continued survival of medicinal herbs and place great importance in sharing knowledge about cultivation. I encourage everyone who uses herbs to grow some! After all, if we take plants from the earth, an important balance to sustain and renew our resources is maintained by establishing more plants. This act of reciprocity is an aspect of ancient wisdom followed by many of our ancestors. Cultivation not only maintains balance, it is also an expression of our deep gratitude to the Earth for the gift of life. Gardening offers us the opportunity to be cooperative participants with Nature in creating more plant life and beautifying our backyards and the earth. Growing our own herbs becomes more important as the cost of pharmaceutical medicine rises, legislation to restrict consumer access to herbs fluctuates, and increasing commercial demand for many herbs leads to dwindling supplies from naturally occurring stands. Growing herbs empowers us with greater independence, providing the opportunity to produce the highest quality and most potent herbal remedies for responsible and effective health care.

> *Cultivating herbs is an expression of deep gratitude to the Earth for the gift of life.*

My favorite aspect of herbalism is spending time in the garden and countryside with the plants. It is delightful to plant seeds and roots, weed, water, harvest, and simply stop to admire the beauty of the herbs, while appreciating their healing gifts and comforting presence. On one level, the plants are my "kids" to whom I help Nature give birth by propagating, watering, and nurturing them until they are mature. On another level, they are wise beings manifesting the perfection, beauty, and abundance of life, offering balance and wholeness to anyone willing to partake. Healing comes to us at even more profound levels when we are in the physical presence of live plants, allowing us to develop a more personal relationship with them and embrace their healing energies. Having a garden promotes calm stability and mental health, and I enthusiastically encourage everyone to grow medicinal herbs whenever possible! Even apartment dwellers can grow a few potted herbs by a window or on a porch, or ask a friend who has gardening space to plant herbs on their property and share the harvest. Start by growing a few medicinal herbs that appeal to you and fit your needs, and then expand over time.

Specific information is provided in the Materia Medica for the successful cultivation and special needs of each herb. Before planting, please read the "Cultivating Medicinal Herbs" chapter in Section One for an in-depth discussion of basic cultivation principles and techniques.

Sustainable Harvesting

This section offers information on the correct times and methods of harvesting herbs to provide the most potent medicinal preparations. Before harvesting, please read the "Sustainable Harvesting of Medicinal Herbs" chapter in Section One for guidelines. Remember the importance of ethical and sustainable wildcrafting practices, which are vital for the continued survival of plants on our planet.

Preparation of Plant Medicine and Dosages

Creating your own herbal remedies is an empowering and earthy experience connecting us to the plants and the vast circle of ancient and modern herbal healers. I fondly remember the first time I saw herbal salve being made. My friend Laura, a registered nurse and midwife, was working over a huge pot in her oven that was nearly overflowing with chopped pieces of roots, leaves, and flowers floating in olive oil. The whole thing looked like a dark, soupy mash. Watching her stir this brew, I felt an air of enchantment and antiquity that captivated my attention and became the initial spark igniting my interest in making herbal salve.

You can process herbs in your kitchen to create teas, tinctures, pills, capsules, oils, salves, douches, eyewashes, ear drops, fomentations, poultices, and liniments. Specific information on the best methods of extraction and preparation is given for each herb listed in the Materia Medica. For complete instructions, refer to the chapters in Section One titled "Drying and Storing Medicinal Herbs" and "Creating Herbal Preparations." Using these chapters as references will greatly enhance usability of the Materia Medica. Instructions for preparing **flower essences**, often mentioned in the Deva readings, are found on pages 128-9.

This section also provides recommended dosages for adults weighing 120-150 pounds. Children's doses are always smaller and best determined by the weight of the child. Refer to "How to Calculate Dosages" in Section One for specific instructions and guidelines used to calculate dosages for children and the elderly. The "Weights and Measures for the Herbalist" chapter can also be helpful when figuring dosages.

Chemical Constituents in Herbs

Chemical constituents are the major compounds, or phytochemicals, in plants that are responsible for their healing properties and physiological effects on humans and animals. Under this heading, the primary constituents are listed with some of their pharmacological actions determined by scientific research. Plant chemistry analysis is a complex science that continuously expands our knowledge base. Considering that most plants contain hundreds of different chemicals, this section is a cursory exploration of the major chemicals known to date; it is not intended to be a complete synopsis of all the chemical constituents in each herb. Identifying phytochemicals provides rational explanations as to how herbs heal, and scientific research often confirms their historical folk uses.

The chapter on "Chemical Constituents in Plants" in Section One provides information about the more common chemicals found in medicinal herbs. Many thanks to herbal expert and authority James Duke, Ph.D., whose extensive phytochemical database (available online at www.ars-grin.gov/duke/) is one of my primary reference sources. Another excellent reference on phytochemicals is David Hoffmann's *Medicinal Herbalism: The Science and Practice of Herbal Medicine.*

Safety, Contraindications, and Drug Interactions

This section offers information on the overall safety of each herb listed in the Materia Medica. This includes possible side effects, contraindications when it should be avoided, interactions with pharmaceutical drugs, and restrictions during pregnancy and lactation. The safety of each herb is evaluated by assessing traditional and current knowledge, historic use, chemistry, pharmacology, and laboratory and clinical research findings. The most reliable and time-tested evidence supporting herbal safety is typically a long history of human use without serious problems. Current scientific investigation and identification of specific chemical constituents in herbs also sheds light on safety and toxicity issues.

Refer to "The Safety of Medicinal Herbs" in Section One for more specific information and guidelines to make wise choices when using medicinal herbs.

Medicinal Uses

The medicinal uses of each herb are presented under four categories; *History of the Plant, Healing Qualities, Traditional Chinese Medicine (TCM) Perspective,* and *Primary Actions.*

History of the Plant

Just as people have a fascinating and unique history to divulge, so do the plants! The history of each herb incorporates the globally accumulated knowledge and experience of many people. Human interaction with most medicinal plants spans hundreds or thousands of years and can involve different cultures from various regions of the world. Historical information about traditional uses of herbs is relevant to modern times because it reveals aspects about the healing potential of herbs and provides a strong source of empirical evidence as to their efficacy and safety.

Interesting and pertinent historical accounts are provided for each herb listed in the Materia Medica. Many references and citations are included from well-known ancient and modern herbalists, whose records and experiences laid the foundation for our current knowledge and use of herbs. Current trends regarding each herb are discussed, including their popularity, research investigations, availability on the commercial market, and "at risk" status.

Read "The History of Herbalism and Early Medicine" in Section One to become familiar with many of the significant people, organizations, and movements that created and molded medical and herbal history. This chapter provides a greater understanding and context for appreciating the history of individual herbs in the Materia Medica.

Healing Qualities

Over the ages, specific terms have been established to describe the healing qualities of medicinal herbs according to their physiological actions and effects on the human body. Terms such as astringent, emetic, diuretic, emmenagogue, or nervine define specific aspects of biological activity. Familiarity with the definitions of these healing qualities is beneficial for a more precise understanding of the nature of herbs. Terms for the healing qualities of herbs offer an abbreviated short-hand language, a quick reference guide to their application for health issues. For example, if you know that American Ginseng (*Panax quinquefolius*), Astragalus (*Astragalus membranaceus*), Holy Basil (*Ocimum sanctum*), and Licorice (*Glycyrrhiza glabra*) are adaptogens that help the body handle stress and strengthen immunity, you can safely assume that these herbs are appropriate for people experiencing stressful losses, life changes, hectic lifestyles, adrenal burn-out, and anxiety. Understanding that antispasmodic herbs such as Catnip (*Nepeta cataria*), Rosemary (*Rosmarinus officinalis*), Peppermint (*Mentha x piperita*), and Oregano (*Origanum vulgare*) relax nerves and muscles to ease spasms, you would know that these herbs are helpful for headaches or stomach and intestinal spasms.

For complete definitions of the terms used to describe herbal qualities, refer to "Healing Qualities of Herbs" in Section One and the Glossary in the Appendix

Traditional Chinese Medicine (TCM) Perspective

I have profound appreciation for the ancient and holistic system of Traditional Chinese Medicine (TCM), which has refined the process of restoring equilibrium within the body to a fine art. In my nursing practice, the TCM model is blended with my background in Western medicine and the holistic paradigm with wonderful results. TCM serves as a guide to identifying underlying characteristics of illness and points to logical solutions. The TCM perspective is included in this Materia Medica because, although this medical system is complex, it is based on a very simple, commonsense understanding of our world. Like many other healing systems, including early Western medicine, TCM acknowledges that all things are composed of the elements of nature: fire, water, earth, and air. The basic qualities of hot and cold, dry and damp, excess and deficiency are also recognized in TCM. Understanding these relationships refines the art of herbalism by matching the constitution of each person and the characteristics of their illness with corresponding herbs to encourage balance and promote health.

Incorporating TCM wisdom into the practice of medicinal herbalism is very helpful. For example, every illness is classified as a cold, neutral, or hot condition. If a person has symptoms of heat, such as heartburn, fever, excessive thirst or a flushed face, then moisturizing and cooling herbs are chosen to promote balance for the same reason that water is used to put out fires. However, if warming herbs like Ginger (*Zingiber officinale*) or Garlic (*Allium sativum*) are given to a person who is already excessively hot, they can create further imbalance and worsen symptoms. Giving a hot-natured person warming herbs without balancing them with cooling remedies is like throwing gasoline on a fire.

The following brief discussion highlights the fundamentals of TCM to assist the reader.

Basic Principles of Chinese Medicine

Chinese medicine evolved from ancient Taoist philosophy in which the universe and all life arise from that which is formless and invisible, called the eternal Tao. The Tao is the life force and energy flowing through all things.

The Tao gave birth to one source,
The one gave birth to two things,
Then to three things,
Then to 10,000 . . .
Tao Te Ching (third century B.C.)

The basis of Chinese medical theory includes the concepts of Yin and Yang, the Five Elements, and Qi, which roughly translates as energy.

Yin and Yang

Yin and Yang are the two polar-yet-complementary qualities of energy that make up all life and cycles of movement. They are expressions of duality arising from the "one source," the Tao. The development and existence of all phenomena and life forms result from the interplay of these polarities. Everything exists as a dynamic and constantly changing equilibrium of Yin and Yang, female and male, darkness and light, and one cannot exist without the other.

When considering the four elements, water and earth are Yin, with water being the most extreme Yin element. Earth holds or contains water. Fire and air are Yang, and fire is the most extreme Yang element. Air contains and holds fire.

Comparison of Yin and Yang Qualities

Yin	Yang
female	male
dark	light
cold	hot
water	fire
damp	dry
soft, yielding	firm, resilient
passive, resting	aggressive, active, working
contractive	expansive
descending and inward movement	ascending and outward movement
earth	heaven

Comparison of Yin and Yang Qualities	
Yin	**Yang**
night	day
winter	summer
stillness	movement
substance/structure	function

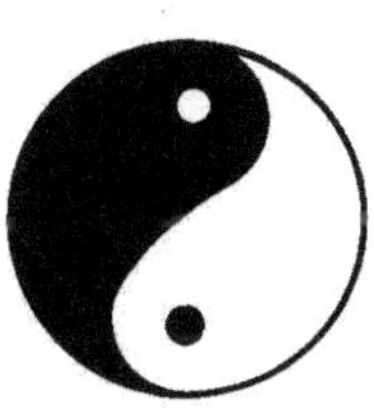

The Yin-Yang Symbol, Tai Ji

The relationship and interdependence of Yin-Yang is represented by the symbol called the "Supreme Ultimate," or *Tai Ji*. This symbol reflects that 1) although they are opposites, Yin-Yang complement each other and create complete unity; 2) Yin contains the seed of Yang and Yang also contains Yin, represented by the small black and white dots; 3) nothing is completely Yin or completely Yang, but rather a combination of the two; 4) life is a dynamic waxing and waning of Yin-Yang, and the two polarities are not stagnant; and 5) under certain conditions, extreme Yin transforms into Yang and vice versa.

When applying Yin-Yang to healing, Yin relates to the substance and structure of the tissues and fluids, and to the nourishment and structure of the body. Yang relates to the function and activity of the tissues and organs, and to warmth and movement of blood, hormones, and other elements within the body. A dynamic balance of Yin and Yang promotes health and well-being. Illness and disease arise from imbalance between these two polarities.

There are four possible states of Yin-Yang imbalance:

Excess Yin can cause fluid retention, sinus drainage, coolness, sluggishness, lack of energy and activity, and Yang deficiency.
Excess Yang can result in excess heat, hyperactivity, agitation, anxiety, dry tissues, and Yin deficiency.
Deficient Yin causes malnutrition, anemia, weakness, fatigue, and dryness.
Deficient Yang can result in sluggishness, exhaustion, lack of motivation, coolness, and poor digestion.

TCM treatment is designed to:

Tone and nourish Yin with nourishing fluids and food.
Tone and nourish Yang with warming and stimulating foods and herbs.
Reduce excess Yin with drying, warming, and stimulating foods and herbs.
Reduce excess Yang with cooling, moisturizing, and calming foods and herbs.

The major organs, fluids, and energies in the body are classified according to Yin and Yang.

Solid organs are Yin and include the heart, liver, spleen, pancreas, kidneys, and lungs.

Hollow organs are Yang and include the gallbladder, stomach, urinary bladder, small intestine, and colon.

Blood and other body fluids such as lymph, vitreous humor within the eyeball, and amniotic fluid are Yin due to their watery nature. Blood and lymphatic fluids transport nutrients responsible for growth and maintenance. Fluids nourish and moisturize all tissues and are responsible for the form and structure of bones, nerves, skin, muscles, and organs.

Qi (pronounced *chee*) is best defined as vital energy, vital force, or life force. It is considered to be Yang in nature. Qi exists within our bodies and permeates the space around us. Everything in the universe is composed of and defined by its Qi. The basis of all life, Qi takes many different qualities and forms as both energy and matter. It is the animating force that manifests as warmth and activity such as walking, thinking, feeling, or working. It is the energy that gives life to the body and consciousness to the brain. Qi flows in, around, and through the human body via pathways called channels or meridians. Qi protects the body from invading bacteria, viruses, and other pathogens. The Qi, or energy, of each organ is referred to as Liver Qi, Kidney Qi, etc. According to TCM, the body is healthy when Qi moves through and nourishes the cells and tissues without restrictions or imbalances. Pain, illness, and disease arise when Qi becomes deficient (causing underactivity, weakness, prolapsed organs, or poor immunity), obstructed or stagnant (causing constipation, arthritis, aches and pains, tumors, or cysts), or excessive (causing hyperactivity, hypertension, anxiety, insomnia, tumors, or cysts).

The qualities of medicinal herbs are classified as Yin or Yang.

Yin herbs are typically mild-tasting, nutritious, moistening, gentle in action, and can be taken as tonics over long periods of time. Examples are Stinging Nettle, Marshmallow, Licorice, the Mints, Red Clover, Burdock, and Chickweed.

Yang herbs are stronger-tasting "movers and shakers." Exerting strong actions that create changes in the body, they are used for short periods of time. Examples include Goldenseal, Isatis, Blue Vervain, Boneset, Horehound, Poke, Sage, and Yellow Dock.

The Five Elements in TCM

The five elements constituting the material world are water, wood, fire, earth, and metal (or air). They are dynamic qualities of nature in constant motion and change, providing the ground substance and building material for everything in the universe. Each of the five elements is a manifestation of varying degrees of Yin and Yang. Each element represents a specific body part, sense organ, emotion, and a season of the yearly cycle.

Element	Body Part	Sense Organ	Season	Yin-Yang Relationship	Emotional Correspondence
Water	kidneys/bladder	ears	winter	extreme Yin	fear
Wood	liver/gallbladder	eyes	spring	lesser Yang	anger
Fire	heart/small intestine	tongue	summer	extreme Yang	excessive joy
Earth	spleen/stomach	mouth	summer's end	balanced Yin-Yang	worry
Metal (Air)	lung/large intestine	nose	autumn	Yin	grief and sadness

Water corresponds to winter and is associated with storage. The winter season brings stillness and extreme cold and is a time of rest when energy is conserved, condensed, and stored. Water is extreme or full Yin. In the body, water is associated with all fluids, including blood, lymphatic fluids, urine, hormones, enzymes, and amniotic fluids. In nature, water is dissipated by excess heat and condensed and constrained by excess cold. Water is associated with the kidneys.

Wood corresponds to spring and is associated with birth, development, vigor, and youth. The wood element arises from the potential energy of water. Wood energy is expansive, explosive, and Yang in nature. Wood energy requires free expression and space for expansion. Blocking wood energy promotes anger, frustration, jealousy, and stagnation. Wood is associated with the liver.

Fire corresponds to summer and is associated with growth and maturation. Due to its intense heat and expansive nature, fire represents extreme Yang. Fire provides the body with life-giving energy that stimulates and sustains all metabolic processes, makes the nervous system function and the heart beat, and is necessary for the production of digestive enzymes and food absorption. The fire element is associated with the heart, generosity, joy, abundance, and the upward and outward movement of energy. If blocked, it gives rise to repression, hypertension, heart and circulatory problems, and nervous and digestive disorders.

Earth corresponds to late summer and is associated with transformation. This is the seasonal time when Yin and Yang energies are in a state of balance. The earth element is associated with the stomach, spleen, and pancreas, which digests food to nourish and support the entire body. Deficient earth energy results in an impaired and sluggish digestive system, physical weakness, and inability to feel grounded and connected with the earth.

Metal corresponds to autumn and is associated with harvest and gathering. Autumn is the time of year when the energies of nature begin to condense, contract, move downward, and store energy. Metal energy refers to the element of air and controls the lungs, which extract and store Qi from the air and expel gases from the blood. Autumn is the time to get rid of excess, to rest and reflect inwards. When metal or air energy is blocked, it can result in breathing problems, chest pain, toxicity, and skin problems.

Applying Yin-Yang and the Five Elements to healing:

In TCM, treating illness is the process of balancing Yin-Yang and the five elements through diet, herbs, acupuncture, therapeutic massage, exercise, rest, and meditation. Medical treatment consists of assessment by inquiry, observing tongue and body appearance, and pulse diagnosis to determine the pattern of disharmony underlying illness.

Illness and disease are regarded as conditions caused by deficiency or excess.

Deficiency conditions are caused by a lack of nutrients, fluids, warmth, or Qi (energy and vitality). Deficiency conditions cause weakness, coolness, and diminished movement. They are treated by restoring, nurturing, warming, and stimulating the body with specific foods and herbs.

Excess conditions occur from an over-abundance of fluids, dryness, heat, or cold. Conditions of chronic excess can eventually cause obstructions and stagnation in organs, tissues, and fluids. Conditions of excess are treated by draining, dispersing, detoxifying, and relaxing the body with foods and herbal remedies.

Pathological conditions are caused by imbalances of hot, cold, dryness, dampness, and wind.

In nature, extreme heat, cold, dryness, dampness, or wind can create havoc in the world. These same forces, when out of balance, can also create problems in the human body. The degrees of hot/cold and dry/damp are used to describe the nature of pathological conditions and the qualities of medicinal herbs in TCM.

Heat excess leads to inflammation, pain, headaches, red rashes, fevers, or excessive thirst. Sometimes the word "fire" is used to describe intense heat, such as Stomach Fire, which manifests as heartburn or ulcers. Excess heat can also affect the emotions and promote restlessness, agitation, explosive anger, or insomnia.

Heat deficiency can result in cool extremities with poor circulation, diminished digestive enzymes with resulting sluggish digestion, and lack of energy.

Cold excess conditions can also affect the digestive system causing sluggishness, gas, bloating, and constipation. Excessive cold slows down all activity in the body, promoting stagnation of Qi energy and circulatory problems.

Excessive dampness can cause edema, abundant phlegm, sinus congestion, swelling, and heaviness.

Deficiency of dampness causes constipation and dry hair, skin, and mucous membranes.

Excess dryness in the gastrointestinal tract can reduce digestive juices and enzymes, promote constipation, or cause dry skin.

Wind is excessive movement of Qi in the body and can manifest as vertigo (dizziness), trembling, tics, tremors, and unsteady movements.

TCM Perspective of the Yin Organs

Heart: The functions of the Heart are to govern the blood, control the blood vessels and circulation, and house the Mind (Shen). If the Heart is constitutionally strong, a person will have good circulation, warm extremities, a rosy complexion, vigorous energy, and calm thoughts and emotions. Heart weakness and deficient Blood potentiates fatigue, weakness, skin pallor, cool extremities, anemia, and menstrual problems. Blood stagnation causes a pale or bluish tinge to the complexion. Excess heat in the Heart induces an excessively red complexion. In TCM, the meaning of Mind or Shen includes a person's emotions, mental faculties, and spirituality. The strength of the Heart and nourishment from the Blood affect Shen. Heart-Qi deficiency weakens Heart function and can cause palpitations, shortness of breath, pallor, fatigue, and spontaneous sweating. These problems also result from Heart-Yang deficiency, and the lack of heat causes cool limbs and poor circulation. Heart-Blood deficiency is very similar to Heart-Yin deficiency because Blood is very Yin (moisturizing and nourishing). These deficiencies cause anemia, palpitations, shortness of breath with exertion, dizziness, insomnia, poor mental function, anxiety, weakness, fatigue, decreased circulation, pale complexion, and night sweats. Heart-Fire is an excess of heat and deficiency of water resulting in palpitations, racing pulse, thirst and dryness, restlessness, agitation, headaches, insomnia, and a red complexion.

Liver: The Liver stores Blood, regulates its circulation through the vessels, and provides Blood to nourish the Heart. One of the most important jobs of the Liver is to ensure the smooth movement of Qi throughout the body. This includes the smooth flow of blood, lymphatic fluids, hormones and enzymes, and the movement of bile for normal digestion and elimination. A healthy Liver also promotes the smooth flow of emotions, but restrained Liver-Qi gives rise to emotional repression, depression or anger, further weakening the Liver. Due to its control of blood flow and reproductive hormones, the Liver also regulates menstruation and reproduction. Deficient Liver-Blood can cause anemia, scanty or late periods, or amenorrhea (abnormal cessation of periods).

If Liver-Qi becomes restrained or stagnated, circulation and bile flow are reduced, and excess heat can build in the body. Liver-Qi Stagnation is a very common problem caused by poor diet, excessive and harmful emotions, and lack of exercise. This can result in joint problems, depression, volatile emotional and psychological states, reduced circulation, painful periods with blood clots, PMS, toxicity, high cholesterol, gallstones, and sluggish digestion with nausea, abdominal distention, indigestion, gas, or constipation. Liver-Fire is caused by excess heat in the Liver and can cause explosive emotional outbursts, tinnitus, dizziness, headaches, insomnia, dryness, constipation, and a red complexion. The Liver is also responsible for healthy muscles, tendons, and joints. If there is Liver-Blood deficiency, the muscles, tendons, and joints are deprived of moisture and nourishment, which can cause pain, impaired movement, cramps, numbness, tremors, and weakness. Liver-Blood deficiency also causes a pale complexion, insomnia, brittle nails, and dry skin and hair. Liver-Wind results from extreme heat that generates Wind, a deficiency of Liver-Yin with excess Liver-Yang, or deficiency of Liver-Blood. Liver-Wind manifests as dizziness, numbness, uncontrollable movements such as tremors, tics, spasms and convulsions, and paralysis.

Lungs: The Lungs govern respiration and Qi derived from air, control circulation in the energy channels and blood vessels, and influence body fluids. If Lung-Qi is strong, circulation will be adequate and provide warmth to the extremities. Lung-Qi deficiency manifests as shortness of breath, coughing, pale complexion, excess coolness, and fatigue. The aspect of Lung-Qi that protects the body against invading pathogens is called Wei-Qi, which is similar to the Western concept of the immune system. The Lungs are easily damaged by dryness and depend on moisture to function properly. Lung-Yin deficiency causes dry coughs and dry skin, thirst, spontaneous sweating, and feelings of excess heat.

Spleen/Pancreas: The Spleen filters blood and is a primary organ of the immune system. The Pancreas produces insulin to regulate blood sugar levels and enzymes to digest food. However, in TCM these two organs are regarded as one and referred to as the Spleen. The Spleen transforms food into Qi and blood, providing nourishment and energy for all cells and organs. The Spleen promotes production of body fluids and regulates and maintains all body functions. When Spleen-Qi is strong, the digestive system works well to provide nourishment, strength, and energy from food. Spleen-Qi deficiency results in poor digestion, abdominal bloating and gas, loose stools, low energy, and muscle weakness. Since the Spleen regulates the transformation and movement of fluids and blood, weak Spleen-Qi results in the accumulation of fluids with excess dampness or phlegm, edema, and abnormal bleeding. Spleen-Yang deficiency is similar to weak Spleen-Qi, but there is also a general lack of warmth throughout the body.

Kidneys: The Kidneys store a vital Essence that determines our basic constitution, vitality, physical strength and endurance, reproductive ability, and will power. Kidney Essence deficiency can result in birth defects, physical and mental retardation, osteoporosis, premature aging and graying of hair, and senility. Kidney Essence controls the growth of bones and bone marrow, and in TCM, the brain is viewed as a type of marrow regulated by the Kidneys. Strong Kidney Essence nourishes the brain, promotes clear mental function and cognition, supports the reproductive system, and nourishes bones and teeth.

The Kidneys are the foundation of Yin and Yang for the other organs. Kidney-Yin is the fundamental substance necessary for birth, growth, and reproduction. It is the origin of water in the body and regulates all types of fluids. Kidney-Yin deficiency causes dizziness, tinnitus, memory loss, night sweats, backaches, general dryness, or constipation. Kidney-Yang provides the energy and heat necessary for all body functions, and is the source of fire and warmth in the body. Kidney-Yang deficiency results in coldness, weak legs, sore back, edema, fatigue, infertility and other reproductive problems, excessive urination, or loose stools.

Although it is a radically different perspective compared to Western medicine, TCM invites us to open our minds to another way of viewing and understanding our bodies. If you wish to dive deeper into the fascinating study of Traditional Chinese Medicine, I highly recommend reading books by Giovanni Maciocia, beginning with *The Foundations of Chinese Medicine*, an extraordinary classic explaining TCM in a very simple and easy-to-understand manner.

Primary Actions

This section of the Materia Medica provides the medicinal uses and specific indications for each herb, from the most popular uses to those that are more antiquated. Specific health issues are underlined to assist the reader with quick references. Pertinent research studies are cited from clinical trials involving human subjects and from laboratory research, including *in vitro* lab experiments conducted in test tubes and petri dishes and *in vivo* or animal-based trials.

Laboratory experiments involving animals are often employed for research studies. Scientists find animal research to be helpful in understanding how herbs work, but many animals suffer and die in these trials. There are definitely ethical considerations to experimenting with animals. Many years ago, an animal rights activist asked me not to cite animal studies in my book as a protest against animal testing. Although I agreed with many of his views, I decided that since the animals had already been sacrificed, it is reasonable to benefit from what was learned so that their sacrifice might not be in vain. Let us be grateful to the animals sacrificed for human benefit, and attempt to purchase products made without animal testing.

Teachings from the Plant Devas

Deva is a Sanskrit word meaning "being of light." Master gardener Machaelle Small Wright describes a deva as "an intelligent level of consciousness within nature that functions as the architect within all form." Devas are the underlying, innate substance of life, the etheric blueprint or design of material form and structure. Just as plants have the amazing ability to transform sunlight into roots, stems, leaves and flowers, devas are intelligent beings of light who transform their etheric essence into form and structure. One may think of devas as the Creator's angels that assist in creating and sustaining all forms of life.

When the mind is still and the heart abides in compassion, there is an open portal into the devic realms where communication with the plants is possible.

When writing about each herb in the Materia Medica, I requested teaching from the deva of that plant and recorded what I heard. Some of the information I received was familiar, but much was original and brought me to a more profound and expanded understanding of the plants' core essences. This aspect of the book has certainly been the most interesting and illuminating one for me because the deva teachings are a unique and poetic insight that few herbals offer.

Spending time with plants in the wilds and in gardens, growing them, watching them mature and move through their life cycles, and preparing and using them for healing naturally opens the "doors of perception," offering us greater understanding and closer relationships with the medicinal herbs. Getting acquainted with the plant devas involves an open heart and mind, trust in one's intuition, and eventually the experiential "knowing" that plants are conscious beings that reside and resonate in a more etheric, subtle vibrational capacity than most humans possess in this day and age. It has only been through continual interaction with the herbs over many years that I have come to understand and live this reality. I would venture to say that almost everyone has the ability to listen and hear the messages of the plants if we practice and choose to open ourselves to this possibility.

Prior to industrialization, when people depended exclusively on Nature for all their needs and lived in close contact with their environment, our ancestors were innately in tune with the subtle energies of life. The ability to hear teachings of the plants was more of a commonplace and accepted reality. The plants certainly choose to interact and communicate with us, and are happy to do so, for part of their purpose of being on earth is to assist animals and humans. Most of us struggle with our fears and limited, deluded views of reality. I always encourage people to trust the wisdom of their intuition and allow Nature to show us a rational, life-affirming approach to existence. Realize that when the mind is still and the heart abides in compassion, there is an open portal into the devic realms where communication with the plants is possible.

The best way to practice communication with plants is two-fold. First, simply relax and allow the smooth, unhampered flow of energy to move through your body. Help this process by nourishing your body with healthy organic food, developing calm emotions and mental stability, engaging in meditation and prayer, and using sound techniques like singing and chanting to "tune up" to the higher frequencies and intelligence of the plant devas. The idea that plant deva awareness and intelligence exceeds that of most humans may be an unusual and humbling thought, but in my own experience it is quite true. The second ingredient in communicating with the devas is to spend time enjoying Nature and being with the plants. Play in the garden, take walks, and speak your heart-felt truth and needs to the plants. Feel gratitude for all the gifts they offer. Open your heart and mind to the possibility of receiving their blessings and hearing their teachings. Then sit with a quiet and receptive mind, a calm heart, be still, and listen. Take time and have patience . . . .

As I met the devas of the medicinal herbs, it became obvious that they each express a unique message, presence, and personality. For the purpose of writing this book, I asked the plant devas to describe who they are, and the following explanation was the response. For those who may not accept or know the reality of the plant devas, enjoy reading these sections as parables or stories to illustrate the diverse qualities of the herbs and provide insight into their healing actions.

Teachings from the Mother Guardian of the Plant Kingdom

"I am the mother and guardian of the plant kingdom who speaks to you now. Creator put the plants and healing herbs here eons back in time, in part for survival of the animals and humans, and in part because plants are the natural manifestation of my Being of abundance and generosity. The green ones are a blueprint of Creator's patterns, showing the unity and grace arising from Creator's mind. The plants are for food, healing, and shelter, and they serve as a pattern or pathway for humans to follow in the ways that lead to happiness and peace in life.

"Plants are intelligent beings. That is to say, we have genetic encoding, as do humans, that guides our evolution and existence on the planet. Plants are indeed the messengers of light and healing, bringing harmony and balance to all who partake of our benefits by growing us, observing our life cycles, using us for food and healing, and by simply enjoying our beauty.

"The plant devas wish people to know that we do not push ourselves on anyone, and all who come to learn do so voluntarily and of free will, for this is a planet of free will. Therefore, we do not wish to scare or startle people, but our presence is real. We are of a different form or vibration than humans and do not have the physical structure of humans. However, we do have what you would call heart, mind, and soul capacity, and it is just like yours, except ours is more perfectly balanced and aligned. Therefore, we resonate on a different level than the physical plane. But it is quite easy for humans to experience us in different sensual, mental and intuitional ways, according to each person's capabilities and awareness. All that is necessary is to have an open mind to the possibility, and learn to still the mind so thoughts are not chattering and fluttering every which way. This may be a major first step for many, but it is quite necessary for a peaceful and happier life, so it is well worth the time to sit quietly, learn a meditation of some kind, and practice stilling the mind and cultivating the ability to focus the attention one-pointedly, to stay focused for a period of time. Then, with a still mind, come sit by us. Smell, feel, and see us in our physical forms as the plants. Open your heart to us and we are here for you at all times. You simply have to invite us in and be still enough to experience and acknowledge us. We are all gentle, though some, especially the protector trees, are more masculine and mighty, but all are benevolent beings whose only purpose is to bless the earth with our presence, glorify Creator, and serve the living beings who have need of us. Thus, we are all interconnected as one family, all from Creator.

"Sitting next to a growing herb, being quiet and listening, is one of the best ways to learn the lessons of the plants. Most people lack this relationship at this time, which is one reason for the current confusion and lack of balance in the modern world. The secrets of the plants ultimately will never be learned by examination under the microscope, but by examination through the heart and senses, through smelling, touching, tasting, and sitting quietly to listen. All who approach and dwell with the plants in this way will receive deep healing emotionally, mentally, and spiritually. The heart especially will be touched, and these people will experience the deep love of the plants and the Earth Mother for all her children. Yes, the plants are an intermediary between Creator and the people. The plants point the way to beauty, balance, grace, and healing for all who will rest and listen to these 'little ones.'

"The plants are your friends and serve in many ways. They heal vibrationally, which means that the energetic vibrations of the plant body resonate to the patterns of the human body to heal and balance. Know that the plant kingdom resonates and vibrates the color green and the qualities of the heart, which are compassion and love. It is from this quality that the plants are enduring and tenacious in their growth, and the abundance of their gifts provides all the sustenance and materials people and creatures need to survive on this planet. Plants connect the earth and the heavens, just as the human heart connects and integrates the earthly personality with the higher energies of generosity, love, and wisdom. In this way, the plants serve as intermediaries and guides through the journey of wholeness and completion (the 'enbrightening' of each individual) simply by following the patterns and rhythms flowing from Creator. The earth must be treated as a huge garden, and my plants tended and nurtured to continue the symbiotic relationship of life.

"Because all plants reflect the qualities of the heart, the plant devas also emanate compassion and love, and many other qualities also. But at their core is always the heart, the heart of the Great Mother. In the footpath of all who have tread before, you continue the journey of healing through the herbal plants. Blessed be your journey, for this is the journey of the heart which returns you to the Mother, the great heart and healer of all life. We plants are the torch-bearers. We are a way to a quiet mind, a peaceful heart, and gentle steps that do no harm to the planet or the creatures upon it. To all people who follow this path, we offer love, gentleness, protection, and health."

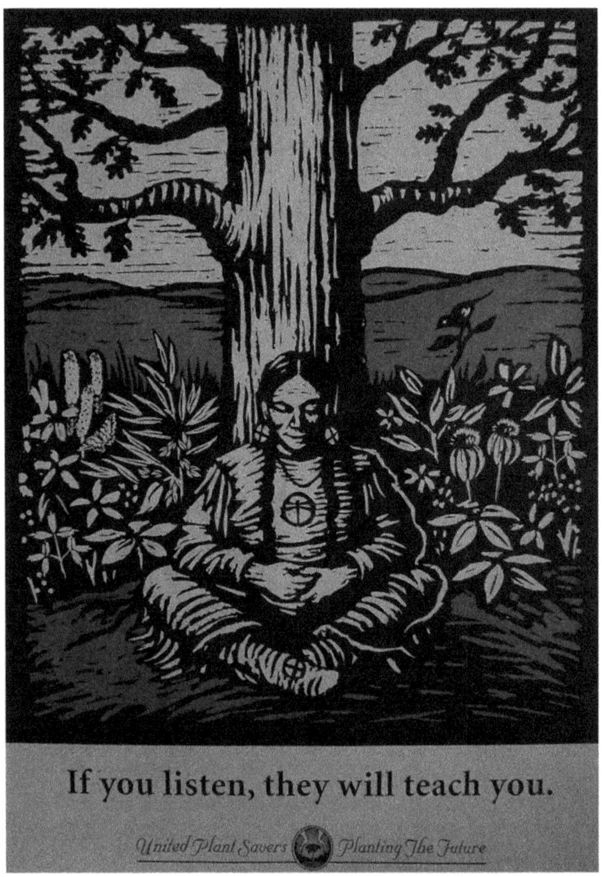

If you listen, they will teach you.
United Plant Savers
Planting The Future

Kevin Morgan, artist
Courtesy of United Plant Savers

In their teachings about medicinal herbs throughout the Materia Medica, the devas share their unique and vast perspective of life in a language of their own, often making references to the astrological signs and planets, the vibrational frequencies of the color spectrum, and the chakras or energy centers in the human body. Further study into these subjects will help to understand the devas' insights and messages.

The devas also frequently mention the "essence of flowers" (meaning flower essences) and invite the reader to prepare an essence of flowers to use for subtle energetic healing and alignment of the body, mind, and emotions. Flower essences are easy and enjoyable to prepare (see instructions on pages 128-129), and many people experience transformational healing at deep, core levels when ingesting this type of flower preparation.

How to Use Herbs for Healing and Daily Health Care

This chapter offers helpful suggestions and safety guidelines for incorporating herbs into your daily life. **By following the holistic perspective and model, you will gain the greatest benefits from using medicinal herbs and experience more success in establishing health and healing root causes of problematic conditions and disease.** Refer to **"The Holistic Perspective ~ Living and Healing in Holism"** at the beginning of this book (pages xiii-xv) for a thorough explanation of the meaning of holism and its application in health care and the practice of herbalism.

The wise use of herbal remedies can drastically reduce the need for doctor appointments, antibiotics, and other pharmaceuticals with potential side effects. Botanical medicines offer improved physical and emotional well-being, empower us to be more responsible for our own health, and support us with their healing potential. There are many ways to receive their benefits, from enjoying a cup of tasty herbal tea to treating serious illness. Herbs touch our lives in subtle ways as culinary delights and ingredients in many shampoos, hair conditioners, body lotions, soaps, deodorants, toothpaste, perfumes, and aromatherapy.

It is my wish that the following pages will guide you in exploring the healing path of the medicinal herbs and partaking of their gifts. May you embrace the plants with an open heart and mind to fully benefit from them, and share your experience with others. In this manner, the ancient healing ways of the plants and those who lived according to this wisdom will continue to flourish. Enjoy the journey!

Health Depends on Good Nutrition and a Strong Digestive System

"Let your medicine be your food, and your food be your medicine."
Hippocrates, the father of Western medicine

Nutritious food is the foundation of health and well-being. The saying, "you are what you eat," is true because foods and fluids that we consume are broken down by enzymes in the digestive system to provide raw materials for the creation and maintenance of every cell in the body. Conscious eating not only promotes greater vitality, emotional calm and mental acuity, it also optimizes the healing potential of herbs. Nourishing foods and medicinal herbs work together and increase each other's effectiveness. People with chronic health issues often suffer from poor diet and problems with digestion and elimination. Repairing a weak digestive system is a primary step on the road to all recovery. As dietary choices, digestion and elimination improve, more nutrients from food and medicinal herbs become available to restore and heal the body and mind.

The most basic, health-promoting diet is the "**ancestral diet**" of organic, unrefined and unprocessed meat, fish, dairy, whole grains, legumes, raw nuts and seeds, and sun-ripened fruits and vegetables. People should adjust this ancestral diet according to individual needs, such as being vegetarian, avoiding gluten and dairy foods, and eliminating problematic foods. Most importantly, **avoid all foods** that are genetically modified (GMO), grown with herbicides and pesticides, and contain chemical preservatives, flavors, and colors. Scientific studies confirm that these are hazardous to human health and the environment. When indigenous people change from their ancestral diets to modern processed foods, it is well documented that their health deteriorates and chronic, degenerative conditions develop. **Remember these important dietary guidelines:**

1) Eat a wide variety of raw fruits and vegetables daily, and lightly steam or sauté additional vegetables.

2) Avoid excess sugars (especially cane and corn syrup sugars); use honey, agave, and stevia (a plant).

3) Cook with coconut and olive oil, eat healthy fats from raw nuts and seeds, avoid hydrogenated oils and deep fried foods. Heated fats and oils become rancid over time and damage cells. Eat healthy EPA-DHA oils.

4) Protein occurs in dairy products, greens and other vegetables, nuts, seeds, beans, legumes, grains (especially quinoa and amaranth), and spirulina and chlorella (fresh water algae high in chlorophyll). Plant proteins are easier to digest than meat. Red meat is more acidic and tends to promote inflammation.

5) Remember that dairy, sugar, and gluten in many grains increase mucous production and inflammation. More people are becoming sensitive to milk and gluten, and feel better after eliminating these.

6) Increasing levels of heavy metals and radiation in oceans now make eating sea fish and seaweeds risky and detrimental to health!

7) A high-potency natural vitamin and mineral supplement provides nutrients you may not be getting in your diet because soil has become depleted and modern-day stresses deplete nutrients from our body.

All too often, food choices are determined by the dictates of our desires, addictions, and mental attitudes rather than by the nutritional requirements of our bodies. An interesting experiment to try for a few days is to ask yourself, before taking a bite of each different food, "Will this nourish me or weaken me?" Eat only what nourishes you. Discover how much your diet does or does not change.

Be Wise and Balanced in Your Health Care Choices

Do not embrace the extremist attitude that herbs are the only source of healing and decide to abandon the medical system, physicians, and pharmaceutical drugs! The best health care system is one that encompasses many different modalities. Use common sense and maintain balance when combining herbal therapy and modern medicine. Do not try to heal a serious infection or disease with herbs alone, especially if herbal therapy is not initiated until the intermediate or more advanced stages. Infections can be damaging and occasionally life-threatening, and antibiotics may be necessary. Diagnostic tests available through medical doctors and hospitals can provide vital information to identify problems, which may then be treated with herbal therapies or may require pharmaceutical medicines. Herbal remedies can often be taken in conjunction with pharmaceutical medicines for specific problems. Herbs can reduce many side effects of drugs or medical therapies such as chemotherapy and radiation. For the most comprehensive health care, blend herbal healing with the benefits offered by the modern medical system.

Check your community resources for knowledgeable, compassionate, and trustworthy health care professionals. When locating a medical doctor, choose one who is open to herbal and other complementary modalities, allowing a comfortable patient-doctor relationship in which you can honestly communicate your ideas, needs, and activities. If you visit holistic practitioners, be sure to inquire about their training, credentials, and experience. There is a rising number of holistic health professionals who are adequately educated in herbal and holistic therapies, including holistic nurse practitioners and naturopathic doctors trained in four-year post-graduate schools. Always remember that you hire your doctor and other health professionals – they work for *you*. Never allow yourself to be disempowered or coerced by overbearing authority figures. Choose health professionals who are respectful of you and your choices, willing to take time to talk and answer your questions, and who are interested in working with you to develop a successful plan of care.

Gather Reliable Information

Take advantage of valuable resources that are available to expand your knowledge of the healing properties and correct application of medicinal herbs. There are many excellent herb books and magazines on the market. The best ones are typically written by professional organizations that produce herbal monographs and by herbalists and professional health practitioners who use herbs in their clinical practice and personal lives. Libraries, bookstores, herbal organizations, and the Internet are good sources of information.

Search your community for people involved with herbs who are willing to share their expertise. Look for herbalists and holistic health care professionals, and ask your friends if they have any experience with herbs. Visit your local health food stores, ask the clerks for assistance, and check out their books and research information. Herbal classes and apprenticeship programs offer some of the best educational and experiential opportunities. If you are fortunate enough to locate elderly folks who used herbs during their youth, or Native Americans willing to share their knowledge, you can gain wonderful information and hear great stories of their healing experiences.

Start Using Herbs Slowly and Do Not Be Overwhelmed

If you are new to the awesomely extensive world of herbs, there is no need to feel overwhelmed by all the possibilities and initial confusion. Relax and start slowly by getting acquainted with a few herbs at a time. Gradually expand your knowledge and use of different herbs. If you proceed slowly and experience the herbs with regular use, you will accumulate wisdom and expertise over time. After reading about the herbs in the Materia Medica, you may find a few that particularly "call to you" and fulfill your medical and health needs. Start working with these. Most importantly, have fun with the herbs while being respectful of their healing potential.

Obtaining Medicinal Herbs

Essentially, there are three options for obtaining medicinal herbs. The most enjoyable and exciting way is to grow and process them yourself (see the chapters on "Cultivating Medicinal Herbs" and "Creating Herbal Preparations"). This obviously requires time and effort, but the benefits of gardening, knowing the plants through a more personal relationship, and making top-quality herbal teas and preparations in your kitchen are so worthwhile! Creating your herbal medicines is not only fun and empowering, but cost-effective. Wildcrafting, the art of harvesting plants growing in the wild, is another way to obtain herbs (refer to the chapter on "Sustainable Harvesting of Medicinal Herbs"). Purchasing botanicals is the third option.

Be selective when purchasing herbs or other supplements – you get what you pay for. I always encourage people to buy from health food stores, health professionals, or manufacturers who sell reliable brands produced with high standards of quality control. Top-quality herbal products are more expensive, but the cost is worth the superior potency and healing activity. People who buy cheaper brands of discount herbs often discover that they do not work and come to the erroneous conclusion that herbs are ineffective. Read all herbal and supplement labels carefully before making your purchases. Unfortunately, many supplement manufacturers sell inexpensive herbal products loaded with unnecessary fillers, artificial colors and flavors, and use poor-quality herbs that have not been grown or processed in ways that optimize their medicinal properties. Be careful of some mail-order catalogs and multi-level marketing that make misleading statements about their products, claiming that they are "cure-alls." There are many high-quality herbal products on the market, so be sure to make wise choices.

Remember that herbs slowly deteriorate and lose potency after being harvested. The amount of time in which they maintain effective biological activity is called their "**shelf life**." Many herbal preparations on the commercial market provide their shelf life, also known as the expiration date, on their labels. Always check the expiration date when purchasing herbs. Dried leaves and flowers have a shelf life of 6 months to 2 years before they start losing their potency. Dried roots are most potent for 2-4 years. Salves last 1-3 years before the oils start smelling rancid, and tinctures (alcohol extracts) last indefinitely due to the alcohol content.

Drink Herbal Teas as Part of Your Daily Routine

Sipping a cup of tasty herbal tea is a refreshing way to start the day. It provides an opportunity to pause during our busy daily activities, and can be calming in the evening. With each sip of tea, the warmth settles in the stomach and the pleasant odor elicits deep inner feelings of comfort and contentment. Drinking tea can provide a time of pleasant social interaction or a chance for quiet relaxation to reflect and be still. The Japanese have refined tea drinking to a wonderful art form called the Tea Ceremony, in which tea is prepared and served as a meditation in peaceful silence.

Harvesting herbs from your own garden is an amazing luxury! Fresh garden herbs brewed into tea offer delicious flavors and aromas. An ever-expanding variety of dried herbal teas can be purchased at health food stores in bulk, which is the most cost-effective form, or prepackaged in tea bags. Even major supermarkets carry packaged herbal teas on their shelves, and most are fairly inexpensive.

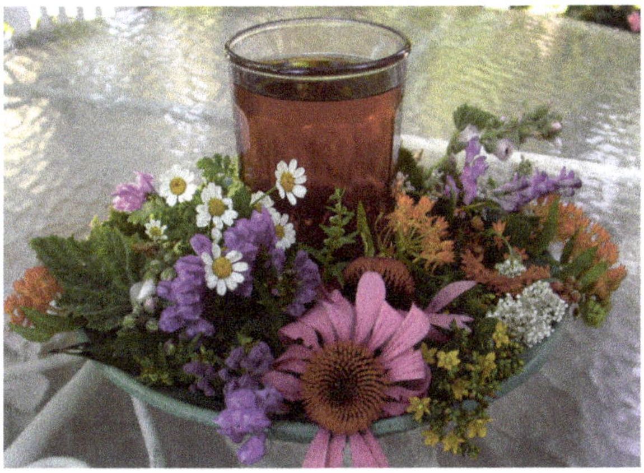

Herbal teas offer excellent replacements for coffee, soda, and fruit juices. The mild teas are delicious, packed with vitamins and minerals, and especially beneficial for children. Current research confirms that highly sweetened fruit juices and soda pop contribute to tooth decay, weaken immunity, and promote sugar craving resulting in excessive sugar intake and unhealthy blood sugar levels. Additionally, soda is very acidic, depleting calcium, magnesium, and other minerals from bones, and it has absolutely no nutritional value (confirm this by reading the label).

Herbal teas can be enjoyed as tasty beverages or employed for healing specific ailments. When used for medicinal purposes, teas are usually more concentrated and stronger tasting, although a light and delicate-tasting tea can also have valuable medicinal effects. Ingesting tea allows herbs to have direct contact with the throat and lining of the stomach and intestines, which can be particularly helpful for sore throats and digestive problems.

Some herbal teas that are especially tasty and mild enough to use on a regular basis include Stinging Nettle (*Urtica dioica*), Chamomile (*Matricaria recutita*), Licorice (*Glycyrrhiza glabra*), Raspberry leaf (*Rubus idaeus*), Chicory (*Cichorium intybus*), Green tea (*Camellia sinensis*), Ginger root (*Zingiber officinalis*), Rose Hips (*Rosa* spp.), and mints like Peppermint (*Mentha x piperita*) and Lemon Balm (*Melissa officinalis*). Many companies offer delicious teas combining several different herbs. Try a variety of herbal teas to discover which ones you like best, and incorporate them into your daily routine. Mother Nature invites you to drink her herbal nectars!

Do Not Use Herbs as a "Quick Fix"

Like anything else, herbs can be used inappropriately. Rather than being employed as part of a holistic program that includes dietary and lifestyle considerations, herbs are sometimes taken as a temporary "quick fix" that does not necessarily contribute to long-term health. Unfortunately, it has become too easy to simply take a pill to "cure" or cover up distressing symptoms of illness, while neglecting to identify and heal the underlying causes. How many television commercials advertise drugs for pain, anxiety, depression, arthritis, digestive problems, high cholesterol and hypertension, but fail to suggest addressing the fundamental causes of these problems? Hopefully, more physicians and other health care professionals are talking to their patients about the importance of nutritious food, regular exercise, happy relationships, and relaxing and reducing stress, all necessary for the creation of strong bodies and vibrant health.

An example of moving beyond the "quick fix" solution can be illustrated by the experience of a young woman who came to my office many years ago complaining of distressing stomach pain, indigestion, and nausea on a daily basis for several months. She had been to different doctors and spent several thousand dollars on medical tests, only to be told that her tests showed nothing wrong. During all this testing, no one had inquired about her diet. When I asked what she generally ate during the course of her day, she replied that her breakfast consisted of a Pepsi and sweet roll. Lunch and dinner were frequently fast foods with more Pepsi, a lot of fried foods, and very few fruits and vegetables. Rather than giving her a "quick fix" attempt at herbal therapy, it was obvious that the first line of business was to improve the terribly deficient diet that caused her so much suffering. After a few weeks of improved nutrition and drinking Peppermint, Chamomile, and Stinging Nettle teas, she was delighted to be free of pain and all other previous complaints.

People often come to my office complaining of depression, wanting St. John's Wort *(Hypericum perforatum)* to "make it go away." I first like to congratulate them and say that their body is responding appropriately! The depression is a signal that something is out of balance and in need of resolution. It is the body's way of bringing awareness to an inner problem that might otherwise go unnoticed. Although pharmaceutical and herbal medicines can help relieve depression, complete healing usually comes with the willingness to explore and resolve the deeper causes of the problem. I always encourage people to follow this sensible route and seek counseling while they are using St. John's Wort or other herbal and pharmaceutical support for depression, anxiety, and other mood disorders.

Most dedicated herbalists assert that our ecological stewardship to the plants requires us to use them in responsible and respectful ways by taking good care of ourselves when we elicit their assistance for healing. Herbs promote wellness by their ability to restore balance in the body. This balance is regulated and determined by our lifestyle, eating habits, exercise, relationships, and emotional and mental states. Be mindful of working at this deeper level, and always address the underlying causes of health concerns when using medicinal herbs.

How to Use Herbs for Acute Health Problems

Acute illnesses and injuries are those of short duration and include the common cold, flu, fevers, bacterial and viral infections, and hive-like rashes. Herbal treatments for acute problems are often remarkably effective and can greatly accelerate the healing process while reducing the severity of symptoms. Suggestions for treating acute problems include the following:

*Have an herbal first aid kit at home and for travel that is handy for emergencies and initial signs of illness.

*Start using the appropriate herbs as soon as you feel yourself getting sick. Parents can teach their children to let them know as soon as they start feeling bad. Herbs have much greater ability to eliminate bacterial and viral infections when taken during the initial stages of illness instead of trying to subdue a full-blown infection.

*Herbs must be taken in substantial quantities several times throughout the day for best results. When symptoms of illness are subdued, taper off the amount and frequency of herbal preparations, but continue to use smaller amounts twice a day for 3-5 more days. When the invading pathogen starts losing its strength and is killed off, symptoms improve and people tend to stop using herbal remedies. But just as prescription antibiotics are to be taken for the full course, herbal preparations should be continued to ensure complete elimination of the pathogen and full recovery.

*Symptoms should improve within 1-3 days if you are using the appropriate herbal formula. If they do not, notify your health care practitioner and start a different formula.

*Do not take tonic formulas during acute illness. Tonics strengthen the body over a period of time and are used for chronic problems. For acute ailments, treatment is focused on moving and releasing infectious pathogens to the exterior of the body, not on toning the body or treating chronic problems. In Traditional Chinese Medicine, it is believed that tonic herbs can "lock" fever and pathogens in the body and therefore should not be used during times of acute fevers and infections.

*Eat a light diet of organic, sun-ripened fruits and vegetables and plant-based proteins when sick. Avoid dairy products, fatty and fried foods, sugar, gluten, and red meat because they increase mucous production and inflammation throughout the body, and tend to have a clogging and constipating effect. A light diet during illness promotes cellular cleansing and restoration for faster recovery and increases the therapeutic potential of herbal remedies. A vegetarian diet is usually most effective for healing digestive and other problems.

How to Use Herbs for Chronic Health Problems

Chronic diseases continue over long periods of time and do not necessarily improve or completely resolve. Examples are asthma, emphysema, allergies, hypothyroidism (low thyroid function), herpes, arthritis, psoriasis, cancer, HIV/AIDS, lupus, diabetes, heart disease, and hypertension. Herbal treatment for chronic problems often consists of a formula of tonic herbs combined with other herbs that address specific issues. Formulas are taken over a period of time to restore greater balance within the body and create gradual improvement of symptoms. The herbal preparation, whether taken as tea, tincture, pill or capsule, is usually ingested a few times each day.

The Western medical system and physicians tend to focus on drugs that reduce the severity of symptoms associated with chronic disease, but are often at a loss when it comes to identifying and healing the underlying causes and re-establishing balance within the body. Herbal therapy has much to offer in this area. When addressing chronic health issues, it is wise and often necessary to develop a protocol incorporating several complementary modalities such as dietary and lifestyle improvements, exercise, adequate rest and play, emotional and psycho-spiritual counseling, acupuncture, massage and other bodywork, and calming techniques like yoga, Tai Chi, Qi Gong, meditation, visualization, and breath work. Combining herbal therapy with this type of protocol allows far greater potential for healing. It is important to remember that chronic health problems develop over time and naturally require time to resolve. While it is best not to expect immediate results, always be open to the possibilities that herbs and a healthy lifestyle offer in balancing and healing the body and mind.

How to Take Herbal Preparations and Times of Administration

It is best to take herbs on an empty stomach to allow for optimal absorption. In this way, herbs do not have to compete with food in the digestive tract. Exceptions to this rule are Cayenne (*Capsicum annuum*) and any other strong or spicy herb that may irritate the stomach or intestines. In these cases, ingest Cayenne and other irritating herbs after eating a little food.

After taking herbal preparations, wait 15-20 minutes before eating to ensure maximum effectiveness. One of the best times to take herbal supplements is first thing in the morning before breakfast when the stomach is empty, and supporting ourselves with herbs is a productive way to start the day.

When taking a tincture, pill or capsule, swallow it with water or herbal tea. Children and adults who are sensitive to strong flavors can take herbs with diluted juices, but avoid tomato and citrus juices because their acidity can negatively affect the biochemistry of herbs. For similar reasons, avoid taking herbs with coffee, soda pop, or alcohol.

Always remove alcohol from tinctures for children, pregnant women, people with liver or kidney problems, recovering alcoholics, and others not wanting to ingest alcohol. Add the dose of tincture to a cup of boiling water, stir, and let it cool. Most of the alcohol evaporates off.

Take vitamin and mineral supplements with food during meals. An easy way to swallow vitamin and mineral pills is to thoroughly chew a bite of food, and just as you are ready to swallow, put the pill in your mouth and swallow it with the food.

If you are using prescription drugs, be sure to take these at different times than herbs and other supplements to reduce possible herb-drug interactions. Space them at least one to two hours apart. Do some research to verify that your prescription drugs are compatible with the herbs and other supplements being taken. Seek information from an herbalist, health care practitioner, or pharmacist if necessary. Since relatively little research has been done on herb-drug interactions, information may not be available. If this is the case, be sure to proceed slowly with small doses.

Take One New Supplement at a Time

Be cautious when starting new supplements or introducing additional herbs and other medications into your existing program. It is best to take each new supplement one at a time, unless you are under the supervision of a health care practitioner and instructed otherwise. This is a smart safety measure that helps prevent complications. After introducing a new herb for a few days without experiencing problems, other herbs or supplements can be added to your regimen.

Increase Dosages Gradually

Although most commercially sold herbs are generally regarded as safe when used in normal doses, it is important to remember that everyone is unique and some people experience food and plant sensitivities. Therefore, when taking an herb for the first time, be safe and begin with small dosages, gradually increasing to the dose recommended on the supplement label or by your health care practitioner. This safety precaution reduces the likelihood of adverse reactions, and is a good rule whenever taking herbs and other supplements for the first time. If an herb causes unpleasant side effects, discontinue it immediately until the problem can be resolved.

Give Yourself "Days Off" and Alternate Herbs

Do not take the same herbs over extended periods of time unless otherwise instructed by a health professional. It is wise to give the body a rest and allow yourself to take short breaks. This is usually not a problem since most people tend to be forgetful and naturally go through an occasional day without taking supplements. Use different herbs by alternating them every month or two. This reduces any tendency for the body to develop a diminished or heightened response to an herb. Tonic remedies are typically taken over time, but even they should be alternated with other formulas occasionally.

Combine common sense with the intention of healing when employing plant medicines. Be flexible enough to avoid rigid regimens that tend to be frustrating, while also being disciplined in remembering to take the herbs of your choice on a regular basis.

Do Not Detoxify When the Body Is Weak or Malnourished

This is an important consideration. Detoxifying or purging an already malnourished person can cause further complications, deterioration, and imbalance. The first step in healing is to nourish and strengthen the system by incorporating a nutritious diet and tonifying herbs such as Stinging Nettle (*Urtica dioica*), American Ginseng (*Panax quinquefolius*), Burdock root (*Arctium* spp.), or Astragalus (*Astragalus membranaceus*). After strengthening a weak system, the body has greater ability to detoxify, and the organs and channels of elimination have greater capacity for optimal function.

When Choosing Herbs, Consider the Qualities of the Illness and Match Them with the Corresponding Herbal Qualities

Deciding which herbs to take for specific problems involves an understanding of the dynamic energies of the human body and the medicinal plants. The energetic qualities of a disease (which is always the result of imbalance in the system) are matched with the appropriate qualities of herbal plants to re-establish balance and improve health. For example, with conditions of excess heat and dryness that can manifest as fevers, heartburn, menopausal hot flashes or red irritated skin rashes, avoid warming and drying herbs like Garlic (*Allium sativum*), Ginger, or Cayenne because they will further increase excess heat in the body. Instead, cooling herbs like Chickweed (*Stellaria media*) and the roots of Marshmallow (*Althaea officinalis*), Burdock, or Dandelion (*Taraxacum officinale*) would be a better choice for diminishing heat and increasing moisture to regain balance. Conversely, if a cold-natured person with poor circulation had the chills, warming herbs would be perfect to reduce the cold. Another example is Ginseng, which is often recommended for the relief of menopausal hot flashes. American Ginseng has cooler qualities than Asian Ginseng (*Panax ginseng*) and would be a wiser choice for relieving hot flashes.

The Traditional Chinese and Ayurvedic medical systems implement this art of balance at a high level of refinement. All herbal remedies in their pharmacopoeia and treatment modalities are based upon the system of energetic dynamics. For further study into these fascinating and enlightening traditions, refer to the Bibliography references for the chapter titled "The History of Herbalism and Early Medicine." The chapter on "Healing Qualities of Herbs" offers explanations of the various healing qualities of plants and their biological activity in people. In the Materia Medica section, the energetic qualities of each herb are provided and discussed to help the reader understand and make correct choices when working with herbs for specific health issues.

Confidence increases as you gain more experience with the plants.

Drinking herbs as daily teas and tonics or taking herbal remedies for acute illness becomes second nature and a welcome addition to a vibrantly healthy lifestyle!

American Centaury

Sabatia angularis

Gentianaceae (Gentian) Family

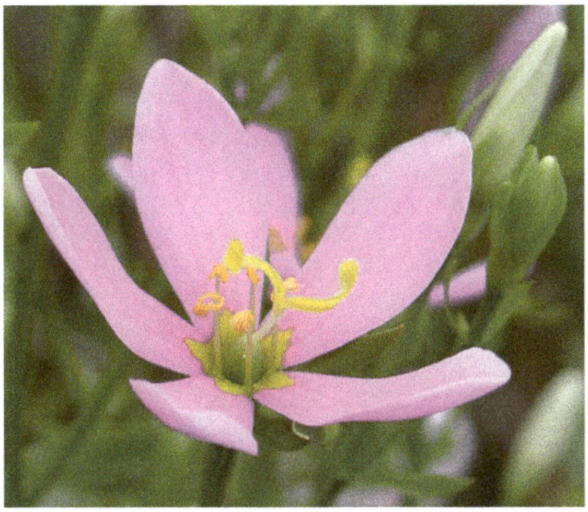

Common Names

Rose pink and rose gentian are common names descriptive of the lovely pink flowers. Bitterbloom, bitter clover, feverwort, felwort, and wild succory are antiquated names.

Medicinal Part of the Plant

Although the entire plant is medicinal, the leaves and flowers are the most frequently used parts.

Range and Habitat

There are several species of Centaury growing throughout North America, Europe, western Asia and North Africa, including *Sabatia angularis, S. stellaris, S. campanulata*, and *S. dodecandra*. European species also include *Centaurium umbellatum* (with pinkish-purple flowers), *C. pulchellum, C. minus,* and *C. erythraea* (also known as *Erythraea centaurium*). Several European varieties have naturalized in the United States. These different species are similar in appearance and medicinal properties, and can be used interchangeably.

American Centaury (*S. angularis*) grows in many parts of the United States. Most species of Centaury like damp, rich soil and grow in moist and swampy places. However, *S. angularis* also grows in drier areas under full sun in open fields and along roadsides.

Description of the Plant

American Centaury is an annual or biennial plant growing 1-2′ tall. The small fibrous root sends up an erect, stout, multi-branching square and angular stem, hence the species name *angularis*. The light-green leaves are ¼-1″ long, ovate in shape, hairless, and entire. The leaves and branching stems are opposite. Sessile leaves clasp the stem so tightly that they almost look joined together. Beautiful, delicate-looking pink flowers are radially symmetrical and have a yellow and pale green center. The leafy calyx at the base of each flower has 5 linear green sepals. Each flower is 1-1½″ wide and consists of 5 pink petals surrounding a central pistil. The pistil consists of a light-green ovary rising into an elongated yellow style that divides and ends in 2 twisted stigmas. Five long yellow stamens circle the pistil. The base of each pink petal is bright yellow, creating a lovely star-shaped pattern in the center of each flower. The multi-branching stems each bear a single flower at their tip, forming a loose corymb cluster of flowers towards the top of the plant. Flowers appear in varying shades of pink, from almost white to dark pink. They are sensitive to sunlight and open wide in daylight and close a bit at night.

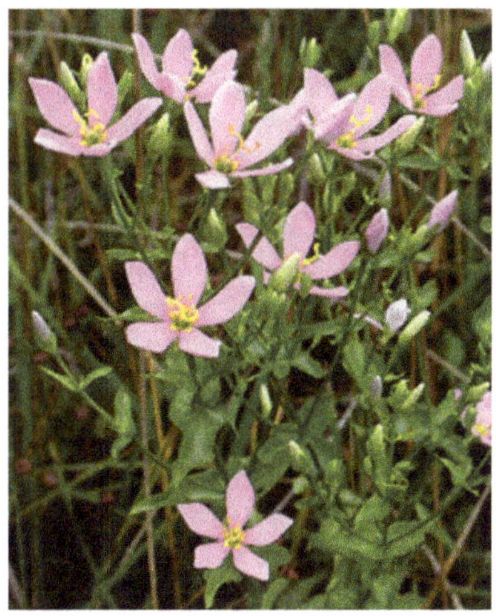

The plant blooms from June through September and is a lovely wildflower creating beautiful pink splashes of color in green fields and meadows. The fruit is a rounded capsule full of tiny seeds that fall close to the parent plant or can be blown further away by the wind. Plants tend to grow together in clustered communities.

The field in front of my log cabin is often adorned with the colorful beauty of American Centaury. I consider it somewhat of an "elusive" herb because it comes and goes, growing abundantly some years and completely disappearing at other times.

Cultivation

Cultivation of Centaury can be challenging because germination tends to be rather poor. Since it is not a widely commercialized medicinal, only seed companies specializing in herbs are likely to sell it. If the plant grows in the wild where you live, a good way to obtain seed is to harvest it from these plants.

Centaury likes to grow in full sun and fertile, moist soil. It prefers temperatures between 65-75°F for germination. For best results, plant the seeds on top of potting soil in a planting tray in early spring after danger of frost has passed. The tiny seeds are light dependent, so gently pat them into the soil without covering. Keep soil consistently moist and move the tray to full sunlight after germination. Use a fine mist to spray the germinating seeds, making sure not to damage them with an excessively forceful spray. Transplant the seedlings into a garden bed when they are 3-4″ high and space them about 10″ apart. Mulch around the plants with dry grass clippings, keep the roots moist, and pamper the babies! When the plants eventually mature and grow seeds, expand your garden by collecting these seeds and planting them.

Harvest

Harvest flowers and upper leaves for medicinal use when plants are in full bloom. Since this herb is becoming increasingly scarce, be sure to leave some flowers so they will develop seeds for future plants. Conservatively prune the aerial portions and refrain from harvesting the roots. By ensuring the continuation of the plant, there will be more to harvest in the future for you and others who follow in your path. Seeds can be collected when their pods are brown and dry if you wish to attempt growing them in a garden.

Preparation of Plant Medicine and Dosages

The freshly harvested leaves and flowers can be tinctured, made into tea, or dried for future use. Centaury yields its healing virtues to water and alcohol, so tea and tincture are good preparations. Tinctures are preferable because they retain their potency and have a much longer shelf life than the dried herb. All Centaury species taste very bitter, so taking a few swallows of the concentrated tincture diluted in water, rather than an entire cup of tea, is much easier on the palate for most people.

PREPARATIONS

Tea: Add 1-2 teaspoons of finely chopped fresh or dried leaves and flowers to 1 cup of boiling water and steep for 10-15 minutes. Dosage: ¼-1 cup of tea every few hours as needed.

Tincture: Stuff the finely chopped fresh herb into a glass jar and cover it with 60% 190-proof grain alcohol and 40% distilled water. Dosage: ¼-1 teaspoon in water 3 times a day as needed.

Chemical Constituents

The medicinal properties of American Centaury are similar to European Centaury. Most chemical analysis and research has been on the European species, *Centaurium erythraea* and *C. minus*. These contain phenolic acids, which include caffeic (anti-inflammatory, cholagogue, hepatoprotective), coumaric, ferulic (cholagogue, anti-inflammatory, hepatoprotective, immunostimulant), hydroxybenzoic (antibacterial), protocatechuic (antibacterial, hepatoprotective, immunostimulant), sinapic (antibacterial, hepatoprotective), syringic (antioxidant), and vanillic (anthelmintic, antibacterial, choleretic) acids.

Alkaloids include gentianine (analgesic, anti-inflammatory), gentianidine, and gentioflavine. Bitter glycosides are amarogentrin (hepatoprotective, sialogogue), erythrocentaurin, gentiopicrin (antimalarial), sweroside (antibacterial), and swertiamarin (antibacterial, cholagogue, hepatoprotective, pancreatic, sialogogue). Oleanolic acid is antimalarial, hepatoprotective, and anti-inflammatory. Sitosterol is also anti-inflammatory and hepatoprotective. Essential oils, flavonoids, magnesium, and potassium have also been identified in European Centaury.

Safety, Contraindications, and Drug Interactions

There are no known reports of toxicity when Centaury is taken in recommended dosages. Excessive amounts may cause gastrointestinal irritation, including nausea, vomiting, and diarrhea (Skenderi, 2003). It may be best to avoid use in cases of excess stomach acid and ulcers. The German Commission E herbal regulatory agency determined that it has no known side effects, contraindications, or interactions with drugs (Blumenthal, 1998). **Avoid Centaury during pregnancy because of its stimulating effect on the uterus.**

Medicinal Uses

History of the Plant

Many species of Centaury have been used medicinally throughout history, and some were believed to be powerful protectors against evil spirits. European species derive their genus name *Centaurium* from the name of the ancient centaur, Chiron, who was famous in Greek mythology for his skill in using medicinal herbs. Chiron used Centaury to heal a wound he suffered from a poisoned arrow. The plant was called "fel terrae" or "gall of the earth" due to its extremely bitter taste. The old English name "felwort" has the same meaning and was assigned to many plants in the bitter-tasting Gentian family.

Ancient Egyptians used Centaury to treat kidney stones and high blood pressure. It was a favorite medicine of the Greek physicians Dioscorides (*circa* A.D. 40–*c.* 90) and Galen (*c.* A.D. 131–*c.* 200), and the English herbalist and apothecary Nicholas Culpeper (1616–1654). They used Centaury for digestive ailments, obstructions and diseases of the liver, gallbladder and spleen, for fevers, parasites, wounds and poisonous bites, as a blood purifier, and to promote menstruation. Father Sebastian Kneipp (1821–1897), a famous German herbalist, recommended the herb for depression and calming the nerves. Eclectic physicians in the United States used American Centaury during the late 1800s–1930s for digestive problems, liver and gallbladder ailments, fevers, parasites, to promote menstruation, and to stimulate circulation. Eclectic doctor William Cook, M.D., wrote, "Its chief power is exerted upon the stomach, gall-ducts, and spleen; and the general circulation and uterus feel it moderately. A warm infusion gently promotes the menstrual secretion, in cases of debility. Cold preparations increase appetite and digestion in weak and flaccid conditions of the stomach, and may be used for chronic dyspepsia and general debility . . . . Its sustaining influence is shown to excellent advantage in the treatment of night sweats, and exhaustion from excess purulent discharges" (Cook, 1869).

European varieties of Centaury have the longest historic use and more scientific documentation because research has focused on these species. There are no clinical studies to date, only laboratory research. Centaury is more popular in Europe than in the United States, where it is not usually commercially available in medicinal preparations. Though not currently listed as an "at risk" herb, it is becoming rare in many areas due to loss of habitat.

Healing Qualities

Antibacterial, anti-inflammatory, antilithic, antiperiodic, aperitive, bitter tonic, carminative, cholagogue, depurative, diaphoretic, digestive stimulant, diuretic, emmenagogue, exanthematous, febrifuge, hepatic, laxative, nephritic, stomachic, vermifuge, and vulnerary. American Centaury belongs to the same family as Gentian (*Gentiana* spp.) and has similar, but slightly milder, properties.

Traditional Chinese Medicine (TCM) Perspective

Centaury affects the liver and spleen meridians and influences the stomach, spleen, pancreas, liver, gallbladder, and intestines. It is a bitter, drying, and cooling herb that clears heat and is stimulating and decongesting. It exerts Yang activity by promoting the smooth movement of Qi throughout the body and resolving stagnation.

Primary Actions

I primarily use American Centaury in formulas for stomach and digestive problems with excellent results. I regard it as a "kicker and mover" herb, whose superb stimulating properties create much movement throughout the body, especially in the throat, gastrointestinal, urinary, and circulatory systems. It is specific for problems caused by congestion, stagnation, and toxic excess.

Digestive System: The bitter flavor of all Centaury species promotes production and secretion of digestive enzymes and bile, which help digest and move food through the gastrointestinal tract, allowing normal digestion and absorption of nutrients. The herb is used for problems resulting from slow and sluggish digestion, including loss of appetite, indigestion, abdominal distension and bloating, flatulence (gas), and constipation. Centaury has a tonic effect and should be used over a period of time (3-5 weeks) for gradual improvement. Always take it on an empty stomach for best results. Drink ½-1 cup of tea or a dose of the tincture (¼-1 teaspoon in water) 5-10 minutes before each meal to stimulate the appetite and secretion of digestive enzymes, and to gradually improve function of all the digestive organs.

Stomach: Centaury is a common ingredient found in Swedish Bitters, a preparation of bitter-tasting herbs specific for stomach problems. The herb promotes gastric production of hydrochloric acid and pepsin to break down minerals and protein (Brinker, 2001). It increases gastric mobility to move stomach contents and is antiseptic to protect the stomach lining from infection. One research study found that a water and alcohol extract of *Centaurium erythraea* (European Centaury) reduced the size and severity of aspirin-induced stomach damage and ulcers by 77% in rats (Tuluce, 2011).

The lukewarm tea or tincture are excellent for dyspepsia (indigestion) and nausea, and stimulate a poor appetite during convalescence or in cases of anorexia. Centaury is not to be used in cases of excess stomach acid or ulcers caused by excess acid.

Pancreas: Centaury helps tone and strengthen the pancreas to enhance production and secretion of pancreatic enzymes necessary for digestion of carbohydrates, fats, and proteins. It also supports production of the pancreatic hormone insulin, which maintains normal blood sugar levels. Thus, it is beneficial for both hypoglycemia (low blood sugar) and diabetes (hyperglycemia).

Liver and Gallbladder: Like many bitter herbs, Centaury stimulates liver activity, bile production, and the flow of bile into the gallbladder. It clears excess dampness, heat, toxins, and congestion from the liver, and is helpful for indigestion, nausea, jaundice, constipation, elevated cholesterol and estrogen levels (both controlled by liver function), and the prevention of gallstones.

A group of researchers evaluated an alcohol extract of the leaves of *C. erythraea* for hepatoprotective activity against acetaminophen-induced liver toxicity in rats. An oral dose of 300 mg/kg/day for 6 days or a single dose of 900 mg/kg for one day exhibited a significant protective effect by lowering aspartate aminotransferase (AST), which is also called serum glutamic-oxaloacetic transaminase (SGOT); alanine aminotransferace (ALT), known as serum glutamic-pyruvic transaminase (SGPT); and lactate dehydrogenase (LDH) (Mroueh, 2004). These enzymes are markers of liver function and health. AST enzymes are found in tissues of the liver, heart, kidneys, brain, and muscles. ALT enzymes occur in the liver. LDH enzymes are present in most of the body's cells and help produce energy. When liver and other cells are damaged, these enzymes leak out in blood, resulting in increased levels.

Intestines: By stimulating bile flow and production of the other digestive enzymes, Centaury assists in breaking food down into small particles for easy absorption through the wall of the small intestines. It relieves abdominal bloating and gas, promotes intestinal mobility, and exerts a mild laxative effect reducing constipation.

As a vermifuge, the tea or tincture can help eliminate parasites from the gastrointestinal tract, and is especially effective against tape worms. It has been used to kill head and body lice by soaking the afflicted area in strong tea, tincture, or oil. For best results, combine Centaury with other antiparasitic herbs such as Wormwood (*Artemisia absinthium*), Black Walnut (*Juglans nigra*), Feverfew (*Tanacetum parthenium*), and Cloves (*Syzygium aromaticum*).

Kidneys, Detoxification, and Blood: The bitter alkaloids in Centaury alkalize the blood with minerals, reduce excess acids in the body, exert a tonic effect on the elasticity of blood vessels to enhance circulation, and stimulate blood flow through the kidneys. This promotes normal circulation and detoxification. The herb gently stimulates the ureters to contract and propel kidney stones out of the urinary tract. Researchers have observed that European Centaury (*C. erythraea*) exerts diuretic effects (Haloui, 2000).

Centaury has long been considered a blood purifier due to this cleansing and tonifying action on the liver, kidneys, and blood vessels. An old historical use of the herb was for the treatment of poisonous bites and stings. The plant can help relieve headaches, acne, and skin rashes caused by excess heat and toxins in the blood, liver and kidneys, which can manifest as headaches and skin eruptions.

Researchers in Portugal reported that infusion teas of European Centaury exhibit antioxidant properties (Valentao, 2003), which have a protective effect on cells throughout the body.

Women's Health: Centaury helps normalize menstrual cycles. It is an emmenagogue that promotes menstruation by stimulating the liver, uterus, and blood circulation. It relieves congestion, stagnation, and excess heat in the pelvis, and promotes estrogen clearance by the liver, which is beneficial for conditions of excessive estrogen such as uterine fibroids, endometriosis, and premenstrual syndrome (PMS).

Do not take this herb when pregnant due to its emmenagogue properties, which stimulate menstruation and can potentially cause a miscarriage, especially during early pregnancy.

Infection, Fevers, and Other Conditions of Excess Heat: The bitters and other constituents in Centaury exert a cooling effect throughout the body to reduce excess heat and inflammation (Berkan, 1991). It is a diaphoretic herb that reduces fevers by stimulating perspiration, which draws internal heat to the surface where it is released. It is especially helpful for people with a ruddy complexion suffering from conditions of excess heat. Ancient European physicians and the American Eclectic doctors used the herb to treat intermittent fevers and malaria, and it was substituted in place of quinine (Mabey, 1988). A group of Algerian researchers reported chemical constituents in European Centaury that reduce fevers (Lacroix, 1973).

A research team from the United Kingdom found that two glycosides occurring in the aerial parts of European Centaury, swertiamarin and sweroside, inhibit the growth of several bacteria, including *Bacillus cereus* (responsible for some types of food poisoning), *Bacillus subtilis* (found in soil and water), *Citrobacter freundii* (causing respiratory and urinary infections), and *Escherichia coli* (causing urinary tract infections, intestinal infections, and diarrhea). Swertiamarin was also found to be active against *Proteus mirabilis* (which can infect the kidneys and lead to the formation of kidney stones, and also cause wound, blood, and pneumonia infections) and *Serratia marcescens* (which can lead to urinary, respiratory, gastrointestinal, and wound infections). Sweroside also inhibited the growth of *Staphylococcus epidermidis*, which infects the skin (Kumarasamy, 2003).

For fevers and infection, combine Centaury with other febrifuge and antibacterial herbs such as Sage (*Salvia officinalis*), Yarrow (*Achillea millefolium*), Goldenseal (*Hydrastis canadensis*), or Boneset (*Eupatorium perfoliatum*) for best results.

Arthritis and Gout: Bitters in Centaury are cooling, anti-inflammatory, and reduce excess acid in blood and tissues. These qualities are helpful in relieving hot, swollen, painful joints. According to Traditional Chinese Medicine, joint problems are often related to liver imbalance, and the restorative action Centaury exerts on the liver also helps ease joint discomfort. Centaury can be combined with Feverfew (*Tanacetum parthenium*), Yucca (*Yucca* spp.), Turmeric (*Curcuma longa*), and other anti-arthritic herbs.

Wounds and External Uses: Since ancient times, Centaury has been ingested and applied externally to heal infected wounds, skin ulcers, varicose veins, poisonous animal bites and stings, poison ivy, eczema, rashes, hives, and other eruptive skin problems involving hot, red, inflamed tissues.

Teachings from the American Centaury Deva

"Greetings. I have been on this planet for quite a long time. My nature is gentle and quiet, and the pink and yellow colors of my flowers attest to my happy and joyful nature. I am rather gypsy-like; for I like to go from place to place, to appear and disappear. I am a wild thing and do not always grow well in gardens. The yellow color in the center of my flowers points to my affinity with the solar plexus in the center of the body that radiates the vibrational frequency of yellow. My primary influence is on the digestive system. My activity is that of movement, to move the energy of the solar plexus, to release constriction and stagnation, to stimulate enzymes of digestion, and to move food through the system. I am a nourishing being that helps the body accept nutrients to grow and prosper. The reddish-pink color of my petals is an indication of my action on the blood to improve its movement and circulation throughout the body. I also cleanse and stimulate the skin to remove blemishes. The cooling and drying nature of my being helps cool excess heat from the heart, blood and liver, and my free-flowing nature helps to move blood and other fluids. In fact, you may call me a 'free-flowing' herb. I am beneficial for all types of inability to move forward and for stagnation in the soul, emotions, and physical body. People of old knew and used me for many things, including the movement of poisons from the body.

"Although not commonly known, I work with the throat chakra and help movement come through the throat and voice. Thus, I can be helpful for the thyroid gland, and for difficulty with expressing and voicing one's truth. I assist with manifestation, not only of the voice but also of physical form, by helping to assimilate nutrients into form and structure. My work, therefore, is to help bring physical form and structure onto the planet. I also like to show humans the strength and benefit of living in communities, as I usually grow in communities with my brother and sister plants."

Throat and Voice: Shortly after learning from the plant deva about the influence American Centaury has on the throat and voice, I had an opportunity to test this information. A young woman, who confided that she was a victim of incest by her father several years earlier, came to my office complaining of depression, anxiety, nightmares, chronic soreness in her shoulders and neck, and feelings of insecurity and inability to express herself. She continued having an uncomfortable and unresolved relationship with her family, especially her father, and reported feeling extremely inhibited and unable to talk or express herself in his presence. We discussed the underlying emotional and psychological causes of her complaints, and I sent her home with American Centaury tincture, hoping it would help open the blocked energy in her throat and neck to relieve the chronic soreness and inhibition. After two weeks of taking three drops of the tincture three times daily, she noticed some major changes when she visited her family. For the first time, she was able to confront her father and tell him what she felt and thought about their history. A few weeks after this visit with her family, she shared with me that confronting her father helped her feel good about herself in refreshing and surprising ways. She experienced a new confidence and inner strength at her parent's home that continued to last, and she was obviously much happier than the first time I saw her. She reported that the chronic feelings of restriction locked in her throat, which made self-expression so difficult, had eased up, and the constant soreness in her neck and shoulders was fading. I was very impressed with the plant's ability to move energy through the throat and assist this woman in expressing herself more fully.

A few years later, I had another opportunity to observe American Centaury's beneficial actions on the throat and voice. A 27-year-old man came to my office complaining of depression. This was a chronic problem since childhood, primarily resulting from emotional trauma inflicted by his raging, abusive stepfather. Any show of fear or anger made his stepfather even more abusive, so the young man learned to stay quiet and maintain a "monotone" existence in which he did not dare express himself. He suffered from chronic fatigue, constant congestion, and excess mucous in his throat. I gave him American Centaury tincture and had him take 15 drops in water twice daily. Two weeks later, he reported developing a "tickling" cough in the back of his throat, and he experienced a few days of anger bordering on rage, which he confessed was "more anger than I have experienced in a long time." I felt that the American Centaury was probably doing its work by stimulating the flow of energy in the throat area, breaking up mucous and bringing up old emotions locked in his system. I recommended that he continue with the herb. When I saw him one month later, he reported that the tickle and cough in the back of his throat were completely gone and his voice was stronger and louder than ever before. He was able to speak more freely without feeling cautious and afraid. He reported that his relationship with his girlfriend was consequently going through many positive changes, for he was able to open up and finally express himself freely instead of always feeling inhibited. He was delighted with his progress and "new" voice, and he and his girlfriend are now happily married.

Astragalus

Astragalus membranaceus
Leguminosae (*Fabaceae*) (Legume or Pea) Family

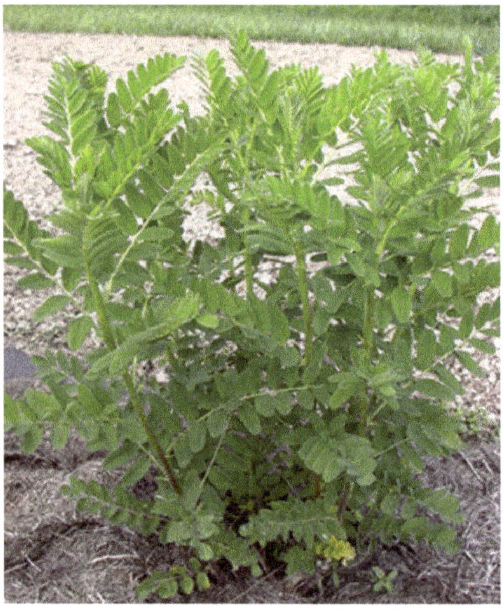

Common Names

Astragalus membranaceus and *Astragalus membranaceus* var. *mongholicus* are the official species used in Traditional Chinese Medicine (TCM) and are commonly known as Huang-Qi in China. Astragalus is called Ogi in Japan and Hwanggi in Korea. The North American Astragalus species known as milk-vetch and yellow vetch are not used medicinally.

Medicinal Part of the Plant

The roots are used for medicinal purposes.

Range and Habitat

Native to Mongolia, *Astragalus membranaceus* has naturalized in Northern China, Tibet, Siberia, Japan, and Korea where it grows along edges of forests, in open woodlands, grasslands, and on mountainsides. It is cultivated in many parts of the temperate world, including North America. There are over 1,750 species of Astragalus found in northern temperate zones throughout the world, and almost 400 North American species. They vary in their medicinal effects. Some are toxic and only a few have medicinal applications.

Description of the Plant

Astragalus membranaceus is a perennial that grows into an attractive, bushy plant up to 4′ tall. The rhizome root is long and branching with yellowish-brown outer skin. The yellowish-white interior is very tough and fibrous. Many rounded, angular, fibrous, erect stalks emerge from the root. The stalks are green and tinged with a dark-maroon hue. Pinnately compound leaves climb the stalk in an alternating pattern. The numerous leaflets are oblong, entire, pinnately veined, and sessile. The leaflets usually grow in 12-24 pairs with a terminal leaflet. Although the stem and leaves feel smooth, they are actually covered with soft, downy hairs visible under a 16X magnifying glass.

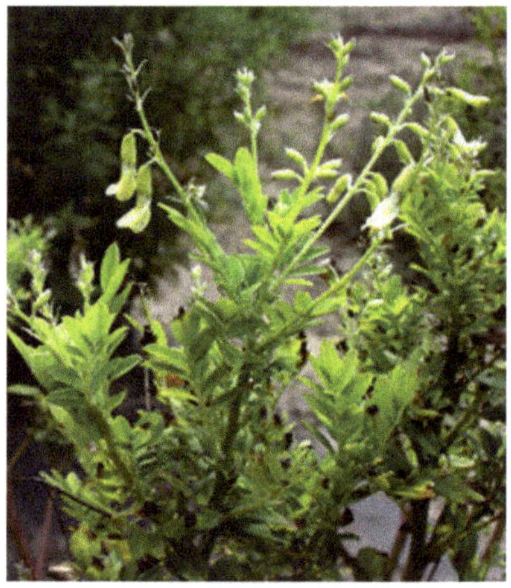

The small, creamy-yellow flowers are ½-1″ long and shaped like pea flowers. A yellowish-green calyx forms a cup that holds the tubular corolla, which opens into a bi-lobed upper lip and a tri-lobed lower lip. The flowers have very short stems attaching to the ends of stalks and form clusters of loose racemes. Flowers grow in an alternating pattern, and as few as 2 or as many as 22 appear on the stems. They mature into hairy, papery pods about 1″ long that turn brown when dry. These pods enclose several 1/8″ long seeds that are dark brown, hard, and kidney-shaped.

Astragalus membranaceus var. *mongholicus* has darker yellow flowers and hairless seedpods.

Cultivation

Astragalus is easy to cultivate because the seeds germinate well and the plant is hardy. It is very tolerant and able to survive in poor soil, drought, and extreme cold. For medicinal purposes however, high-quality roots are desired, which require sandy, slightly alkaline soil that is loose and loamy. Compact clay soil stifles root growth and poorly drained soil encourages root rot. Excessive fertilizing actually produces inferior roots. The Chinese consider cultivated Astragalus roots superior to wildcrafted roots, partly because preparing beds with loose soil encourages faster growth and larger roots.

Sow seeds in nursery flats containing a 6″ depth of sandy soil to allow for full and unimpeded root development. Plant seeds in spring after the soil warms up and cover them with about ¼″ of soil. Seeds may also be planted directly into the garden in autumn for spring germination. The hard seed coat can prolong germination, so scarification is helpful. Scratch the seed coat by rubbing seeds between fine sandpaper and then soak them in water overnight. Germination usually occurs within 2-3 weeks. When seedlings are about 3-4″ tall, transplant them to a sunny area in loose, well-drained, sandy soil of average fertility to promote optimal root growth. Plant the seedlings 1-1½′ apart and keep them watered, mulched, and weeded.

Harvest

When Astragalus plants are 3-6 years old, the Chinese traditionally collect the roots in spring before leaves appear or in autumn after the first frost. In TCM, roots harvested in the fall are believed to be superior for medicinal uses. There are different opinions about the actual qualitative markers of Astragalus. Most research authorities report increased medicinal potency in the larger roots, and this seems to be the standard belief in China. In contrast to this popular opinion, comparative chemical analyses of different aged roots have shown that isoflavone and astragaloside concentrations, which exert biological activity, decrease as the diameter size of the root increases (Anetai, 1994). Testing done by the American Herbal Pharmacopoeia also demonstrated that larger and older roots contain smaller concentrations of most constituents. Herbalist Richo Cech had his 2-year-old roots analyzed, and they contained the highest concentration of astragaloside IV and all other detectable compounds compared to other samples of 4-6-year-old plants (Upton, 1999). In light of this research, it may be wise to harvest the roots of healthy, well-developed 2-3-year-old plants in autumn to obtain the greatest concentration and potency of medicinal properties. Collect the seeds for cultivation purposes in late summer and early autumn when the pods are brown and dry.

Preparation of Plant Medicine and Dosages

In China, the roots are cleaned and graded according to size and are typically dried in the sun. Yellow roots are thought to be superior to those with a pale interior. Some roots are first cut and sliced, and others are dried whole. Before drying is complete, the sliced roots are traditionally pounded into long, flat, thin slices shaped like a wooden tongue depressor. The roots are sometimes soaked, baked, or stir-fried in honey and water. The addition of heat and honey is an ancient process used to enhance the tonifying and nourishing Yin aspects of the plant medicine. However, current research indicates that soaking roots in water and applying excessive heat reduces the medicinal constituents and their beneficial biological properties.

After harvesting the root, clean it with a hard spray of water. Astragalus preparations can be made with fresh or dried roots, but as with most herbs, fresh roots yield the most potent medicines. If dried roots are desired, they will dehydrate faster if sliced or chopped into pieces rather than left whole, especially in climates with high humidity. Place root pieces on a screen in a shady area with good ventilation. When thoroughly dry, store roots in a glass jar out of light for up to two years. They begin to lose their potency after a few years. The fresh or dried roots may also be stored in the freezer for an extended shelf life.

Astragalus is traditionally ingested as a decoction (root) tea in China, combined with other herbs rather than used alone. Liquid preparations are considered to be most potent, and the healing constituents dissolved in tea are more bioavailable compared to tablets or capsules. Hot water extracts (teas) are preferred over the standard tincturing method using cold water and alcohol because the medicinal polysaccharides in the root are best extracted with hot water.

PREPARATIONS

Tea: Astragalus root tea has a pleasant, mild, and slightly sweet flavor. The chopped fresh or dry root is made into a tea by gently simmering 2 teaspoons in a cup of water for 15-30 minutes. A stronger, more concentrated decoction tea is made using 1-3 ounces of root in a quart of water that is simmered for 40-60 minutes. Keep a lid on the pot while simmering to prevent evaporation. Allow the tea to cool, infuse for 2 more hours, and strain. Large amounts of tea can be prepared and refrigerated or frozen to preserve for future use. Dosage*:* In Traditional Chinese Medicine, the recommended daily dose of Astragalus is 9-15 grams of the root prepared as tea. Drink up to 2 cups of tea daily as needed.

Tincture-like preparation: This is a good method of preparing a potent Astragalus product with an extended shelf life due to the addition of alcohol. Gently simmer a very strong decoction tea for 15-30 minutes, allow the tea to cool and infuse for a few hours, then strain out the roots and any sediment. Add 25-30% of 190-proof grain alcohol to preserve the tea and pour it into clean glass containers to store. Dosage: 1-3 tablespoons in water can be taken 1-3 times daily as needed.

Tablets or Capsules: The dried pieces of root are ground into fine powder and made into pills or capsules according to the standard process. Dosage: 8-9 capsules or tablets in divided doses throughout the day.

Culinary Uses

Astragalus roots are nutritious and mild-tasting. They can be chewed raw but are very tough and fibrous. In Asia, large pieces of the sliced or chopped root are traditionally cooked in soup for 30-60 minutes, which allows the medicinal constituents to leech out into the soup, and then the roots are removed prior to eating.

Chemical Constituents

Polysaccharides, triterpene glycosides (saponins), amino acids, and flavonoids are the main phytochemicals possessing biological activity in Astragalus root. Polysaccharide components are collectively called astragalans or astragaloglucans, and are involved in the immunostimulant activity of the herb. They seem to work by binding to cholesterol on the outer membrane of viruses to weaken and destroy them. Saponins are a large group of phytochemicals that include astragenol and the related compounds, astragalosides I-VII.

Flavonoids include quercetin, kaempferol, and isorhamnetin. Various amino acids (proteins) include alanine, arginine, aspartic acid, GABA (gamma-aminobutyric acid), glutamic acid, and proline. GABA is one of the principle inhibitory neurotransmitters in the central nervous system that has beneficial anticonvulsant, anti-anxiety, antihypertensive, and cardiovascular effects. Lignans include lariciresinal and syringaresinol. Studies have shown that lignans protect the liver, stimulate immunity, and have anti-inflammatory and antiviral effects (Skenderi, 2003).

The root also contains coumarin (a blood thinner), folic acid, nicotinic acid, phenolic acids (ferulic, caffeic, and chlorogenic acids), choline (hepatoprotective, hypotensive, lipotropic), betaine (hepatoprotective, lipotropic), and essential fatty acids. Linoleic acid (anti-arteriosclerotic, antihistamine, anti-inflammatory, anticancer, hepatoprotective), linoleinic acid, and beta-sitosterol are all beneficial for the heart. Beta-sitosterol is antibacterial, anticarcinogenic, anti-inflammatory, antioxidant, antiviral, and hepatoprotective. More than 20 trace minerals are present in the roots, including calcium, magnesium, potassium, manganese, selenium, zinc, iron, copper, vanadium, and chromium.

Safety, Contraindications, and Drug Interactions

Based on current research and historical validation from centuries of use by thousands of Asians, Astragalus is classified as a very safe and gentle herb for human consumption. No toxicity, side effects, or adverse reactions have been reported in the literature (McGuffin, 1997). There are no special precautions during pregnancy or lactation, and the herb has a long historic use in TCM in treating many childhood diseases, which also confirms its safety.

Astragalus, like most tonic herbs in TCM, is primarily used for non-acute conditions. It is typically not taken alone during a high fever or severe inflammation. Unless it is combined with other herbs to create a balanced formula, Astragalus is contraindicated for conditions of excess and congestion such as constipation, bowel obstruction, and Qi (energy) stagnation. Its sole use is also contraindicated for conditions of excess heat and Yin deficiency heat signs such as high fevers, inflammation, or hot, toxic skin rashes. Yin deficiency heat is an imbalance caused by a deficiency of fluids and nutrients resulting in excessive heat. Conditions of excess should be cleared before Astragalus is introduced. Astragalus is traditionally combined with other herbs in TCM, which may explain why some classic references cite its use for reducing excess heat in the heart and lungs, treating fevers, and draining Yin deficiency heat.

Astragalus may be incompatible with corticosteroids or other immunosuppressive drugs and inappropriate for people with autoimmune disease and organ transplants because it stimulates the immune system. Research has shown it increases the immune-stimulating effects of interleukin-2 (a cancer therapy) and acyclovir, an antiviral drug for herpes (Upton, 1999). Ingesting Astragalus may aggravate allergic symptoms in some people due to the immune-stimulating polysaccharides, which may increase histamine release and resulting allergic reactions.

Medicinal Uses

History of the Plant

Astragalus has been a revered herb throughout Chinese history and was listed in the ancient herbal classic, *Shen Nong Ben Cao Jing* (*The Divine Husbandman's Classic of the Materia Medica*), which is at least 2,000 years old. In China, the root is called Huang-Qi, meaning "yellow leader," referring to its popular use as a superior class of herbal tonics in both ancient and modern Chinese Medicine. It is currently listed in the pharmacopoeias (drug listings) of China and Japan. European botanists have known about Astragalus for hundreds of years. Recorded literature about the herb can be traced back to the time of the first-century Greek physician and botanist Dioscorides (Foster, 1992). It was introduced in the United States in 1925, and has become a popular herb in Europe and the United States, where it is grown commercially. The herb has undergone much research and many clinical studies in the West and China, validating its ability to protect against the common cold, boost immunity, and reduce water retention, high blood sugar, and hypertension. It continues to be one of the most popular herbs employed in TCM.

Healing Qualities

Adaptogen, antibacterial, anticarcinogenic, antihydrotic, anti-inflammatory, antioxidant, antiviral, cardiotonic, diuretic, hepatoprotective, hypotensive, immunomodulator, nephritic, nutritive, pectoral, restorative to the nervous and female reproductive systems, stomachic, tonic, vasodilator, and vulnerary.

Traditional Chinese Medicine (TCM) Perspective

Long regarded as a "superior" Qi tonic that provides vital essence and energy, Astragalus is highly esteemed for its energizing and tonifying activity throughout the body, and is helpful for most deficiency conditions. It is used as a Yin tonic taken daily over a period of time to produce gradual but dependable results. As an adaptogen, Astragalus improves general weakness, replenishes vital Qi, and helps the system deal with stress and "burn-out." It increases the body's overall vitality, endurance, and resistance to illness.

The root has a mild flavor classified as sweet-tasting in TCM. It is slightly warming and primarily affects the spleen and lung meridians. Astragalus tones and strengthens the spleen and is used for conditions related to Spleen Qi deficiency (spleen/pancreas weakness) such as general fatigue, muscle weakness, lack of sufficient body heat, indigestion, abdominal bloating, poor appetite, edema, loose stools, excessive and spontaneous sweating and night sweats, and abnormal uterine bleeding. It is known as a "lifting" herb used for problems related to deficiency and eventual collapse of Qi, manifesting as muscle weakness that allows organs to prolapse and blood vessels to expand into varicose veins and hemorrhoids.

Astragalus is also specific for Lung Qi deficiency that can eventually lead to poor resistance against illness, shortness of breath, asthma, fatigue, poor circulation, cool extremities, or depression. The herb strengthens and stabilizes the *Wei Chi,* which is the exterior protective energy centered around the lungs that is known as the immune system in Western terminology.

As a nourishing Yin tonic, Astragalus builds and strengthens the body and immune system, treats debilitating and chronic degenerative diseases, childhood illness and diabetes, and improves function of the liver, stomach, spleen, lungs, heart, and kidneys. It nourishes the blood and is used to treat anemia. In China, it is commonly given to cancer patients in conjunction with radiation and chemotherapy to reduce their side effects and increase longevity.

In TCM, Astragalus is usually combined with other herbs like Ginseng (*Panax ginseng)* for fatigue, general debility, spontaneous perspiration, and loss of appetite, or with Codonopsis (*Codonopsis pilosula*) to strengthen the heart and improve circulation. In modern TCM, Astragalus is often prepared as an injection and is used in many clinical studies and medical treatments.

Primary Actions

Astragalus is an adaptogen herb specific for chronically weak and fatigued people with depleted immune systems, frequent illness, adrenal exhaustion, digestive problems, and chronic degenerative illness.

Immunity: Astragalus is a primary herb used to enhance immunity in TCM. The majority of research has focused on its ability to activate immunity and restore a depleted or suppressed immune system. Long historic use, clinical trials, and pharmacological data provide evidence of its excellent ability to prevent and treat the common cold, flu, and other viral infections. It is currently being researched and given to restore immunity in people with cancer and HIV/AIDS (Chu, 1998; Huang, 1999). Clinical studies in the United States demonstrate that cancer patients using Astragalus while receiving chemotherapy or radiation experience faster recovery, fewer side effects, and longer life expectancy (Chevallier, 1996; Upton, 1999).

The polysaccharides, saponins, and flavonoids in Astragalus root enhance all aspects of the immune system, including cell-mediated and humoral immunity (Du, 2011), the complement system, and cytokine activity (Nalbantsoy, 2012). Researchers report that Astragalus tea stimulates production of white blood cells called leukocytes and increases macrophage activity of engulfing and destroying infectious organisms (Zhao, 2011). The tea also stimulates production of natural killer cells, interferon, tumor necrosis factor, and antibodies (immunoglobulins), which all serve to inhibit cancer, viral, and bacterial infections (Chang, 1987; Hou, 1981; McCaleb, 1991; Upton, 1999; Zhao, 1992). The herb stimulates generation of red blood cells and blood platelets in bone marrow, and the proliferation of splenocytes, which destroy pathogens (Rou, 1983; Verotta, 2001). Astragalus promotes DNA and RNA synthesis for cell regeneration in the thymus and spleen, which are immune organs (Upton, 1999).

The herb protects against Lyme's disease and treats early stages when taken in daily doses of 2,000 mg. Stephen Buhner provides an extensive herbal protocol for both preventing and treating Lyme's disease in his book *Healing Lyme* (Buhner, 2005).

In China, it is often combined with Ginseng, Licorice (*Glycyrrhiza* spp.), and Codonopsis to treat immune system disorders. It may be helpful for autoimmune conditions, but should be monitored closely to ensure that it improves rather than worsens symptoms.

Adaptogen: Astragalus is an adaptogen herb because it helps the body cope with stress, exerts a normalizing and restorative effect on the endocrine system and major organs, and increases energy and physical stamina. Research indicates that polysaccharides in Astragalus normalize and stimulate activity of the pituitary gland and adrenal cortex. The herb has been used for the treatment of chronic leukopenia (low white blood cell counts) caused by steroids and anticancer drugs (Chang, 1987). Astragalus helps reduce fatigue by increasing oxygen uptake and utilization (Chen, 2002). It is beneficial for chronic degenerative diseases, adrenal exhaustion, chronic fatigue, poor appetite, digestive problems, muscle weakness, and fibromyalgia. It helps regulate blood glucose levels in cases of hypoglycemia and diabetes. In animal experiments, the herb improves survival of mice subjected to toxins and swimming stress tests, and enhances their cell growth, metabolism, and longevity.

Colds, Flu, Infections: One of the main applications of Astragalus in TCM is to treat chronic and recurrent infections, colds, influenza (flu), bronchitis, and other upper respiratory infections. Resistance against seasonal allergies also improves (Matkovic, 2010). The herb strengthens the lungs, stimulates immunity, and reduces viral and bacterial infections. Research demonstrates its effectiveness against several bacteria, including *Shigella dysenteriae* (causing dysentery), *Streptococcus haemolyticus, Diplococcus pneumonia, Corynebacterium* (causing diphtheria, a very serious and contagious respiratory infection), *Staphylococcus aureus, Bacillus subtilis,* and *Bacillus anthracis,* which causes anthrax (Chang, 1987). An epidemiological study in China involving 1,000 people demonstrated that the root has prophylactic effects against the common cold, decreasing its occurrence and hastening recovery. White blood cells were shown to increase their production of interferon, which attacks viral infections. Beneficial levels of IgA and IgG antibodies that fight against bacterial infections also improved after ingesting Astragalus for two months (Chang, 1987). The herb significantly reduces seasonal allergy symptoms of runny nose, sneezing, nasal congestion, and watery, itchy eyes (Matkovic, 2010). It is beneficial for treating encephalitis, a serious inflammation of the brain often caused by viruses (Zuo, 1995). Research using mice demonstrates the ability of Astragalus roots to potentiate the effects of the pharmaceutical drug acyclovir when treating the *Herpes simplex* virus after 5 days of use (Upton, 1999). I have successfully used Astragalus in combination with other herbs to reduce symptoms and speed recovery in several cases of mononucleosis, which is caused by the Epstein-Barr and cytomegalo viruses.

Cardiovascular System, Lungs, and Hypertension: Astragalus is a mild heart tonic used to treat and prevent heart palpitations and arrhythmia (irregular heartbeats). It is beneficial for shortness of breath, pulmonary diseases, including emphysema and asthma (Lin, 2011), and blood deficiency diseases like anemia. Antioxidants in Astragalus protect cells from damage and discourage blood platelet aggregation (clumping) leading to thrombosis (blood clots) and other circulatory problems. Saponins in the roots increase the ability of the heart muscle to contract and blood vessels to dilate, which benefits circulation and helps lower high blood pressure (Hikino, 1976; Skenderi, 2003). Clinical evidence shows that Astragalus can improve congestive heart failure and angina (heart pain) caused by ischemic (lack of oxygen) heart disease, and enhance recovery after acute myocardial infarct (heart attack) (Chen, 1995; Li, 1995; Upton, 1999).

Chinese researchers found Astragalus to be effective against Coxsackie B virus, which causes myocarditis, a serious inflammation of the heart muscle. The root protects heart cells from viral damage and from changes in electrical impulses resulting in irregular heartbeats. In *The Green Pharmacy*, herbal authority James Duke cites a Chinese study on 10 people infected with Coxsackie B virus who had low levels of natural killer cells (NKCs), which are specific white blood cells that attack invading organisms. After 3-4 months of receiving injections of Astragalus extract, the patients' symptoms improved and blood tests showed substantial increases in blood levels of NKC and another antiviral component called interferon (Yuan, 1990).

Liver: Astragalus protects and restores the liver, and is given for chronic liver diseases, including cancer and fibrosis (Chen, 2000). It is popular in China for the treatment of hepatitis, and studies show that it has normalized elevated SGPT (serum glutamic-pyruvate transaminase) levels in patients with chronic hepatitis within two months of treatment (Fan, 1996; Tang, 1992 & 2009). Astragalus protects the liver from toxic exposures, and laboratory experiments demonstrate that it can protect the livers of animals against hepatitis, acetaminophen (Tylenol) toxicity, carbon tetrachloride, and other toxins (Cui, 2003; Zhang, 1992). It promotes RNA and DNA synthesis for cell regeneration in the liver, spleen and thymus, and mineralizes the blood in cases of anemia. The flavonoids in the plant have protective antioxidant activity, and the saponins also help protect the liver and cardiovascular system (Upton, 1999; Wang, 2001). Polysaccharides can reduce cholesterol without the potential side effects of statin drugs (Cheng, 2011). In TCM, Astragalus is typically combined with Ginseng, Atractylodes (*Atractylodes macrocephala*), and Licorice for liver problems.

Kidneys and Bladder: Astragalus tea promotes normal kidney function, tissue regeneration, and blood flow (Jin, 2001). Research validates its ability to increase the flow of urine and reduce edema and high blood pressure caused by fluid overload (Chevallier, 1996). It is helpful for treating bladder and kidney infections and inflammation, bloody urine, urinary incontinence, and bladder prolapse caused by weak muscles. In China, it is used for chronic nephritis (kidney inflammation) and to treat albuminuria (excess proteins in urine) occurring with chronic nephritis and diabetes.

Laboratory studies confirm its diuretic effects. One human study demonstrated that ingesting 200 milligrams of Astragalus root extract for every 2.2 pounds of body weight increased urine output by 64% and sodium excretion by 14.5% (Duke, 2000).

Stomach and Pancreas: Astragalus reduces excess secretion of hydrochloric acid, making the tea helpful for treating indigestion, acidosis, heartburn, stomach ulcers, and acid reflux. The root helps normalize and restore pancreatic function to improve digestion. It is also used as a treatment for diabetes in TCM.

Cancer and HIV/AIDS: Results of Chinese clinical studies published during the 1970s and early 1980s demonstrated the ability of Astragalus to enhance immunity in patients receiving chemotherapy for various types of cancers (Foster, 1992). Astragalus has been widely used in the treatment of cancer in China since 1975, both as a primary treatment and in combination with conventional medical treatments. Chinese physicians prescribe it to cancer patients receiving radiation and chemotherapy because the adaptogen qualities of the roots reduce many debilitating side effects of these therapies, including muscle weakness, nausea, vomiting, decreased appetite with weight loss, fatigue, hair loss, and secondary infections (Duan, 2002). Astragalus helps the body and immune system recover from radiation and chemotherapy by stimulating increased production and circulation of immune-enhancing factors in the blood and lymphatic fluid. It also protects adrenal cortical function during stressful cancer treatments, decreases bone marrow suppression to prevent anemia, and is helpful for recuperation from all debilitating illnesses.

Many studies validate the herb's anticancer and antiviral properties. A study done in Houston, Texas, found that an Astragalus extract restored T-cell (white blood cells involved in immunity) function in 19 cancer patients (Mavligit, 1979). In laboratory research, water extracts of the root were able to protect cells from mutation, indicating chemoprotective activity (Foster, 1992 & 1998). A research group studied a galactose-binding lectin present in Astragalus for its anticancer and antiviral activities. The lectin induced apoptosis (programmed cell death) in leukemia cells, and the researchers concluded that this lectin could act as a potential anticancer drug (Huang, 2012). One *in vitro* study showed that polysaccharides in Astragalus inhibited the proliferation of breast cancer cells (Ye, 2011).

Researchers have found that the combination of Astragalus and Ligustrum (*Ligustrum lucidum*) teas can significantly inhibit the growth of kidney carcinoma in mice. Studies of people with breast cancer, cervical cancer, lung cancer, and chronic leukopenia (low counts of white blood cells) have shown improvement with the use of Astragalus and Ligustrum teas (Wei, 2003; Chang, 1987).

Research shows that Astragalus can increase survival time in some people with cancer, HIV, and AIDS. According to herbal authority James Duke, it is safe to use in cases of HIV and AIDS "based on its known potent antiviral activity against a wide range of viruses" (Duke, 1997). Historic use and evidence show that Astragalus can be safe and effective when used in conjunction with other cancer and HIV/AIDS therapies.

Women's Health: Astragalus can nourish and normalize the endocrine glands to promote fertility and tonify, strengthen, and restore the blood and body following pregnancy and childbirth. It is excellent for postpartum depression, anemia, muscle weakness, uterine prolapse, and hemorrhoids, and is especially valuable for older mothers who have greater need of its wonderful regenerative and restorative energies. As a Yin tonic, the roots help restore the general loss of moisture occurring with menopause, and can help normalize excessive and spontaneous sweating from hot flashes.

Wounds and Inflammation: Astragalus root has been used since ancient times in Asia to heal old, persistent sores, ulcers, and wounds. It helps eliminate infections of the mucous membranes, encourages release of heat and toxins from the skin, and promotes discharge of pus followed by tissue regeneration. Saponins in the roots reduce inflammation, and their effectiveness has been comparable to hydrocortisone in research studies. It can be helpful for eczema and other types of inflammatory dermatitis. An Astragalus ointment, poultice, or fomentation made from the tea may be externally applied to the skin, and the tea is also taken internally to fortify the blood and stimulate immunity to fight infections.

Teachings from the Astragalus Deva

"Greetings, dear one. I am strong in the earth element and have an affinity with the number 4, which has a grounding impact that elicits physical form and manifestation. I contribute to the form of human beings by nourishing and tonifying the cells. I am a strong, resilient and protective herb, guarding the body against illness. I have moisturizing qualities and protect the spleen and kidneys, helping to normalize the flow of water and fluids. I help regulate digestion by stimulating digestive juices and encouraging the flow of bile from the liver. I am a mild and enduring plant to be used as a tonic over time. My nature is comforting, loving, abundant, and expanding. Although my home is in China, I am very adaptable and grow easily in many different places. My purpose is to heal and stabilize the energies that sustain and nourish the body. Therefore, I have a very solidifying and concrete effect upon the system. I am good for people with difficulty in concentrating, sitting still, and being quiet; for my roots go deep into the earth and elicit stillness within my being, which is comforting. I incorporate the female quality of the earth and am nourishing. I can be of benefit to all age groups, though most young people do not need me because their bodies are strong and stable. However, if a child suffers from deep, underlying or hereditary weakness, I am appropriate to use in the healing process. People who are strong and earth-bound do not have as much need of my energies as those who suffer from weakness and need grounding. Please consider me a nourishing, grounding, and solidifying herb that helps provide the foundation of life and health."

Black Cohosh

Cimicifuga racemosa (*Acteae racemosa*)
Ranunculaceae (Buttercup or Crowfoot) Family

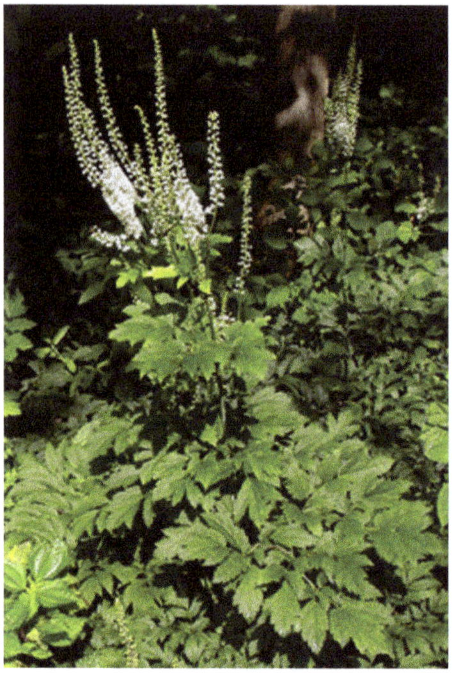

Botanical Name

Taxonomists have had a difficult time deciding whether the genera *Cimicifuga* and *Acteae* should be separated or combined into one genus, and opinions have varied as to which genus Black Cohosh belongs. The earliest botanical classifications for Black Cohosh include *Christopheriana facie, Christopheriana canadensis,* and *Herba spicata*. Swedish botanist Carolus Linnaeus (1707–1778) classified Black Cohosh as *Actaea racemosa* in his 1753 work, *Species Plantarum,* but later determined that *Cimicifuga* should be a distinct genus from *Acteae* based on the differences in their fruit. In other circles it was called *Cimicifuga serpentaria,* and Thomas Nuttal (1786–1859) named the herb *Cimicifuga racemosa* in his 1818 book, *The Genera of North American Plants*. The American botanist Rafinesque (1783–1840) proposed placing it in a different genus, and for a while it was called *Macrotrys racemosa,* often misspelled as *Macrotys*. The early American Eclectic physicians adopted the common name of "Macrotys" for Black Cohosh. *Cimicifuga racemosa* has been the accepted nomenclature for many years, but recent studies on the plant's morphology and DNA structure have elicited another shift in opinion. Based on results of these studies, some investigators believe that the entire genus *Cimicifuga* should be returned to its original placement under *Actaea,* and Black Cohosh should be called *Actaea racemosa* once again (Compton, 1998; Foster, 1999).

Common Names

Black snake root, rattleroot, rattlesnake root, and rattleweed are old names referring to the dark color and snake-like appearance of the thready rootlets, to its historic use in Native American healing of snake bites, and to the rattling sounds of the dried seeds when shaken in their pods. Squaw root, macrotrys, and macrotys are older names for the plant. The leaves and flowers of some *Cimicifuga* species (excluding *C. racemosa*) have a strong, unpleasant odor that repels bugs. The genus name *Cimicifuga* comes from the Latin genus name for the common bed bug, *cimex,* and from *fugare,* meaning "to drive away." Bugwort and bugbane are antiquated names reflecting this bug repellent quality.

Medicinal Part of the Plant

The entire rhizome with its thready rootlets is used for medicinal purposes. The flowers can be taken to calm the nervous system and be of assistance during difficult times of transition.

Range and Habitat

There are approximately 18 species in the genus *Cimicifuga* and all are indigenous to northern temperate zones. One species is native to Europe, six to North America, and the remaining species to Asia. *Cimicifuga racemosa,* indigenous to deciduous forests of the middle and eastern United States, is the popular species sold commercially for medicinal preparations. Other eastern North American species include *C. americana* and *C. rubifolia*, and western varieties are *C. arizonica, C. elata,* and *C. laciniata*. Several species of *Cimicifuga* indigenous to Asia are used medicinally in Traditional Chinese Medicine and have been the subject of Chinese research, including *C. heracleifolia, C. dahurica,* and *C. foetida*.

Cimicifuga racemosa grows in rich, moist, well-drained, loamy woodland soils ranging from Ontario, Canada as far south as Georgia, and west to Missouri and Wisconsin. It is most abundant in the Ohio River Valley and Appalachian Mountain region. Indigenous plants grow under a canopy of Oak, Maple, Sycamore, Beech, Poplar, Ash, Sassafras, Walnut, and Buckeye trees. It once grew in abundance, but over-harvesting and decreasing habitat due to urban development have greatly reduced wild populations.

Description of the Plant

C. racemosa is a beautiful and stately perennial herb that is easy to recognize in the forest when clusters of small, creamy-white flowers bloom along the ends of tall stalks. The medicinal roots are a knotted and gnarly cluster of dense, hard, bulbous, and irregularly-shaped rhizomes that send out many slender, smooth, thready root fibers. Rhizomes are brown on the outside with creamy-white interiors that become grayish black

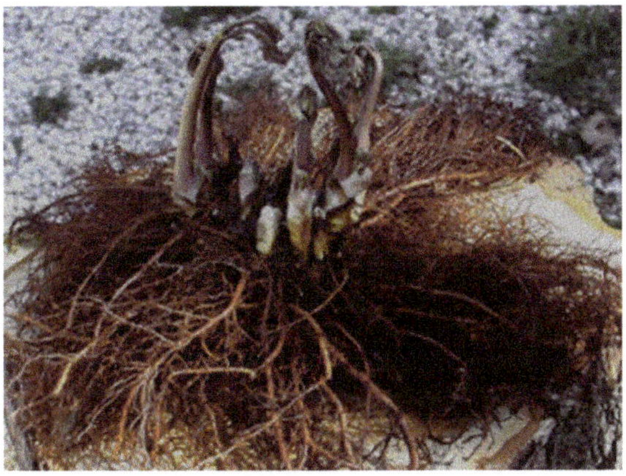

Root rhizomes with sprouting stalks

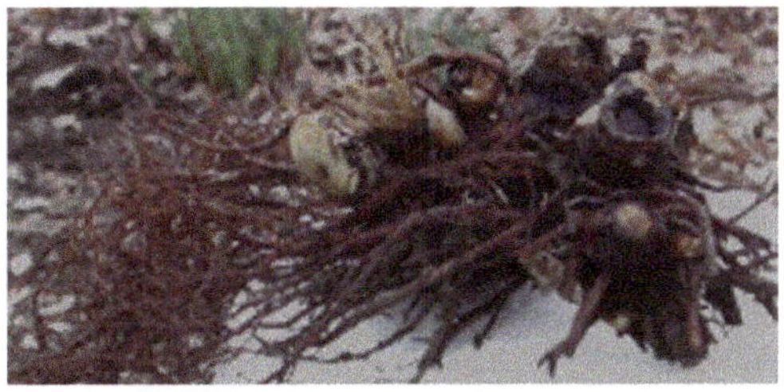

Root rhizomes with scars

when they are dried. The upper surfaces of the rhizomes have circular scars that are remnants of dead stalks from previous years' growth. One or several new stalks shoot up from the rhizomes every spring.

The erect green stalks are smooth, round, and furrowed with maroon-colored nodes where leaves attach to stems. Each stalk divides into 3 long-stemmed, pinnately compound leaves consisting of several pairs of leaflets. The smooth, deep-green leaflets are 1-4″ long and ovate to lance-shaped with sharply pointed tips. They are pinnately veined and have deeply serrated teeth along their margins. The leaflets have 3 lobes with the largest lobe in the middle. The bushy mass of leaves reaches a height of 1-3′.

The flower stalk emerges from the base of the plant and typically reaches a height of 4-5′, but under ideal conditions it can grow up to 8′. The stalks are sometimes covered with a whitish-blue film. Before flowers open, they are small, tight, white balls with a short petiole attaching to the stalk in an alternating pattern. As each flower opens, 4-5 white sepals quickly fall away, and the flower looks like a round ball composed of numerous creamy-white stamens sitting atop long filaments that surround a single white pistil. The delicate-looking flowers are ½-¾″ across and form a long, wand-like raceme 6-24″ long on top of the tall stalks. The pure-white flowers have a pleasant earthy and musky fragrance. Flowers at the base of the raceme bloom first and proceed upward, and lower flowers begin to mature into seedpods while flowers at the top of the raceme are opening. The plant blooms beginning in June in southern ranges and later in the north. Flowers mature into little dark-brown oval pods containing numerous flat, dark-brown seeds.

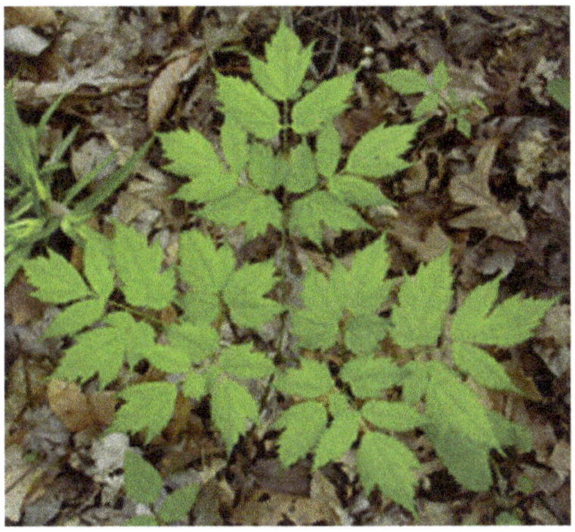

Pinnately compound leaves

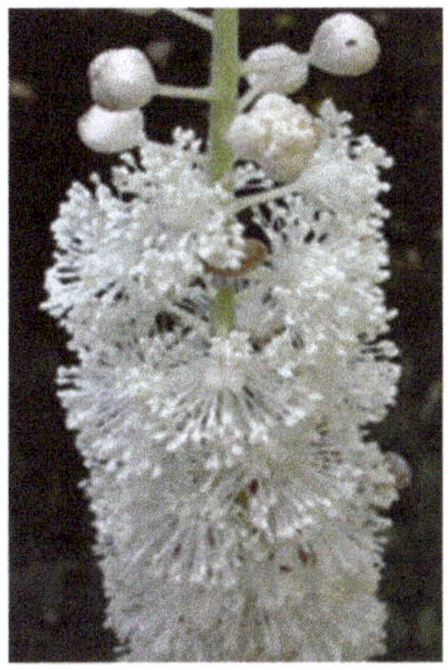

Flower stalk

Cultivation

Until recently, all commercially sold Black Cohosh was obtained by wildcrafting native stands. For many years, thousands of roots have been harvested from the woodlands of eastern North America to be marketed in the United States and Europe. Indigenous stands cannot possibly meet this huge commercial demand, so this beautiful plant is now listed as "at risk" of extinction. Cultivation is paramount to its survival and is underway in Europe and the United States.

Black Cohosh grows in rich woodland soils that are loamy and moist but well drained. The plant is susceptible to fungal infections and root rot, so there must be adequate drainage and airflow in garden beds. The soil should be loose and high in humus content to allow maximum root growth. Optimal pH is slightly acidic at 5.0-6.0, which humus provides. This herb typically grows under shade trees, but growers are discovering that it tolerates more open sunlight than previously thought.

I cultivate Black Cohosh in southern Indiana woodlands with great success. I have experimented growing it in two slightly different environments: shaded woodland gardens and along the edges of fields under shade trees where the plants get morning sun but are shaded from the more intense heat of the afternoon sun. For the shaded woodland gardens, I utilize fertile areas with adequate space between trees to allow rototilling and the creation of nursery beds. The other type of garden plot is made by rototilling along the edges of fields under trees. In my experience, Black Cohosh roots and foliage grown in areas receiving morning sun and afternoon shade develop considerably faster than those growing in complete shade.

The plant is easy to grow from root division and more difficult to germinate from seed. Live roots can be dug up or purchased (preferably from other growers instead of wildcrafted) in autumn after the foliage has died back and roots have developed buds for next year's growth. Divide roots into 1½″ pieces with a sharp knife. Be sure to divide roots so that each piece includes a bud. Invite the Black Cohosh to come live on the land, thank it for its healing gifts, then plant it 2″ deep and 2′ apart in a prepared bed. Be sure that the buds are pointing upward in the direction they will grow. Keep the patch weeded and moist. I experience about 95% success with this method. Although the root is considered to be fairly slow growing, I have been quite amazed and encouraged at the accelerated growth rate made possible by cultivation in loose, loamy soil and morning sunlight. I discovered that after 4 years of growth, pieces of root that were divided into sections weighing 24-50 grams grew into mature roots weighing an average of 324.5 grams each. This was an increase of about 81 grams per year of growth.

Growing from seed is more difficult than root division and requires some patience. Seeds quickly lose viability when dehydrated, so immediate planting after their harvest is recommended for best germination. They can be cold-stored in a bag of moist sand in the refrigerator if immediate planting is impossible. Left alone without human intervention, Black Cohosh seeds drop to the earth and go through alternating freezing and thawing over winter and spring. They naturally require this preparatory stratification sequence of warm autumn weather, cold winter temperatures, and warm spring weather to germinate. Whenever possible, attempt to mimic Mother Nature, and plant these seeds as soon as they are ripe and ready to drop in August or September. Plant the seeds about ¼″ deep and 2-3″ apart in well-prepared, shaded, woodland nursery beds. The seeds must be kept moist over autumn and winter, which occurs naturally if rainfall is adequate. Seeds often germinate at different times. In my experience, about 10-15% of seeds planted in autumn germinate the following spring after the soil has warmed up. However, about 95% of several hundred seeds planted in a nursery bed in September 2001 germinated in April 2003 (a total of about 600 days), which was a thrilling success!

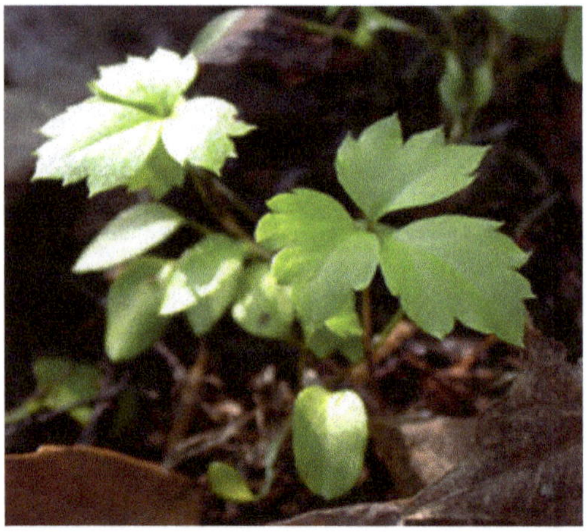

First-year seedlings with cotyledons

The first-year seedlings have 2 rounded cotyledons (the first leaves to emerge from the seed) and a compound leaf composed of 3 tiny leaflets with very large serrated teeth. Allow at least one year of growth, then dig up the young plants and move them to a permanent bed, spacing them 1½-2′ apart. Plants grown from seed can take up to 3-4 years to flower and 6-7 years to develop roots big enough for harvesting.

Compared to root division, cultivation of Black Cohosh from seed is more challenging and requires time before roots are large enough to harvest. Explore both methods – getting those seeds to sprout and eventually mature into flowering plants is a wonderful and satisfying accomplishment!

Harvest

Pick flowers when they are in full bloom. Harvest the root in late autumn at the beginning of dormancy when leaves have died back and chemical constituents in the root are most potent. It is also ecologically prudent to harvest in autumn after seeds have matured and dropped, allowing the plant to self-sow. Dig up the root and always remember to cut off a 1½″ piece of the crown containing a sprout or bud, and replant it in the hole about 2″ deep with the bud pointing upward. It will grow into a mature plant and you will be able to return for another harvest after 3-4 years. Using this method, the crop can be maintained, expanded, and harvested on a regular basis, and you will be a cooperative gardener with Nature and a friend to the Cohosh plants by ensuring their continued survival.

If you must wildcraft Black Cohosh, be extremely careful not to confuse it with the related and more common species, Baneberry (*Actaea pachypoda, A. alba*) which is potentially toxic. The leaves of both plants are nearly identical, although the flowers and seeds are very different in appearance. Baneberry seeds are a fleshy berry, compared to Cohosh seeds that grow in dry pods. Baneberry roots are rounded, smooth bulbs lacking the many fibrous rootlets and gnarled lumps of Cohosh roots.

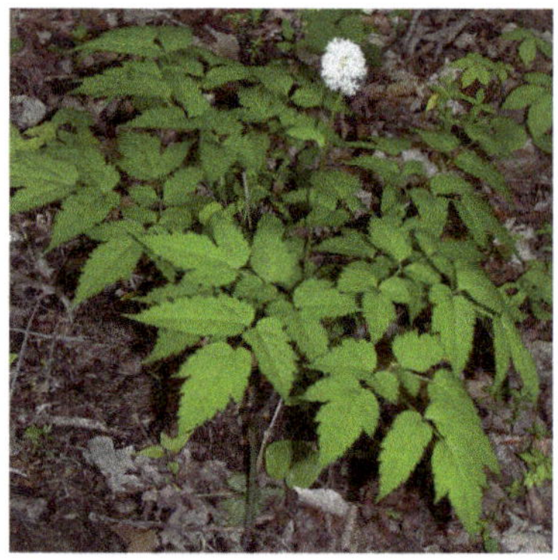

Poisonous Baneberry

Collect Black Cohosh seeds in late summer after their pods have dried. This can be challenging because once dry, they pop out of their pods, falling and disappearing on the ground. A good collection method is to wrap and tape cheesecloth around the seedpods at the end of flower stalks as they start to turn brown. The cheesecloth will allow airflow to discourage mold and rotting, and it will catch the seeds as they mature and dry, making collection easier and more successful. Seeds are damaged by mold, which detrimentally affects germination, so be sure to collect seeds that are not moldy and plant them immediately.

Preparation of Plant Medicine and Dosages

Wash fresh roots and chop them into small pieces. Boiling water and alcohol both extract medicinal phytochemicals from the roots, but tincturing is my favorite way to preserve and ingest this herb. Although most dried roots tend to deteriorate over time, Black Cohosh root seems to retain potency over many years. An illuminating study comparing an 85-year-old dry Black Cohosh root with a freshly harvested root revealed similar amounts of the primary medicinal constituents: phenols and triterpene glycosides (Jiang, 2005).

PREPARATIONS

Tincture of Roots: Stuff a glass jar with the freshly harvested, finely chopped root and cover with 80% 190-proof grain alcohol and 20% distilled water. Dosage: 20-40 drops of tincture in water 1-3 times a day as needed. Black Cohosh is marketed in Germany as a standardized extract called Remifemin. This is prepared as tincture, which physicians recommend to take in doses of 40 drops twice daily, or in pill extract form taken in doses of 40 mg daily.

Decoction Tea: Gently simmer 1-2 tablespoons of chopped root (fresh or dry) in a quart of water for 10-20 minutes, allow tea to cool, and then strain. Dosage: 1-2 cups a day as needed. The root tea has a sharp, bitter taste that lingers on the tongue.

Flowers: These can be prepared as tincture or tea. To make tincture, use 50% 190-proof grain alcohol and 50% distilled water. Dosage: 2-10 drops 1-3 times a day. For tea, steep 1 teaspoon of fresh flowers in 1 cup of hot water. Dosage: 1-2 cups a day.

Buy Black Cohosh products made with cultivated rather than wildcrafted roots!

Chemical Constituents

Active constituents of Black Cohosh have not all been identified, but three major classes of phytochemicals known to exert biological effects include triterpene glycosides, phenolic compounds, and flavonoids.

Triterpene glycosides include actein, cimicifugoside (also called cimigoside), racemoside, and cimicifugin, which was called "macrotin" by the Eclectic physicians and may exert estrogenic activity. Actein has vasodilating (relaxes and opens blood vessels), hypotensive, and anticarcinogenic effects. Cimicifugoside is thought to have a normalizing influence on the hypothalamus-pituitary axis that regulates the reproductive and nervous systems. Remifemin, the German preparation of Black Cohosh root, is standardized on the basis of these triterpenoid glycosides. Formonetine is a weak estrogenic isoflavone.

Phenolic compounds are anti-inflammatory. These include ferulic and isoferulic acids, acetic acid (antibacterial, expectorant), butyric acid (anticarcinogenic), cimicifugic acid A and B, gallic acid (analgesic, anticarcinogenic, bronchodilator), oleic acid (anticarcinogenic), palmitic, and salicylic acid (analgesic, anti-inflammatory). The bitter taste of the roots is thought to come from a crystalline principle called racemosin. N-methylserotonin has calming serotonin effects and has been identified in the herb.

Nutrients include calcium, potassium, magnesium, iron, chromium, beta-carotene, ascorbic acid (vitamin C), inositol, riboflavin (vitamin B2), niacin (vitamin B3), pantothenic acid (vitamin B5), and silicon.

Safety, Contraindications, and Drug Interactions

The efficacy and safety of Black Cohosh has been confirmed by many years of pharmacological and laboratory research, by documented clinical studies of more than 1.5 million menopausal women (primarily in Germany), and by the American Eclectic physicians. Research shows that there are no long-term toxic, mutagenic, carcinogenic, or teratogenic (causing birth defects) effects, and no significant drug interactions are reported to date (Blumenthal, 2000). Occasional mild stomach discomfort is the primary side effect. The German Commission E herbal regulatory agency has confirmed that Black Cohosh root has no contraindications other than during pregnancy (Blumenthal, 1998).

Due to the stimulating and estrogen-like influence on the uterus, very large doses can induce miscarriage at the beginning of pregnancy. Therefore, **the herb should not be taken until the last 2-3 weeks before the expected due date**, at which time it is traditionally used to tone uterine muscles and enhance labor. No adverse effects during lactation are noted in the literature, but stomach discomfort is possible with nursing infants since this is an occasional complaint of some adults taking the herb (Brinker, 2001).

The use of Black Cohosh by women who are at risk of breast cancer or who suffer from this disease has been a concern because synthetic estrogens are known to stimulate and increase tumor growth. Recent studies have shown that this herb has the opposite effect and protects the breast by inhibiting carcinogenic effects of estradiol and other estrogens on breast tissue (Bodinet, 2002). Black Cohosh is appropriate and safe for women who should not take hormone replacement therapy (HRT) due to history or risk of breast cancer, fibrocystic breast disease, abnormal uterine bleeding, fibroids, endometriosis, liver and gallbladder disease, or pancreatitis.

The literature cites that excessively large doses of Black Cohosh root taken over time may cause hypotension, nausea, vomiting, dizziness, frontal headaches, tense and rigid muscles, and nervous trembling. These symptoms have primarily occurred from homeopathic preparations given over a long period of time in minute doses that will eventually cause symptoms identical to the problems for which it is given. People using Black Cohosh while taking medications for hypertension should monitor their blood pressure since the herb has a tendency to lower high blood pressure. The German Commission E agency has recommended limited use for only six months because this is the maximum length of most clinical trials. However, many women safely and effectively ingest the herb for long-term treatment of menopausal complaints.

Over the past few years, there have been several reports of possible liver toxicity associated with use of Black Cohosh, and European, Canadian, and Australian regulatory agencies have established warnings about possible liver problems. To determine the validity of these reports, researchers from the Hospital of Johann Wolfgang Goethe University of Frankfurt in Germany analyzed all 42 case reports of liver toxicity. Researchers concluded that there was no proof of toxicity due to lack of scientific evidence, insufficient documentation, and because several people took Black Cohosh in addition to medications with known liver toxicity. Therefore, evidence of toxicity was never validated (Blumenthal, 2006; Teschke, 2009 & 2011).

Problems have emerged in the industry due to adulteration of Black Cohosh mainly with *Actaea* species from China (Foster, 2013; American Botanical Council staff, 2016), so purchase it from reliable companies.

Medicinal Uses

History of the Plant

Black Cohosh was widely used by native people of the North American woodlands. It was an important remedy in the healing traditions of the Iroquois, Hurons, Cherokees, and the Algonquian groups, including the Potawatomi, Delaware, Miami, Shawnee, Kickapoo, Sac, Fox, Ojibwa, Penobscot and Mohegan, among others. "Cohosh" is an Algonquian word meaning "rough and gnarly," which describes the appearance of the root. The antiquated and rather derogatory name "squaw root" reflects the widespread use of the root among many native women. Although there is a lack of reliable ethnobotanical data, some written accounts describe Native use of the root boiled as a tea and primarily employed to ease childbirth pains, treat menstrual problems, and relieve painful arthritic conditions. Other applications were for colds, coughs, sore throats, and kidney problems. It was taken in tea form as an antidote for poisons and venomous snake bites, and the root was ground into powder and applied externally as a poultice on wounds. Native Americans introduced early European trappers, traders, and immigrants to the plant, which eventually became a popular medicine among the early settlers and frontier herb doctors who called it "black snakeroot" (Foster, 1999).

> *Black Cohosh was an honored remedy in the healing traditions of Native Americans and was especially revered among the women.*
>
> *Today, scientists are investigating the effects of Black Cohosh root in human physiology.*
>
> *Many modern women use the herb to help with reproductive and hormonal problems, and have experienced improvement in many of their symptoms.*

In 1844, John King, M.D., introduced Black Cohosh to his fellow Eclectic physicians, referring to it as his "favorite remedy." King, one of the most prominent and influential Eclectic physicians, specialized in obstetrics and gynecology, which provided him with ample opportunities to observe the effects of Black Cohosh on women. It became one of the popular herbs of the Eclectics, who called it "macrotys," meaning "long raceme" or "spike." It was their primary remedy for treating muscle and nerve pain, inflammation, arthritis, and disorders of the female reproductive system. It was also employed for lung ailments, scarlet fever, whooping cough, lack of glandular secretions, headaches, and as a heart tonic. They believed the primary action of macrotys was a relaxing effect on the nervous system, working secondarily on the organs and tissues of secretion and reproduction. William Cook, M.D., wrote, "It is almost purely relaxant, leaving behind only a trifling astringent impression on mucous membranes. Its power is expended chiefly upon the nervous structures, beginning at the peripheries and extending to the brain, including the ganglionic system; through the sensory nerves influencing the heart and pulse, and through the sympathetic nerves making a decided impression upon the uterus. It manifests a distinct action upon the whole class of serous tissues, and a milder action on the kidneys, lungs, and skin. Upon this large range of organs its impression is always relaxant" (Cook, 1869). King and other Eclectic physicians found it to be very helpful for many female reproductive problems, including ovarian and uterine inflammation, menstrual irregularities such as amenorrhea (lack of menses), dysmenorrhea (painful periods), menorrhagia (excessive bleeding), infertility, and threatened abortion. Prompted by King's enthusiastic endorsement, Black Cohosh was routinely used by Eclectic doctors during the 1880s–1930s. It was listed as an official medicine in the *U.S. Pharmacopoeia* from 1830–1936, and in the *National Formulary* until 1950. The advent of pharmaceutical medicines and demise of the Eclectic physicians during the 1930s put an end to the use of Black Cohosh by American physicians. However, many rural midwives, who were often herbalists, continued using it in their practice throughout the 1900s.

The early popularity of Black Cohosh spread to Europe where it was introduced into Germany during the late 1800s. It was primarily administered as a homeopathic remedy in Europe and later became available in herbal preparations. Over the past 50 years, many German physicians have prescribed the root to treat premenstrual syndrome (PMS), painful menses, and menopausal symptoms. Currently, the popularity of Black Cohosh continues to grow throughout Europe and has been rekindled in the United States as a top-selling herb for menopausal complaints.

There has been substantial research on Black Cohosh over the years. Early Eclectic pharmacists analyzed and identified some of the chemical components in the root. Eclectic physicians initially based their knowledge of the herb on Native American traditions, and after many years of clinical use they provided a wealth of documentation demonstrating the herb's physiological activities. Since the 1950s, Black Cohosh has been the subject of much research in Germany, where it is manufactured and marketed as the popular standardized extract known as Remifemin. Research has focused on either validating or disproving the plant's apparent estrogen-like activity and remarkable ability to improve menopausal hot flashes, depression, insomnia, and other hormone-related problems. Almost all clinical and lab studies validate the plant's traditional uses among Native Americans and the Eclectic physicians, but a few studies have resulted in conflicting outcomes and assumptions that are the subjects of continuing controversy. So the plant shrouds itself in some mystery!

Healing Qualities

Abortant (in excessively large doses), alterative, analgesic, anti-inflammatory, antispasmodic, antivenom, mild astringent, cardiac, diaphoretic, diuretic, emmenagogue, exanthematous, expectorant, hypotensive, nephritic, nervine, oxytocic, pectoral, peripheral vasodilator, restorative, sedative, and nerve and uterine tonic.

Traditional Chinese Medicine (TCM) Perspective

Chinese varieties of *Cimicifuga* are collectively called Sheng Ma and exert similar medicinal properties as *C. racemosa*, the North American species. In TCM, Sheng Ma is employed to raise Qi (vital energy) and move energy upward, which helps prolapsed or "fallen" organs regain muscle tone. The roots are indicated for prolapsed uterus and bladder and for hemorrhoids. The herb regulates the circulation of Qi and stimulates blood circulation throughout the pelvis and entire body. This vitalizing quality is helpful for stagnant Uterine Qi and Uterine Qi deficiency, which are the root causes of many menstrual and reproductive problems. Sheng Ma is beneficial for treating constrained Kidney Qi causing edema and kidney stones, and for constrained Lung Qi giving rise to lung congestion, coughs, and difficult breathing. It tones the Yin and is specific for Heart, Lung, and Kidney Yin deficiency commonly occurring during menopause and causing increased dryness in the tissues. Sheng Ma clears internal wind to relieve spasms. Its cooling and mildly drying nature reduces heat and inflammation. The Chinese ingest the root at the onset of eruptive rashes, such as measles, to drive out the rash and fever and hasten recovery. Sore throats, mouth irritations, headaches, bronchial infections, coughs, and ulcers also respond well to this treatment.

Primary Actions

Black Cohosh's primary impact is on the nervous and female reproductive systems. The root exerts a calming influence on the nerves, which tones and benefits the entire body, especially the uterus, cardiovascular system, and lungs. A multitude of research shows that the roots contain constituents having estrogen-like action. I have recommended it to many women who have found it to be helpful for reproductive problems related to hormonal imbalances, nervous irritability, and achy muscles. It excels in its capacity to improve all aspects of menopausal problems, including hot flashes. *Cimicifuga* is specific for premenstrual or menopausal women who experience mood swings of irritation and anxiety with deep, dark, brooding depression, and who feel disconnected to themselves and the world in general.

Women's Reproductive Health: Black Cohosh is one of the most valuable herbs known for normalizing and restoring the female hormonal system and treating menopausal complaints (Beer, 2013; Wuttke, 2014). Its nervine and sedative qualities relieve emotional and physical tension, and help relax and tone pelvic muscles and organs. The root is especially indicated for reproductive problems related to uterine tension, congestion, and inflammation resulting in menstrual irregularities, pain and cramps, deficient or excessive bleeding, muscle aches, headaches, nervousness, emotional irritability, or depression. It is used for amenorrhea (failure to menstruate) and delayed menses. I have recommended Black Cohosh to many women over the years with successful results. Time and again, it has proven to be helpful in treating premenstrual syndrome (PMS) and irregular and painful menstrual cycles. The Eclectic physicians employed it for these conditions as well as for mastitis (breast infection and inflammation) and muscle atony (loss of muscle tone) causing the uterus, bladder, and other organs to fall or prolapse from lack of support. Black Cohosh also influences the reproductive system by its beneficial action on the pituitary gland (Mitchell, 2003).

> *The most effective herbal hot flash remedy I have found is prepared with equal amounts of tinctured Black Cohosh root and leaves and flowers of Blue Vervain and Sage.*

Helping to balance hormone levels, Black Cohosh is used for estrogen deficiency contributing to menopausal complaints and infertility. The late German physician Rudolf Weiss, M.D., prescribed it for many problems caused by deficient estrogen (Weiss, 1988). Thousands of women have experienced Black Cohosh to be a safe and effective alternative to potentially dangerous hormone replacement therapies (HRT). It helps normalize the hormones following a hysterectomy and after discontinuing birth control pills or

HRT. The herb is also indicated for conditions of estrogen excess, including endometriosis, uterine fibroids, fibrocystic breasts, and PMS.

A study involving 62 women suffering from menopausal complaints and uterine fibroids compared the ability of 40 mg Remifemin (the German preparation of Black Cohosh root) with 2.5 mg tibolone (a synthetic drug prescribed for fibroids and endometriosis that increases levels of estrogen and progesterone) in reducing the size of the fibroids. The women were divided into two groups and took daily doses of either the herb or drug for 12 weeks. Those using the Black Cohosh experienced less menopausal symptoms and a 30% reduction in the size of their fibroids, while those taking tibolone had no reduction in fibroids (Xi, 2014).

Especially effective for menopausal complaints, I recommend the tinctured root for hot flashes, anxiety, mood swings, sleep disturbances, and vaginal thinning and dryness. Black Cohosh is excellent for headaches caused by low estrogen levels that occur before and during menstruation and with menopause.

The most effective hot flash remedy I have found is a combination of equal parts Black Cohosh, Blue Vervain (*Verbena hastata*), and Sage (*Salvia officinalis*) tinctures. If extra help is needed, Chasteberry (*Vitex agnus-castus*), St. John's Wort (*Hypericum perforatum*), Hops (*Humulus lupulus*), Motherwort (*Leonurus cardiaca*), and American Ginseng (*Panax quinquefolius*) may be added to this formula.

Research on Hormonal Effects: Since the 1950s, the identity and activity of chemical constituents in Black Cohosh root have been the subject of much research, especially in Germany, and there have been more than 20 clinical trials involving over 3,500 women. A wealth of clinical trials and pharmacological studies consistently demonstrate that the roots exert estrogen-like effects. It has proven to be superior to placebos and comparable to pharmaceutical estrogens for treating menopausal symptoms without causing side effects (McCaleb, 2000). These symptoms include hot flashes, sleep disturbance, vaginal dryness, mood swings, irritability, depression, and psychological disturbances associated with hormone imbalance. Researchers from the University of Gottingen in Germany reviewed research abstracts and publications written about Black Cohosh since 1980, determining that laboratory and clinical evidence shows that it exerts beneficial properties of estradiol (an endogenous form of estrogen produced by the ovaries), including reduced serum luteinizing hormone (LH) levels and osteoporosis prevention. Research also establishes the roots to be an effective alternative to HRT (Wuttke, 2003).

> *A wealth of clinical trials and pharmacological studies consistently demonstrate that Black Cohosh exerts estrogen-like activity in the human body.*
>
> *It has proven to be superior to placebos and comparable to pharmaceutical estrogens for treating menopausal symptoms without causing any significant side effects.*

Researchers have consistently used Remifemin tincture or pill preparations in their studies. The first pharmacological studies that demonstrated estrogenic effects of Black Cohosh began in 1944 with animal experiments. In 1959, J. Foldes conducted studies to determine the estrogenic activity of Remifemin in mice. The mice given the Remifemin showed an increase in uterine weight, and Foldes concluded that this was evidence of the herb's estrogenic action (Foldes, 1959; Foster, 1998). By 1960, there were 1,256 case reports published in 11 studies by health professionals who validated the ability of Remifemin to effectively treat menopausal symptoms without adverse side effects (Foster, 1999). Since the 1980s, many more clinical trials have been conducted to determine the efficacy of Black Cohosh root in responding to complaints of perimenopausal and postmenopausal women, and to compare the herb with hormone therapy drugs (Blumenthal, 2000). These clinical findings further confirm its beneficial influence in restoring hormonal levels and relaxing the nervous system.

A large clinical study conducted in 1982 by 131 physicians and gynecologists evaluated the results of 629 menopausal women who took 40 drops of Remifemin extract twice daily for 6-8 weeks. More than 80% of the women experienced improvement and relief from hot flashes, anxiety, insomnia, headaches, dizziness, tinnitus, and heart palpitations. Almost half of the women enjoyed complete relief from symptoms. Temporary upset stomach was the only side effect reported by 7% of the women, but it was not severe enough to prevent them from continuing the herbal treatment (Stolze, 1982).

Results of a multi-center placebo-controlled study involving more than 300 postmenopausal women confirmed findings of previous studies by demonstrating the effectiveness and safety of Remifemin in relieving menopausal complaints. For 12 weeks, half of the participants took one Remifemin tablet twice a day and the other women received a placebo. The Black Cohosh was significantly more effective in reducing hot flashes and other symptoms, and was comparable to HRT. The herb appeared to be most helpful during early menopause (Osmers, 2005). Another multi-center clinical study involving 304 postmenopausal women clearly indicated the efficacy and safety of the Black Cohosh extract (Remifemin) in addressing menopausal symptoms, especially hot flashes (Ross, 2012).

Several studies have shown the herb to be as effective as pharmaceutically conjugated estrogens and estriol used in HRT, but without the potentially dangerous and widely publicized side effects (Wuttke, 2006). In 1985, the results of a 12-week German study were published comparing Remifemin (40 drops twice daily) to 0.625 mg of conjugated estrogens and 2 mg of Valium in 60 menopausal women. The Remifemin and estrogens both stimulated growth of vaginal mucosa and reduced vaginal dryness and discomfort. They also relieved depression, mood swings, anxiety and hot flashes, demonstrating Black Cohosh to be superior to synthetic estrogen and HRT in relieving menopausal complaints (Warnecke, 1985). Another German clinical study by Willenbrock and colleagues in 1988 compared Remifemin (8 mg daily) with the pharmaceutical drugs estriol (1 mg daily) and conjugated estrogens (1.25 mg daily) for treating menopausal symptoms in 60 women younger than 40 years of age. The benefits of Black Cohosh were found to be equal to the estrogen drugs in relieving hot flashes, mood swings, and sleep disturbances (Foster, 1998). A German trial published in 1995 reported that Black Cohosh used in combination with St. John's Wort was 90% effective in improving menopausal hot flashes, insomnia, mood swings, and depression in 812 women after 12 weeks of use. Almost all of the women (98%) denied experiencing side effects, while the remaining 2% reported slight nausea as the only inconvenience (Beuscher, 1995). Other researchers concluded that this combination was effective for menopausal complaints after a study involving 77 perimenopausal and postmenopausal women (Chung, 2007). A study in China investigating the efficacy of Black Cohosh in mice and human breast cancer cells demonstrated several estrogenic results, including increased uterine weight, while blood levels of estrogen remained unchanged (Liu, 2001). In a German study, 62 postmenopausal women were given either Black Cohosh, pharmaceutical estrogens, or a placebo. Results showed that Black Cohosh was equal in potency and effectiveness to the pharmaceutical estrogens in protecting against osteoporosis and relieving menopausal complaints like mood swings, memory loss, hot flashes, sleep disturbances, loss of libido, vaginal dryness, and urinary incontinence (Wuttke, 2003).

Evidence derived from many clinical trials and testimonials of hundreds of women confirms the ability of Black Cohosh roots to help normalize estrogen levels.

The herb eases many menopausal symptoms including hot flashes, depression, anxiety, mood swings, heart palpitations, headaches, and sleep disturbances.

As ovarian function declines during menopause, estrogen and progesterone production also diminish. These lower hormone levels cause increased follicle stimulating hormone (FSH) and luteinizing hormone (LH) release from the pituitary gland, which normally induces ovulation. Sporadic spurts of LH are associated with hot flashes and heart palpitations. Animal studies on rats have shown that Black Cohosh extracts suppress LH, and clinical studies involving 110 menopausal women demonstrated that 8 mg of Remifemin taken daily inhibited LH secretion (Duker, 1991). This resulted in decreased incidence and severity of hot flashes and other menopausal complaints, while raising hormone levels in the blood. Unlike synthetic estrogens, Black Cohosh does not affect FSH or prolactin release.

In 2007, a very large clinical observation study was conducted in 1,287 gynecologic practices throughout Germany. Participants consisted of 6,141 menopausal women. This study compared the results of using Remifemin alone or combined with St. John's Wort to improve psychologically related menopausal symptoms. Following 3 months of treatment, the outcomes revealed improvement in all psychological symptoms with both herbs. However, the combination of Black Cohosh and St. John's Wort was found to be superior in alleviating mood symptoms (Briese, 2007).

Although Black Cohosh acts like a phytoestrogen, it is presently not clear whether or not it binds to estrogen receptors in human tissues. The German Commission E herbal regulatory agency confirmed that it does bind to receptor sites in breast, ovarian and uterine tissues, stimulating estrogen-like activity. Research has shown that it binds to estrogen receptors in specific tissues and exerts estrogenic activity on the vaginal lining similar to estriol, one of the milder estrogens produced by women (Murray, 1997). Several *in vitro* studies and animal experiments with rats have shown that Black Cohosh extract competes with 17-beta-estradiol for estrogen receptor binding sites in cells (Duker, 1991). However, other researchers have documented that the herb has very little receptor-binding activity (Zava, 1998).

Research findings plus many clinical trials involving menopausal women indicate that Black Cohosh helps normalize hormone levels and treat estrogen insufficiency. It appears to have a balancing effect on the reproductive and hormonal systems, and is helpful in treating problems related to excess or deficiency of estrogen. But how can the plant do both? One explanation involves estrogen receptor sites in specific tissues to which estrogen hormones attach, somewhat like a lock and key system. The cell receptors are like a lock with a specific shape that only allows estrogens with a similar structure to enter and attach to the receptor. Once estrogen binds to the receptor, it stimulates estrogenic activity in the tissues. Synthetic and pharmaceutical estrogens bind to cell receptors and exert much stronger activity than endogenous estrogens naturally produced by the ovaries and adrenal cortex. Phytoestrogens in herbs also fit into cellular receptor sites, but they exert the weakest estrogen activity. Thus, if there is an excess of estrogen in the system, Black Cohosh constituents are thought to bind to receptor sites and block out the biologically stronger endogenous estrogens. This effectively decreases overall estrogen activity. On the other hand, during menopause when estrogen levels are low, the phytoestrogens simply bind to empty cell receptors and stimulate an overall increase in hormonal activity.

Some people have expressed concern about the dangers of estrogen-like components in Cohosh roots promoting growth of estrogen-dependent cancer cells in the breast, uterus, and ovaries. In response, lab tests confirm that unlike pharmaceutically produced synthetic estrogens, Black Cohosh extracts have shown to be protective against cancers and actually inhibit the proliferation of breast carcinoma cells (Bodinet, 2002; Rebbeck, 2007; Henneicke-von Zepelin, 2007; Fritz, 2014; Li, 2011). One study investigating the effects of Black Cohosh on samples of human breast cancer cells discovered that triterpene glycosides (the main active components of the root) seemed to change the structure of the cancer cells and initiate their programmed cell death, known as apoptosis. The triterpene glycoside actein (isolated from Black Cohosh root and administered separately) was found to be particularly active at inhibiting breast cancer growth (Einbond, 2008).

Phytoestrogens (estrogen-like substances occurring in different plant species) offer protection against estrogen-dependent conditions like uterine fibroids, endometriosis, and cysts, tumors, or cancers in the breasts, ovaries, and uterus.

These weaker plant estrogens protect breast, uterine, and ovarian cells from the stronger effects of estrogens produced by the body.

Especially important is the protection phytoestrogens provide against the dangers of powerful synthetic estrogens produced by pharmaceutical companies and occurring in many toxic yet widely used environmental chemicals.

The ability of Black Cohosh to inhibit breast and other reproductive cancers may also be related to its capacity to bind to estrogen receptors in the cells and block out stronger estrogens made by the body or introduced from environmental sources. The herb has demonstrated antagonistic effects against estradiol, a form of estrogen associated with increased risk of breast, ovarian, and uterine cancers. The root also exhibits similar activity as tamoxifen, a pharmaceutical drug prescribed to treat breast cancer by lowering estrogen levels to prevent proliferation of estrogen-dependent cancer cells. In a study examining the effects of Black Cohosh on hot flashes caused by tamoxifen therapy in young premenopausal breast cancer survivors, the herb significantly reduced the number and severity of hot flashes. Almost 50% of the women were free of hot flashes after 12 months of herbal therapy (Hernandez, 2003).

In addition, Black Cohosh extract exhibits a binding affinity for the aryl hydrocarbon receptor. Substances that activate this receptor (including resveratrol from grapes) can help reduce growth of breast and prostate cancer cells. One *in vitro* test confirmed that Black Cohosh displays significant inhibition of cancer cell production, even in the presence of dihydrotestosterone and estradiol. These are both known to stimulate growth of prostate cancer, and estradiol can also potentiate female cancers (Jarry, 2005). One of my male clients diagnosed with prostate cancer experienced severe hot flashes while receiving drug therapy to reduce his testosterone levels. The hot flashes were greatly reduced when he took regular doses of Black Cohosh, Sage, and Blue Vervain tincture.

Elevated levels of androgens (male hormones), and testosterone in particular, can cause hirsutism, which is excessive hair growth on the face, neck, chest, abdomen, and back experienced by some menopausal women. Research shows that Black Cohosh can reduce excess androgens to treat hirsutism.

Osteoporosis: Metabolic changes during menopause can lead to mineral loss in bones, and several studies confirm osteo-protective properties of Black Cohosh. In one clinical trial involving 62 postmenopausal women, the herb exerted estrogenic activity on bones by stimulating specialized cells, called osteoblasts, to generate new bone cells. This maintains bone density to prevent or treat osteoporosis. Black Cohosh was tolerated well by trial participants and there were no known adverse effects on the liver (Wuttke, 2003 & 2006). Animal research has also confirmed the herb's ability to inhibit mineral loss in bones and increase bone density (Seidlova-Wuttke, 2003 & 2012; McCaleb, 2000).

Menstruation: Black Cohosh helps to regulate the menstrual cycle. It normalizes irregular or delayed menses and scanty menstrual flow and is used for amenorrhea (absence of menses), dysmenorrhea (painful and difficult menses), fluid retention, and premenstrual syndrome (PMS). It is an emmenagogue that stimulates uterine contractions to help initiate menstruation. For this purpose, 20-40 drops of tincture are taken in water every 6 hours until bleeding starts. As an antispasmodic, nervine and sedative, the herb is effective in relieving ovarian pain, menstrual cramps, and premenstrual symptoms of depression, brooding, emotional "heaviness," irritability, joint and muscle pains, backaches, and breast tenderness. It is excellent for headaches and migraines occurring in the late luteal phase of the reproductive cycle when estrogen levels drop just prior to menstruation. One double-blind study involving 49 women showed that those who took daily supplements of 50 mg of Black Cohosh, 100 mg of Dong Quai (*Angelica sinensis*), and 60 mg of soy isoflavones (plant estrogens) experienced a significant reduction in migraines associated with menstruation (Burke, 2002). Black Cohosh is valuable for women who stop using the birth control pill because it helps restore normal menstrual cycles, hormonal activity, and ovarian function.

Black Cohosh can be a beneficial treatment for polycystic ovarian syndrome (PCOS) caused by hormonal imbalances of excessive testosterone, insufficient progesterone, and elevated prolactin resulting in failure to menstruate, ovulate, and become pregnant. In a study involving 50 women diagnosed with PCOS, 20 mg of a Black Cohosh extract was ingested for 3 months. Outcomes revealed improvements in luteinizing hormone and progesterone levels, which promoted increased ovulation (Kamel, 2013).

Pregnancy and Childbirth: Black Cohosh can stimulate uterine contractions and is **not to be used during pregnancy until the last 2 weeks before the expected due date**. Used at this time, it is quite safe and is an excellent short-term tonic that strengthens, tones and prepares the uterus for delivery, halts premature labor, and relieves false labor pains. It is traditionally administered in combination with Blue Cohosh (*Caulophyllum thalictroides*) for their synergistic actions. The usual dose is 10-30 drops of each tincture in water taken twice daily until labor begins.

Black Cohosh has a long history of use by Native American women, early American Eclectic physicians, and many midwives who report its excellence in preparing the uterus, facilitating labor, and reducing complications of childbirth. Years ago when I assisted with homebirths, I frequently observed Black and Blue Cohosh establish regular, strong contractions, while reducing pain and calming the mother during childbirth. To promote labor and relax and dilate the cervical os (the opening from the womb into the birth canal), ½ teaspoon of each tincture is diluted in water and ingested every 30 minutes until contractions are strong and productive. A small amount (only 3-5 drops) of Lobelia (*Lobelia inflata*) tincture can be added for its ability to open the cervical os.

After birth, Black Cohosh stimulates uterine contractions that expel the placenta and reduce bleeding. To halt uterine hemorrhage after childbirth, combine Black Cohosh with herbal astringents such as Shepherd's Purse (*Capsella bursa-pastoris*), Cranesbill (*Geranium maculatum*), or Cinquefoil (*Potentilla* spp.). Black Cohosh helps relieve "after-pains" following delivery, and encourages recovery of the uterus by toning the muscles so that it returns to its normal pre-pregnancy size and placement in the pelvis. The herb facilitates postpartum recovery by toning pelvic muscles to prevent uterine and bladder prolapse, reducing anxiety, and restoring hormonal balance. It can be especially helpful for older postpartum women.

When I was pregnant with my two sons, I drank Black and Blue Cohosh tinctures as a pre-labor tonic. When assisting homebirth mothers, I had many fortunate opportunities to witness how wonderfully these herbs worked to safely and gently assist women during labor and post-partum.

Abortant: Black Cohosh is a known abortant when taken during the first 3 months of pregnancy. I personally know several women who have chosen to terminate their pregnancies by fasting and using large amounts of Black Cohosh tincture with other abortive herbs. This is a delicate and highly charged issue, and if herbs are used for this purpose, it must be understood that the decision cannot be reversed and fetal damage is possible if the abortion attempt fails. The abnormally large amount of herbs needed for this purpose has an accumulating reaction and should not be used without medical assistance or ingested for more than three days. Discontinue if uncomfortable symptoms such as hypotension, nausea, vomiting, dizziness, or headaches arise. If the herbs are not effective, medical intervention is absolutely essential.

Nervous System: Black Cohosh is an excellent nervine and sedative herb that helps calm, tone, and restore the central nervous system. It promotes muscle relaxation in addition to mental and emotional peace. Research studies validate its anti-inflammatory and antispasmodic properties, making the herb suitable to relieve anxiety, hyperactivity, muscle tension, traumatic injury, irritated nerves, and general restlessness. The roots contain salicylic acid, an analgesic that relieves nerve and muscle pain. Black Cohosh has a long history of use for treating premenstrual and menopausal anxiety, nervous tremors, muscle spasms, seizures and epilepsy, sciatica and neuralgia (nerve pain), arthritic pain and stiffness, spinal meningitis (a bacterial infection and inflammation of the spinal cord), and delirium tremens related to alcohol and drug withdrawal. It is specific for tinnitus (ringing in the ear) and vertigo (dizziness). Black Cohosh can be combined with Kava Kava (*Piper methysticum)* and Ashwagandha (*Withania somnifera)* for problems involving inflammation and pain.

The early American Eclectic physicians used Black Cohosh root to treat acute and chronic arthritis, childhood epilepsy, and chorea (an old term describing constant rapid, jerky, and involuntary muscle movements). Eclectic physician John King, M.D., wrote that "Black Cohosh uniformly lessens the force and frequency of the pulse, soothes pain, allays irritability, and lessens the disposition to irritation and congestion of the brain" (King, 1864). In his *Book of Herbal Wisdom,* Matthew Wood writes that Black Cohosh root has an affinity for the cerebrospinal system, recommending it for congestion of cerebrospinal fluid, spinal stiffness, whiplash, fibromyalgia, nervous spasms, and to heal damage caused by high fevers and meningitis (Wood, 1997).

As previously mentioned, Black Cohosh is specific for depression of a dark, brooding, and heavy nature, especially when related to PMS and menopause. It helps repair the psychological wounds caused by emotional and sexual abuse, substance abuse, and feelings of despair, loneliness, and hopelessness. A tincture or flower essence made from the white flowers brings a deep harmony and wholeness to the entire system by creating an even flow of energy between the physical body, emotions, mental thoughts, and the subtle, energetic etheric body. The flowers are especially useful during periods of emotional crisis when people need grounding and stabilization. They help calm the emotions and the mind, and assist people in connecting with their calm center. A few drops of the flower essence or tincture made from the flowers or roots may be taken 2-3 times a day for several weeks to assist with this type of emotional healing.

When treating problems arising from the nervous system, Black Cohosh may be combined with other nervines and muscle relaxants such as Valerian (*Valeriana officinalis*), Scullcap (*Scutellaria lateriflora*), Lobelia (*Lobelia inflata*), and Ginger (*Zingiber officinale*).

Interesting research offering an explanation of the herb's relaxing influence on the nervous system reveals its involvement in the neurotransmitter system. Neurotransmitters are crucial chemicals in the brain and peripheral nervous system that regulate body processes. Serotonin is one of the primary inhibitory neurotransmitters that calms the central nervous system, and is also involved in thermo-regulation. N-methylserotonin has been identified in crude root extracts, and *in vitro* studies demonstrate that it binds to serotonin cell receptors creating calming serotonin activity (Burdette, 2003; Powell, 2008).

Other pharmacological *in vitro* studies have confirmed that Black Cohosh produces dopaminergic effects. Dopamine is a stimulating neurotransmitter responsible for providing energy, motivation, and a sense of well-being. The herb has a moderating influence on gamma-aminobutyric acid (GABA) receptors. GABA is another inhibitory neurotransmitter especially calming for anxiety, panic attacks, and obsessive thinking. Black Cohosh has also been shown to diminish the hypothalamic-pituitary-adrenal axis (HPA axis) stress response by decreasing corticosterone levels (Nadaoka, 2012; Reame, 2008). The herb's influence on these neurotransmitters and the HPA axis appear to be important mechanisms contributing to the reduction of hot flashes, anxiety, depression, and other menstrual or menopausal complaints.

Cardiovascular System: The nervine and sedative properties of Black Cohosh exert a relaxing influence on the cardiovascular system. The smooth muscles within blood vessels relax to allow increased vasodilation. This improved circulation benefits all organs, including the heart, and helps reduce high blood pressure (Richard, 2005). Black Cohosh tones the heart, strengthens the force of contractions, and normalizes the pulse rate. The antispasmodic and relaxing properties of the herb can help relieve angina pain. It combines well with other cardiac tonics such as Hawthorn (*Crataegus* spp.), Motherwort (*Leonurus cardiaca*), and Cayenne (*Capsicum annuum*).

Respiratory System: Black Cohosh treats spastic and congested lung conditions by improving blood circulation and relaxing the central nervous system and muscles. Thus, breathing is enhanced when the bronchials relax, dilate, and expel mucous. The roots are a remedy for many lung problems, including dry or wet coughs, whooping cough, wheezing, asthma, and bronchitis.

Liver, Kidneys, and Lymph: Black Cohosh has a tonic effect on mucous membranes and promotes normal secretions of the liver, kidneys, and lymphatic fluids. Its diuretic properties activate kidney function and antispasmodic properties relax nerves and spasms in the urinary tract and ureters, allowing for easier and less painful urination and passing of kidney stones.

Teachings from the Black Cohosh Deva

"Greetings, dear one. I will teach you the nature of my healing plants. My roots go deep into the earth drawing minerals, nutrients, and the power and energy of the Great Mother into my being. This power within my roots moves into the female body and into the womb to balance, nurture, and bring the female system into its beingness, and to promote the birth of other beings in a safe way. I restore and strengthen the womb to receive life, to sustain life, and at the right time, to propel life forward into the world. I am an ally to women; for I have been used for many years upon this land, and indeed, the Native Americans who once walked here in great beauty and stature knew of my virtues by sitting with me. For I also talked to those people, and this is how wisdom of myself and other plants spread. At that time, people were much more in tune with Nature and open to receiving and hearing her voice. Their livelihood and survival depended on close contact with Mother Nature and nature energies, and gathering information from them. In this way, people have sat before me and asked for information that I have given freely to all those with good hearts and the wish to heal. This is what I have told them in the past, and I tell you now.

"Yes, my roots go deep into the earth just as they touch the most earthy place in women, which is the womb. In the same way that the power of the earth is absorbed into my roots, these roots give strength to the womb. The energetic vibration of my roots is a golden orange hue that nourishes, balances, and sustains the womb. The womb is an organ of relationship; its fullness and purpose come into being when the polarities of man and woman dance and merge to create another human being. The energy of the golden orange helps to sustain and enliven the infant, and in this way promotes life and birth. As the energy of my roots enters the fertile womb, it helps sustain the second chakra of the mother and of the infant as it develops. It is not necessary to ingest the herb during the gestational period, but simply to be close to the plant and the energies of the earth. If the woman has used the herb before pregnancy, its energy will continue to work in sustaining the uterus and the growing fetus. Using my roots just before birth will provide strength to the womb and help to enliven the infant. I assist in the transition of birth, as the infant moves from womb time (which is time in the ocean of life when the vibrational frequencies of the earth and mother are absorbed by the infant) into the world of form. Using the herb at this time actually helps the infant embody the world of form in a strong and grounding way.

"My energy is grounding and calming throughout the entire body. My white flowers appear at the very top of the plant and indicate that my energy affects the very highest centers of the brain and nervous system. When one is disconnected from the earth, emotions get flighty with agitation or depression. Being a very earthy plant, I help ground the nervous system to connect with the energetics of the earth. I strengthen and stabilize the first and second chakras, and also balance and calm the seventh and higher chakras. In this way, a balanced and harmonious current of energy is established which flows through the system, touching the very base of the womb and connecting and aligning with the highest centers of the mind. This serves to connect the body via the energetic and nervous system to promote very pure, flowing, peaceful energy that soothes out all energetic wrinkles, spasms, and constrictions.

"I am calming to women going through menopause. During this time, the hormonal system moves through many fluctuations that affect the nerves and the basic reptilian ability to maintain body temperature. I am able to stabilize and ground women at this time. I am especially called upon to help women return to the "wombness" and "cave" of their being, to sit quietly and reclaim oneness with the earth, and to remember their ability to co-create with the Earth Mother.

"I am also useful for men, because not only do women need this connection with the Earth, but also men. I am able to help men connect with their feminine nature and to the Earth Mother so they can be complete and balanced within themselves. Just as in women, the energy of my white flowers also benefits and aligns the flow of energy from the seventh chakra down to the first chakra, helping men connect to the earth and calm the higher centers of their brain and nervous system. When there is imbalance in men's hormonal system, I can help the prostate gland by grounding and releasing excessive energy and relaxing spasms.

"My earthy, cooling roots bring these qualities into the human body. In this way, I relieve excess fire to reduce nervous hyperactivity and agitation. My nature is calming and quieting, and coming into my presence is somewhat like going into a cave, just as the womb of a woman is like a cave in which the developing child is protected and nurtured. So when seeking healing through me, sit quietly and go into the being of your inner cave where all is silent, cool, comfortable, and safe. I offer protection to the womb and to the nervous system, and the opportunity to feel at one with the earth and the ability to sit in powerful solitude upon the earth. For this reason, I am a great ally to all women in their menopausal years, the time when women retreat further into their inner "cave," when women need to understand their own sense of power, of being, and of their connection with the earth. In this way, being in the cave is invigorating and comforting, and is in itself a preparation for death. For death invites us to feel at peace with being alone, to feel connected with the earth and sky. My white flowers sitting so high up on the plant help people connect with this sky energy.

"In my greatest capacity, I am a plant ruled by the astrological sign of Scorpio. Like Scorpio, I exert much influence on the reproductive system, and I connect and balance extremes – the dark recesses and energy of the womb and the earth with the higher energies of the sky and light beings. It is the line of energy between the first and seventh chakra that connects the whole being to prepare for birth and for death. The healing power of my flowers is helpful support when going through all major transitions of life including birth, menstruation, menopause, losses, and traumatic events. Although it has not been well known that I may be used at the time of death as well as at birth, I share this with you now. At the time of death, use my flowers as a tincture or flower essence. The flowers calm the brain and nervous system, and are an ally at the time of death during the transition of the dissolution of the physical body and the continuing existence of the spirit vehicle. Remember to use me at the time of your death so I may be of help during your journey."

Black Walnut

Juglans nigra
Juglandaceae (Walnut) Family

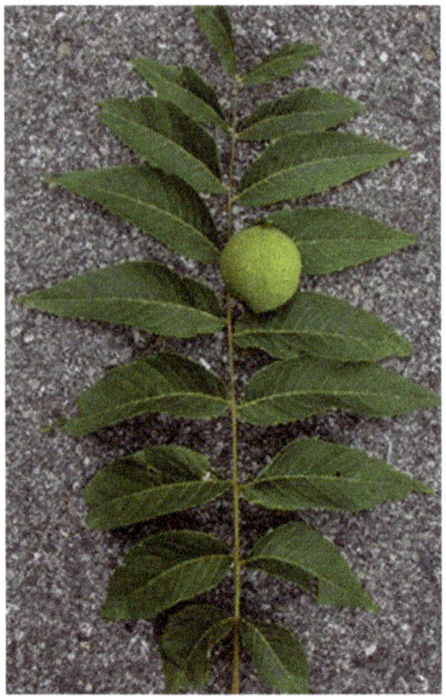

***Juglans nigra* leaf and hull**

Common Names

Juglans nigra is American Black Walnut.
J. regia is known as English, European, and Persian Walnut.
J. cinerea is White Walnut, better known as Butternut. The leaves of this tree have similar chemical constituents and medicinal properties as its cousins, *J. nigra* and *J. regia*.

Medicinal Part of the Plant

The bark, leaves, and light-green hull surrounding the edible walnut contain medicinally active phytochemicals. The unripe hulls and leaves are currently the most commonly used parts of the tree.

Range and Habitat

Juglans nigra (American Black Walnut) grows throughout much of central and eastern North America. *Juglans regia* (English, European, and Persian Walnut) is indigenous to the Middle East and Asia, including India, Nepal, and China. It was introduced into Europe and England hundreds of years ago, where it has naturalized. There are about 40 species of Walnut trees that produce edible nuts and have been cultivated in temperate zones throughout the world.

Description of the Plant

Black Walnut is a resinous, aromatic, deciduous tree growing to a height of 60-100′. Trees can live to be over 200 years old, and in the early 1900s, Walnut trees having a diameter of 3-4′ were common in the midwestern United States. The leaves are alternate and pinnately compound, reaching up to 2′ in length. Each compound leaf has 7-11 pairs of simple leaflets and a terminal leaflet that is often missing or reduced in size. The sessile leaflets have pinnate venation, finely serrated teeth, and are lance-shaped to ovate with pointed tips. Topsides of leaflets are glabrous (smooth without hairs) and lightly pubescent (hairy) underneath. Oil glands on the underside of the leaflets give off a citrus-like odor when they are cut or crushed.

Male and female flowers are unisexual, meaning that they grow separately on the same tree, and appear in early spring from April through May before leaves fully emerge. Male flowers appear in catkins that hang down from branches, and have a calyx of 5-6 scales surrounding many stamens. Female flowers have 4 sepals and no petals. The calyx surrounds and is fused to the ovary, which has 2-3 fleshy stigmas. The ovary matures into a fruit that is a single, round, hard-shelled nut with a bumpy, lumpy surface, and grows up to 3″ in diameter. The inner seed, which is the edible walnut, is oily with a distinctive delicious flavor. The fleshy but tough hull is a light-green color when it falls from the tree in late summer and turns dark brown while on the ground.

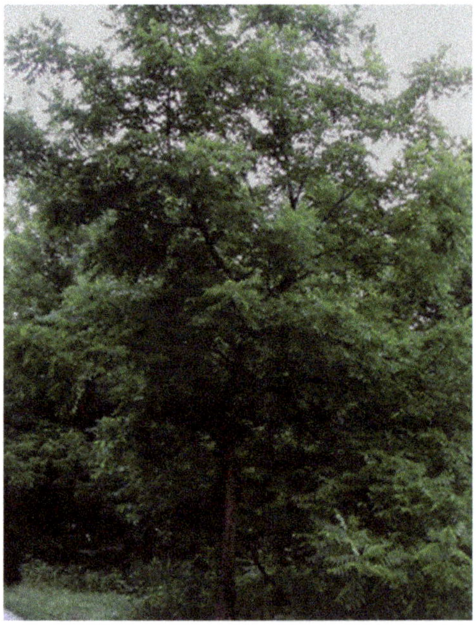

***Juglans nigra* tree**

Cultivation

Black Walnut prefers full sun and grows in a variety of soils, but thrives best in deep, fertile, moist soil with good drainage. Adequate airflow around the growing area is necessary to prevent mold and fungal diseases.

The easiest, fastest, and most reliable way to cultivate Black Walnut is to purchase seedlings that are at least 2- or 3-years-old from nurseries. Prepare a deep hole in fertile soil and plant them 20-35′ apart. They start producing nuts when about 10 years old, but the best nuts come from mature trees that are 25-30 years old.

Trees may also be started by planting the nuts containing the edible kernels. First, remove the nuts from their hulls and put them in a bucket of water. Those nuts that sink to the bottom have a more mature kernel and should be planted for best chances of germination. The nuts need to be stratified, so plant them 2″ deep in prepared soil in late summer or early fall, allowing the freezing and thawing over the winter and spring months to prepare them for germination. Some nuts will germinate the following spring and some may require a complete year. After 1-2 years of growth, the seedlings should be transplanted to a permanent location.

The roots and leaves of Black Walnut trees secrete juglone and other chemicals into the soil which can inhibit plant growth, so keep your gardens at least 10-20 feet from the tree's drip line.

Harvest

Harvest the leaves in early summer around June or July by pruning the lower branches of trees. Harvest the hulls when they are immature and still light green in color. They often fall from the trees at this stage, allowing for easy harvest, and can also be knocked off tree limbs using long poles or rakes. Although our ancestors harvested the bark, it is best not to collect the inner bark because this can inflict damage or death to the tree unless it is done by an expert. Leaves and hulls make excellent medicine and are much easier to collect than the inner bark.

Preparation of Plant Medicine and Dosages

Freshly harvested leaves may be prepared as a tincture, tea, or poultice. They can also be dried in the usual manner to make tea and poultices, or ground into fine powder to prepare as pills and capsules.

To prepare the light-green hull, it must be smashed to separate it from the inner, edible Walnut seed and then chopped into small pieces. This is a job requiring some effort, a good hatchet, and care to keep all your fingers! The hulls are made into a tincture preparation.

If the inner bark is collected, it is traditionally dried for a year before being ingested as tea because the fresh bark tends to cause intestinal spasms and cramping. However, as previously mentioned, harvesting the inner bark is not recommended due to potential damage to the tree.

Black Walnut is a potent herb requiring close attention to dosage, and is not recommended for long-term use. Start ingesting the herb in small doses and gradually build up to the desired dose. If loose stools, diarrhea, or stomach and intestinal upset occur, stop use completely or cut back on the dosage until you can find a maintenance dose that does not cause symptoms. For treating parasites and other health problems mentioned in this section, take preparations of the leaves or hulls for 14 days and then stop for 14 days. Alternate this on-and-off cycle for 2-4 months, then stop taking the herb for at least 2 months.

All parts of the plant taste extremely bitter, so most people prefer taking Black Walnut in the form of a pill, capsule, or tincture rather than tea. Topical application stains the skin a yellowish-brown or blackish-green color for a few days, so wear gloves when working with the hulls.

PREPARATIONS

Tincture of Leaves and Hulls: I highly recommend making tincture when working with Black Walnut, especially when using the green hulls. They tend to be quite moist and hard, making them more difficult to dry and grind into powder. Since the tea is very bitter, tinctures are preferred.

Prepare the tincture in the standard way by filling a glass jar with chopped fresh leaves or green hulls, and covering them with 60% 190-proof grain alcohol and 40% distilled water. Dosage: 10-40 drops 1-4 times a day as needed.

Tea of Leaves: Steep 1-2 teaspoons of finely chopped fresh or dry leaves in 1 cup of water for 10 minutes and strain. Dosage: 1-2 cups a day as needed.

Tea of Hulls: Gently simmer 1-2 teaspoons of chopped fresh or dry hulls in 1 cup of water while covering the cooking pan with a lid. Dosage: 1-2 cups a day as needed.

Pills: Grind dried leaves or hulls into a fine powder. Add water to make a thick paste that can be rolled into round pills and then dried in the usual manner. Dosage: 1-2 pills up to 3 times a day, or up to 495 mg of commercially purchased pills 1-3 times a day.

Capsules: Grind the dried leaves or hulls into a fine powder and put it into capsules. Dosage: 2 "00" sized capsules up to 3 times a day as needed.

Culinary Uses

The fruit of Walnut trees is a popular and delicious nut loaded with valuable nutrients. One signature of the tree is the shape of its nut, which looks like the two large lobes of the brain contained in the hard shell resembling a human skull. Walnuts have long been regarded as "brain food," and the vitamins, minerals, proteins, and especially the essential fatty acids they contain are excellent nourishment for normal brain and nerve function. The nuts are also a good dietary source of serotonin, a neurotransmitter or brain chemical that relaxes the nervous system and promotes sleep. Eat walnuts raw because heat increases oxidation and begins to diminish the benefits of their health-promoting essential fatty acids.

Chemical Constituents

Tannins and juglone are the primary phytochemicals in the leaves and hulls. The tannins, called ellagitannins, are formed from ellagic acid, which has been of interest in cancer research (Trease, 1989; Harborne, 1993). Ellagic acid has been shown to be antibacterial, anti-HIV, anti-inflammatory, antioxidant, antiplaque, antiseptic, antiviral, astringent, detoxant, and a pesticide. Juglone (also called nucin or juglandic acid) is a naphthoquinone derivative that is a bitter antifungal, antiseptic, astringent, antiviral, and antiparasitic. It is considered to be the major vermifuge (parasite killer) of the plant and occurs in the immature light-green hulls and leaves (Yarnell, 2003). Juglone induces apoptosis (the body's process of programmed destruction of cancer cells) and inhibits proliferation of various malignant cells (Chae, 2012). Leaves also contain flavonoids (quercetin and kaempferol), juglandine, alkaloids, malic, citric and oxalic acids, essential oils including germacrene D (Blumenthal, 2000), and organic iodine which is antibacterial, antiseptic, antigoiter, antiviral, and a fungicide. Phenolic acids include caffeic, chlorogenic, ferulic, and gallic acids (Skenderi, 2003).

The hulls contain ascorbic acid (vitamin C), beta-carotene (vitamin A), calcium, and chromium. Myricetin in the hull is antibacterial, anticancer, antihistamine, anti-HIV, anti-inflammatory, antimutagenic, antioxidant, antiplaque, antiviral, and a candidicide. Sakuranetin is antibacterial, antiseptic, and a fungicide and pesticide. Iodine in the hulls is a known antibiotic, antiseptic, and protects against radiation damage.

Walnut seeds contain protein, essential fatty acids, calcium, magnesium, manganese, potassium, iron, boron, zinc, and many trace minerals. Walnuts are an excellent source of serotonin, but nuts from the Butternut tree (*Juglans cinerea*) are thought to be one of the best plant sources of this important calming neurotransmitter involved in brain, nerve, and digestive function.

Safety, Contraindications, and Drug Interactions

Black Walnut is a relatively safe herb lacking side effects when taken in small doses over short periods of time (McGuffin, 1997). There are no reports of contraindications or drug interactions when used properly (Blumenthal, 1998; Skenderi, 2003). Doses of juglone have caused genetic mutations in test tube and animal experiments (Duke, 2000). Some literature states that chronic use may have carcinogenic effects in people, but there is no clinical evidence or historical data supporting this hypothesis. The hulls and leaves may cause temporary contact dermatitis or irritation with prolonged external application. The American Eclectic physicians prepared Walnut syrup to treat constipation in nursing mothers and for bowel complaints of infants and children (Ellingwood, 1919), and the **German Commission E herbal regulatory agency stated that there are no contraindications during pregnancy. However, I recommend against ingesting Black Walnut during pregnancy and lactation** because it is a strong herb for the delicate system of infants. It is best for mothers to use Black Walnut prior to pregnancy for parasites, conditions of toxicity, or sluggish digestion and elimination in order to prepare a strong, healthy, and vibrant body to grow a baby.

Medicinal Uses

History of the Plant

Wherever it grows, the Walnut tree has been revered and valued over thousands of years for its beautiful dark wood, potent medicine, and delicious, nourishing nuts. The early Greeks and Romans extensively used the nuts and oils of *Juglans regia* for culinary and medicinal purposes. Pliny the Elder (A.D. 23–79), a naturalist during the Roman Empire, recorded that Walnut trees were introduced from Persia and cultivated in Italy by the first century B.C. The Greek physician and botanist Dioscorides (*circa* A.D. 40–*c.* 90) wrote about the European varieties of Walnut in his journals. He used the plant as an antidote against poisons, combined it with Rue (*Ruta graveolens*) to expel worms, and applied it externally to inflamed breasts, carbuncles, and gangrenous wounds (Dioscorides, 1959). Another famous Greek physician, Galen (*c.* A.D. 131–*c.* 200), recommended Walnut preparations "to drive worms forth from the belly . . . comfort the stomach, and expel poisons," and he also applied the oil to skin disorders, including bruises, carbuncles, and gangrenous wounds. He used the hull for its binding and astringent properties (Gerard, 1633).

Herbalist Maude Grieve wrote that the Romans called the tree *nux,* referring to its edible nuts. Walnut is an English name partly of Teutonic origin, and in Germany it was called *wallnuss* or *welsche nuss, welsche* meaning "foreign." The genus name *Juglans* comes from the Latin words *Jovis* (Jupiter) and *glans* (acorn or nut), meaning "Jupiter's nuts." According to old legends, ancient people once lived on bitter acorns while the gods indulged and feasted on delicious Walnuts, and hence the name Jupiter's nuts (Grieve, 1971).

Native Americans used their indigenous species, *Juglans nigra,* and its cousin the Butternut tree (*J. cinerea*) for food, dye and medicine, and taught European explorers and settlers about the value of these trees. A tea made with the inner bark acted as a cathartic laxative, and the bark was chewed to relieve toothaches by several Indian tribes, including the Cherokee, Comanche, Delaware, Iroquois, Dakota, Fox, Menominee, and Potawatomi (Moerman, 1998). The hull surrounding the nut was applied externally to treat ringworm and inflammations. A tea of the leaves was used as an astringent to stop bleeding wounds and diarrhea.

During America's colonial period, Butternut was the favorite of the two trees. But Black Walnut's popularity increased due to the influence of herbalist Samuel Thomson (1769–1843), who combined Black Walnut with small amounts of Cayenne (*Capsicum annuum*) to purge and cleanse the body, a common medical treatment of that period. Black Walnut is an old folk remedy for fungal infections like ringworm and athlete's foot, and was ingested to rid the body of parasites. During the 1880s–1930s, it was a popular herb used by the Eclectic physicians for conditions of toxicity, skin rashes, eczema, fungal infections, and parasites. Master herbalist and naturopath John Christopher (1909–1983) continued to promote the herb for these conditions in addition to intestinal cleansing, wound healing, skin diseases, inflammations, boils, acne, abscesses, shingles, excessive mucous discharge, hemorrhage, hemorrhoids, dysentery, ulcers, tumors, cancers, and severe dandruff due to toxic overload.

> *Walnuts are historically known as "brain food." According to the Doctrine of Signatures, the plant gives us this clue by the shape of the inner nut, which resembles the lobes of the brain contained in a hard hull similar to the human skull.*
>
> *Modern research confirms that the vitamins, minerals, protein, and especially the essential fatty acids in the nuts are excellent nourishment for normal brain and nerve function.*

Today, Walnut hulls continue to be a reputable treatment for parasites and fungal infections. They are commercially available in tincture, pill, and capsule preparations. Much of the current research on Black Walnut has been focused on the European variety, *Juglans regia*.

Healing Qualities

The entire plant is antibacterial, antifungal, anti-inflammatory, anti-hemorrhagic (stops bleeding), antiseptic, antiviral, astringent, depurative, detoxifying, emetic (in large amounts), laxative, and vulnerary.

The leaves have alterative, detergent, lymphagogue and vermifuge actions, and are more stimulating and effective in reducing spasms than the hulls. The leaves are excellent for treating digestive problems caused by a sluggish system and lack of digestive enzymes resulting in stagnation and constipation.

The hulls have diaphoretic, vermifuge, and exanthematous (treats skin diseases and eruptions) actions. They kill intestinal parasites and reduce chronic inflammation and infections, especially chronic digestive and genitourinary infections occurring with discharge. The bark is alterative, cathartic, and detergent.

Traditional Chinese Medicine (TCM) Perspective

The Walnut fruit is a Yin tonic food providing exceptional nutrients and oils to treat emaciation, malnutrition, and conditions of dryness. The strong medicinal bark, leaves, and hulls are bitter, drying and cooling, and exert very powerful and stimulating Yang energies that promote movement and purge heat, infections, and parasites. These medicinal parts of the tree stimulate bile flow in cases of Liver Qi Stagnation and improve conditions of Intestinal Qi Stagnation manifesting as abdominal distention, gas, pain, and chronic constipation. As a Kidney Yang herb, it stimulates strong movement and purging of impurities via the kidneys. The plant is dissolving to toxins, parasites, fungi, warts, tumors and infections, and stimulating to open the bowels and promote detoxification. The astringent quality reduces secretions, bleeding and diarrhea, and raises central Qi to improve conditions of prolapsed organs.

Primary Actions

The Walnut tree is a strong-acting warrior herb that forcefully purges infection, parasites, and toxic accumulation of waste products out of the body. Its powerful cathartic action opens the portals of elimination for their release through the skin, bowels, and kidneys. It is specific for <u>toxic</u> <u>conditions</u> in the intestines, blood, and skin caused by sluggish activity and stagnation in the gastrointestinal tract. This congestion causes gas, slow transit of food, chronic constipation, and eventual build-up of waste products and toxins that are unable to be eliminated through normal channels. Instead, skin rashes, boils, pimples and acne develop, and wounds become infected and resistant to healing. This condition stresses the immune system and provides an inviting opportunity for microbial invasion resulting in chronic parasites, fungal and Candida yeast infections, and eventually even tumors and cancers caused by stagnation and toxicity. The leaves and immature green hulls of Black Walnut trees are specific for this type of congested and toxic condition, and serve to stimulate, open, and purge the body.

The delicious nuts inside the hulls nourish the body by fortifying and strengthening the blood, bones, tissues, and nerves with an abundance of vitamins, minerals, proteins, and essential fatty acids. All seeds contain these nutrients essential to the lives of plants and humans, making nuts and seeds one of nature's "perfect foods." Eating a daily assortment of raw nuts and seeds promotes optimal health, both physical and mental.

Always be aware of the power of this herbal tree, and be sure to use the recommended dosages and instructions. Small to medium doses have an effective but gentle cleansing action.

Parasites: Black Walnut has a notable reputation and long history of use for eliminating parasites. Modern research has identified juglone, found in the leaves and green hull, to be the primary vermifuge in the plant that kills many types of mites and parasites, including amoebas, tapeworms, and giardia. It is especially effective against roundworms and pinworms. For mites and scabies that burrow under the skin, apply tincture or tea directly on the skin and allow the area to soak. Remember that it will temporarily stain the skin.

To kill internal parasites, their breeding and hatching cycle must be taken into account. Parasites enter the body, locate a place of residence, and lay eggs or cysts. The protective walls of the cysts can make them difficult to kill, and often they must first hatch. Parasites typically increase their activity around the time of the full moon, and use of Black Walnut and other vermifuge herbs should revolve around this moon cycle. For best results, ingest these herbs for 2 weeks, beginning a week before the full moon and continuing until a week after. Stop taking the herbs for 2 weeks around the new moon, then start again a week prior to the full moon. Considering that parasites lay their eggs in cycles, it is most effective to use this 2-weeks-on and 2-weeks-off schedule for 3-4 months to ensure that all parasites and their eggs are destroyed.

Be sure that the bowels are open to facilitate complete passage and elimination of parasites. Black Walnut has a strong laxative effect, but if constipation is a problem, take it with other laxative herbs such as Cascara Sagrada (*Rhamnus purshiana*) and Senna (*Senna marilandica,* spp).

Combining other vermifuge herbs with Black Walnut produces a more effective, broad spectrum ability to kill parasites, and include Wormwood (*Artemisia absinthium*), Cloves (*Syzygium aromaticum*), Pau D'arco (*Tabebuia impetiginosa*), Yarrow (*Achillea millefolium*), American Centaury (*Sabatia angularis*), Elecampane (*Inula helenium*), Mugwort (*Artemisia vulgaris*), Cayenne (*Capsicum annuum*), Garlic (*Allium sativum*), and Feverfew (*Tanacetum parthenium*).

I highly recommend using food grade diatomaceous earth in addition to herbal therapy when treating parasites. Diatomaceous earth (DE) is a powdered sedimentary rock composed of the fossilized remains of microscopic shells of ocean algae, called diatoms. DE consists of 80-90% silica, which has a sharp crystalline structure that pierces through the bodies of intestinal parasites and kills them, but does not damage intestinal tissues. DE does not kill parasite eggs, so it must be taken in 2-week cycles as described above. Although DE is not absorbed through the intestinal walls into the bloodstream, it does pull heavy metals and other toxins out of the intestinal tract. The recommended dose is 1-3 teaspoons of the powdered food grade DE in liquid, applesauce, yogurt, or other suitable food once a day. Do not breathe the powder into the lungs because it can damage delicate membranes lining the respiratory tract. Food grade DE can be taken by cats, dogs, and other animals as well as humans. My cats used to be infested with parasites on a regular basis, but no longer have this problem when given very small amounts of DE periodically. DE is gentle to the digestive system, non-toxic, and completely safe to ingest. Since antiparasitic herbs tend to be very potent, especially for children and adults with sensitive systems, I recommend DE to clients, including children, with good results.

Candida Yeast, Fungal, Bacterial, and Viral Infections: Many research studies demonstrate that juglone's antimicrobial properties include antifungal (Ali-Shtayeh, 1999; Heisey, 1992), antiviral (Harborne, 1993), and antibiotic activity (Blumenthal, 2000; Clark, 1990; Omar, 2000; Tripathi, 1988). It is beneficial for treating all types of fungal infections, including ringworm, athlete's foot, and internal and external Candida yeast. It can be effective against warts, which are viral infections. Ellagic acid and juglone in Walnut trees have demonstrated inhibitory effects on some types of cancers in mice, such as decreased tumor growth and size, while increasing weight in the mice (Bhargava, 1968; Chae, 2012). A tincture of Black Walnut hulls contains large amounts of iodine, which is well known for its antibiotic and antiseptic properties and ability to protect against radiation damage. The hulls are able to inhibit of several types of bacteria, including *Klebsiella pneumonia, Proteus vulgaris, Salmonella, Shigella, Staphylococcus aureus, Bacillus subtilis,* and *E. coli* (Brinker, 1995).

For warts and external fungal and yeast infections, Black Walnut tincture or tea can be applied to the affected area 2-3 times during the day (remember that it temporarily discolors the skin). It is also beneficial to take small doses of the tea, tincture, capsules, or pills internally for 2 weeks, stop for a couple of weeks, and then continue this on-and-off schedule (described above) for 2-3 months.

Digestion and Elimination: The potent bitter quality of Black Walnut leaves, hulls, and bark have a very stimulating effect on the organs of digestion and elimination. Eclectic physicians recognized this and Finley Ellingwood, M.D. (1852–1920) wrote, "Experiments with the drug have ascertained that it influences, with great energy, the liver, small intestine, colon and rectum, causing an increased manufacture and elimination of bile, as well as increased activity of the glands of the intestinal tract. Full doses produce large bilious evacuations, without much pain or griping" (Ellingwood, 1919). Walnut leaves and hulls are beneficial for liver congestion, and Eclectic doctors used these as a laxative for chronic constipation due to a deficiency of bile, which causes the stool to be clay-colored. They used Black Walnut in small doses to treat chronic jaundice, dysentery, diarrhea, intestinal and blood toxemia (toxins in bowels and blood), and intestinal problems involving bleeding, inflammation, and hemorrhoids. In her book, *Health from God's Garden,* Austrian herbalist Maria Treben recommended sipping 2-3 cups of the leaf tea over the course of a day to treat jaundice (Treben, 1986). Black Walnut is helpful for chronic diarrhea or constipation caused by parasites, Candida yeast infection, or disruption of beneficial intestinal flora.

The astringent property of Walnut leaves and hulls helps stop diarrhea and bleeding throughout the digestive tract. Astringents tone weak, flabby, atonic muscles and help prolapsed organs return to their normal positions. Astringents also reduce excessive secretions, discharges, and bleeding from atonic, boggy membranes. The Eclectic physicians combined Black Walnut with Cayenne (*Capsicum annuum*) for these types of sluggish and debilitated conditions. Small amounts of Walnut leaves and hulls can be beneficial for the treatment of peptic ulcers, gastroenteritis (inflammation of the stomach and intestinal lining), colitis, and other irritable bowel syndromes.

Detoxification and Skin Conditions: The ability of Black Walnut to eliminate parasites, fungal, bacterial and viral infections, plus its stimulating action on the liver and intestines, make it a wonderful herb for many types of toxic conditions of the blood, intestines, skin, and other organs. It is specific for toxicity caused by a slow, sluggish system with resulting stagnation and constipation. The German Commission E regulatory agency has endorsed Walnut leaves for treating skin inflammation and to stop bleeding from wounds. The herb has antiseptic and detergent (cleansing) actions on the skin and mucous membranes. Research shows that it has a vasorelaxant effect (relaxes blood vessels), which improves blood flow and elimination of toxins (Perusquia, 1995). Black Walnut leaves encourage the normal flow and detoxification of lymphatic fluids, reduce congestion, and eliminate bacteria and viruses responsible for enlarged, inflamed lymph nodes. Black Walnut works well combined with 2-5 drops of Poke (*Phytolacca decandra*) root tincture. Poke is an excellent and very potent herb for lymphatic infection and congestion that should be taken 1-2 times a day in small amounts of 2-5 drops due to potential for toxicity.

Use Black Walnut externally as a wash or poultice, and in small amounts internally for all conditions of blood and metabolic toxicity with poor elimination, including chronic dermatitis, skin rashes, oozing or irritated skin conditions such as eczema, impetigo (a staph infection on the skin) and other infections, abscesses, boils, acne, tumors, ringworm, athlete's foot, herpes and shingles lesions, and chronic, slow-to-heal wounds and ulcers. The tincture may be used full strength or diluted, and applied to the affected area 2-3 times a day. The tea may be used as a wash in the same way. A cotton gauze or piece of cloth may be dipped and saturated with the tincture or tea, placed over the area, and secured with tape or ace wrap. The dried leaves may also be made into a poultice for external application.

In her book, Maria Treben recommended a tea of the leaves to purify the blood. For dandruff, cradle cap, hair loss and head lice, she bathed the scalp with a tea of the leaves. She wrote, "Even the most stubborn rashes and pus-filled eruptions can be healed by bathing the affected area with a Walnut leaf wash" (Treben, 1988). In Germany, the leaves are approved for skin inflammation and excessive perspiration of the hands and feet. In France, they are topically applied for the treatment of itchy scalp and dandruff, superficial burns and skin disorders, and in India for malignant sores and pustules (Blumenthal, 2000). In one research study, Black Walnut protected rat livers from arsenite (a very toxic and carcinogenic mineral) poisoning, and prevented chromosomal damage and mutation (Owumi, 2013).

Women's Health: This herbal tree is effective for the treatment of vaginal infections and discharge, Candida yeast, and cervical ulcers or erosion. For these problems, make a lukewarm tea of Walnut leaves or green hulls and administer it as a douche on a daily basis for 7-10 days, or until all symptoms are absent for 5 days. Other herbs to combine with Walnut for this purpose include Goldenseal (*Hydrastis canadensis*), Yarrow (*Achillea millefolium*), and Marshmallow (*Althaea officinalis*) root.

Cardiovascular System: The nuts of the Walnut tree are especially beneficial in protecting against cardiovascular disease due to their high content of omega-3 fatty acids, antioxidants, and arginine. Clinical research confirms that daily consumption of one ounce of Black walnuts (*Juglans nigra*) can reduce total cholesterol and increase beneficial high-density lipoprotein cholesterol (HDL) (Fitschen, 2011).

Thyroid: Thyroxine, called T4, is a thyroid hormone containing iodine and the amino acid tyrosine. It is one of the important thyroid hormones that acts as a catalyst exerting a wide range of influence throughout the body. It increases metabolic rate and is necessary for general growth and development, the digestion of food, reproduction, and resistance to infection. Underactivity of the thyroid gland, or hypothyroidism, is very common and undiagnosed in many people.

In his book *Green Pharmacy*, herbal authority James Duke notes that in Turkish folk medicine, Walnut hulls are remedies for various glandular problems, including thyroid imbalance and underactivity. He cites a study in which the fresh juice of green Walnut hulls doubled thyroxine levels to improve hypothyroidism. A tea made by boiling the green Walnut hulls for 20 minutes increased thyroxine levels by at least 30% (Duke, 1997).

Teachings from the Black Walnut Deva

"Greetings, dear one. I am the Black Walnut Tree Deva. It would be good for you to sit on the ground at my base with your back leaning against my trunk. Then you will more closely feel, both physically and intuitively, the strength and firmness of my body and my being.

"I have lived on this land for a long time. I was a favorite of the indigenous people who once populated and thrived on this land, which they called Turtle Island. They used me for a dye and as an astringent to tighten the skin and heal wounds, and yes, they knew to use me to protect against and combat internal worms and parasites. I have tannins in my bark, leaves and seed hulls, which is excellent medicine to tighten the skin and stop bleeding. For this purpose, my fresh leaves were pulverized into a mash and placed upon wounds after the skin had been sewn together with sinew. I decrease inflammation and wound pain, as well as prevent and treat infections.

"Today, I am primarily used to combat worms and parasites by your people. For this purpose, I must be used with caution and for short intervals over a period of time, as my action is powerful, and excessive use can actually bring imbalance to the system. You wonder how I can be a treatment for worms and parasites when tiny worms eat and live in my decaying hulls? This is because some creatures have adapted to my toxins and strong chemicals, but the parasitic creatures that cause disruption to animals and humans are not so adapted. And thus, I eat away and dissolve the soft bodies of parasites with my harsh chemicals.

"I am a tree, a large herb, and just as my roots travel deep into the earth, so my medicine power naturally moves down into the bowels of the body to clean and empty. I have a stimulating effect on the liver and quickly move bile into the gallbladder and out into the intestines, stimulating contractions and movement to propel waste and parasites out of the body. My hulls purify and cleanse to destroy and expel invasive creatures. Respect my power by using small amounts with caution.

"My energies resonate with the color yellow. This is the color of my juices that stain the hands deep yellow after handling my hulls. Yellow is the vibrational quality that generates and governs the solar plexus nerves and digestive system. My gifts to the digestive system are the perfect foods of my seeds that build and maintain the body structure, which benefit many animals and humans alike. When eaten raw, my seeds provide all the nutrients essential to life: protein, carbohydrates, vitamins, minerals, and fats. These are the core and radiance of my feminine nature, offering nourishment to provide structure to the body. My hulls are the embodiment of masculine energies, and like warriors they surround and protect the seeds. When living in a balanced way, people must eat nourishing foods that produce healthy bodies. Then the wrathful power of my hulls to kill parasites and stir up the system is rarely required. In this way, I will be used in balance and do no harm to those who use my medicine.

"This is the message of the Black Walnut: Walk in balance upon this land, which is Creator's gift to people and animals. Be in community with your brothers and sisters, and exist in a peaceful way. Look at the Black Walnut trees and follow our example, as we naturally grow in communities when left undisturbed. All of life is intrinsically interconnected and sacred to Creator. This is my voice and my song. When you see a Black Walnut tree, remember this song and sing it to your family of brothers and sisters on the earth. We invite all humans to sit next to us and lean against our strong, supportive trunk. And if you sit with an open heart and still your mind to hear the silence, we will be here to teach you and grace you with a deep sense of well-being!"

Parting Thoughts

Black Walnut is certainly a "protector plant" and is the strongest, most forceful of all the deva personalities I have yet had the pleasure to meet. The presence and feeling of the Black Walnut Deva was like standing under the tallest and oldest of trees, whose wise, powerful, and somewhat stern presence towered above and protected all creatures — the younger, smaller trees and herbs below, the woodland animals, and me.

Bloodroot

Sanguinaria canadensis
Papaveraceae (Poppy) Family

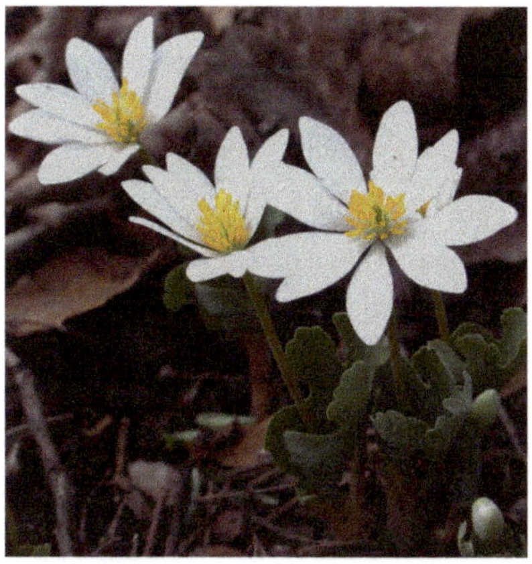

Common Names

Red root, red puccoon, Indian plant, Indian paint, and red paint root are older names descriptive of the bright-red roots and their historic use by Native Americans. Strongly colored plants like Bloodroot that were used as dyes were commonly called "puccoon." Tetterwort is another old name. Tetter is an antiquated term for skin eruptions like fungus and warts, which Bloodroot has been known to heal.

Medicinal Part of the Plant

The root is the official and most potent part, although the whole plant contains medicinal constituents.

Range and Habitat

Bloodroot is a perennial herb indigenous to the rich, moist, loamy deciduous woodlands of central and eastern United States and Canada. It grows in similar habitats as Goldenseal (*Hydrastis canadensis*), Ginseng (*Panax quinquefolius*), Mayapple (*Podophyllum peltatum*), Wild Ginger (*Asarum canadense*), Black Cohosh (*Cimicifuga racemosa*), and Blue Cohosh (*Caulophyllum thalictroides*).

Description of the Plant

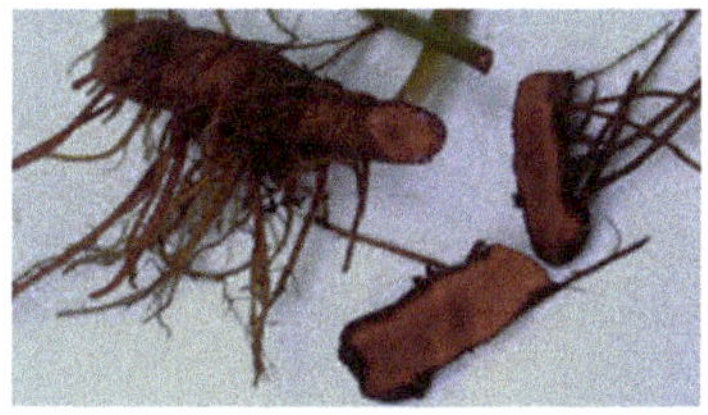

Red roots

Bloodroot is a beautiful ornamental herb and one of the earliest spring flowers to grace the woodlands. The plant grows 6-12″ tall. The root is 1-5″ long and is a horizontally growing rhizome that can spread out into short, branching sections. This unusual fleshy, succulent root is round and about as thick as a woman's pinky finger. Circular bands cover the outer surface and probably reflect the age of the plant. Thread-like rootlets grow off the main rhizome. The end of the rhizome typically looks like it is broken or cut off. The roots have a brownish-red exterior and a juicy, brilliant reddish-orange interior. This characteristic is described by the plant's common name "Bloodroot" and by the botanical name *Sanguinaria,* which in Latin means "bloody." The stems and leaf veins all exude red juice when broken.

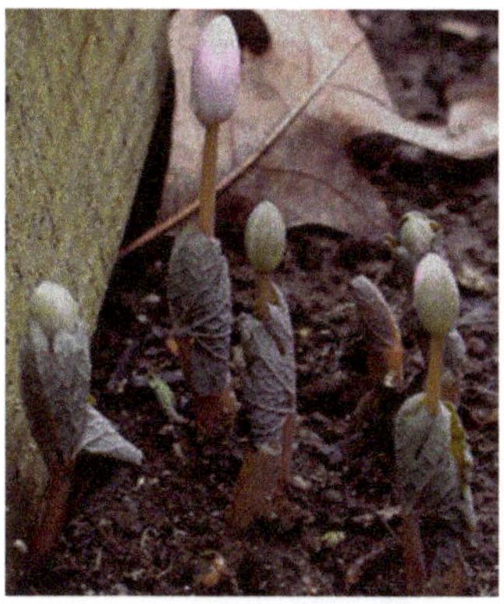

Sprouting flower heads and leaves

A leaf stalk and a separate flower stalk emerge from buds on the rhizome in very early spring, beginning in March in southern ranges to May in northern woodlands. The flower bud is completely enclosed by a developing leaf when it first emerges from the root. As the leaf unwraps, the flower opens on the terminal end of its stalk. The erect stems are round and smooth. Each has one single flower or one leaf at its tip. The lovely, shiny-white flowers grow 1-2″ in diameter and are odorless. They usually have 8-12 narrow petals and about 24-35 stamens with large, flat, yellow anthers surrounding the central pistil, which consists of a pale-green ovary and yellow stigma. The short-lived flowers only last a few days before the petals and stamens fall off, leaving the ovary.

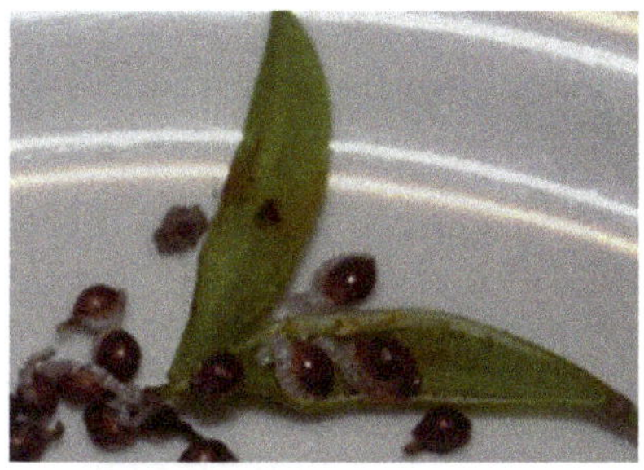

Seeds with white arils

About four weeks after blooming, the ovary matures into a pointed, oblong, green pod. This turns brown as it dries, and many round, shiny, dark-brown seeds pop out of the pod. Each seed has an appendage, which is a distinctive white, fleshy crest called an aril or raphe. Ants are attracted to the sweet flavor of the aril and carry the seeds considerable distances from the plant to their nests for future meals, leaving seeds in the soil to germinate. Bloodroot plants and ants have an interesting symbiotic relationship in which the plants provide food and ants disperse the seeds.

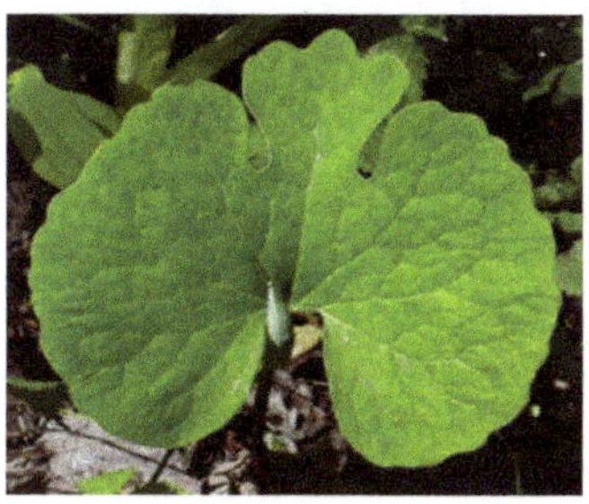

Leaf with seedpod

Each simple, palmately-shaped leaf is deeply lobed with 3-9 deep, rounded indentations. Leaves emerging from older roots can reach 8-12″ across towards the end of their growing season. The palmately veined leaves are smooth with an entire, wavy margin. The veins on the underside have a reddish-orange cast due to the presence of the brightly colored juice. The leaves have a distinctively unique appearance that, in addition to the red juice, provides an easy way to identify the plant.

Years ago, I spent many hours with friends hiking and playing in the woods. We were drawn to this unique-looking plant and, discovering the red root, we instinctively painted our faces and arms with the juice, feeling very "earthy" and primal. Many years later, my friend Dark Rain Thom of the Shawnee Nation told me that Native American people used to paint their bodies with the red juice of Bloodroot to keep insects away, and she wondered if that was why the "boat people" (as she calls the European immigrants) called Native Americans the "red man."

Cultivation

Bloodroot can be propagated from seed or by root division. The plant naturally self-propagates when the seeds ripen in late spring and drop to the ground. Seeds do not require stratification to germinate. Once they are blanketed in moist soil, they absorb and swell with water, split in half, and the embryonic root establishes itself by autumn or the following spring. Some seeds remain dormant for two years until the second spring before germinating.

Seed cultivation can be challenging because they quickly lose viability with dehydration. Freshly harvested seeds and roots may be purchased from nurseries specializing in herbs or, if you have access to woodlands where the plant grows, the seeds can be harvested and immediately planted before drying out. Seeds can be stored in moist sand in the refrigerator for a short time only, since they have a tendency to rot in this environment.

Sow the seeds ¼" deep and 2-4" apart in a prepared woodland bed or another shady area such as the north-facing side of a house or garage. The soil must be rich in humus, loose, and moist with good drainage. After germinating, seedlings can remain where they are or be transplanted to a permanent shady bed after a few years of growth. Using this method, I generally have a 75-85% germination rate. Plants will start flowering 3-4 years after germination and require at least 5-6 years to grow roots large enough to harvest for medicine or use for root divisions.

Root division is the easier and faster way to propagate this herb. Dig up the roots of mature plants in summer after the seeds have matured and dropped, but before the leaves die back. Divide roots into 1" pieces that each have a bud, and immediately replant them about 1" deep with the bud pointing upward in the direction it will grow. Water and mulch the divided roots, and keep a watchful eye for flowers and leaves to emerge the following spring.

Harvest

Roots may be harvested in spring or autumn. One study showed that the highest alkaloid content occurs during the flowering and seed-forming stage (Foster, 1993). However, I suggest harvesting the root right after the plant has blossomed and dropped its seeds, giving it the opportunity to re-seed. When digging up the root, take most of it, but be sure to break off a 1" piece containing a bud and replant it. This should grow into a new plant the following spring and contribute to the herb's survival.

Seeds can be harvested and immediately planted for cultivation purposes. Timing is essential when harvesting seeds. The green seedpod begins to develop after flower petals fall off in early spring. Staying green for 2-4 weeks, the seedpod then starts to dry and turns brown. The seeds are mature 5-7 weeks after the blossoms fade. When the pod is sufficiently dry, it bursts open and the shiny, dark-brown seeds pop out and land close to the parent plant. The pods must be carefully watched and the seeds collected when they are mature, but before the pod pops open. Regular visits to the plant as the pods dry and turn brown are helpful.

Preparation of Plant Medicine and Dosages

After harvesting and thoroughly washing the roots, they can be prepared fresh as tincture, tea or salve, or chopped into pieces and applied directly to the skin. These preparations are much more potent if made with fresh rather than dried roots, which deteriorate rapidly. Active properties of Bloodroot can be extracted by alcohol or boiling water. Tincturing the roots is the best form of preparation because alcohol is the superior solvent and tinctures remain potent medicines with a long shelf life. It is also much easier to take a few drops of tincture in a little water than to drink the very bitter tea.

Sometimes Bloodroot is needed as powder for external application. In this case, the roots must be dried and ground into powder. Chop the fresh roots into pieces and place them on screens to dry in a shaded, well-ventilated area. Do not chop the root into excessively tiny pieces when drying because the medicinal juice leaks out from the severed roots and is lost. Store dehydrated roots in jars away from light and do not grind them into powder until you are ready to use them, because grinding increases oxidative damage and hastens deterioration. Although not nearly as strong as fresh roots, dried roots retain potency for at least two years. When taking Bloodroot tea or tincture internally, be sure to drink large amounts of water to dilute it and carry it through the system. Be *extremely cautious* of the strong effects this herb can induce and use *very* small amounts!

PREPARATIONS

Due to its potential toxicity, only use Bloodroot with the supervision of a health professional!

Tincture: Chop freshly harvested roots into small pieces and stuff them into a glass jar. Cover with a mixture of 60% 190-proof grain alcohol and 40% distilled water, and prepare in the usual manner. Dosage: 3-6 drops diluted in water taken 1-3 times daily for acute conditions and lung infections. For treating cancer and other chronic problems, take 1-3 drops once a day. Some herbalists recommend as many as 25 drops of tincture per dose, but I always encourage smaller doses until each person's sensitivity to this very potent herb is determined.

Small doses of 1-3 drops have a stimulating effect on circulation, heart activity, and secretion of digestive enzymes. Medium doses of 4-6 drops are used as a lung expectorant. In larger doses, Bloodroot acts as an emetic to induce vomiting, lowers blood pressure, and is sedating to the heart (Felter, 1922). Various herbalists suggest different dosages of the tincture. My recommendation of 1-5 drops is conservative compared to the dosages of the Eclectic physicians, which ranged up to 15 drops. Acclaimed herbalist and naturopathic physician John Bastyr used 10 drops 3 times a day for infections (Mitchell, 2003). Due to the powerful activity and potential toxicity of Bloodroot, respectful caution is recommended. For chronic problems, only take small doses and alternate use by taking it for 3 weeks and then skipping a couple of weeks before continuing again. This cycle can be repeated several times. It is usually best to take Bloodroot with other herbs appropriate for the problem being addressed.

Tea: Follow the example of the Eclectic physicians and simmer 1 teaspoon of the chopped root in a cup of water for 4-5 minutes, then let it steep for 10 minutes. Dosage: The Eclectics recommended small doses of 1 teaspoon every 2-3 hours as needed (Felter, 1922). The fresh root and tea have a harsh, sharp, bitter, and peppery (acrid) flavor that lingers on the tongue and throat for several minutes.

Paste and Salve for External Application: Bloodroot can be made into a water- or oil-based paste by grinding dried roots into a fine powder (with a small coffee bean grinder) and adding enough water or oil to make a thick paste. Or prepare salve by chopping fresh roots into small pieces, placing them in a stainless steel pan, barely covering them with olive oil, and baking the mix at 220°F for 2 hours. Cool and strain the oil from the pieces of root. Beeswax may be added to solidify the oil into an ointment. Apply the dark-brown paste or salve to the skin to draw out and reduce cancers, tumors, warts, moles, and fungal infections. **Warning: *Only* cover ½-2" of the skin with Bloodroot paste or salve, and *never* cover large areas of skin since it can leave an open wound.**

Chemical Constituents

Bloodroot contains several isoquinoline alkaloids found in other members of the Poppy family. The most abundant alkaloid is sanguinarine (about 50% of the alkaloid content), which has broad-spectrum antibacterial, antiviral, antifungal, anti-inflammatory, antioxidant, antitumor, and expectorant properties. It binds to plaque on teeth and kills most bacteria that promote tooth decay. It can reduce gum inflammation and infection occurring with gingivitis. Sanguinarine is also known to increase respiration, raise blood pressure, and have laxative effects by stimulating intestinal movement.

Other alkaloids include protopine (abortifacient, analgesic, antibacterial, anti-arrhythmic, antitussive, anti-inflammatory, uterine tonic), sanguidimerine (antitumor), coptisine (anti-inflammatory and antitumor), chelirubine (antibacterial and pesticide), and chelerythrine (analgesic, antibacterial, antiviral, anti-inflammatory). Allocryptopine is analgesic, anti-arrhythmic and oxytocic, and berberine (also found in Goldenseal) is analgesic, antibacterial, anticarcinogenic, anticonvulsant, anti-inflammatory, cholagogue, and hypotensive. The root also contains chelidonic acid, citric acid, and malic acid (sialogogue and antibacterial).

Safety, Contraindications, and Drug Interactions

Bloodroot is a powerful plant that should always be used with much respect and caution. **Due to its potential toxicity, only use Bloodroot with the supervision of an experienced herbalist and health care practitioner.** When taken internally, small doses of 1-3 drops of the tincture are stimulating and warming, and some sensitive people experience symptoms of hyperactivity, pounding heart, feeling faint, vertigo (dizziness), burning sensations in the stomach and intestines, increased salivary and bile secretions, nausea, vomiting, and visual disturbances for several hours. These symptoms have occurred in two of my clients, and were rather frightening for them. Although many people have reported these side effects, there are no published reports of the plant causing toxicity in humans. Due to the strong potency of the alkaloids, however, large amounts of Bloodroot are not recommended under any condition.

Animal studies show that excessive doses of Bloodroot initially stimulate and accelerate heart activity and blood pressure, and then depress the entire system. When the system is depressed, the muscles relax, the skin becomes cold and clammy, pupils dilate, activity of the nervous system diminishes, and heart rate and blood pressure decrease. Animal research indicates that continual high doses can cause liver toxicity and pitting edema, although the plant is traditionally only used for short periods of time. **Bloodroot is absolutely contraindicated during pregnancy and lactation, and is not given to small children** (Brinker, 2001; McGuffin, 1997).

One of my apprentices, an elderly man, shared his experience of interesting symptoms after using Bloodroot. He had a problem tooth where the gum had receded, and he squirted several drops of the tincture around the tooth and surrounding gum. He immediately felt a strong pulsation of blood in the tooth area that lasted two to three hours. His nasal sinuses became dry and the herb stimulated a productive cough expressing yellow phlegm, which was the last symptom of a cold he was trying to shake off. He reported feelings of lassitude, lethargy, loss of motivation, and difficulty articulating his speech for about four days. He also experienced confusion from distorted visual perceptions, and had difficulty recognizing two women he had known for years. Sharing with me, he said that his overall feeling was that his body was "shutting down." He fully recovered after four days, but his story is a good example of the extreme side effects this herb can induce, emphasizing the need for prudence and small doses.

External use of Bloodroot also demands much caution. Its caustic ability to dissolve tissue with prolonged contact is helpful for dissolving warts, tumors, and some types of cancers. However, it can cause incredible damage and actually eat away at the skin when used incorrectly or combined with other caustic materials such as zinc chloride. Although the possible side effects of Bloodroot seem daunting, 1-3 drops of the tincture or external application can be very effective when used as recommended and with the supervision of an herbalist experienced in using this herb.

Medicinal Uses

History of the Plant

Bloodroot was commonly used for medicine, dye, and body paint by Native American people living in the eastern and central deciduous forests of North America. The Cherokees used small amounts of the root to treat lung inflammation, coughs and excessive mucous discharge, breast cancer, and externally as a wash for skin ulcers and sores. The Iroquois used the roots as an emetic to purge toxins, as a remedy for colds, intestinal problems and parasites, and externally for wounds and skin cancers (Foster, 1993). The Mohegans steeped the root to use as a blood purifier and emetic. Menominees added it to other medicines to increase their strength. The Potawatomis and Ojibwas squeezed juice from the root onto maple sugar lumps and sucked them for sore throats. The Delaware and other tribes employed the plant for gastrointestinal and respiratory problems, coughs, bronchitis, and for conditions involving the blood, including hemorrhage, wounds, and toxic conditions. A paste was externally applied for swellings, aches, and joint pain. The Delaware also used it for gynecological problems (Moerman, 1998).

The early trappers, explorers, and settlers in North America learned about Bloodroot from the indigenous people. By the 1800s, the herb was a favorite of the early American Eclectic physicians, who prescribed the root as a stimulating expectorant for coughs, bronchitis, pneumonia, whooping cough, and other lung diseases. Medical doctors used it to treat gonorrhea, syphilis, vaginal yeast infections, menstrual irregularities, amenorrhea (abnormal absence of periods), painful menses, male impotence, jaundice, chronic hepatitis, otitis media (ear infection), and lupus. They applied the pulverized root to treat eczema, wounds, warts, and fungal growths like ringworm. The tea was applied as a wash on tumors and ulcerated skin, and taken as a snuff for nasal polyps. During the 1800s, a London physician named Dr. Fells mixed the powdered root with flour, water and zinc chloride, and applied it to breast cancers with good results. Bloodroot was listed as an official medicine in the *U.S. Pharmacopoeia* from 1820–1926 and in the *National Formulary* from 1925–1965.

Since it is a very powerful and potentially toxic herb, Bloodroot is not in large demand commercially. Due to loss of habitat caused by human sprawl, it is becoming increasingly scarce and is on the "at risk" list for plants in danger of becoming extinct. Cultivation is encouraged to ensure the continued survival of this beautiful woodland herb.

Healing Qualities

Antimicrobial activity includes antiseptic, antibiotic, antiviral, and antifungal properties. Roots are also anticarcinogenic, anti-catarrahal, anti-inflammatory, antispasmodic, antitumor, cardio-active, cathartic, caustic, emetic, exanthematous, expectorant, pectoral, rubefacient, sialagogue, sedating in large doses, and stimulating in small doses.

Traditional Chinese Medicine (TCM) Perspective

Bloodroot is bitter, hot, and potentially toxic in large doses. It is a very powerful Yang herb that stimulates a lot of heat, activity and movement, and is useful for conditions of Qi stagnation throughout the body.

Primary Actions

Bloodroot exerts primary activity on the blood. Its broad-spectrum antimicrobial capacity helps purify the blood and tissues. The herb stimulates vigorous movement throughout the body, purging whatever gets in its way. It increases circulation and secretions of the mucous membranes, glands, and digestive enzymes. It can dissolve and draw out tumors and toxins and eliminate fungal infections and viral warts. It is used to treat sluggish, atonic conditions of the nasal sinuses and lungs that cause increased mucous production, and for poor circulation eventually leading to toxic accumulation.

I mainly use the tinctured root for treating coughs, bronchitis, and resistant lung infections. Most research on Bloodroot pertains to its use in dentistry, investigations concerning its antibacterial and antiviral properties, and its ability to treat cancer.

> *Bloodroot is potentially toxic and should only be used in small doses with supervision of a health professional.*

Infections and the Respiratory System: Bloodroot has a stimulating effect on circulation in the lungs. On the bronchial muscles it exerts a relaxing, antispasmodic action that resolves spasms and coughs and reduces phlegm. Bloodroot is specific for burning, itching, and irritated mucous membranes in the nasal sinus cavities and lungs, and helps normalize excessive mucous secretions causing sinus drainage or congestion. American Eclectic physicians used the herb for the treatment of acute and chronic respiratory problems, including lung congestion and hemorrhage, coughs (especially indicated for dry, harsh coughs), whooping cough, bronchitis, croup, pneumonia, sore throat, laryngitis, and emphysema.

Extensive research investigations have identified sanguinarine as the major alkaloid in Bloodroot. It possesses broad antimicrobial activity against both bacterial and viral infections, and it is also an anti-inflammatory and expectorant (Karlowsky, 1991). Animal studies have shown that the alkaloid is active against both Gram-positive and Gram-negative bacteria, Candida yeast, fungi, and *Trichomonas*, which is a genus of protozoa parasites (Godowski, 1989). In laboratory research, sanguinarine induced cell death in methicillin-resistant *Staphylococcus aureus* (MRSA) (Obiang-Obounou, 2011).

I have noticed substantial improvement in several cases of stubborn coughs, bronchitis, and other acute lung infections after using 3-5 drops of the tincture twice a day for a few days. For respiratory problems, it should always be combined with other herbs lacking potential toxicity, such as Horehound (*Marrubium vulgare*), Pleurisy Root (*Asclepias tuberosa*), Elecampane (*Inula helenium*), Goldenseal (*Hydrastis canadensis*), and Sage (*Salvia officinalis*). For coughs and bronchial asthma, Bloodroot works well when blended with small amounts (3-5 drops) of Lobelia (*Lobelia inflata*) tincture.

Dental Applications for Periodontal Problems: Bloodroot's ability to reduce plaque, which promotes cavities, and gingivitis (gum disease) have been scientifically demonstrated. For many years, sanguinarine in Bloodroot was marketed as an anti-inflammatory and antimicrobial ingredient in dental hygiene products such as anti-plaque toothpastes and mouthwashes. Sanguinarine chemically binds to dental plaque, preventing it from adhering to teeth and inhibiting 98% of bacterial growth (Dzink, 1985; Harkrader, 1990).

Several clinical studies have shown Bloodroot extract to be safe and effective in promoting healthy gums and preventing plaque formation, cavities, and periodontal disease (Godowski, 1989; Frankos, 1990). It has been used to fight gingivitis and was added to commercial toothpastes such as Viadent and Dentifrice, which are recommended by dentists to treat periodontal disease. Viadent reduced plaque by 57%, gum inflammation by 60%, and bleeding gums by 45% in a 6-month clinical study involving 24 people (Hannah, 1989). In another clinical trial, 30 people suffering with gingivitis and bleeding gums used toothpaste and oral rinse containing sanguinarine for 12 weeks. The test group reported diminished gum bleeding and inflammation and reduced reoccurrence of gingivitis (Tenenbaum, 1999).

A 1990 review of clinical trials revealed that people using dental preparations containing Bloodroot consistently experienced positive reductions in plaque, cavities, gum inflammation, and bleeding. With the exception of only one person out of 260 people tested, there were no adverse tissue effects (Kuftinec, 1990). However, the herb is no longer added to commercial dental preparations after data entered the media indicating that continual use may cause leukoplakia, which are precancerous lesions caused by irritation on the inside of the cheek or tongue.

Cancer: Bloodroot has a long historic use in treating different types of tumors and cancers. It is taken internally and for many years has also been marketed as a salve for topical application on skin cancers and tumors. Bloodroot exerts a cleansing effect on the blood and stimulates sluggish circulation to move and disperse toxins and excess heat, which is always beneficial in treating tumors and cancers.

Many studies indicate that the herb's primary mechanism to reduce cancer cells is the ability of sanguinarine to stimulate apoptosis. Apoptosis is the biological "time clock" process of programmed cell death that protects the body by destroying damaged or dysfunctional cells. Apoptosis protects against uncontrolled cell division and proliferation, which is one of the main characteristics of cancerous cells.

Researchers performing *in vivo* studies on the effects of sanguinarine on prostate cancer found that after 24 hours of contact, sanguinarine initiated death of prostate cancer cells by apoptosis and inhibited growth of new cancer cells. The researchers concluded that sanguinarine may be developed as an agent for the management of prostate cancer (Adhami, 2004). Sanguinarine induces apoptosis in leukemia, a cancer of the white blood cells (Han, 2008), in lymphoma cells (Hussain, 2007), and in human breast cancer cells (Kim, 2008). Researchers have also observed that sanguinarine treatment induces a dose-dependent increase in apoptosis of human colon cancer cells (Lee, 2012).

Naturopathic physician and herbalist John Bastyr, N.D., used Bloodroot to treat cervical erosion and dysplasia (precancerous cells in the cervix) by applying 3 drops of the tincture to the cervix. His student, William Mitchell, described his experience of applying Bloodroot salve on a patient with suppurative (discharging pus) breast cancer: "This patient refused allopathic treatment and wanted only natural, traditional earth medicine. The tumor suppurated and eventually the body healed itself. The cancer destroyed the breast itself, and when the wound healed all that was left was the chest wall with scar tissue and skin on it. It looked remarkably like the breast had been removed surgically" (Mitchell, 2003).

I have seen a few cases in which external applications of Bloodroot salve removed tumors. When thick applications of the ointment are placed on the skin for several hours, the caustic and irritant qualities of the herb create an open wound by dissolving the skin. If cancer or tumors are present, Bloodroot penetrates into deep tissue layers and draws cancerous cells out of the body. This treatment should only be done under medical supervision.

For further information and instructions for applying Bloodroot in this way, refer to the excellent book *Cancer Salves: A Botanical Approach to Treatment* by Dr. Ingrid Naiman, Seventh Ray Press, 1704-B Llano St, Suite 227, Santa Fe, NM 87505.

HIV: In 1992, a combination of Bloodroot and Celandine (*Chelidonium majus*) was given to 13 HIV patients as an experimental study (D'Adamo, 1992). Improvements were noted in persistent generalized lymphadenopathy, a disease of the lymph nodes. Although it is not traditionally used for HIV, it might be worth trying small daily doses of Bloodroot tincture, considering its broad antimicrobial activity and ability to cleanse the blood.

External Applications: Bloodroot has a long history of external use for removing warts, moles, tumors, cancers, and for treating skin ulcers, chronic wounds, and fungal infections manifesting as ringworm, athlete's foot, and Candida yeast. The powdered root was once used as a snuff for treating nasal polyps. External application of Bloodroot must be done very carefully because it is so caustic. The herb contains chelerythrine, sanguinarine, and proteolytic enzymes that irritate, inflame, and eventually burn away and dissolve any tissue it touches. It will create an open sore when applied in a thick wad and left on the skin for 6-12 hours. As an escharotic, it destroys tissue and causes it to slough off.

To treat fungal infections, the tea or tincture may be applied full-strength or diluted, or a very small amount of salve can be rubbed over the area. A thick salve or paste is applied over warts, moles, and tumors. It can take up to 3 weeks for warts to fall off with daily application, and Bloodroot is not as effective for deep plantar warts (Duke, 1997).

Apply Bloodroot salve only to the affected area. To protect healthy tissues, put tape on the skin surrounding the affected area so that it forms a doughnut shape around the application site. By this method, the salve only touches the desired skin while the tape protects the surrounding tissues. If working with a very small area like a wart, simply cut a hole in a piece of tape, stick it on the skin so the wart pops through the hole, and cover the wart with salve or a small piece of the fresh root. Salve should be applied 1/8" thick and kept moist to remove small cancers and warts. Cover it with tape to keep it in place. The salve or piece of root can be left on for 5-12 hours. People can usually feel the herb working after a few hours and report that it makes the skin feel itchy, hot, irritated, or painful. The external use of Bloodroot is a delicate and serious process that should be executed very carefully, and only with the assistance of a qualified herbalist or health professional.

Teachings from the Bloodroot Deva

"Yes dear one, we are the spirit of the Bloodroot. We dwell deep in the forest absorbing the red ray of the earth into our roots. Just as this red ray is the energetic essence of the earth, it is also the essence, nourishment, and life support for the first root chakra in the human body. This energy center is located at the base of the spine. It anchors the spirit into the physical body and is associated with red blood as the essence of the physical body. The aura of my roots is a golden reddish-yellow color.

"As the juicy red color of my root indicates, I act on the blood deep within the body to nourish and purify this essence. I can be healing to people with weakness or imbalance in the first chakra, which leads to fundamental insecurities and feelings of being disconnected from the earth. By strengthening and being grounded in the root chakra, the will to live is enhanced and feelings of connection and security of one's place on the earth become more firmly established. I can also help normalize the second chakra, which influences the reproductive and eliminating organs, but my primary action is on the root chakra.

"When you use me for healing, do so with the acknowledgment of my red color, my affinity with blood, and my ability to purify the blood and stimulate the first chakra, which radiates a red vibration. I affect the heart, but because I am such a powerful plant you only need very small amounts of me. I must be used carefully, for to use too much of me is to be in excess. I am a good teacher to remember how to stay in balance, for using only small amounts of powerful medicine is quite sufficient and maintains balance.

"People suffering with cancer may benefit from using me. For I act on the very basic cellular framework of the body to detoxify and release major imbalances originating in the blood stream. It is wise to be close to the earth and work directly with nature in a fulfilling way when using me. Those who have cancer need to re-ground and re-connect with the earth to heal and strengthen the first chakra. By balancing the first chakra, alignment with all the other chakras is possible. My lily-white flowers point to my affinity with the crown chakra (which radiates the white vibration) and with the nervous system, and to my ability to help connect the crown and root chakras. Bloodroot can be beneficial for those who have weakness in the first chakra, usually originating from childhood trauma or from the deeper past. Using me in small amounts helps mend rents in the first chakra, which heals the very fundamental structure of the human body originating in the blood. The blood is the life support, the 'river of life' so to speak, that nourishes all cells in the body. When blood becomes toxic, excess heat moves through the body, toxic conditions arise in the tissues, and cancer can follow. This is one of the mechanisms of this disease. Ingesting my medicine in small doses is cooling to the blood, but using me in large doses brings heat and imbalance into the system. Therefore, very small amounts such as 1-2 drops taken on a daily basis, while connecting with the earth, is very helpful for healing and purifying the blood and the first chakra in a profound way.

"When ingested, I travel through the body using the blood as the vehicle for my healing power. Within the blood, I am able to dissolve and move through stagnation, hard constrictions and tumors, because stimulating movement and flow are a basic part of my nature. When placed on the skin for a period of time, I can dissolve the tissue and move through the body to do my healing work. I am a plant of movement and am able to dissolve and purge whatever gets in my way.

"The red juice flowing through my stems and leaves indicates the connection of the blood flowing through all the vessels of the human body, even up into the head as it nourishes the brain and nervous system. My white flower indicates the purity that the blood can establish within all the tissues, the purity to relieve the body of cancerous cells and establish a whole vehicle that can walk on the earth in peace and balance. The shape of my leaves, having many lobes, points to my affinity with the lobes of the lungs. I am able to move blood through the lungs to remove stagnation and congestion, and initiate cleansing. I am useful for serious lung infections and coughs.

"It is wise to remember the proper use of me, for I am a *heyoka* [a Native American word meaning 'trickster'] plant, by being healing in small doses and detrimental in large doses. And so you must walk in balance to use me, just as you must walk in balance to have a good life upon the earth, and to keep connected with the earth and with the soil itself. Remember where your roots are. Go now in peace this day, and walk in grace and purity."

Parting Thoughts

Bloodroot is certainly a dynamic and powerful herb that stimulates change in the body, being a "mover and shaker" even to the point of dissolving tumors. It is interesting to note the correlation between information given by the plant deva and historic uses of the plant. The deva stated that Bloodroot's primary affinity is with the root chakra, which influences blood, followed by the second chakra that regulates the reproductive and eliminative systems. Native American Indians and Eclectic physicians were aware of the plant's purifying and stimulating action on blood, and used it for venereal disease, yeast infections, impotence and menstrual problems, which are all related to the first and second chakras in the pelvic area.

If you choose to use Bloodroot for your healing, employ the aid of a knowledgeable herbal practitioner if possible, follow suggestions for starting with small doses, and do what the deva recommends by connecting with the earth. This can be accomplished by pleasant outdoor activities such as gardening, hiking, camping out in nature, or lying on the ground and absorbing the energies of the earth. It would also be helpful to take other steps to detoxify and nourish the blood, such as eating food and drinking fluids that are free of chemical additives, and drinking chlorophyll and Stinging Nettle (*Urtica dioica*) tea.

Above all, realize that this is a very powerful herb that can affect people in many different ways, which are sometimes strange and uncomfortable. Please be very cautious when using it!

Blue Cohosh

Caulophyllum thalictroides
Berberidaceae (Barberry) Family

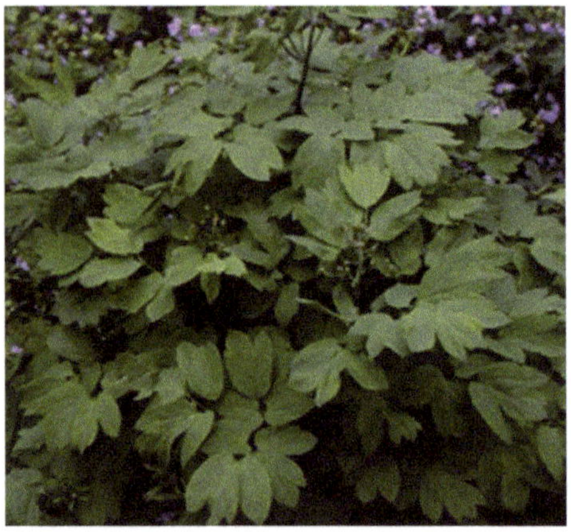

Common Names

Blue berry, blue ginseng, and beechdrops are old names for the plant. Squaw root and papoose root are names that reflect its historic use among Native American women.

Medicinal Part of the Plant

Only the root is used medicinally. **Do not eat the poisonous blue berries.**

Range and Habitat

This attractive plant is indigenous to the fertile, moist, deciduous woodlands of eastern and central United States and Canada. Blue Cohosh grows naturally on slopes, low ground, and along streams. There are several *Caulophyllum* species in North America and regions of Japan and eastern Asia. In North America, *C. thalictroides* is the most popular species for medicinal purposes and *C. giganteum* is a larger plant with more vigorous flowers. These two species are difficult to distinguish and are used interchangeably in herbal medicine. *C. robustum* is indigenous to Asia and has similar medicinal uses as the North American varieties.

Description of the Plant

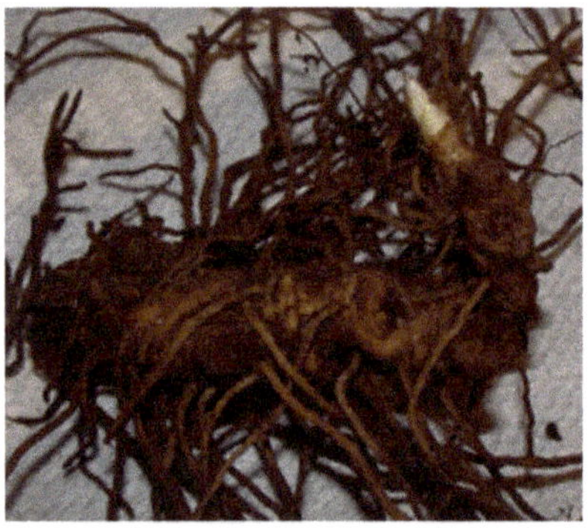

Rhizome with sprouting stem

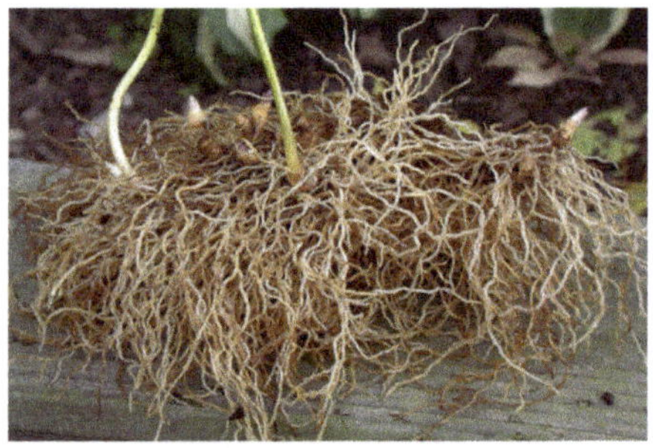

Rhizome covered with stringy rootlets

Blue Cohosh is a showy perennial reaching a height of 1-2′. The roots are gnarly, knotted, irregularly-shaped rhizomes that look like a crooked finger with many long, cream-colored, matted rootlets growing out of them. The outer rhizome is tan with a creamy-white interior. The stem and leaves typically dry up and disappear in mid-to-late summer, especially when conditions are dry. When the stem dies back, it leaves a crater-like scar on the upper side of the rhizome.

Several round, smooth, erect stems emerge from the rhizome in early spring. Each stem branches into a whirl of 4 compound pinnate leaves. Each leaf is triternate, meaning that it divides into 3 sections, and each section has 3 leaflets (occasionally 5), so each compound leaf typically has 9 leaflets. The leaflets look like mittens or paws and have 2-3 unequal and deeply indented lobes. They have long stems and toothless margins with 1-2 deep notches at their tips. The leaflets are velvety smooth, bluish green in color and pale underneath, and grow 1-3″ long. The leaves and stems are sometimes coated with a light-blue film. The shape of the leaves resembles Meadow Rue (*Thalictrum*), hence the species name *thalictroides*.

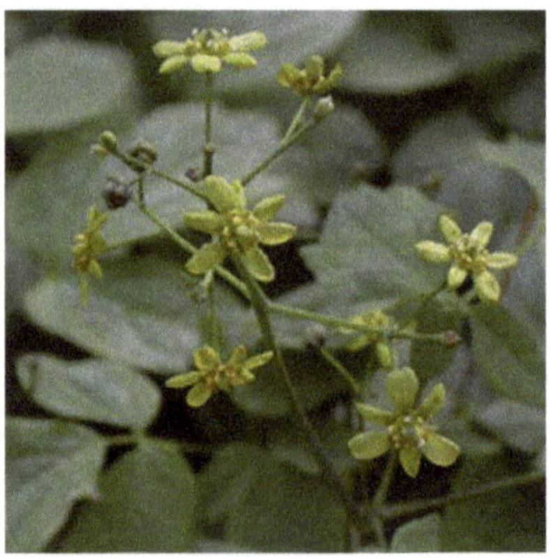

Flowers

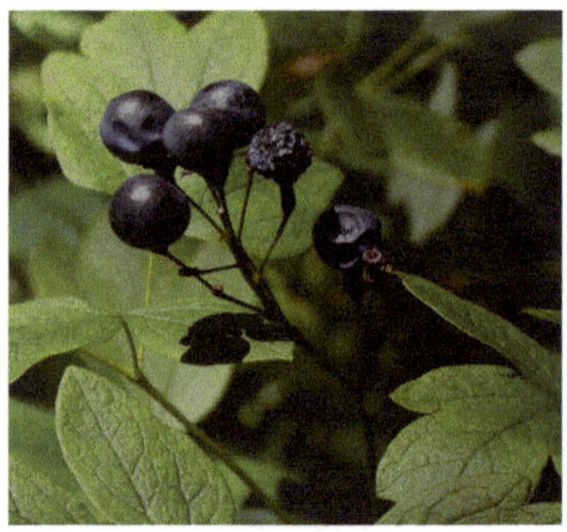

Poisonous blue berries

The small, inconspicuous star-shaped flowers are yellowish green. They appear in early spring from April to May soon after the stems sprout from the roots and while the leaves are still small. Several flowers grow in panicles (loosely branched terminal clusters) from one of the compound leaves. The flowers are only ¼-½″ wide and have 6 pointed sepals, 6 smaller hood-shaped petals, and 6 stamens. About 4 weeks after blooming, they mature into hard, perfectly round green berries the size of a pea. Each poisonous berry turns blue within several weeks and contains one large round seed.

Cultivation

Blue Cohosh naturally grows in moist, well-drained, loamy woodland soil. Spend ample time preparing a garden or nursery bed that fits this description prior to planting. Be sure to mix plenty of humus, rotted leaves, and compost into the soil. This greatly enhances germination, prolific foliage, and root development. The herb normally grows under a shaded forest canopy but will tolerate some partial sunlight. It can do well on the north side of a house, along the edge of a yard or field that is shaded under trees, or in a woodland garden.

The herb propagates by self-sowing its seeds. It can be started by seed germination or root division, but root division is easier, faster, and more productive. Blue Cohosh rhizomes may be purchased, although most seed companies do not sell the seeds because they must stay moist to be viable.

Midsummer is the best time for root division because the plant has time to mature and drop its seeds before its roots are disturbed. Rhizomes that have been purchased or dug up are divided into 1-1½″ pieces. Each piece of rhizome should have a bud on it. Plant the pieces about 2″ deep and 1′ apart with the bud pointing upward. As long as they are consistently kept moist and covered with mulch, the pieces of divided rhizomes usually grow into new plants the following spring. Pieces lacking a visible bud may take up to 2 or 3 years to develop roots and foliage. New plants are typically very small the first year and experience rapid growth the second year. Plants started by root division usually require at least 3 or 4 years before they mature to produce seeds and have roots large enough to be harvested for medicine or divided to cultivate more plants.

Once Blue Cohosh is established, it is fun and rewarding to encourage larger populations by harvesting and planting the mature seeds. Immediately after harvesting the ripe, dark-blue berries, soak them in water overnight and then peel away their blue skin to uncover the inner seed. Do not allow them to dehydrate, which drastically reduces their viability. Sow the seeds close to the parent plant to grow a larger patch or put them in a separate woodland bed. Bury the seeds ½″ deep and place them 4-5″ apart. Mulch the bed with well-rotted leaves or grass clippings and keep the soil moist during the autumn and winter period of stratification. Seeds germinate slowly, growing 1-4″ rhizomes the first year and sending up stems and leaves the second year. Allow at least 2-3 years to let the seedlings grow 2-3″ high before transplanting them to a permanent bed. Then plant them 1′ apart and allow at least 5-6 years of growth before harvesting the rhizomes. The longer the rhizomes stay in the ground, the bigger they get.

If you are fortunate enough to find a patch of Blue Cohosh growing in the wild, know that it transplants easily into a cultivated garden. Keep moist dirt around the roots to prevent shock and dehydration when transplanting. Never harvest an entire patch of herbs. Always leave some of the well-established and larger plants in the patch to ensure their continued survival in the wild. A good friend living in southern Michigan, where this herb covers the woodland slopes like a blanket, allowed me to transplant several plants into my forest gardens, and these have grown into mature plants bearing seeds that I harvest and plant each year to continually increase their population.

Harvest

Harvest seeds for replanting in late spring or early summer after the berries have turned dark blue. Keep a watchful eye to harvest them when they are mature, but before they drop to the ground. Plant them immediately after harvesting and do not let them dry out. If a prepared bed is not available, simply bury the seeds around the parent plant and let nature take its course.

Harvest the rhizomes in mid-to-late summer after the seeds have matured and dropped and the leaves have begun to die back. A good way to harvest part of the rhizome without killing the plant is to dig away the dirt around the rhizome to expose it. Use a very sharp knife to slice off a section of the rhizome behind the emerging stem, leaving 1-1½″ of rhizome attached to the stem. Carefully harvest the larger section of rhizome, then push the soil back around the remaining rhizome and stem. Water and mulch the plant, and it will stay alive and emerge the following spring. Or you can dig up the whole rhizome, cut off a few of the rhizome sprouts with buds on them, and replant these. Then take the remaining rhizome for medicine. In this way, sustainable harvesting and planting become companion activities to ensure the survival of this precious and increasingly scarce woodland beauty. Using these methods, it is eventually possible to harvest yearly while propagating more plants to expand gardens and wild populations.

Preparation of Plant Medicine and Dosages

Blue Cohosh roots are significantly more potent when prepared as a tincture compared to tea or pill preparations, which deteriorate faster with age. Eclectic pharmacist John Uri Lloyd wrote that Blue Cohosh roots partially yield their virtues to hot water and fully to alcohol. Analytical tests confirm that freshly harvested roots contain more active components than the dried ones, so using fresh roots is always preferred to produce a more concentrated tea or tincture (Cech, 2000). Wear a mask if grinding the dried root into powder because the dust is irritating to the lungs. Do not chew on the fresh root because it can irritate the mouth and throat.

PREPARATIONS

Tincture: Clean and chop the fresh root into very small pieces, stuff them into a glass jar, and cover with 90% 190-proof grain alcohol and 10% distilled water. Dosage: 5-30 drops in water up to 3 times a day as needed. It is best to use in small frequent doses to avoid any side effects.

Tea: Gently simmer 1-2 tablespoons of finely chopped fresh root or powdered dried root in a quart of water for 8-10 minutes. Keep the pan covered with a lid and allow the tea to cool for 30 minutes. Dosage: 1-2 cups a day as needed. The tea made from freshly harvested roots has an earthy, slightly bitter taste and an astringent drying effect on the membranes of the mouth that lingers for a short time.

If purchasing Blue Cohosh, get products made from cultivated roots rather than wildcrafted!

Chemical Constituents

Blue Cohosh root contains the quinolizidine alkaloid caulophylline, which is identical to N-methylcytisine and is one of the primary constituents exerting biological activity. Its actions of vasoconstriction, increasing blood pressure, and stimulating the small intestines are similar to nicotine but much weaker. Other alkaloids found in the root are anagyrine (cardiotonic, anti-arrhythmia, diuretic, oxytocic) and magnoflorine (antibacterial, antispasmodic, central nervous system depressant, hypotensive, vasodilator). Caulosaponin and caulophyllosaponin are glycoside saponins having oxytocic (uterine stimulating) properties that promote contractions of uterine smooth muscles and increase circulation to the pelvic area (Skenderi, 2003). Daucosterol is a phytosterol. The saponins and phytosterols have been found to promote hormonal activity (Costello, 1950). The root also contains hederagenin (diuretic, anti-inflammatory) and resins. Minerals include potassium, magnesium, calcium, iron, manganese, silicon, chromium, selenium, phosphorous, and zinc. Vitamins in the roots include ascorbic acid (vitamin C), beta-carotene (the plant source of vitamin A), thiamine (vitamin B1), riboflavin (vitamin B2), and niacin (vitamin B3).

Safety, Contraindications, and Drug Interactions

Blue Cohosh is a safe herb when used cautiously according to recommended small doses. **It is contraindicated during pregnancy until the final two weeks before delivery.** Like many compounds with strong biological activity, **excessive amounts can be dangerous.** There are no known drug interactions.

Like its synergistic partner Black Cohosh (*Cimicifuga racemosa*), Blue Cohosh stimulates the uterus, and large repeated doses can cause miscarriage in early pregnancy and possible premature labor during later pregnancy (Brinker, 2001). The Eclectic physicians and obstetricians of the 1880s–1930s and some modern-day herbalist midwives have successfully recommended small amounts of Blue Cohosh and Black Cohosh during pregnancy for threatened miscarriage due to its ability to ease uterine contractions. However, most professional and clinical herbalists currently discourage using Blue Cohosh and Black Cohosh during pregnancy until the very end of term (McGuffin, 1997).

Blue Cohosh is a potent herb that must be used cautiously in small doses.

Historical evidence shows that Blue Cohosh and Black Cohosh are safe to use during the last two weeks of pregnancy when combined and ingested in normal doses (10-20 drops of the tincture of each herb per day) to prepare the uterus for childbirth. **Do not use Blue Cohosh alone** because it can cause precipitous labor and adversely affect fetal heart rate during labor (Weed, 1985).

There have been confusing cases reported concerning the use of Blue Cohosh during labor. One instance involved a pregnant woman whose obstetrician advised her to take Blue Cohosh to induce labor. The baby was born with congestive heart failure and had seizures and a stroke shortly after birth. The infant was critically ill for several weeks but eventually recovered. The baby's urine and meconium (first stool) tested positive for the cocaine metabolite benzoylecgonine. The mother's bottle of Blue Cohosh was tested and also came back positive for benzoylecgonine. These findings indicate that either benzoylecgonine is a metabolite of both cocaine and Blue Cohosh, or that the Blue Cohosh was contaminated with cocaine, which is extremely unlikely (Jones, 1998; Finkel, 2004). However, there is no published evidence that Blue Cohosh contains benzoylecgonine or that it contains compounds that are metabolized to benzoylecgonine (Potterton, 2004). In light of these facts, doubts arise about possible faulty lab testing on the Blue Cohosh, and it seems probable that the pregnant woman was using cocaine during her pregnancy. She also ingested excessive amounts of Blue Cohosh (3 tablets a day for 3 weeks prior to birth) and took it alone without its traditionally recommended partner, Black Cohosh. Allegations of Blue Cohosh causing the infant's problems were never substantiated.

An overdose of Blue Cohosh can cause nausea, vomiting, dull nagging headaches, increased blood pressure, muscle weakness, or sore throat due to irritation of the mucosal surfaces. When researchers isolated caulophylline from the roots and injected it into animals in abnormally large doses, it caused a toxic reaction on heart muscle, constriction of coronary blood vessels, increased respiration, and hypertension.

From this finding it was concluded that the herb can damage the heart and cause hypertension (Newall, 1996; Gladstar, 2001). However, these test results and assumptions do not accurately reflect the biological activity of the herb when used under normal conditions and dosages. Instead, they were derived from results of large-dose, isolated chemical injections rather than a tea or alcohol extract of the entire root ingested orally, which are the traditional preparations used by herbalists.

Medicinal Uses

History of the Plant

Blue Cohosh was a favorite herb of many Native American woodland groups, including the Menominees, Potawatomis, Chippewa and Ojibwa, who drank it for indigestion, as an analgesic for stomach cramps and painful menstruation, and for lung problems. Several tribes prepared a tea of the root to treat profuse menstruation, urinary tract infections, coughs, fevers, rheumatism, backache, joint pain, and inflammation. The Cherokee made a syrup or tea of the root to treat convulsions and hysteric fits. The Iroquois ingested the tea for fevers and soaked in a bath of the tea to soothe rheumatism (Moerman, 1998; Vogel, 1970). Pregnant women often drank the root tea two or three weeks before birth and during labor to facilitate easier and less painful childbirth. Blue Cohosh is not botanically related to Black Cohosh (*Cimicifuga racemosa*), although their roots look very similar and they are often used together because they share common biological properties. *Cohosh* is an Algonquian word meaning "rough," reflecting the rough and gnarled appearance of these roots. Native Americans introduced Blue Cohosh to the European colonists, who adopted it into their medical systems. The roots became a folk remedy for women's health and birthing, uterine inflammation, cramps, arthritis, and epilepsy.

Peter Smith, a traveling minister who advertised himself as an "Indian herb doctor" (which meant that he used herbs traditionally employed by Native American Indians), wrote in his book, *The Indian Doctor's Dispensatory:*

> The blue berry root is said to be the great medicine that the squaws use at the birth of their children. It is said to be made use of in the following manner – take a handful of green or dry roots, make it into a tea (say half a pint), give the half of it and fill it up with hot water; repeat the drinking every ten minutes or oftener, until it has its effect. When a woman finds she is in labor, let her drink as above and if it is not her time, she will probably get easy and be well; but if it is her time, expect the delivery will be facilitated with much safety . . . . The great benefit is the state of safety and of speedy and sure recovery that the mother experiences afterward. The squaws, I have heard, drink a little of a tea of this root for two or three weeks before the expected time. (Smith, 1813)

In 1835, Smith's writings describing Native American use of Blue Cohosh caught the attention of Eclectic physician John King, M.D., who promoted its use. It became a popular herbal remedy among Eclectic medical physicians, obstetricians, and midwives. Following the example of the Native American woodland tribes, the Eclectics used the root in small doses for chronic uterine problems such as ovarian inflammation and pain, menstrual cramps, delayed menses, prevention of miscarriage and premature labor, and to relieve the pains of false labor and after-birth. The Eclectics extolled Blue Cohosh as one of the best nervines and antispasmodics in their herbal materia medica, using it for treating nervous irritability, spasms, involuntary muscle tremors and twitching, epilepsy, bronchitis, whooping cough, and pneumonia.

The plant was listed in the *U.S. Pharmacopoeia* from 1882–1905 and in *The National Formulary* from 1916–1950 as a labor inducer, antispasmodic, and diuretic. The Eclectic pharmacists did some scientific investigation of Blue Cohosh, and further studies were conducted in the 1950s and 1970s, but there has been very little clinical research since then.

Blue Cohosh is a slow-growing root that is becoming increasingly scarce and is included in the United Plant Savers "at risk" list of endangered herbs. It is not nearly as popular as Black Cohosh, and is more difficult to find in the commercial market. Blue Cohosh is occasionally recommended by midwives, clinical naturopaths or herbalists, and dosages and safety precautions are emphasized. Although the herb's relaxing nervine properties were historically used for digestive, respiratory, urinary and muscular problems, it is now almost exclusively used as a woman's aid two weeks before and during childbirth.

Healing Qualities

Abortifacient, anti-inflammatory, antispasmodic, diaphoretic, diuretic, emmenagogue, expectorant, hypotensive, nephritic, nervine tonic, oxytocic, parturient, pectoral, stomachic, uterine tonic and stimulant, and vasodilator.

Traditional Chinese Medicine (TCM) Perspective

Blue Cohosh influences the liver, lung, and Ren (conception vessel) meridians. It is stimulating, restoring, relaxing, and decongesting to the nervous system and reproductive organs. The invigorating activity of the roots circulate and release constrained Qi (vital energy) to induce relaxation by relieving tension, irritability, pain, and spasms. It is warming and drying in nature and indicated for cold, damp, and deficiency conditions.

Primary Actions

Blue Cohosh is first and foremost a relaxing herb to the nervous system and is excellent for muscle tension and all types of spasms. Its affinity with the nervous system has a marked effect on the female reproductive system, and it is best known as a "woman's herb" that tones and normalizes the female hormones and reproductive system.

Blue Cohosh is traditionally used in combination with other herbs rather than alone. It is most often combined with its synergistic partner Black Cohosh (*Cimicifuga racemosa*) because they complement each other and exert similar properties on the female reproductive and nervous systems. Blue Cohosh and Black Cohosh have been the main ingredients in my "Female Hormonal Regulator" tincture for many years, and numerous women have experienced relief from premenstrual syndrome (PMS), hormonal imbalances, menopausal hot flashes, and other female complaints when using it on a regular basis.

Nervous System: Blue Cohosh exerts a calming and relaxing influence on the nervous system that benefits the whole body. It is especially indicated when nervous tension and irritability are caused by general debility and weakness. The root's antispasmodic activity is helpful for muscle tightness, spasms, and chronic inflammation. The herb helps relieve neuralgia (nerve pain), headaches (especially dull headaches around the forehead), hysteria (an old term describing the emotional ups and downs caused by fluctuating hormones), and hypertension. It is anticonvulsant and has been used for epilepsy in the past. Eclectic physician William Cook, M.D., wrote, "It is a moderate diffusive, stimulating and relaxing in about equal degrees, spending its main powers upon the nervous system. These qualities make it one of the best antispasmodics to relieve nervous feebleness with irritability, as in cramping of the bowels, twitching of the muscles in typhoid and parturient [childbirth] cases . . ." (Cook, 1869).

Blue Cohosh combines well with other nervines and antispasmodics such as Black Cohosh, Scullcap (*Scutellaria lateriflora*), and Valerian (*Valeriana officinalis*) for problems stemming from nervous tension and hyperactivity.

Kidneys and Bladder: In the urinary system, Blue Cohosh eases tense muscles, relaxes and expands blood vessels to allow improved circulation, and opens the kidney and bladder ducts, ureters, and urethra to promote easier passage of urine. The herb is a mild diuretic. Eclectic physicians used it for kidney weakness and albumin in the urine, which indicates malfunctioning kidneys (Cook, 1869). The herb can be soothing for muscle spasms during the agonizing passage of kidney and bladder stones, allowing easier and less painful elimination. It reduces tissue irritation and can be used in the treatment of cystitis (bladder infection) and nephritis (kidney inflammation).

Respiratory System: Blue Cohosh's nervine and antispasmodic properties relax lung and bronchial tissues to enable easier breathing and normal mucous secretion. It has traditionally been employed for treating bronchitis, pneumonia, asthma, and coughs, including whooping cough.

Muscle and Joint Pain: Blue Cohosh helps dispel cold and dampness in the joints and muscles, increases circulation, and reduces inflammation. It was commonly used by the Eclectic physicians for cases of rheumatoid arthritis and for muscle and nerve pain, now called fibromyalgia. Researchers have found that the herb reduces inflammation by suppressing COX-2 and cytokines (Lee, 2012).

Women's Health: Blue Cohosh exerts a normalizing effect on the reproductive system and uterine muscles. It is a uterine vasodilator (dilates and opens blood vessels) that increases circulation to bring warmth and nutrients to the womb. It acts as a uterine stimulant to catalyze normal function, drain fluid congestion, and warm achy, cold muscles. As a uterotonic, it normalizes uterine muscle tone. Its antispasmodic quality relieves nervous tension and irritation in the pelvic organs, and is specific for chronic inflammation and uterine cramps and spasms. Not only does Blue Cohosh relax tight and rigid muscles, it is also beneficial for the reverse condition of muscle atony (sluggishness and weakness) caused by general debility and nutritional deficiencies. The herb's ability to strengthen weak muscles lacking tone makes it an excellent remedy for prolapsed (fallen) organs, including uterine and bladder prolapse. It is also used for hemorrhoids occurring from increased pressure on weak veins in the anus that causes them to expand into large, painful varicose veins.

> *Blue Cohosh is a wonderful plant ally for women that has historically been used with Black Cohosh to promote reproductive health and facilitate easier childbirth.*

Research using *in vitro* testing has confirmed that compounds in the roots bind to estrogen receptor sites in breast, uterine and ovarian tissues, and exhibit estrogenic activity without causing uterine cells to proliferate (Costello, 1950; Fackelmann, 1998). This action helps to balance and normalize estrogen levels without potentiating the risk of uterine cancer. Blue Cohosh is specific for heavy, aching pains, pressure, and spasms in the uterus, pelvis, lower back, and thighs. It is indicated for chronic and acute uterine problems with pain and tenderness, endometriosis, uterine fibroids, ovarian and breast pain, Candida yeast infections, and other types of vaginitis (vaginal infections) with leucorrhea (vaginal discharge). It has also been used for problems of infertility. To strengthen and normalize the uterus, combine Blue Cohosh and Black Cohosh with Motherwort (*Leonurus cardiaca*), Yarrow (*Achillea millefolium*), and Blue Vervain (*Verbena hastata*) to take as a tincture or tea over a period of several weeks.

Menstruation: As an emmenagogue, Blue Cohosh relaxes nervous tension and promotes blood flow in the pelvis to help bring on delayed or suppressed menstruation. It helps to normalize estrogen activity and is used to regulate the menstrual cycle and reduce excessive menstrual bleeding (menorrhagia) or normalize a scanty flow. The antispasmodic property of the root reduces cramping and painful menses. It is specifically indicated for menstrual cramps that are most painful the first day of bleeding. These qualities make it helpful for premenstrual syndrome (PMS) and many menstrual difficulties. A combination of Blue Cohosh with Cramp Bark (*Viburnum opulus)* is very reliable for easing menstrual cramps.

Pregnancy and Childbirth: Eclectic physician William Cook, M.D., who used this herb in his medical practice, wrote that it "is of special service in strengthening and relieving painful functional difficulties of the female generative organs. It is one of the most valuable parturients [used during childbirth] when the uterine action is becoming weary" (Cook, 1869). To be completely safe, Blue Cohosh should only be taken in small doses the last two or three weeks of pregnancy to tone the uterus and facilitate labor. Historically, it is almost always used in combination with other herbs, most notably Black Cohosh, and is not given alone. The usual dose is 10-30 drops of each tincture in a little water twice a day until the birth. Its use is especially indicated when the uterus is fragile due to muscle weakness or multiple births. It can ease false labor pains while relaxing the mother, and stalls premature labor by halting uterine contractions.

> *Blue Cohosh is only taken in small doses 2-3 weeks before the due date, and always in combination with Black Cohosh.*

Ingesting Blue Cohosh and Black Cohosh tincture during childbirth stimulates labor and promotes strong, regular, and productive contractions that allow for an easier and less painful labor. It is most valuable in cases of delayed birth and stalled, painful, or difficult labor especially due to debility, fatigue, or lack of muscle tone. To induce and support labor, the dose is 10-30 drops of each tincture every 30 minutes until contractions are strong and consistent. Herbalist Susun Weed notes, "If fetal heart tones are monitored, there may be a noticeable elevation as the Blue Cohosh starts to work. Also remember that Blue Cohosh tends to lower blood pressure" (Weed, 1985).

At several home births, I have seen a combination of Blue Cohosh and Black Cohosh with Lobelia (*Lobelia inflata*) tincture successfully soften the cervical os to allow full dilation and induce strong uterine contractions. Following the birth, Blue Cohosh and Black Cohosh can be taken to expel a retained placenta, reduce excessive bleeding, and relieve "after-pains," which are severe uterine cramps. The herbs help uterine muscles contract back to pre-pregnancy state and strengthen pelvic muscles to prevent postpartum uterine or bladder prolapse.

A national survey involving 500 members of the American College of Nurse-Midwives documented their use of herbs for cervical ripening, labor induction, and successful childbirth management. Out of 500 members, 90 who used herbs for childbirth returned their survey questionnaires showing that 64% used Blue Cohosh and 45% used Black Cohosh to successfully stimulate labor (McFarlin, 1999).

Miscarriage Prevention and Abortant Properties: The ability of Blue Cohosh to reduce nervous irritation, spasms, and premature uterine contractions, which can induce miscarriage, was recognized by the Eclectic physicians, who reported several cases of successfully prescribing the herb to stop threatened miscarriages. It was typically combined with Black Haw (*Viburnum prunifolium*) to promote this action. However, modern researchers and herbalists discourage this use due to Blue Cohosh's emmenagogue and abortifacient abilities. It carries the potential to cause miscarriage when taken in consistently high doses, and is currently contraindicated during pregnancy until the last 2-3 weeks, when it serves as a uterine toner.

I know of several women who have used large doses of equal parts Blue Cohosh, Black Cohosh, American Pennyroyal (*Hedeoma pulegiodes*), and Tansy (*Tanacetum vulgare*) several times a day for 3-4 days to induce an abortion. These large, continuous doses can stimulate uterine contractions that expel the fetus and cause unpleasant symptoms of nausea, dizziness, and headaches in women. Only attempt an herbal abortion under the supervision of a knowledgeable herbalist. Understand that medical intervention is absolutely necessary if the herbs do not successfully promote the desired results.

Menopause: Due to its uterine and nervine properties, Blue Cohosh benefits women moving through the transition of menopause. It can increase estrogen activity, help relieve symptoms such as hot flashes, and has a calming effect on the nerves. It works best when used in combination with other estrogenic herbs, especially its synergistic partner, Black Cohosh.

Men's Prostate Health: Excessive levels of testosterone can contribute to prostate enlargement and other problems. The estrogenic, anti-inflammatory, and nervine properties of Blue Cohosh were used by the Eclectic physicians to reduce testosterone levels and treat chronic prostate problems (Cook, 1869). Combine it with Black Cohosh for prostate issues.

Teachings from the Blue Cohosh Deva

"Greetings. I am your woodland friend, the Blue Cohosh Deva. My sister and partner, the Black Cohosh, is my companion to aid and benefit women, but we can also be used by men for some purposes. In the old times when the indigenous people in this country were strong and prosperous, I covered the ground like a rich carpet of green in many areas of moist, fertile, shady woodlands.

"My large medicinal roots live in the earth and resonate to the rhythms of the womb of the Great Mother. My gift to people is the ability to bring balance and normalize the rhythmic pulsations of the nervous system at deep levels. My nature is soothing and calming. I relax and quiet spasms and jerky movements caused by nervous strain and stress upon the body, and especially upon the emotions and mind. For this purpose, I serve both men and women.

"I am most powerful in my female attributes and embody the qualities of the creative Mother. I am a grandmother among the plants, and my benefits are not for young and immature girls, but rather for women who are fertile and for those who have moved beyond their cycles of fertility. I am womb medicine for women, and just as I normalize jerky, spastic movements of the nerves into a relaxed and rhythmic flow, I also normalize the rhythmic cycles of the bleeding times and relax spasms of the womb. During birth, I create strong, rhythmic contractions. I stimulate and tone the womb. When taken for a short while before birth, I prime the uterus to move and contract in a forceful way, but also with a regularity and strength of purpose that helps open the mouth of the womb. I also provide a time of deep rest between contractions so the birthing mother has a few moments of space to re-charge for the oncoming waves. When used in conjunction with my sister, the Black Cohosh, I bring balance and rhythm to the rising and falling of the waves of contractions and bring strength to the laboring mother. The Native women of the eastern woodlands knew to use us during childbirth, and also to stimulate contractions of the womb and the final expulsion of the placenta after its job of sustaining the infant is complete.

"I incorporate the radiance of female qualities. My large bulbous rhizomes of creamy-colored, fleshy pulp are rooted firmly in the ground, saturated with the energies of the moist, dark, living soil that is the womb of the earth. My roots also resonate with the fertile ground or womb within women. My bushy mass of deep-green leaves look like a multitude of open hands reaching out, just as the hands of midwives reach out to receive children emerging from the womb. Hands open to care for children, to receive all that life offers, to give nourishment, healing, and perform many tasks. My large, round, beautiful blue seeds may be called my crowning glory, and like all seeds, they are the living and life-giving culmination of creative forces.

"I assist with transitions and new beginnings: the transition of giving birth, the transition into menopause with the cessation of fertility, and the transition into new avenues of creativity. Women may sow many kinds of seeds throughout their lives: the seeds that beget children, the seeds that grow into loving relationships and fulfilling work, and the seeds that manifest into the experiences of a woman's life. Tend carefully to your seeds. Be aware and responsible for what you create with the seeds of your thoughts, intentions, and actions. For the seeds that you plant in the activities of each day will influence the unfolding of your life. Let your intention be for the happiness and good of many people and creatures, rather than to harm. This lesson of honoring and caring for one's seed and creative abilities is also an important lesson for all men. A good beginning for men is to honor the placement of their seed into women, and to do so only in a loving way that does no harm or violence. Let all our seeds come forth with good and kind intention.

"As a grandmother plant, I also offer assistance to women whose creative energies have subsided, when the womb is complete in its purpose. I help balance the womb energies, relaxing tightness and tension, and toning and strengthening where there is weakness. By adjusting the nervous energies, I offer menopausal women greater peace and comfort at deep, inner levels. Know that although the womb no longer has the power to create new life, this time of transition offers new opportunities for creativity. For when the menses cease and the door closes to birthing children, another door opens and much creative power moves from the womb to higher centers of vision, wisdom, and latent abilities. Opportunity presents for further fulfillment, connection with the earth, oneself and all others, and for walking one's path. It is a time to question, 'What makes my heart happy, and what do I need to do or create to feel peace, contentment, and wholeness?' Take the time for reflection from deep within, to discover the answers to these questions. For this is where your happiness is born."

Blue Vervain

Verbena hastata
Verbenaceae (Verbena) Family

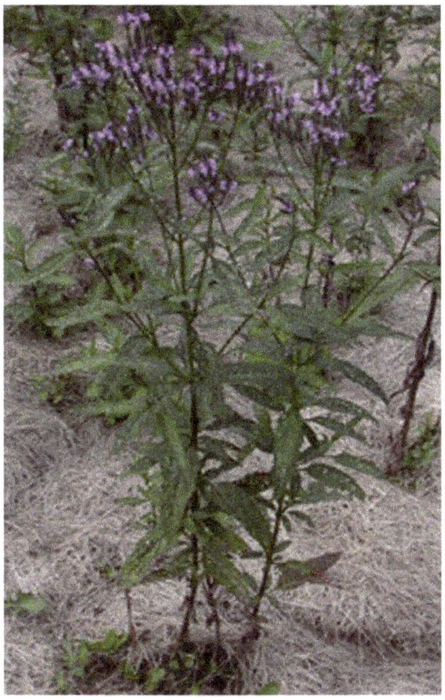

Botanical Name

Verbena hastata is the North American species commonly called Blue Vervain. *Verbena officinalis* is the European species. Both possess similar medicinal properties and can be used interchangeably. *Verbena hastata* is a more beautiful plant with larger, more ornately colorful flowers, and is considered to be superior in medicinal qualities than its milder-acting European cousin.

Common Names

American vervain, Herb of Grace, Herbe Sacrée, Herb-of-the-cross, Herba veneris, Indian hyssop, wild hyssop, iron weed, purvain, simpler's joy, traveler's joy, enchanter's herb, and wild verbena are all antiquated names for *Verbena hastata*.

Medicinal Part of the Plant

The roots, leaves, and flowers provide excellent medicine. However, when wildcrafting, please harvest only the leaves and flowers rather than the roots so that these increasingly rare plants can continue to survive.

Range and Habitat

There are an estimated 200-352 varieties of *Verbena* growing in northern temperate climates, and many are medicinal. *V. hastata* is indigenous to North America. Although it is native to the Mediterranean region, *V. officinalis* has become established in North America. Blue Vervain likes growing under full sun in open fields and meadows. In the past, it was commonly found growing along roadsides and in fields, but is becoming scarce in due to human sprawl and loss of habitat.

Description of the Plant

V. hastata is a tall, showy perennial growing up to 4-6′. A few erect stems emerge from the fibrous root system. The distinctly square and furrowed stems are very tough and fibrous with opposite branches. Simple, petiole leaves are 3-8″ long with pinnate venation and large serrated teeth. They grow opposite each other along the stems. They are linear to lance-shaped with very pointed (acuminate) tips. The larger leaves close to ground level sometimes have an up-turned hastate (arrow-shaped) base that inspired its botanical name *hastata*, a Latin word meaning "armed with a spear." Stems and leaves are covered with short hairs that give them a rough texture. As summer progresses, leaves often become partially covered with a white, powdery-looking film giving them a rather splotchy appearance. Unlike most herbs, insects like to eat Blue Vervain and typically nibble many small holes in the leaves.

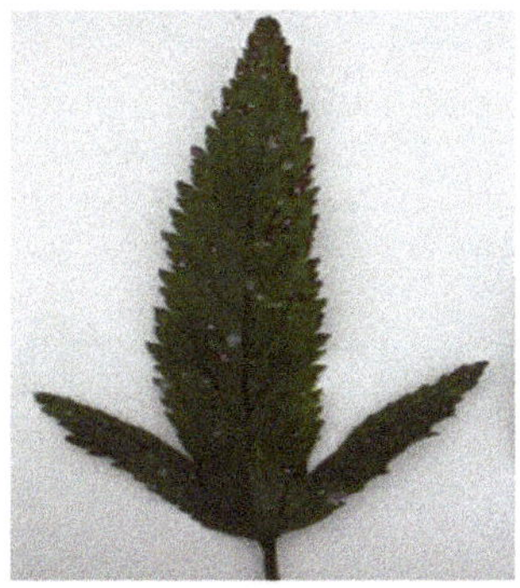

Hastate leaf

The tiny violet-blue flowers are 1/6-1/3″ long and form numerous beautiful, tight clusters of thin, erect, 6-8″ long panicle spikes at the ends of the tall stems. Flowers have 5 petals that form a tubular corolla and are sessile (lacking stems). They bloom from June to September a few flowers at a time, beginning with the lower flowers that open first, and progressively bloom upwards to the tip of the spike. Flowers mature into hundreds of round, very tiny brown seeds.

The European variety, *V. officinalis*, is a smaller, more spindly and loosely branched plant. It is an annual that grows 2-4′ tall. The smooth leaves are opposite with deeply cut lobes and sharply serrated teeth. The tiny flowers are purple to pinkish mauve in color and arranged in slender spikes.

Other varieties native to many parts of North America include White Vervain (*V. urticifolia*) (with white flowers and very slender spikes), the purple-flowered Narrow-leaf Vervain (*V. simplex*), and Hoary Vervain (*V. stricta*), which occasionally has pink flowers.

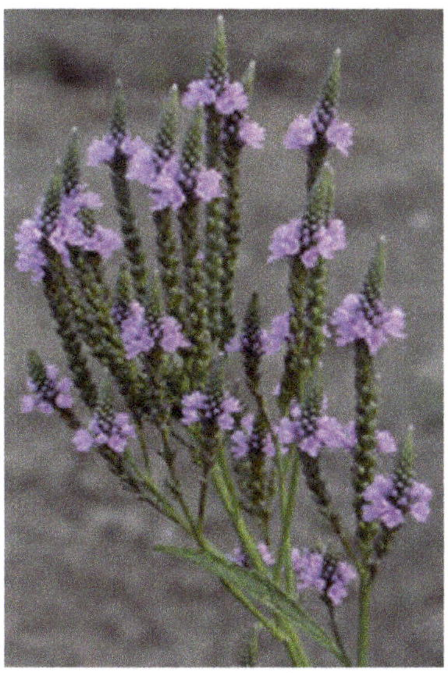

Blue Vervain (*Verbena hastata*)

Cultivation

An established garden of Blue Vervain creates an intensely vibrant bluish-purple cloud of flowers, making this one of my favorite garden herbs. Gazing at a cluster of Blue Vervain from a short distance, brilliant bluish-purple waves of dancing energy can be seen radiating out and upward from the flowers. A strikingly beautiful and inspiring vision!

This herb is typically a prolific germinator and easy to grow. It does best in full sun and prefers medium to well-fertilized soil with adequate drainage. The seeds usually have better germination with cold conditioning. This is accomplished by either planting them in a prepared garden bed in autumn to allow winter stratification, or by refrigerating (33-38°F) the seeds in moist sand or paper towel for 2-4 weeks before planting in spring. The seeds are tiny, so barely cover them with only 1/8″ of soil. Keep soil moist with a light spray of water. Transplant seedlings when they are 3-4″ tall and space them about 1′ apart in a permanent bed. Water and mulch well to keep roots moist and protected. Blue Vervain may also be propagated by stem cuttings taken in springtime.

Once matured plants are established in cultivated beds, they self-sow by dropping their seeds. These usually germinate the following spring in abundance and can be transplanted or thinned out to create larger beds. Larger, mature plants generally do not like to be transplanted.

Harvest

Harvest the leaves and flowers for medicinal purposes when the herb is in full bloom. Avoid killing the plant by carefully and conservatively pruning no more than 25% of the foliage. Collect mature seeds for planting when they are brown and dry in late summer or early autumn. Roots should be harvested only after the seeds have matured. However, help preserve this increasingly scare herb and *only* collect the roots if there is an abundance of plants in the area or in your garden.

Preparation of Plant Medicine and Dosages

Alcohol and boiling water both extract medicinal constituents from Blue Vervain, providing potent tincture and tea preparations. Tinctures are usually preferred over tea due to the bitter flavor. The herb can also be prepared as a salve or poultice for external application. Freshly harvested leaves and flowers provide better quality medicines than the dried plant, which deteriorates over time.

PREPARATIONS

Tincture: Chop fresh leaves and flowers into small pieces and pack them into a glass jar. Cover with 60% 190-proof grain alcohol and 40% distilled water. Blue Vervain makes a very dark, blackish tincture. Dosage: 20-90 drops in water up to 4 times a day.

Tea: Steep 2-3 teaspoons of fresh or dried herb in 1 pint of boiling water for 20 minutes. If the roots are used, gently simmer 2 teaspoons per pint of water for 10 minutes. Dosage: 1 cup up to 3 times a day. A fomentation of the tea may be applied to wounds, ulcers, skin eruptions, and swollen glands.

Salve: The freshly harvested leaves and flowers are chopped, covered with olive oil, and baked in the standard way to make a salve for external healing. To enhance potency of the salve, combine Blue Vervain with other vulnerary (wound healing) herbs (refer to those listed under "Skin Problems" in the "Index of Health Issues and Herbal Recommendations").

Poultice: This can be made by pulverizing or cooking fresh or dried leaves into a moist mash for external application.

Chemical Constituents

Most of the research and analytical studies have been on *V. officinalis* (European Vervain), and although very little research has been conducted on *V. hastata*, it is reasonable to assume that it contains many similar constituents as its European cousin.

Primary active principles of *V. officinalis* are iridoid glycosides that include verbenin (hemostatic, galactagogue), verbenalin (also called verbenaloside) (galactagogue, uterine tonic, and oxytocic), aucubin (antibacterial, anti-inflammatory, antioxidant, diuretic, hepatoprotective, galactagogue), and hastatoside (analgesic, anti-inflammatory). These iridoid glycosides have a calming and restorative effect on the parasympathetic nervous system, which is involuntary and automatically functions without our conscious control. Parasympathetic stimulation by iridoid glycosides can decrease heart rate and increase gastrointestinal secretions and movement. Iridoids are also bitter, choleretic, laxative, antiviral, and immunomodulating. Verbascoside is a phenylethanoid glycoside demonstrating anti-inflammatory and liver protective properties.

Volatile oils include citral (antibacterial, antihistamine, broncho-relaxant, expectorant, sedative), geraniol, limonene, verbenone, and lupeol (anti-inflammatory, antilithic, antimalarial, antioxidant, antiviral, and hypotensive). *V. officinalis* also contains mucilage (soothing and cooling), saponins, beta-sitosterol, caffeic acid (analgesic, antibacterial, anticancer, anti-inflammatory, antioxidant, antispasmodic, cholagogue, hepatoprotective, sedative, vulnerary), tannins (anthelmintic, antibacterial, anticancer, hepatoprotective), ursolic acid (analgesic, anti-arthritic, anticancer, antihistamine, anti-inflammatory, antimalarial, antiviral), adenosine (analgesic, anti-arrhythmic, antihypertensive, antispasmodic, immunomodulating, laxative, sedative, vasodilator), beta-carotene (anti-asthmatic, anticancer, antioxidant), and the flavonoids luteolin, scutellarin, artemitine, sorbifolin, pedalitin, and nepetin.

Safety, Contraindications, and Drug Interactions

Blue Vervain is **contraindicated during pregnancy** because its emmenagogue properties have a direct effect on the uterus and can stimulate menstruation and contractions (McGuffin, 1997). There is no documentation of toxicity, drug interactions, or side effects when moderate dosages are ingested (Blumenthal, 1998). Very large doses can cause gastrointestinal symptoms of nausea, vomiting, or diarrhea (Skenderi, 2003).

Medicinal Uses

History of the Plant

The Vervains have been revered over the centuries, and much lore and magic revolve around the European and Mediterranean varieties. Many cultures have regarded Vervain as a heal-all. The ancient Egyptians, Druids, and Romans used it medicinally and believed it to be endowed with magical powers. According to Egyptian mythology, Vervain grew from the tears of Isis, the goddess of fertility, as she mourned for her murdered husband, Osiris. It was one of the most important herbs used by Druid priests in their healing rituals. *Verbena* was a classical Roman name given to plants placed on sacred alters. "Herba Sacra" and "Herba veneris" were common names for this sacred ally of magicians, sorcerers and priests, who often used it during ceremonial rituals and incantations. In Christian legends, it is believed that Vervain leaves were pressed into Jesus' wounds on Calvary to stop the bleeding, hence its old name, "herb-of-the-cross." During the Middle Ages and Inquisition, when rampant belief in witchcraft perpetuated great fear, Vervain was a popular ingredient in magical charms made to protect people from harm. It was also used as a symbol of mutual trust and good faith.

The Greek physician Hippocrates (*circa* 460–*c.* 377 B.C.) recommended European Vervain for infectious plagues and ague, an old term for malaria. Dioscorides (*c.* A.D. 40–*c.* 90) employed it for treating fevers, edema, jaundice, ulcers, wounds, and snakebites. A tea of Vervain and vermouth was prescribed for blood toxicity, infections, and toothaches by the German abbess and herbalist Hildegard of Bingen (A.D. 1098–1179). The English apothecary and surgeon John Gerard (1545–1612) gave Vervain for headaches, nervous disorders, inflammation, painful wounds, and ulcers. Nicholas Culpeper (1616–1654) declared Venus to be the planetary ruler of this herb, and encouraged its use for "the womb" and female problems, liver and spleen obstructions, jaundice, gout, coughs, wheezing and shortness of breath, fever, plagues, parasites, kidney stones, and wounds. The name Vervain is derived from the Celtic word *ferfaen. Fer* means "to drive away" and *faen* is a word for "stone," referring to its historic use in treating bladder afflictions and kidney stones.

When the colonists arrived in North America, they grew European Vervain in their gardens and it eventually naturalized in the new land. The Europeans also learned the medicinal uses of the native species, *V. hastata*, from Native American Indians who drank tea made from the leaves for coughs, colds, intestinal problems and dysentery, bladder infections, and as a female tonic. The Menominee made a root tea to treat the kidneys and cure cloudy urine indicative of infection. The Delaware used the root tea for fevers and chills, the Dakota made a tea of the leaves for stomach aches, and the Cherokee drank the tea to relieve pain and diarrhea (Moerman, 1998). Native Americans living on the west coast of North America roasted and ground the seeds into flour for culinary uses.

During the Revolutionary War when drugs were scarce, surgeons often harvested Blue Vervain leaves from the battlefields where they grew, preparing them into poultices for soldiers' infected and painful wounds and as tea for respiratory infections and coughs. The American Eclectic physicians of the 1880s–1930s used the herb in similar ways as the Native Americans, holding it in high esteem for many conditions caused by nervous anxiety and spasms, including epilepsy, tics, headaches, and depression. It was also used to treat digestive problems, menstrual complaints, colds, flu, fevers, malaria, kidney stones, and parasites. The Eclectics preferred the root to the leaf, and it was sometimes used as a substitute for Boneset (*Eupatorium perfoliatum*) because they share similar healing properties.

V. hastata and *V. officinalis* have a long folk history of use demonstrating their value as potent medicinals. *V. hastata* was listed as an official medicine in the *National Formulary* from 1916–1926 as a diaphoretic and expectorant. However, both species are currently under-utilized and have not received much attention from the scientific community. Most information comes from historic references, clinical observations, and research on the pharmacology of *V. officinalis*.

The Council of Europe regulatory agency has classified European Vervain (*V. officinalis*) as a natural source of food flavoring, allowing it to be added to foods in small amounts. In the United States, the Food and Drug

Administration (FDA) lists Blue Vervain (*V. hastata*) as an herb of "undefined safety." Although it is not a well-known medicinal herb, commercial preparations are usually available in tincture form.

Healing Qualities

Alterative, analgesic, antibacterial, anti-inflammatory, antilithic, antiperiodic, antispasmodic, antiviral, aperitive, astringent, bitter tonic, carminative, cholagogue, diaphoretic, diuretic, emetic in large doses, emmenagogue, expectorant, febrifuge, galactagogue, hepatic, hypotensive, mild laxative, nephritic, nervine, oxytocic, parturient, pectoral, sedative, stomachic, vasodilator, vermifuge, and vulnerary.

Traditional Chinese Medicine (TCM) Perspective

Blue Vervain's properties are bitter and cooling. It is relaxing to the nervous system and restores normal nerve function. Its bitter, stimulating activity disperses excess and stagnated Qi (vital energy), heat and fluids, and dissolves obstructions throughout the system. Its ability to invigorate and promote movement of Qi benefits the nervous system, circulation, and all organs of the body, especially the lungs, uterus, stomach, liver, and kidneys. Blue Vervain helps strengthen weak Kidney Yin, resolve Kidney Qi Stagnation, restore Kidney Essence, and resolve Liver Qi Stagnation. Thus, it is helpful for many kidney, liver, and reproductive problems. It calms Liver Wind that can give rise to spasms, tremors, numbness, dizziness, and seizures.

Primary Actions

Blue Vervain is a valuable medicinal herb that addresses a wide variety of health issues. Although quite bitter, it is relatively mild in action but very effective for acute conditions like infections and fevers. It is also an excellent tonic for chronic health problems and imbalances. Its primary relaxing and restorative action on the nervous system benefits the entire body. The bluish-purple flowers are a signature of the plant's calming influence on the nervous system.

This is one of my favorite medicinals to grow and use, and for many years it has been an important and dependable ingredient in several of my tincture combinations for colds, flu, coughs, fevers, normalizing liver function, promoting menstruation and normal reproductive function, and for gently calming the nervous system. It exerts wonderful healing capacity for external wounds and inflammation, and has long been one of the ingredients in my "Herbal Healing Salve." Taken daily as tea or tincture over a period of time, Blue Vervain restores vitality while calming the nervous system, and detoxifies and strengthens the whole body.

Nervous System: Blue Vervain's relaxing and restoring influence on the nervous system benefits the entire body by its action on the parasympathetic, or involuntary, nervous system regulating the organs, glands, and everything that automatically functions without our awareness. This parasympathetic dominance promotes generalized relaxation. The herb strengthens a debilitated nervous system and restores normal energy levels while reducing tension and stress. It is a nervine and mild sedative specific for chronic and acute nervous tension, anxiety disorders, nervous twitches, and all types of muscle spasms, especially in the neck and back. Researchers have confirmed the presence of several constituents in the plant with noticeable anti-inflammatory and analgesic properties (Deepak, 2000; Oliver-Bever, 1986; Sakai, 1963; Speroni, 2007). An interesting study showed European Vervain to have a protective effect on nerve cells (Lai, 2006).

Blue Vervain can be an excellent remedy in the treatment of depression, insomnia, headaches and migraines, nervous tics and tremors, seizures and epilepsy, numbness, dizziness, tinnitus (ringing in the ears), neuralgia (nerve pain), fibromyalgia, neurasthenia (lack of energy, fatigue, listlessness), obsessive compulsive disorders, and other neurological conditions. It helps calm and restore the nervous system during alcohol and drug withdrawal, and eases delirium tremens. Blue Vervain may be combined with other nervines and sedatives such as Passion Flower (*Passiflora incarnata*), Valerian (*Valeriana officinalis*), and Scullcap (*Scutellaria lateriflora*). For depression, blend it with Lavender, Scullcap, Lemon Balm (*Melissa officinalis*), and St. John's Wort (*Hypericum perforatum*). It also combines well with St. John's Wort for relieving nerve pain.

Digestive System: The extreme bitterness of Blue Vervain makes it a wonderful digestive remedy that stimulates production and secretion of digestive enzymes necessary to break down fats, proteins, and carbohydrates. It contracts smooth muscles in the digestive tract to promote normal muscle peristalsis, which moves food through the stomach and intestines (Mowrey, 1986). The herb's calming, antispasmodic, and anti-inflammatory qualities help relax rigid abdominal muscles and organs, relieve abdominal cramps, spasms and pain, and promote normal digestion.

Liver and Gallbladder: Blue Vervain acts specifically on the liver to strengthen and restore balance. As a cholagogue, it promotes the formation of bile in the liver and stimulates bile secretion into the gallbladder. This action helps digest fats, prevent the formation of gallstones, and dissolve pre-existing stones. Vervain's relaxing, antispasmodic effect on the nerves and muscles allows ducts in the liver and gallbladder to open, promoting smooth movement of bile and passage of stones. The herb is beneficial for a sluggish liver, jaundice, high cholesterol levels, toxicity, and liver and gallbladder inflammation.

Pancreas: The herb stimulates secretion of pancreatic enzymes and relaxes pancreatic ducts. This allows optimal flow of enzymes into the small intestine, where they reduce food into tiny particles to be absorbed through the walls of the small intestine into the bloodstream.

Large and Small Intestines: Blue Vervain also relaxes the intestinal nerves and muscles, making it helpful for cramps, spasms, constipation, pain, gas, colitis, and other inflammatory irritable bowel syndromes. Its stimulating action on the liver and gallbladder to secrete bile promotes intestinal movement that is beneficial for chronic constipation. Iridoid glycosides in the leaves also have a laxative effect (Inouye, 1974). The tannins in the leaves provide astringent properties that help arrest diarrhea, especially when used in conjunction with other astringent herbs such as Cranesbill (*Geranium maculatum*), Shepherd's Purse (*Capsella bursa-pastoris*), or Cinquefoil (*Potentilla* spp.). Large amounts of Blue Vervain tea taken while fasting can help eliminate intestinal parasites.

Kidneys and Bladder: Blue Vervain normalizes kidney function and has a long historic use for treating diseases, infections, inflammation, and weakness of the kidneys and entire urinary tract. The alkalizing properties of the herb help eliminate excess acids via the kidneys. It is a mild diuretic useful for fluid retention. As it calms the nervous system, it helps relax muscles and ducts of the kidneys, ureters, and bladder to allow smooth flow of blood and urine, and easier, less painful passage of kidney stones. Researchers think that the beneficial effect on passing kidney stones is due to the presence of saponins (Grases, 1994).

Detoxification: This is an appropriate herb for treating metabolic toxicity resulting from kidney and liver congestion, poor circulation, and excess acids and heat in the bloodstream. The tea or tincture is helpful for red, irritated eruptive skin rashes, hives, and illnesses that are triggered by toxic conditions.

Heart and Circulation: The sedative, nervine, and antispasmodic qualities calm the heart and help stabilize normal cardiac rhythm. Blue Vervain can be beneficial for tachycardia (excessively fast heart rate) and toning the system during convalescence from heart disease. The plant relaxes muscles in the blood vessels, allowing for vasodilation and increased blood circulation. It is helpful for hypertension due to its properties of relaxing the nerves, dilating blood vessels, and reducing fluid retention. Animal studies have documented the ability of Vervain to lower high blood pressure (Oliver-Bever, 1986).

Bacterial and Viral Infections: Blue Vervain is one of my favorite and most dependable remedies for bacterial and viral infections, the common cold, flu (influenza), fevers, coughs, and respiratory infections. It is most effective when taken at the onset of illness and is safe for children when given in smaller doses. This herb has antibiotic properties, and as a diaphoretic it induces sweating, which lowers elevated temperatures. The early American Eclectic physicians used it for treating influenza, the common cold, respiratory infections, and intermittent fevers. They considered it to be as efficient as quinine for treating malaria and related spleen enlargement (splenomegaly). Blue Vervain is a powerful expectorant, anti-inflammatory, and antispasmodic that decreases excessive mucous secretions and breaks up congestion in the throat, bronchioles, and lungs. It helps relieve lung spasms and tightness, shortness of breath, wheezing, asthma, coughs (including whooping cough), pneumonia, and bronchitis. *In vitro* studies show that leaves of European Vervain (*V. officinalis*) exhibit excellent antifungal activity (Casanova, 2008), and the essential oils are antioxidant, antibiotic, and antifungal (De Martino, 2009).

For infections and fevers, Blue Vervain works in combination with Boneset (*Eupatorium perfoliatum*), Yarrow (*Achillea millefolium*), Thyme (*Thymus vulgaris*), Goldenseal (*Hydrastis canadensis*), Echinacea, and Sage (*Salvia officinalis*). For respiratory remedies, add Horehound (*Marrubium vulgare*), Pleurisy Root (*Asclepias tuberosa*), and Elecampane (*Inula helenium*). It can be helpful for severe fevers that dry up body fluids when taken as ½-1 cup of hot tea or 30-40 drops of tincture ingested every hour until the temperature drops.

Cancer: Researchers have discovered that Vervain may be helpful in treating leukemia (cancer of the white blood cells) by stimulating apoptosis. Apoptosis is the innate biological process of programmed cell death that protects the body by destroying damaged or dysfunctional cells. Apoptosis prevents uncontrolled cell division and proliferation, one of the main characteristics of cancerous cells. Several researchers found that *V. officinalis* essential oil and its main component citral stimulated apoptosis on lymphocytes collected from patients with chronic lymphocytic leukemia (De Martino, 2009; Dudai, 2005).

Women's Health: Blue Vervain is appropriate to use for all types of menstrual and menopausal problems. Recent *in vitro* studies on intact human breast cancer cells revealed that *V. officinalis* extracts can bind to estrogen and progesterone receptors on cells, indicating that it may mimic estrogen and progesterone activity in the body (Owen, 2002). This may be one mechanism of action on the female reproductive system.

As an emmenagogue, the herb stimulates delayed menstruation. Antispasmodic properties relieve cramps and pain. It helps regulate menstrual flow by normalizing circulation to the pelvis and uterus to improve a scanty flow, or by reducing profuse bleeding with the astringent property of its tannins. Vervain is used to treat amenorrhea (lack or cessation of menses) and dysmenorrhea (painful menses), and combines well with Motherwort (*Leonurus cardiaca*) for these imbalances (Oliver-Bever, 1986). Its nervine qualities address anxiety and mood swings of the premenstrual phase (PMS) and menopause.

> *The combination of Blue Vervain, Black Cohosh, and Sage is remarkable in relieving menopausal hot flashes!*

I have found the combination of Black Cohosh (*Cimicifuga racemosa*) and Blue Vervain to be excellent for normalizing hormones, regulating menstrual cycles, and alleviating symptoms of premenstrual syndrome (PMS,) including mood swings and pain. The best herbal formula I have found for menopausal hot flashes is a tincture prepared with equal amounts Blue Vervain, Black Cohosh, and Sage. Dosage is 60 drops every 4-5 hours or as needed.

Blue Vervain is contraindicated during pregnancy because it is an emmenagogue that stimulates the uterus and promotes menstruation. Animal studies confirm that it contracts smooth muscles of the uterus (Oliver-Bever, 1986). However, it can be used during labor because its oxytocic property strengthens uterine contractions (Farnsworth, 1975) and nervine actions relax the mother. Vervain is a galactagogue that stimulates lactation to increase milk supply in nursing mothers. Research studies attribute this activity to aucubin found in the leaves (Bingel, 1994; Oliver-Bever, 1986).

Gout and Arthritis: In folk medicine, Vervain was ingested as tea and externally applied as a poultice or fomentation for gout and joint pain. Its anti-inflammatory and analgesic constituents contribute to the healing actions, while the bitter alkalizing properties help eliminate excess acids promoting inflamed and painful joints. Blue Vervain's stabilizing and healing effects on the kidneys also reduces painful gout.

Wounds and Skin Diseases: Blue Vervain's antibiotic, anti-inflammatory, and pain-relieving qualities are beneficial for treating wounds and skin diseases. Its stimulating and detoxifying action on the kidneys, liver, and blood help relieve toxic conditions, skin diseases, and eruptive rashes. The herb is applied externally as a salve, poultice, or fomentation to heal old sores and fresh wounds, sprains, bruises, abscesses, burns, ulcers, swollen glands, eczema, hives and other hot, irritating eruptive rashes. Vervain tincture or tea should also be ingested to resolve the internal causes of toxic or infectious conditions. A sitz bath made with strong tea can be employed to shrink and reduce the pain of hemorrhoids.

Teachings from the Blue Vervain Deva

"Greetings, dear one. I am the deva of the Blue Vervain who speaks to you now. My gifts to humans are many. The bluish-purple color of my flowers affects the mind and nerves to calm disruptions in the system and to 'soothe out the wrinkles.' My expression is of joy, and though the texture of my leaves and stem is rough, my nature is gentle and soothing to the nerves and soul. Yes, I am 'soul food,' useful for those who are grieving and despondent of life, and for wounded and joyless souls. Taken as a tea, I am bitter and soothe the bitterness sometimes encountered in life. Underneath my bitterness there is sweetness, joy and contentment, which are my gifts to you. This is one reason I am useful to menopausal women, who these days are so often despondent and full of remorse. I help uplift these souls to reach outward for love and light, and to reach inward for joy and compassion. There is great healing in learning to love oneself as a part of creation, to embody oneself as the Great Mother, and to acknowledge that the blood and consciousness of the Great Mother flows through us all. This is our common bond and strength; for there is great strength in union with the Mother.

"I help heal the distress of the soul that manifests as pain, guilt, loss, and many illnesses. I bring fullness where there is emptiness, joy where there is sorrow, and I bring movement where there is stagnation. My flow of movement is upwards, connecting the heart to the heavens, and I sing for joy.

"Within my flowers are cures for nervous afflictions, deep internal weakness, and loss of confidence. My water element is a purifier and mover of blood, improving the quality and circulation of blood through the body. And just as I assist the blood in flowing freely, I also bring clarity to the mind and encourage uninhibited and courageous thoughts free of fear or reservations. For fear has a freezing, stagnating quality, and I am a plant that promotes movement. This also includes moving through life's transitions of menopause, grief, and losses with joy and expanded wisdom.

"I increase movement in the digestive and elimination systems, and assist in releasing emotional pain and suffering to be replaced with deep internal joy and peace. I am calming to the heart and help it to rest in peace. From a peaceful heart arises a peaceful mind and great generosity. I am a teacher of generosity, and each one of my plants produces thousands of tiny seeds that germinate quite readily. For in my genetic coding, I am to bear fruit and multiply upon the earth to bring great beauty and healing to humans and the animals. Use me for many illnesses and for a heavy heart and clouded, dark thoughts. Allow me to brighten your day and increase your peace of mind and body. All who use me in a good way are blessed."

Boneset

Eupatorium perfoliatum

Compositae (*Asteraceae*) (Sunflower or Aster) Family

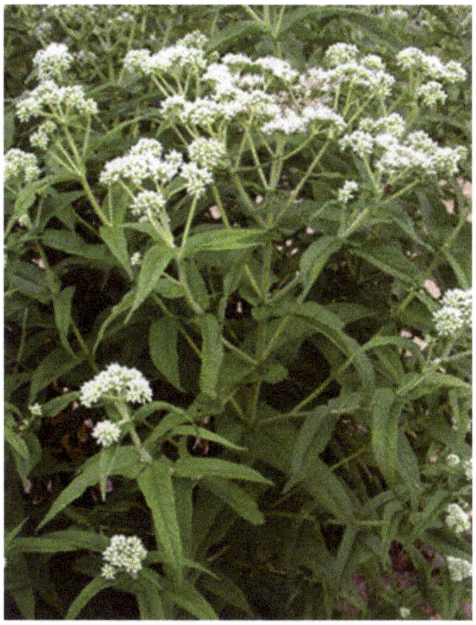

Common Names

Agueweed, feverwort, and sweat weed are antiquated names referring to the herb's diaphoretic property and historic use to reduce fevers. Ague is an old term for the intermittent fevers and chills of malaria and influenza (the flu). Other common names include thoroughwort (alluding to its thorough healing potential), vegetable antimony, crosswort, and Indian sage.

Medicinal Part of the Plant

The flower heads and upper leaves are used medicinally.

Range and Habitat

Boneset is indigenous to many areas of North America. Preferring a moist, sunny habitat, it is often found on low ground around swamps, marshes, ponds, lakes, or streams. It is a hardy plant that can also thrive on higher ground in fairly dry fields.

Description of the Plant

Boneset is a handsome perennial herb growing to a height of 2-5′. Several fibrous, stout, and erect stems emerge from the fibrous root system. The round stems are densely covered with long, white, downy hairs.

Many leaves climb the length of each stem, and their unique appearance makes identification of this herb easy. Rather than two separate leaves connecting at the stem, they are joined at their bases to create one long leaf, which the stem pierces or perforates. This perforation through the middle of each leaf inspired its Latin species name, *perfoliatum*. Leaves are elliptical to linear in shape, and both ends of the long, perforated leaf taper into sharp (aristate) points. Leaves are simple with a pronounced mid-rib vein and deeply matted pinnate vein pattern that gives it a rough, wrinkled (rugose) texture. Leaf margins are finely serrated with rounded teeth. Both sides of the leaves are covered with fine, short hairs, which are found in greater concentration on the underside. Leaves on mature plants can grow 8-14″ in length.

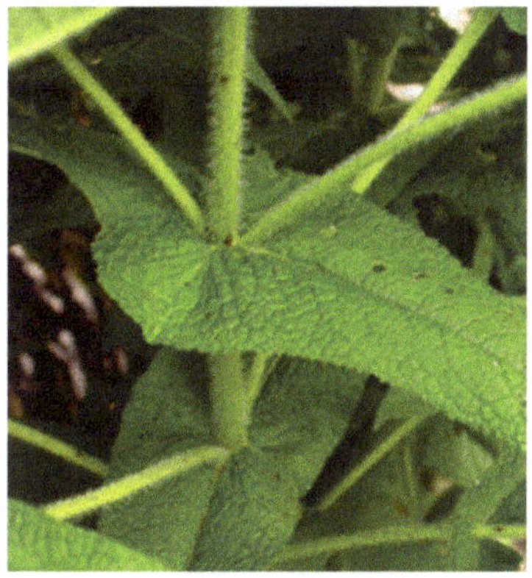

Stem piercing through Boneset leaves

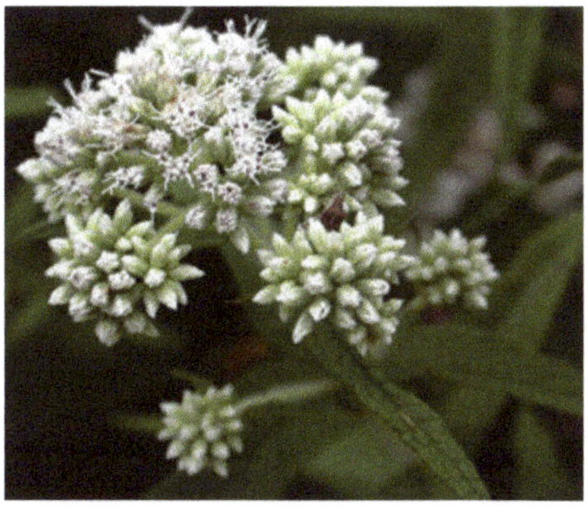

Upper stalks of the plant branch out, and bone-white flower heads emerge from the end of each stalk. These form umbrella-shaped corymb clusters of compound umbels. The flower heads contain a mass of complexly formed tiny flowers that are 1/5-1/4″ long and held within a green cup-shaped calyx. Looking through a magnifying glass, each calyx is seen to hold 7-15 minute, white, tubular florets. Each floret opens into 5 lobes and has 2-5 long, protruding stamens. The attractive flower heads bloom toward the end of summer from late July through October. The seeds mature into brown achenes with several coarse hairs attached like parachutes to carry them in the wind.

Cultivation

Boneset prefers growing in rich, moist soil under full sun, although it tolerates partial shade. In many regions, the plant grows abundantly in undeveloped areas and can be wildcrafted rather than cultivated. However, Boneset is such a wonderful medicinal ally that it is convenient to grow a few of these attractive plants to grace your garden. It can be germinated easily from seed or propagated by stem cuttings and root divisions.

The seed has a short life span and is often viable for only a year. Planting seeds in autumn or very early spring provides cold stratification that encourages better germination rates. Plant the seeds in greenhouse trays or outdoor nursery beds. This is a light-dependent germinator that should be sown on the soil surface, patted down, and barely covered with soil. Keep the seeds moist until germination occurs, usually within 1-2 weeks after soil temperatures have warmed. When seedlings are 3-4″ tall, transplant them to an area of full sun in moist soil containing plenty of humus, spacing them 2′ apart. Eventually, the flowering plants drop their seeds and many new seedlings appear around the adults. The seedlings may be thinned out or transplanted.

Stem cuttings are pruned in late spring before flowering occurs. Cuttings will grow roots when placed in a wet mix of potting soil, sand, and vermiculite. Root divisions are made in early spring before stems emerge or in late autumn after they have died back. Mature roots may be dug up, divided into sections containing sprouts, and replanted 2-3′ apart.

Harvest

Shortly after the plant starts blooming, harvest the flowering tops and upper leaves by pruning off 12-18″ lengths of the upper stems. Collect seeds for planting in late summer when flower heads have turned brown and the hairy seeds are clumped together in a loose mass.

Preparation of Plant Medicine and Dosages

Based on the widely publicized statement that fresh Boneset contains the potentially toxic constituent tremerol, I always followed the recommendation that the leaves and flowers must first be dried to eliminate the toxicity of tremerol before they are prepared as tea or tincture. However, according to master herbalist Stephen Harrod Buhner's research (Buhner, 2000) and my own investigations, tremerol occurs in White Snakeroot (*Eupatorium rugosum*) and not in Boneset (*E. perfoliatum*), making the precaution to dry the leaves unnecessary. According to Buhner, many herbal clinicians report that tincture is best prepared with the fresh herb and that dried Boneset should be used for tea. To dry Boneset, tie 12-18″ lengths of the upper stems into small bundles and hang them upside down in a well-ventilated, shady area. The leaves and flower heads may also be placed on trays or screens to dry.

PREPARATIONS

Tea: The dried leaves and flowers may be ingested as tea, but it is exceptionally bitter, reflecting Boneset's powerful punch as a potent medicine! Cold tea is best to use for the mucous membranes and as a liver tonic. Steep 1 ounce of the herb in a quart of hot, boiled water for 30-60 minutes. Dosage: Sip on the quart of cold tea throughout the day. Hot tea is best to use for acute infections and recurring chills and fevers, and acts as a diaphoretic to induce sweating. Steep 1-2 teaspoons of the herb in 1 cup of hot, boiled water for 15-30 minutes. Dosage: 4-6 ounces up to 4 times a day.

Tincture: Due to the very bitter flavor of this herb, many people prefer using ½-1 teaspoon of the tincture in a few ounces of water rather than drinking a cup of the tea. To prepare tincture, chop fresh leaves and flowers into small pieces and stuff them into a glass jar. Cover the plant material with 60% 190-proof grain alcohol and 40% distilled water. Dosage: 30-60 drops in water up to 5 times a day for acute problems and infections. This can be given every 30 minutes or over longer time intervals. For chronic problems, use Boneset as a tonic by taking 30-60 drops of tincture 1-2 times a day on an alternating schedule of 14 days on and 7 days off for a few months as necessary.

Pills or Tablets: These can be handmade by grinding dried leaves into a fine powder and adding enough water and Slippery Elm powder (*Ulmus rubra*) to make a thick paste. Slippery Elm powder is a thickening agent containing healing mucilage that holds the wet, powdered leaves together in a ball. Roll the mix between the palms of the hands into pill-size balls, then dry them. Dosage: 3 tablets 3-4 times a day for acute conditions and 2-4 tablets daily for chronic problems.

Syrup: Boneset can be used alone or combined with other herbs to make syrup for coughs, sore throats, and hoarseness. Other appropriate herbs for syrups are listed under "Lung and Bronchial Problems" in the "Index of Health Issues and Herbal Recommendations." Dosage: 2-3 teaspoons of syrup up to 4 times a day.

Chemical Constituents

Several constituents have been identified in Boneset. Sesquiterpene lactones include eufoliatorin, euperfolitin, euperfolin and eufoliatin, which all demonstrate immunostimulant activity in research studies. Eupatorin is antibacterial, anticarcinogenic, antimalarial, and antiparasitic. Helenalin is analgesic, anti-arthritic, antibacterial, anticarcinogenic, anti-inflammatory, diuretic, immunostimulating, and antiparasitic. Flavonoids include quercetin, rutin and kaempferol, which are antibacterial, anticarcinogenic, antihistamine, anti-inflammatory, antileukemic, antioxidant, antispasmodic, and hepatoprotective. Astragalin is a flavonoid that is antileukemic, expectorant, hypotensive, and immunostimulating.

Glucuronoxylan, the primary immunostimulating polysaccharide, is phagocytic, meaning that it seeks out, surrounds, and destroys infectious pathogens. Gallic acid is analgesic, anti-asthmatic, antibacterial, anticarcinogenic, anti-inflammatory, antiviral, bronchodilating, choleretic, hepatoprotective, and immunostimulating. The herb contains inulin and the sterols sitosterol and stigmasterol.

Safety, Contraindications, and Drug Interactions

The prolific folk use of Boneset goes back several hundred years, confirming its reputation as a safe medicinal herb. There are no cases of toxicity or drug interactions reported in the current literature. It is **contraindicated during pregnancy** due to possible abortant properties, and also during lactation because it is too strong and stimulating for infants (Brinker, 2001). Excessively large doses can have an emetic effect causing vomiting or diarrhea, but considering the extremely bitter taste, overdosing is usually not a problem.

As previously mentioned, it is erroneously cited that Boneset contains tremerol, a toxin that often causes fatal muscle tremors when grazing animals eat the fresh leaves. People who drink the milk of these animals can contract "milk sickness," which is characterized by nausea, vomiting, loss of appetite, constipation, and weakness. However, these problems are caused by *E. rugosum*, a different *Eupatorium* species containing tremerol, and not by Boneset.

Most members of the *Eupatorium* family contain pyrrolizidine alkaloids that can be damaging to the liver when taken in large doses over an extended period of time, but their presence has not been confirmed in Boneset (Smith, 1981; Skenderi, 2003).

Medicinal Uses

History of the Plant

Eupatorium perfoliatum was a popular remedy among many Native Indian groups throughout North America. It was used for treating colds, sore throat, flu, fevers, malaria, typhoid, stomachaches, menstrual irregularities, gonorrhea, kidney problems, rheumatic pains, snakebites, and parasites. Boneset was harvested and used by the Delaware, Fox, Menominee, and Iroquois people for these purposes, and by the Mohegans as a panacea for general debility (Moerman, 1998). Some tribes combined it with Goldenseal (*Hydrastis canadensis*) to heal skin cancers. Boneset was one of the many herbs Native Americans introduced to the early explorers, trappers, and immigrants from Europe. The herb was so closely identified with Native Americans that it was once called "Indian sage."

A white man named Joe Pye learned about medicinal plants from Native Americans and called himself an "Indian doctor." He taught New England colonists the virtues of Boneset and its relative, Gravel Root (*Eupatorium purpureum*), also known as Joe Pye Weed. Experiencing its remarkable healing properties, the colonists enthusiastically adopted Boneset into their medical pharmacy and it became one of the most popular herbal remedies in early America. The colonists used it for so many ailments that it was regarded as a healing panacea, especially for acute and chronic fevers, flu influenzas, and dangerous epidemics. By 1699, Boneset was so popular that it was exported to England for medicinal purposes.

During the late 1700s, an influenza epidemic called "break bone" fever spread throughout the United States. Medical historians later identified this as dengue fever, a mosquito-transmitted virus causing such deep, intense joint and muscle pain that people feel like their bones are breaking. This herb was so successful in reducing the fever that patients felt like it re-set their bones, and consequently the plant was called Boneset. After discovering this successful treatment for break bone fever, American physicians and herbalists began using Boneset for other types of flu and feverish conditions. It became a substitute for quinine in treating malaria and other infectious diseases. Quinine was a popular antibiotic of that era made from the bark of the Peruvian Cinchona plant that had to be imported from South America, making it more expensive and less available than Boneset, which was easily attainable from meadows throughout the United States.

Dr. Benjamin Barton, an authority on herbs and a renowned professor at the University of Pennsylvania, reported that Boneset was helpful in combating the yellow fever epidemic of 1793 in Philadelphia, and in treating ringworm and herpes. Boneset was listed in almost every botanical book of North American medicinal plants, and was one of the few herbs used by all schools of herbalism and medicine of the time, which included the Thomsonian, Eclectic, Homeopathic, and Allopathic systems. It was a common remedy of people living in the countryside and among African-Americans.

In 1887, Dr. Charles Millspaugh extolled the healing gifts of this common herb and wrote, "The attic, or woodshed, of almost every country farm-house, had its bunches of the dried herb hanging tops downward from the rafters during the whole year, ready for immediate use should some member of the family, or that of a neighbor, be taken with a cold. How many children have winced when the maternal edict: 'drink this boneset; it'll do you good' has been issued. The use of a hot infusion of the tops and leaves to produce diaphoresis [profuse sweating] was handed down to the early settlers of this country by the Aborigines, who call it by a name that is equivalent to ague-weed" (Millspaugh, 1887). Millspaugh also wrote about a friend who was a physician suffering from an intermittent fever, which was probably malaria, for three years. He gradually became extremely weak and emaciated even after using quinine and all other medicines known at the time. One day, an old woman told him to drink Boneset for a cure. He took a dose and went to bed, and in the morning felt noticeably better. He continued to improve without further doses, and the fever never returned (Wood, 1997).

The Eclectic physician William Cook, M.D., stated, "The leaves and flowers of this plant are among the truly valuable remedies of our native Materia Medica. They have long been employed in family practice, and deserve to be esteemed as one of the most useful medicines of the people" (Cook, 1869). Finley Ellingwood, M.D., wrote, "No more popular remedy has ever stood the test of time, since America's settlement. It unlocks internal secretions, eliminates the emunctories [excessive mucous discharge], equalizes circulation, and stimulates any depressed activity of the vital organs. Thus it is indicated in any form of fever and influenza, for headaches, severe muscle aches and backaches which often accompany fever" (Ellingwood, 1919). Eclectic physicians and other medical practitioners of that era also used Boneset in the treatment of colds, bronchitis, pneumonia, arthritis, gout, inflammation, spasms, indigestion, constipation, general debility, skin diseases, epilepsy, malaria, and typhoid fever.

The plant was an official medicine listed in the *United States Pharmacopoeia* from 1820–1916 and in the *National Formulary* from 1926–1950. Despite its great popularly in early colonial America, Boneset fell from use with the advent of modern medicine and production of aspirin and antibiotics. Although modern herbalists continue using Boneset in the traditional ways, it is not widely sold in the commercial market and there has been little scientific investigation of the plant.

Boneset is still a common herb found growing in many areas and is not listed as an endangered species. Considering its many powerful healing gifts, availability, and low degree of toxicity or side effects, this herb is a valuable ally that deserves a place in everyone's medicine cabinet!

Healing Qualities

Analgesic, antibacterial, anti-catarrhal, antifungal, anti-herpes, anti-inflammatory, antiperiodic, antispasmodic, antiviral, aperitive, astringent, bitter tonic, carminative, cholagogue, diaphoretic, diuretic, emetic (in large doses), expectorant, febrifuge, hepatic, immunostimulant, mild laxative, nervine, pectoral, restorative, stimulant, and stomachic.

Traditional Chinese Medicine (TCM) Perspective

Boneset's nature is bitter, cooling, and drying. It is a Yang-acting herb that stimulates and harmonizes the movement of Qi throughout the body, especially in the liver, stomach, pancreas, spleen, kidneys, intestines, lungs, and uterus. This stimulation disperses stagnation, obstructions, excess Qi, heat, and Liver Fire resulting from Liver Qi Stagnation. It dispels Wind Heat to reduce fevers. The herb also stimulates and normalizes the Wei Chi (immune system) and the lungs. It is restoring to the nervous, digestive, respiratory, and urinary systems.

Primary Actions

Boneset is one of my favorite and most trusted herbs, always kept close at hand in my medicine cabinet for fevers, colds, flu, infections, and sluggish digestion. For many years, it has been a dependable ingredient in my "Cold & Flu Relief" and "Cough & Lung Relief" tinctures, which have helped countless friends, family members, and clients. This versatile herb is an excellent remedy for both acute and chronic ailments. For acute illness and infections like colds and flu, it works best when taken as tincture or hot tea in frequent, large doses for up to seven days. It is taken as a tonic in smaller doses over several weeks for chronic conditions and low-grade infections that settle in the body and slowly drain the system to exhaustion. I have found Boneset to be a soothing and relaxing tonic for long-term indigestion, liver problems, and constipation. It works slowly and persistently to restore normal function throughout the body. In my experience, this herb is a true gem that can benefit everyone!

The Common Cold, Flu, Infections, and Immunity: I consider Boneset to be one of the most reliable herbs to treat all stages of viral and bacterial infections, and the general debility, fever, chills, and muscle aches that often accompany these illnesses. It helps break up the common cold, flu, and long-term chronic infections that seem to hang on. Historically, Boneset has been one of the most frequently used herbs to treat influenza. It was also given for epidemic diseases, malaria, and other intermittent fevers and infections that periodically come and go (Maas, 2011).

When taken hot, the herb's diaphoretic property lowers fevers by inducing sweating, which moves heat from the core of the body to the surface, where it is released. After the fever breaks, Boneset should be continued in smaller doses. The combined diaphoretic and laxative properties stimulate the release of toxins. As an anti-catarrhal and tonic to mucous membranes, Boneset reduces the production of phlegm and decreases mucous drainage and congestion occurring with the common cold, sinusitis, and influenza. Nervine and anti-inflammatory qualities also ease discomfort during illness (Hensel, 2011; Maas, 2011).

Research studies initiated in the 1980s confirm Boneset's ability to stimulate immunity, reduce inflammation, and treat the common cold and flu (Wagner, 1985). Its polysaccharides and sesquiterpine lactones stimulate immunity by targeting specific white blood cells, called granulocytes and monocytes, to increase phagocytosis. This is an immune process in which white blood cells engulf and destroy viral and bacterial pathogens (Wren, 1989; Wagner, 1991; Hensel, 2011). This is similar to the action of Echinacea; however, one German study found that **Boneset is about ten times more potent than Echinacea in stimulating immunity** (Wagner, 1985). Several sesquiterpene lactones and flavones isolated from Boneset have demonstrated anticarcinogenic and antitumor activity in animal studies (Woerdenbag, 1992). An extract of the herb showed potent cytotoxicity (ability to destroy cancer cells) comparable to a standard cytotoxic drug used to treat leukemia, chlorambucil. Research also shows that Boneset has mild antibacterial action against *Staphylococcus aureus, Bacillus megaterium,* and *E. coli* (Habtemariam, 2000; Mitchell, 2003).

Boneset is excellent as a first line of defense at the initial signs of illness, during the mid-stage, or as a preventative following exposure to illness. The bitter tea works wonders when used as a gargle and swallowed for sore throats. Time and again, I have experienced Boneset's dual ability to prevent infections from taking hold and to complete the healing process during active infections while reducing fever, aches, and mucous congestion.

In his clinical newsletter for herbal practitioners, *Medical Herbalism*, herbalist Paul Bergner has eloquently explained his understanding of the etiology of the common cold and influenza (flu):

> A person becomes first run down, with their digestion not quite right, their liver possibly sluggish, and their adrenals and energy level not up to par. This would be a 'deficiency' condition in Chinese medicine. A person can exhibit some symptoms of a cold, such as chronic cough, fever, or loss of appetite from this condition alone. In this state, a person's resistance to environmental fluctuations – cold, wind, heat, etc. – is reduced. Maintaining the steady-state temperature and other parameters of the body is a lot of work, and when the system is run down, it is harder to accomplish. After exposure to cold, usually a cold wind – we do call them 'colds' after all – the system becomes overwhelmed, and the cold penetrates past the normal temperature barriers in the body. The result is further derangement of the flow of energy in the system, especially a weakening of the immune system at the surface of the body, and of the flow of energy in parts of the nervous system. This is the point where an actual viral infection – which requires the above 'fertile ground' before it can infect – might begin. In a simple cold or mild flu, most of these symptoms stay at the surface of the body, such as a runny nose, fever, chills, and general fatigue. In a more complicated condition, if the cold has penetrated the system to a deeper level, and especially if the underlying deficiency state was more serious, deeper symptoms appear, such as muscle aches, headache, nausea, a longer infection, and chronic 'periodicity' of feverish symptoms as the body repeatedly but inefficiently tries to cast off the cold condition. Boneset earned its fame as a remedy for 'intermittent fever' because it is so effective in such conditions. (Bergner, 1995)

Boneset combines well to work synergistically with Echinacea, Goldenseal (*Hydrastis canadensis*), Yarrow (*Achillea millefolium*), Sage (*Salvia officinalis*), Elderberry (*Sambucus canadensis*), and Blue Vervain (*Verbena hastata*) for infections, colds, and the flu.

Cough and Lungs: Boneset is helpful in treating viral and bacterial lung infections and coughs. It has been a traditional folk remedy in treating acute and chronic coughs, laryngitis, bronchitis, pleurisy, pneumonia, asthma, and emphysema. It exerts a specific toning, soothing, and healing action on the mucous membranes of the sinuses, bronchioles, and lungs. The herb helps clear up excessive mucous discharge, drainage, and congestion throughout the entire respiratory tract. As an expectorant, it promotes the expulsion of mucous, and its anti-inflammatory and antispasmodic properties also help relieve coughs and the irritation they cause. Boneset is especially beneficial for the elderly when they have a lot of phlegm in their lungs and lack the power to cough it out. For sore throat, coughs, and all upper respiratory tract infections, it can be taken as tea, tincture, or made into a sweetened cough syrup for children and others who have difficulty with the bitter taste. Boneset works well for all types of bronchial and lung problems when combined with Pleurisy Root (*Asclepias tuberosa*), Elecampane (*Inula helenium*), Elderberry, Wild Cherry bark (*Prunus serotina*), and Horehound (*Marrubium vulgare*).

Herpes simplex and Herpes zoster (Shingles): Several herbalists have reported success in using Boneset for both oral and genital herpes (Bergner, 1995). I have personally seen several severe cases of herpes simplex and shingles heal more quickly and with less pain using Boneset tincture combined with the other two superb anti-herpes herbs, St. John's Wort (*Hypericum perforatum*) and Lemon Balm (*Melissa officinalis*). Take 30 drops of each of these tinctures in a little water 4 times daily for a herpes outbreak, or 5 drops of each on a daily basis for prevention. This blend consistently eases herpes pain and speeds recovery!

It is interesting to note that Boneset, which is known for helping intermittent fevers, is also good for herpes, an intermittent or recurring viral infection of the spinal and peripheral nerves. Boneset also works well to reduce symptoms and speed recovery from mononucleosis, which is caused by the Epstein-Barr and cytomegalo viruses, both members of the herpes family.

Digestion: Boneset's bitter nature makes it a wonderful digestive aid that activates the production and secretion of stomach acids and pancreatic enzymes necessary to digest food. The herb also stimulates the liver by promoting the production of bile, and its relaxing influence on liver and gallbladder ducts allows for easy bile flow. Bile promotes intestinal contractions, called peristalsis, that push food through the digestive tract, and Boneset exerts mild laxative action on the bowels that is beneficial for treating constipation and jaundice. Eclectic physician William Cook, M.D., reported that Boneset's action on the liver is "slow and mild, but persistent and very reliable" (Cook, 1869).

Small doses of cold Boneset tea or tincture are traditionally taken 10 minutes before meals over a period of time as a stimulating tonic for weak, sluggish digestion, poor appetite, and constipation. This helps heal the mucosal lining of the stomach and intestines, and is beneficial for all types of indigestion, gas, and bloating. It is especially suited for the elderly, who often suffer from these problems. Boneset's soothing and relaxing action on the nervous system supports the entire gastrointestinal tract by reducing inflammation, spasms, and digestive problems perpetuated by nervous anxiety. Eclectic physician Finley Ellingwood, M.D., wrote about an intractable case of hiccups that he treated with 15 drops of Boneset tincture mixed with Cayenne (*Capsicum annuum*) tea given every hour for a permanent cure (Ellingwood, 1919). Boneset is effective against parasites and gastrointestinal bacterial and viral infections. It helps restore digestion and normalize mucous membranes and enzyme secretions after damage from high fevers. For digestive problems, it works well combined with Gentian (*Gentiana lutea*), American Centaury (*Sabatia angularis*), Goldenseal, and Cayenne. Boneset is excellent for chronic liver disease, including all types of hepatitis.

Urinary Tract: Boneset is a mild diuretic promoting movement of blood and urine through the kidneys, making it helpful to treat edema (water retention). Its bitter alkaline properties help remove toxins and acids from the blood to relieve painful gout. I have found the plant's antibiotic activity, especially against *E. coli*, to be an effective treatment for all types of urinary tract infections, including cystitis. Thirty drops of the tincture added to a little water and taken 4 times a day is recommended for urinary infections, and it should be combined with other antibiotic herbs, most notably Yarrow and Goldenseal.

Nervous System: William Cook, M.D., wrote in his 1869 edition of *The Physiomedical Dispensatory*, "Boneset is almost a pure relaxant, with stimulating properties scarcely noticeable. It acts rather slowly and persistently. Its greatest power is expended upon the more inward muscular structures, as those of the stomach, gall-ducts, bowels and uterus, but it impresses the nervous peripheries, and also influences the skin decidedly" (Cook, 1869).

The herb is a nervine that helps restore the nervous system and decrease spasms throughout the body. As an analgesic, Boneset relieves pain. The late clinical herbalist Dr. John Christopher recommended using equal parts Boneset, Blue Vervain (*Verbena hastata*), and Chamomile (*Matricaria* spp.) for epilepsy. He made a tea by steeping one teaspoon of each herb in a cup of boiling water, and administered adult doses of one cup taken three times daily (Christopher, 1976). Boneset helps reduce anxiety, neuralgia (nerve pain), neurasthenia (nervous exhaustion), and myalgia (deep-seated muscle pain, aching, and spasms). In the past, herbal physicians gave it to their patients in small tonic doses for arthritic joint pain and muscular rheumatism. People with fibromyalgia who experience nerve and deep muscle pain may benefit from trying Boneset. It can also be used to treat chronic headaches that come and go over a period of time.

Heart and Spleen: Although not considered a cardiac herb, Boneset's bitterness has mild, normalizing actions on the heart and circulation. As a calming nervine, it helps normalize heart contractions and relax the muscular layers of the blood vessels, allowing for vasodilation (dilation or expansion of blood vessels) and increased blood flow. Boneset's stimulating and tonic properties also benefit the spleen by stimulating blood flow and exerting a cleansing action on the spleen and the blood moving through it.

Skin: Many of the herb's properties contribute to healing skin problems, fungal infections, and wounds. It is anti-inflammatory and antiseptic, and the diaphoretic action helps release toxins and excess heat from the interior. Its beneficial influence and detoxifying activity on liver and kidney function also reduces toxicity and promotes healthy skin.

Broken Bones: Conventional literature denies that Boneset heals broken bones. But in his *Book of Herbal Wisdom*, herbal expert Matthew Wood discusses several Native Americans and other people living in rural Appalachia and Ozark Mountain areas who have reported much success using the plant for this purpose. Wood says that he has repeated experience of broken bones healing better and faster with Boneset (Wood, 1997). Try combining it with Solomon's Seal root (*Polygonatum* spp.) and small amounts of Comfrey root (*Symphytum officinale*) for bone healing.

Teachings from the Boneset Deva

"Greetings, dear one. Long have I been here upon this land. Your ancestors, the Native American Indians, knew me well and used me in a multitude of ways for healing. I was used externally and internally as a healer of wounds. I am powerful and my effects are felt strongly in the body. My qualities are more masculine in nature due to my powerful activities of movement and stimulation. For this reason, I am not to be ingested constantly, but periodically to heal imbalances. My masculine energies are strong enough that it is wise to combine me with more gentle-acting plants when preparing a balanced medicine. I am a good springtime tonic to take in small doses over a period of 5-6 days to clear the congestion and old energies of the winter months. I stimulate the blood and body into activity, just as the energy of spring stimulates new growth after the long hibernation period of the winter snows.

"I am a pusher and mover. My bitter-tasting properties are one cause of this action. I stimulate the liver and flow of bile, as most bitters do, and in turn, improve the natural movements of the digestive system. Stagnation in this area of the body causes obstructions in the flow of energy and food, and inability to absorb nutrients from foods. Therefore, I provide an emptying quality; for as I move food though the system and relieve congestion and excess, in my wake there remains emptiness and spaciousness. This is the natural flow, to fill up and empty out. One cannot exist without the other. So in this way, my ability to stimulate and create movement brings balance and ease to the digestive system.

"I also activate movement to balance the spleen and pancreas. I have a cleansing effect on the spleen and the blood moving through it. Within the pancreas, I normalize the secretion of enzymes that break down food. In the kidneys, I promote movement of fluids, and my minerals and bitter properties help remove toxins and acids from the blood. For the heart, I offer stimulating and harmonizing action. I encourage movement of nervous energies and blood flow, and normalize rhythmic contractions. In balancing the flow in this way, I actually relieve the heart of excess so it may function in a more relaxed, less restricted way. Again, I bring the element of spaciousness to the heart where there was once restriction and congestion.

"My white flowers reflect my tendency to ultimately calm the nerves and brain. Although my initial effect on the nervous system involves movement and stimulation that influences the entire system, after this action has removed obstructions and excesses, the body rests in a more relaxed and balanced state. And so in the wake of my stimulating activity, there is calm and greater stability. The white color of my flowers also reflects the unification of all colors in the rainbow and is the essence of purity and unity. And so my ultimate gift to humans is assisting in movement toward pure and balanced bodies and minds.

"Part of my activity to maintain purity in the human body is to destroy invasive creatures like viruses, bacteria, fungi, and yeast. Even parasites have a difficult time surviving in my strong and bitter presence. My powerful strength assists in this ability to cleanse and purify. Therefore, I am to be used during times of infection and contamination. But know that the other side of my bitterness is the sweetness I leave in my wake. For when impurities, imbalance, and disease are freed from the system, there remains the sweetness of cleanliness, balance, and space to be filled with light, health, and normal function.

"I am also a balance of the four elements; fire, water, earth, and air. My fire element initially stimulates the nervous system, sparks the heart, promotes fire in the digestive system, and provides heat for the acids and enzymes that digest food. Fire helps burn infection and clear away stagnation in the tissues that causes conditions of coolness or excess heat, poor circulation, indigestion, edema, and even cancer. Once this stagnation clears and movement resumes, the tissues and organs resume more normal function. My water element moves my healing potential through the fluids of the body–the blood, lymph, digestive juices, and urine. Water cools hot, feverish, and inflamed tissues. The earth element contributes strength and endurance to my healing qualities. This nourishing element makes my stems grow strong and upright, and also provides human bones with this solidity and strength. My air quality allows swift and cutting movement throughout the body, and my medicine also aids the lungs in combating infection, congestion, and lack of airflow.

"And so I act on many levels, but remember that my main attributes are movement, directness of action, purifying abilities, and a strong bitterness that cuts through all congestion, obstruction, and impurity. Just as my stems pierce through the center of my leaves, remember that my warrior action moves with swiftness and pierces through the core of illness.

"The lesson I teach is one of purity. For during the bitter and rough times of life, there is also the opportunity for healing and peace. My medicine offers balance and brings understanding of this law of nature, which is the polarity of opposites. Know that opposites do not have to oppose each other in conflict, but can more easily complement each other to bring peace and balance to the whole. The difference in what appears to be opposites or similarities is only a matter of perception, but this perception determines how people live and use their gifts in conflicting or peaceful ways. This is a planet of choice, and so the choice within the two extremes is available to all. The wise person sees unity within all life and lives accordingly, no matter how opposite or antagonistic things appear to be. For appearances are deceptive, and the underlying, indestructible truth rests in the unity, inter-dependence, and inter-connection between all things and all of life. To live in this reality of oneness brings much relief from the suffering that is universal in the existence of humankind."

Burdock

Arctium lappa (Great Burdock)
Arctium minus (Common Burdock)
Compositae (*Asteraceae*) (Sunflower or Aster) Family

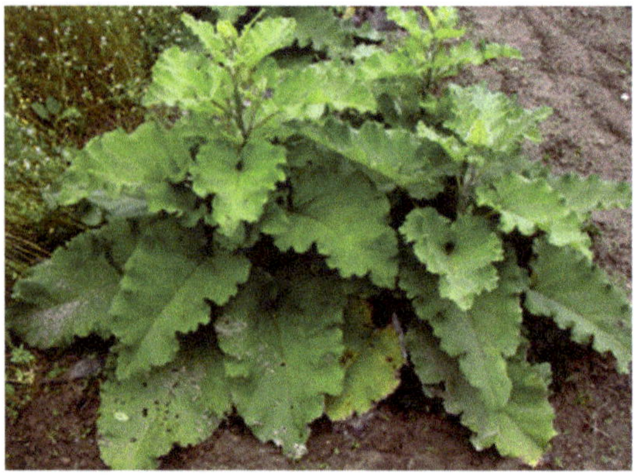

Common Names

Cocklebur, clotburr, bardana, harebur, turkey burr seed, and beggar's buttons are common names descriptive of the hooked burrs on the seedpods that cling to clothing and animal fur.

Medicinal Part of the Plant

Roots, leaves, and seeds of *Arctium lappa* and *A. minus* are all medicinal. Roots and seeds are used internally, and the very bitter leaves are primarily applied externally.

Range and Habitat

Native to Asia and Europe, Burdock was introduced into North America by the early European explorers and colonists. It tolerates a wide range of climates and has naturalized in central and eastern North America and throughout many areas of the temperate world. This is a common plant found growing in uncultivated fields and gardens, along the edges of woods and roadsides, and in waste areas. Burdock can be so plentiful that many people, unaware of its healing virtues, consider it to be an annoying weed.

Description of the Plant

Arctium lappa and *A. minus* are very similar in appearance. The primary ways to distinguish between the two species are to determine 1) whether the stalk is solid or hollow; 2) if flower heads are on a long stalk or no stalk; and 3) the size of the flower heads.

Arctium lappa is called Great Burdock and is a larger plant than *A. minus*, growing 2-9′ tall. The stalk is solid, stout, round, deeply grooved, and hairy with many wide-spreading branches. Flower heads are 1-1½″ wide and grow on long stems called petioles.

A. minus or Common Burdock grows 2-5′ tall. The stalk is stout and hairy like *A. lappa*, but is hollow and lacks the deep grooves. Flower heads are smaller, about ½-1″ wide, and are either stemless or appear on short petioles. There are interbred varieties of Burdock that all have similar healing properties. *A. lappa* and *A. minus* are used interchangeably for medicinal purposes and both have a rather striking appearance, especially the two-year-old plants with their huge leaves and tall stalks.

Both species have potentially large, thick, fleshy, and somewhat succulent conical taproots that can grow up to a couple of feet in length. Smaller lateral roots grow out of the main taproot, which is grayish brown on the outside and creamy white inside. Older roots lose moisture to become fibrous and woody.

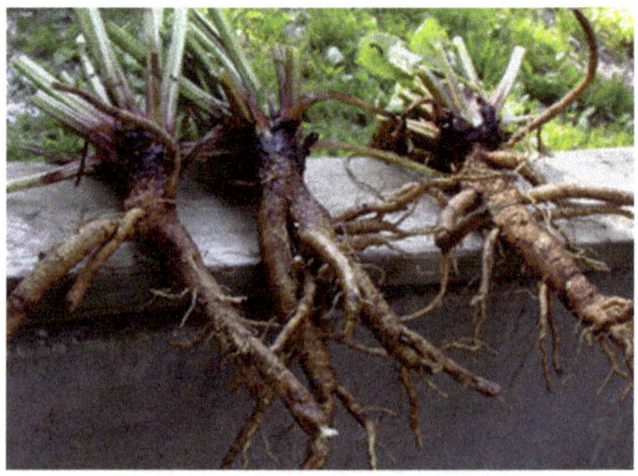

Arctium lappa taproots

All Burdocks are biennials. During the first year of growth, the plant appears as an attractive basal rosette of large leaves. Several erect, fibrous, dark maroon and green stems emerge from the crown of the taproot, each stem supporting one leaf.

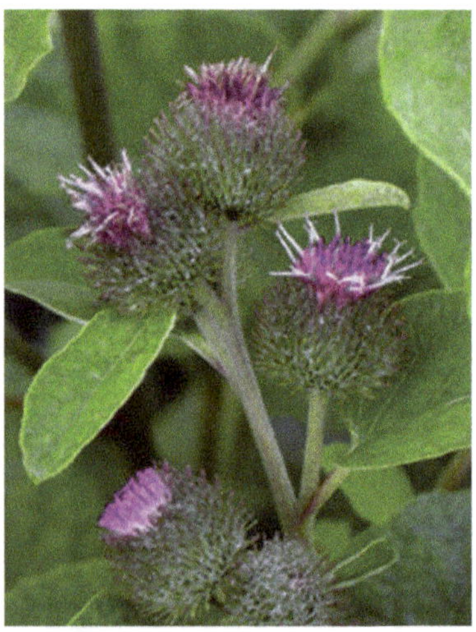

Arctium lappa flowers

During the second year of growth, a long stalk rises above the basal leaves and branches out, developing many smaller leaves and flowers. Flowers and seeds appear during the second year of growth, characteristic of all biennial plants.

The simple cordate (heart-shaped) leaves at the plant base can be huge, growing up to 2′ long and 1′ wide, and resemble elephant ears. The leaf margins are curved in wave-like ripples with crenate (rounded) edges. Leaves have a matted, pinnate vein pattern. They are pubescent (covered with a smooth, fuzzy, hairy down) and are a lighter greenish-white color underneath. Leaves on the tall flower stalk grow in an alternating pattern and become smaller and more egg-shaped (ovate) towards the top of the stalk.

From July through October, bristly, thistle-like flower heads appear in loose clusters along the ends of the upper stalks. The globular-shaped flower head is composed of many long, pointed, overlapping green bracts that hold numerous tubular, pinkish-lavender florets. Each minute floret has 5 tiny sepals and 5 petals that are fused together. The bracts terminate in tiny, curved, hooked tips and mature into seedpods known as the Burdock burr or cockle burr. The hooked tips are like Velcro and cling to anything they contact, such as clothing, hair, and animal fur. This provides an excellent mechanism for seed dispersal, allowing the seedpods to "hitch" rides a distance away from the parent plant, resulting in wide distribution. The small black seeds inside the burr are curved and quadrangular (four-sided).

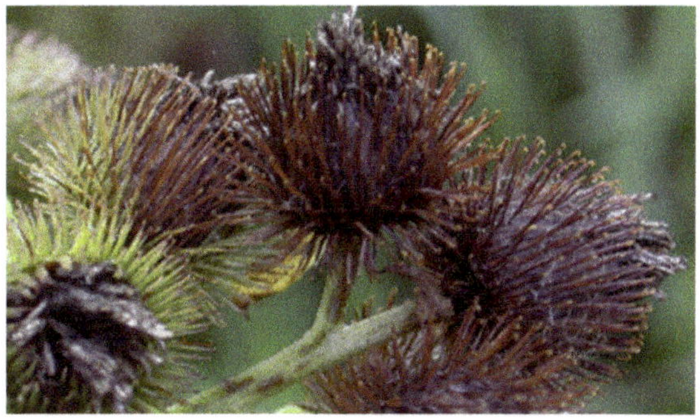

Arctium lappa **cockle burr seedpods**

Cultivation

Cultivation is often unnecessary because Burdock is a very common plant that can usually be found growing in the wild. Although farmers who labor to eradicate it may shake their heads in disbelief, I enjoy cultivating this herb in loose, loamy garden soil that makes it easy to dig up the long taproot. The plant accepts partial shade and will grow in almost any soil, but thrives best in full sun and fertile, well-drained soils for maximum root growth.

Burdock can be grown easily from seeds by sowing them into a garden bed in autumn or very early spring. When planted in autumn, the seeds lay dormant over winter and germinate as the soil warms in spring. Seeds may also be started in the greenhouse during early spring. The taproot grows deep, so trays must be 4″ deep to allow for unhampered root growth. Plant the seeds ¼″ deep and they will usually germinate in 2-4 weeks with warm weather. When seedlings are 4″ tall, they can be transplanted 8-12″ apart in permanent beds. Growing them tightly together encourages development of long, straight roots. Burdock is a vigorous self-seeder, and if allowed to grow to maturity and drop its seeds, many new plants appear around the parent plant the following year.

Harvest

Collect mature, clean leaves in spring or early summer. When harvesting, allow several inches of stem to stay attached to the leaves in order to tie them into bundles if drying is desired. Modest pruning of leaves will not kill the plant or stunt root growth.

Only one-year-old roots are used as medicine, so harvest them in autumn of the first year after the leaves have died back, or in spring of the second year before much leaf growth begins. Second-year roots tend to get fibrous and woody or rot by the time the seedpods mature, making them unsuitable for medicine. Digging the long taproot requires muscle, a good shovel, and some endurance. Chop off the leaves and dig a hole around the root, going deep enough to harvest the entire root without cutting off its end.

The seeds are mature and ready to harvest when the cockle burr seedpods are brown and dry and can easily be pulled off the stems. To get seeds out of their pods, put the pods in a paper bag and shake, punch, hammer, or stomp on the bag to break them open and dislodge their seeds. Then shake the bag upside down while holding the open end tightly closed, allowing only a small space for the dislodged seeds to fall out. When handling the burrs and seeds, wear gloves and clothing that fully covers your body. In addition, wear a face mask and protective eyeglasses or goggles to avoid the tiny irritating seedpod hairs that can sliver into the skin and irritate your eyes or lungs (if inhaled). If these hairs do get on your skin or in the eyes, wash them off with lots of water rather than wiping them, which will push them further into the skin.

Preparation of Plant Medicine and Dosages

Burdock leaves are most potent when used fresh, but they may be dried in a well-ventilated, shady area for future needs. To dry them, tie the stems of a few leaves into bundles and hang them upside down. Or, to speed up dehydration time, remove the stems, cut the leaves into small pieces, and spread them out on screens. Burdock leaves have an extremely bitter flavor compared to the mild-tasting root. For this reason, I typically only use leaves for external healing in a poultice or salve. They are a valuable and long-time ingredient in the herbal salve that I have been producing for many years.

For internal use, the root is the most commonly used portion of the plant. After harvesting, it is thoroughly washed and chopped into small pieces. The healing chemical constituents are readily extracted by boiling water or alcohol, making it ideal for teas and tincturing. The root can also be used to make salves.

The fresh root contains about 75% water plus volatile oils that evaporate quickly at ordinary temperatures when exposed to air. To prevent loss of these medicinal oils, it is best to use the fresh root rather than dried, and to extract the chemical constituents in a stable alcohol tincture. The alcohol makes inulin (a carbohydrate in the root) separate out into thick, white, dust-like sediment that settles on the bottom of the jar. This should not necessarily be filtered out since it has medicinal value and promotes intestinal health.

If drying is desired, spread the chopped roots on screens in a well-ventilated area out of direct sunlight. Fans may be used during humid weather to speed up the drying process and prevent molding. Dried roots maintain maximum potency for only about one year. The mucilaginous roots have a pleasantly mild, neutral to slightly sweet flavor, and tea made from freshly harvested roots has a milder, sweeter taste than one made from dried roots.

Seeds should be ground or bruised and prepared as a tincture to obtain the maximum effect of their very potent healing phytochemicals. Seeds have a pungent flavor and make the tongue tingle. There are tiny slivers on the fresh seeds that are very irritating, so be sure not to put the seeds into your mouth. When preparing tincture or tea, carefully strain the seeds through coffee filter paper to remove the slivers.

PREPARATIONS

Tincture of the Root: Stuff the finely chopped fresh root into a glass jar. Cover with 65% 190-proof grain alcohol and 35% distilled water. Dosage: 20-60 drops in water 1-4 times a day as needed.

Tincture of seeds: Put seeds in a small plastic bag, crush them with a hammer, put them in a glass jar, and cover with 65% 190-proof grain alcohol and 35% distilled water. The seeds may also be pulverized using a blender with the appropriate amount of fluids. Dosage: 10-30 drops in water 1-3 times a day as needed.

Decoction (Root) Tea: Put 2 tablespoons of chopped fresh root in a pan with a quart of water. For dried roots, use 1 tablespoon of chopped pieces or powdered root. Cover the pan with a lid, gently simmer for 15 minutes, and strain. My favorite way to use Burdock is in a tea made from powder because the entire root is ingested and the full benefit of the plant obtained. Dosage: 1-3 cups of tea a day. Use for 3-4 months for chronic conditions.

Infusion (Leaf) Tea: Put 1 teaspoon of dried leaves or 2 teaspoons of fresh leaves in a cup of boiling water and steep for 10 minutes. Dosage: Sip on ½-1 cup of tea throughout the day for digestive problems. The tea is extremely bitter and should only be used in small doses.

Capsules of dried Root: Dry and grind the root into fine powder (inexpensive coffee bean grinders are excellent for this) and pack into capsules. Unless used fairly quickly, this preparation is not as effective as tinctures or teas prepared from the fresh plant due to deterioration caused by drying. Dosage: Take up to 6 capsules throughout the day as needed.

Pills of dried Root: Dry and grind the root into fine powder, and add water to make a thick paste. Roll the paste into pill-size balls and dry. Dosage: Take up to 6 pills throughout the day.

Poultice: Leaves are used externally for skin problems such as inflammation, dermatitis, burns, wounds, gout, and hemorrhoids. Fresh leaves can be thinly sliced (allowing juices to leak out), placed over the affected area, and wrapped to keep in place. When using dried leaves, crumble them into tiny pieces and add enough water to make a paste.

Wash: Use strong, concentrated tea prepared from the root or leaves as a soak for external problems.

Salve: To treat external wounds and skin problems, Burdock leaves and/or roots are chopped and baked in olive oil using the standard method. For a list of other vulnerary herbs (healing to skin and wounds) to add to your salve, refer to "Skin Problems" in the "Index of Health Issues and Herbal Recommendations."

Culinary Uses

Burdock root has traditionally been eaten as a vegetable by Europeans, Asians and Native Americans, and continues to be sold in Oriental markets as "Gobo." The fresh, tender young roots of one-year-old plants can be grated or chopped into thin pieces like a carrot and simmered until tender for a mild, pleasant-tasting and nutritious addition to soups, stews, and vegetable dishes. It is a popular food in Japan, where Gobo is considered to be a mild aphrodisiac and source of strength and endurance.

Chemical Constituents

Burdock root contains an abundance of vitamins, including vitamin C, quercetin, beta-carotene (plant source of vitamin A), thiamine (vitamin B1), riboflavin (vitamin B2), and niacin (vitamin B3). Easily digested minerals consist of calcium, magnesium, phosphorus, potassium, iodine, selenium, chromium, zinc, silicon and iron, making this herb valuable for enriching blood and treating anemia.

Roots contain several acids, including acetic (antibacterial, expectorant, fungicide, mucolytic), butyric (anticancer, antitumor), caffeic (allergenic, analgesic, antibacterial, anticancer, antihistamine, anti-inflammatory, antimutagenic, antioxidant, antitumor, antiviral, cholagogue, hepatoprotective, immunostimulant), chlorogenic (allergenic, analgesic, antibacterial, anticancer, antihistamine, anti-inflammatory, antioxidant, antiviral, cholagogue, immunostimulant, vulnerary), lauric (antibacterial, antiviral), linoleic (anti-arthritic, anti-eczema, antihistamine, anti-inflammatory, hepatoprotective, immunomodulator), myristic (cancer preventative), oleic (allergenic, anti-inflammatory, cancer preventative, choleric), and propionic (fungicide) acids. Arctigenin also occurs in the root (Predes, 2011).

Proteins found in the root include the amino acids alanine (antioxidant, anticancer), arginine (diuretic, vasodilator), glutamic acid (antilithic), histidine (antioxidant, anti-ulcer), lysine (anti-herpes), methionine (anti-eczema, antioxidant, cancer preventative, hepatoprotective), serine (cancer preventative), and tryptophan (analgesic, anti-anxiety, hypoglycemic).

Phytosterols in the root include sitosterol and stigmasterol (hepatoprotective, anti-inflammatory, antiviral, estrogenic). Arctiopiricin demonstrates antibiotic activity against Gram-positive bacteria in lab tests. The bitter compound artipicrin is antibacterial. Guanidinobutyric acid may have hypoglycemic activity. Tannins, volatile oils, and carbohydrates that include mucilage, pectin, and inulin are also present.

Burdock root contains up to 50% inulin, a complex polysaccharide commonly found in plants of the *Compositae* family. Inulin is a non-digestible prebiotic that promotes growth of beneficial intestinal bacterial flora necessary for optimal digestion.

Seeds have a more dynamic, concentrated, and rapid effect compared to the root, and are beneficial for both acute and chronic conditions. A total of 14 lignans have been identified in Burdock seeds, but only trace amounts were found in the roots (Liu, 2012). Lignans are antibacterial, antioxidant, anticancer, antitumor, antiviral, and anti-HIV. The majority of *A. lappa* research has focused on arctigenin and arctiin extracted from the seeds, although they are present in other parts of the plant as well.

Arctigenin is a lignan phytoestrogen with amazing capacity to regulate immune response and reduce oxidative stress and inflammation (Fan, 2012; Hyam, 2013). Numerous lab studies reveal arctigenin's vasodilating (properties and ability to treat viruses, HIV, and several types of cancers and tumors. Arctiin also demonstrates cancer and tumor cytotoxicity. It is a diuretic and a bitter that stimulates digestion and liver function. Research indicates that arctiin protects skin cells from ultraviolet radiation damage (Lee, 2014). Arctiin is transformed into a number of estrogenic metabolites by human intestinal bacteria (Xie, 2003).

Burdock seeds also contain phenolic acids (caffeic acid, chlorogenic acid, cynarin, and dicaffeoylquinic acid), matairesinol (antileukemia), isolappaol A, and lappaol F, which exhibits strong anti-inflammatory and antitumor activity (Sun, 2014). Higher concentrations of lignans and caffeoylquinic acids occur in Burdock seeds than in the roots (Liu, 2012).

Several phytochemicals in the leaves contribute to wound healing. Arctiopicrin, costic acid, isochlorogenic acid (antioxidant) and lauric acid (antioxidant and candidicide) are all antibiotic. Taraxasterol is anti-inflammatory. Arctiin, arctigenin, phenolic acids, quercetin, and luteolin have also been detected in the leaves (Ferracane, 2010).

Safety, Contraindications, and Drug Interactions

Burdock root is very safe when used in normal dosages (McGuffin, 1997; Skenderi, 2003). No toxicity, side effects, or drug interactions have been reported, and the German Commission E herbal regulatory agency reported no known risks (Blumenthal, 1998). Historically, the root has been considered safe to ingest during pregnancy and lactation in moderate amounts, although there is speculative concern now because researchers have reported oxytocic tendencies that stimulate uterine contractions in animal tests (Brinker, 2001). To be safe, **use Burdock root in small amounts only after the first trimester and small doses of the stronger-acting seeds only during the last three months of pregnancy.** The Council of Europe regulatory agency has listed Burdock as a natural source of food flavoring, which allows it to be added to food in small quantities (Newall, 1996).

Burdock seeds are more potent than the root, and should be ingested in smaller amounts.

Medicinal Uses

History of the Plant

Burdock was extensively used in ancient Europe by the early Greeks, the medieval and Renaissance herbalists, and in Asia, where it continues to hold a prominent place in Japanese and Traditional Chinese Medicine and cuisine. The name "Burdock" is a combination of *burr*, referring to the seedpod that tenaciously clings to clothes and hair, and *dock*, an Old English word meaning "large-leafed plant." The name of the genus, *Arctium*, is derived from the Latin word *arktos*, meaning "bear," referring to the coarseness of the burrs and their resemblance to bear fur. The species name *lappa* means "to seize or hold tightly," which describes the clinging nature of the burrs.

During the Middle Ages, people believed that stone-like qualities in plants pointed to their ability to cure stony ailments in people. The stone-like appearance of Burdock seeds and seed heads was one basis of its original use in remedies for kidney stones. Dioscorides (*circa* A.D. 40–*c.* 90) was a famous Greek botanist and physician who used it for "those that spit blood and corrupt matter," and for toothaches and inflammation (Dioscorides, 1959). Galen (*c.* A.D. 131–*c.* 200) wrote that it was a popular remedy to increase urination and treat bladder pain, stomachaches, and bites of poisonous snakes. The English herbalist and apothecary Nicholas Culpeper (1616–1654) also used the plant for snake and dog bites, bladder problems, kidney stones, and healing burns, ulcers, and other wounds. Later European herbalists prescribed it for cancer, fevers, gout, syphilis, gonorrhea, acne, eczema, psoriasis, ringworm, and other skin infections.

European colonists brought Burdock to the New World, where they grew and introduced the plant to many Native American Indian tribes who adopted it for their own culinary and medicinal purposes. Plains tribes utilized Burdock for ceremonial purposes, and the Ojibwas prepared the root in a tonic formula for stomach pain. The Potawatomi made a root tea for purifying the blood (Vogel, 1970). Historic accounts report that Native Americans used Burdock leaves and roots in tea, poultices, and powder preparations for wounds, infections, boils, abscesses, rashes, swollen glands, arthritis, fevers, stomach pains, lung problems and coughs, and cancer.

Early American herbalists and the Eclectic medical doctors (1880s–1930s) extolled Burdock root as an excellent diuretic and treatment for kidney and urinary tract infections, skin infections, arthritis, gout, scurvy, venereal disease, and scrofula (tuberculosis of lymph glands in the neck). They prescribed a tincture of the seeds as a diuretic for kidney diseases and bladder infections (cystitis) occurring with symptoms of burning urine containing mucous. Seed preparations were also given to treat boils, styes (inflammation of sebaceous glands on the eyelid), lung irritations and coughs, muscular aches, rheumatism, aphthous ulcerations (small, white blisters) in the mouth and digestive tract, indigestion, and skin ailments, especially psoriasis and eczema. An ointment made from the leaves was used externally for skin diseases and ulcers. Burdock appeared in the *U.S. Pharmacopoeia* from 1831–1842 and in *The National Formulary* from 1916–1947, where it was listed as a diuretic and a diaphoretic remedy to reduce fevers by promoting perspiration.

Burdock's global popularity as a medicinal herb continues to grow, and it is commercially available in a variety of preparations. Most of the research has been *in vivo* and *in vitro* lab studies on the biological activity of only two constituents, arctigenin and arctiin, and there have been very few human clinical trials in which all chemical constituents in the plant are assessed.

Healing Qualities

The root is alterative, antacid, antibacterial, anticarcinogenic, antifungal, anti-inflammatory, antilithic, antiscorbutic, anti-uric, cholagogue, depurative, diaphoretic, diuretic, exanthematous, expectorant, febrifuge, hepatic, immunomodulator and stimulant, mild laxative, lymphagogue, mucilaginous and demulcent, nephritic, nutritive, pectoral, resolvent (for tumors), restorative, stomachic, tonic, and vulnerary.

The very bitter leaves have cholagogue, depurative, diuretic, stomachic, and vulnerary properties.

Seeds possess similar properties as the root but are much stronger, faster, and temporary in their actions. They contain high concentrations of arctigenin and arctiin, and potent antioxidant, anti-inflammatory, and anticarcinogenic constituents. Seeds are diaphoretic, diuretic, expectorant, pectoral, and relaxant. They are employed for inflammation, upper respiratory infections, sore throats, chronic skin conditions and eruptions, kidney and bladder problems, and to prevent or treat tumors and cancers.

Traditional Chinese Medicine (TCM) Perspective

Arctium lappa is native to northern China. Known as Niu Bang Zi, it has a long history of use in TCM. I generally regard Burdock as a Yin tonic because of its ability to nourish, balance, restore, and clean the body to maintain the structural integrity of cells and organs. The cooling quality of the moist roots is beneficial for treating hot, inflamed Yang conditions and to clear internal heat. The root enhances the flow of body fluids, including blood, lymph, urine, and menstrual blood. It also normalizes perspiration and secretions from glands and mucous membranes that lubricate and moisturize the skin and tissues. These are definitely Yin attributes. However, the diaphoretic and diuretic properties of Burdock have a drying influence. When used in conditions of dryness, such as dry cough or dry skin, combining Burdock with moisturizing herbs such as Marshmallow root (*Althaea officinalis*) prevents exacerbating underlying constitutional dryness. The ability of Burdock to increase oily secretions of the skin combined with dehydrating actions may sometimes produce contradictory results.

Burdock dissolves and eliminates wastes, toxins and abnormal masses, and is beneficial for lymphatic congestion, swollen glands, kidney stones, gallstones, cysts, and tumors. The herb is stimulating to the digestive system, liver, gallbladder and kidneys, while reducing Uterine Qi Stagnation and raising Qi in prolapsed organs. It has a restoring influence on the digestive, urinary, reproductive, blood and lymphatic systems, and is healing to wounds and rashes. It primarily affects the kidneys, liver, blood, and lymph. The herb is a superior kidney tonic that fortifies Kidney Essence. It treats Bladder Qi deficiency, Liver Qi Stagnation with excess heat, and clears conditions of damp heat.

TCM traditionally employs Burdock root and the dried seedpods for blood and lymphatic detoxification, cancers and tumors, hypertension, hepatitis, vertigo, constipation, arthritis, gout and other inflammatory disorders, the common cold, sore throat, pharyngitis, tonsillitis, cough with yellow phlegm, fever, pneumonia, influenza, boils, mumps, measles, chicken pox, and other hot, inflamed rashes and skin diseases.

Primary Actions

Burdock root is a gentle tonic that can be taken daily as food, tea, or tincture for several weeks or months to improve chronic conditions. It corrects multi-layered imbalances in the body that manifest as a variety of conditions involving digestive, urinary, and skin problems. The roots and seeds primarily affect the liver, kidneys, blood, lymphatic, and immune systems. Burdock gradually but persistently strengthens the body and immunity, builds and replenishes energy, and supports a calm nervous system. The roots reach deep into the earth, absorbing nutrients and alkalizing minerals. When we ingest the root, those nutrients and minerals nourish the blood and organs deep within the body. I often combine Burdock roots with Yellow Dock (*Rumex crispus*) and Dandelion (*Taraxacum officinale*) roots for the above purposes, creating the herbal trio I affectionately call "the three sisters." These three herbs have similar properties and act synergistically to potentiate their biological activity.

The root is appropriate for both internal and external use, and its milder action is beneficial to use as a tonic for chronic conditions. Alcohol extracts of the seeds show outstanding potential for treating oxidative stress, inflammation, and several types of cancers and tumors.

Kidneys, Liver, Blood, and the Lymphatic System: Burdock root is a valuable alterative that restores normal health and organ function by stimulating removal of waste products and other impurities from the kidneys, liver, spleen, blood, lymphatic fluid, and lymph nodes. The abundance of minerals in the root enriches blood by neutralizing excess acids and providing easily absorbed iron and other minerals.

The herb's gentle diuretic action increases urine output to eliminate excess acids and other waste products of metabolism. Cholagogue properties stimulate liver and gallbladder activity to increase bile flow. Bile carries cholesterol from the liver into the intestines for elimination. Bile also encourages peristaltic movement in the intestines, enhancing healthy bowel function and complete elimination.

Ample research validates that Burdock's protective actions on the liver are linked to its strong antioxidant properties of reducing free radical damage and inflammation to cells (Chan, 2011). One study involving rats, whose livers were damaged by a 28-day diet of alcohol and an injection of toxic carbon tetrachloride, showed that they recovered within 7 days of treatment with *A. lappa*. Researchers concluded that the herb's antioxidant properties were partially responsible for the liver protection (Lin, 2002). Earlier trials showed that *A. lappa* decreased elevated liver enzymes SGPT (serum glutamic-pyruvic transaminase) and SGOT (serum glutamic-oxaloacetic transaminase) induced by carbon tetrachloride and acetaminophen (Tylenol), and alleviated the severity of liver damage (Lin, 2000). In another study on rats fed with high fat and cholesterol diets, constant ingestion of *A. lappa* root resulted in significantly lowered systolic blood pressure and protection against vascular inflammation (Lee, 2012).

Burdock soothes inflamed tissues in the urinary tract and cools painful burning with urination. Tea or tincture made from the root or crushed seeds is specific for acute and chronic problems, including kidney and bladder infections (cystitis), nephritis (kidney inflammation due to infection, toxins, or auto-immunity), and kidney stones. The herb's ability to prevent or reduce kidney stones is attributed to saponins in the roots (Grases, 1994). Diuretic activity is helpful for edema and hypertension caused by water retention. A study designed to assess the effect of arctiin on rats with kidney damage due to diabetes revealed that arctiin decreased abnormal levels of urinary albumin (protein), prevented sclerosis (hardening) of glomeruli in the kidneys, and effectively restored glomerular filtration (Ma, 2013).

The roots and seeds are employed to treat ailments caused by excessive toxins and acids due to insufficient liver and kidney function, including blood and lymphatic disorders, cancers, anemia, canker sores in the mouth, and skin rashes and eruptions. Burdock also normalizes the opening and closing of skin pores, which contributes to the normal elimination of body heat and sweat, along with the waste products sweat may contain.

A wonderful tonic that mineralizes the blood and eliminates toxins is made with Burdock root, Yellow Dock root, Dandelion root, Red Clover blossoms (*Trifolium pratense*), Stinging Nettle (*Urtica dioica*), and St. John's Wort (*Hypericum perforatum*). Combine some or all of these herbs in equal amounts and drink 1-2 cups of tea or 50-60 drops of tincture in water daily for several weeks. When using herbal teas or tinctures to detox chronic conditions, always start with small doses and gradually increase to gently stimulate the process. Drink plenty of pure water and combine Burdock with stronger diuretics such as Dandelion or Cleavers (*Galium aparine*) to encourage release of toxins through the kidneys and urine. For vascular headaches, the "three sister" combination of Burdock, Dandelion, and Yellow Dock roots can be combined with Feverfew (*Tanacetum parthenium*) and Scullcap (*Scutellaria lateriflora*).

Immunity, Infections, Fevers, and Inflammation: The presence of arctigenin and arctiin in the plant contributes to Burdock's effectiveness in moderating and strengthening the immune system, reducing oxidative stress, and fighting infections and inflammation. The cooling and diaphoretic properties of the root and seeds promote perspiration to assist in reducing fevers, inflammation, and other conditions of toxic excess heat in blood and tissues. The seeds work especially well for acute fevers.

Researchers have identified several chemical constituents in the plant that demonstrate activity against pathogens. Several substances, including polyacetylenes, kill bacteria and fungi (Schulte, 1967; Holetz, 2002). Components in the leaves and flowers show antimicrobial activity against Gram-positive bacteria (*Staphylococcus aureus, Bacillus subtilis, Mycobacterium*) and Gram-negative bacteria (*E. coli* and *Shigella*), and the roots are active against Gram-negative bacteria (Moskalenko, 1986). Phenolic constituents, including caffeic and chlorogenic acids, demonstrate antiviral activity against herpes viruses and adenoviruses. Arctiin and arctigenin show potent *in vitro* antiviral activities against influenza A virus in mice (Hayashi, 2010). *In vitro* and *in vivo* studies also confirm that arctigenin inhibits the replication of human immunodeficiency virus (HIV) (Eich, 1996; Vlietinck, 1998).

Oxidative stress occurs when our cells generate dangerous by-products known as free radicals. These are highly reactive molecules with unpaired electrons that roam the body in search of other electrons to "steal." In the process, these free radicals seek out and destroy healthy cells. Thus, free radicals and resulting oxidative stress are primary causes of cellular damage and aging, inflammation, scar tissue formation, and many chronic degenerative diseases. Burdock is an antioxidant herb capable of reducing oxidative stress and inflammation via several pathways. An alcohol extract of the root can elicit powerful antioxidant activity by increasing levels of superoxide dismutase (SOD) and glutathione, which are primary antioxidants produced by the body to protect cells from damage (da Silva, 2013). Arctigenin inhibits the body's production of several pro-inflammatory substances such as nitric oxide, cytokines, leukotrienes, and COX-2 (Cho, 2004; Hyam, 2013; Zhao, 2009). Studies also indicate that arctigenin has anti-inflammatory activity against Alzheimer's disease, ischemic stroke, and complications of diabetes (Fan, 2012). One trial demonstrated that water and alcohol extracts of the roots exhibit the strongest free radical scavenging activity when compared with other preparations (Predes, 2011). Along with arctigenin, inulin has also demonstrated anti-inflammatory and immunoregulatory activity, and both may be helpful for underactive or overactive immune response, and possibly autoimmune conditions.

Arthritis and Gout: For the past 200 years, American herbalists have testified to Burdock's capacity to reduce the pain, inflammation, and some of the underlying causes of arthritis and gout. The cooling, anti-inflammatory, blood purifying and alkalizing properties of the roots, with their normalizing action on kidneys and liver, contribute to the reduction of gout and arthritic symptoms. Burdock stimulates kidney elimination of acids, including uric acid, which promotes inflammation and gout. The oils and starches in the root also have a lubricating, moisturizing, and soothing influence on tissues and joints.

Cancer and Tumors: Burdock root has a long folk history as a cancer treatment in Europe, China, India, Russia, and the Americas. In medieval times, Hildegard of Bingen (1098–1179), a German Benedictine nun and famous herbal healer, used this herb to treat cancerous tumors. Native Americans also used the herb for tumors. Burdock root is an ingredient in the herbal cancer treatment promoted and marketed in America by Harry Hoxsey during the 1930s–1950s, and also in the Essiac formula that continues to be a popular cancer treatment in Canada and the United States. Rene Caisse (Essiac spelled backwards) was a nurse who promoted the formula and attributed its origins to the Ojibwa Indians. The data from one study indicates that Essiac tea possesses potent antioxidant and DNA-protective activity, which are properties common to natural anticancer agents (Leonard, 2006).

The traditional use of Burdock in treating cancer has been validated in laboratory tests. Many modern researchers have identified several phytochemicals demonstrating strong immune-stimulating properties with anticancer, antitumor, and antimutagenic activity (Foldeak, 1964; Dombradi, 1966; Newall, 1996).

As previously mentioned, arctigenin is a potent immune regulator, antioxidant and anti-inflammatory, all of which enhance cancer prevention and treatment. *In vitro* and *in vivo* studies reveal arctigenin's ability to inhibit several types of cancer and tumors, induce apoptosis (cancer cell death), inhibit tumor necrosis factor production, and minimize mutations in cells exposed to carcinogenic chemicals. Several trials have demonstrated arctigenin's ability to inhibit growth of breast cancer cells (Hsieh, 2013), human lung adenocarcinoma (Susanti, 2013), and pancreatic cancer (Tezuka, 2013). Arctigenin specifically inhibited the proliferation of cancer cells in the lungs, liver, and stomach without damaging normal cells (Susanti, 2012). Another study verified cytotoxic properties of alcohol extracts containing arctigenin to induce apoptosis of leukemia cancer cells (Matsumoto, 2006; Wegiera, 2012). Matairesinol found in seeds is also antileukemia.

Other phytochemicals in Burdock have been studied for their cytotoxic activity. Arctiin isolated from the seeds demonstrated protection against breast and liver cancers in rats (Hirose, 2000). Polysaccharides in the root have shown immune-stimulating and antitumor potential (Belkin, 1961). Japanese researchers discovered a substance called the B-factor (for "Burdock factor") with unique capabilities for reducing cellular mutation (Morita, 1984). Benzaldehyde is another constituent in the herb that elicits antitumor activity (Yance, 1999).

Studies on mice showed that L-asparagine derived from the root had strong antimetastatic activity against malignant lung carcinoma and melanoma cancers. L-asparagine also increased antimetastatic activity of cyclophosphane, and partially reduced the toxic side effects of this chemotherapy drug without diminishing its antitumor and antimetastatic activities (Urazova, 2011).

Another phytochemical, Lappaol F, induced cell death (apoptosis) in several types of cancer cells while exhibiting minimal damage on healthy epithelial cells. Lappaol F was well-tolerated in treated animals without significant toxicity (Sun, 2014).

Modern science points to Burdock's potential as a treatment for cancer and other diseases of oxidative stress. It is interesting that research validates the historic use of the plant for these issues.

Digestive System: Burdock root neutralizes excess acids and eliminates toxins from the digestive tract, and is a cooling, soothing demulcent to inflamed, irritated tissues. It benefits the stomach, pancreas, liver, and gallbladder. The root tea is especially helpful for indigestion, gastritis (stomach inflammation), glossitis (inflamed tongue), canker sores in the mouth, and excess stomach acid leading to heartburn and acid reflux. Burdock root helps the liver break down fats, and is a mild tonic that normalizes liver and gallbladder function over time. It gently stimulates bile flow and exerts a laxative response in the intestines. It is beneficial for inflammation, congestion, and other problems of these organs, including high cholesterol and gallstones. A decoction of root tea is specifically indicated for stomach and intestinal ulcers, irritable bowel syndrome, Crohn's disease, ulcerative colitis (de Almeida, 2013), and colon cancer. Small, frequent doses of the tea or tincture of the bitter leaves also increases bile flow.

One research study evaluated the curative ability of a tincture extract of *A. lappa* root in healing chronic gastric ulcers in rats and investigated the possible mechanisms underlying this action. Oral administration of the extract reduced ulcerated stomach lesions by as much as 59% (according to dosage) and promoted significant regeneration of stomach mucosal lining. Vascular permeability improved, along with decreased volume and acidity of stomach secretions. Burdock also stimulated increased levels of the antioxidants superoxide dismutase (SOD) and glutathione (da Silva, 2013).

High concentrations of inulin, found in the roots, contain fructo-oligerosaccharides (FOS). These are prebiotic food nutrients that stimulate growth and activity of beneficial *Lactobacilli* bacteria in the intestines. This bacteria promotes optimal digestion and elimination, and reduces pathogenic organisms in the intestines, including Candida yeast. Inulin is beneficial for intestinal inflammation, diarrhea or constipation, protective against colon and breast cancers, helpful in reducing high blood sugar, and has immunostimulating activity in the intestines.

A study investigating amounts of FOS in different herbs discovered that the raw roots of *A. lappa*, Chicory (*Cichorium intybus*), Jerusalem artichoke (*Helianthus tuberosus*), Garlic (*Allium sativum*), and Dandelion leaves all contained over 10% FOS per fresh weight. Trials involving FOS and inulin showed similar benefits on intestinal microflora (Hawrelak, 2002).

Inulin has a mildly sweet taste and is filling like starchy foods. It is only slightly soluble in cold water or alcohol but dissolves in hot water, so Burdock decoction teas contain substantial amounts of inulin. Human clinical trials show that 15 grams of inulin taken for 15 days can increase healthy intestinal *Lactobacillus bifidobacteria* up to 10%. Bifidobacteria digest inulin, producing acetic, propionic, and butyric acids. Acetic and propionic acids may be utilized for energy production in the liver (Spiller, 1994). Animal studies show that inulin and butyric acid prevent precancerous conditions in the large intestines (Reddy, 1997).

Diabetes: Animal studies demonstrate that Burdock root has strong hypoglycemic activity. It promotes long-lasting reductions in blood sugar concentrations in rats, along with increased carbohydrate tolerance and reduced toxicity levels (Lapinina, 1964; Bever, 1979). Herbalist Matthew Wood has found that the roots help stabilize blood sugar levels in people with adult onset diabetes. Inulin is sometimes recommended for diabetes because it does not raise blood sugar levels, but it has no connection with insulin even though the names sound similar.

In vivo research has shown that arctigenin helps regulate blood sugar levels by activating muscle uptake of glucose and inhibiting the production of sugars and fats by the liver. Arctigenin improved glucose and lipid metabolism in diabetic mice (Miele, 2012).

Respiratory System: The roots and seeds soothe and moisturize lung tissue, reduce inflammation, and their antibiotic components are beneficial for bronchial and lung infections. Researchers have discovered that arctigenin relaxes bronchial tissues to expand the airway and ease labored breathing (Zhao, 2013), and it helps treat adenocarcinoma lung cancer (Susanti, 2013).

Use Burdock roots and seeds as tea or tincture on a daily basis to treat either dry coughs or excessive mucous, bronchitis, pneumonia, sore and swollen throat, asthma, emphysema, and other chronic lung problems, including those caused by smoking or chemical exposure. Combine Burdock with other respiratory herbs for best results (Refer to "Lung and Bronchial Problems" in the "Index of Health Issues," page 579).

Reproductive System: Burdock root works specifically on the ovaries and may be used to restore their normal function and regulate the menstrual cycle. It can be beneficial to reduce tumors and cysts in the ovaries and breasts. The root's gentle tonic influence on the liver also contributes to normal menstrual cycles and absence of premenstrual syndrome (PMS). As a mild diuretic, it reduces excess fluids and can be helpful for bloating, tender and swollen breasts, and feelings of pelvic fullness and congestion that may occur around the menses. A formula to aid elimination and provide nutrients during menstruation is made by combining equal parts Burdock, Yellow Dock, Red Clover, and Stinging Nettle in a tea or tincture.

Ancient European herbalists employed Burdock to strengthen a weak, prolapsed uterus and to aid childbirth. Cherokee and other Native American women ingested the root to strengthen the uterus before and after childbirth. Some modern midwives recommend the root tea during pregnancy for its exceptional mineral and nutritional content. Burdock seed tea or tincture helps reduce water retention during the latter part of pregnancy. Research shows that Burdock has minimal stimulating effects on the uterus, and some people speculate that it should be avoided during pregnancy. However, there are no known reports of problems and so many pregnant women have safely ingested the root over the centuries that it is reasonable to consider it to be safe when taken in normal amounts. For the lactating mother, the tea can be helpful for treating mastitis (breast inflammation and infection). A poultice of the crushed root and leaves may be applied on the breast to relieve heat and inflammation.

Men can drink Burdock tea or tincture to treat prostate swelling and inflammation. It should be combined with Saw Palmetto (*Sabal serrulata*) and Stinging Nettle root (*Urtica dioica*) for best results.

Skin and External Healing: The detoxifying, nourishing, antioxidant, and anti-inflammatory qualities of the whole plant promote healthy skin. Both seeds and root contribute to normalizing sweat glands and sebaceous oil-secreting glands of the skin. As a diaphoretic, Burdock increases perspiration, allowing excess heat and toxins to be released through the pores of these glands. Burdock's regulation of the opening and closing of skin pores makes it helpful in reducing night sweats and normalizing profuse sweating (hyperhydrosis) or lack of perspiration (hypohydrosis).

The root or seeds are taken internally as tea or tincture to address deep-seated internal imbalances causing chronic skin problems. Due to its cooling, soothing mucilaginous and demulcent properties, the root can also be applied externally. Prepare it as a poultice, wash, or salve for hot, dry, itchy or inflamed skin conditions. The same types of preparations made from the leaves are excellent for external application for both chronic and acute skin problems. When directly applied to the skin, the leaves have a "drawing" action that pulls toxins, infection, and pus to the surface for elimination. This is helpful for mumps and many types of skin eruptions such as boils, abscesses, acne, hives, measles, and chicken pox.

Burdock inhibits fungal and bacterial growth (Vincent, 1948; Schulte, 1967), and is helpful for athlete's foot, ringworm, and infectious wounds. It has long been used for old sores that are slow to heal, burns, bruises, ulcers, rashes, tumors, cysts, hemorrhoids, venomous bites, inflammations, and dry, scaly skin conditions. The herb has a long tradition as a specific treatment for psoriasis and eczema when used for an extended period of time. For internal treatment of psoriasis, combine Burdock root with equal parts Yellow Dock root, Red Clover blossoms, Cleavers (*Galium aparine*), and Sarsaparilla (*Smilax aristolochiifolia*) root. For eczema, combine Burdock with Stinging Nettle and Chamomile (*Matricaria recutita*).

Regular ingestion of Burdock root tea can help reduce dandruff by addressing possible liver imbalance, mineral deficiencies, and excessive toxins that can be causal factors. Because Burdock normalizes the oil-secreting sebaceous glands on the scalp and skin, it is specific for conditions of dry skin. The famous German physician and herbalist Rudolf Weiss, M.D., recommended massaging oil made from Burdock root into the scalp on a daily basis for 1-3 months. The oil can be applied externally for cradle cap in infants.

Teachings from the Burdock Deva

"Greetings, dear one. I am the deva of the Burdock tribe who speaks with you. My essence is primarily of the earth element, and my healing energies originate from deep within the soil and are drawn into my roots. My healing gift is to build and nourish the form and structure of the physical body. I help people to be grounded and firmly rooted in their own body and upon the earth, to live comfortably, peacefully, and securely. I am specific for those who are ill-at-ease, who feel weak and lost because they lack connection with the earth, and those who, like leaves in the autumn wind, are blown to and fro, lacking stability and direction in their lives.

"My huge leaves, substantial roots, and tall stature reflect the generous abundance and lush richness of Nature. Just as my strong, solid roots grow deep to absorb the healing and nurturing energies and minerals of the earth, I am a pillar of strength. I offer this endurance and fortitude to all those who use me. The white flesh of my roots works deep in the human body, tending to the needs and nourishment of the inner organs, including the liver, kidneys, spleen, and pancreas. Although I grow in abundance in many areas and appear to be a persistent and tenacious weed to some people, this quality actually reflects the intense, foundational strength of my being. Wise people value and use me in a respectful way, and receive this strength by ingesting my roots.

"My watery nature helps dissolve and disperse toxins and excess acids from the organs and tissues. I promote gentle movement and flow of fluids and energies throughout the body, cleansing and nourishing the cells. The curly edges of my leaves, appearing like rising and sinking waves on the ocean's surface, reflect this gentle mobility and fluidity. My heart-shaped leaves, pinkish flowers, and the reddish-maroon color of my stems and leaf veins all point to my calming, nourishing effect on the heart and blood. I establish normal fluid movement of blood, lymph, urine, and menses.

"With the removal of impurities comes freshness, vitality, joy, playfulness, and a deep, quiet calm. Yes, I am a plant that likes to play and delights in children. A tea of my roots can be safely given to children to nourish them, build strong bones, develop their physical strength, and provide the security of being grounded within their own bodies and on the earth. My humble gifts are powerfully strong and consistent, yet gentle and safe to be used by all."

Calendula

Calendula officinalis
Compositae (*Asteraceae*) (Sunflower or Aster) Family

Common Names

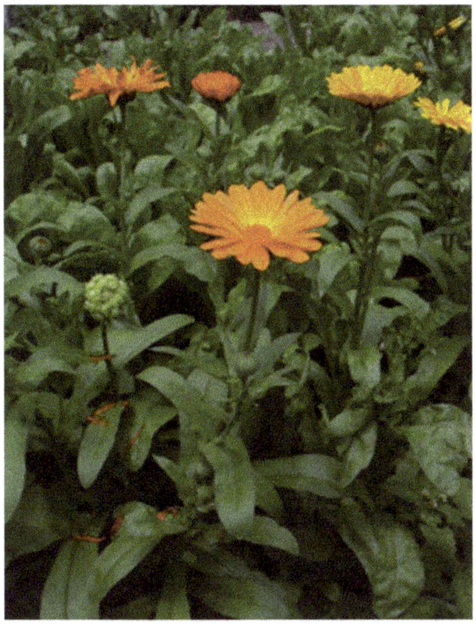

Calendula is sometimes called pot marigold, but it is not the same plant as the common garden marigold (*Tagetes* spp.). Holigold, goldbloom, Marybud, and Marygold are older names referring to the flower's golden hues and association with holy and feminine qualities. My friend Chunpay, a Tibetan Buddhist monk, once told me that the Tibetan name for Calendula is "Meido Dolma" or "Tara's Flower." Meido means "flower" and Dolma is the Tibetan name for Tara, the Great Compassionate Mother. According to Buddhist tradition, Tara was born from the tears of Avalokiteshvara, the Bodhisattva of Compassion, when he contemplated the sufferings of the world. Tara is the goddess of compassion in its most sacred, feminine, gentle, and heartfelt capacity, encompassing the pure qualities of nature, maternal nurturing, and protection.

Early Christians called Calendula "Marybud" or "Marygold" because it bloomed during the Catholic festivals honoring Mary, the mother of Jesus, and the flowers were used to adorn statues of her image. It is interesting that both Christian and Buddhist traditions associate Calendula with Mary and Tara, two archetypes of the all-compassionate and sacred mother. This is a beautiful reflection of Calendula's healing qualities.

Medicinal Part of the Plant

The flower heads contain the primary medicinal constituents, although the leaves may also be used.

Range and Habitat

Calendula is native to Europe and northern Africa. It naturalizes effortlessly in temperate zones, where it has spread throughout the Americas and Asia and is widely cultivated for its vibrant beauty. Several years ago, I was pleasantly surprised to find the familiar and colorful yellow and orange Calendula flowers growing abundantly in a university garden in Hangzhou, China. They looked exactly like the ones in my own garden. I picked some of the seeds to bring home, and the flowers are now flourishing in Indiana soil.

Description of the Plant

Calendula is an annual herb and popular ornamental garden plant. There are about 20 species in the genus, plus many hybrid cultivars that have questionable medicinal properties. *Calendula officinalis* grows up to a height of 2′. A rounded but angular, fairly erect, and multi-branching stem grows from a fibrous root system. The pale-green stems, leaves, and calyx are densely covered with short, erect, soft pubescent hairs. The simple, alternate leaves are rather thick and succulent, and are entire with wave-like and irregular margins. The sessile leaves are lanceolate with pointed or rounded tips. The base of each leaf clasps around the stem.

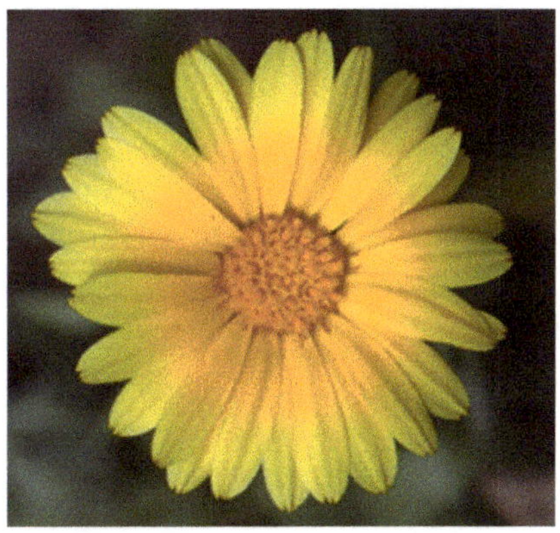

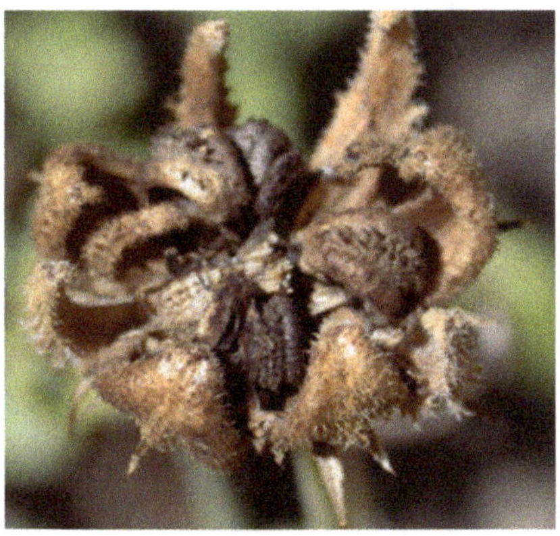

Dry seeds

Brilliantly colored, solitary, daisy-shaped flower heads are typically 1½-2″ in diameter and appear on the ends of branching stems. The cheerful flowers are painted in bright, sunny shades of golden yellow, amber, and orange. Typical of the *Compositae* family, flower heads consist of long ray petals surrounding a central cluster of disc flowers that are tiny tubular florets. The tip of each ray petal has two or three notches. The calyx holding the base of the flower head consists of many narrow, leaf-like sepals. The flowers and leaves emit a sticky resin that can be felt when handling the plant. Under a 16X magnifying glass, oil droplets can be seen "oozing" out of the green parts of the plant, especially visible on a sunny day. Flowers mature into brown achene seeds that are distinctively curved like crescent moons.

Calendula (*Calendula officinalis*)

Calendula begins blooming in June and continues throughout summer. Flowers are sensitive and respond to light by partially closing with the setting sun and on overcast days, and fully opening in sunshine. The delicate-looking flowers are tougher than they seem and are able to withstand the first mild frosts of autumn.

Cultivation

Calendula is a hardy, easy-to-grow annual that is started from seed. Be sure to get your *C. officinalis* seeds from a company that provides the Latin name to avoid horticultural strains that may not have the desired resin content and medicinal properties. The high resin content in *C. officinalis* will make your fingers sticky after handling the flowers and leaves.

The plant likes full sun and fairly rich, well-drained soil. It will tolerate partial shade, but sun increases the amount of medicinal resins. Calendula may be started in greenhouse trays, although the easiest way is to sow the seeds directly into a weed-free outdoor garden bed in early spring after the last frost. Cover the seeds with ¼″ of soil and keep moist. Germination usually requires 10-15 days of warm soil temperatures. If allowed to go to seed, Calendula self-sows freely and new seedlings appear the following spring. These can be transplanted or thinned out to allow 8-10″ between plants. Deadheading (picking off flower heads after they have faded) stimulates constant blooming until the first hard frost.

Harvest

Gather the flower heads when in full bloom. To ensure maximum resin content, harvest on a sunny day in the late afternoon. Calendula is a continual bloomer, so flowers can be gathered on a regular basis every 4-5 days during the summer and early autumn. A colorful basketful of vibrant, freshly harvested Calendula flowers is a visual delight! The leaves are collected when young and tender. Harvest seeds for future planting by allowing some flower heads to dry out and turn brown. The crescent moon-shaped seeds are large and easy to collect before they fall off the flower heads.

Be sure to maintain a constant supply of Calendula flowers. Harvest flowers for making salve and tinctures, but be sure to leave plenty of flowers to develop into seeds that can be collected for planting the next year.

Preparation of Plant Medicine and Dosages

Calendula flowers and leaves yield their properties to boiling water, alcohol and oil, and can be prepared as tea, tincture, and salve. Typically, the more potent flower heads are used for healing rather than the leaves, and most Calendula products on the market are salves produced from the flowers. For external use, freshly harvested flower heads can be heated in oil with other vulnerary herbs and made into salve. Fresh or dried flowers can also be prepared into a moist mash for poultice application. The tea or diluted tincture can be applied as a topical wash or fomentation.

Rather than drying Calendula flower heads for future use, I always recommend making tincture, oil, or salve with the fresh flower heads. The dried herb is potent for no longer than a year, while the tincture has an unlimited shelf-life. Another method of preservation is to chop up the fresh flower heads and store them in the freezer for several months.

Sometimes drying may be desirable. To dry the flowers for culinary purposes, pick the edible petals off the green center. For medicinal uses, chop the entire flower head into small pieces. Place flowers on screens and dry in a well-ventilated, shady area. Care must be taken to dry the petals thoroughly and quickly or they will lose their color and medicinal properties. Store them in an airtight glass jar out of direct sunlight.

PREPARATIONS

Tea: Steep 2-4 teaspoons of chopped fresh or dried flower petals or leaves in 1 cup of water. Dosage: 1 cup daily or every 1-2 hours as needed. The plant has a mild, pleasant flavor.

Tincture: Make with freshly harvested flower heads using 50% 190-proof grain alcohol and 50% distilled water. Dosage: 30-60 drops in water up to 4 times a day.

Oil and Salve: Chop flower heads, cover with olive oil, and bake at 200°F for 2-3 hours. Add beeswax to solidify oil into ointment. Calendula is typically combined with other vulnerary herbs (refer to "Skin Problems" in the "Index of Health Issues and Herbal Recommendations").

Wash or Fomentation: Saturate a cloth with strong tea or tincture diluted with 5 parts water (1:5) and apply to the skin. Freshly squeezed juice from the leaves and flower heads may also be used.

Poultice: Fresh flowers or leaves are macerated into a paste and spread over the problem area. If the dried plant is used, grind or blend it into a powder and add enough water to make a thick paste.

Culinary Uses

Calendula flower petals and leaves have been used to garnish and flavor food since the days of the Roman Empire. The flowers were known as "poor man's Saffron," and their appetizing color and mild flavor were a common addition to soups, stews, salads, omelets, cakes, cookies, and to color cheese. The flowers and leaves can be eaten fresh or dried. Create a beautiful presentation by decorating cakes and salads with the flowers, or put a few petals in ice cube trays to make a colorful and unique addition to iced drinks.

Chemical Constituents

The primary medicinal constituents in the flower heads of C. *officinalis* are flavonoids, volatile oils, terpenoids, and polysaccharides, which are immunostimulants. Flavonoids are vasoprotective (protect blood vessels) and antioxidant, and include isoquercitrin, isorhamnetin (hepatoprotective, antibacterial), kaempferol (antibacterial, anticancer, anti-inflammatory, antimutagenic, antiseptic, anti-ulcer, choleretic), quercetin (anti-inflammatory, anti-allergenic), rutin, narcissin, and neohesperidoside.

Caryophyllene is a volatile oil that is anti-acne, anti-asthmatic, antibacterial, anticancer, anti-inflammatory, antispasmodic, antitumor, diuretic, fungicide, and sedative.

Terpenoids include lupeol (antiviral, anti-inflammatory, antilithic, antimalarial, antioxidant, antitumor, diuretic), oleanolic acid (antibacterial, antimalarial, antitumor, antiviral, cardiotonic, diuretic, hepato-protective), calenduladiol, and alpha- and beta-amyrin (anti-inflammatory, antitumor, diuretic).

Phytosterols include sitosterol (antibacterial, anticancer, anti-inflammatory, antileukemic, antilymphomic, antimutagenic, antitumor, diuretic, hepatoprotective), stigmasterol (anti-inflammatory, antiviral, anticancer, estrogenic), and campesterol (antioxidant, lowers cholesterol). A triterpene glycoside known as calendulozide B exerts a marked ability to heal ulcers and calm the nerves.

Carotenoid pigments are antioxidant and promote healthy eyesight. These include lutein (anticancer, antitumor in breast and colon cells), carotene, lycopin, zeaxanthin, and calendulin. Lycopene is antioxidant and demonstrates anticancer activity in bladder, breast, cervical, and prostate tissues.

Acids include lauric (antibacterial, antiviral, choleric), caffeic (analgesic, antibacterial, anticancer, antiviral, antihistamine, anti-inflammatory, antimutagenic, antioxidant, antiseptic, antispasmodic, diuretic, vulnerary), malic (antibacterial, antiseptic, antitumor, sialogogue), gentisic (analgesic, antibacterial, antirheumatic, antiviral), and chlorogenic acid (analgesic, antibacterial, anticancer, antihistamine, anti-HIV, anti-inflammatory, antimutagenic, antiseptic, antitumor, choleretic, hepatoprotective, immunostimulant, vulnerary). Myristic and palmitic acids demonstrate anti-inflammatory activity and reduce edema. Salicylic acid occurs in the fresh plant and is analgesic and anti-inflammatory. Calendula also contains mucilage, vitamins C and E, calcium, and phosphorous.

Safety, Contraindications, and Drug Interactions

Calendula is a gentle herb that can be used safely by all ages, including young children and the elderly. The authoritative German Commission E herbal regulatory agency has reported no known toxicity, side effects, contraindications or drug interactions, and has approved the herb as safe and effective for wound healing, burns, eczema, and other inflammatory skin conditions (Blumenthal, 1998). Some people assume that the plant causes allergies similar to Ragweed, Marigolds, and other members of the Aster family, but Calendula does not seem to contain the allergenic sesquiterpenoid lactones (Skenderi, 2003). It is best to **avoid use during early pregnancy** due to its mild emmenagogue properties (Brinker, 2001).

Medicinal Uses

History of the Plant

The history of this colorful and cheerful herb is full of poetry and symbolism. Calendula received its name from the ancient Romans, who noticed that it usually bloomed on the first day, or "calends," of every month. The species name *officinalis* identifies it as the official variety used for medicinal purposes. The ancient Egyptians revered it as a rejuvenating tea, and it was valued by gypsies, monks, and other herbal healers of Old Europe.

Calendula was believed to possess magical properties. It was used in charms and talismans enabling people to see fairies and nature spirits, and to give women foreknowledge of the man they would marry. If people were robbed, they wore an amulet of Calendula, thinking the herb would bestow power to recognize the thief. Because of its association with Mary, the mother of Jesus, people believed the power of this holy plant was so great that by simply gazing upon it, the eyes would be strengthened and evil driven away.

English herbalist, apothecary, and surgeon John Gerard (1545–1612), who used Calendula in his medical practice, wrote, "It strengthens and comforts the heart . . . and is for inflammation and pain" (Gerard, 1633). During this era, the herb was also taken for headaches, jaundice, toothaches, and malaria. A tea of the flowers was administered as eye drops for sore and inflamed eyes. Nicholas Culpeper (1616–1654), the famous European herbalist and astrologer, claimed that it was an herb of the Sun and ruled under the fiery astrological sign of Leo.

The ancient Romans introduced the plant and its medicinal applications to England and the rest of Europe, and eventually Calendula naturalized throughout Asia and across the ocean in the Americas. During its long history of medicinal use around the world, Calendula flowers have traditionally been employed to treat cancers, fevers, swollen and sore lymph glands, suppressed menstruation, spasms, stomach ulcers, indigestion, and most especially as an external application for burns and all types of wounds and skin problems. During the American Civil War and World War I, the flowers were applied as a hemostatic (to stop bleeding) and antiseptic dressing for wounds. The American Eclectic physicians (1880s–1930s) prescribed it for these conditions as well as liver complaints including jaundice, liver and spleen congestion, headaches, varicose veins, endometriosis (inflammation of uterine tissue), vaginitis (vaginal infection and inflammation), gonorrhea, urethritis (inflammation of ureters), torn perineum during childbirth, toothaches, traumatic injuries to eyes and ears, conjunctivitis (eye infection), mucous congestion or drainage of the sinuses, typhoid fever, and tuberculosis.

Calendula continues to be a popular herb and garden ornamental around the globe. In the United States and Europe, it is a common ingredient in most herbal salves. Current research and animal studies confirm many of its traditional medicinal uses.

Healing Qualities

Alterative, antibacterial, antifungal, anti-inflammatory, antioxidant, antiseptic, antispasmodic, anti-tumor, antiviral, astringent, cardiac, cholagogue, demulcent, depurative, diaphoretic, emmenagogue, exanthematous, febrifuge, hemostatic, hepatic, immunostimulant, lymphagogue, nervine, opthalmicum, stomachic, tonic, and vulnerary.

Traditional Chinese Medicine (TCM) Perspective

Calendula is a neutral herb encompassing a harmonious blend of warming and cooling properties. The plant's ability to stimulate and normalize circulation generates warmth. The diaphoretic and febrifuge qualities cool feverish and inflammatory conditions. Calendula primarily affects the liver, stomach, lymphatic system, blood, heart, uterus, skin, and blood vessels. It influences the liver, heart and lung meridians, and the conception (Ren) vessel. It is calming to the nervous system, stimulating and decongesting to the liver, blood and lymphatic circulation, and dissolving to tumors and pathogens. The flowers clear toxic and Damp Heat from the internal organs, blood, and lymph. They revitalize the Blood, resolve Liver and Uterine Qi Stagnation, and Heart Qi deficiency. Calendula strengthens Wei Qi (immunity) and is used for Wind Heat conditions of fever, sore throat, the common cold, and flu.

Primary Actions

Calendula is a potent herb that decreases oxidative stress, stimulates immunity and wound healing, and promotes blood and lymphatic cleansing and circulation. Traditional uses of the herb for cancer, fungal, bacterial, and viral infections have been validated by modern research, which has specifically focused on its antioxidant and anti-inflammatory properties. For many years, Calendula has been a valuable and reliable addition to my tincture combinations for cleansing and detoxifying the blood, lymph and liver, and for stomach ailments. The flowers have also been a primary ingredient in my "Herbal Healing Salve."

I have always regarded Calendula as a plant capable of generating balance in our lives. The cheerfully radiant orange-yellow flowers express the vibrant masculine quality of the sun, while the crescent moon-shaped seeds reflect the nourishing and calming feminine qualities of the moon. In its lovely way of manifesting both polarities of male and female energies, the plant points us toward the healing ways of balance and harmony, both physically and emotionally.

Antioxidant and Inflammatory Protection: Calendula's extensive history as a folk remedy for infections, cancers, and tumors has prompted many research studies to investigate the herb's antioxidant properties. Alcohol extracts of the flower heads enhance production of the body's three most important antioxidant enzymes: superoxide dismutase (SOD), catalase, and glutathione. These enzymes are responsible for eliminating free radicals, which damage cells and are a root cause of inflammation, scar tissue formation, diminished immunity, degenerative diseases, and cancers. The herb reduces levels of cytokines, C-reactive protein and COX-2 (cyclooxygenase-2), which are all markers of inflammation (Preethi, 2009 March).

Cigarette smoke causes free radical damage and reduces antioxidant levels of SOD, glutathione, beta-carotene, and vitamins A and C. In a study exploring the activity of Calendula on rats exposed to cigarette smoke, investigators found that the herb protected against cellular injury and maintained normal levels of these antioxidant enzymes and vitamins (Ozkil, 2012). In another study, rats were given monosodium glutamate (MSG), a flavor enhancer used in food industries, to induce nerve toxicity. Treatment with Calendula significantly raised antioxidant levels and demonstrated neuroprotective action by reducing brain damage in the rats (Shivasharan, 2013). These potent antioxidant and anti-inflammatory properties contribute to Calendula's immune support and healing effects throughout the body.

Immune Protection for Infections and Cancer: Calendula is helpful in combating bacterial and viral infections, and fungal infections such as ringworm, Candida yeast, and thrush. Many studies validate the herb's ability to activate the immune system and increase efficacy of white blood cells. Polysaccharides, flavonoids, and volatile oils in the flower heads are partially responsible for these attributes (Wagner, 1985). Several researchers have reported that the polysaccharides stimulate the beneficial TH1 immune response leading to cell-mediated immunity, which responds to allergies, fungi, viruses, and cancers (Danilets, 2010). In mice studies, the flowers also stimulated the humoral immune response involving phagocytic and antibacterial activity (Borsuk, 2009). Alcohol extracts of the flowers demonstrate excellent antimicrobial activity against Gram-negative and Gram-positive bacteria and fungi (Efstratiou, 2012). Another *in vitro* study showed that essential oils in Calendula are effective against 23 clinical strains of fungi (Gazim, 2008).

The tea is used as a mouthwash for inflamed mouth sores and gingivitis (gum disease), and as a gargle for sore throats. The flowers have demonstrated mild antimicrobial activity against oral *Streptococcus*, *Staphylococcus*, *Pseudomonas*, enterobacteria, and thrush (Candida yeast) when used as a daily mouthwash (Faria, 2011). The tea or tincture can be given for the common cold, influenza (flu), laryngitis, and cystitis (bladder infection). The flowers act as a febrifuge to reduce fevers, while diaphoretic properties increase perspiration to flush poisons from the body and reduce body heat. The herb decreases congestion and excess discharge of mucous from the nasal sinuses and is soothing to raw, irritated mucous membranes.

Oil made from the flowers may be dropped into the ears to treat earaches and infections (Brown, 2002; Sarrell, 2001). For best results, combine this with Garlic oil and place 1-2 drops in each ear 2-3 times a day. For eye inflammation and infections like conjunctivitis (pink eye), make a tea of the flower heads, filter out all sediment, and apply this as eye drops or eyewash several times a day. Combine Calendula with filtered Goldenseal tea for exceptional results in resolving eye infections.

Several *in vitro* studies have not only demonstrated Calendula's antiviral activity against the common cold and stomach infections, but also against some cancers, tumors, and HIV/AIDS (Boucaud-Maitre, 1988; Loggia, 1990 & 1994; Kalvatchev, 1997). The herb's powerful antioxidant properties contribute to cancer prevention and treatment. Calendula exerts cytotoxic action against target cancer cells and promotes apoptosis, the programmed death of cancer and mutated cells (Matic, 2013; Abdel-Aziem, 2013).

When scientists investigated the effects of a *C. officinalis* flower extract on melanoma lung cancer metastasis in mice, they discovered that the herb reduced lung tumor nodules by 74% and increased the life span of the mice by 43.3%. The herb inhibited key enzymes involved in processes of cancer metastasis (Preethi, 2010). In a 32-week study investigating the ability of alcohol extracts of Calendula to treat skin cancer in mice, the herb diminished inflammation, promoted apoptosis, and reduced the number, incidence, and proliferation of tumors (Ali, 2013).

Due to its gentle non-toxic nature, Calendula tea or tincture may safely be taken over a long period of time as part of a protocol for treating cancers, tumors, and HIV. Austrian herbalist Maria Treben, author of *Health Through God's Pharmacy*, cited a mixture of 10.5 ounces of dried Calendula and 3.5 ounces each of Stinging Nettle (*Urtica dioica*) and Yarrow (*Achillea millefolium*) as a cancer preventative and treatment. She recommended drinking two quarts of this tea daily for an extended period of time. Her combination for treating leukemia included Calendula, Speedwell (*Veronica officinalis*), Cleavers (*Galium aparine*), Yarrow, Wormwood (*Artemisia absinthium*), Elderberry shoots (*Sambucus nigra*), Celandine (*Chelidonium majus*), Stinging Nettle, St. John's Wort (*Hypericum perforatum*), Dandelion root (*Taraxacum officinale)*, and Goat's Beard (*Aruncus dioicus*). These herbs may be used in conjunction with other cancer therapies, but are not intended to replace medical treatment.

Blood, Lymphatic Fluids, and the Heart: Calendula is a gentle but powerful tonic for the cardiovascular and lymphatic systems. It has a long history of use for heart health, although adequate clinical research on this is lacking. English herbalist and apothecary Nicholas Culpeper regarded it as a beneficial tonic that strengthens the heart. Maria Treben used the flowers for cardiac asthma caused by a weak, congested heart resulting in labored breathing (Treben, 1988). British herbalist Maude Grieve mentions in her book, *A Modern Herbal,* that it was often used by the common people "to strengthen and comfort the heart." For the lymphatic system, Calendula has traditionally been used to promote lymphatic drainage and circulation, and to treat swollen lymph nodes, tonsillitis, lingering low-grade infections, and lymphoma (cancer of lymph tissue and nodes).

American Eclectic physicians noted its calming influence on the nervous system and ability to relax muscles in the blood vessels, allowing vasodilation and increased blood flow to normalize circulation. Astringent properties help strengthen and restore normal tone to weak, protruding blood vessels, reduce bleeding, and benefit conditions of venous blood stagnation, including varicose veins and phlebitis (inflamed blood vessels). A placebo-controlled, double-blind study found that this formula increased circulation and extended the time of pain-free walking in people with intermittent claudication (Smulski, 1995).

In an interesting study, researchers observed that Calendula was cardioprotective against ischemic heart disease due to its antioxidant and anti-inflammatory properties. The herb stimulated left ventricular pressure and aortic flow in rat hearts, reducing the size of the myocardial infarct (the area of dead cells caused by oxygen deprivation) (Ray, 2010).

Although I have not heard other herbalists comment on Calendula's ability to treat mild depression and seasonal affective disorder (SAD), I have found it to be beneficial for some people with these conditions. Growing Calendula in one's garden, being outdoors in nature, and enjoying the beauty of this delightfully cheerful plant is certainly a great way to lift the spirit.

Wound Healing: External applications of Calendula excel at healing wounds and many other skin ailments. Ingesting the herb also benefits external healing from the inside out by reducing oxidative stress, improving immunity, and cleansing the blood and lymphatic fluids. For external use, apply Calendula as an oil, salve, poultice, or wash made from tea or tincture. The flowers are used most often for this, but the leaves are also beneficial. The plant may also be put through a juicing machine and the expressed juice applied externally.

Calendula was greatly valued by the American Eclectic physicians, who prescribed it as tea or diluted tincture for internal use and external applications for skin rashes, diaper rash, eczema, burns, cancers, ulcers, tetanus, gangrene, and lacerated and post-surgical wounds. William Clary, M.D., an Eclectic physician from Ohio during the 1800s, wrote that "as a local remedy after surgical operations, it has no equal . . . . Its forte is its influence on lacerated wounds . . . . If applied constantly, gangrene will not follow, and there will be but little danger, if any, of tetanus. When applied to a wound it is seldom that any suppuration [pus] follows. It has been tested by several practitioners, and by one, is used after every surgical operation with the happiest effect. You need not fear to use it in wounds, and I would not be without it for a hundred times its cost. It is made into a saturated tincture with whiskey, and diluted with one-third its quantity of water; lint is saturated with this, applied to the parts, and renewed as often as it becomes dry" (Felter, 1898).

Several research studies validate the herb's wound-healing abilities (Fronza, 2009; Markvicheva, 2009; Preethi, 2009) and anti-inflammatory benefits (Akihisa, 1996; Loggia, 1994). Oleanolic acid isolated from the flowers inhibited growth and survival of several Gram-positive skin bacteria (Szakiel, 2008). Other antimicrobial constituents in the herb attack bacteria and fungi to allow clean wound healing and reduce incidence of infections, gangrene, and tetanus (Foster & Leung, 1996). During the process of wound healing, Calendula promotes repair and growth of new cells and capillary blood vessels (Patrick, 1996; Parente, 2011) and stimulates the formation of granulation tissue, which fills in and seals over wounds and ulcers (Kiouchek-Popova, 1982).

One study explored the therapeutic efficacy of the flowers on 21 patients suffering from venous ulcers on their lower legs. Patients were treated with an ointment containing Calendula extract that was applied twice a day for 3 weeks. Upon completion of this regimen, the total surface area of all the ulcers was reduced by 41.71%, and complete healing occurred in 7 patients (Duran, 2005).

Calendula soothes the skin and mucous membranes by reducing pain, inflammation, discharge of pus (indicative of infection), and formation of scar tissue. I have found it to be quite helpful for all acute and slow-healing wounds and cuts, bruises, eruptive skin conditions such as eczema, hives, boils, abscesses, pimples and acne, hemorrhoids, fungal infections including athlete's foot and ringworm, impetigo (a staphylococcus skin infection), and insect stings and bites. Rubbing the fresh juice on warts several times a day for an extended period of time may eradicate them. As a hemostatic and astringent, it helps stop bleeding, bruising, and nosebleeds.

The herb not only helps heal first-degree burns and sunburns, but in an 8-month clinical trial involving 254 women undergoing radiation treatment for breast cancer, Calendula oil significantly reduced mild to severe radiation-induced dermatitis and pain (Pommier, 2004). The herb may also be applied externally to treat skin cancers and pigmented brown spots.

Calendula is an excellent first-aid remedy and is typically prepared as a salve in combination with Comfrey (*Symphytum officinale*) and Goldenseal (*Hydrastis canadensis*). For more than 35 years, these three illustrious wound healers have been primary ingredients in the highly effective salve I produce to treat all types of external problems.

Digestive System: I first witnessed the wonderful healing potential of this herb many years ago, when my youngest son suddenly bent over in severe pain from stabbing stomach spasms. I quickly gave him a couple teaspoons of Calendula and Wild Ginger (*Asarum canadense*) tincture in water, and within a minute or two the pain had dramatically subsided.

Calendula flowers protect the inner mucosal lining of the stomach and intestines to soothe and heal inflamed tissues. As a calming nervine, the herb eases indigestion and spasms (Bashir, 2006). Antimicrobial activity eliminates infectious viruses, bacteria, and yeast throughout the digestive tract. A tea or tincture of the flowers is wonderful for many gastrointestinal problems, including cramps, nausea, vomiting, heartburn, acute and chronic stomach inflammation (gastritis), stomach and intestinal ulcers, diarrhea, colitis, and other inflammatory intestinal conditions.

Several clinical studies confirm the herb's efficacy in treating digestive problems. Drinking the flower tea or diluted tincture is healing for stomach and intestinal ulcers and colitis (Chakurski, 1981; Krivenko, 1989). *C. officinalis* has also been used as a homeopathic preparation to successfully reduce *Heliobacter pylori* bacteria in treating patients suffering from gastritis and gastric ulcers. (Cwikla, 2010; Hofbauer, 2010). Japanese researchers found that an alcohol extract of the flowers lowered blood sugar levels and protected the stomach lining in rats (Yoshikawa, 2001).

Calendula stimulates and detoxifies the liver. Larger doses of the tincture (one tablespoon daily), taken over time, act as a cholagogue to promote formation of bile and its excretion from the gallbladder into the small intestines. This action improves liver and gallbladder function and is helpful for sluggish digestion, difficulty digesting fats, jaundice, hepatitis, constipation, gallstones, and high cholesterol.

Flower extracts protect both the liver and kidneys from chemically induced toxicity. Animal trials confirm that administration of the herb prior to toxic exposure resulted in diminished levels of liver enzymes normally increased by toxins, including serum glutamic-pyruvic transaminase (SGPT), serum glutamic-oxaloacetic transaminase (SGOT), and alkaline phosphatase (ALP). Elevated lipid peroxidation and bilirubin are also markers of liver damage, and Calendula reduced these. Kidney function markers, including urea and creatinine, were also significantly increased in the animals exposed to toxins. However, these levels were found to be lowered in animals pretreated with Calendula. Researchers believed this protection of both liver and kidneys was due to antioxidant activity (Preethi, 2009 March).

Women's Health: Calendula promotes blood and lymphatic circulation in the pelvis, eases inflammation, and helps regulate the menstrual cycle. As an emmenagogue, it stimulates delayed menstruation to begin, reduces premenstrual syndrome (PMS) and painful menses, and can help correct amenorrhea (abnormal cessation of menses). By reducing uterine and venous blood congestion, Calendula is appropriate for copious menstrual bleeding or clotting, fluid retention, breast tenderness, uterine fibroids, varicose veins, leg cramps, hemorrhoids, phlebitis, and ovarian cysts and tumors. Ingesting the tea and using it as a douche is recommended for yeast infections and other vaginal infections and discharge. Eclectic physicians administered this herb to treat swollen inguinal lymph nodes, gonorrhea, endometriosis, and torn perineum from childbirth (Felter, 1898). The tea is used as a douche and the flower heads made into vaginal suppositories to treat abnormal cervical cells and uterine cancer. A poultice or ointment may be applied to heal cracked nipples from breast feeding, mastitis, breast lumps and cysts, and poor lymphatic drainage (Loggia, 1994). It is excellent for use after a mastectomy. Research on women with lymphedema (chronic fluid retention of the lymphatic system) following mastectomies showed that external application of Calendula significantly reduced pain and swelling in the arms and chest (Casley-Smith, 1983).

Teachings from the Calendula Deva

"Greetings, dear one. I am the deva of the Calendula. My radiant flowers bring joy and light to the darkness of the heart isolated from the love of Creator. In my gradual yet powerful way, I gently melt the hardness of ignorant beliefs and disruptive, hurtful emotions. This process allows the energy to flow through the body and heal imbalances from distorted views and afflicted emotions that create sickness and suffering.

"My blessings to humans are vast. The beauty of my colorful flowers draws people, insects, and animals to my resinous nectars. My sweetness draws and connects to the inherent goodness of all things. Yes, I am a reflection of love, beauty and balance, and these are my gifts and blessings.

"My nature is of expansive joy and radiance. These drive darkness from the human soul. Take the tea and tinctures of my leaves and flowers to make you whole, to heal a broken and ruptured heart, to heal the stomach and nervous system. On a very physical level, my gentle movement penetrates through the body into very old, deep wounds, traumas, and emotional pain that become locked in the tissues and engulfed by rigid, dense, and stagnated energy. I am powerful medicine to relieve stagnation, release toxins and toxic emotions, and to bring light into dark spaces. For it is in dark spaces, where harmful thoughts and emotions shut out the life force, that cancer cells find a hold and dwell, sometimes to contaminate the whole body.

"The radiance of my flowers potentiates the radiance of the heart and mind, this being my greatest gift to people. On more mundane levels, the physical body will heal as the mind and emotions heal and 'lighten up.'

"I am, in a sense, a reflection of the Christos bringing light to the world. The Tibetans call me Tara's Flower because I embody the heart of the Divine Mother, and joy radiates from my flowers just as joy radiates from the heart of the Mother. I embody the nourishing, bountiful, loving attributes of the female principle, the Earth Mother. I rest in the heart of life and offer the blessings of a strong and loving heart to all who grow me in their gardens, who adorn their homes and sacred spaces with my flowers, and who ingest me for healing. These are my humble gifts offered as a reflection of the benevolence of Creator. For Creator loves all and offers many tools and flowers of beauty to guide people back home to an existence of peace, beauty, and kindness.

"I am strong and hardy, as evidenced by my ability to stay green even in briefly freezing temperatures. I am enduring, as manifested in the power and abundance of my seeds that germinate easily in the warmth of spring.

"My message to humanity is to walk peacefully and gently upon the earth. Life is a blessing not to be taken for granted. Each person has responsibility for his or her actions, and each life unfolds as a result of previous choices and actions. Let my beautiful flowers point the way to a gentle and simple life that radiates loving kindness to all beings. For just as the sun shines on me, it also indiscriminately shines on all people. Each person is responsible to shine love, humility, and compassion on all who cross their path. Yes, I am a pointer of the beauty way. To all those who follow my heart-felt guidance will come peace, love, and serenity. Go now and dwell in peace and beauty on the earth, the Creator's most beautiful garden."

Catnip

Nepeta cataria
Labiatae (*Lamiaceae*) (Mint) Family

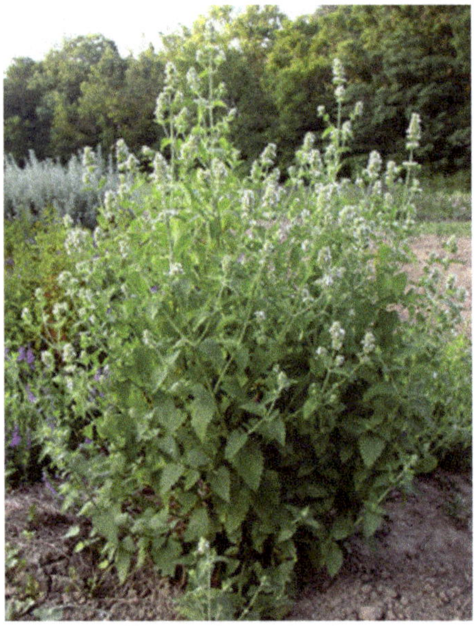

Common Names

Catmint, catrup, cat's-wort, catnep, nip, nep, and field balm are common names for this herb.

Medicinal Part of the Plant

Flowers and upper leaves are used for culinary and medicinal purposes.

Range and Habitat

Catnip is indigenous to temperate regions of Europe, Asia, southern Siberia, China, and Africa. The plant has been introduced and naturalized in North America and other temperate zones around the world. There are over 250 species of *Nepeta*.

Description of the Plant

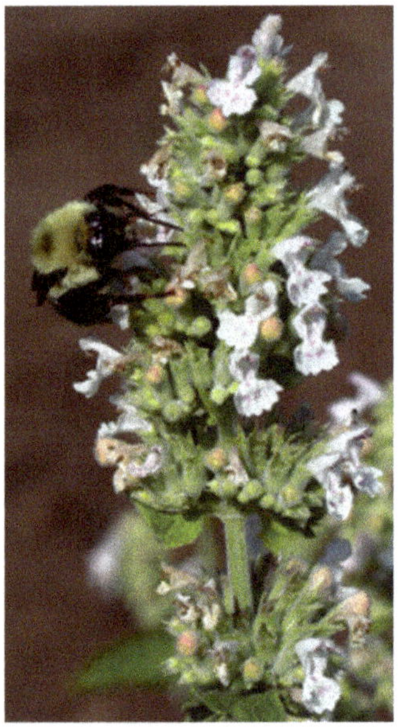

Catnip is an attractive, hardy perennial reaching a height of 3-5′. The whole plant has a strong but pleasant minty fragrance. Roots are fibrous and older plants develop a small, horizontally growing taproot. Several erect stalks with multiple opposite branches emerge from the root system. The square stems are characteristic of members of the Mint family. Many lightly colored, grayish-green leaves grow opposite each other along the length of the stems. The petiole leaves are somewhat deltoid (triangular-shaped) with a pointed tip, pinnate veins, and coarsely serrated teeth. Stems, leaves, and flowers are covered with short, white, pubescent hairs that give the plant a very soft, downy texture. Catnip matures into an attractive bushy mound of grayish-green foliage.

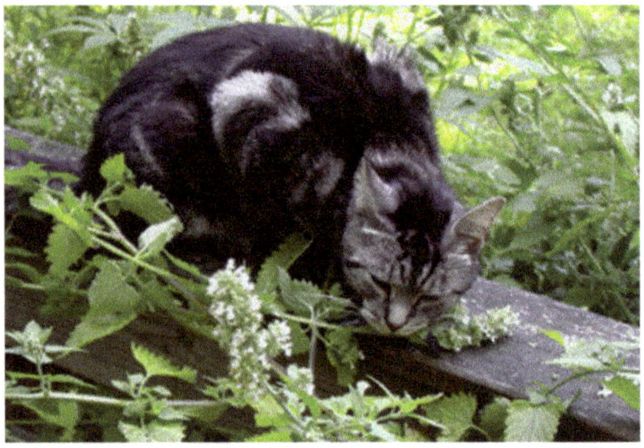

Numerous tiny flowers are 1/5-1/4″ long and arranged in several dense clusters of short whorled spikes that grow along the ends of branching stalks. The bilabiate (two-lobed) flowers are whitish pink or lavender and speckled with light purple to reddish spots. The corolla and 5-toothed calyx are both tubular. Four stamens ascend under the corolla. Flowers bloom in early spring and continue into autumn with warm weather. Bees love Catnip flowers and are attracted to their pollen and nectar, which they work diligently to harvest. Many cats are attracted by the fragrance of the volatile oils and enjoy nibbling and rolling around on the leaves.

Cultivation

Catnip is fairly hardy and easy to grow. It thrives in a variety of habitats, including poor, dry soils as well as rich, loamy humus. It does best in full sun, which stimulates production of the medicinal aromatic oils, but will tolerate partial shade. Plants grown in full sun and fertile, sandy soil have more fragrance than those grown in heavy clay under shade. This type of mint only propagates by seed and does not spread by underground root runners like its cousins, Peppermint (*Mentha x piperita*) and Spearmint (*Mentha spicata*).

Propagate Catnip by root divisions, stem cuttings, or seeds. Dig up and divide mature fibrous roots, transplanting 2′ apart in early spring or late autumn. Take stem cuttings in spring prior to blooming and they will readily develop roots when placed in a wet mix of potting soil, sand, and vermiculite.

Propagation by seeds is easy and reliable. Plant seeds in greenhouse flats or directly into the garden in spring, after the soil warms up. Cover them with 1/8″ soil. They usually germinate within a couple of weeks and can erratically germinate for up to five years. When seedlings are about 4″ tall, thin or transplant them 2′ apart. Catnip does not like excessive moisture, and over-watering or mulching with wet material too close to the plant encourages the crowns to rot and leaves to wilt. I learned this the hard way – I once lost a beautiful patch of first-year plants after applying a mulch of freshly mown grass clippings too close to the base of the plants.

Harvest

Harvest the upper leaves and flower spikes when they are in full bloom during the early flowering stage. Collect seeds for planting in late summer and autumn when the spikes are dry and brown.

Preparation of Plant Medicine and Dosages

Freshly harvested leaves and flowers are always preferred for preparing tea, tincture, salve, or a poultice. They can also be dried for future teas or poulticing material, but remember that dried herbs lose much of their potency after one year. Dried Catnip leaves are a pleasant addition to herbal smoking mixtures and can be helpful to people trying to stop smoking cigarettes.

PREPARATIONS

Tea: Steep 1-3 teaspoons of fresh or dried herb in 1 cup of hot water for 5-10 minutes. Excessively hot water destroys the valuable oils in Catnip leaves and flowers, so never boil them. Keep the pan covered with a lid while steeping to prevent steam loss of volatile oils.

Clinical herbalist and Eclectic physician William Cook, M.D., wrote that "Catnip infusion is best made by digesting half an ounce of the herb for ten minutes in a pint of water much below the boiling heat, and then straining with pressure. The most desirable properties of the article are wasted by the usual plan of pouring boiling water on the herb, and then steeping it on a hot stove. A bitter infusion remains, which is unpalatable, and possesses no carminative nor antispasmodic virtues" (Cook, 1869). Dosage: 1-4 cups daily. When properly made, the leaves make a pleasant-tasting tea with a mild mint flavor. A little honey makes the tea even tastier, especially for children.

Tincture: Chop the freshly harvested leaves and flowers, stuff them into a glass jar, and cover with 60% 190-proof grain alcohol and 40% distilled water. Dosage: 30-90 drops in water 1-4 times a day as needed.

Salve, Poultice, Fomentations: Catnip leaves are a beneficial addition to salves and poultices. External problems can also be treated with a diluted tincture or a fomentation or wash of the tea.

Smoking Mixture: Smoking dried Catnip leaves calms the nerves and provides a menthol flavor when combined with other herbs such as Mullein (*Verbascum thapsus*) and Sage (*Salvia officinalis*) leaves. Try smoking only a little at first, since some people may experience headaches. In the past, people with breathing difficulties like asthma and bronchitis smoked Catnip leaves. When people want to stop smoking cigarettes, I often recommend rolling and smoking nicotine-free herbal cigarettes to replace tobacco.

Culinary Uses

Since ancient times, Catnip leaves and young sprouts have been added to teas, sauces, soups, vegetables, meats, and stews for their minty fragrance and flavor.

Chemical Constituents

Volatile oils are the major active ingredients in *N. cataria*. Nepetalactone and its isomers make up 70-99% of the volatile oil and are responsible for many of the plant's medicinal properties. Nepetalactone causes the intoxicating effect on cats and repels insects (Skenderi, 2003). Additionally, it is analgesic, anti-inflammatory, antispasmodic, antibacterial, and antifungal. Nepetalactone and valeric acid in Catnip are similar to the valepotriates in Valerian in their structure and sedative actions.

Volatile oils also include thymol (analgesic, anthelmintic, anti-acne, anti-arthritic, antibacterial, anti-inflammatory, antispasmodic, antitussive, carminative, expectorant), carvacrol (anthelmintic, anti-atherosclerotic, antibacterial, anti-inflammatory, antioxidant, antispasmodic, antitussive, candidicide, carminative, expectorant, fungicide, vermifuge), citral (anti-allergenic, antibacterial, antihistamine, antiseptic, broncho-relaxant, cancer preventative, expectorant, fungicide, sedative), nerol (antibacterial, antiseptic, sedative), valeric acid, nepetalic acid, camphor (analgesic, anti-acne, anti-emetic, antiseptic, antispasmodic, cancer preventative, carminative, expectorant), citronellol (antibacterial, antiseptic, sedative), elemene (cervical anticarcinogenic), geraniol (antibacterial, anticancer, antispasmodic, antitumor, candidicide, expectorant, fungicide), pulegone (anticholinesterase, antihistamine, antipyretic, cancer preventative, sedative), and humulene (antitumor, aromatic).

Other constituents include caryophyllene (anti-acne, anti-asthmatic, antibacterial, anticancer, anti-inflammatory, antispasmodic, antitumor, candidicide, diuretic, fungicide, sedative), linoleic acid (anti-atherosclerotic, anti-arthritic, anti-eczema, antihistamine, anti-inflammatory, hepatoprotective, immunomodulator), and rosmarinic acid (anti-atherosclerotic, antibacterial, anticoagulant, hepatoprotective, anti-inflammatory, antioxidant, immunostimulant). Beta-sitosterol and campesterol have been identified. The leaves are rich in beta-carotene, vitamins C and E, iron, calcium, magnesium, manganese, phosphorus, chromium, selenium, and zinc.

Safety, Contraindications, and Drug Interactions

Catnip is a mild herb that is extremely safe for both infants and the elderly. It may cause nausea if taken in very large doses, but in normal amounts it can relieve this problem and ease stomach distress. **Catnip should not be ingested by pregnant women** due to its stimulating action on the uterus and emmenagogue properties promoting menstruation (Brinker, 2001; McGuffin, 1997), but mothers who are breast feeding can safely drink the tea. Large doses of Catnip may intensify the effects of prescription sedatives or tranquilizers.

Medicinal Uses

History of the Plant

The alluring fragrance of Catnip has captured the attention of people from many cultures, and the plant has a long tradition of medicinal and culinary use wherever it grows. The ancient Greeks, Romans, and Europeans cultivated Catnip. The plant has primarily been employed to aid digestion, calm the nerves, and promote menstruation. Equal parts of Catnip and Saffron were once given to treat smallpox and scarlet fever. Fresh Catnip leaves were chewed to relieve toothaches and dried to smoke as a remedy for bronchitis and asthma. John Gerard (1545–1612), the English apothecary, herbalist and surgeon, recommended it for headaches, stomachaches, and lung congestion (Gerard, 1633). Another English herbalist and physician, Nicholas Culpeper (1616–1654), who was also an astrologer, assigned Venus as the ruling planet of Catnip and used it to regulate women's cycles and treat headaches, stomachaches, wounds, and hemorrhoids (Potterton, 1983). He wrote that "It is effectual for any cramp, or cold aches, to dissolve cold and wind that afflicteth the place; and is used for colds, coughs, and shortness of breath" (Culpeper, 1992). The minty leaves were a favorite domestic tea of the British, who brought it to America. The colonists introduced the plant to Native American Indians, who in turn adopted Catnip into their herbal pharmacy and used it for infant colic, colds, flu, and fevers.

During the 1880s–1930s, the early American Eclectic physicians employed the herb for its diaphoretic and carminative actions. The hot tea was used to stimulate perspiration when treating colds, flu, and fevers. It was a favorite for stomachaches and indigestion, spasms, insomnia, irritability, and nervous headaches. It was included in formulas for treating typhus, measles, and other eruptive and feverish illnesses. Catnip was considered to be a beneficial uterine tonic for normalizing women's cycles, and was given to children to soothe the pains of colic and teething. The Eclectic physicians applied a poultice of the leaves to painful and inflamed skin conditions. Harvey Felter, M.D., wrote, "If less ridiculed and more used in place of far less safer remedies, a 'catnep' tea would be found a very useful medicine for women and children" (Felter, 1922).

Catnip earned its name because many members of the feline family, including the common house cat, display intoxicated and comical reactions to the plant. The aroma of the volatile oils, which escapes when the leaves are bruised, attracts many cats who love to roll around on the leaves and cover themselves with the pungent odor. They sometimes nibble the leaves and damage small plants. The plant does not have this intoxicating effect on people. Curiously, rats are said to be repelled by Catnip, perhaps because cats are apt to be lurking nearby.

The herb was listed as an official medicine in the *U.S. Pharmacopoeia* from 1842–1882 and in the *National Formulary* from 1916–1950. Currently, it is still a popular herb that is widely cultivated and sold commercially as tea, tincture, and in pills and capsules. Research has identified several of the chemical constituents (most notably nepetalactone) in the plant that explain many of its activities, but human clinical studies are lacking.

Healing Qualities

Analgesic, antacid, anti-emetic, antioxidant, antiseptic, antispasmodic, aperitive, aromatic, astringent, carminative, diaphoretic, mild diuretic, emmenagogue, exanthematous, expectorant, febrifuge, galactagogue, nervine, opthalmicum, pectoral, mild sedative, stomachic, tonic, mild vasodilator, and vulnerary.

Traditional Chinese Medicine (TCM) Perspective

Catnip is classified as a warming herb because of its calming and relaxing properties on the nerves and muscles and its ability to stimulate circulation. It also has secondary cooling properties due to the diaphoretic potential of releasing and dispersing internal heat to the exterior. It benefits the nervous system, stomach, intestines, and uterus. Stimulating effects of the herb remove stagnation, release constrained Qi, and restore circulation of Qi. Catnip is used for Wind Heat and Wind Cold illnesses such as fevers, colds, coughs, and the flu.

Primary Actions

The prominent therapeutic benefits of Catnip revolve around its ability to relax the nervous system, relieve muscle spasms, and normalize digestion and menstruation. It is a gentle herb specific for infants and young children. I have given the tea to my own children and grandchildren, and recommended it to many others with satisfying results of happy babies and relieved parents. I usually encourage parents to take Catnip along with their children, especially when the kids are cranky and restless, so that everyone can relax.

Nervous System: Catnip is a gentle sedative and nervine that helps calm, normalize, and restore the nervous system. Essential oils, including nepetalactone, are analgesic to reduce pain and antispasmodic to relax muscles, cramps, and spasms throughout the body (Aydin, 1999). Catnip has traditionally been employed to treat inflammatory conditions. When investigating this mode of action, researchers discovered three glycosides: teucrioside, verbascoside, and lamiuside A (teupolioside). These reduced the inflammatory response by inhibiting calcineurin, which is an important regulator of T-cell mediated inflammation (Prescott, 2011).

The plant relieves energetic congestion and muscle tightness resulting from pent-up emotional tension, and is helpful for anxiety, stress, tense and rigid muscles, and nervous headaches. In the past, it was included in remedies for convulsions. Catnip helps to induce sleep and reduce the incidence of nightmares. It is helpful when the nervous system needs nourishing and calming during withdrawal from nicotine, alcohol, and other types of drugs. Catnip tea or tincture is excellent for all nervous conditions, headaches, and insomnia, especially when combined with Valerian (*Valeriana officinalis*), Passion Flower (*Passiflora incarnata*), Hops (*Humulus lupulus*), and Scullcap (*Scutellaria lateriflora*).

Stomach and Digestive System: Catnip is specifically indicated for indigestion caused by anxiety and nervousness. Its relaxing, anti-inflammatory actions on smooth muscles throughout the digestive tract relieve cramps, spasms, hiccups, and abdominal pain. The carminative qualities of the warm tea or tincture are helpful for most stomach problems, including indigestion, nausea and vomiting, gas, colic, and gastritis (stomach inflammation). Catnip helps reduce excess secretion of hydrochloric acid from the stomach to ease heartburn and acid reflux. Drinking a cup of the lukewarm tea or diluted tincture before meals stimulates a poor appetite.

This herb benefits the small and large intestines by restoring normal bowel tone. The astringent property is helpful for diarrhea and abnormal bleeding. Catnip may be included in formulas to treat stomach and intestinal ulcers, and inflammatory, spastic, irritable bowel syndromes. Nepetalactone exhibits antimicrobial activities against food-borne pathogens in research studies (Zomorodian, 2012). Catnip is beneficial after chemotherapy to treat side effects of nausea, pain, and anxiety.

Colds, Fever, Flu, and Bronchitis: Catnip is a traditional cold and flu remedy, especially helpful for fevers, coughs, and acute bronchitis. When taken hot, it is a diaphoretic that induces perspiration to reduce fevers. It also relaxes and dilates blood vessels to enhance circulation and move heat out of the body. The herb is an expectorant that loosens phlegm and eases coughing spasms (Gilani, 2009). Its ability to relax rigid muscles in the chest and lungs can be helpful to relieve asthma.

Several of the volatile oils in the leaves and flowers are antioxidants that exhibit antimicrobial activity against fungi, Candida yeast, and Gram-positive bacteria, including *Staphylococcus aureus* strains responsible for MRSA (methicillin-resistant *Staphylococcus aureus*) (Abascal, 2002; Nestorovic, 2010; Nostro, 2001). Nepetalactone has been most investigated for these properties (Adiquzel, 2009; Zomorodian, 2013).

When treating colds, flu and coughs, I always combine Catnip with strong antibacterial and antiviral herbs, such as Echinacea, Boneset (*Eupatorium perfoliatum*), Elderberry (*Sambucus canadensis*), Yarrow (*Achillea millefolium*), Cayenne (*Capsicum annuum*), Isatis (*Isatis tinctoria*), and Thyme (*Thymus vulgaris*).

Children: Catnip tea has a long tradition as one of the best herbs specifically for infants and children, and I have seen it work wonders. It is excellent for infant colic with stomach and intestinal cramps, gas, and pain. The leaves and flowers are calming for restlessness and irritability, help with teething and persistent crying, and safely promote sleep. The herb is particularly beneficial for hyperactive children and has a history of use for childhood convulsions. It is very safe to use for childhood fevers, colds, flu, infections, nausea, and vomiting. An enema of the tea reduces fevers in infants and young children, and restores fluids in cases of dehydration. Eclectic physician Harvey Felter, M.D., wrote that Catnip is "a splendid quieting agent for fretful babies, and carminative and antispasmodic for abdominal pain with flatulence" (Felter, 1922).

Give 1-3 teaspoons of mild tea to infants every 20 minutes as needed, and more to older children. Small amounts of a natural sugar (avoid cane sugar) or maple syrup may be added to encourage children to drink the tea. Administer the tea through a plastic dropper or bottle to infants. Catnip works well when combined with Fennel (*Foeniculum vulgare*), Chamomile (*Matricaria recutita*), Marshmallow root (*Althaea officinalis*), Calendula (*Calendula officinalis*), Peppermint (*Mentha x piperita*), or Lemon Balm (*Melissa officinalis*) for children's needs. Always use smaller doses for children and taste the herbal preparation before giving it to your child. (Refer to "How to Calculate Dosages" on page 148 to determine pediatric dosages.)

Women's Health: Catnip is a mild emmenagogue that stimulates suppressed menstruation. It is beneficial for premenstrual syndrome (PMS) when taken as tincture or hot tea. It relaxes nervous tension in the pelvis, normalizes circulation, and is an effective analgesic and antispasmodic for painful menstrual cramps and uterine spasms. The Eclectic physicians regarded Catnip as a superior remedy for atonic amenorrhea (failure to menstruate) and dysmenorrhea (painful menses). Atonic conditions are caused by lack of muscle tone resulting in weakness and sluggishness of the organs, blood vessels, and circulatory system. Harvey Felter, M.D., wrote that "When marked nervous agitation precedes menstruation in feeble and excitable women and the function is tardy or imperfect, this simple medicine gives great relief. It is especially valuable for the nervous irritability of dyspeptics [stomachache], nervous headache . . . and wards off nervous and hysterical attacks" (Felter, 1922). (During this era "hysteria" was the term coined for severe premenstrual and hormonally related mood swings, anxiety, and depression).

Catnip works especially well combined with Motherwort (*Leonurus cardiaca*), Blue Vervain (*Verbena hastata*), and Mugwort (*Artemisia vulgaris*) for PMS and other menstrual problems.

Childbirth: New mothers benefit from drinking 1-2 cups of tea or 30-40 drops of tincture immediately after birth to help expel the placenta. The herb normalizes postpartum bleeding, reduces blood clot formation, and helps relieve uterine spasms known as the "after-pains of birth." Use it in combination with Shepherd's Purse (*Capsella bursa-pastoris*) to control postpartum bleeding.

Lactation: Catnip is a known galactagogue, and mothers who breast-feed can enjoy a cup of the tea before nursing to increase flow of breast milk. Its relaxing influence encourages the "let-down" response. It can reduce jaundice in the newborn, benefit the infant's immature digestive system, and calm restlessness. The herb may also be externally applied as a poultice or salve on sore breasts and nipples of nursing mothers.

Cataracts: Damage to the eyes and cataracts are partially caused by oxidative damage to the tissues. Respected herbal authority James Duke believes that the generous amounts of antioxidants in Catnip, including beta-carotene (the plant source of vitamin A), vitamin C, vitamin E, selenium and zinc, can help prevent cataracts (Duke, 1997). The tea should be used on a regular basis for this purpose.

External Uses: When applied as a poultice or ointment, Catnip relieves painful swelling, cools inflamed tissues, and reduces pain. The volatile oils are antiseptic. It is used on wounds, sprains, bruises, acne, poison ivy, insect stings and bites, hives, hemorrhoids, and arthritic joints. Nepetalactone in the volatile oil have insect repelling properties, and rubbing Catnip oil on the skin helps keep away irritating bugs.

Teachings from the Catnip Deva

"Greetings, dear one! I am the deva of the Catnip plant, and I contain the qualities of a youthful, jovial and light-hearted being, as well as the wise and radiant grandmother. I like to play, especially with the children, and have a special affinity for their young and playful natures. I am good medicine for many of the bumps and grinds of little ones, and can be given as a mild tea in moderate amounts to the youngest of children, to mend them and heal them to become playful and happy again.

"I have much fire and air element in my being, and my spicy nature is warming and stimulating. The medicine within my plants encourages secretions and creates movement and activity within the body. As I move toxins, infections, phlegm, and fevers out of the body, in my wake there is relaxation and greater balance. I am helpful for illness in the lungs and sinuses, and ease congested and labored breathing. My soft, pale, silvery-green leaves point to my gentle nature and safe use with children and the elderly. My tiny white flowers are a reflection of my purity and a signature of the pure quality of my medicine for fragile little ones and elders.

"Like many of the medicine plants, I assist in harmonizing the energies and movements within the body. My teaching is to balance the playful and light-hearted nature of children with adult work and tasks. Bringing play, fun, and laughter into one's life also brings more vibrant health and a stronger and radiant heart. Allow children, with their trusting and childish ways, to remind you to enter into the play, laughter, and joy of life; for this is good medicine."

Cayenne

Capsicum annuum
Solanaceae (Nightshade) Family

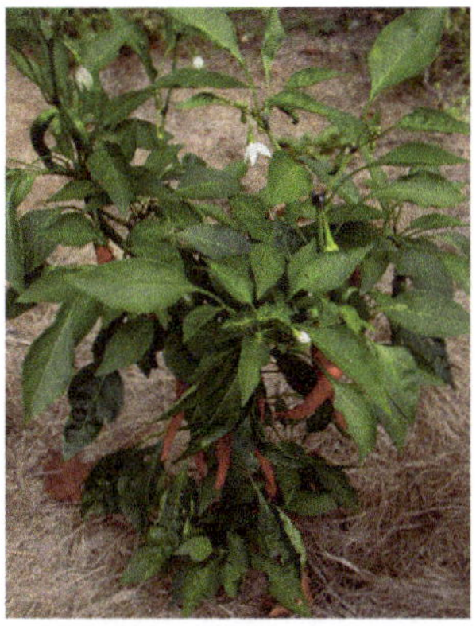

Capsicum annuum

Common Names

Capsicum annuum consists of many cultivars, including Cayenne, Bell, Chili, Banana, Red, Mexican Chili, and Jalapeno Peppers. *Capsicum frutescens* includes Tabasco Pepper, African Capsicum, and several other hot Peppers.

Medicinal Part of the Plant

The red fruit and white pith surrounding the seeds are the medicinal portions.

Range and Habitat

All *Capsicum* species are indigenous to the tropical regions of Central and South America. They have been cultivated worldwide in warm climates for the past several hundred years and have naturalized in many tropical areas. There are about 20 species and over 1,700 varieties of *Capsicum*. *C. annuum* and *C. frutescens*, the two primary species used in Western herbalism, are cultivated in American gardens as a culinary spice.

Description of the Plant

In its native tropical habitat, Cayenne is a perennial shrub that develops woody stems that can grow up to 4′ tall. In temperate zone gardens, *Capsicum* species are grown as annuals and only reach a height of 2-3′. *C. annuum* and *C. frutescens* are similar in appearance. Their stems are smooth, angular, furrowed, and branch out near the top. The shiny, smooth, deep-green leaves are simple, entire, and oval to lance-shaped. Having long petiole stems, leaves grow 1-5″ in length and end in a pointed tip.

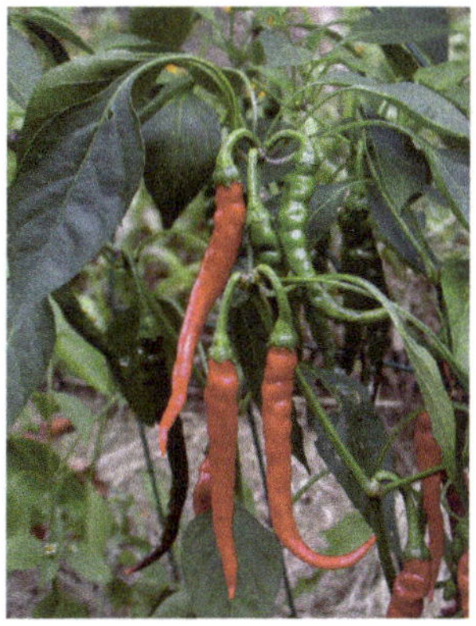

Capsicum annuum

The drooping, star-shaped flowers are usually white, or sometimes light creamy yellow, and grow from leaf axils on long petioles. Flowers of *C. annuum* are solitary, while those of *C. frutescens* appear in small clusters of 2 or 3 flowers. The calyx of *C. annuum* is angular, has 6 short lobes, and holds a short, tubular corolla with 5 spreading lobes and 5 stamens. Flowers bloom from June through September and mature into pendulous, pod-like, capsular fruits that are strikingly brilliant in color. The fruit of *C. annuum* is bright red, while fruit of other cultivars appears in colors ranging from scarlet red to orange, yellow, green, and even deep blue. Shapes of *Capsicum* fruit pods vary from round, oblong, horned, or cordate (heart-shaped). *C. annuum* pods are long with pointed tips, while pods of *C. frutescens* tend to be smaller. Numerous seeds inside the pods are whitish yellow, flat, and reniform (kidney-shaped).

Cultivation

Capsicum species need a rich, light, sandy loam. They thrive with long, hot summers and full sun, but will tolerate some shade. Cayenne Pepper is very easy to grow by seed germination. The seeds have a fairly short period of viability and are best planted within a year of harvest. In tropical zones, the seeds may be directly sown 1½′ apart into a prepared bed. In cooler temperate areas, they can be started indoors or in a greenhouse 7-8 weeks before the last expected frost. When seedlings are 2-3″ tall and danger of frost is past, transplant them into a well-prepared garden bed, spacing each one 1½′ apart. A consistent water supply with good drainage encourages optimal growth. The roots develop near the surface, so mulching with grass or other organic compost is helpful.

Harvest

Harvest Cayenne when the fruit is completely ripe and turns a brilliant, deep red color. Keep the green stem attached to the fruit to retard spoilage if the pods are to be dried. Seeds from mature pods can be dried and stored for next season's planting.

Preparation of Plant Medicine and Dosages

The Eclectic pharmacists and physicians discovered that Cayenne's medicinal resins are completely extracted in 98% alcohol, partially in diluted alcohol, and to a considerable extent by vinegar and boiling water (Cook, 1869). Tinctures are excellent preparations that maintain potency for a long time and can be used both internally and externally. The fresh fruit contains greater amounts of medicinal constituents than the dried and is always preferred for making medicines, but either may be prepared as a tincture, tea, poultice, liniment, oil, or salve. **When handling the fresh pepper, wear gloves for protection from the hot resins**. After touching fresh Cayenne, the potent oil absorbs into fingers and causes a burning sensation to any tissues they touch, especially the eyes. Handle this herb with care!

To dry Cayenne, wear latex or rubber gloves to cut the fruit into strips or small pieces, place on a screen, and dry in a shaded, well-ventilated area. In dry desert climates, the whole pepper may be threaded with string and hung to dry. Store fully dehydrated peppers in a glass jar out of direct sunlight and grind them into a fine powder (a small electric coffee bean grinder works well) when ready to use. Peppers may also be stored fresh in a freezer to preserve potency. Remember that capsaicin, one of the primary phytochemicals, is present in highest concentrations in the white pith around the seeds, so **include the pith with the fruit when making medicinal preparations**.

Always start with a small dose of Cayenne and increase it gradually to determine individual tolerance levels, allowing the stomach and intestines to adjust to the hot sensation. Taking it during meals is highly recommended because having food in the stomach reduces the feeling of heat. Eating some yogurt or drinking a cup of soy milk, almond milk, or regular dairy milk can also ease intense burning. When using the herb externally, first apply a modest amount to a small area of skin to ascertain sensitivity, and dilute it if necessary.

When taking Cayenne internally, always remember that its hot taste and warmth increase heat in the body. It naturally dilates capillary blood vessels, promoting blood flow and causing the skin to become warm and flushed. People who are naturally warm-blooded, or who have health problems involving an excess of heat with conditions like fever, inflammation or flushed skin, must be sure to balance Cayenne's intense warming properties with cooling herbs (see *Primary Actions* below).

PREPARATIONS

Tincture: Wear gloves to chop fresh peppers into small pieces and stuff them into a glass jar along with the seeds. The medicinally active resins in Cayenne are soluble in alcohol and only slightly soluble in cold water, so the tincture is made with 100% 190-proof grain alcohol. Dosage: 2-20 drops up to 3-5 times a day. Start with low doses and **always dilute the tincture in water.**

Infusion Tea: In a covered pot, steep 1/8-1/4 teaspoon of the dried powder or 1/2 teaspoon of finely chopped fresh pepper in a pint of boiled water for 10 minutes. Dosage: One tablespoon at a time, up to 1-2 cups a day. The tea may be diluted with more water if necessary. Children may need help with the hot taste, so the tea may be added to a little grape or apple juice diluted with water.

Capsules: This is a good way to take Cayenne because the hot taste bypasses the tongue. The ripe pods must be dried, ground into powder, and stuffed into small size "00" gelatin capsules. Dosage: One small "00" capsule every 3-4 hours as needed. Cayenne capsules are available commercially in doses ranging from 30-500 mg, and are taken 1-3 times a day. **Always have a little food in your stomach when taking Cayenne capsules** to reduce the burning sensation.

Liniment: This is for external application and prepared by combining the tincture with water. **Do not put tincture on open cuts or wounds** – it will sting and burn!

Oil and Salve: To prepare oil for external application, chop fresh Cayenne into small pieces and cover with olive oil. If using dried pods, grind them into powder and then add oil. Bake at 200-225°F for one hour, cool, and strain. Add bees wax to the hot oil if salve is desired. Due to its hot, burning quality, do not combine Cayenne with other herbs when making oil or salve, just use it by itself.

Poultice: Chop fresh Cayenne into small pieces, simmer in a little water for a few minutes to make a soft mash, and apply a small amount to the affected area. The dried powder may also be made into a thick mash by adding a little water or oil. Cover and check on the area every 10-20 minutes. Remove the poultice if the burning sensation gets too intense.

Culinary Uses

Cayenne is a popular seasoning in tomato sauces, salsa, and many foods enjoyed throughout the world. Paprika is prepared from Cayenne and other members of *C. annuum*. Ripe Peppers are generally dried and ground into powder for a spicy, sizzling hot addition to foods. However, the raw pods contain higher amounts of vitamin C and antioxidant compounds. Studies have shown that the best cooking methods to preserve vitamin C and antioxidants are stir-frying or roasting. The greatest loss of these nutrients occurs with boiling or steaming (Hwang, 2012). Peppers are often a staple in the diets of people in warm climates. Prior to electricity and refrigeration, people ate Cayenne and other hot peppers to prevent bacterial and parasite infestation after eating contaminated or spoiled foods.

Chemical Constituents

Cayenne fruit contains capsaicinoids that cause the burning sensation characteristic of all hot Peppers and are largely responsible for the herb's biological and medicinal activities. The most important and researched capsaicinoid is capsaicin, a pungent alkaloid resin and one of the primary active components. All members of the *Capsicum* genus, with the exception of Bell Peppers, contain capsaicin. Contained in both the fruit and white pith surrounding the seeds, capsaicin is antibacterial, antioxidant, anti-inflammatory, and a topical analgesic. Its strong alkaline properties produce the initial burning and discomfort.

The plant also contains steroidal alkaloid glycosides (solanine, solanidine, solasadine, and capsicosides), scopoletin (a blood-thinning coumarin), aspirin-like compounds called salicylates that contribute to the plant's analgesic and anti-inflammatory activity, and capsicidins, which are steroidal saponins found in the seeds and roots. Carotenoids are antioxidants and include carotene, lutein, capsanthin, and capsorubin. Fatty acids include oleic, palmitic, ascorbic, and stearic acids. Notable amounts of beta-carotene (plant source of vitamin A) and vitamin B1 (thiamine), B2 (riboflavin), and B3 (niacin) are present. Cayenne also contains proteins, fats, sodium, potassium, magnesium, calcium, iron, zinc, and lecithin.

Safety, Contraindications, and Drug Interactions

Confirmed by modern research findings and by hundreds of years of medicinal and culinary use by people all over the globe, Cayenne is regarded to be a safe herb. There are no contraindications during pregnancy or lactation when taken in normal, moderate doses (Blumenthal, 2000; McGuffin, 1997). It is safely used by children and the elderly, but is generally too strong for children under two years of age. This herb is "hot going in and hot coming out," and although it causes an intense burning sensation, most authorities agree that it does not damage the skin, mucous membranes, or eyes (Fetrow, 1999). However, prolonged application on the skin may irritate mucous membranes and cause temporary hives, rash, or raised blisters in some people (Brinker, 2001). To avoid discomfort, do not put Cayenne on sensitive tissues or in the eyes. Capsaicin, the heat-inducing phytochemical, does not dissolve in water, making it difficult to wash off the skin. **If it gets in the eyes or on other sensitive tissues, flush with cold water or milk until the burning subsides.** Vinegar may also be used to reduce burning on the skin because it is very acidic and neutralizes capsaicin, which is alkaline, but vinegar should never be put in the eyes.

Eating large amounts of Cayenne in capsules and drinking the tea or tincture may create a hot, burning sensation in the stomach, so it is best taken with food to diminish this possibility. Excessive and prolonged consumption may cause damage to the stomach lining, liver, intestines or kidneys, but these complications are rare even in countries where hot peppers are a dietary staple. Internal use is contraindicated in cases of irritable bowel and other inflammatory conditions in the digestive tract because the stimulating and peristaltic actions of Cayenne can worsen these problems (Brinker, 2001). For high fevers and other symptoms of excessive heat, avoid using Cayenne, or combine it with cooling herbs like Marshmallow (*Althaea officinalis*) and Dandelion (*Taraxacum officinale*).

Cayenne may increase the absorption and activity of some pharmaceutical medicines due to its ability to stimulate circulation and enhance drug delivery to tissues. High doses have anticoagulant (blood-thinning) effects that may increase pre-existing bleeding tendencies or potentiate anticoagulant drugs, which are given to people with blood clots and cardiovascular blockages. People using these drugs may ingest Cayenne in moderate amounts, but should be aware of possible increased bruising or bleeding. Cayenne has been reported to interfere with monoamine oxidase (MAO) inhibitors and with some drugs that lower blood pressure, such as ACE inhibitors.

Medicinal Uses

History of the Plant

Archeologists estimate that Cayenne was used as food and medicine at least 9,000 years ago by people living in the tropical regions of the Americas, and excavations provide evidence that it was cultivated in Mexico at least 7,000 years ago. Artifacts show that ancient Mayans used it to treat sores and inflammation of the mouth and gums. The Aztec name for Cayenne Pepper is "chili," and a reference in a 1552 Aztec herbal, known as the *Badanius Manuscript*, indicates that it was used to eliminate toothaches and scabies.

This unique-tasting plant was introduced to the rest of the world by the Caribbean Indians, who shared it with Christopher Columbus when he voyaged to their islands. In his book *Herbal Renaissance*, Steven Foster writes that it was initially introduced into Europe by Dr. Diego Chanca, who accompanied Columbus to the West Indies. In 1492, Columbus journaled in his log book that he longed to find a source of Pepper (*Piper nigrum*), the popular spice enjoyed by Europeans that had to be imported from the Far East. Instead, he was introduced to the *Capsicum* hot Pepper by the Arawak Indians, and he called this new spice "Red Pepper." He brought the Pepper seeds back to Italy, where cultivation was established, and Cayenne's popularity quickly spread throughout Europe, Africa, and Asia via established trade routes. Other historical accounts claim that Cayenne was introduced into England from India around 1548, and was being cultivated throughout northern Europe by 1650. Over time, *Capsicum* was incorporated into the medical systems of Europe, China, Japan, Korea and India, where it was employed for similar ailments, including digestive problems, spasms, and muscle and nerve pain. The genus name *Capsicum* comes from the Greek word *kapto*, meaning "to bite," referring to the hot, pungent taste of the fruit and seeds.

Herbal practitioner Samuel Thomson introduced Cayenne into North American medicine during the late 1700s and early 1800s. At that time, the practice of purging with strong emetic drugs to induce vomiting was a popular medical intervention to treat cases of food poisoning and other ailments. Lobelia (*Lobelia inflata*) was a favorite emetic that Thomson combined with Cayenne to improve circulation and to keep warmth in the stomach after it had been emptied of food. This herbal combination became a popular hallmark of Thomsonian herbal medicine and was widely used by the early American Eclectic physicians (1880s–1930s) as a balanced formula to stimulate perspiration, restore normal digestion, and reduce muscle spasms. The Eclectics used Cayenne's stimulating qualities to treat colds and mucous congestion, fevers, sluggish digestion, heart problems, nerve and muscle pain, and as an antibiotic for serious infectious wounds and diseases. John King, M.D. (1813–1893) wrote, "It may be used in all cases of diminished vital action, and is frequently combined with other medicines to promote their action" (King, 1864). It was once listed as an official medicine in the *U.S. Pharmacopoeia* and *National Formulary* as a carminative, stimulant, analgesic, and rubefacient.

Currently, Cayenne continues to be a popular herbal remedy and is one of the most widely consumed spices in the world. It was approved as an herbal medicine by the German Commission E herbal regulatory agency and is a main ingredient in several commercially sold ointments for the treatment of pain and spasms. Numerous clinical and laboratory research studies validate the plant's healing abilities.

Healing Qualities

Adjuvant, alterative, topical analgesic, antibacterial, anti-catarrhal, anti-inflammatory, antioxidant, antiscorbutic, antiseptic, antispasmodic, aperitive, cardiac, carminative, cholagogue, depurative, diaphoretic, emetic, expectorant, febrifuge, hemostatic, pectoral, restorative, rubefacient, sialagogue, stimulant, stomachic, tonic, vasodilator, vermifuge, and vulnerary.

Traditional Chinese Medicine (TCM) Perspective

Cayenne is an extremely Yang herb with hot, drying, and stimulating qualities that promote warmth and movement throughout the body. It is a classic remedy for cold, deficiency conditions in people with low vitality, debility, sluggishness, depression, congestion, poor circulation, or a weak pulse. It circulates and disperses warming Yang Qi, and dispels conditions of cold, wind, and dampness occurring with the common cold, respiratory illness, indigestion, nerve and muscle pain, and stiff joints. The herb stimulates Kidney Yang and is beneficial for the lungs, spleen, stomach, intestines, kidneys, heart, and blood vessels. Its stimulating properties relieve congestion and stagnation throughout the body, including chronic respiratory, abdominal and pelvic congestion, and Qi stagnation in the liver, heart, blood, lungs, kidneys, and uterus.

Primary Actions

Cayenne is a wonderful healing herb that provides well-documented health benefits. It can be used as a general tonic and is one of the most stimulating herbs that reaches all tissues of the body by normalizing and improving blood circulation. It is specific for the digestive, respiratory and cardiovascular systems, and for pain reduction. Cayenne is traditionally used as an adjuvant remedy, meaning that it is combined with other herbs because it carries them to tissues and increases their biological effects due to its ability to promote circulation.

> *Cayenne is indicated for exhausted people who are sluggish, debilitated, and cool-natured.*
>
> *It is specific for those with poor circulation who feel better with exercise, and whose aches and pains are worse in cold and damp weather.*

Although hot to taste and touch, Cayenne exerts cleansing and healing actions on tissues both internally and externally. When using this herb for healing, always keep in mind its qualities of extreme heat and stimulation, and apply the principle of balancing the herbal remedy with the person's ailment and basic constitution. Cayenne is indicated for exhausted people who are sluggish, debilitated, cool-natured, or have weak, sagging (atonic) muscles. It is specific for those with poor circulation who feel better with exercise, and whose aches and pains are worse in cold and damp weather. It is especially indicated for people with a pale tongue and weak, irregular pulse. It should not be taken by those with a rapid, full pulse, unless it is irregular, indicating congestion in the vessels. In this case, Cayenne is appropriate. People having a hot constitution and who are naturally hot-blooded, highly stimulated, and energetic can be pulled further out of balance and their symptoms worsened if given a hot, stimulating herb, especially in the presence of high fevers or hot inflammatory conditions. Warm-blooded people often have a flushed, ruddy complexion and should not use Cayenne without cooling herbs. However, a reddish-purple complexion is usually due to blood stagnation causing broken blood vessels and discoloration, especially on the cheeks and nose, rather than being caused only by excess heat. In this case, Cayenne is indicated to improve circulation and remove the stagnation. An assessment to determine the correct herbal remedy is important in promoting balance and reducing symptoms. Hot conditions call for cooling remedies, and Cayenne's extreme heat and resulting dryness may be adjusted by combining it with cooling, moisturizing herbs such as Chickweed (*Stellaria media*), Marshmallow (*Althaea officinalis*), or Slippery Elm (*Ulmus rubra*). Other herbs such as Isatis (*Isatis tinctoria*), Stinging Nettle (*Urtica dioica*), Burdock (*Arctium lappa*), Boneset (*Eupatorium perfoliatum*), Dandelion (*Taraxacum officinale*), and Yarrow (*Achillea millefolium*) are not moisturizing, but they are very cooling. When people with fiery temperaments or anxiety need to use Cayenne, create a balancing formula by adding calming, sedating herbs such as Scullcap (*Scutellaria lateriflora*) and Chamomile (*Matricaria* spp.).

Stimulant: The Eclectic physicians regarded Cayenne to be a pure, energetic, and reliable stimulant that surpassed any other remedy when a strong, prolonged stimulant was needed for problems like chills, heart failure, or sudden drop in blood pressure. Finley Ellingwood, M.D. (1852–1920) stated, "It produces an increase in tone and a marked and comfortable sensation of warmth in the entire system, and a glow and sensation of increased nerve influence and more active circulation" (Ellingwood, 1919). William Cook, M.D., wrote that "the fruit is one of the purest known stimulants, of great intensity, very permanent in its action, spreading through the system rather slowly, but ultimately reaching every organ of the frame . . . . It acts mainly on the circulation, but also upon the nervous structures" (Cook, 1869). Cayenne's stimulating influence helps counteract shock and revive sudden hypotension, and removes congestion and stagnation throughout the system. It helps reduce fatigue and addresses chronic fatigue syndrome. In one of the most important Eclectic works, *King's American Dispensatory*, Harvey Felter, M.D. (1865–1927) wrote, "Capsicum meets the debility of young and old, but is particularly useful in old people when the body-heat is low, vitality depressed, and reaction sluggish. Tired, painful muscles, stiffened joints, and relaxation of any part are common conditions in the elderly that are, in a measure, rectified by capsicum" (Felter, 1898).

Cayenne's warming and stimulating properties increase circulation to all tissues of the body. The herb reduces inflammation, spasms, and pain.

Although Cayenne is warming, its vasodilating ability to relax and expand blood vessels increases circulation and brings internal heat to the skin surface where it dissipates. This results in an overall cooling response. People living in tropical climates actually eat the fruit to help them tolerate the heat. The hypothalamus gland in the brain regulates temperature control in the body, and current research shows that Cayenne stimulates hypothalamic secretions, which lowers body temperature (Dib, 1992). The herb stimulates activity and secretions in all the glands and organs, and has a restorative influence on a sluggish, underactive endocrine system. Stimulation of the stomach, pancreas, and liver results in increased digestive enzymes allowing optimal digestion. Stimulation of sudoriferous (sweat) glands on skin increases perspiration to cool the body and induce elimination of toxins. Although the hot quality of Cayenne is basically drying, activation of sebaceous glands increases oily secretions on the skin and has a moisturizing effect.

Nervous System and Pain Relief: Potent antioxidant and analgesic activities of several constituents in Cayenne, including capsinoids and carotenoids, provide protection against inflammation and cellular damage throughout the body (Rosa, 2002; Hernández-Ortega, 2012; Loizzo, 2013). When applied to the skin, Cayenne is an excellent analgesic pain reliever for neuralgia (nerve pain), myalgia (muscle pain), spasms, arthritis, rheumatism, and cramps.

Cayenne contains higher concentrations of salicylates (the source of aspirin) than other foods, which contributes to pain relief when taken internally. Capsaicin has analgesic effects, and research shows that it increases the production of specific prostaglandins that reduce pain and inflammation (Partsch, 1990 & 1991). When applied externally, capsaicin acts as a temporary counterirritant, causing irritation to tissues where it is applied, and thus distracts the original pain or irritation. The exact mechanism of this analgesic activity is not fully understood, but researchers believe that capsaicin interferes with the action of substance P, a neurotransmitter in the peripheral nerves that sends pain sensations from the skin to the brain. When topically applied, capsaicin initially stimulates a release of substance P, causing the characteristic burning sensation. Continual application eventually depletes substance P from peripheral sensory neurons, desensitizing nerve endings and interfering with the brain's ability to feel pain (Blumenthal, 2000; Scheffler, 1991). Several days of external application are necessary for pain relief to become effective, so it works best when used daily for chronic pain. Cayenne also decreases pain transmission and inflammation in joint tissues, while increasing blood flow to painful joints and cold extremities.

The United States Food and Drug Administration (FDA) has approved several creams, including Zostrix and Capzasin-P (which contain 0.025-0.075% capsaicin), for the treatment of herpes, shingles, arthritis, and rheumatism. Many clinical studies confirm Cayenne's effectiveness when externally applied as a liniment or ointment for lower back pain (Gagnier, 2006; Keitel, 2001), chronic and post-surgical pain (Ellison, 1997), neuralgia (nerve pain), trigeminal neuralgia (severe pain of the face), painful herpes lesions, sprains, rheumatoid and osteoarthritis, gout, bursitis, carpal tunnel, and post-amputation phantom pain syndromes (Fusco, 1992; McCarthy, 1992; Blumenthal, 2000).

One study involved 23 patients suffering from chronic post-herpetic neuralgia (pain following a severe herpes outbreak) uncontrolled by medications. Patients received 4 daily applications of a 0.025% capsaicin cream over the painful areas. After 4 weeks of treatment, 56% reported good or excellent results, and 78% noticed significant reduction of their pain (Watson, 1988). Several clinical tests have validated Cayenne's ability to reduce diabetic neuropathy (chronic and painful nerve damage) in over 360 people using daily applications of 0.025-0.075% capsaicin cream (Chad, 1990; Ross, 1989; Tandan, 1992; Capsaicin Study Group, 1992). In one test, the cream was significantly more effective than a placebo in relieving diabetic neuropathy in 49 patients with moderate to severe pain. By the eighth week of treatment, 90% of the Cayenne group reported reduction in their pain, including an average of 49% decrease in pain intensity (Scheffler, 1991). A study of 14 women afflicted with post-mastectomy pain syndrome, who found no relief from their medications, reported significant improvement after 4 weeks of topical application of 0.025% capsaicin cream. Twelve women reported improvement in their pain reduction and eight had good to excellent results (Watson, 1989). Another research study assessed 98 people with psoriasis who applied a capsaicin cream to their skin lesions, compared with 99 others who used a placebo cream. The capsaicin group had a marked reduction in skin redness, dry scales, and discomfort compared to those using the placebo (Ellis, 1993).

When initially trying Cayenne for external problems, test it by applying a little on a small area to determine individual sensitivity. For many systemic problems like arthritis, gout, fibromyalgia, bursitis and diabetes, the herb should also be ingested to address internal causes of these issues by improving circulation and normalizing organ and glandular function (McCarty, 1994).

Cayenne tea, tincture, oil, ointment, or liniment can be applied externally and diluted if necessary. It is often recommended to avoid direct contact on open skin and cuts because of its hot, burning sensation, but Cayenne can actually be put on open wounds and is very healing. The herb's antiseptic action and ability to stimulate circulation to wounds greatly contributes to healing. Dr. John Christopher successfully packed deep cuts and wounds with Cayenne powder to arrest bleeding, kill infection, and promote healing (Christopher, 1976). The Eclectics extolled its virtues as "one of the most powerful arrestors of mortification" due to its antiseptic and circulatory properties, and administered the herb to prevent and treat necrotic (dead) tissue, including gangrene (Cook, 1869).

Clinical studies verify Cayenne's benefit for headaches and migraines. It has been shown to prevent and relieve the pain of cluster headaches (extremely severe pain on one side of the head) and migraines when tiny amounts of the powder or cream are snorted up the nose (Marks, 1993). This is hot and can be irritating to the mucous membranes lining the nose, so it takes a real warrior to snort Red Pepper! An easier way is to apply Cayenne oil, ointment, or tincture to the forehead or temples. I would also recommend ingesting the herb to help correct the underlying causes of the headaches.

Painful toothaches and inflamed gums can be treated by saturating a small piece of cotton with Cayenne oil or tincture and applying it to the affected area. Dip a pointed toothpick into the oil or tincture and rub it between the tooth and gum, allowing the herb to touch and saturate the tissues. Mixtures of powdered Cayenne, Myrrh (*Commiphora molmol*), Goldenseal (*Hydrastis canadensis*), and Clove oil (*Syzygium aromaticum*) are excellent for painful toothaches or pyorrhea (gum inflammation and infection).

The Eclectic herbal physicians considered Cayenne to be invaluable in treating delirium tremens, an acute toxic state caused by alcohol or drug withdrawal marked by spastic tremors in the arms and legs, hallucinations, mental confusion, restlessness, and digestive disturbances. Eclectics observed that Cayenne helps remove the alcohol and drug craving, reduce nausea and vomiting, restore stomach tone and function, and promote appetite and normal digestion. It was used for treating opium, cocaine, and alcohol addiction (Felter, 1898). For detoxing from drug withdrawal, combine Cayenne with nervine herbs such as Scullcap (*Scutellaria lateriflora*), Hops (*Humulus lupulus),* and Valerian (*Valeriana officinalis*) to support and calm the nervous system.

As an excellent cardiovascular tonic, Cayenne dilates blood vessels to increase circulation.

By normalizing the activity of blood platelets, the herb inhibits the formation of dangerous blood clots leading to strokes, heart attacks, and pulmonary emboli.

Cardiovascular System: Long ago, herbalists noticed that the inner Cayenne Pepper is divided into four chambers, just like the human heart. They interpreted this structure, along with the crimson-red color of the fruit, as the plant's "signature" pointing to its beneficial actions on the blood and heart. Hundreds of years of folk use and modern research validate this ancient "doctrine of signatures."

Cayenne is an excellent cardiac tonic whose stimulating action can be felt immediately. Taken over time, it helps to normalize heart function, tone and strengthen muscles of the heart and blood vessels, and is quite exceptional in increasing and normalizing circulation in the heart and throughout the entire body. It has long been used for an irregular and weak heartbeat, and when taken in normal doses it increases contractile force of the heart muscles without dangerously increasing heart rate. Studies validate its ability to help reduce hypertension (Toh, 1955).

Cayenne eases muscular spasms and as a vasodilator it dilates capillaries to allow increased blood flow (La, 1993). It equalizes circulation by opening areas of depleted or stagnated blood flow and moving blood to the surface. This has a warming influence that promotes sweating, and as capillaries fill up with blood, the skin becomes warm and pink. Because Cayenne increases peripheral circulation to cold hands and feet, "old timers" sprinkled powdered Cayenne in their shoes to keep their feet warm in winter. Used internally or externally, it can increase blood flow to arthritic joints and sprained, achy muscles. Cayenne's hot, stimulating qualities are helpful for Raynaud's disease, a painful condition in which blood vessels in the hands and feet contract, causing diminished blood flow and oxygen to the tissues, making them cold and blue. Along with a good magnesium supplement, this herb also improves intermittent claudication, a problem of insufficient circulation to the legs causing severe leg cramps and restlessness.

Capsaicinoids and other components in Cayenne have a normalizing action on blood platelets (Wang, 1984; Tsuchiya, 2001), which coagulate to form blood clots that prevent blood loss from injuries. The herb decreases excessive or abnormal blood platelet aggregation (clumping together) that can lead to heart attacks, strokes, abnormal blood clots, and thrombophlebitis (inflammation of a vein caused by blood clots). Another way Cayenne thins the blood and contributes to the inhibition of platelet aggregation is by stimulating the enzyme destruction of fibrin, a protein essential for blood clotting (Brinker, 1999). In a controlled study involving 16 healthy medical students who consumed 2 teaspoons of ground fresh Cayenne in noodles at one sitting, researchers found that the destruction of fibrin (fibrinolysis) was immediately detectable (Wasantapruek, 1974).

Research validates that Cayenne helps reduce blood levels of cholesterol and triglycerides due to its stimulating and normalizing effects on liver and gallbladder function that promote the secretion of bile (Mowrey, 1986; Wang, 1984). Lab studies show that Cayenne can reduce fat deposits in arteries by stimulating liver enzymes and bile responsible for breaking down fats (Kawada, 1986). All these qualities are beneficial for treating and preventing blood clots, strokes, heart attacks, hypertension, arteriosclerosis (the hardening and thickening of artery walls that occludes blood flow), and atherosclerosis (a type of arteriosclerosis in which deposits of plaque containing cholesterol and other materials form in medium and large-sized arteries and block blood flow).

Master herbalist and naturopathic doctor John Christopher wrote that "this herb is a great food for the circulatory system in that it feeds the necessary elements into the cell structure of the arteries, veins and capillaries so these regain elasticity of youth again, and blood pressure adjusts itself to normal. Cayenne regulates the flow of blood from the head to the feet so that it is equalized; it influences the heart immediately, then gradually extends its effects to the arteries, capillaries, and nerves" (Christopher, 1976). Cayenne tones blood vessels and helps varicose veins, hemorrhoids, and all types of peripheral vascular disease. It has a long history of use for treating conditions caused by poor circulation, including heart murmurs, irregular heartbeats, heart attacks, shortness of breath, and congestive heart failure. Dr. John Christopher and herbal practitioner Samuel Thomson reported using it many times to stop and treat heart attacks. Hawthorn (*Crataegus* spp.) acts synergistically with Cayenne to maximize their potential for cardiovascular problems.

Blood Cleanser: Cayenne's ability to promote circulation and remove vascular stagnation and congestion make it an excellent blood cleanser. As a diaphoretic, it stimulates excretion of waste products by increasing perspiration. It helps maintain normal metabolic function by stimulating the vital organs, including the liver, intestines and kidneys, all of which are essential in eliminating waste products and toxins. Combine Cayenne with other depuratives such as Echinacea, Red Clover (*Trifolium pratense*), Burdock root (*Arctium lappa*), Yellow Dock root (*Rumex crispus*) or Dandelion root, using equal amounts of each herb.

Hemorrhage: Cayenne is a hemostatic that normalizes and equalizes blood flow. Although it helps prevent blood clots, it is also known for its ability to stop internal and external bleeding. It is applied externally to halt hemorrhage from wounds and is ingested for internal bleeding. This herb is appropriate for any hemorrhaging organ, hemorrhoids, bloody stools and urine, nosebleeds, and bleeding uterine fibroids. It may be combined with other hemostatic herb such as Cranesbill (*Geranium maculatum*), Cinquefoil (*Potentilla* spp.), Shepherd's Purse (*Capsella bursa-pastoris*), and Yarrow (*Achillea millefolium*).

Infections and Respiratory System: Cayenne contains antimicrobial compounds and is an excellent remedy for bacterial and fungal infections throughout the body. Researchers at Ohio University tested antimicrobial activities of the most widely used *Capsicum* species and found that alcohol extracts exhibited varying degrees of inhibition against *Bacillus*, *Clostridium*, and *Streptococcus* bacteria (Cichewicz, 1996). Further *in vitro* studies have shown that peptides and other chemicals in *C. annuum* fruit effectively inhibit activity and growth of several yeast strains, including Candida, in addition to the bacterial species *Escherichia coli*, *Staphylococcus*, and *Pseudomonas aeruginosa* (Iorizzi, 2002; Keskin, 2011; Taveira, 2014).

As a diaphoretic and febrifuge, the herb reduces fevers by stimulating perspiration and bringing internal heat to the surface of the body. Cayenne also contains salicylates, aspirin-like chemicals that reduce pain and inflammation.

Cayenne is specific for lung ailments and is anti-catarrhal, meaning that it decreases mucous production. Catarrh is an old term for excessive amounts of mucous. The herb is an expectorant that thins and expels mucous and reduces coughing, muscle spasms, and chest tightness. It is appropriate for both acute and chronic inflammatory lung problems and infections. Cayenne protects the lungs by reducing vascular permeability (the ability of fluids to leak out of blood vessels) and edema caused by allergic reactions and cigarette smoke (Tilgner, 1999). Antioxidants reduce inflammation, relax bronchioles for easier breathing, and help protect lung tissue from irritants and cellular damage (Brinker, 2000; Jang, 2011).

This herb is highly recommended to prevent sickness in people exposed to cold, damp weather. It works best when taken at the onset of illness, and is excellent for the common cold, chills, coughs, pleurisy (lung inflammation due to infection, injury, or tumors), sinusitis, tonsillitis, laryngitis, lung infections and congestion including bronchitis and pneumonia, and lung hemorrhage. Cayenne can also improve chronic problems such as emphysema, asthma, and hay fever. The Eclectic physicians once used it for treating serious infectious diseases such as typhus, smallpox, scarlet fever, diphtheria, yellow fever, cholera, and meningitis. A mild tea or diluted tincture may be employed as a gargle for sore, infected throats. It may be combined with cooling and soothing Marshmallow root (*Althaea officinalis*), Plantain leaves (*Plantago* spp.), or Slippery Elm (*Ulmus rubra*) for colds, coughs, and bronchial problems. For asthma and chest tightness, combine Cayenne with a few drops of Lobelia (*Lobelia inflata*) tincture.

> *Cayenne tincture or tea is an effective remedy for colds, flu, and bacterial infections.*
>
> *It decreases mucous production and is a superb remedy for deep coughs with thick mucous.*

Many years ago when I was a home health aide working night shifts, I had the opportunity to observe Cayenne's amazing effect on coughs. On separate occasions, two elderly women in my care were suffering from constant deep, productive coughs that continued even after taking their prescription cough medicine, making sleep impossible. At the time, I always carried a small bottle of Cayenne tincture with me and used it as a type of "rescue remedy." After a few doses of their ineffective cough medicine, I offered each woman several drops of the Cayenne tincture in water, warning that it would taste and feel hot. They accepted my offer and, after only one dose, each of them stopped coughing and was able to have a peaceful night's sleep.

Cancer: Several *in vivo* and *in vitro* research studies document the ability of capsaicinoids in Cayenne to inhibit cancer (Nick, 2002), including T-cell leukemia cells that are resistant to conventional chemotherapy (Zhang, 2003). An interesting study demonstrated that injecting capsaicin into preexisting tumors in animals retarded further growth of the tumor, regardless of whether it was in an early or late stage. In addition, capsaicin significantly inhibited growth of non-injected tumors in the same animal. Capsaicin-elicited immunity proved to be T-cell mediated and tumor-specific (Beltran, 2007). Capsaicin has been shown to cause cell death of colon and pancreatic cancers, and in 2016 a German study also found it effective against several types of breast cancers (Weber, 2016). Cayenne's anti-inflammatory and antioxidant properties protect cellular membranes from damaging oxidation that can lead to cell mutation and cancer.

Digestive System: Cayenne is stimulating to a slow-moving, sluggish digestive system and improves both absorption and elimination of food when taken with meals or shortly after eating. The herb promotes normal appetite and digestion by increasing blood flow to the abdominal area and increasing secretions of saliva in the mouth, hydrochloric acid in the stomach, and pancreatic enzymes (Brinker, 2001). The herb normalizes atonic muscles lacking tone and strength, and stimulates peristalsis, which are wave-like contractions that propel food through the intestinal tract. Cayenne helps relieve indigestion, gas, bloating, nausea, vomiting, cramps, spasms, pain, and constipation. As an antibacterial herb, it may be taken for diarrhea, dysentery, and other gastrointestinal problems caused by bacterial infection. Adding the powder to foods and eating capsules containing Cayenne helps prevent and treat intestinal parasites.

> *Cayenne stimulates liver and gallbladder activity that helps reduce excessive blood levels of cholesterol and triglycerides.*
>
> *This is another way the herb keeps the blood flowing and the blood vessels and heart healthy.*

Human clinical studies have shown contradictory results of Cayenne's effect on stomach and intestinal ulcers. Several studies demonstrate that it actually helps prevent and heal ulcerated stomach lining and inhibits overgrowth of *Helicobacter pylori* bacteria associated with ulcer formation (Jones, 1997). Researchers in the medical department of the National University of Singapore conducted a study involving 103 Chinese patients with peptic ulcers, and their data showed that Cayenne exerted protective action on the stomach mucosa (Kang, 1995). In a study of 18 volunteers who ingested 20 grams of Cayenne 30 minutes before taking 600 mg of aspirin, endoscopies showed reduced damage to the stomach lining compared to a later test when aspirin was given without Cayenne. This indicated that the herb protected the stomach from adverse effects of aspirin (Yeoh, 1995). A study determined that the herb also protected the stomach from alcohol-induced damage by 92%. Researchers found that Cayenne decreased stomach contractions and increased mucous secretion, protecting the stomach lining from damage (Takeuchi, 1991). Another study, in which people with duodenal ulcers ate 10 grams of Red Chilies in wheat cereal, found no significant difference on the secretion of acid or pepsin in their stomachs (Pimparkar, 1972). In contrast, other studies have found that Cayenne increased stomach acids (Locock, 1985; Solanke, 1973), worsened ulcer symptoms, and initiated exfoliation and bleeding of the stomach lining (Myers, 1987; Viranuvatti, 1972). Therefore, people with stomach or intestinal ulcers should start with very small doses.

Cayenne is a cholagogue, promoting optimal liver and gallbladder function by stimulating a sluggish liver to increase the production and release of bile. Bile breaks down fats and stimulates peristaltic movement in the intestinal tract. This action benefits all conditions of liver stagnation by reducing high cholesterol blood levels and enhancing its fecal excretion, preventing the development of gallstones, and treating jaundice and constipation (Sambaiah, 1980).

The herb may also assist in managing diabetes type 2. A small clinical study consisting of 12 healthy volunteers demonstrated that ingesting 5 grams of Capsicum provided an adequate amount of capsaicin to reduce blood sugar levels and help normalize insulin levels (Chaiyasit, 2009).

Kidneys: Cayenne's stimulating action increases blood circulation through the kidneys to assist in the formation of urine and excretion of waste products. Eclectic physician Harvey Felter, M.D., wrote that "capsicum in very small doses is said to control kidney irritation and stimulate renal capillary activity in chronic renal congestion" (Felter, 1922).

Women's Health: Cayenne's ability to increase circulation and stimulate glandular secretions in the pelvis helps normalize a sluggish and congested reproductive system and promote normal menstrual bleeding. It is warming and relaxing to the tissues and helpful for painful uterine cramps. Taken internally, it is beneficial for treating vaginal infections and discharge. Eclectic physicians prescribed it for profuse menstrual bleeding and uterine hemorrhage, including uterine fibroid bleeding. Herbalist midwives have given it for postpartum (after childbirth) hemorrhage, and combine it with Lobelia for relief from the intense postpartum uterine contractions called "after-pains."

Teachings from the Cayenne Deva

"Greetings, dear one. I am the Cayenne Deva, a joyful plant of light! My nature is of heat and fire, and my movement is swift and piercing like the wind and rays of the sun. The fire nature of my hot fruit creates stimulating movement throughout the body. Just as fire travels quickly, consuming all in its path, so too, my fire essence consumes and purifies all putrid, toxic, and infectious substances in the body. My essence purges all that is impure and leaves in its wake transformation and fresh vitality.

"In this way, I am a cleansing herb for the tissues, blood, and lymph fluids. The red color of my fruit points to my beneficial actions on the heart and blood. The long pointed shape of my pod resembles a spear capable of piercing through obstructions.

"I possess Aries warrior energy of dynamic, expansive movement with strong and determined action that is powerful but balancing. As symbolized by the astrological sign of Leo, I also embody the fiery intensity of the sun.

"As an herb of the heart, I am beneficial for emotional suffering and physical problems. My fruit is helpful for sluggish, depressing conditions when vitality, enthusiasm, and the spark of life are diminished. People who feel weak and frail, who have lost hope and feel despondent, have need of my gifts. In small doses, I will clear stagnant, dark, brooding thoughts and feelings. Just as the sun dispels all darkness, I can lift the spirit and lighten the heart. So use me for heavy, deep emotions that have frozen into the heart and mind. A few drops of the essence of my white flowers will also brighten and clear emotional gloom and dark thoughts.

"I am warming and expansive to cold, rigid, painful, shut-down areas in the physical body such as frozen joints, immovable bowels, and tight blood vessels. For I will warm and open passageways, allowing the flow of energy, blood, and fluids throughout the body.

"I am a little plant, but I encapsulate tremendous light, warmth, and movement of the wind to stimulate cleansing and equilibrium throughout the body and mind. We are all beings of light. This is my message to humans: Remember your light and the light of all. You are invited to partake of my fruit for medicine, and to move freely, purely, and joyfully in the light!"

Chamomile, German

Matricaria recutita

Compositae (*Asteraceae*) (Sunflower or Aster) Family

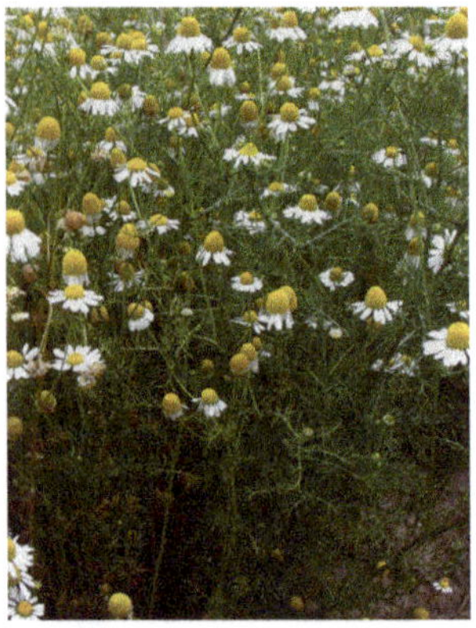

German Chamomile
Matricaria recutita

Botanical Names

German Chamomile and Roman Chamomile are the two species used interchangeably for beverages and medicines since ancient times. German Chamomile is currently the more popular variety for medicinal purposes. Botanists have bestowed this herb with several Latin names. *Matricaria recutita* and *Matricaria chamomilla* are older names, while *Chamomilla recutita* is the most recent.

Roman or English Chamomile is called *Anthemis nobilis*, and *Chamaemelum nobile* is the most recent name.

Common Names

Common names of German Chamomile are Hungarian Chamomile, common Chamomile, and wild Chamomile.

Medicinal Part of the Plant

The flower heads are used medicinally and as a tasty tea.

Range and Habitat

German Chamomile is indigenous to Europe and Western Asia. It has naturalized in North and South America, northern and eastern Africa, and Australia. Roman Chamomile is indigenous to England and Italy, and has also naturalized in the Americas. Both species are popular garden herbs that grow in sunny areas, open fields, and along roadsides.

Description of the Plant

German and Roman Chamomile flowers and leaves are almost indistinguishable from each other in appearance. Roman Chamomile (*Anthemis nobilis*) is a creeping perennial ground cover that droops and lays almost prostrate on the ground. It grows up to 12″ tall and appears as two subspecies, one with single flowers and the other with double flowers. Roman Chamomile emits less fragrance and seems to thrive when stepped on.

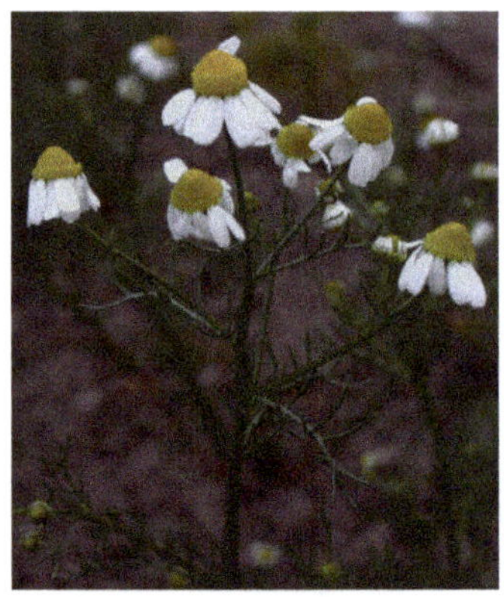

German Chamomile
Matricaria recutita

German Chamomile (*Matricaria recutita*) is a fragile, wispy-looking annual reaching 8-24″ in height, growing erect rather than prostrate. The rounded stem is grooved, lacks hairs, and is alternately branching. The pale-green leaves have a somewhat feathery appearance and are finely incised or divided into tiny leaflets that are linear, smooth, and pinnate. The cheerful and attractive daisy-like flowers grow in loose clusters of cymes at the tips of each branching stem and emit a pleasant, apple-like fragrance. All species of Chamomile have the typical flower head characteristic of the *Compositae* family. The small flowers reach a diameter of ½-¾″. Several white ray petals surround a brightly colored, button-shaped center of tightly compacted yellow disc flowers tinged with a hint of light green. The receptacle and disc flowers of German Chamomile form a cone that is hollow inside, a characteristic that separates it from Roman Chamomile. Chamomile flowers start blooming in spring and can last into the summer months.

Be sure not to mistake Pineapple Weed (classified as *Matricaria discoidea*, *Matricaria matricarioides*, or *Chamomilla suaveolens*) for German or Roman Chamomile. It is similar in appearance, but Pineapple Weed flowers lack the white ray petals.

Cultivation

German Chamomile is an attractive garden ornamental easily grown from seed. Although it has a delicate appearance, it is a hardy plant. It thrives in a sunny location in fertile, sandy loam soil that is moist but well-drained. Seeds can be planted directly in a garden bed in late autumn or early spring, or in greenhouse flats in early spring. Chamomile is a light-dependent germinator, so scatter the tiny seeds on the soil surface and, rather than covering with dirt, gently tap them down onto the soil. Keep soil moist and germination will occur within 2 weeks when weather and temperatures are favorable. Space the seedlings about 6″ apart. The flowers bloom for several weeks.

Chamomile plants are very prolific without human intervention. When left undisturbed, the tiny seeds that mature and drop to the ground will germinate in late autumn or the following spring to create a cheerful carpet of sunny flowers.

Harvest

Harvest the flower heads when in full bloom during late spring and early summer. This can be tedious, but pick the flowers with your fingers or use scissors.

Preparation of Plant Medicine and Dosages

The flower heads are used fresh or dried, but fresh is always more potent. If drying is desired, place flowers on screens, a clean sheet or piece of cardboard, and leave them in a shady, well-ventilated area. The flowers are often ingested as tea because of their pleasant flavor. Alcohol tinctures also have an agreeable taste and extract the medicinal volatile oils in greater amounts than hot water. Steeping Chamomile flowers for tea only extracts 10-15% of the medicinal essential oils. When using this herb for medicinal purposes, remember that alcohol extracts produce much stronger effects.

A strong tea can be prepared for different types of external applications to treat a variety of skin problems, rashes, injuries, and infections. An oil or salve of the flowers is also excellent for external application. The volatile oil should be used cautiously in small amounts if ingested, and only 1-2 drops in a cup of water is taken per dose.

PREPARATIONS

Tea: For a mild tasting tea, steep 2-3 teaspoons of fresh or dried flowers in a cup of boiled water for 10-20 minutes. A stronger tea can be prepared by stepping ½ ounce of flowers in a pint of boiled water. While steeping, cover the cup or pan with a lid to prevent loss of volatile oils through steam. Dosage: 1-3 cups a day as needed.

Tincture: Prepare the flower heads in the usual manner using a mix of 70% 190-proof grain alcohol and 30% distilled water. Dosage: ½-1 teaspoon of tincture in water taken 1-3 times a day.

Pills and Capsules: Grind dried flowers into fine powder and prepare it as pills or pack it into capsules. Dosage: 2-3 pills or capsules 1-3 times daily as needed.

Poultice: Apply a poultice of crushed flower heads directly to inflamed and injured skin. Keep it moist and secure the flowers with an ace wrap or bandage material.

Fomentation, Wash, Bath, Sitz, Gargle, and Douche: A strong tea of the flower heads is used for these applications. Tea may be added to bath water for an aromatic, relaxing, and luxurious experience.

Oil and Salve: Chop freshly harvested flowers into small pieces, place in a pan, and cover with olive oil. Bake in the usual manner and add beeswax if a salve consistency is desired.

Chemical Constituents

German Chamomile is considered medicinally superior to the Roman variety. Essential oils and flavonoid glycosides in the flowers of German Chamomile are believed to be responsible for most of the medicinal properties. The two primary constituents in the essential oils are bisabolol and azulene (and chamazulene which is a derivative of azulene), which have strong anti-inflammatory and antispasmodic effects. Studies show that bisabolol is anti-oxidant (Mamalis, 2013), analgesic, anti-arthritic, protects against and treats peptic ulcers, reduces fevers, promotes faster healing from burns, and inhibits bacterial, yeast, and fungal infections (Der Marderosian, 1998). Azulene is a compound in the essential oil of both species that is brilliant blue in color. It is highly valued for its ability to reduce inflammation, inhibit bacterial growth, and reduce pain. Several researchers have found that azulene blocks histamine release, reducing inflammation and allergic responses (Farnsworth, 1972; Mann, 1986). Many preparations of German Chamomile on the European market are standardized to azulene and bisabolol content. Farnesene (carminative) and matricin are other components found in the volatile oils. Matricin, necessary for the synthesis of chamazulene, is analgesic and anti-inflammatory.

Flower heads contain 6-8% flavonoids, which are antioxidant and antispasmodic. Apigenin is a flavonoid and mild sedative that reduces anxiety and is analgesic, anti-inflammatory, antibacterial, antihistamine, antioxidant, anti-ulcer, choleretic, a vasodilator, and reduces blood platelet aggregation. Chamomile flowers are one of the best sources of apigenin, shown to inhibit growth of cancer cells, sensitize cancer cells to destruction by apoptosis (programed death), and retard the development of blood vessels that feed growing tumors (Lefort, 2013).Other flavonoids include luteolin (antioxidant, anti-inflammatory, neuroprotective, and blocks mast cells to reduce allergic reactions), rutin (strengthens capillaries), patuletin, isorhamnetin, and quercetin (anti-inflammatory, anti-allergenic).

Coumarins are antispasmodic and thin blood to reduce thrombus or blood clot formation. The primary coumarins in Chamomile are herniarin (hemostatic, anthelmintic, antibacterial, antifungal, candidicide, cholagogue, hepatoprotective, anticonvulsant, spasmolytic) (Ahmad, 1997) and umbelliferone (antibacterial, antihistamine, anti-inflammatory, candidicide, choleretic). Herniarin and umbelliferone have been reported to be anticoagulant *in vitro* (Booth, 2004).

The flower heads contain up to 10% mucilage polysaccharides, amino acids, fatty acids, phenolic acids, and small amounts of vitamins and minerals that include choline, niacin (vitamin B3), riboflavin (vitamin B2), ascorbic acid (vitamin C), calcium, magnesium, phosphorus, and silicon.

Safety, Contraindications, and Drug Interactions

Chamomile is a nontoxic herb that is safe for young children and the elderly. The literature contains many cautions about allergic reactions to the herb, but this has only been observed in a small percentage of people who are allergic to ragweed and other members of the *Compositae* family. Any symptoms of runny nose, itchy eyes, or sneezing are short-lived. A global literature search discovered 50 reports of allergic reactions from ingesting Chamomile from 1887–1982. Five cases were attributed to German Chamomile and the others were caused by the Roman species (Hausen, 1984). Avoid washing eyes with the tea because it has caused eye inflammation in some people.

Due to its mildly stimulating effect on the uterus, **German Chamomile is sometimes contraindicated during pregnancy**. This is a hypothetical assumption that is unsubstantiated by real-life evidence, and for hundreds of years pregnant women have benefited from the tea's abundant mineral content, calming effects, and ability to ease morning sickness. The American Eclectic physicians prescribed the tea to women during the later months of pregnancy for nervous twitching, restlessness and anxiety, coughs, and false labor pains. Excessive consumption, especially of the oil, may induce vomiting or uterine contractions. While German Chamomile is safe to use in small amounts, **Roman Chamomile is very stimulating to the uterus and should not be taken during pregnancy due to its abortifacient actions.**

Although no drug interactions have been reported, natural coumarins in the flower heads could possibly enhance the potency and activity of pharmaceutical blood thinners. Possible interactions with warfarin have been reported, so it is best not to use Chamomile while taking blood thinners.

Medicinal Uses

History of the Plant

Chamomile has been a favorite tea and valuable medicine for over 2,000 years in ancient Egypt, Europe, and India. The Egyptians used it to treat fevers and malaria. They called it "plant of the sun" and dedicated it to their deities because the plant was so revered. The name "Chamomile" is derived from the Latin word *chamos* or *kamai*, meaning "on the ground," because the plant grows low and thickly covers the ground, and *melos*, which means "apple," referring to the apple-like fragrance of the flowers. *Matricaria* comes from the Latin *matrix*, meaning "womb," because it was used historically to treat female problems.

The Greek botanist and physician Dioscorides (*circa* A.D. 40–*c.* 90) and the Roman naturalist Pliny (A.D. 23–79) both recommended the herb for anxiety, headaches, and digestive, kidney, and liver ailments. The Greek physician Galen (*c.* A.D. 131–*c.* 200) used it for colic and as a diuretic. European healers employed Chamomile oil for external applications, and baths of strongly brewed tea eased all types of aches and pains, bruises, swellings, and inflammation. The tea was sometimes mixed with wine and given for stomach problems, indigestion, gas, bloating, expelling phlegm from congested sinuses and lungs, and bringing on monthly menses. The English herbalist and apothecary Nicholas Culpeper (1616–1654) wrote, "A decoction made of camomile [sic], and drank, taketh away all pains and stitches in the side. It easeth all pains of the colic and stone, and all pains and torments of the belly, and gently provoketh urine. The flowers . . . help to expel all colds, aches and pains whatsoever, and is an excellent help to bring down women's courses" (Culpeper, 1992).

Chamomile was introduced into American gardens by European immigrants. The early American Eclectic physicians of the late 1800s and early 1900s applied the herb externally for skin problems and wound healing, and prescribed the tea for digestive problems, anxiety and nervous conditions, earaches, childhood ailments, liver inflammation and congestion, and to promote menstruation and relieve painful menstrual cramps. Chamomile is currently one of the most popular and widely used tea beverages in Europe and the United States. It is listed in the pharmacopoeias of 26 countries as an official drug for its anti-inflammatory, antibacterial, antispasmodic, and sedative properties (Salamon, 1992).

German Chamomile is more popular than Roman Chamomile and has been the focus of extensive scientific research for over 20 years. This research supports the herb's historic uses in reducing anxiety, muscle spasms, inflammation, bacterial and fungal infections, digestive distress, and in treating wounds and problematic skin conditions. Much of the current research also reveals powerful antioxidant and anti-inflammatory actions.

Healing Qualities

Analgesic, antibacterial, mild anti-catarrhal, antifungal, antihistamine, anti-inflammatory, antioxidant, antiseptic, antispasmodic, carminative, diaphoretic (when taken hot), emmenagogue, febrifuge, hemostatic, immunomodulator, nervine, sedative, stomachic, and vulnerary.

Traditional Chinese Medicine (TCM) Perspective

Chamomile flowers are mildly bitter, cooling, drying, and stimulating. These properties are helpful for Liver Qi Stagnation and the resulting excess heat, or Liver Fire, which can cause irritability, tension, mood swings, inflammation, spasms, headaches, indigestion, bloating, and menstrual problems. The flowers stimulate blood flow to relieve excess heat, tension, and stagnation in the digestive system and uterus. They clear internal wind to stop spasms and clear damp heat in the intestines, sinuses, and lungs.

Primary Actions

The smooth, calming action of Chamomile flowers upon the central nervous system, and specifically the solar plexus, is felt throughout the entire body. The herb is specific for conditions involving nervous tension and anxiety that affect the digestive tract, and is excellent for indigestion, gas, ulcers, muscle spasms, and all types of inflammation. It is a tasty and relaxing tea, pleasant to drink during the day to ease anxiety or before bedtime to enhance peaceful and restful sleep.

Nervous System: For physical tension and pain or emotional stress, treat yourself to a cup of delicious Chamomile tea or take the convenient tincture. Chamomile is a gentle nervine and mild sedative that relaxes and tones the nervous system. It excels in reducing tension and anxiety throughout the body, first in the nerves and then in the muscles and tissues. A strong tea or tincture acts as a muscle relaxant to ease muscle cramps and spasms, headaches, and migraines. The herb also brings calm to the mind and emotions by soothing irritability, restlessness, moodiness, and all types of stress disorders caused by inner tension that "locks up" the system. As a mild sedative, the herb induces restful sleep and can be helpful for insomnia and subduing nightmares when taken shortly before bedtime. This sedative effect is very calming for excessive stimulation of the nervous system manifesting as hyperactive behavior. The volatile oils have analgesic properties helpful for mild neuralgia (nerve pain) and increased sensitivity to pain. Some people have found Chamomile to be helpful for vertigo (dizziness) and motion sickness.

> *The gentle calming action of Chamomile flowers on the nervous system, and specifically upon the solar plexus, relaxes muscle pain and tension throughout the body, while relieving emotional stress and irritability.*

The herb's long history of use in traditional medical systems to soothe the nerves has been substantiated by modern research. In one study, mice were given Chamomile infusions in amounts comparable to human consumption, and their drowsiness and diminished movement confirmed that the herb induced mild depression of their central nervous system (Della Loggia, 1982). In another trial designed to observe Chamomile's influence on the heart, 10 out of 12 patients undergoing cardiac catheterization fell into a deep sleep within 10 minutes of drinking 6 ounces of the tea. There were no cardiac effects from ingesting the herb except a slight increase in the average brachial artery pressure. Patients continued to sleep until the procedure was finished (Gould, 1973).

Several chemical constituents in the flower heads contribute to the herb's sedating and relaxing properties. Laboratory research indicates that the flavonoid apigenin binds to benzodiazephine receptors in the brain, which reduces anxiety and promotes nervous system sedation (Viola, 1995; Brown, 1997). Studies also show that apigenin is about three times more effective for pain than papaverine, an opiate drug (Kunde, 1980). Other flavonoids and coumarins have been shown to relax smooth muscle tissue found in blood vessels and organs (Mann, 1986; Forster, 1980). Studies have documented antispasmodic effects when alcohol extracts of Chamomile reduced muscle contractions and spasms caused by histamine and acetylcholine release (Forster, 1980). Chamomile's antispasmodic effects are due to flavonoids, such as apigenin, and volatile oils like bisabolol and chamazulene.

The effects of Chamomile in treating generalized anxiety disorder (GAD) were explored during an 8-week randomized, double-blind, placebo-controlled study involving 57 people suffering from mild to moderate GAD. People receiving Chamomile experienced significantly greater relief than those taking a placebo (Amsterdam, 2009).

Digestive System: Chamomile flowers have a strong affinity with the solar plexus, the network of nerves controlling functions of the liver, stomach, pancreas, kidneys, and adrenal glands. By regulating and maintaining the relaxed flow of nerve impulses throughout the solar plexus, muscles within the abdominal cavity relax to allow easy movement of digestive enzymes and food through the stomach and intestines. Thus, Chamomile promotes optimal digestion and can ease stress and tension, including a nervous, unsettled stomach that feels like "butterflies." The tea and tincture are soothing to the stomach and are a valuable remedy for people whose nervous tension seems to originate in the solar plexus.

Studies reveal that the essential oils and flavonoids contained in the flower heads exert a relaxing effect on the smooth muscle and mucous membranes that line the entire digestive tract (Kunde, 1980). The anti-inflammatory, antispasmodic, and carminative properties of Chamomile are excellent for all types of gastrointestinal problems that include indigestion, gas and bloating, colic, abdominal cramps and spasms, hiccups, and diarrhea. The mild bitter principle in the herb has stimulating effects on the liver to promote normal function and bile production. Essential oils stimulate the liver and kidneys to eliminate waste products and toxins. Chamomile is especially helpful for gas, colic, and sluggish digestion when combined with Ginger (*Zingiber officinale*) or Peppermint (*Mentha x piperita*).

> *Chamomile flowers have a strong affinity with the solar plexus, which is the network of nerves controlling functions of the liver, stomach, pancreas, kidneys and the adrenal glands.*
>
> *By regulating and maintaining the relaxed flow of nerve impulses of the solar plexus, this herb promotes optimal digestion and eases all stress and tensions, including a nervous stomach.*

Chamomile reduces excess secretion of hydrochloric acid from the stomach, and is widely used in Europe for treating heartburn, stomach and intestinal ulcers, and reducing inflammation throughout the gastrointestinal tract, including the mouth and throat. It is beneficial for the treatment of gastritis (stomach inflammation), ulcerative colitis, and other irritable and inflammatory intestinal problems. Rudolf Weiss, M.D., the late, well-known German physician and herbalist, recommended that large doses of Chamomile be taken over a period of time as the remedy of choice for long-term healing of stomach and intestinal ulcers, and for inhibiting inflammation. He wrote, "Chamomile does not merely give symptomatic relief in these cases, but directly effects a cure, influencing the pathological process" (Weiss, 1988).

Several scientific studies have investigated the herb's activity in healing ulcerated tissues. In lab studies, apigenin inhibited growth of *Helicobacter pylori*, the bacteria causing stomach ulcers, and demonstrated potent protection against stomach cancer (Kuo, 2013). Animal studies revealed that the essential oil bisabolol also protected against the development of stomach ulcers and enhanced their healing (Szelenyi, 1979; Isaac, 1975). Researchers have found that Chamomile heals ulcers and inhibits their development by strengthening the mucosal layer of the stomach and decreasing the secretion of pepsin (Thiemer, 1972). Irritable bowel syndrome (IBS) patients experience improvement using Chamomile (Agah, 2015).

A mouthwash of strong Chamomile tea is effective in treating ulceration and swelling of the mucous membranes of the mouth caused by gingivitis (gum inflammation) and painful toothaches. This has been under investigation by several researchers, and mouthwashes of Chamomile tea were found to be beneficial for cancer patients suffering from inflamed and ulcerated tissues in the mouth following radiation and chemotherapy (Carl, 1991). In one clinical trial, Chamomile mouthwashes reduced bleeding associated with gingivitis and demonstrated antimicrobial and anti-inflammatory properties similar to that of chlorhexidine 0.12%, considered the gold standard of antibacterial mouthwashes (Batista, 2014). Two other clinical trials involving mechanically ventilated patients in intensive care units compared the antibacterial actions of Chamomile and chlorhexidine 0.2% mouthwashes. Accumulation of bacteria in the pharynx is one of the risk factors of pneumonia due to ventilation. Bacterial colonies of *Staphylococcus aureus* and *S. pneumoniae* significantly decreased in 50 patients after 6 treatments of chlorhexidine 0.2% mouthwash and, to a lesser extent, in 50 patients given Chamomile mouthwash (Baradari, 2012; Darvishi, 2013).

Kidneys: German research has demonstrated that 120 drops of the tincture taken 3 times daily reduces blood urea nitrogen (BUN) levels over time (Mitchell, 2003). BUN is a breakdown product of protein metabolism. Urea is formed in the liver and is the primary nitrogen end product of protein metabolism and breakdown. The urea is carried to the kidneys via the blood for excretion in urine. Most kidney diseases cause reduced urea excretion leading to elevated BUN levels. Thus, the BUN level is directly related to the metabolic function of the liver and the excretory function of the kidneys, and serves as an index of the function of these organs.

Blood and Circulation: Coumarins from the flower heads demonstrate hemostatic properties that exert blood-thinning activity. Researchers have found that these coumarins inhibit platelets in the blood from clumping together, which is a potentially dangerous condition that makes the blood too thick, reduces circulation, and increases the possibility for blood clots and thrombosis (Landolfi, 1984). Blood platelet aggregation is an underlying cause of atherosclerosis and other cardiovascular diseases. Polysaccharides and polyphenols isolated from German Chamomile decreased platelet aggregation in blood obtained from healthy donors and from patients receiving anti-platelet drug therapy (Bijak, 2013).

The herb has a relaxing and dilating action on the smooth muscle within blood vessels, allowing greater blood flow throughout the body, especially to the digestive system and uterus. *In vivo* tests revealed that apigenin, luteolin, and bisabolol extracted from Chamomile flowers produced slow relaxation of isolated coronary blood vessels (Roberts, 2013).

Protection from Inflammation and Oxidation: Chamomile has been employed for its powerful anti-inflammatory properties for hundreds of years. Bisabolol and flavonoids, specifically apigenin, possess antioxidant properties that protect against cellular damage and minimize inflammation. Rat studies have validated the herb's ability to reduce oxidative stress and maintain healthy levels of the primary antioxidant enzymes: superoxide dismutase (SOD), catalase, and glutathione (Sebai, 2014). Phenols occurring in Chamomile tea have demonstrated the ability to reduce free radical damage and inhibit growth of colon cancer cells (Kogiannou, 2013). Researchers have identified an important mechanism vital for antioxidant production, which is Chamomile's ability to induce Nrf2 activation. Nrf2 (nuclear factor-like 2) is a protein occurring in all cells that is necessary to stimulate production of antioxidants (Bhaskaran, 2013).

The flower heads are beneficial for skin inflammation and hemorrhoids when applied externally and ingested. They are also helpful for all types of internal inflammation. Both German and Roman Chamomile have traditionally been used to treat sciatica, gout, lower back pain, and arthritic conditions. Patients diagnosed with carpal tunnel syndrome have reported significant decline in pain by applying Chamomile oil to their wrist twice daily for one month (Hashempur, 2015).

Current research substantiates the presence of several chemical constituents in the flower heads responsible for reducing inflammation (Yakolev, 1969; Jakavlev, 1979). Research from the University of Munich in Germany has shown that the essential oils inhibit production of prostaglandins in laboratory experiments. Prostaglandins are chemicals in the body that promote inflammation. Flavonoids in the herb inhibit arachidonic acid production, which also decreases the inflammatory response (Van Rietshoten, 1990). Some studies have shown that Chamomile is a better anti-inflammatory than indomethacin, a commonly prescribed non-steroidal anti-inflammatory drug (Duke, 2000). A study compared the effects of a topical application of Chamomile extract with the anti-inflammatory drug benzydamine for the treatment of edema and inflammation in the middle ear. The topical application of Chamomile extract in the ear produced a reduction of fluid and inflammation similar to the activity of the drug (Tubaro, 1984).

Bacteria, Colds and Flu, Fungi, Immune Stimulation, and Allergy Relief: Volatile oils contained in the flower heads are antibacterial and antifungal. Several doses of Chamomile tincture or a strong brew of the tea can ease the symptoms of the common cold and flu. Taken hot, its diaphoretic action stimulates perspiration and is cooling for fevers. The herb is helpful for coughs by reducing inflammation and spasms in the lungs. It is also a mild anti-catarrhal that helps reduce and eliminate excess mucous in the nasal sinuses and lungs. The steam from a big pot of strong tea may be inhaled to relieve congestion from colds. Chamomile is also beneficial for treating Candida yeast (Aggag, 1972).

Research shows that the herb strengthens the immune system. Polysaccharides in the flower heads stimulate phagocytosis, which is the activity of specialized immune cells to search out, engulf, and destroy pathogenic organisms (Wagner, 1984).

Chamomile contains several flavonoids and essential oils with antihistamine activity that can reduce allergic reactions, such as hay fever and hives. However, since some people may have allergic reactions to the plant itself, Chamomile should be used cautiously when treating allergies. Research studies have led scientists to believe that azulene and chamazulene in the oil help prevent allergic responses by blocking histamine release from tissues throughout the body. Histamine release triggers the immune response and inflammation, giving rise to allergic symptoms such as sinus drainage, sneezing, itchy eyes, wheezing, and facial edema. Although the mechanism of action is still in question, it is thought that azulene stimulates the pituitary and adrenal glands to release cortisone, a hormone that inhibits histamine production (Mann, 1986).

Children: Chamomile tea has a long history of use as a remedy for many typical childhood problems and may be given safely to babies and young children. It is soothing for fussy, whining, or angry children. The herb promotes restful sleep and is excellent for colic, tummy aches, diarrhea and other digestive problems, and for croup, fevers, earaches, and infant convulsions. It is beneficial during the painful teething period, and for the restlessness and hyperactivity accompanying attention deficit disorder (ADD) and attention deficit hyperactivity disorder (ADHD).

Chamomile tea is gentle and tasty for infants and young children.

It is calming and provides relief from stomachaches, earaches, fevers, colds, the flu, and eases the pain of teething.

In a clinical trial involving 79 children between the ages of 6 months and 5.5 years, the efficacy of Chamomile and pectin liquid extract was investigated for the treatment of acute diarrhea. After three days of treatment with the extract, diarrhea in the Chamomile/pectin group had significantly resolved compared to the placebo group. Parents documented their child's well-being twice a day and, compared to those receiving the placebo, a trend of continuous improvement was observed in those given Chamomile and pectin (de la Motte, 1997).

Women's Health: The flower heads have stimulating and tonic actions on the uterus that relieve pelvic congestion and increase blood flow. Mild emmenagogue properties encourage delayed menstruation to begin, and antispasmodic properties relax muscles to reduce uterine cramps. The anti-anxiety influence of Chamomile is beneficial for premenstrual syndrome (PMS), mood swings, irritability, and breast pain associated with PMS. This was validated in studies involving 90 college students experiencing severe PMS symptoms. Half of the women received a 100 mg capsule of Chamomile, while the other half took 250 mg of mefenamic acid (a prescription drug for PMS symptoms) 3 times a day. There was a greater reduction of intense emotional symptoms and breast pain in the students taking Chamomile after two menstrual cycles of daily supplementation compared to the control group (Sharifi, 2014).

Over the centuries, many pregnant women have enjoyed drinking German Chamomile tea to ease morning sickness, anxiety, insomnia, headaches, spasms, and inflammation. In an 8-year study of 8,058 pregnant women, the essential oils of Chamomile and Clary Sage (*Salvia sclarea*) were found to be effective in alleviating pain during childbirth (Burns, 2000).

External Uses for Skin and Wounds: Chamomile's analgesic, anti-inflammatory, antibacterial, antifungal, and vulnerary properties make it an excellent remedy for external skin problems. The flower heads have traditionally been employed for the treatment of inflamed tissues and mucous membranes, wounds, acne, ulcers, burns, bruises, varicose veins, and all types of rashes such as hives and eczema. The herb can be applied externally as a salve, poultice, or wash. It is also wise to ingest the tincture or tea to help heal these conditions from the inside out.

Several research studies have investigated the herb's external wound-healing abilities. Lab tests demonstrate that Chamomile oil is very effective for healing burns (Zita, 1955), and the herb accelerates wound healing by reducing inflammation and promoting tissue granulation and regeneration (Carle, 1987). A German study compared the efficacy of a Chamomile ointment (Kamillosan) with an ointment containing 0.25% hydrocortisone for the treatment of eczema in 166 patients. After a period of 3-4 weeks, researchers found that the Chamomile ointment was equal to or better than hydrocortisone for reducing skin inflammation and treating eczema (Aertgeerts, 1985).

Chamomile is widely used in Germany and other European countries, and the German Commission E herbal regulatory agency approved the herb for external treatment of bacterial skin diseases and irritation and inflammation of the skin and mucous membranes lining the throat, gastrointestinal tract, respiratory system, and urinary system. The volatile oils kill bacterial and fungal infections. The flowers can be made into a strong tea and used as a bath or sitz bath to heal hemorrhoids and other types of anal and genital inflammation. The tea can also be used as a hair rinse and imparts a beautiful sheen to blond hair.

Teachings from the Chamomile Deva

"Greetings, dear one! I am the deva of the merry little plants you call Chamomile. Many of us grow together in large communities, reflecting the constant abundance that is our natural way of being. We are of the air element and are blessed with an open, free-flowing, and playful nature. Just as the wings of birds allow flight through the air, the feathery appearance of our leaves indicates our affiliation with the element of air. Like the air sign Gemini, our movement radiates outward, initiating flow in all directions, and there is lightness in our activity and influence. Our outer petals, arranged in a circular pattern surrounding the yellow center, reflect movement radiating outward like a spinning wheel. This movement initiates gentle, rippling waves of calm, and thus we help establish a smooth flow of energies and movement throughout the body to bring great comfort.

"The bright sunny-yellow color shinning from the center of our flowers specifically points to our cheerfully calming yet energizing influence upon the nerves and digestive organs of the solar plexus area. The solar plexus, in the center of the human body, radiates the yellow ray of light and is a central power area of the personality and physical body. Anxious thoughts, harmful emotions, and stresses of daily life all contribute to building inner anxiety, especially in the area of the solar plexus. Our ability to promote smooth flow of nervous energy allows calm relaxation that untangles tight knots of tension. Thus, the smooth flow of energies through the digestive system relieves nervous tension manifesting as inflammation and stagnation, allowing optimal absorption of nutrients to strengthen and provide vitality. Throughout the physical body, we promote the free flow of energy allowing calm nerves, unrestricted blood flow, and comfortable muscles. Just as the bright rays of the sun dispel darkness, our cheerful flowers dispel dark thoughts and brooding emotions, allowing a sunny disposition to shine forth. The white color of our outer petals indicates this cleansing and purifying activity.

"Our rounded petals and flowers offer good medicine to those having sharp spikes of anger and who need their rough edges smoothed out. Our flowers provide the calming flow of energy that helps people integrate with life rather than suffering in isolation with sharp, angry, rigid thoughts and bitter feelings that create tension in the heart, mind, muscles, and organs.

"Just as our flowers grow in a dense carpet covering the earth, allow us to blanket you with ease and comfort to soften the bumps and grinds and sharp points of life. We offer the gift of deep inner peace and stillness, allowing the light of inner joy to shine and radiate outward."

Chasteberry

Vitex agnus-castus
Verbenaceae (Verbena) Family

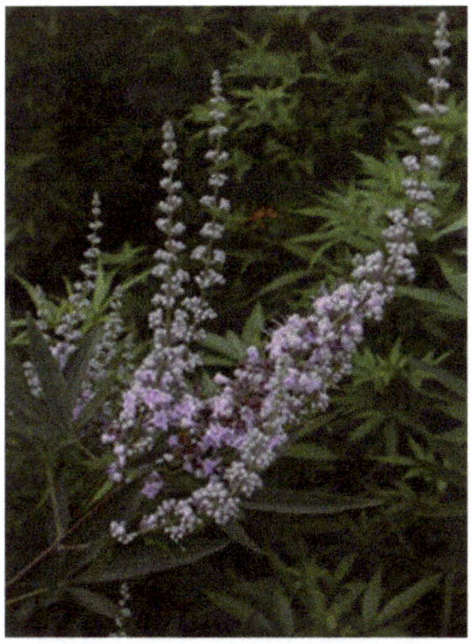

Common Names

Chasteberry and Vitex are the most commonly used names for this herb. Chaste tree, chastity bush, and monk's pepper are older names reflecting the plant's use among Catholic monks in Europe. Indian spice and wild pepper are names referring to the spicy, pungent flavor of the berries.

Medicinal Part of the Plant

The ripe fruit is a berry and the medicinal part of the plant.

Range and Habitat

The genus *Vitex* consists of more than 250 species of shrubs and trees. Most are tropical and a few species, including *Vitex agnus-castus,* grow in temperate climates. Chasteberry is native to western Asia. It has naturalized in Europe, where it is commonly found throughout the Mediterranean region, and in the southern United States. Often found along ponds and riverbanks, it can also grow in very dry desert soils, and I have seen plants thrive in southern Arizona.

Description of the Plant

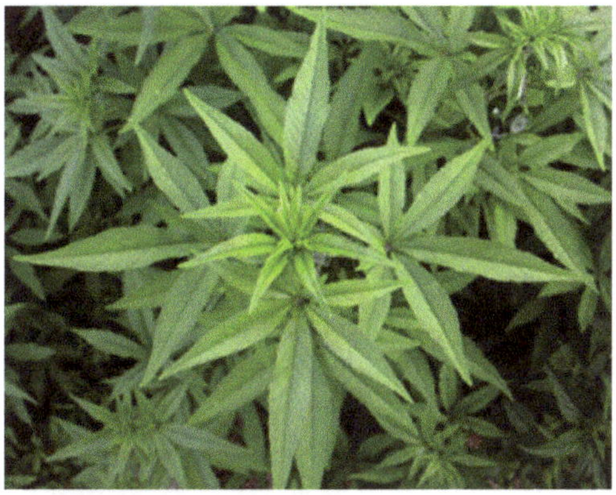

Chasteberry is a perennial bush and tree growing 9-16′ in height. The attractive leaves and flower clusters make this a striking ornamental for gardens and hedges. Several woody stalks grow from the large, fibrous root system and gradually become soft and herbaceous at their ends. Leaves grow opposite along the entire length of the stalks and are compound palmate in shape, usually consisting of 5 large leaflets, and occasionally 3 or as many as 9 appear. Leaflets are linear in shape, pinnately veined, and smooth. The topside of leaves is deep, rich green with a lighter, silvery-green tone underneath.

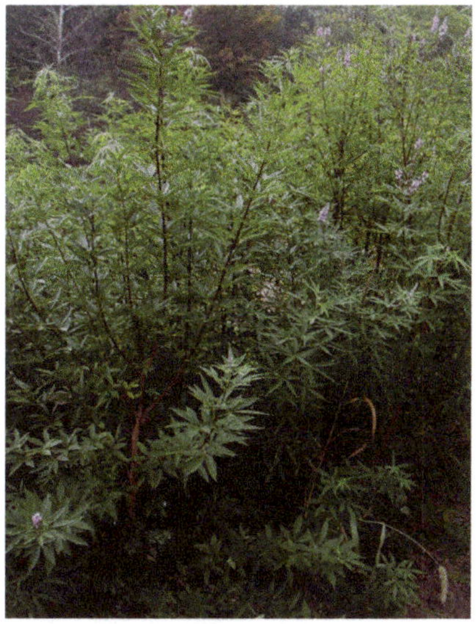

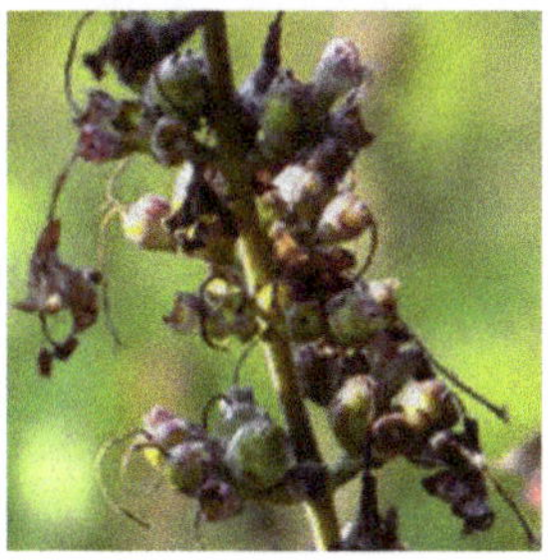

Immature berries

Many small lavender-colored flowers form beautiful spikes of whorled clusters on the tips of leaf stalks. Flowers are 1/3-1/2″ long with a pale-green cup-shaped calyx holding a tubular corolla that opens into 5 lips. A central pistil and 4 surrounding stamens protrude out. Flowers usually bloom from June through August, and later in cooler climates. They mature into small round berries that are initially green and turn dark with maturity. Berries are about the size of peppercorns. The entire plant emits a strong, unique, and somewhat spicy aroma.

Cultivation

Chasteberry thrives in a variety of soils ranging from dry and sandy to moist and fertile. The plant needs good drainage and prefers full sun. It grows slowly in cold regions and requires a thick mulch to protect the roots and crowns during winter freezes. It is easy to cultivate by seed, layering, or stem cuttings. Seeds do not require stratification and may be planted during spring in deep flowerpots and covered with 1/8″ of soil. After a year of growth, transplant the seedlings to a prepared garden area and plant them 5-10′ apart.

To propagate by layering, place a few outer branches of the bush flat on the ground and pin them down with stakes. Cover the middle of the branches with soil. Eventually, when adventitious roots grow from the leaf nodes along the buried stem, cut off the rooting branch from the parent plant and transplant it. Another method, nearly 100% successful, is to cut off long stems in spring when leaves are present, but prior to flowering, and put the cuttings in a bucket with a mix of equal parts sand, vermiculite, and potting soil. Punch holes in the bottom of the bucket for drainage and keep the mix very moist. Keep shaded, and over several weeks the stems develop roots and can eventually be planted in a permanent garden bed.

Plants become established after 3-4 years. Dead growth can be pruned away in spring after leaves have appeared on the stalks. The long, spreading roots of older plants make them very difficult to transplant.

Harvest

Chasteberry plants bear their first flowers in late summer and autumn of their second or third year of growth. Harvest the dark berries from September to November when fully mature, but before they dry out.

Preparation of Plant Medicine and Dosages

After harvesting the berries, strip them away from the stem. I have consistently found tincture produced from freshly harvested berries to be far superior in potency than preparations containing dried berries, such as tea or capsules. A well-prepared tincture retains the unique and pleasant odor of the berries.

The amount of Chasteberry typically used in research studies is 40 drops of standardized extract taken once or twice daily. In clinical studies, this dosage restored progesterone levels in women when used for 3 months (Newall, 1996). This is a safe tonic herb that must be taken over a period of time (6-24 months) to normalize pituitary and reproductive function. During the first month of treatment, the length of the menstrual cycle may temporarily shorten or lengthen before normalizing. Many women notice benefits within 2 months, but it may take more time for Chasteberry to resolve long-standing health issues.

PREPARATIONS

Tincture: Grind fresh berries into a coarse powder or crush them by placing them in a plastic bag and hammering them. Put the ground or crushed berries in a glass jar and cover with 70% 190-proof grain alcohol and 30% distilled water. Another method that works well is to combine the berries with the alcohol/water mix and grind everything together in a blender or food processor. Tincture and decant in the usual manner. Dosage: 40 drops in water once or twice daily.

Tea: Prepare from fresh or dried berries that have been crushed or powdered. Steep 1 teaspoon of berries in 1-2 cups of boiled water for 20 minutes and strain. Dosage: 1-2 cups a day.

Fresh Berries may also be chewed and eaten. Dosage: ½-1 teaspoon a day.

Chemical Constituents

Chasteberry contains many flavonoids that are anti-inflammatory, antispasmodic, antibacterial, antifungal, anti-yeast, antioxidant, and anticarcinogenic (Hirobe, 1997). Flavonoids include kaempferol, quercetin, penduletin, chrysosplenol, vitexin (destroys leukemia cells by the process of apoptosis) and isovitexin. Casticin is a flavonoid that regulates and supports the immune system and is toxic to cancer cells (Mesaik, 2009). Iridoid glycosides include aucubin, which is antibacterial, antioxidant, antiprolactin (prolactin excess causes hormonal problems), diuretic, galactagogue, and a phytosterol. Diterpenes include rotundifuran and clerodadienols, which stimulate dopamine activity and reduce prolactin levels (Wuttke, 2003). Volatile oils include cineol (antibacterial, anti-inflammatory), pinene (anti-acne, antibacterial, anti-inflammatory), limonene, sabinene, castine, eucalyptol, myrcene, linalool, citronellol, cymene, camphene, carophyllene, farnesene, cardinene, and ledol. Cell culture experiments have shown that the flavonoid glycosides orientin, apigenin, vitexin, and penduletin bind to estrogen receptors and mediate estrogenic activity. These significantly increased blood levels of progesterone and estrogens, and reduced prolactin levels (Ibrahim, 2008; Jarry, 2003; Wuttke, 2003).

Safety, Contraindications, and Drug Interactions

Clinical studies and an extensive history of folk use validate Chasteberry's safety, even when taken over long periods of time. However, it is not an herb for children. Side effects are rare and have not been observed in my clinical practice, but may include minor skin irritations and itchy rash, stomach upset, dry mouth, headaches, agitation, fatigue, or bleeding between menstrual periods (Brown, 1996). When depression is a predominant premenstrual complaint, estrogen deficiency may be the cause. In this case, Chasteberry could worsen this type of depression and should not be taken.

Chasteberry influences pituitary activity and hormonal balance and may affect or counteract birth control pills and hormone replacement therapy (HRT), so should not be taken in conjunction with these (Brinker, 2001). Due to its ability to bind to dopamine receptors, it is not given with dopamine-related medications because of possible interaction (Jarry, 1991 & 1994; Skenderi, 2003). Although references often recommend avoiding it during pregnancy due to its emmenagogue effect of stimulating menstruation, I (and other practitioners) have seen Chasteberry successfully prevent miscarriages during the first trimester in women with progesterone deficiency. Some references also state that it is contraindicated during lactation, but the berries have historically been used as a galactagogue and several German researchers conducting clinical studies found that the berries safely help maintain adequate levels of milk production (Brown, 1994; Mohr, 1954; Weiss, 1988).

Medicinal Uses

History of the Plant

Chasteberry has been used as a medicinal herb since antiquity and is mentioned in the writings of Hippocrates, Dioscorides, and Theophrastus. Hippocrates (*circa* 460–*c.* 377 B.C.) recommended the herb for injuries, inflammation, and enlarged spleen. He steeped the berries and leaves in red wine to ease female reproductive problems and to treat hemorrhage following childbirth. Dioscorides (*c.* A.D. 40–*c.* 90), the Greek physician who lived during the time of the Roman Empire, used the berries for snake bites and stimulating milk flow in nursing mothers. A decoction of leaves and seeds was given for uterine inflammation and to lower libido in men. Pliny the Elder (A.D. 23–79) prescribed the herb for women's reproductive complaints and to promote normal menstruation and lactation. The Greek physician Galen (*c.* A.D. 131–*c.* 200) wrote in his herbal, "Agnus-castus is a singular remedy and medicine for such as would willingly live chaste, for it withstands all uncleanliness, or desire to the flesh, consuming and drying up the seed of generation. The seeds and leaves are good against pain and inflammation of the uterus." He recommended the seeds for stomachaches and gas, and to open obstructions of the liver and spleen. According to one of the most famous Arab pharmacists and physicians, Avicenna (*c.* A.D. 980–1037), who used the seeds in sitz baths, "Sitting in a decoction of chaste tree seed is effective against pains and tumors in the uterus." Arab physicians also prescribed it as an analgesic, anti-inflammatory, and cure for insanity (Alakbarov, 2003).

The species name *agnus-castus* is derived from the Latin word *agnus*, meaning "lamb," and *castus*, which translates as "chaste." As the name "chaste tree" suggests, this plant has a reputation for helping quell sexual passions and was believed to inspire chastity in both men and women. In ancient Greece, the leaves of Chasteberry were associated with priestesses of the goddess Demeter, who took vows of chastity. During the Middle Ages, when European monasteries regularly served monks the spicy berries to flavor food and help them remain chaste, the herb was commonly called "monk's pepper." The leaves were often sown into their robes or scattered on monastery pathways and floors as novice monks entered monastic life. When parted from each other, wives often placed the herb upon their husband's bed as a promise of fidelity. In Europe, a tea of the berries has long been given for the pain of rheumatism and arthritis because it decreases spasms and relaxes muscles. It also has traditional uses for treating coughs, colds, and stomach problems.

During the early 1900s, the American Eclectic physicians prescribed a tincture of the fresh berries to women with menstrual problems and to improve inadequate milk production in nursing mothers (Blumenthal, 2000). After the demise of Eclectic medicine in America during the late 1930s, Chasteberry continued to be a popular phytomedicine in Europe. Since the 1950s, the Madaus Company in Germany has produced a commercially available alcohol extract of the ripe berries called Agnolyt. Many German researchers have investigated the biological effects and chemical constituents in the berries and leaves. About 32 clinical trials were conducted on Chasteberry between 1943–1997 to evaluate and validate its effectiveness in treating menstrual problems, mastitis, fibrocystic breast disease, menopausal symptoms, insufficient lactation, and abnormal uterine bleeding (Hobbs, 1998). It remains a popular herbal remedy that is highly recommended by many herbalists to normalize the female reproductive system by balancing hormonal output.

Healing Qualities

Chasteberry is alterative and tonic to the hypothalamus, pituitary gland, ovaries and uterus, anticarcinogenic, anti-inflammatory, antimicrobial, emmenagogue, and galactagogue.

Traditional Chinese Medicine (TCM) Perspective

TCM physicians use the dried fruits of the Asian species, *Vitex trifolia* and *V. rotundifolia*, both referred to as Man Jing Zi, for medicinal purposes. The berries are bitter, drying, and slightly cooling. They are relaxing to the nervous system while stimulating and normalizing to the reproductive system. Vitex helps resolve Liver Qi Stagnation and tones and circulates Uterine Qi to harmonize reproductive hormones and the menstrual cycle. It resolves congestion, drains fluids, and stimulates glandular activity. In TCM, the herb is used for wind and heat problems of fever, headache, dizziness, and neuromuscular pains.

Primary Actions

Vitex agnus-castus is one of my favorite and most reliable herbs to help normalize hormone levels and regulate the female reproductive system. It promotes increased progesterone levels and is an excellent treatment for women experiencing an imbalance in the estrogen-to-progesterone ratio, with an excess of estrogen and deficiency of progesterone. For hundreds of years, the berries have been used to treat reproductive problems caused by this imbalance. Chasteberry's action is slow but sure. To restore the hormonal system, it is best taken as a tonic for an extended period of time, up to 12 months or more.

Over the years, many women have come to me seeking help for menstrual problems, infertility, miscarriages, fibrocystic breasts, uterine fibroids, endometriosis, and menopausal symptoms, including hot flashes. I have experienced the greatest satisfaction witnessing Chasteberry's amazing ability to relieve so many of these problems without side effects. Several women who were heart-broken because they had suffered miscarriages or could not get pregnant became happy mothers by using this herb.

Dynamics of the Menstrual Cycle: The menstrual cycle is regulated by complex interactions between the ovaries and hormones of the hypothalamus and pituitary glands in the brain. The hypothalamus secretes a gonadotropin-releasing hormone (GnRH) that stimulates the anterior pituitary to produce and release **follicle stimulating hormone (FSH)** and **luteinizing hormone (LH)**. The menstrual cycle has two distinct phases called the **follicular phase** and **luteal phase**. At the start of the **follicular phase**, FSH is released by the pituitary and finds its way to the ovaries. FSH stimulates ovarian follicles containing an ovum, or egg, to mature and move toward the surface of the ovary. During this phase, the follicles secrete estrogen, which promotes release of LH from the pituitary. Over a period of two weeks, the levels of FSH and LH increase to stimulate maturation and rupture of a follicle through the ovary at the time of ovulation. FSH is the primary hormone responsible for the maturation of follicles into fertile eggs, and for the increased production of estrogen by the ovaries. LH causes the release of an egg from the ovary at ovulation and stimulates development of the corpus luteum, which produces progesterone.

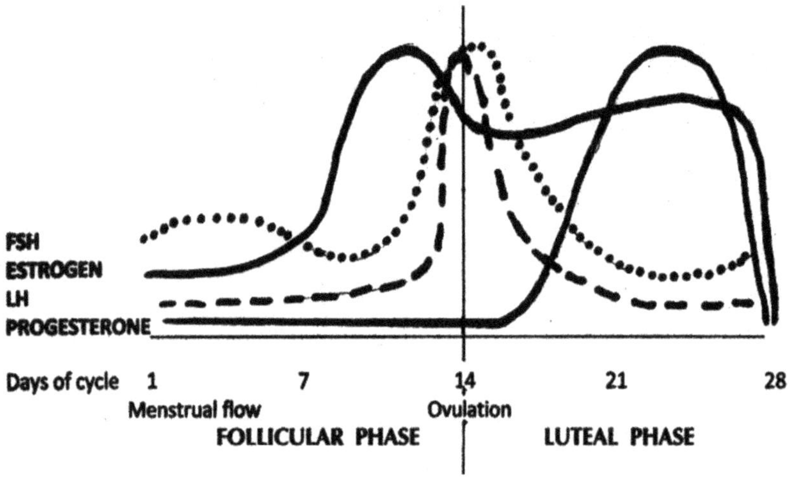

Representation of Hormone Levels During a Menstrual Cycle

The **luteal phase** begins after ovulation, when cells from the ruptured follicle remaining in the ovary undergo a rapid increase in size to become the corpus luteum. If the egg becomes fertilized and pregnancy occurs, the corpus luteum grows and primarily secretes progesterone and some estrogen until the end of pregnancy. If there is no fertilization, the corpus luteum secretes these hormones and reaches maximum development within about ten days, and then rapidly deteriorates.

Estrogen is the primary hormone secreted by ovarian follicle cells during the follicular phase, typically the first 14 days of the menstrual cycle. As the size of the follicle increases, it progressively secretes more estrogen. **Progesterone is the primary hormone secreted by the corpus luteum during the luteal phase during the last 14 days of the cycle**. When there is a progesterone deficiency, estrogen continues to dominate the luteal phase and promotes menstrual irregularities, including amenorrhea (absence of periods), menorrhagia (abnormally heavy or long menstruation), anovulation (lack of ovulation), mid-cycle bleeding and abnormal spotting, premenstrual syndrome (PMS), fluid retention, breast swelling and pain, uterine fibroids, endometriosis, infertility, miscarriage, and menopausal complaints. This condition of excess estrogen and deficient progesterone is known as **luteal phase defect**.

Another problem frequently associated with luteal phase defect is overproduction of **prolactin**. Prolactin is a hormone released by the pituitary that has numerous target organs, including mammary glands and the corpus luteum in the ovaries. Prolactin promotes the growth of breast tissue and stimulates milk production in lactating women. In non-lactating women, prolactin should be in balance with FSH and LH. Excessive prolactin inhibits maturation of eggs in the ovary and the corpus luteum's release of progesterone, potentially causing progesterone deficiency, infertility, short menstrual cycles, PMS, breast pain, and other symptoms of luteal phase defect.

Menstruation and Premenstrual Syndrome (PMS): Chasteberry affects the female reproductive system by its stimulating and normalizing action on hypothalamus and pituitary gland function, which in turn regulates estrogen and progesterone levels. The herb is exceptional in adjusting hormonal imbalances, specifically estrogen dominance and progesterone deficiency, as described in the luteal phase defect.

Early scientific evidence showed that Chasteberry increases secretion of LH and inhibits the release of FSH levels, producing a net effect of increased progesterone secretion from the corpus luteum (Amnon, 1965). More recent studies have focused on the herbs' ability to reduce high prolactin levels during the luteal phase (Milewicz, 1993). Prolactin tends to be abnormally high in approximately 70% of women with symptoms of luteal phase defect (Muhlenstedt, 1978). When investigating how Chasteberry diminished elevated prolactin levels, several research teams conducting clinical and *in vitro* studies found that diterpenes in the berries bind directly to dopamine receptors on the pituitary gland. This stimulates dopamine secretion, which suppresses release of abnormally high prolactin levels (Jarry, 1991 & 1994; Klaus-Jurgen, 1997; Sliutz, 1993; Wuttke, 2003). Short menstrual cycles are often related to insufficient progesterone secretion by the corpus luteum, and Chasteberry can prolong the luteal phase of the cycle (Schulz, 1998). In a double-blind, placebo-controlled

> *Chasteberry normalizes female hormones by safely balancing levels of estrogen and progesterone.*

clinical study focusing on 52 women with luteal phase defects due to elevated prolactin, participants received daily doses of one capsule (20 mg) of Chasteberry or a placebo. After 3 months, women taking the herb experienced lower prolactin levels, increased progesterone levels, and normalized menstrual cycles. No side effects were reported, and two women treated with the herbal preparation succeeded in becoming pregnant (Milewicz, 1993).

Due to all these actions, Chasteberry is helpful for many menstrual problems and PMS symptoms, including irregular periods, cramps, mood swings and irritability, excessive bleeding, mid-cycle spotting, fluid retention, breast pain, headaches, and food cravings. European women often use the herb to normalize menstruation and ovulation after discontinuing birth control pills. An abundance of clinical trials validate many of these attributes.

A large study of 1,571 women with low progesterone and elevated estrogen levels revealed that 90% of the women who took 40 drops of a standardized Chasteberry extract daily for 4.5 months experienced good results in reducing PMS and other menstrual problems. Only 2% of the women experienced minor side effects (Feldmann, 1990). Another clinical study involved 551 women who experienced menstrual disorders and PMS. After taking 40 drops of Chasteberry extract daily for about 4 months, 32% of the women reported improvement in their symptoms within the first 4 weeks. Following 3 months of treatment, 84% of the women reported improvement. During the trial, 33 women (42%) with infertility problems became pregnant (Peters-Welte, 1994).

A 3-month, double-blind clinical study of 127 women revealed that 77% of those who ingested daily doses of Chasteberry had greater reduction in PMS symptoms compared to the group taking only vitamin B6. Noticeable improvements in breast tenderness, fluid retention, fatigue, tension, headaches, and constipation were reported by participants receiving Chasteberry (Lauritzen, 1997).

Several clinical studies concur that 40-80 drops of Chasteberry extract taken daily for 3 months can reduce blood levels of prolactin and significantly alleviate breast pain (Carmichael, 2008; Halaska, 1999; Wuttke, 2003). A trial involving 104 women with menstrual breast pain demonstrated that those who took 30 drops of the liquid extract twice daily for 3 months experienced pain reduction and improvement of other menstrual complaints, including cramps, edema, headaches, and mood swings (Wuttke, 1997).

Efficacy of a Chasteberry extract was investigated in a multicenter trial involving 1,634 women suffering from PMS. After a treatment period lasting 3 menstrual cycles, 93% reported decreased depression, anxiety, food craving, and water retention. Analysis of frequency and severity of breast pain as the predominant symptom showed that 3 months of therapy diminished much of the pain without problematic side effects. While no women were pregnant at the start of the study, 23 conceived while on Vitex treatment. Nineteen of these women were from a group of 126 women who had been unsuccessful at becoming pregnant (Loch, 2000). In a placebo-controlled clinical study, 170 women with PMS were divided into two groups, one receiving an alcohol extract of Chasteberry and the other taking a placebo daily for 3 menstrual cycles. Interestingly, 11 women receiving the herb also took oral contraceptives with no reported adverse interactions. Those using Chasteberry reported reduced headaches, breast tenderness, irritability, and other PMS symptoms (Schellenberg, 2001). Acne that flares up around menstruation is often caused by estrogen dominance and progesterone deficiency, in which case Chasteberry can also be beneficial (Amann, 1975; Feldmann, 1990).

> *Problems with menstruation, menopause, infertility, fibroids, and endometriosis can be due to estrogen excess and progesterone deficiency.*

Amenorrhea is the abnormal cessation of menstruation frequently associated with high blood levels of prolactin, which inhibits maturation of eggs. Chasteberry's ability to reduce excessive prolactin helps regulate this imbalance when taken over a period of time. In a small clinical study, 10 out of 15 women with amenorrhea resumed their periods after 6 months of taking Chasteberry daily. Lab tests revealed that they all experienced a beneficial increase in LH and progesterone levels (Loch, 1990).

Endometriosis and Uterine Fibroids: Endometriosis is an abnormal build-up of the endometrium, or inner lining, of the uterus. Uterine fibroids are non-malignant tumors growing in or on the uterus. Both conditions can originate from excessive estrogen, causing significant pain and abnormal bleeding. Chasteberry's ability to normalize the estrogen-to-progesterone ratio makes it helpful for all estrogen dominance problems. The berries also have an anti-inflammatory effect (Choudhary, 2009) on the uterus and endometrium, and regular use for 1-2 years can reduce endometriosis and the size of uterine fibroids.

Infertility, Miscarriage, and Pregnancy: Low progesterone and high prolactin levels are often underlying causes of infertility and miscarriages. Chasteberry restores balance to these hormones and provides sufficient progesterone necessary to initiate and maintain pregnancy. I have given Chasteberry tincture to several women experiencing infertility or a history of miscarriages with successful outcomes of full term pregnancies and healthy babies. One woman with a history of two miscarriages came to my office because she was one month pregnant and desperately wanted to have a baby. I recommended that she keep her progesterone levels elevated by ingesting 40 drops of Chasteberry tincture every morning and applying ½ teaspoon of a high quality Wild Yam progesterone cream on a daily basis. Following these suggestions, she successfully carried to full term without any complications and gave birth to a beautiful baby girl 8 months later.

A clinical study involving 45 women between the ages of 23-39 who were diagnosed with infertility demonstrated that after daily use of Chasteberry for 3 months, 7 women became pregnant and progesterone levels were restored to normal in 25 women. Seven other women had a rise in progesterone that did not completely reach normal levels, but researchers stated their belief that continued use of the herb would eventually promote normal levels (Propping, 1987). In another clinical study investigating 96 women with fertility problems, a placebo or a dose of 30 drops of a Chasteberry extract called Mastodynon were given twice a day over a period of 3 months. Women receiving Mastodynon experienced improved progesterone and prolactin levels, and 57% either resumed menstrual periods or became pregnant (Gerhard, 1998).

Lactation: Chasteberry also balances hormones by promoting high prolactin levels when necessary for lactation, while decreasing prolactin levels when they are pathologically or abnormally high. For many centuries, Chasteberry has been used as a galactagogue to stimulate milk production in nursing mothers without altering the composition of breast milk, and there is scientific validation for this tradition. In a large study, 353 new mothers with poor milk production experienced significant improvement using Chasteberry after only 7 days, compared with 362 other women taking a placebo (Mohr, 1954). The best way to stimulate milk production is to take Chasteberry immediately after birth. It can also be ingested to re-establish regular menstrual cycles following pregnancy and lactation.

Fibrocystic Disease, Breast Tumors, and Cancer: Most tumors, cancers, and cysts of the breast, uterus, and ovaries are estrogen-dependent. Estrogen dominance with progesterone deficiency promotes these abnormal growths, as well as precancerous cells lining the cervix, known as cervical dysplasia. Long-term use of Chasteberry can be beneficial in the treatment of these conditions.

Research shows that the berries exhibit anticarcinogenic properties (Ohyama, 2003). Casticin is a flavonoid in Chasteberry with potent immunomodulatory and cytotoxic activities (Mesaik, 2009). When a university team in Florida evaluated 374 herbal extracts for their efficacy in destroying tumor cells, data demonstrated Chasteberry to be one of the strongest plants that inhibited tumors (Mazzio, 2009). *In vitro* studies confirm that Chasteberry extract specifically inhibits growth of breast cancer cells (Dixon-Shanies, 1999).

Chasteberry also has potential for treating colon cancer. The proliferation of a human colon carcinoma cell line was effectively suppressed through apoptosis induced by flavonoids in an extract of *Vitex agnus-castus* berries. Researchers concluded that the herb activates a pathway to restore apoptosis, the programmed self-destruction of cells when they become cancerous (Imai, 2009). Researchers have documented that vitexin in the berries exhibited antitumor activity in liver cancer cells by inducing apoptosis (Wang, 2014).

Menopause: Regular use of Chasteberry extract helps restore dwindling progesterone levels that naturally drop during menopause. The herb helps restore thickness and moisture to vaginal walls, and is beneficial for reducing menopausal symptoms of hot flashes, mood swings, headaches, and dizziness. The herb is also helpful for women who experience uncomfortable menopausal symptoms following a hysterectomy.

The efficacy and safety of a formula containing standardized extracts of Chasteberry, Black Cohosh, Dong Quai, Milk Thistle, Red Clover, and American Ginseng was evaluated for its ability to relieve menopausal hot flashes and sleep-depriving night sweats. In a placebo-controlled trial, 50 healthy pre- and postmenopausal women, aged 44-65 years, ingested this formula or a placebo twice daily for 3 months. Those receiving the herbal formula reported significant reductions in menopausal symptoms compared to the placebo group. The effect of treatment improvements increased over time, and by 3 months there was a 73% decrease in hot flashes and a 69% reduction of night sweats, accompanied by a decrease in their intensity and significant benefit in terms of sleep quality. Hot flashes completely ended in 47% of women in the study group compared with only 19% in the placebo group (Rotem, 2007).

The phytoestrogen activities in Chasteberry's flavonoids promote strong bones and mineral uptake, as evidenced by animal studies in which ingestion of *Vitex agnus-castus* extracts increased bone mass and promoted healing of fractures (Oztürk, 2008; Sehmisch, 2009). In a small clinical trial, about 25 women who took 4 mg of dried Chasteberry extract daily for 8 weeks experienced improved healing of their bone fractures compared to those who did not use the herb (Eftekhari, 2014). Chasteberry can be beneficial for prevention and treatment of osteopenia and osteoporosis (conditions of bone loss and brittleness) when combined with a nutritious diet, plenty of physical activity, and high quality calcium, magnesium, boron, and vitamin D supplements.

Men's Health: Much mythology and historic use of Chasteberry was based on the belief that the berries reduce sexual urges in men, although this notion is questionable. In the male reproductive system, luteinizing hormone (LH) stimulates development of interstitial cells in the testes and their secretion of testosterone. Most experts consider excessive levels of testosterone to play a role in benign prostatic hypertrophy (BPH) and prostate cancers, and allopathic treatment focuses on reducing testosterone levels. Interesting research has shed some light on the plant's influence on males.

In one animal study, a Chasteberry extract significantly decreased LH and testosterone serum levels, indicating potential use in treating BPH (Nasri, 2007). Data derived from other research suggest that the herb contains components that induce apoptosis and inhibit proliferation of human prostate cancer cells (Weisskopf, 2005).

Nervous system: Chasteberry has a calming effect on the nervous system and is beneficial in relieving mood swings and anxiety associated with PMS, menopause, and mid-life crisis. British herbalist Maude Grieve wrote, "The fresh ripe berries are pounded into a pulp and used in the form of a tincture for the relief of paralysis, pains in the limbs, and weakness" (Grieve, 1971). One practitioner found that the berries have significant ability to decrease drug cravings, especially withdrawal from heroin (Yarnell, 2003). This may be due to Chasteberry's ability to bind to dopamine receptors. Dopamine, a neurotransmitter that elicits comfortable feelings of well-being, is usually depleted during heroin addiction.

Teachings from the Chasteberry Deva

"Greetings, dear one. I am the keeper of the Chastity bush. I am of a feminine nature and my action on the body is steady and gentle. My bluish-purple flowers reflect my beneficial influence on the brain and nervous system, and I am calming to the mind, emotions, and even the soul. Being especially helpful for women, my berries help normalize the reproductive system by affecting the brain centers that control the workings of the ovaries and cycles of fertility. I help women flow through the cycles of nature, the seasons, and all transitions at very deep levels within the physical, emotional, and awareness being. For like the Black Cohosh, I am also ruled by the astrological energies of Scorpio that regulate creativity, reproduction, birth, death, and all transitions. I am most strongly aligned to female energies, and my very expansive essence nurtures and brings freedom for the full expression of feminine qualities.

"How interesting that the name people gave me, Chasteberry, refers to my influence upon men rather than on women, whom I primarily serve. Celibate monks once ingested me to diminish their masculine sexual drive. In women, however, my energies serve to balance the male and female energies; for all humans contain both male and female essence. And so my offering to humans is mainly for women. I offer the seeds of my being to balance and bring regularity to the life of the seeds in women's ovaries and womb, and also breathe life into the seeds of your creativity at a very deep level. This is our connection.

"I help to instill balance between the heart and mind, and when this is fully complete, great peace, contentment, and oneness with nature and all women are experienced. I may be used in all phases of reproductive life, and resonate with older women who pass through the transition from fertile beings to non-fertile – as you would say, the time of menopause. At this time, I help balance and stabilize the chemistry of the brain and ovaries. I assist in the natural transition during menopause when the reproductive powers of the womb diminish, and creativity becomes more established in the higher centers of the brain. New dimensions of creativity are available to women when the bleeding times have ceased. When women relax and move into this new but very natural dimension, there is a feeling of expansion, adventure, and yes, some exhilarating wildness! My qualities allow for much expansion and movement of energies into new growth cycles, and I am good medicine for moving into this higher octave and new cycle of female creativity.

"So come sit by me and feel my presence close to you. Allow me to make your journey easier and more gentle. My lessons are to move through each transition of your life with acceptance and celebration, and to learn the wisdom each one has to offer. Know that the flow of life moves through all things, through billions of women before you and billions that will come after you. Know that this pulse of life flowing through womankind is a sacred seed entrusted to you. Be yielding, accepting, and trusting of this life that flows through you. Do not mistakenly think you are in charge of the flow — all is the activity of Creator. The flow of life cannot be controlled or grasped, for it has its own movement and purpose. As you learn to trust and accept its flow through your body and your being, rather than tenaciously clinging or fearfully running away, if you gently rest in the hand of the Mother and life itself, your way will be easier with less suffering. Know that all aspects of your life, the joyful and difficult, can bring wisdom and wholeness to your being.

"Therefore, use me during times of movement and transition to help maintain your center. For your physical body, like all of life, comes into being, constantly changes, and grows older. Find peace in this truth and cling to love, kindness and light, rather than to things that eventually pass away into nothingness . . . .

"Look outside yourself and observe the flow of life in Nature, and then look within yourself and observe the same flow and natural cycles. For there is no separation between you and Nature. All arise from the same seed of life contained in the womb of the Great Mother. Each transition offers new and exciting insights into your true nature, which is radiance, love, and awareness. Through each journey you traverse, may you relax and open to this core and womb of your being, which is always present to be fully lived and experienced."

Chickweed

Stellaria media
Caryophyllaceae (Carnation or Pink) Family

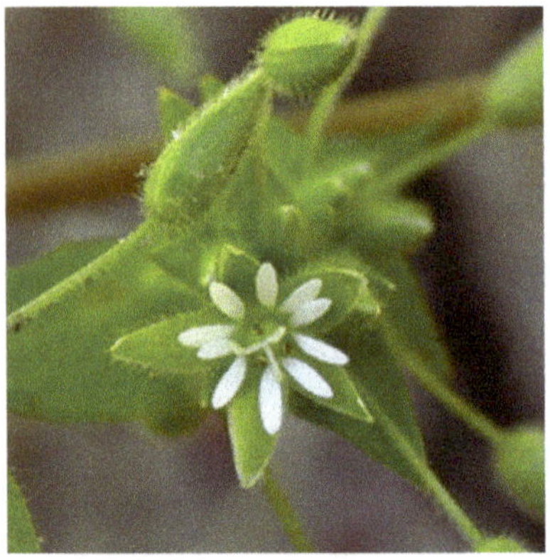

***Stellaria media* flower**

Common Names

Starwort, star chickweed, starweed, white bird's eye, stitchwort, satin flower, adder's mouth, winter weed, tongue-grass, and mouse-ear are antiquated names descriptive of the flower's appearance.

Medicinal Part of the Plant

The entire aerial portions, including leaves, stems and flowers, are used for medicinal applications.

Range and Habitat

There are an estimated 90-120 species of Chickweed. *Stellaria media* is indigenous to vast areas of Europe and Asia. One of the most common "weeds" that takes up permanent residence in a wide variety of soils, it has naturalized in North America and temperate regions all over the world, even in the Arctic. It grows abundantly in many fields, wastelands, and woodlands in moist, shady places and under full sun. It often finds its way into cultivated fields and gardens where it appears every spring.

Description of the Plant

S. media is a small annual or biennial plant, usually growing no taller than 6-12". The fibrous, thready roots develop close to the ground surface. Weak, tangling stems are decumbent and diffuse, lying on the ground and spreading outward from the center. Many plants often form massive mats of foliage. The round stems are green and tinged with maroon. *S. media* is easily identified by the single line of fine hairs extending along one side of each stem in a single band. All other species in the family *Carophyllaceae* have hairs uniformly covering their entire stem. The sepals of *S. media* are also covered with the fine hairs. Simple, ovate leaves are entire and arise opposite along the stems. Lower leaves have petioles (stalks) attaching to stems, and upper leaves are sessile (lacking stalks). The fleshy leaves are smooth with pinnate venation, growing ½-1" long. The entire plant, including the stems, is a juicy succulent.

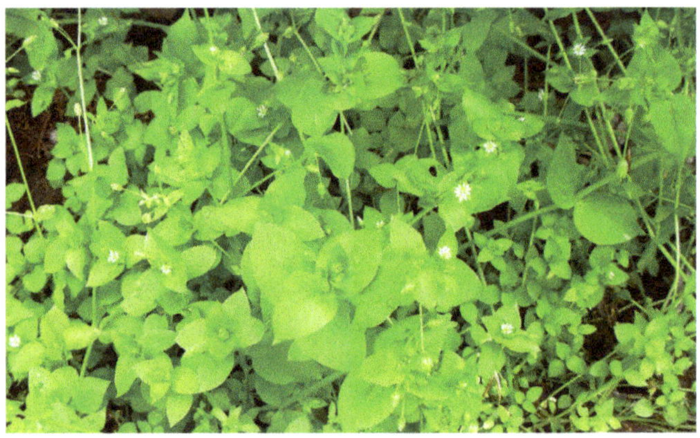

***Stellaria media* plants**

Tiny white flowers are ¼" across, emerging singly or in terminal clusters at the ends of stems. The 5 petals are so deeply divided into two parts that they appear to be 10. The 5 light-green sepals are hairy and longer than the petals. The number of stamens varies from 3, 5, or 10. Varieties of Chickweed in the genus *Stellaria* contain 3 styles emerging from the ovary, while those in the closely related genus *Cerastium* have 5 styles. Flower petals open on sunny days and close at night and on cloudy days. The plant appears in early spring and blooms into the summer months.

Cultivation

Chickweed is one of the most prolific and hardy herbs, often misunderstood to be a useless weed. The plant grows in most conditions but prefers cool, moist soil high in humus content. Cultivation is seldom necessary because it freely self-seeds and grows as a ground cover in so many areas. Once established, it hardly ever disappears. However, if cultivation is desired, the seeds can be planted in rich soil in late autumn or very early spring. Press the tiny seeds into the soil without covering them, and keep them moist.

Early every spring, some of my gardens are full of two varieties of *Stellaria*. After harvesting sufficient amounts for food and medicine, I used to work like a wild woman trying to weed them out, but eventually realized that it was more productive and less frustrating to change my attitude about this persistent plant rather than trying to get it out of my garden. Now I regard it as "beneficial green manure" that gets mixed into the soil to add nitrogen and become humus. What is not worked into the soil usually dies out in late spring after it completes its cycle. So the lovely and tenacious Chickweed is embraced as a welcome gardening companion that enriches the soil, offers a wealth of nutrients, and provides good medicine. It has been an interesting teacher!

Harvest

S. media leaves, flowers, and stems are all succulent and can be harvested when blooming begins in early spring. Chickweed can be gathered into the summer months as long as the plants retain vitality. To harvest the seeds, collect the seedpods formed after flowering and store them in a bag or box. As the pods dry, the tiny seeds will spill out into the container for easier collection.

Preparation of Plant Medicine and Dosages

Freshly harvested Chickweed, significantly more potent than the dried, is preferred for medicinal use. Water and alcohol both extract the chemical components, so the fresh plant may be tinctured, prepared as tea or salve, or used externally as a poultice or fomentation. It may also be dried or frozen for future use. I encourage people to use Chickweed tea rather than tincture because the medicinal emollient properties are left intact when brewed in water, while alcohol tends to greatly reduce them. The tea may be freely ingested, and daily use is encouraged for chronic problems and excessively dry conditions.

PREPARATIONS

Tea: Steep 1-2 tablespoons of fresh or dried leaves, flowers, and stems in a cup of boiled water for 10-15 minutes. To make a stronger infusion, gently simmer 6-8 heaping tablespoons of the herb in a quart of water for 4 minutes and then steep for 30 minutes. Dosage: 1-3 cups daily. The tea is mild and pleasant-tasting, resembling the flavor of spinach.

Tincture: Prepare in the standard way by combining the fresh herb with a mix of 40% 190-proof grain alcohol and 60% distilled water. Less alcohol is used to extract and preserve the healing mucilage. Dosage: 1-2 teaspoons in water up to 3 times a day.

Salve: Due to their high water content, allow the stems and leaves to dry out partially before baking them in oil. Chickweed is a wonderful addition to salves and should be combined with other vulnerary herbs (refer to "Skin Problems" on page 591 in the "Index of Health Issues and Herbal Recommendations" for suggestions).

Poultice: Bruise, chop, or blend fresh leaves into a pulpy mash and apply this as a poultice for external problems. Dried leaves can be used by crumbling them into little pieces, or grinding into powder, and adding enough water to make a paste. Apply over the affected area, bind the poultice in place with ace wrap, and keep the herbs moist. Change the poultice 2-3 times during the day.

Bath or Fomentation of the strong tea can soothe inflammation, itchiness, rashes, and encourage tissue repair.

Juice: The fresh plant can be juiced or mixed in a blender and ingested or applied for external healing. For a nutritious and soothing drink, add it to fruit or vegetable juices.

Culinary Uses

The fresh leaves and flowers have a mild, pleasant flavor and can be used as salad greens or steamed and eaten like spinach. They are full of vitamins and minerals, making a nutritious addition to soups, stir-fry vegetables, scrambled eggs, and casseroles. Try steaming or sautéing Chickweed with other greens like Plantain (*Plantago* spp.), Stinging Nettle (*Urtica dioica*), and Dandelion (*Taraxacum officinale)* greens in early spring when the leaves are tender.

Chemical Constituents

Chickweed is an incredibly nutritious herb containing vitamins, minerals, and even protein. Nutrients include beta-carotene (the plant form of vitamin A), several of the B vitamins (B1, B2, B3), vitamin C, tocopherols (vitamin E), and easily digested minerals, including calcium, iron, magnesium, potassium, phosphorus, copper, manganese, chromium, cobalt, silicon, selenium, and zinc. Other compounds include coumarins, fatty acids such as gamma-linolenic and oleic acids, polysaccharide mucilage, and stearic and palmitic acids.

Other chemical groups identified in Chickweed consist of glycosides, phytosterols, and flavonoids, including rutin and apigenin. Flavonoid components promote antioxidant activity (Budzianowski, 1991). Genistein is a phytosterol thought to act as a cancer-preventative by preventing blood vessels from delivering nutrients to developing tumors. Saponins also diminish tumor formation (Duke, 1996).

Safety, Contraindications, and Drug Interactions

Stellaria media has a long tradition of folk use and is generally regarded as very safe and non-toxic. It is a mild herb that can be safely used in large doses and combined with other herbs. There are no known contraindications, side effects, or problematic interactions with drugs (Skenderi, 2003).

Medicinal Uses

History of the Plant

Native American Indians used indigenous varieties of Chickweed as a poultice for wounds, skin diseases, inflammation, and itching. The Chippewa made tea from the leaves as a wash for sore and irritated eyes. It was ingested for respiratory problems, coughs, sore throats, and the flu. Ancient Europeans employed *S. media* in similar ways and prescribed it for tuberculosis. The tasty leaves were often a welcome addition to foods among country people. Nicholas Culpeper (1616–1654), the English apothecary and astrological herbalist, wrote that it is "a fine, soft, pleasing herb, under the dominion of the Moon" (Culpeper, 1992). John Gerard (1545–1612) and other European medical herbalists used it for wound healing, ulcers, inflammation and arthritic pain, as did the American Eclectic physicians in the late 1800s and early 1900s. The Eclectics also used it for acute eye inflammation and erysipelas (a streptococcal skin infection).

The Swedish botanist Carl Linnaeus (1707–1778) named this herb *Stellaria,* meaning "little star," in reference to the star-like appearance of the delicate white flowers. *Media* is Latin for "in the midst of," which creates an image of being in the midst of little stars when standing in a patch of Chickweed. Wild birds, chickens, and other domesticated birds eat Chickweed seeds, and some of the common names of this plant are derived from its use as bird feed.

Although people continue to enjoy Chickweed as food and medicine, it is not a popular or commercially sold remedy. Researchers have identified chemical components in several *Stellaria* species indicating the plant's biological activity, but clinical studies are lacking.

Healing Qualities

Alterative, antacid, anti-inflammatory, antioxidant, antiscorbutic, antitumor, carminative, demulcent, mild diuretic, emollient, expectorant, febrifuge, hepatoprotective, laxative, lymphagogue, mucilage, nutritive, opthalmicum, pectoral, resolvent, and restorative.

Traditional Chinese Medicine (TCM) Perspective

Chickweed is a classic Yin tonic, as it is extremely moistening, lubricating, cooling, and nourishing. It is indicated for all Yin deficiency conditions of heat and dryness, especially Lung, Stomach, Kidney, and Heart Yin deficiency. It clears excess heat caused by Yin deficiency, restores moisture, and softens tissues throughout the body. *S. media* is a traditional Chinese medicine that has been used for over 2,000 years, mainly for the treatment of dermatitis and other skin diseases. It has also been used as an anti-viral agent (Ma, 2012).

Primary Actions

Chickweed is a cooling and soothing herb traditionally given for dehydration and "hot" problems associated with blood toxicity, fevers, or inflammation. It helps any form of internal and external inflammation, and is healing and moisturizing to all mucous membranes and tissues upon contact. Due to its abundance of nutrients, Chickweed is a nourishing tea and food for all ages, including young children. This plant is very mild and is often combined with stronger herbs or to balance effects of heat-promoting herbs when treating specific health problems.

Respiratory System: Chickweed's demulcent and emollient qualities soothe and moisten dry, inflamed, irritated tissues, making it beneficial for most bronchial and lung problems. The herb is an excellent expectorant that helps to liquefy and dislodge thick, congested mucous. Its cooling property reduces fever and inflammation. It is indicated for dry coughs, including smoker's cough, bronchitis and other lung infections, asthma, and emphysema. Drinking 2-4 cups of the tea every day for several months can help heal chronic lung problems involving dryness and irritation, which are perpetuated by dry air and smoking. Gargle and drink the tea for sore throats and hoarseness. Use it sparingly, if at all, for conditions involving excessive fluids in the lungs. I always combine Chickweed with other herbs appropriate for specific lung and bronchial conditions.

> *Chickweed's valuable moisturizing, lubricating, and cooling qualities are excellent for treating many respiratory problems.*

Digestive System and Liver Protection: The soothing, cooling, and moisturizing nature of this plant also benefits the digestive organs. It is excellent for weak and debilitated people with poor nutrition and malabsorption problems. An abundance of alkaline minerals helps restore normal stomach function, reduce excess acidity, and nourish the blood. The plant heals and protects the inner mucosal lining of the stomach and intestines, and is wonderful for excess stomach acid causing heartburn and acid reflux, as well as gastric and intestinal ulcers and inflammation.

Chickweed soothes liver irritation and inflammation while increasing bile flow. For these reasons, and because it moistens the intestines, it can help remedy chronic constipation. The leaves contain rutin, a bioflavonoid that strengthens weak blood vessels, making it helpful for hemorrhoids.

A few scientific studies have shed some light on the herb's antiviral action and ability to protect the liver from damage caused by hepatitis. When researchers evaluated the activity of *S. media* against hepatitis B virus in human liver cells, they demonstrated that a preparation of fresh Chickweed juice effectively suppressed the hepatitis B virus *in vitro*. Flavonoid C-glycosides, polysaccharides, and proteins were identified in the fresh juice and exhibited diverse antiviral activities (Ma, 2012). In another study involving rats infected with the hepatitis virus, water-soluble polysaccharides isolated from Chickweed helped normalize liver enzymes adversely affected by the hepatitis. Liver inflammation and incidence of liver cell death due to hepatitis diminished with the herbal treatment. Blood levels of liver enzymes also stabilized, including serum glutamic oxaloacetic transaminase (SGOT), serum glutamic-pyruvic transaminase (SGPT), alkaline phosphatase, and bilirubin (Gorina, 2013).

Urinary Tract: Chickweed tea is beneficial for acute or chronic bladder and kidney weakness, infection, and inflammation. Several cups of tea may be ingested daily for the treatment of cystitis (bladder infection) and burning, scanty urine. The herb soothes urethral irritation and is a mild and safe diuretic to reduce water retention. For best results, always combine the tea or tincture with other appropriate herbs for urinary tract infections, such as Goldenrod (*Solidago* spp.), Yarrow (*Achillea millefolium*) and Goldenseal (*Hydrastis canadensis*).

Blood, Lymphatic, and Glandular Systems: An abundance of vitamins, minerals, and green chlorophyll in Chickweed nourishes the blood and tissues, contributes easily digested iron to improve anemia, and produces an alkalizing effect on blood and lymphatic fluids. This is useful in treating excess acidity throughout the system, in addition to cooling and detoxifying "hot" blood. Overly acidic, hot, toxic blood and lymphatic fluids are often underlying causes of cancers, tumors, swollen lymph nodes, and eruptive or chronic skin problems such as pimples, acne, boils, eczema, psoriasis, hives, and other rashes. The herb's cleansing and nourishing qualities improve glandular function, and the tea, tincture, and salve may be used to reduce swollen glands and lymph nodes.

Ability to Soften and Dissolve Cysts, Tumors, and Tissue Swelling: Chickweed contains saponins which have a soapy quality that increases permeability of tissues allowing more fluid and nutrient movement through the body. Saponins can soften and dissolve thick fibrous membranes, cysts and tumors, neutralize toxins, and weaken bacterial cell walls in preparation for destruction by the immune system. Chickweed is indicated for the treatment of mastitis and breast, ovarian, and uterine cysts and cancers in women. For men, the herb is helpful for prostate and testicular cancers and inflammation. The tea or tincture is taken internally, and a poultice may be applied externally for these purposes on a daily basis over a period of time.

Interestingly, an antiviral protein, designated as stellarmedin A, was isolated from *S. media* and inhibited the herpes simplex virus type 2 (the cause of genital herpes) during *in vitro* testing. The protein also inhibited proliferation of leukemia and colon carcinoma cells (Shan, 2013).

Arthritis and Gout: Chickweed soothes and lubricates painful and inflamed joints while also drawing out excess heat. The abundance of minerals and chlorophyll in the leaves neutralizes excess acids in the blood, which can be associated with joint pain, inflammation, and gout.

Skin, Wounds, Inflammation, and Eyes: Chickweed may be ingested as tea or tincture, or applied externally as a salve, poultice, or fomentation for hot, dry skin conditions and wounds. The demulcent and emollient constituents moisturize, lubricate, and cool tissues that are irritated, inflamed and damaged, including burns. It is very effective to relieve itching. The herb is cleansing and draws out infection, splinters, and venom. *In vitro* tests have shown that the plant possesses antioxidant properties that reduce oxidative stress along with the resulting tissue inflammation, damage, and cellular aging (Pieroni, 2002). Chickweed is helpful for most skin problems such as acne, boils, insect and animal bites, abscesses, ulcers, hives, poison ivy and poison oak, eczema, chicken pox, measles, mumps, diaper rash, and other rashes. It also soothes rashes caused by brushing against Stinging Nettle.

The herb is healing to both internal and external wounds. It can help prevent painful adhesions after surgery when a quart of tea is ingested daily for one week following the procedure. In *King's American Dispensatory*, one of the authoritative herbal manuals of the Eclectic physicians, Harvey Felter, M.D., wrote, "I have seen the fresh leaves bruised and applied as a poultice to indolent, intractable ulcers on the legs, of many years' standing, with the most decided and immediately beneficial results, to be changed 2 or 3 times a day" (Felter, 1898).

To treat eye inflammation or dryness, prepare Chickweed tea and strain it through coffee filter paper with care to remove all particles. Use the sterile tea as an eyewash. For best results, combine it with Goldenseal root tea, my favorite and most dependable remedy for eye infections or a stye (an inflamed swelling of a sebaceous gland on the margin of an eyelid usually caused by the *Staphylococcus aureus* bacteria). This formula is safe and quite effective for red, itchy, pus-filled eyes occurring with conjunctivitis (pink eye) and other bacterial infections, ulcerated eyelids, or irritation from pollen and allergies.

Bone Health and Osteoporosis: Considering the high mineral content of Chickweed, which includes calcium, magnesium, phosphorus and silica, the herb is beneficial in maintaining strong bones. According to Traditional Chinese Medicine, osteoporosis involves a fluid deficiency known as "Yin deficiency," allowing bones to become increasingly drier, brittle, and more breakable. This Yin, or fluid, deficiency is also part of the spectrum occurring during menopause, when tissues become more dehydrated and lose their elasticity, vaginal fluids dry up, and osteoporosis often progresses. Since *Stellaria* provides so much moisture to the body, it may be helpful in counteracting this aging process.

Weight Loss: Chickweed's folk tradition includes its reputation to promote weight loss. This may be related to its mild diuretic activity, possible regulatory effect on the thyroid gland, and tendency of saponins to dissolve fat. For best results, be sure to use Chickweed in addition to other weight loss methods, including calorie reduction, lots of exercise, and eating less at night.

Teachings from the Chickweed Deva

"Greetings, dear one. I am the deva of the Chickweed people. We are primarily of the water element and also contain a bit of the earth element. Our leaves and stems are juicy and succulent. When eaten or taken as tea, we influence fluids and secretions to move through the tissues, just as water seeps through the soil. We keep tissues clean, moist, and cool by washing away debris and offering life-giving water and nourishment. For in the human body, just as in plant bodies, nutrients and wastes are carried through watery fluids like blood, lymph, and urine. My action is gentle and requires time to bring change to the body. I lack the fire element and am not stimulating to the nervous system or warming to the tissues. I am cleansing and nourishing, and my white flowers reflect this aspect of purity.

"My water element is ruled by Pisces, the force of water that dissolves and washes away impurities and that which is no longer needed, so that freshness of health and new life may emerge. Taurus, the energy of springtime's fertility and abundance, rules my earth element. Just as water naturally flows into empty spaces, my roots easily take hold in fallow soil. In areas where I grow, I appear abundantly in a thick carpet of little green leaves speckled with tiny white flowers in early spring. Like the flavor of my leaves, my spirit is light, gentle and soft, not bitter or overpowering in any way. I am mild enough to be used for food as well as medicine.

"I am soothing and ease tightness throughout the tissues. I cleanse impurities not by harshness, but by the gentleness of my flowing, watery nature. My tea is best for this washing and dissolving action. Use me also with the bitter, stronger herbs that fight infections and harmful substances, and as they kill these things, I will wash and remove them from the body.

"I am a simple plant with a simple message: Be fluid in the flow of life. Honor and partake in the gifts of abundance, simplicity, and purity. Like water diffusing through the earth, be yielding, smooth and gentle, while constantly moving with intention and direction towards purification and nourishment on all levels of the heart, mind, and physical body. For this is the foundation of vibrant health and happy hearts."

Cinquefoil

Potentilla spp.
Rosaceae (Rose) Family

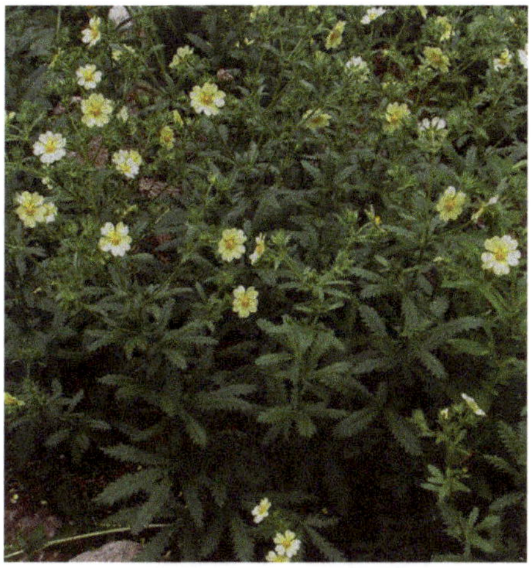

Potentilla recta

Common Names

Potentilla is a large genus containing over 300 species, several of which are medicinal. Cinquefoil plants are sometimes called Tormentil. Some of the medicinal species and their common names include:

Potentilla recta (Sulphur Cinquefoil or Rough-Fruited Cinquefoil);
P. reptans (Creeping Cinquefoil or Creeping Tormentil);
P. anserina (Silverweed);
P. norvegica (Rough Cinquefoil); and
P. tormentilla, P. erecta, Tormentilla erecta (This plant has several species names. Its common names include Tormentil, Septfoil, Erect Cinquefoil, Thornmantle, and Shepherd's Knot).

Medicinal Part of the Plant

Cinquefoil species, and the Rose family in general, contain large amounts of astringent tannins used in healing. When using the medicinal species, remember that the roots have the greatest concentration of tannins, but the leaves are also quite potent.

Range and Habitat

Potentilla species are native to Europe, temperate Asia, and North and South America. *P. recta* is native to Eurasia but was introduced into North America, where it grows throughout most of the continent, excluding the northernmost parts of Canada and Alaska. *P. tormentilla* and *P. reptans* are European species that have also naturalized in the United States. Cinquefoil plants grow in a variety of habitats, including dry fields and meadows, along roadsides, and by bodies of water.

Description of the Plant

Most plants in the genus *Potentilla* are hardy perennials, although a few are annuals and biennials. The root systems are fibrous and usually quite vigorous, sometimes sending out runners that can become invasive. Stems are rounded, hairy, and branched. Some stems are stout and others wiry. Some species (*P. reptans*) are creeping ground covers with prostrate stems reaching up to 1′ in height, while others (*P. recta*) have erect stems and grow up to 3′ tall.

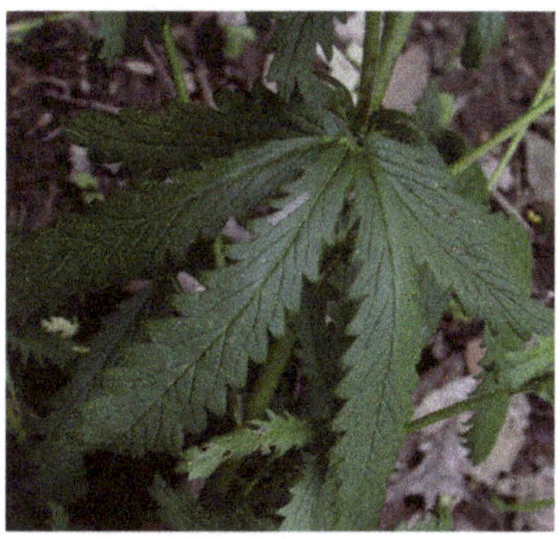

Potentilla recta

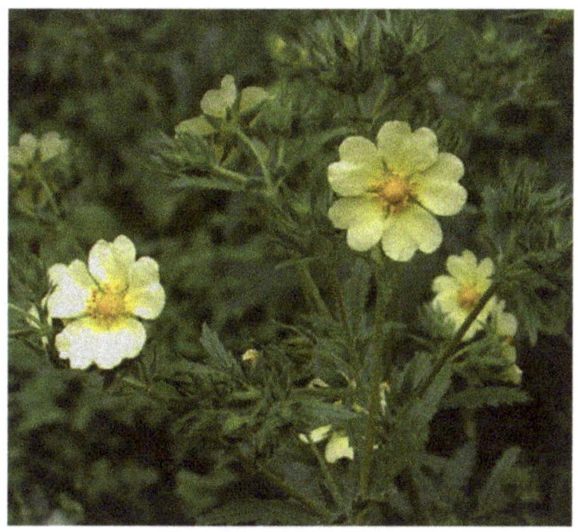

Potentilla recta

The majority of Cinquefoil species have palmately compound leaves usually consisting of 5-7 leaflets. *P. norvegica* and *P. tridentata* have only 3 leaflets. Cinquefoil means "five-parted leaf," but this is somewhat misleading since the number of leaflets can vary from 3-9 per leaf, even in the same species. The lance-shaped, coarsely toothed, serrated leaflets are hairy, pinnately veined, and different shades of green varying from a rich, dark hue to a light silvery green.

Most Cinquefoil flowers range from bright yellow to cream-colored and have 4 or 5 petals, a calyx of 5 green hairy sepals, and 5 green bracts (small modified leaves at the flower base). Flowers can bloom from May through September and are sensitive to light, fully opening in sun and partially closing on cloudy days and overnight. The fruits are clusters of dry achenes, partly enclosed by the calyx.

Cultivation

Due to their resilient and prolific nature, Cinquefoil plants often grow abundantly in the wild or find their way to disturbed garden soil. This makes wildcrafting fairly effortless, and cultivation is often unnecessary. However, the plants are easy to start from seed and by the standard methods of stem cutting or layering. Plant seeds in early spring in a greenhouse or directly sow them into the garden. They are light-dependent germinators, so barely cover them with soil and keep them moist until germination. When seedlings are 2-4″ tall, transplant them 1′ apart in a sunny, moist garden area.

Harvest

Gather leaves when the yellow flowers are in full bloom. Harvest roots in late summer or autumn. To harvest seeds for future planting, gather the seedpods when they become dry and turn brown.

Preparation of Plant Medicine and Dosages

Cinquefoil plants yield their medicinal virtues to water, alcohol, and oil. The leaves and roots can be used fresh or dried, but the fresh herb is preferred because it is more potent. The plant has a bitter flavor, and the astringent tannins leave an interesting sensation in the mouth as the mucous membranes constrict and pucker, making the mouth feel drier. Medicinal species may be ingested several times during the day for acute diarrhea or bleeding, but should not be used for more than 5-7 consecutive days due to their very astringent nature, which has a constricting effect on tissues. For chronic problems, it should be taken a few times a day for one week, discontinued for 10 days, and started again for another week. Alternating in this on/off schedule works well and is safer than continual use.

PREPARATIONS

Decoction Tea: Gently simmer 1-2 teaspoons of fresh or dried chopped root in 1 cup of water for 7-10 minutes in a pot covered with a lid. Dosage: ½ cup every 30 minutes as needed.

Infusion Tea: Steep 1-2 teaspoons of fresh or dried leaves in 1 cup of boiled water. Dosage: ½ cup every 30 minutes as needed. This is milder than the decoction tea made from roots.

Tincture: Chop the freshly harvested roots and/or leaves into small pieces and cover with 60% 190-proof grain alcohol and 40% distilled water. Dosage: 30-60 drops 3 times daily in water, or 30 drops every 30 minutes as needed for up to 5 doses.

Salve: Prepare in the usual way by placing the chopped plant material in a glass or stainless steel bowl, covering it with olive oil, and baking it in an oven at 200-225°F for 2-3 hours. Combine and bake Cinquefoil with other herbs for best healing results (refer to the "Index of Health Issues and Herbal Recommendations" for suggestions).

Poultice: Chop or grind the fresh or dry leaves and/or roots into small pieces and simmer them with a little water to make a moist, pasty mash. Apply the mash to the affected area and kept it in place with a cloth or ace wrap.

Wash: Prepare a strong decoction or infusion tea to soak or bathe the affected skin.

Fomentation: Soak a cloth in the decoction or infusion tea, place it on the problem area, and hold it in place with tape or ace wrap.

Chemical Constituents

Cinquefoil species contain up to 20% tannins in the form of tannic acid, the strong astringent responsible for many of the herb's medicinal attributes. Researchers have found that *P. recta and P. tormentilla* contain flavonoids, including kaempferol (antioxidant and anti-inflammatory), tormentol (a triterpine alcohol), tormentillin, gallic acid, ellagic acid, catechol gallates, and essential oils. A bitter compound called quinovic acid is present and also occurs in Peruvian bark (*Cinchona officinalis*), the source of quinine, which was the first effective medicine given for malaria and other intermittent fevers.

Safety, Contraindications, and Drug Interactions

Medicinal species of Cinquefoil are regarded as safe herbs with no known drug interactions. Due to the constricting nature of the tannins on tissues, large amounts should not be ingested for more that 5-7 consecutive days, because long-term use may damage the lining of the gastrointestinal tract. European sources recommend avoiding large amounts in cases of gallstones or liver disease. All astringent herbs are **contraindicated during lactation** because they have a drying effect on milk production (McGuffin, 1997).

Medicinal Uses

History of the Plant

Various species of Cinquefoil have a rich tradition of use in European folk medicine, and they continue to be employed for similar conditions by modern herbalists. Hippocrates (*circa* 460–*c.* 377 B.C.), the Greek physician known as the "father of medicine," used Cinquefoil to treat intermittent fevers and malaria, common ailments for people living in marshy areas. The Greek physician and botanist Dioscorides (*c.* A.D. 40–*c.* 90) used the herb for toothaches, ulcers and inflammation of the mouth and throat, dysentery, bleeding, edema, skin eruptions, and stomach and liver problems, including jaundice. Galen (*c.* 131–*c.* 200) also prescribed it for these ailments and for prolapsed organs. Nicholas Culpeper (1616–1654), the English herbalist and apothecary, wrote, "It is a special herb used in all inflammations and fevers, whether infectious or pestilential or, among other herbs, to cool and temper the blood and humours in the body. As also for all lotions, gargles, and infections; for mouth sores, ulcers, cancers, fistulas, and other foul and running sores" (Culpeper, 1992). He claimed that Cinquefoil is ruled by Jupiter, and he used it to expel venom and poisons, and treat coughs, fevers, jaundice, plagues, malaria, and quinsy (infection and abscess of the tonsils). Culpeper also packed the root around painful teeth.

The name Cinquefoil is derived from the Latin word *quinque*, meaning "five" (referring to the typical five leaflets comprising each leaf) and *foil*, which means "leaf." "Tormentil" comes from the Latin *tormentum*, signifying the tortuous gripping of the intestines and painful toothaches that the herb relieves. Cinquefoil was used as a magic herb in love divinations and included in many concoctions prepared for spells and charms during the European Middle Ages. Following the Doctrine of Signatures, Cinquefoil leaves resemble an outstretched hand, and they were believed to offer protection against witchcraft and harmful interference in one's life.

In North America, many Native Indian groups used indigenous Cinquefoil species in similar ways as the Europeans. A tea of the pounded roots was prepared to treat weak bowels, diarrhea, dysentery, bleeding, fevers, and to heal external wounds. A gargle was administered for sore throats. The Cheyenne and other tribes also regarded the plants as protective medicine against their enemies and witchcraft.

Early American colonists brought European species of Cinquefoil to the new world, and many of the species naturalized in North America. Although it was not a popular herbal remedy during the 1880s–1930s, the American Eclectic physicians included the root of *P. tormentilla* in their pharmacy for its astringent properties. They used the tea to treat chronic diarrhea, dysentery and hemorrhages, and applied it to skin ulcers (Felter, 1898). William Cook, M.D., wrote, "The herb five-finger was at one time in high repute as a medicine, and was accredited with almost miraculous powers . . . . The common mode of exhibition is by infusion. The tormentil roots are quite purely and actively astringent, and though much employed in some sections of Europe, are scarcely known or used in this country" (Cook, 1869). John Christopher (1909–1983), a clinical herbalist and naturopathic doctor who used Cinquefoil in his practice, called it "a powerful astringent beneficial for all types of bleeding."

Although several varieties of Cinquefoil have been popular healing remedies in European history, it remains an under-appreciated and under-utilized herb in the United States. Very little scientific research has been conducted on this genus.

Healing Qualities

Alterative, antihydrotic (reduces excessive perspiration), anti-inflammatory, antioxidant, antiseptic, antispasmodic, powerful astringent, febrifuge, hemostatic, and vulnerary.

Traditional Chinese Medicine (TCM) Perspective

Cinquefoil species exert a cooling influence. Their tannins are drying and restoring to normalize secretions and reduce excess fluids and discharges. These astringent and drying properties bring balance to damp heat or damp cold conditions in the abdominal and pelvic areas that cause multiple problems, including diarrhea, dysentery, colitis, peptic ulcers, genitourinary infections, vaginal discharge, incontinence, and hemorrhage.

The Cinquefoils tone weak digestive Qi and are indicated for chronic and constitutional Stomach, Intestinal, and Spleen Qi deficiencies, which cause indigestion, diarrhea, and fatigue. These herbs relieve congested Liver and Kidney Qi, and raise Central Qi to reduce organ prolapse. They tone Heart Qi and clear toxic heat responsible for infections, inflammation, burns, boils, skin eruptions, septicemia (bacterial infection in the blood), venereal infections, headaches, arthritis, and gout. An Asian species, *P. discoloris*, is used in TCM to treat enteritis (intestinal inflammation), dysentery, pharyngitis, bleeding in the gastrointestinal tract, and diabetes (Yang, 2010). *P. multifida* is another species given to treat diabetes (Xue, 2007).

Primary Actions

The exceptional astringent property of tannins found in the roots and leaves is responsible for Cinquefoil's primary medicinal actions. Astringents tone and normalize the body by tightening and constricting boggy, overly relaxed, leaky tissues, muscles, and blood vessels. Astringents reduce abnormal bleeding, diarrhea, and excessive secretions and perspiration. Members of the genus *Potentilla* also beneficially influence the mind and emotions by relieving deep internal tension, strain, frustration, and rage that can get "locked" into cellular memory and torment people for long periods of time.

Cinquefoil is high on my list of favorite and most dependable herbs for all abnormal bleeding and diarrhea. I usually combine two varieties growing in southern Indiana, *P. recta* and *P. reptans*, with Cranesbill (*Geranium maculatum*), another strong astringent. The different species of Agrimony (*Agrimonia* spp.) also belong to the Rose family and have similar astringent properties. Cinquefoil, Cranesbill, and Agrimony can be used interchangeably or combined for heightened potency.

When using strong astringents to arrest bleeding or diarrhea, be aware that the underlying causes of the problem must always be addressed for complete healing to occur. Do not use Cinquefoil and other astringents as a "band-aid treatment" while ignoring the underlying issues. For example, if a person has diarrhea caused by eating spoiled food, it is best to allow the diarrhea to expel the tainted food from the intestines to resolve the problem, instead of medicating with astringents that can turn off this natural healing response of expelling the toxins quickly and efficiently.

I often combine Cinquefoil with other herbs specific for different health issues, especially when working with infections and the digestive, urinary, and female reproductive systems.

Abnormal Bleeding: Cinquefoil is wonderful to reduce all types of hemorrhage. The tea or tincture is ingested for internal bleeding, hemorrhoids, and nosebleeds. Externally, the herb can be applied to injured skin as a salve, fomentation, or poultice to retard bleeding and treat painful wounds, burns, and hemorrhoids. For varicose veins, it can be taken internally and applied externally to constrict the weak muscular walls that allow veins to enlarge. Cinquefoil also has a cleansing action on the bloodstream and is excellent for toxic conditions of the blood and tissues. A Swedish research team found *P. recta* to be an active anti-inflammatory, and validated its ability to promote clotting of blood platelets and stop abnormal bleeding (Tunon, 1995).

Digestive System and Diarrhea: The astringent property of Cinquefoil tones the membranes of the gastrointestinal tract to normalize secretions of digestive enzymes and arrest bleeding, diarrhea, and abnormal discharges. The herb is specific for diarrhea caused by atonic tissues, infections and dysentery (bloody diarrhea due to intestinal infection), stomach ulcers, spastic colon, Crohn's disease, and ulcerative colitis. It is excellent when treating chronic infections in the digestive tract involving inflammation. I have used Cinquefoil in many cases of diarrhea with excellent results and rely on its consistent actions.

By toning and strengthening muscles and tissues, Cinquefoil benefits atonic, overly relaxed, boggy tissues lacking the tone and strength necessary to maintain their proper support and positions. It helps prevent and treat uterine, bladder, and intestinal prolapse, and assists in the prevention and treatment of hernias resulting from muscle weakness.

Dr. John Christopher used *P. tormentilla* to treat organ prolapse. In his book *School of Natural Healing*, he noted, "It is a very powerful astringent and is useful in toning relaxed bowels and in checking abnormal discharges. It heals relaxed and atonic mucous membranes. It relieves any gripping pains of the stomach or intestines, and it opens up obstructions of the lungs, spleen, etc" (Christopher, 1976).

The herb has a long history of use in relieving abdominal cramps, spasms, pain, and colic. Cinquefoil works well when combined with Chamomile (*Matricaria recutita*) for digestive problems. Both herbs ease the physical, psychological, and emotional tension that contribute to digestive problems.

In vivo studies have found that the antioxidants in Cinquefoil species are helpful for inflammatory bowel diseases (Langmead, 2002). Research validates the herb's safety and usefulness as an alternative medicine for disorders like ulcerative colitis (Huber, 2007). *P. erecta* has been safely used as an herbal remedy for inflammation and gastrointestinal disorders (Shushunov, 2009). Turkish researchers evaluated tea made from *P. reptans* leaves for its traditional use in treating peptic ulcer symptoms such as stomachache and heartburn. The study documented that the oral administration of the tea to rats showed significant protection against the development of stomach ulcers (Gurbuz, 2005).

Another research test evaluated the effectiveness of *P. tormentilla* root extract for the treatment of rotavirus diarrhea in 40 children. Rotavirus is one of the most widely spread pathogens responsible for acute dehydrating diarrhea, causing an estimated 800,000 deaths a year in children living in developing countries. In a randomized, double-blind, placebo-controlled study, 20 children were given 3 drops of the root extract per each year of their life, 3 times a day. The other 20 children received a placebo. In the group taking the extract, 8 of 20 children (40%) were free of diarrhea after 48 hours, compared to 1 of 20 children (5%) receiving the placebo (Subbotina, 2003).

Sore Throats: Astringent herbs are helpful in treating sore throats. Cinquefoil tea or diluted tincture may be used as a mouthwash or gargle to heal inflamed, ulcerated mouths and throats, laryngitis, and gum disease, including infection and bleeding. A clinical study in Russia involving 53 patients with lichen planus, an inflammatory skin ulceration on the inner buccal cheek of the mouth, demonstrated that mouth ulcers (known as canker sores) healed faster by gargling with *P. tormentilla* tincture (Volodina, 1997). Gargling with Cinquefoil tea shrinks an elongated uvula (the little flap of tissue at the very back of the throat) that can occur during surgery when an airway tube is placed down the throat and pushes against the uvula.

Kidneys and Bladder: The Potentilla genus is beneficial for bladder ulceration, inflammation and bloody urine, especially when combined with Yarrow (*Achillea millefolium*), Goldenseal (*Hydrastis canadensis*), Goldenrod (*Solidago* spp.), and Gravel Root (*Eupatorium purpureum*). Cinquefoil may be helpful for urinary incontinence and bed-wetting, while helping to relieve the nervous tension that incontinence can cause in children and adults.

Women's Health: Cinquefoil's astringent property is consistently helpful for excessive menstrual bleeding, called menorrhagia, and reduces the blood flow without completely stopping it, which is the desired effect. I have given a combination of Cinquefoil and Yarrow tincture to many women complaining of menorrhagia and uterine bleeding due to fibroids, and typically see exceptional results. Cinquefoil can be combined with

Shepherd's Purse (*Capsella bursa-pastoris*) to stop uterine hemorrhage following childbirth. Cinquefoil also helps relieve the tension and anxiety many women experience with their menstrual cycles.

A tea of the roots or leaves can be administered as a douche for vaginal infections and discharge, including Candida yeast, and Cinquefoil has a long historic use for this purpose. Douche 1-2 times daily until relief is obtained. Combine Cinquefoil with equal parts Goldenseal, Yarrow, Blue Vervain (*Verbena hastata*), and Sage (*Salvia officinalis*), which are excellent antibiotic and antifungal herbs. Marshmallow root (*Althaea officinalis*) or Plantain (*Plantago* spp.) may be added to the blend for their demulcent property that soothes inflamed and irritated tissues.

Infection, Fever, and Inflammation: Herbal practitioners of the past used Cinquefoil to treat arthritis, gout, and other joint and muscle inflammation and stiffness. They also combined it with other herbs to reduce fever and treat malaria, whooping cough, cholera, and gonorrhea. Cinquefoil's cleansing action on the bloodstream makes it appropriate for cases of septicemia and toxemia, which are conditions involving toxins in the blood. The herb can sometimes produce rashes as it eliminates old toxins, but it should be continued in reduced doses to complete the cleansing process.

Studies have demonstrated that *P. tormentilla* has immunostimulant, anti-allergic, antioxidant, antiviral, and antihypertensive properties, although these are not its traditional uses (Bos, 1996).

External Healing: Cinquefoil helps heal new and slow-to-heal wounds and injuries. When applied immediately after an injury, it will reduce inflammation and stop bleeding and bruising. I always add Cinquefoil (*P. recta*) and Yarrow to my herbal salve, and many times I have witnessed their remarkable ability to completely stop the bruising process. It should be stressed that immediate application is necessary to avoid bruising, but it does work!

Cinquefoil has been used to treat ulcerated skin and infectious gangrene in wounds. Application of tea or tincture relieves the pain of burns. Its ability to reduce toxins in the blood makes it helpful for clearing skin conditions caused by a toxic overload, including rashes, skin eruptions like boils and acne, alopecia (hair loss), and swollen glands.

Teachings from the Cinquefoil Deva

"Greetings, dear one. So you want to know a few of my secrets? Yes, I will share with you. I radiate the vibration of the life-giving color red, which reflects my relationship with the blood and vessels. I have a constricting nature that draws together, tightens, and mends all that is too loose and expansive. My healing energies ride through the body with the in-breath as I promote movement flowing inward and upward. In the blood vessels, this inward, drawing movement pulls blood particles together to clot and repair holes in the vessels, thus preventing the sacred blood from leaking out.

"My inward constrictive nature joins and glues torn and damaged tissues together to reconnect, strengthen, and become a stable part of the whole body once again. Fragmentation and weakness are stabilized. My healing action is like knitting the tissues together and works well with my sister, the Comfrey plant, known among some people as 'knitbone.'

"My upward flow of movement contracts and draws together weak, flabby muscles. This action helps prolapsed, or fallen, organs to maintain or return to their normal positions, especially those organs in the lower abdomen and pelvis.

"So, rather than being expansive, my offering promotes balance by constricting elements of the physical body. Think of me as useful for drawing torn, wounded, fragile fragments together to create strong, cohesive tissues and bonds.

"My yellow flowers reflect affinity with the solar plexus, which radiates and is nourished by the yellow rays of light. My constricting flow of movement in the human body draws inward, centering upon the solar plexus and all the tissues and organs contained in this center.

"I am under the rule of Virgo, and like Virgo, I am of the Earth element that draws in upon itself to condense and solidify. Just as pieces of rock, fallen plants and leaves, broken tree limbs, and decaying animals all consolidate and harden together into earth, so do I draw together and heal all torn, wounded, and fragmented parts.

"Use my flowers for emotional and spiritual healing. I am helpful for people who are 'spaced out' and lack the security of being grounded. I offer solidity and wholeness to those feeling torn apart or beside themselves. I am able to draw all the fragments back together, allowing balance and harmonious flow of energy with the experience of oneness. I help heal gaping holes in the emotional energy field when the heart feels ripped apart in pain or grief. I integrate and settle all parts of the whole. Even though I am a little plant, I offer protection. My action on the human body and psyche is strong and dependable in drawing together and bonding that which has been loosened or torn apart."

Comfrey

Symphytum officinale
Boraginaceae (Borage) Family

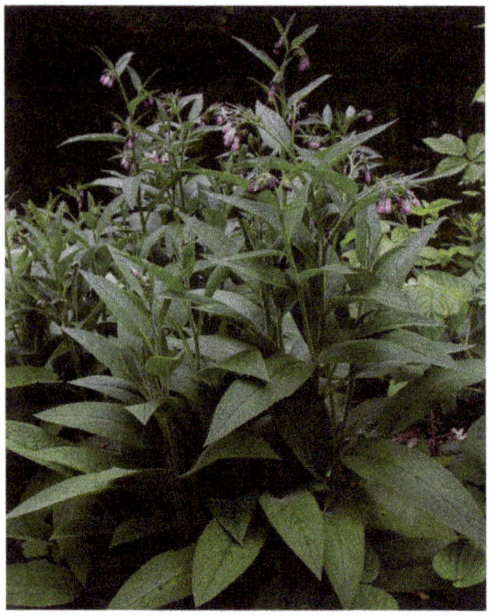

Common Names

Knitback, knitbone, boneset, nipbone, healing herb, carpenter's herb, and bruisewort are names reflecting the plant's historic ability to heal broken bones and injured tissues. Gum plant, slippery root, blackwort, and blackroot are old names descriptive of the slimy texture of the inner root and the dark color of the outer root. Salsify and consound are other antiquated names.

Medicinal Part of the Plant

The root and leaves are both used medicinally, but the roots are the most potent part of the plant.

Range and Habitat

There are about 35 species in the genus *Symphytum*, most of which are native to Europe and temperate Western Asia. *Symphytum officinale* has naturalized extensively throughout Europe, Canada, and the United States. It grows in moist areas, grasslands and lowlands, and continues to be widely cultivated by many gardeners and herbalists.

Description of the Plant

Comfrey (*S. officinale*) is a hardy perennial growing up to 4′ tall under ideal conditions. It is an attractive, bushy plant with rich, deep-green foliage of large, curving leaves and delicate-looking, bell-shaped drooping flowers. The large branching taproot has a black exterior and the fleshy creamy-white interior is moist and slimy due to a tasteless mucilage. Roots can penetrate deep into the soil, growing 1-3′ long and up to 1½″ in diameter. The erect stalks and 8-16″ long leaves are densely covered with rough, bristly white hairs that can cause skin irritation and itching when rubbed against the skin of sensitive people. The fibrous stem is hollow, juicy, and rounded but angular.

Many leaves, each having a stem, grow directly from the root crown. Several tall stalks branch out to develop flowers. Single leaves climb the entire length of these flower stalks in an alternating pattern, becoming progressively smaller towards the top of the plant. Leaves have a pinnate and webbed vein pattern, creating a rugose (wrinkled) texture. They are oblong to lanceolate in shape, and lower leaves are petiole (having stems) while the upper are sessile (lacking stems). It is interesting to note that the base of the leaves attaching to the stalk actually continue downward in longitudinal, leaf-like ridges, adding to the stalk's angular appearance. Leaf margins are entire (lacking teeth) but have a curly, wavy structure.

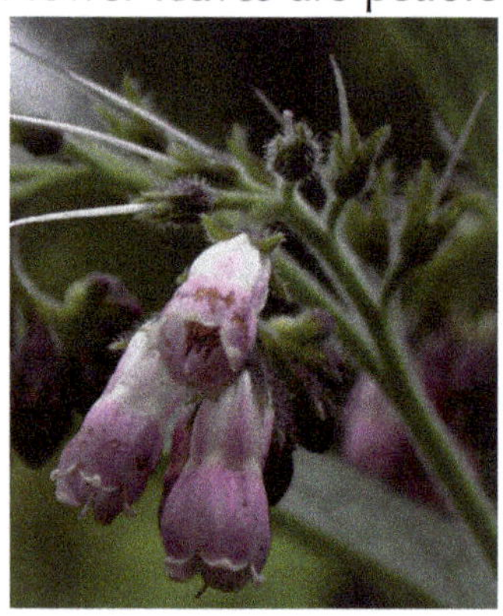

The small, bell-shaped flowers are ½-1″ long and hang in clusters at the ends of the upper leaf stalks. They blossom from April through September and range in colors from white to creamy yellow, pink, light blue, and purple. The tubular corolla has 5 slightly outward-curving lobes. The green calyx has 5 pointed tips and is hairy like the stem and leaves. There are 5 stamens in each flower.

British herbalist Maude Grieve stated in her book *A Modern Herbal* that plants with whitish-yellow flowers are *S. officinale* proper, and those with purple flowers are *S. officinale* var. *patens*. They are considered to be equal in medicinal value. The species of Comfrey from Russia is *Symphytum x uplandicum,* a hybrid of *S. officinale* and *S. asperum* (Prickly Comfrey). Both *S. officinale* and *S. x uplandicum* are commonly grown in North America. Russian Comfrey is a large perennial growing up to 4-6′ in height. At the base of the plant the leaves are rounded or heart-shaped, and larger flowers vary in shades from dark purple to blue or pink. *S. asperum* and *S. x uplandicum* contain more of the potentially toxic pyrrolizidine alkaloids than *S. officinale* and other varieties.

Cultivation

Due to lower concentrations of pyrrolizidine alkaloids, *S. officinale* is the best variety to cultivate. Comfrey grows in almost any soil under shade or full sun, but thrives and produces larger roots in full sun and moist, fertile, loamy soil. Adequate drainage is imperative to prevent roots from rotting. The plant rarely produces viable seeds, so propagation is always by root division. Plants with older roots are dug up in early spring or late fall when flowers are not present, or the root may be purchased. Divide roots into 1-2″ pieces and plant horizontally 2-3″ deep, spacing each piece 1½-2′ apart. The roots are very prolific and a small piece sprouts leaves in a short time. Keep in mind that Comfrey may be difficult to eradicate once established, so plant it where it has plenty of room to grow.

Harvest

Collect leaves in summer when they are mature and deep green in color. Several cuttings of leaves can be made during the growing season, and if plants are conservatively pruned, the cuttings will not harm or weaken them. Harvest roots in spring or fall when levels of the healing compound allantoin are highest. Before harvesting the root, cut the leaves from the crown to make the job easier. Dig a hole around the root large enough to prevent chopping off the bottom root. To propagate another plant, cut off 1-2" pieces of the root and replant them. A small piece of root attached to the crown will quickly grow leaf stems.

A group of phytochemicals in Comfrey called pyrrolizidine alkaloids (PAs) can have a toxic effect on the liver when ingested in large doses over an extended period of time. Consideration of PA concentration in the leaves and roots should be taken into account when harvesting the plant. In his book, *Herbal Renaissance*, herbalist Steven Foster cites a 1987 study by Gary Steuart (Steuart, 1987) indicating that the undesired PA content in the leaves is affected by the growth stage of the plant and time of harvest. In the study, the first spring leaf cuttings contained the highest amount of PAs (0.026% of dry weight), while cuttings taken in late summer had minute amounts averaging 5 parts per million. This study suggests that it is best to use later cuttings for medicinal purposes rather than the first leaves of spring. PAs in the dried root of *S. officinale* measure around 0.3-0.4% (McGuffin, 1997). Other studies demonstrate that the root contains up to 10 times more PAs than the leaf, and young leaves may contain up to 16 times the level of PAs compared to mature leaves (Foster, 1993).

Preparation of Plant Medicine and Dosages

The roots and leaves are used fresh or dried, although freshly harvested herbs are more potent. Roots contain the greatest concentration of healing mucilage, which is best extracted by water but damaged by alcohol. For this reason, Comfrey tea is much more effective than tincture for internal use, and I do not recommend tincturing this plant. Comfrey roots and leaves can be prepared as a salve, poultice, or fomentation (a wash of the tea) for external uses. The leaves and roots have a mild flavor.

The freshly harvested leaves and roots can be chopped and stored in a freezer, or dried in a shady, well-ventilated area. Tie a few leaves together by their stems and hang them up, or spread them in single layers on screens. Thoroughly wash the fresh roots, chop them into pieces, and place them on a screen to dry. In humid weather, use a fan to increase airflow and hasten the drying process. Store dried materials in a glass container, but recheck them after a few days to ensure that drying is complete and mold is not growing.

The presence of pyrrolizidine alkaloids (PAs) has caused quite a controversy over safety. **If you decide to take Comfrey internally, do so in small doses over a short period of time.** Drinking 1-2 cups of tea daily over 1-3 weeks at a time, for no longer than 6 weeks in a year, is considered safe for adults.

PREPARATIONS

Infusion Tea: Steep 1 tablespoon of dried leaves or 2 tablespoons of finely chopped fresh leaves in 1 cup of boiled water for 15-20 minutes. Dosage: 1-2 cups a day for 1-3 weeks at a time.

Decoction Tea: Unlike most root teas, Comfrey roots do not need to be boiled or simmered because the medicinal mucilage extracts well when allowed to steep in hot or warm water. Put 2 tablespoons of the finely chopped root in a quart of hot water for 1-4 hours and cover the pan with a lid while it steeps and cools. It may be allowed to steep overnight. Dosage: 1-2 cups a day for 1-3 weeks at a time.

Fomentation: Saturate a wash cloth with a strong tea of the root or leaves and apply externally.

Poultice: This can be made from fresh Comfrey leaves or roots, or from the dried plant. When using the freshly harvested plant, slash the leaves several times to allow the healing juices to seep out, then wrap them around the injured area. The fresh leaves are rather scratchy and irritating to the skin, but this can be remedied by chopping the leaves into small pieces and gently simmering them in a little water until they turn into a mash. Apply the mash to the skin and bandage it to stay in place. The fresh or dried leaves and roots can all be prepared by this method. The dried root must be ground into a powder and mixed with enough water to produce a thick paste.

Ointment or Salve: Put pieces of root and leaves in a pan and cover with olive oil. Bake at 200-225°F for 3 hours. Comfrey releases gas as it sits in oil, but this is normal and does not indicate spoilage.

Culinary Uses

The fresh leaves are tasty when steamed like spinach. They have a long traditional use as food, but in light of current knowledge about potential liver toxicity, only eat moderate amounts of leaves, and only those harvested in summer or autumn. I once watched a young man walk over to my flowering Comfrey patch and start eating the fresh leaves right off the plant! Most people object to the scratchy hairs on the leaves, which are eliminated with steaming, but he seemed quite content with his raw salad.

Chemical Constituents

Comfrey contains allantoin, a cell proliferate (stimulates new cell growth and repair) and primary constituent involved in bone and tissue healing. Allantoin is anti-inflammatory, antioxidant, anti-ulcer, immunostimulating, keratolytic (prevents scar formation), and is concentrated in the root (0.6-2.5%). The root contains up to 29% mucilage (a mucopolysaccharide of fructose and glucose), a greater concentration than in any other known plant. Mucopolysaccharides demonstrate immunostimulant properties. Also present are tannins (astringent), inulin, resin, and essential oils. Triterpenes include the phytosterols sitosterol and stigmasterol (anti-hepatotoxic, anti-inflammatory, antioxidant, estrogenic). There are also steroidal saponins (including asparagine) in Comfrey.

Phenolic acids include rosmarinic (anti-inflammatory, antibacterial, antioxidant, protects capillary blood vessels in the heart and lungs), chlorogenic (analgesic, antibacterial, anti-hepatotoxic, antihistamine, anti-inflammatory, antioxidant, antimutagenic, cholagogue, immunostimulant), caffeic (analgesic, antibacterial, anticarcinogenic, antihemolytic, antihistamine, anti-inflammatory, antioxidant, cholagogue, vulnerary), salicylic (analgesic, anti-inflammatory), and lithospermic acids.

The leaves are highly nutritious, containing protein and easily assimilated vitamins and minerals such as thiamine (vitamin B1), riboflavin (B2), niacin (B3), cobalamine (B12), choline, vitamin C, beta-carotene, vitamin E, calcium, potassium, iron, magnesium, manganese, phosphorous, selenium, sodium, chromium, zinc, and silicon in the form of silicic acid. Silicic acid dissolves in water, allowing for easy absorption from the tea. Silicon is essential for the normal development of connective tissue, cartilage, elastin, and bone. It is an important factor in the formation of the collagen matrix of bone, and facilitates bone repair and the uptake of minerals into bone.

Comfrey also contains the controversial pyrrolizidine alkaloids (PAs) that have been linked to hepatotoxicity (liver toxicity). More than 200 different PAs have been identified in many plants, primarily from the Borage, Aster, and Pea families. Other herbs containing PAs include Coltsfoot (*Tussilago farfara*) leaf and flower, Borage (*Borago officinalis*) leaf, and several species of *Eupatorium*. The PAs in Comfrey include symphytine, echimidine, symlandine, echinatin, lycopsamine, acetyllycopsamine, lasiocarpine, intermidine, and myoscorpine (Duke, Phytochemical Database; Newall, 1996). According to research conducted by Dr. Dennis Awang, former research director of natural products for the Drugs Directorate of the Canadian government, the most toxic alkaloids found in Comfrey are symphytine and echimidine. Echimidine is considered to be the most toxic and occurs in Prickly Comfrey (*S. asperum*) and Russian Comfrey (*S. x uplandicum*), but is undetectable in *S. officinale*. Symphytine is the primary PA in *S. officinale* (Foster, 1993).

Safety, Contraindications, and Drug Interactions

The safety controversy surrounding Comfrey revolves around the potentially harmful pyrrolizidine alkaloids (PAs). **Internal use is contraindicated for children and pregnant or nursing women** due to the delicate liver of the fetus and infants. No drug interactions are known (Blumenthal, 1998).

Comfrey's renowned reputation as a superb wound healer, established over 2,000 years of popular use, has been undermined by recent documentation of potential toxicity associated with large doses and long-term use. PAs are metabolized in the liver and converted into toxic metabolites called pyrroles. These can damage liver cells and cause abnormal cellular growth leading to blood clots and obstruction in the capillaries of the liver. This process can promote cirrhosis and a serious condition known as hepatic veno-occlusive disease (HVOD). HVOD is difficult to diagnose without a liver biopsy, and people with strong, healthy livers are just as susceptible as those with liver weakness. Symptoms that may not be obvious for several months or years include abdominal pain, vomiting, diarrhea, liver and spleen enlargement, jaundice, accumulation of fluid in the abdominal cavity (ascites), cirrhosis, and liver failure (Mattocks, 1968). Toxicity of PAs is related to the size of the dose and length of time consumed, and Comfrey must be consumed in large doses over an extended period of time for the PAs to build up and cause harm. Critics have been quick to attack this ancient healing plant. Although a study published in the prestigious *Lancet* medical journal estimated that one cup of Comfrey root tea may be a "significant health risk," it should be noted that **consumption of normal, reasonable amounts of Comfrey has never been linked to liver problems**.

The question of Comfrey's safety due to PAs originated following the publication of a Japanese study (Hirono, 1978 & 1979). Lab rats were fed abnormally large amounts of Comfrey leaf and root for 600 days, resulting in liver toxicity and tumors in all the animals. Other lab animals were injected with isolated PAs with similar damaging results. Since the 1980s, at least 6 cases of Comfrey poisoning in people have been documented, although none specified which varieties of Comfrey were ingested (Awang, 1991; Bergner, 1989 & 1993). In all these cases, Comfrey was consumed in excessively large quantities over long periods of time. In one case, a 49-year-old woman developed HVOD after 6 months of ingesting 6 Comfrey/pepsin capsules daily (Ridker, 1985). In another, a 13-year-old boy with a 3-year history of Crohn's disease was treated with prescription drugs and developed HVOD after ingesting Comfrey root tea on a regular basis for 2 years. A 47-year-old woman who drank up to 10 cups of Comfrey tea a day and took several Comfrey/pepsin capsules daily developed HVOD after 9 years of continual use. And in New Zealand, a 23-year-old man who died of liver failure had been eating 4-5 fresh young Comfrey leaves daily over an extended period of time (Yeong, 1990).

There is research that sheds more light and logic on the truth of PA danger. A study conducted in the late 1980s found that 29 people who had consumed Comfrey for up to 20 years developed no sign of liver disease (Anderson, 1989). Research performed by cancer authority Bruce Ames, Ph.D., chairman of the Biochemistry Department at the University of California, was published in a 1987 issue of *Science* and offers more realistic perspectives of Comfrey's actual threat to health. Ames studied the average person's lifetime cancer risk from exposure to hundreds of man-made and naturally occurring carcinogens. Based upon outcomes of his study, Ames estimated that one cup of Comfrey tea has:

- ❖ About the same cancer risk as a peanut butter sandwich that contains traces of aflatoxin, the naturally occurring peanut carcinogen.
- ❖ About one-third the risk of eating one raw mushroom containing traces of hydrazine, a natural carcinogen.
- ❖ About half the risk of one diet soda containing saccharin, a known carcinogen.
- ❖ About one-hundredth the risk of a glass of wine or beer that contains carcinogenic ethyl alcohol (Castleman, 1991).

These statistics reflect the fact that many popular foods contain chemicals that are harmful or carcinogenic. However, these chemicals often occur in combination with other substances that act synergistically to alter potential toxicity. Phytochemicals occur in such small amounts that they do not necessarily exert adverse effects. But when chemicals are isolated from their original plant source and fed or injected into lab animals in large doses, tumors and other imbalances are a normal result. Data, outcomes, and hypotheses derived from this type of research are not representative of actual human use or traditional dosages and routes of administration, and should be evaluated appropriately and realistically.

There is no question that long-term use of large amounts of PAs are toxic to the liver and should be avoided. In light of current knowledge, **Comfrey should only be taken internally in moderate doses for short periods of time**. Considering Comfrey's excellent healing ability, it is indeed a shame that it has been judged so severely as dangerous and banned in several countries, promoting a public reaction of fear. It is especially interesting that the U.S. Food and Drug Administration (FDA) has chosen to ban Comfrey after six known cases of liver toxicity, while hundreds of pharmaceutical drugs with known toxicity are approved by the FDA and allowed for public use. According to the U.S. Poison Control Center, acetaminophen (found in Tylenol, Darvocet, Lortab, Percocet, Vicodin, and NyQuil) overdose is the most common cause of liver failure. It can cause liver toxicity when daily dosage exceeds 3,000 mg, which many people with intractable pain take daily for months or years. In 1997, U.S. Regional Poison Control centers treated more than 10,000 cases of acetaminophen overdose. A 1998 study of 47 children suffering from acetaminophen overdose reported that 23 died (Kearns, 1998). And yet, a multitude of acetaminophen products remain on the market and many are over-the-counter drugs not requiring a prescription. Herbs and pharmaceutical medicines are evaluated according to very different criteria and are regulated differently. Ultimately, the decision to use Comfrey, or not, is a personal choice, based hopefully on reason rather than misinformation and fear.

> *Comfrey can damage the liver if taken in large doses for a long period of time.*
>
> *Remember that Comfrey should be taken internally in moderate doses for only one to two weeks at a time.*

Since toxicity of PAs results from highly reactive compounds formed during Comfrey's metabolism in the liver, external use is safe, especially on unbroken tissue (Blumenthal, 1998). Caution should be taken to ensure that all wounds, especially deep punctures, are disinfected before covering with Comfrey preparations to avoid sealing infection into the body. Although some overly cautious people speculate that this herb should not be applied externally for longer than 4-6 weeks, I have personally used a salve and lotion containing a small percentage of Comfrey leaf and root at least once daily for over 35 years without liver problems or other issues. I know of countless other people who safely use it externally for extended periods of time.

Medicinal Uses

History of the Plant

For thousands of years, Comfrey has been a highly esteemed medicinal herb used worldwide. It was one of the most popular herbs in European folk medicine, and its recorded use dates back to the early Greeks and Romans. The name Comfrey is thought to be derived from the Latin word *confervere*, meaning "to heal," or from *conferva*, meaning "to grow together and make firm." The genus name *Symphytum* comes from the Greek word *symphyto*, "to unite," indicating its ability to knit together and repair torn tissues, muscles, and broken bones.

The Greek physician and botanist Dioscorides (*circa* A.D. 40–*c.* 90) prescribed the tea for respiratory and digestive ailments, to staunch heavy bleeding, and to heal wounds and broken bones. Pliny the Elder (A.D. 23–79) and Paracelsus (1493–1541) both recommended Comfrey for its amazing healing power. It was commonly cultivated in British and European gardens during the Middle Ages, when it was a famous remedy for broken bones. In *The Herball or General Historie of Plantes*, John Gerard (1545–1612) stated, "The roots of Comfrey help those that spit blood and healeth all inward wounds and burns" (Gerard, 1633). He recommended a poultice for external wounds and the tea for lung problems, coughs, internal and external ulcers, back pain, inflammation, and hemorrhoids. English herbalist and apothecary Nicholas Culpeper (1616–1654) prescribed the herb for gangrene, fevers, joint and gout pain, hemorrhoids, and lung and menstrual problems. He wrote, "This is an herb of Saturn, and I suppose under the sign of Capricorn, cold, dry, and earthy in quality. Comfrey helpeth those that spit blood or make a bloody urine: the root boiled in water or wine and the decoction drank, helpeth all inward hurts, bruises, and wounds, and ulcers of the lungs, causing the phlegm that oppresses them to be easily spit forth. The roots being outwardly applied cure fresh wounds or cuts immediately" (Culpeper, 1992).

Comfrey was introduced to North America by the European immigrants. Native American Indians recognized the plant's mucilaginous healing properties and incorporated it into their herbal pharmacy, becoming quite adept at employing it for wound healing. It was a favorite of the American Eclectic physicians during the 1880s–1930s, who prescribed the tea for diarrhea, dysentery, bronchial problems including pneumonia and coughs, internal bleeding, stomach and intestinal ulcers and inflammation, sore breasts, and leucorrhea (vaginal discharges). Finley Ellingwood, M.D. (1852–1920) wrote, "Old European writers called attention to this remedy as a vulnerary. It had a great reputation as an external application in the treatment of wounds, bruises, and putrefying sores. They used it for ruptures and applied it where a bone was fractured, believing that it would stimulate the knitting of the bone" (Ellingwood, 1919).

Comfrey remained a popular medicine in the United States and Europe until the late 1970s, when potentially toxic pyrrolizidine alkaloids were discovered in the plant and its use became increasingly controversial. The sale of Comfrey for internal use is currently banned in several countries, including the United States, Canada, Germany, Australia, and Japan. Most leading manufacturers in the United States discontinued Comfrey in the mid–1980s due to concerns about potential toxicity, and Comfrey preparations for internal use were removed from the market in 1992. However, Comfrey continues to be a primary ingredient in most commercially sold herbal salves for external application. Most research has been focused on PA content and toxicity, and on animal tests and human clinical trials investigating the herb's ability to reduce muscle pain, inflammation, and heal wounds, broken bones, sprained ankles, and other injuries.

Healing Qualities

Analgesic, anti-inflammatory, antilithic, slightly astringent, cell proliferate, demulcent, emollient, expectorant, febrifuge, hemostatic, mucilaginous, nephritic, nutritive, opthalmicum, pectoral, stomachic, and vulnerary.

Traditional Chinese Medicine (TCM) Perspective

Comfrey is a classic Yin herb that is cooling and moistening with secondary drying effects due to the astringent tannins that reduce secretions. Its taste is classified as neutral to sweet. It nourishes Yin and the blood, restores fluids, moistens dryness, and clears Yin deficiency heat and damp heat. Comfrey is specific for Yin and fluid deficiency problems that often accompany hot, fiery conditions such as inflammation, dry cough, brittle bones, ulcers, and dry scaly skin. The herb especially influences the lungs, stomach, kidneys, and skin.

In the Ayurvedic medical system of India, Comfrey root is employed in similar ways to promote tissue growth and as a nutritive and rejuvenating tonic for the lungs and mucous membranes.

Primary Actions

Comfrey is specific for healing torn and damaged tissues, making it an excellent remedy for internal and external wounds, injuries, and the mending of broken bones. The demulcent mucilage that is most abundant in the roots, and to a lesser degree in the leaves, has a thick, slimy, gelatinous consistency similar to that of Jell-O water. This mucilage is one of the primary elements responsible for the plant's healing ability. It has a special affinity with the mucous membranes throughout the body, which are specialized tissues lining all the hollow organs and cavities that open to the skin surface, such as the nasal passages, mouth, throat, lungs, stomach, and intestines. Mucous membranes contain many types of glands that secrete sweat, hormones, enzymes, and mucin, which lubricates tissues. Comfrey's mucilage serves to keep these membranes moist, a vital factor for their normal function. The herb is moisturizing and cooling, and reduces dryness, excessive heat, irritation, and inflammation to skin and mucous membranes throughout the gastrointestinal, respiratory, and genitourinary tracts.

Comfrey's moisturizing and demulcent properties have a general cleansing action on the blood and tissues. Rich in proteins, vitamins and minerals, it is very nourishing and has been used for anemia, especially when combined with Stinging Nettle (*Urtica dioica*) leaves, Yellow dock (*Rumex crispus*), and Dandelion (*Taraxacum officinale*) roots. Historically, it has been used as a nutritive and cleansing tonic to gradually strengthen the body over time, but with current research confirming the presence of pyrrolizidine alkaloids it is not recommended for long-term daily ingestion.

Comfrey leaves and roots are one of the main ingredients in the herbal salve I have made and used for over 35 years to successfully heal wounds and rashes, decrease pain and inflammation, and soothe dry, irritated skin. I have personally experienced the healing power of this plant to be consistently amazing for simple and very difficult cases alike. Many people using the salve have shared their healing stories and continually teach me more about Comfrey's therapeutic abilities.

Broken Bones and Wound Healing: Comfrey is one of the most respected herbs for healing all types of problematic skin conditions, wounds, and rashes. It alleviates pain, inflammation, and swelling of muscles and joints in cases of arthritis, acute back pain, sprains, bruises and strains after sports injuries and accidents, and mends broken bones. The older common name of "knitbone" refers to the herb's wonderful ability to stimulate fibroblast and osteoblast activity in bones. Fibroblasts are specialized cells that generate new tissue and osteoblasts. Osteoblasts generate new bone cells and "knit" broken bone cells back together. The moisturizing, mucilaginous components in the plant provide healing and soothing effects on all organs and tissues, relieving irritation, inflammation, swelling, and pain.

Allantoin, occurring in greatest concentrations in the roots, is a cell proliferate encouraging cell growth and regeneration. It is the primary constituent responsible for superb healing. Silicon, in the form of silicic acid, and a multitude of other minerals and vitamins in Comfrey promote normal development of connective tissue, cartilage, elastin and bone, and facilitate uptake of minerals into bone to enhance repair (Bergner, 1998). Comfrey is excellent for chronic skin ulcers. When I worked as a hospital medical/surgical nurse, I was pleased to see that the pharmaceutical ointment I applied to decubitus ulcers on many bed-ridden patients contained allantoin as the only primary ingredient.

Allantoin and the mucilage contained in Comfrey roots, and to a lesser extent in the leaves, are the primary phytochemicals contributing to the herb's vast healing potential.

Comfrey salves, hot fomentations made from tea, and poultices of leaves or ground root may be applied to broken bones, bruises, burns, recent and older slow-healing wounds, ulcers, gangrene, eruptive rashes, diaper rash, insect bites, and most other skin problems. In addition to topical application, the tea may be taken internally to assist in bone repair and tissue healing. Mild astringent properties help reduce bleeding both internally and externally. The astringent quality also restores normal muscle tone to blood vessels and is helpful for treating varicose veins, hemorrhoids, and thrombophlebitis (vein inflammation caused by blood clots), especially when combined with other stronger astringents such as Witch Hazel (*Hamamelis virginiana*), Cranesbill (*Geranium maculatum*), or Cinquefoil (*Potentilla* spp.).

When my former husband broke his leg and had a metal plate screwed into his tibia, I gave him a cup of Comfrey tea daily for about two weeks. His leg healed and remains strong after many years. Maria Treben, the well-known Austrian herbalist, successfully applied Comfrey root powder as a poultice over a decayed spinal disc to strengthen and normalize the cartilage (Treben, 1988). For sprains, backaches, and torn muscles and ligaments, try putting a thick wad of Comfrey salve combined with Tiger Balm (an analgesic ointment available in health food stores) on the affected area. If the live plant is available, slice a few large leaves of Comfrey in several places with a knife to release the healing juice, and wrap them over the salve and Tiger Balm. Cover with plastic wrap to contain the ointment and leaves, and then cover the area with an electric heating pad for 1-2 hours. To avoid any scratchy irritation from the fresh leaves, they may be chopped up, combined with a small amount of water, and simmered for a few minutes. This is then applied to the skin along with the other ingredients. The heat and Tiger Balm open skin pores, allowing the ointment deep penetration to decrease inflammation and regenerate torn and injured tissues. Many years ago, I continually sprained my ankles quite severely and developed this protocol that relieved pain almost immediately and decreased swelling within 24 hours every time!

For red, inflamed, and irritated eyes, use a wash of the filtered tea to soothe and heal injured tissues. It is especially beneficial when combined with Goldenseal (*Hydrastis canadensis*) tea for eye irritation and infection.

Be cautious when using Comfrey for very deep wounds – the herb is such a profound healer that it can promote tissue formation over the wound before it is healed in deeper skin levels. This could encourage incomplete healing or allow infection to be sealed in, which can lead to abscesses and other toxic conditions (Bergner, 2002). It is always best to combine Comfrey with herbs that are strong antiseptics such as Goldenseal root, Yarrow (*Achillea millefolium*), Echinacea (*Echinacea* spp.), Calendula (*Calendula officinalis*), and Sage (*Salvia officinalis*) to prevent these possible complications. The herbal salve I make contains all these herbs and several more, and after continual use for over 35 years by many people and myself on a daily basis, I have not seen a single case of incomplete healing or lingering, trapped infections.

There have been many animal and human studies documenting the wound healing, anti-inflammatory, and analgesic effects of Comfrey (Goldman, 1985; Barna, 2007). Rosmarinic acid in the plant exerts strong anti-inflammatory activity (Gracza, 1985). In a double-blind, multicenter, placebo-controlled, group comparison study on 142 patients suffering from acute ankle sprains, a Comfrey ointment was applied 4 times a day over an 8-day treatment period. Compared to placebo, Comfrey was superior in reducing pain and inflammation and improving ankle mobility (Koll, 2004). Other human clinical trials have shown similar results (Kucera, 2004; Predel, 2005). *In vivo* tests demonstrated significant wound healing with extracts of the leaves. Inflammation subsided and collagen deposits of new tissue were enhanced (Araujo, 2012). In a double-blind, randomized, multicenter trial investigating 215 patients with lower and upper back pain, topical application of Comfrey reduced back pain and allowed improved mobility (Kucera, 2005). Another clinical trial involving 120 patients with back pain showed similar results with the herbal therapy (Giannetti, 2010). Comfrey relieved painful osteoarthritis of the knee and improved joint mobility during a trial involving 220 patients (Grube, 2007). In a double-blind clinical study of 108 children with fresh wound abrasions, applications of Comfrey leaf enhanced wound healing and reduced pain (Barna, 2012).

Respiratory System: The mucilage in Comfrey is moisturizing, soothing, and healing to lung and bronchial tissues. Its cooling influence decreases inflammation and the heat of fevers. As an expectorant, it is a good remedy for lung congestion and excessive phlegm, and is beneficial for coughs (especially dry coughs), bronchitis, sinusitis, pneumonia, whooping cough, bleeding lungs, sore throat, and any ulceration in the throat or lungs. It is primarily used for acute conditions and infections rather than as a long-term tonic for chronic problems.

The allantoin and mucilage in Comfrey soothes and heals tissues in the respiratory, digestive, and urinary systems.

The herb relieves hot inflammation, moisturizes dry tissues, lubricates lungs, eases coughs, and heals damaged and ulcerated tissues.

For respiratory ailments, Comfrey should always be combined with other herbs rather than used alone, and its cooling quality should be taken into consideration. In cases with copious amounts of clear or white-colored phlegm, indicating excess coolness in the lungs, always combine Comfrey with warming herbs such as Ginger (*Zingiber officinale*), Cloves (*Syzygium aromaticus*), Cardamom (*Elettaria cardamomum*), or Cayenne (*Capsicum annuum*). Other excellent herbs for the respiratory system include Horehound (*Marrubium vulgare*), Elecampane (*Inula helenium*), Pleurisy Root (*Asclepias tuberosa*), Hyssop (*Hyssopus officinalis*), and Wild Cherry bark (*Prunus serotina*). These may be blended with Comfrey into a tea, tincture, or cough syrup.

Digestive System: Taken internally as tea, Comfrey is soothing and healing to the entire gastrointestinal tract due to its allantoin and mucilage components. It helps relieve tissue irritation and excessive dryness, and is remarkable for treating all inflammatory bowel diseases and ulceration of the gut wall, including ulcerative colitis, irritable bowel syndrome, Crohn's disease, and stomach and intestinal ulcers. The tea is used as a gargle and mouthwash for sore and ulcerated mouths, throats, and hoarseness. The cooling and moisturizing properties are helpful for heartburn, acid reflux, upset stomach, and constipation.

Years ago, a friend shared with me that she had been having problems swallowing food due to some kind of tightness and constriction in her lower esophagus. This continued for several weeks until she had the idea to drink some Comfrey root tea. After only two cups of tea, she reported the problem resolved and it has not returned.

A soothing tea for stomach problems and a general aid for digestion is made with 1 tablespoon each of Comfrey, Marshmallow root (*Althaea officinalis*), Ginger root, and Fennel seed (*Foeniculum vulgare*). These are gently simmered in a covered pot containing 2 quarts of water for 5-10 minutes. Turn off the flame, steep for 30 minutes, and drink throughout the day. Unless acid reflux is a problem, 1-2 tablespoons of Peppermint leaves (*Mentha x piperita*) may be added. Peppermint is contraindicated for acid reflux because it relaxes the muscle sphincter between the stomach and esophagus, which allows stomach contents to push upward, causing burning sensations.

Researchers conducting human studies found that Comfrey extracts effectively reduce inflammation and lesions on the gums and membranes of the mouth (Suciu, 1988) and exhibit ability to repair gums and tissues in the mouth following surgical procedures (Gafar, 1989). Trials also confirmed that Comfrey tea is helpful for stomach ulcers and gastrointestinal hypermotility that causes fast transit time of food and diarrhea (Culvenor, 1985).

Kidneys, Bladder, and Gallstones: The root tea is especially soothing to inflamed, irritated, or ulcerated kidneys and bladder. It can be taken to treat bloody urine and ease symptoms of urinary tract infections, including cystitis and urethritis. Combine it with antibiotic and diuretic herbs such as Echinacea, Yarrow, Gravel Root (*Eupatorium purpureum*), and Uva-ursi (*Arctostaphylos uva-ursi*) when treating urinary infections. The soothing, mucilaginous quality of the tea makes passage of painful kidney stones less traumatic. However, this herb should be used for acute conditions and not as a long-term tonic.

Women's Health: Comfrey tea may be administered as a douche to treat yeast and other vaginal infections and discharges. The mucilage heals and soothes pain, irritation, and inflammation throughout the reproductive tract. Always combine it with antibacterial herbs such as Goldenseal and Yarrow for best results. One research study found that Comfrey tea enhanced uterine tone (Shipochliev, 1981).

A compress or sitz bath of Comfrey and Plantain (*Plantago* spp.) tea are beneficial for postpartum care and following an episiotomy to heal tears in the perineum. These are administered 2-3 times a day for 5-20 minutes at a time. A hot compress of Comfrey tea, a poultice, or salve soothes sore nipples and heals nipple fissures and bruises. It softens engorged breasts, reduces pain of swollen breasts, helps clear obstructions in milk ducts, and can be used for mastitis. Nursing mothers should use Comfrey externally rather than drinking the tea.

Teachings from the Comfrey Deva

"Greetings. I am the Comfrey Deva that speaks with you now. My earth and water elements are strong and bestow healing potential to humans and animals. The bones, muscles, and tissues of the body emerge from the earth element to form your body's solidity and structure. I heal this structure when there is damage, cuts, and fragmentation that separate broken parts from the whole. As my old name 'knitbone' implies, I knit together the fabric of tissues and bones to heal and make whole. And so I am a strong sustainer and protector of the physical body, holding all together.

"My element of water is present in the thick and slick juices permeating through my roots and veins. And when ingested or laid upon the body, my soothing juices permeate through human and animal tissues just as water gently and persistently seeps through the soil. These cleansing juices wash away all debris and waste, and in their wake there is freshness and vitality. My thick mucilage softens hardness, cools hot, inflamed tissues, and glues together torn fragments of bones and tissues. And so I have a binding and 'holding together' influence on the physical form. Abundant nutrients to heal and sustain the body are offered in my luscious green leaves full of life-sustaining chlorophyll and minerals.

"The old astrologer Culpeper intuited that I am regulated by the sign of Capricorn. But the water element and healing juices within my plants are also influenced by the moon and the astrological sign of Cancer. Cancer is a water sign extremely sensitive to feelings and emotions, and the moon qualities resonate with the deep, hidden emotional energies of the heart.

"My bell-shaped flowers, like little cups, hold the essence of my heart energy. The quality of purity magnified in their white, pink, and bluish-purple colors resonates with the purity of heart, and this purity of heart is such a vast and mysterious space! For the heart is deep open space of pulsating energy in the realm of feeling and emotion. E-motion means 'energy in motion.' There is the aspect of radiant, outward flowing heart energy in search of its own reflection of love. When the space of the heart is open and flowing, there is connection with others and with all of life. There is joy of being, gratitude of abundance, and completeness of merging in loving relationships.

"This is the natural, innate life of the heart when unsullied by pain, despair, anger, or hatred. For all these emotions constrict, harden, and freeze feelings and sensitivities of the heart, and eventually even the muscles and tissues in the heart and body become tight, restricted in movement, and painful. To be open in the flow of life is to choose to have a heart open and accepting to all the joys and sorrows of life, while always remaining in gratitude and compassion. And when people live and abide in this indestructible compassionate heart, magic comes forth as this compassion radiates outward into the hearts of others. Love begets love. Relax into this flow!

"And so, I am a plant of heart healing. My power, though mild and gentle, is strong and resilient, as evidenced by the tenacious nature of my roots, which will sprout new shoots of vibrant leaves even from small broken pieces and transform into large thriving plants. My earth element and powerful roots are so strong that my reproductive forces are held underground in my roots rather than airborne in seeds. For the seeds from my flowers do not develop into fertile maturity.

"Please prepare and use an essence of my flowers to resonate with the open, flowing nature of your own heart and to rest in the radiating joy of compassion. Through the window of your open heart, may you see this radiant heart shining forth in those around you.

"And so, from our flower hearts to yours, we wish you a gentle flow through your life. A journey of the open heart is a journey of awesome wonder and unbounded love. This is the message of the Comfrey beings. Be in peace!"

Cranesbill

Geranium maculatum
Geraniaceae (Geranium) Family

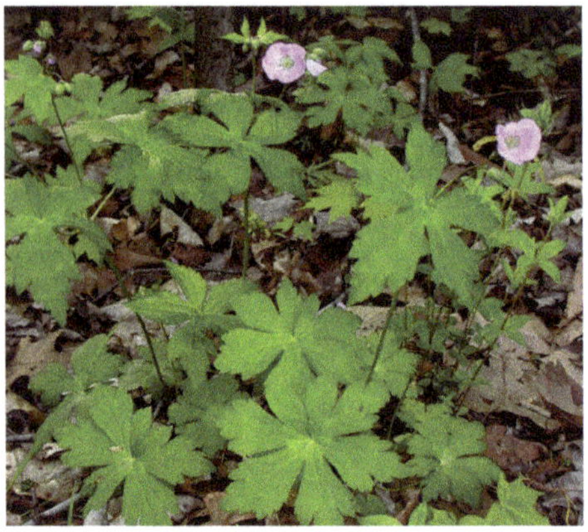

Common Names

Spotted cranesbill, wild cranesbill, and storksbill are common names describing the appearance of the seedpod, which resembles the bill of a crane or stork. Wild geranium, wild alum root, alum bloom, crowfoot, dove's foot, old maid's nightcap, and tormentil (also a common name for Cinquefoil) are older names for the plant.

Medicinal Part of the Plant

The root is the most potent and commonly used part of the plant, but the leaves also contain medicinal astringents.

Range and Habitat

Geranium maculatum is an early spring wildflower native to the woodlands of Europe and eastern and central North America. Flourishing in low areas that are moist and loamy, it is often found on hillsides and along the edges of fields and meadows. It typically grows in large patches, and the showy pink flowers brighten up the forest in early spring. There are several varieties of Cranesbill and some have naturalized from Europe.

Description of the Plant

G. maculatum is a hardy perennial growing 1-2′ tall. The root is a unique-looking rhizome ¼-½″ in diameter that grows horizontally a few inches below the ground surface. Rhizomes typically range from 1-6″ in length depending on the age of the plant, and several smaller branches often divide off the primary rhizome. The rhizome is rough and contorted due to short, stubby protuberances pointing outward along its entire length. It is also covered with scars, showing the remains of stems from previous years' growth. Many thread-like rootlets grow out from the rhizome. The outer root is dark reddish brown and the inner fleshy part is a lighter cream color with a pinkish tinge. Familiarity with the unique appearance of this root is a helpful way to identify the herb after the flowers have disappeared.

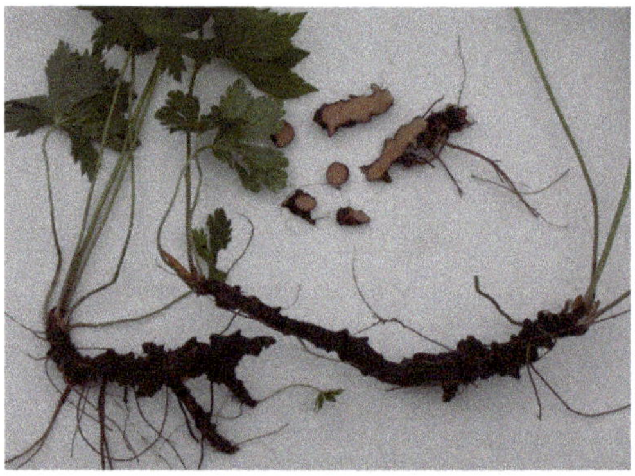

Cranesbill roots

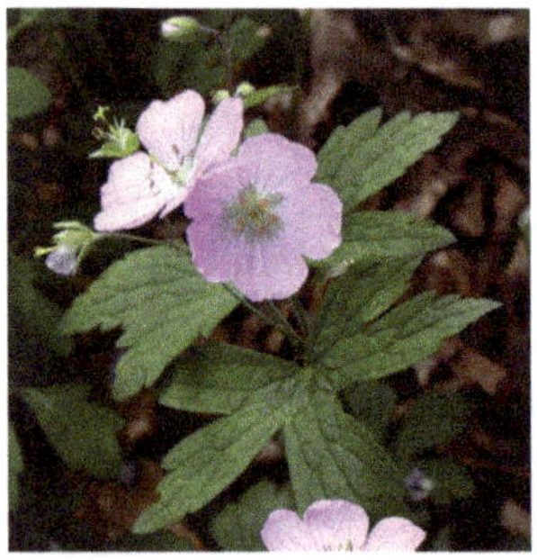

Several erect stems grow from one or both ends of the rhizome. Stems are round and covered with minute pubescent hairs. Leaves emerge singly at the ends of stems or in pairs opposite each other along the stem on long petioles. The simple, palmate leaves are deeply indented into 5 lobes (sometimes 3 or 7) and have serrately toothed margins. They are palmately veined and covered with fine hairs. The leaves are mottled with whitish-green splotches, hence the name *maculatum*, meaning "spotted."

The delicate and attractive pinkish-lavender flowers bloom from April in southern locations and June in northern areas for about 3 weeks. Flowers are 1-1½″ wide, occurring mostly in pairs on long pedicel stalks in loose clusters of 2-5 at the end of stems. Each flower has 5 rounded petals and 5 pointed green sepals. The petals are marked with whitish green at their bases. The 10 stamens curve outward, surrounding a central pistil. As the flower matures and wilts, the pistil develops into the distinctive seedpod resembling a crane's bill, hence its common name. The genus name is derived from the Greek word *geranos*, meaning "crane."

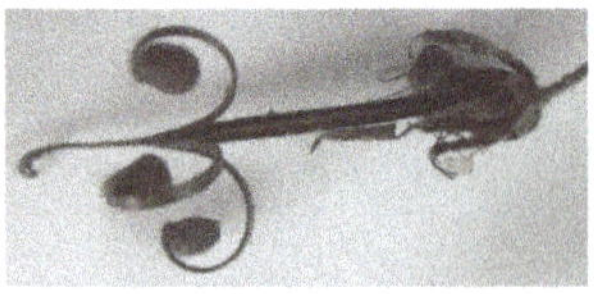

Cranesbill seedpod

Cultivation

Cranesbill readily self-propagates, making cultivation unnecessary in areas where it naturally grows. It is not difficult to establish a patch because it re-seeds itself each year and voluntarily spreads over time. Prepare a bed in partial or total shade with rich woodland dirt containing a lot of humus. The soil should be moist but well-drained.

Cranesbill propagates by seed and root division. Seeds may be collected when they are mature about 6-7 weeks after blooming. Plant the seeds immediately after harvesting or in spring or autumn if they are purchased. Space seeds about 3″ apart and barely cover with dirt. They need a conditioning period of cold stratification and may take 2 years to germinate. Propagating by root division is faster and more dependable. Dig up and cut the roots into pieces at least 1″ long, making sure each has a bud. Replant the pieces horizontally so the bud is pointed in the direction it will grow, and space the root pieces 6″ apart. Cover each piece with 1-2″ of soil and keep the soil moist.

Harvest

Harvest the root and leaves just before or as the plant starts blooming in spring when levels of medicinal tannins are highest. The seeds are not used medicinally but can be harvested for planting in late spring or early summer. Seed collection requires patience and frequent checking of the seedpods because seeds must be harvested after they are mature, but before they fall out of the dried pod.

Preparation of Plant Medicine and Dosages

Preparations are usually made with the more potent root, but leaves are also useful. Water and alcohol both extract the plant's medicinal properties, making tea and tincture appropriate preparations. However, alcohol is the best extractor of the astringent tannins. Leaves and roots may also be used in a salve for external application. The fresh plant is most potent and always preferable, but Cranesbill may also be dried.

PREPARATIONS

Tea: Gently simmer 1-2 teaspoons of chopped or powdered root or leaves in 1 cup of water for 8-10 minutes. Dosage: 1-3 cups a day as needed. The tea has a mildly bitter taste and produces an interesting sensation on the tongue for a few minutes due to its astringent tannins.

Tincture: Chop fresh root or leaves into small pieces, stuff into a glass jar, and cover with 60% 190-proof grain alcohol and 40% distilled water. Dosage: 10-30 drops in water every 1-2 hours or 10-60 drops up to 4 times a day as needed.

Salve: The roots and leaves are excellent additions to salve to decrease bruising and bleeding.

Suppository: This is used to treat hemorrhoids and vaginal infections. Fresh roots and leaves must be dried and ground into powder to prepare suppositories. Cranesbill may be used alone or combined with other appropriate herbs that are also ground onto powder.

Suppositories can be made with water or coconut butter. To prepare with water, add enough water to the ground herb to make a thick paste the consistency of peanut butter. Roll the herbal paste into 2″ pieces for vaginal use and 1″ pieces for rectal use, making sure they are about the thickness of the little finger. Set the pieces on a tray and dry in a low oven at 200ºF. To make suppositories with coconut butter, blend the herbs in enough melted coconut butter to make a thick paste. Roll the paste into 1-2″ pieces and, rather than baking, place the suppositories in a refrigerator to solidify. Store water- and oil-based suppositories in a refrigerator or freezer for the longest shelf life.

Chemical Constituents

Cranesbill contains 12-25% tannic acid (Brinker, 2001), occurring in highest concentrations just prior to blooming. The tannins are very astringent and responsible for the primary healing qualities of the plant. Cranesbill also contains mucilage, small amounts of resin, and large quantities of gallic acid, which is analgesic, anti-allergenic, anti-asthmatic, antibacterial, antiviral, anti-inflammatory, antioxidant, antitumor, astringent, and an immunostimulant.

Safety, Contraindications, and Drug Interactions

Cranesbill is considered to be a safe herb that is well-tolerated by children and the elderly due to its gentle and non-irritating nature. No toxicity, contraindications, or adverse drug interactions have been reported, and it does not upset the stomach (McGuffin, 1997). Since the astringent quality is drying and ideal for treating diarrhea, it may worsen constipation. Astringent herbs are **contraindicated during lactation**.

Medicinal Uses

History of the Plant

Apparently, Cranesbill was not used medicinally by many early Europeans. The English herbalist and apothecary John Gerard (1545–1612), who wrote about *G. maculatum* and other species of Cranesbill in his famous *Herball*, stated that they had no known medical effects. But in North America, the plant was employed by the Cherokee, Chippewa, Choctaw, Iroquois, and other woodland tribes to treat bleeding, diarrhea, hemorrhoids, dysentery, kidney and stomach problems, sore throats, canker sores in the mouth, gonorrhea, cancer, and oral thrush (yeast infection in the mouth) (Moerman, 1998). Cranesbill was dried and used as a powder to control bleeding wounds and was also prepared as tea.

Native Americans taught settlers about the healing properties of this herb, and early American physicians incorporated Cranesbill into their medical practice for similar ailments. It was the favorite astringent of the Eclectic physicians, who regarded it as suitable for both children and adults. They mixed the powdered herb in an infusion of milk for dysentery, diarrhea, infant cholera, and weak, atonic membranes. The roots were used internally and externally for all conditions requiring astringent and toning qualities, including hemorrhage, excessive menstrual bleeding, bleeding hemorrhoids and wounds, hematuria (bloody urine), epistaxis (nose bleeds), eye inflammations, leucorrhea (vaginal discharge), chronic excessive mucous discharges, tuberculosis, cholera, skin ulcers resistant to healing, and night sweats. A gargle of the tea was taken for sore throats, canker sores, and relaxation of the uvula (the little flap of skin hanging down from the back of the throat). It was often combined with Goldenseal (*Hydrastis canadensis*) or small amounts of Cayenne (*Capsicum annuum*) for treating these conditions. Eclectic physicians William Cook, M.D. wrote, "This root is a superior astringent with tonic properties; rather positive, yet not so powerful; operating slowly and persistently, somewhat soothing in its impression, and usually quite acceptable to the stomach" (Cook, 1869). Finley Ellingwood, M.D. (1852–1920) reported excellent results when he used the root in a case of liver cirrhosis with ulceration of the intestinal duodenum (Ellingwood, 1919).

Dr. John Christopher (1909–1983), a clinical herbalist and naturopath who used Cranesbill extensively in his practice, wrote that "Cranesbill is an excellent and effective astringent with pleasant tonic properties. Its astringent action is powerful and non-irritating, well-suited for relieving relaxed, atonic and enfeebled conditions of the mucous tissues debilitated by copious discharges. It is not nauseous, making it useful for infants and persons with sensitive stomachs. Cranesbill is moderately drying in action, strengthening and invigorating the stomach, kidneys, and the other internal organs" (Christopher, 1976).

Cranesbill was listed as an official tonic and astringent medicine from 1820–1916 in the *United States Pharmacopoeia* and in the *National Formulary* from 1916–1936. Currently, it is not a popular herb and there has been little research on the plant. Although rarely sold in health food stores, Cranesbill can be harvested from its natural habitat. Most herbalists who discover its reliable healing capabilities appreciate its value.

Healing Qualities

Cranesbill is antihydrotic (reduces excessive perspiration), antifungal, anti-inflammatory, antiseptic, strong astringent, lactifuge, tonic (restores tone to tissues and mucous membranes), vulnerary, and anti-catarrhal. Catarrh is an old term for phlegm and mucous secreted from irritated membranes, particularly in the respiratory tract.

Traditional Chinese Medicine (TCM) Perspective

This is a classic herb for treating Spleen Qi deficiency characterized by weak, boggy, atonic tissues leading to prolapsed organs, hemorrhage, excessive secretions and perspiration, and diarrhea. It is cooling and drying in nature, and exerts a restoring and toning effect on the mucous membranes and tissues. Cranesbill is given for conditions of damp heat and damp cold such as diarrhea and infectious vaginal discharges, and its cooling action is beneficial for acute inflammation.

Primary Actions

As I have become acquainted with this beautiful forest wildflower, I am grateful for the plant's consistent reliability in arresting diarrhea and abnormal bleeding. Cranesbill's medicinal use stems from its superior astringent and tonic properties. The plant grows plentifully in my woodlands, so I tincture some each year to use for my family and nursing practice. I have recommended a Cranesbill and Cinquefoil (*Potentilla* spp.) tincture combination for numerous cases of diarrhea and abnormal bleeding with successful, fast, and sometimes amazing results.

Astringent for Bleeding, Diarrhea, and Atonic Tissues: Cranesbill's astringent tannins have a constricting action on tissues and mucous membranes throughout the body, including those lining the mouth, throat, lungs, blood vessels, and digestive and genitourinary tracts. Astringents are excellent for normalizing atonic conditions in which weak, overly relaxed tissues, muscles, and mucous membranes lack tone and strength, becoming increasingly dysfunctional. Atonic muscles in blood vessels balloon out into varicose veins and hemorrhoids. Weak muscles allow organs they support to prolapse or fall from their normal position. Atonic tissues and mucous membranes permit fluids to leak out, causing excessive discharge of blood, mucous, water, and other secretions. The astringent properties of Cranesbill are also anhydrotic, meaning that they reduce excessive perspiration, a condition known as hyperhydrosis.

Cranesbill tea or tincture constricts and normalizes tissues to reduce excessive secretions, including diarrhea and all types of internal bleeding, such as hemorrhage, nose bleeds, hemorrhoids, dysentery, ulcerative colitis with bloody stools, and bloody urine (indicative of urinary tract bleeding). The Eclectic physicians found that the herb decreases excess stomach acid and mucous and pus in the intestines and bladder, actions that are healing for heartburn and stomach and intestinal ulcers.

Prepare an excellent blend to help heal bleeding ulcers by simmering 2 tablespoons chopped Cranesbill root and 1 teaspoon Goldenseal root in 1 quart water for 10 minutes. Turn off heat, add 3 tablespoons finely chopped or ground Marshmallow root (*Althaea officinalis*) and allow it to steep for 2-3 hours. Sip this throughout the day. This blend, or Cranesbill alone, may be gargled for sore and ulcerated throats, tissue inflammation and canker sores in the mouth, and thrush, a yeast infection in the mouth most common in infants and immune-compromised people.

An external application of the herb constricts enlarged varicose veins, and daily ingestion of small amounts of tea or tincture can help prevent new ones from forming. Combine Cranesbill with Cayenne when treating varicose veins to increase circulation and thin the blood, which helps prevent blockage in the blood vessels. For hemorrhoids, prepare suppositories by combining equal parts of the dried and powdered roots of Cranesbill and Marshmallow or Slippery Elm (*Ulmus rubra*). Insert a suppository rectally at night before going to bed and continue until relief is obtained.

Women's Health: The astringent properties of this herb are beneficial for excessive or abnormal bleeding. I have seen several women suffering from profuse menstrual bleeding (menorrhagia) and break-through bleeding caused by uterine fibroids, who have been amazed at the quick results from taking 60 drops of Cranesbill and Cinquefoil tincture blend 3-4 times a day to stop the bleeding. It is also useful for uterine hemorrhage after childbirth. As a lactifuge, Cranesbill roots reduce milk secretions in nursing mothers and can be combined with Sage (*Salvia officinalis*) to wean children. Mothers who want to continue nursing should avoid ingesting Cranesbill and other astringent herbs.

Cranesbill tea and tincture are excellent for leucorrhea, a vaginal discharge caused by bacteria or Candida yeast. For vaginal infections, it works best when combined with Goldenseal, Myrrh (*Commiphora myrrha*), Yarrow (*Achillea millefolium*), and Marshmallow root. These can be prepared as a tea for internal healing or used as a douche, or they are ground up and made into suppositories. Insert a suppository high into the vagina before bed and leave overnight. Continue this treatment until all signs of yeast infection are gone.

External Healing: Cranesbill, an excellent vulnerary for healing all types of external wounds, is a welcome addition to the herbal salve I have been making for many years. Salve, powdered root, diluted tincture, or fomentations (the application of a cloth soaked in strong tea) are used externally. Cranesbill is an effective blood coagulant to stop bleeding that, if applied immediately after injury, can constrict damaged blood vessels to prevent bruising. It may be used for chronic ulcers and fungal infections.

Ears: In *Health from God's Garden*, Austrian herbalist Maria Treben recommends putting a few drops of Cranesbill tincture in the ear for complaints of tinnitus (ringing in the ear) and diminished hearing. These conditions are often caused by a build-up of fluids in the ear, and the drying astringent action of Cranesbill may be helpful for this type of edema.

Teachings from the Cranesbill Deva

"Greetings, dear one. I am the deva of the Cranesbill. My plants are of the earth element and are forest dwellers. They grow within the rich, moist humus that releases pungent aromas of fresh new life springing forth after the stillness and cold of winter months.

"Like my friends Comfrey and Cinquefoil, I mend tears, breaks, and fragmentation of muscles and tissues. I blend especially well with Cinquefoil. Our similar constricting actions heal by sealing damaged blood vessels to stop bleeding and by binding intestinal tissues when there is diarrhea. And so my movement, like that of Cinquefoil, is inward and upward to draw together and cement broken pieces back into wholeness.

"The pink color of my flowers and pinkish-tinged roots point to my affinity with the blood itself, and not only to the ability to repair vessels transporting the blood. Just as my plants appear in the early spring amidst the fullness and richness of budding life, my healing energies also bring forth new life and exciting possibilities. I am ruled by the earth sign of Taurus, the phase of fresh, vital life force when solid form emerges from the earth. I offer balance to the physical body.

"My message to humans is to be present in the joy and revelation of each moment of your life as it emerges, just as if each day were the first day of spring, resplendent with the miraculous awe and wonder of new life unfolding. I am a harbinger of hope in the potential of each moment. I provide deep peace and the security of being constantly held in the powerful moment of the eternal now, from whence all arises.

"Use my flowers in an essence to impart these subtle gifts. I ease the mind and soul when they are frustrated and flung about by life's mishaps. Enjoy my gifts to become grounded in the depths of being, where all is held securely in the creative web of life. For just as the fibers of a spider's web can hold torn tissues in place, medicines made from my roots do the same with torn vessels and tissues. My flowers draw together the torn fragments of the heart and mind to calm the soul and bring wholeness. These are my gifts. Please use them wisely to allow the freshness of spring and revelation of each moment to dawn."

Dandelion

Taraxacum officinale
Compositae (*Asteraceae*) (Sunflower or Aster) Family

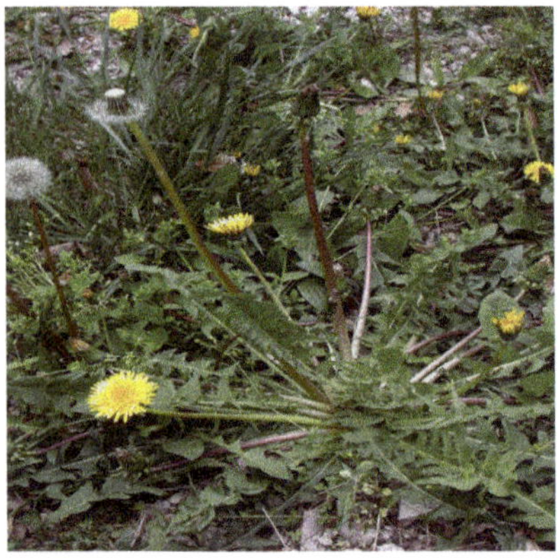

Common Names

Wild endive, white endive, priest's crown, swine snout, cankerwort, and blowball are antiquated names. Pissenlit is a French name that translates as "piss-in-bed," referring to the plant's diuretic action.

Medicinal Part of the Plant

The roots, leaves, and flowers are medicinal.

Range and Habitat

Indigenous to Asia, Europe and northern Africa, Dandelion has prolifically naturalized throughout temperate zones around the world, including North and South America, New Zealand, and Australia.

Description of the Plant

Dandelion belongs to the *Taraxacum* genus, a diverse and complex group encompassing many species and varieties. Most are perennials but some are biennials. All have taproots and the entire plant contains bitter-tasting, milky-white latex that oozes out of broken stems and roots.

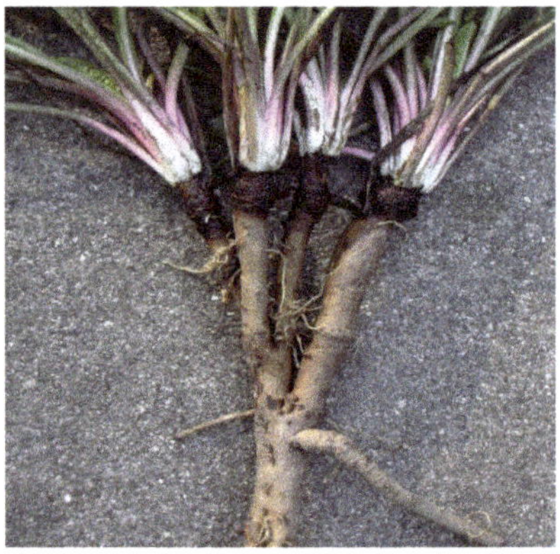

Dandelion grows up to 1′ tall. The cylindrical, fleshy taproot is light brown outside and creamy white inside, with a yellowish and porous central axis. The main taproot can be somewhat branched with a few thready rootlets growing off the sides. Large roots can grow to a foot in length and 1″ in diameter at the crown. Older roots often divide into several crowns.

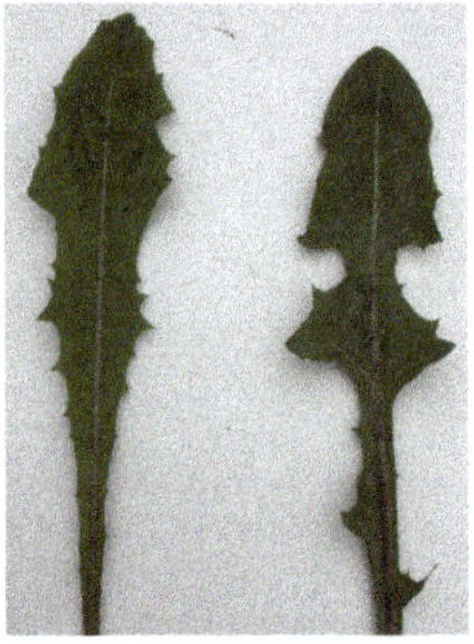

Many long leaves rise directly from the root crown forming a basal rosette. The leaves are simple, glabrous (smooth, without hairs) and somewhat shiny, and have a large, prominent central midrib vein with smaller pinnate veins extending outward. The actual shape of the leaves varies from lance-shaped to spatulate with a tapering, pointed leaf base and a wider, rounded upper tip. Large, jagged, pointed teeth along the leaf margins are widely and irregularly spaced, and deeply indented. The name Dandelion comes from the French name "dent de lion," which means "tooth of the lion," describing the sharp leaf margins resembling teeth.

One or two flower heads emerge from each crown and sit on a long, round, hollow stem that is greenish maroon in color. The flower head is 1-2″ in diameter and looks like a typical *Compositae* flower head, except that it lacks the central disc flowers and is entirely composed of many flat, bright-yellow ray petals. The calyx consists of many green sepals. Flowers bloom from early spring through autumn and provide nectar for bees and other insects. They are light-sensitive, opening fully in sunlight and partially closing in the dark of night and cloudy weather.

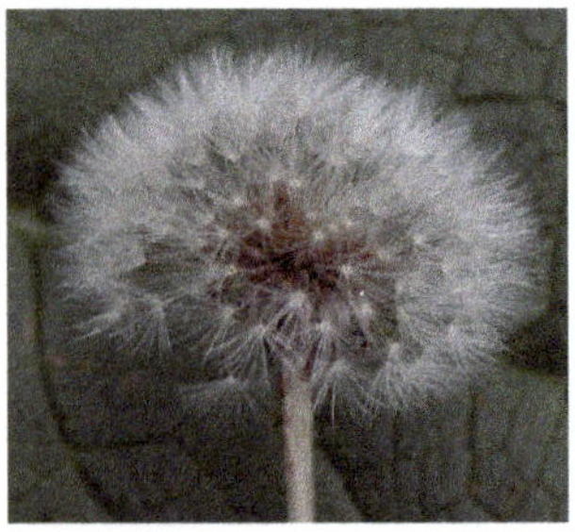

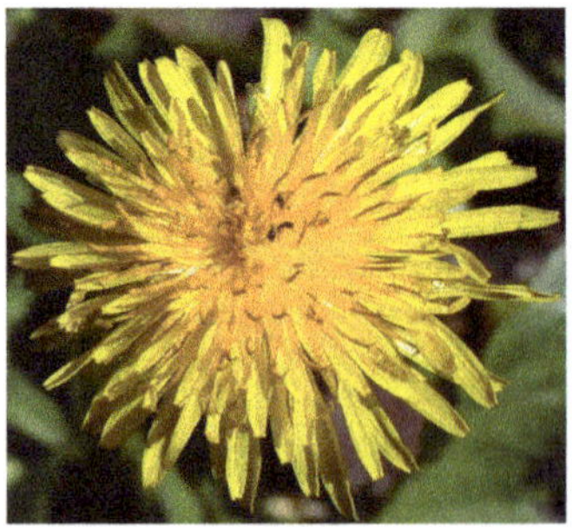

As flowers age, the yellow petals wither and the green sepals of the upper calyx close around the seeds to protect them while they mature. Then the calyx opens, holding a puffball cluster of seeds. Each brown seed is attached to a hair-like tuft that carries it in the wind like a tiny parachute, one of nature's mechanisms for dispersing seeds.

Cultivation

Yes, it may be difficult to fathom, but some people actually cultivate Dandelion, while others go to all lengths of chemical warfare to eradicate it. Since Dandelion readily self-sows its seeds and is a hardy germinator, it is a common weed in lawns, fields and gardens, and propagation is usually unnecessary. But some people like planting it (or allowing it to grow) in their gardens because the roots grow larger and longer in loose, loamy soil and less effort is required to harvest these roots compared to digging them out of compact lawns and fields. The plant is easy to cultivate and grows in sun or shade, but growth rate is greatly increased by full sunlight. Sow seeds directly into garden soil about 1/4-1/8″ deep anytime during the growing season. Space plants 4-6″ apart and keep them watered.

Harvest

Be sure to harvest Dandelion from areas that are free of chemical pesticides and herbicides. For culinary purposes, harvest young leaves in early spring, prior to blooming, when they are tender and mild-tasting. They get increasingly bitter and tough after flowers appear, until autumn, when the bitterness subsides following the first hard frost. Leaves may be harvested anytime to prepare a medicinal tea or tincture since the bitter properties are beneficial.

Harvest roots from plants that are at least 2 years old, fleshy, and substantial in size. They can be gathered in early spring, summer, or fall. However, research indicates that concentrations of desired phytochemicals in the roots vary according to season. For best medicinal potency, collect roots in autumn before the first frost when they contain the greatest amounts of inulin and bitters, which are important biologically active components. Dandelion roots dug up in autumn contain 24-40% inulin, while those harvested in March contain about 2% (European Scientific Cooperative, 1996). Tinctures made from autumn-harvested roots tend to have a milky-opaque color due to the greater volume of constituents, including inulin, compared to spring-harvested roots that produce a dark, clear extract.

Preparation of Plant Medicine and Dosages

Dandelion roots and leaves yield their properties to alcohol and boiling water, making tinctures and teas effective preparations. Teas are the best way to extract the therapeutic water-soluble polysaccharides and inulin. The medicinal bitter principles are more soluble in alcohol than water, so the tincture form is recommended for liver and digestive problems. Dandelion may be dried in the usual manner, but fresh roots and leaves produce the most potent remedies and exert the strongest cholagogue action on the liver and gallbladder.

PREPARATIONS

Infusion Tea: Steep 1 tablespoon of chopped fresh or dried leaves in 1 cup of boiling hot water for 15-20 minutes. Dosage: 1-3 cups a day as needed. Tea prepared from leaves collected in spring has a pleasant taste, ranging from no bitterness to mildly bitter.

Decoction Tea: Gently simmer 1-2 teaspoons of fresh or dried root in 1 cup of water for 10 minutes in a pan covered with a lid to prevent evaporation. Dosage: 1-2 cups a day as needed. The root tea has a mildly bitter flavor.

Tincture: This is prepared with just the root or the root and leaves together. Tincture fresh Dandelion in a mixture of 60% 190-proof grain alcohol and 40% distilled water. Tincturing the roots in brandy produces a tasty cordial. Dosage: 10-90 drops in water up to 4 times a day as needed.

Freshly Squeezed Juice: Extract juice from fresh Dandelion leaves and roots with a juicing machine. Drink the juice immediately. It may be preserved for future use by storing it in a freezer or by adding 25% alcohol. Dosage: 1 tablespoon diluted in water 1-2 times a day.

Tablets: Homemade pills are fun to make with the dried leaves and roots. Grind these into a fine powder, add water to form a thick paste, and roll into pill-sized balls. Powdered Marshmallow root (*Althaea officinalis*) or Slippery Elm bark (*Ulmus rubra*) may be added to the blend for their "gluey" consistency that helps the Dandelion powder stick together. Dry pills in an oven or air-dry, and store in airtight containers in the refrigerator or freezer. Dosage: 3 tablets up to 3 times a day.

Capsules: Dandelion roots and leaves are dried, ground into powder, and packed into capsules. Dosage: 3 capsules up to 3 times a day as needed, or 3-9 grams daily.

Culinary Uses

Fresh Dandelion flowers have traditionally been ingredients in jam, wine, and beer. I love dipping the fresh flowers in an egg-and-flour batter, then frying them in coconut or olive oil. They look like little buttons and are delicious with soy sauce and other condiments. The leafy greens are extremely nutritious with an abundance of easily assimilated vitamins and minerals. Greens collected in spring (before they get bitter) are quite tasty to eat fresh, dried or steamed, and can be added to salads, soups, stews, stir-fried vegetables, scrambled eggs, or quiche. Chopping and marinating fresh leaves in a little olive oil for several hours removes much of their bitterness. The roasted roots provide a healthy and alkalizing coffee substitute.

Many people are hooked on sweet or salty foods and shy away from bitter flavors. However, bitters are so beneficial for the liver and digestive system that it is good to remember that "the liver loves bitters." They are free for the taking, so try some healthy Dandelion flowers and greens!

Chemical Constituents

Dandelion's abundant vitamin and mineral content greatly contributes to its medicinal value. The leaves are considered to be one of the best plant sources of beta-carotene, which converts into vitamin A. According to the U.S. Department of Agriculture, 8 ounces of raw Dandelion leaves contain 14,000 I.U. (International units) of vitamin A, compared to only 11,000 I.U. in the same amount of carrots. Dried leaves hold up to 4.5% potassium and provide traces of protein, ascorbic acid (vitamin C), and several of the B vitamins including choline, an important nutrient for the liver (Broda, 1966). Three ounces of the cooked greens contain approximately 48 mg of ascorbic acid (vitamin C), 140 mg of calcium, 230 mg of potassium, and 1.8 mg of easily digested iron. The yellow flowers are one of the best plant sources of lecithin, which helps normalize elevated cholesterol levels and promotes healthy livers, joints, nerves, and skin. The roots draw minerals out of the soil, providing ample amounts of iron, calcium, magnesium, potassium, phosphorus, manganese, silica, boron, chromium, copper, iodine, selenium, sodium, sulfur, and zinc.

Scientific researchers have identified many phytochemicals in Dandelion and documented their biological activities. Bitter-tasting sesquiterpene lactones (terpenes) are considered to be the primary medicinal constituents and include amyrin, taraxacin, taraxerol, taraxacerin, taraxol, and taraxasterol. These have demonstrated a remarkable inhibitory effect on mammary tumors in mice. Taraxasterol and amyrin are diuretic and anti-inflammatory. These bitter terpenes are distributed throughout the entire plant (Blanchet, 1995). Taraxinic acid may have potential as a therapeutic agent in human leukemia (Choi, 2002). Eudesmanolides and germacranolides also appear to be diuretic. Aesculin in the leaves improves vascular resistance and normalizes capillary wall permeability. Phytosterols include beta-sitosterol (anti-inflammatory, antibacterial, anticarcinogenic, antioxidant, antitumor, antiviral, diuretic, febrifuge), stigmasterol (anti-inflammatory, antioxidant, antiviral, anticarcinogenic, estrogenic, hepatoprotective), and campesterol. Coumestrol is estrogenic, antimicrobial, antifungal, and reduces excess fats in the blood. Cycloartenol is antibacterial, anti-inflammatory, antirheumatic, and reduces cholesterol. Faradiol has been shown to be diuretic and anti-inflammatory.

Flavonoids in Dandelion include apigenin and luteolin (diuretic due to inhibition of aldosterone, anti-inflammatory, antiviral). Lutein is a carotenoid found to be anti-atherosclerotic, anticarcinogenic for breast and colon tissues, and antioxidant. Glutamic acid protects and heals the tissues lining the stomach and intestines and is also antilithic (reduces kidney and gallbladder stone formation). Coumaric acid is hepato-protective, antioxidant, antispasmodic, and diuretic due to its ability to inhibit aldosterone. Fatty acids include myristic, lauric, palmitic (diuretic, antioxidant, hemolytic, lowers cholesterol), stearic, chlorogenic, linoleic (anti-arthritic, anti-eczema, antihistamine, anticarcinogenic, hepatoprotective, lowers cholesterol), and oleic acids (diuretic, anticarcinogenic, stimulates bile production). Caffeic acid protects against blood clotting and is antibacterial, anticarcinogenic, diuretic, hepatoprotective, antihistamine, anti-inflammatory, antioxidant, antiviral, cholagogue, and an immunostimulant (Blumenthal, 2000). Tannins are anticarcinogenic and hepatoprotective. Saponins in Dandelion may ease kidney stone problems (Grases, 1994).

Polysaccharides (carbohydrates) in the root include glucans, fructose, a cooling mucilage, and inulin. Inulin is a form of starch found in roots of the *Compositae* family, including Burdock (*Arctium lappa*), Elecampane (*Inula helenium*), Chicory (*Cichorium intybus*), and a Chinese herb called Dang Shen (*Codonopsis pilosula*). It is a storage food for plants that is not digested well by people. It has a mildly sweet taste and is filling like other starchy foods. Inulin is a soothing demulcent. It helps normalize blood sugar, cholesterol, diarrhea and constipation, protects against breast and colon cancers, and is an expectorant and gastro-stimulant. Sometimes it is recommended for diabetes since it is not absorbed through the intestines and does not elevate blood sugar levels. Inulin is also a prebiotic that feeds and increases populations of beneficial lactobacilli bacteria in healthy intestines. Inulin has no connection with insulin, although the names sound similar. Inulin dissolves in hot water and is only slightly soluble in cold water or alcohol, making the decoction tea the best source.

Safety, Contraindications, and Drug Interactions

Dandelion is a mild and slow-acting herb considered to be safe even in large doses taken over extended periods of time. During pregnancy and lactation moderate amounts of the roots and leaves are beneficial due to the high mineral content. There are no known interactions with drugs.

The German Commission E herbal regulatory agency approved Dandelion root and leaf for treating bile flow problems, water retention, dyspepsia (indigestion, gas, bloating, and nausea), and loss of appetite. Clinical studies confirm the herb's benefit in treating gallstones with acute or chronic bile duct inflammation causing obstruction. However, many sources contraindicate Dandelion for these conditions because it may cause gas, pain, or diarrhea in people with intestinal irritation or inflammation. More importantly, the herb could potentially worsen blockages and obstructions in the abdomen, especially when these conditions are pre-existing. For this reason, Dandelion is generally contraindicated in acute stomach, intestinal, or gallbladder inflammation, intestinal blockage, and paralytic ileus (Blumenthal, 1998 & 2000; Brinker, 2001).

Medicinal Uses

History of the Plant

Although many people consider it to be a common and obnoxious weed, Dandelion is a valuable herb rooted in a long and rich tradition of folk use. People throughout the world have revered and utilized its flowers, leaves, and roots as a source of food and healing medicine. In ancient China, the health benefits of Dandelion were documented in the *Tang Materia Medica* (659 B.C.). Arabian physicians during the 10th century A.D. administered it as a diuretic and introduced the plant to Europeans. Dandelion was highly valued by Nicholas Culpeper, the 17th century English apothecary and astrologer, who regarded it to be under the dominion of Jupiter, writing, "It is of an opening and cleansing quality, and therefore very effectual for the obstructions of the liver, gall, and spleen, and the diseases that arise from them . . . it openeth the passage of urine both in young and old" (Culpeper, 1992). British apothecary and surgeon John Gerard (1545–1612) recognized Dandelion's cooling and drying nature. He used the tea for stomach ailments and dysentery, and wrote that it "doth withall cleanse and open by reason of the bitterness." He prescribed it for "hot burning fevers" and to "helpe the stopping of the gall, yellow jaundice, lacke of sleep, and stopping of urine" (Gerard, 1633). Early European herbalists recommended Dandelion for urinary problems, as indicated by the French name pissenlit, meaning "piss-in-bed." It was thought that the genus name *Taraxacum* was derived from the Latin *taraxos* or *taraxis*, meaning "disorder," and *akos*, "pain." However, now it is believed that the name comes from the Persian words *talk*, meaning "bitter" and *cakuk*, meaning "purslane," referring to the bitterness of the plant. Dandelion was used by the Gypsies, who believed dreaming of the herb to be an omen of ill fortune, and blowing the seeds carries one's thoughts to a loved one.

Native American Indians adopted Dandelion into their healing systems when the early European settlers introduced the plant into North America. The Osage tribe valued it for treating rheumatism and healing the livers of alcohol drinkers, and applied the white latex juice to warts. The Iroquois were known to utilize the root and leaf tea for kidney disease, edema, and skin problems. The Ojibwas prepared a tea of the roots for heartburn and other stomach pains, and the Potawatomi employed the roots as a bitter tonic (Vogel, 1970).

From the 1880s–1930s, the American Eclectic physicians included Dandelion in their pharmacy as a tonic, diuretic and mild laxative, and prescribed the herb for chronic afflictions of the liver, spleen, pancreas, and kidneys. It was administered for stomach weakness and dropsy (an older term for general fluid retention in the tissues usually caused by congestive heart failure). The root was listed as an official medicine in the *U.S. Pharmacopoeia* from 1831–1926.

Dandelion is currently grown and sold throughout Europe and the United States, and remains a popular herb widely used as tea, tincture, tablets, and capsules. In Germany and other European countries, it is a standard treatment for digestive issues, liver problems, gallstones, urinary problems, water retention, and arthritis. In the Ayurvedic medical system of India, it is primarily given as a detoxifying herb for the liver, blood, lymphatic fluids, and is specific for breast and mammary gland problems, swollen lymph glands, tumors, and cysts. The currently approved therapeutic applications of Dandelion are substantiated by long historic use in well-established medical systems and by pharmacological research, animal studies, and clinical trials.

Healing Qualities

Alterative, antifungal, anti-inflammatory, antilithic, antioxidant, antiscorbutic, anticarcinogenic, antitumor, anti-uric, aperative, astringent, bitter tonic, carminative, cholagogue, depurative, diuretic, exanthematous, febrifuge, galactagogue, hepatoprotective, mild laxative, lymphagogue, nephritic, restorative, sialogogue, and stomachic.

The whole plant has diuretic properties, but the leaves are especially strong in this capacity. The leaves also stimulate secretions of stomach acids and enzymes. Dandelion roots exert greater activity on the liver, gallbladder, pancreas, spleen and kidneys, and are traditionally used to support and heal these organs. Laxative actions are also stronger in the roots.

Traditional Chinese Medicine (TCM) Perspective

In TCM, Dandelion is known as Pu Gong Ying, and the entire plant has been used as food and medicine over many generations. It has two primary qualities reflected in the slightly sweet taste of roots and leaves harvested during spring, and in the bitter flavor of roots and leaves collected in late summer and autumn. The slightly sweet flavor is due to carbohydrates called polysaccharides that provide Yin qualities of nourishing and restoring tissues with nutrients and moisture. These specifically enrich and nourish Blood and Liver Yin, support the pancreas and immunity, and benefit all Yin deficiency conditions, including anemia, fatigue, frequent infections caused by weak immunity, blood sugar imbalances, and afternoon and night sweats.

The bitter principles in Dandelion are cooling, drying, and Yang in nature. Bitters stimulate normal function of the tissues and organs and the movement of Qi (life force or vital energy) and fluids (including digestive enzymes, blood, lymph, and urine) through the body. By promoting movement and activity, Dandelion bitters help correct conditions of excess, such as stagnation, congestion, and damp, toxic heat.

According to TCM, a primary function of the liver is to maintain the smooth flow of Qi and blood throughout the body. When Liver Qi becomes congested, a condition known as Liver Qi Stagnation, it creates imbalance throughout the entire system. When Liver Qi cannot flow smoothly, Qi or energy accumulates, causing fullness and distention in the abdomen, and digestion becomes sluggish. Problems may develop such as liver and gallbladder inflammation, gallstones, high cholesterol levels, stomach problems, indigestion, and constipation. The accumulation of excessive Qi also increases internal heat, promoting fevers, inflammation, painful joints, heartburn, or headaches. Liver Qi Stagnation interferes with detoxification of blood and allows excess heat, acids, and toxins to move throughout the body, which can lead to toxemia, chronic skin eruptions, fevers, infections, rheumatism, gout, cysts, breast pain, and tumors. The liver influences the female reproductive system and menstruation by clearing excess estrogen and ensuring the smooth flow of blood through the uterus. Imbalances caused by blood stagnation and diminished circulation may give rise to premenstrual tension, bloating, and irregular or painful periods. A healthy liver promotes the smooth, calm flow of emotions. Liver stagnation and imbalance often manifest as depression, anger, irritability, and mood swings. Dandelion is a classic herb for Liver Qi Stagnation and is beneficial for treating all the resulting imbalances.

The roots and leaves are cleansing, restoring, and rejuvenating to the entire system. Dandelion is specific for people with a bitter taste in their mouth (often a symptom of liver and gallbladder problems), and for tongues that either lack fur or are covered with thick white or yellow fur that comes off in patches, leaving excoriated, red, raw-looking areas. In TCM, the herb is prescribed to treat food poisoning, snakebites, abscesses, eye infections, edema, kidney stones, female reproductive problems, breast cancer and mastitis, and to stimulate milk flow in lactating mothers.

Primary Actions

Dandelion is one of my favorite and most reliable herbs for its normalizing and gently stimulating action on the liver, gallbladder, pancreas, spleen, and kidneys. It promotes general detoxification that cleanses the blood, lymph and liver, and is a good remedy for chronic internal heat and low-grade infections. A classic diuretic, it is beneficial for excess fluids and resulting edema, heart problems, and high blood pressure. Dandelion is slow-acting and primarily used as a tonic herb, exerting mild but dependable action, that is taken daily over a period of several weeks or months to restore balance, replenish energy, and treat chronic conditions. Its abundant vitamin and mineral content nourish the body and contribute to strong bone density, mineral-rich blood, heart health, and a relaxed, well-functioning nervous system.

Dandelion is often combined with other herbs and works especially well with Yellow Dock (*Rumex crispus*) and Burdock (*Arctium lappa*), creating a classic synergistic blend of roots I fondly call "the three sisters." I blend these "three sisters" with Calendula (*Calendula officinalis*) and St. John's Wort (*Hypericum perforatum*) in a tincture formula for supporting liver problems and cleansing the liver and blood. Many years ago after eating a mango for the first time, I turned bright red and could hardly breathe because my throat was constricting. Realizing that I was going into anaphylactic shock from an allergic reaction to the mango, I decided to saturate myself with herbs instead of going to the emergency room. I guzzled a tablespoon of this cleansing formula with lots of water every 5 minutes for about 30 minutes. I went to sleep and woke up several hours later feeling fine, and was very grateful for my herbal allies!

Antioxidant and Anti-inflammatory Support: Several studies have confirmed the presence of phytochemicals in Dandelion that effectively decrease damaging oxidation and inflammation. These actions strengthen immunity and benefit every cell in the body. Researchers isolated taraxasterol from the herb and discovered that it significantly lowered blood levels of cytokines. Cytokines are a group of proteins involved in immune protection that respond to infections, inflammation, sepsis (blood poisoning), and cancer. Blood concentrations of several cytokines, including tumor necrosis factor, interferons and interleukins, were all diminished in the presence of taraxasterol, indicating that Dandelion's strong anti-oxidant and anti-inflammatory activity reduces the body's need to produce cytokines (Zhang, 2014). In another study, polysaccharides from the herb alleviated oxidative stress and inflammation by stimulating Nrf2, a protein occurring in all cells. When stimulated, Nrf2 accelerated the production of the primary antioxidants; superoxide dismutase (SOD), catalase, and glutathione (Park, 2014).

Digestive System: Dandelion's bitter constituents and cooling nature help restore normal function to the digestive system in several ways. The herb reduces oxidative stress and inflammation in the tissues. As a mild bitter, it stimulates the production and secretion of stomach acids, pancreatic enzymes, and bile. This stimulation ensures the smooth flow of digestive enzymes and food through the alimentary canal, providing relief for sluggish digestion. The herb resolves problems of congestion and stagnation resulting in gas, indigestion, stomach distress, excessive internal heat, constipation, toxic accumulation, and poor fat metabolism with clay-colored stools due to insufficient bile. Loss of appetite is also restored.

Liver and Gallbladder: Dandelion is a classic liver and gallbladder tonic highly valued for treating inflammation in the liver, gallbladder and bile ducts, hepatitis, jaundice, cirrhosis, and fibrosis. The American Eclectic physicians prescribed the herb for most liver and gallbladder problems, which included mild cases of chronic liver obstruction with insufficient bile secretion and blood engorgement.

Cholagogue properties increase bile production in the liver and bile secretion into the gallbladder, and promote the smooth flow of blood and fluids through the liver. This has a cleansing influence on the hepatic system. Bitter terpenes stimulate gallbladder contractions to release bile into the intestines, where it digests fats and increases intestinal mobility leading to regular bowel movements. By promoting normal digestion and elimination, Dandelion helps prevent and treat the formation of gallstones (Weiss, 1988). Dandelion exerts a slow, gentle, consistent improvement in chronic gallbladder inflammation known as cholecystitis.

Generous amounts of choline in the leaves help reduce elevated cholesterol levels. Dandelion reduces total cholesterol and triglyceride levels and increases the beneficial high-density lipoproteins (HDL) (Moss, 2002). Treatment with Dandelion root and leaves has improved blood levels of antioxidant enzymes and lipid profiles in rabbits fed a high cholesterol diet (Choi, 2010). An interesting *in vitro* study revealed that a leaf and root extract of Dandelion decreased lipid and triglyceride levels and inhibited lipogenesis, the transformation of nonfat foods into body fat (González-Castejón, 2013).

Many studies investigating the antioxidant properties of Dandelion have determined that it is specifically indicated for conditions of liver and blood toxicity, and it protects liver and gallbladder cells from damage caused by toxins and alcohol or drug abuse. Researchers have validated its ability to increase levels of the protective antioxidant, superoxide dismutase (SOD), and normalize other liver enzymes (Moss, 2002). *In vitro* tests and mice studies have clearly demonstrated the hepatoprotective activity of Dandelion leaf extracts against toxicity and oxidative stress induced by acetaminophen (Tylenol) overdoses (Colle, 2012). Other tests involved mice with induced liver fibrosis. The mice were given a water and alcohol extract of Dandelion root that successfully decreased fibrous deposits in their livers, while also reducing levels of oxidative stress and cell damage (Domitrovi, 2010). In cases of liver toxicity in mice, alcohol extracts of the root normalized liver enzymes and bilirubin levels. Oxidative stress was reduced, allowing blood levels of glutathione to normalize (Mahesh, 2010). A hot water extract of the root was the most effective Dandelion preparation to completely protect mice from alcohol-induced liver toxicity and cellular damage. Levels of the protective antioxidants catalase and glutathione increased, while damaging lipid peroxidation was reduced (You, 2010). Lipid peroxidation results from oxidative stress and occurs when free radicals "steal" electrons from lipids (fats) in cell membranes, causing cell damage or death. Combining Dandelion with Milk Thistle (*Silybum marianum*) is wonderful for added liver protection and detoxification.

> *Dandelion excels as a remedy for the entire digestive system.*
>
> *Its strong affinity with the solar plexus benefits the liver, gallbladder, stomach, pancreas, and the intestines.*

Stomach: Dandelion's bitter properties increase secretions of saliva in the mouth and hydrochloric acid in the stomach to promote optimal digestion of nutrients. It is helpful for chronic and acute stomach problems, including indigestion and gas. Alkalizing minerals and bitters in the leaves and roots reduce excess acids and provide a cooling effect. The herb is traditionally administered in European herbalism to treat heartburn and canker sores in the mouth.

Pancreas and Diabetes: Dandelion root and leaves support both pancreatic functions of regulating digestion and blood sugar levels. Bitter constituents in the plant stimulate production and secretion of pancreatic enzymes to break down food. Rat studies show that the plant offers protection against pancreatitis (Seo, 2005). Polysaccharides tend to normalize blood sugar levels and prevent sudden and severe fluctuations. The root has a long history of use in treating diabetes. This has been validated by research studies demonstrating the herb's hypoglycemic actions in reducing high blood sugar levels in animals (Farnsworth, 1971; Newall, 1996; Moss, 2002) and by its ability to stimulate insulin secretion (Hussain, 2004). Dandelion also helps diabetics by improving kidney function and the ability to filter blood and reabsorb nutrients.

Intestines: The plant's bitter properties that stimulate production of stomach acids, pancreatic enzymes, and bile secretion promote optimal intestinal absorption of nutrients with normal bowel movements. Dandelion is a mild laxative for chronic constipation. Its cooling and anti-inflammatory properties are helpful in treating colitis and other chronic inflammatory bowel conditions. In a 1981 Bulgarian study involving 24 patients with chronic colitis, several herbs that included Dandelion, St. John's Wort, Lemon Balm (*Melissa officinalis*), Calendula, and Fennel (*Foeniculum vulgare*) were given orally on a daily basis. After 15 days of this herbal therapy, 96% of the patients experienced relief from intestinal pain and reported normal bowel movements (Chakurski, 1981).

Spleen: Dandelion stimulates improved blood flow through the spleen. European herbalists and American Eclectic physicians traditionally employed the root to treat spleen ailments, including sluggish circulation, blood engorgement, and chronic enlargement (Bradley, 1992; Mitchell, 2003).

Kidneys, Bladder, and Diuretic Actions: Dandelion leaves are a powerful and frequently employed diuretic that safely and efficiently removes excess fluids and fluid congestion from the tissues of the body. They help reduce all types of edema resulting from kidney, liver, congestive heart failure, and other cardiac or pulmonary problems. High blood pressure caused by fluid overload can also improve. This herb is appropriate for long-term use in treating edema of the extremities, face, and even fluid retention in the middle ear. One of my clients with severe Meniere's disease, which often involves excess fluid in the ear, has been using Dandelion for a few years and claims that it helps reduce her symptoms.

Without over-stimulating the kidneys, the herb corrects urinary tract problems resulting from stagnant damp heat and excess fluids. When combined with antibiotic herbs, it is effective for bladder and kidney infections, including cystitis, because it flushes urine out of the bladder. This diuretic action results from the plant's ability to inhibit reabsorption of sodium and chloride in the kidneys, making urine more dilute and plentiful.

Dandelion's diuretic action can be comparable to that of Lasix (furosemide), the prescription diuretic that causes potassium depletion. However, potassium depletion is not a side effect when using Dandelion because of the high level of potassium contained in the whole plant, especially the leaves. In a 30-day study investigating the diuretic activity of Dandelion on rats and mice, researchers found that oral consumption of a leaf extract (50 ml/kg body weight, equivalent to 2 grams of dried leaf) exerted stronger diuretic action than the root. The diuretic effect of the leaves was equal to that of Lasix given in doses of 80 mg/kg (Racz-Kotilla, 1974). In a small clinical study involving 17 people, all participants ingested a Dandelion leaf water and alcohol extract and experienced a noticeable increase in the frequency of urination during a five-hour period following ingestion (Clare, 2009).

Dandelion reduces inflammation in the kidneys and bladder and is helpful for urethritis (inflamed urethra). Regular ingestion of the leaf tea helps prevent and remove stones and other obstructions from the bladder and kidneys, and reduces inflammation and spasms they cause (Heron, 1998; Weiss, 1988). This action has been documented by studies showing that the herb reduced the formation and occurrence of kidney stones in rats (Grases, 1994).

Blood and Lymphatic Cleanser: Dandelion's antioxidant properties and capacity to protect the liver from destructive alcohol, drug, and toxic overload has a cleansing impact on the quality of the blood and lymphatic fluids. The herb promotes blood and lymphatic detoxification and circulation, and reduces lymphatic congestion. Abundant minerals in the root and leaves enrich the blood and provide easily assimilated iron for the treatment of iron deficiency anemia. In a study investigating the effects of a water and alcohol Dandelion extract on blood cells in mice, administration of the herb for 20 days significantly increased the number of red blood cells and the levels of hemoglobin in the mice, indicating improved iron levels (Modaresi, 2012).

Dandelion is revered as an alkalizing and detoxifying herb that purifies the body.

It protects the liver from alcohol, drugs, and other toxins.

This cleansing action improves the quality of blood and lymphatic fluids, which enhances immunity and supports optimal vibrant health.

Arthritis and Gout: The leaves and roots have a long history of use for joint pain. According to Traditional Chinese Medicine, the liver regulates joints and ligaments, and the herb's beneficial influence on the liver is also helpful for joints. Bitters are cooling to hot, inflamed tissues, and antioxidant and anti-inflammatory constituents in the herb promote joint health and comfort. The substantial alkaline mineral content in the root and leaves reduce excess acids in blood that promote painful inflammation in joints and tissues throughout the body. Dandelion's action on the kidneys stimulates elimination of urea and uric acid, making it helpful for the relief of gout that is caused by an excess of these acids.

Women's Health: Due to its action on the liver and its phytosterol content, Dandelion helps normalize and strengthen the female hormonal and reproductive system. Phytosterols are plant hormones that exert a similar but weaker activity than human hormones. Many female problems such as uterine fibroids, endometriosis, premenstrual syndrome (PMS), and breast and ovarian cysts and tumors can be caused by liver imbalances. These include liver stagnation and congestion, iron-poor blood, and hormonal imbalance due to excessive estrogen. Dandelion supports the liver in clearing excess estrogen out of the body to maintain normal levels of reproductive hormones.

Menstruation and PMS: Dandelion's diuretic action eases breast tenderness, bloating, and pelvic pressure associated with fluid retention. The abundant mineral content replenishes iron and other minerals lost during menstruation. The herb reduces irritability, mood swings, cramps, and pain associated with menstruation.

Pregnancy: Women can safely eat Dandelion leaves or drink a cup of the tea a few days a week during pregnancy. If tincture is used, put it in boiling water to evaporate and reduce the alcohol. Folic acid, iron, and many other nutrients in the roots and leaves offer optimal nutrition, prevent anemia, and tone the system. The tea is safe to use for cases of pre-eclampsia involving hypertension and edema, and is especially recommended for women who previously had infants with jaundice. A few drops of weak tea may be given to a jaundiced newborn (up to a teaspoon throughout the day), and the nursing mother can drink 3-4 cups of the tea. Dandelion tea is a galactagogue, meaning that it promotes milk production in nursing mothers.

Mastitis: During lactation, milk ducts may become congested or infected, causing inflammation, excess heat, and pain. In Traditional Chinese Medicine, an ounce of sliced Dandelion root is boiled in 2-3 cups of water until only half of the water is left, and the tea is soaked in cloth and applied as a compress over the breast. Drinking the tea also helps decrease heat and inflammation.

Menopause: Due to its cooling properties, phytosterols, and beneficial actions on the liver, Dandelion helps improve hormonal levels and decrease hot flashes and mood swings. It works best when combined with other herbs such as Black Cohosh (*Cimicifuga racemosa*) or Chasteberry (*Vitex agnus-castus*).

Osteoporosis: A daily tonic of Dandelion helps prevent and treat osteoporosis. This is due to the presence of many vitamins and minerals in the leaves and roots that are necessary for bone growth, including calcium, phosphorus, magnesium, boron, and silicon.

Skin Health: Dandelion benefits the general health of skin due to its cleansing, nutritive and cooling properties, its normalizing action on the liver and kidneys, and its laxative effects. It is specific for blemishes and chronic eruptions caused by excess toxins, acidity, and heat released through the skin to cause irritation and inflammation. The leaves and root are used to treat the underlying causes of skin diseases, boils, abscesses, cysts, acne, fungal infections, hives, and eczema. For these problems, Dandelion should be taken internally and also applied externally as a poultice or wash. To remove warts, the white latex juice in the stems can be applied directly on the wart several times daily until it disappears.

> *Dandelion cleanses the body from the inside and also keeps the skin healthy.*
>
> *Drink a tea of the roots and leaves to heal pimples, acne, boils, hives, and eczema.*

Immunity, Infections, Sinus Problems, and Allergies:

Several properties of Dandelion support strong immunity, including high levels of nutrients, protective antioxidants, and the ability to detoxify the liver, blood, and lymphatic fluids. Oligosaccharides in the herb have demonstrated strong antibacterial activity against *Escherichia coli* (causing urinary tract infections and diarrhea), *Bacillus subtilis* (responsible for conjunctivitis or pink eye), and *Staphylococcus aureus* (causing skin infections) (Qian, 2014). Large doses of a water and alcohol extract given to mice for 20 days increased the number of white blood cells involved in immunity (Modaresi, 2012).

Dandelion is helpful for sinus infections and allergies related to excessive heat and dampness that create mucous, and for chronic sinus infections in which low-grade heat and infection get "locked" into the tissues and facial bones around the sinuses, ears, eyes, and neck. As a diuretic, it is specific for boggy mucous membranes that are swollen and edematous. During one research study, taraxasterol was isolated from Dandelion and fed to mice with allergic asthma. After 5 days, taraxasterol dramatically decreased inflammation of lung cells, elicited antioxidant protection evidenced by reduced production of cytokines (inflammatory substances), and improved ease of breathing (Liu, 2013).

For best results when taking Dandelion for infections or allergies, combine it with strong antimicrobial herbs that also reduce mucous production such as Goldenseal (*Hydrastis canadensis*), Yarrow (*Achillea millefolium*), Blue Vervain (*Verbena hastata*), Garlic (*Allium sativum*), Isatis (*Isatis tinctoria*), and Echinacea (*Echinacea* spp.).

Cancer: Dandelion root and leaf have a long history of use in Chinese, Islamic, and Native American traditional medicine to treat various types of cancers and tumors. Several *in vitro* and animal studies have demonstrated immunostimulant and antiviral phytochemicals in the root that inhibit some cancers and solid tumors, especially in the breast, colon, and skin (Baba, 1981). In TCM, Dandelion is used in the prevention and treatment of breast tumors generated by excessive estrogen levels. Chinese researchers found that it helps restore the three major types of immunity: cell-mediated, humoral, and non-specific (Moss, 2002).

Taraxasterol in Dandelion has demonstrated remarkable ability to inhibit breast tumors in mice (Takasaki, 1999). This reduction of mammary carcinoma in mice is partly due to the herb's immune activation of tumor necrosis factor and macrophages that destroy cancer cells (Kim, 1998 & 1999). Dandelion tea made from the leaves and roots appears to be the best preparation for treating cancers. Researchers evaluated three water-based extracts prepared from leaves, flowers, and roots for their effects on the proliferation of breast and prostate cancer cells. Dandelion leaf tea decreased the growth and metastasis of breast cancer cells, as well as blocking metastasis of prostate cancer cells. Although the root tea had no ability to deter growth of either cancer, it was able to block metastasis of breast cancer cells. Tea made from the flowers showed no beneficial activity (Sigstedt, 2008). When researchers investigated the effect of Dandelion on eradicating human liver tumors and malignant cells, they discovered that the herb significantly increased tumor necrosis factor and interleukin production, which contributed to apoptosis (destruction) of 26% of the cancerous cells (Koo, 2004). Korean researchers found that taraxinic acid in Dandelion exhibited potent macrophage activity against proliferation of human leukemia (Choi, 2002).

Considering that its historic use in treating cancers is supported by current research, Dandelion is a safe remedy to use for cancer prevention and in conjunction with other cancer herbs or treatments. So many gifts are offered by this little plant. Dandelion teaches us the humble lesson that common and even unwanted plants can offer wonderful healing possibilities. People often consider resources that are scarce to be of greatest value, but it is a blessing to understand the preciousness of things that are common, and even underfoot.

Teachings from the Dandelion Deva

"Greetings, dear one. I am the deva of the Dandelion tribe. I am an ancient elder of the plant kingdom and participate in the ageless evolution of people and animals. For I support and provide the essence and vital nutrients for the substance and growth of bodies. In early springtime, my abundant nature is witnessed by the vast numbers of my plants and their ease in propagating throughout the world.

"I am influenced by the earth sign of Taurus and radiate the colors of red, orange, and yellow to bring strength and vitality to the body. My deep-yellow flowers point to my focus and affinity with the solar plexus and the organs and tissues within this central area of the body. My stem is a hollow tube reminiscent of the hollow tubes of the ureters and urethra in the urinary tract, and of the long tube going through the center of the body, starting at the mouth and continuing through the stomach and intestines. My long roots, extending deep into the earth absorbing minerals, indicate my connection to the organs deep within the body, like the liver, pancreas, stomach, intestines and kidneys; for my nutrients support these organs.

"The color of my flowers, like the color of urine, is also a signature for my beneficial action on the kidneys and bladder. I promote smooth flow of urine through the urinary vessels, and equalize concentrations of water and fluids in the tissues, bringing all into comfortable balance.

"I am a plant providing stability and substance, which is an aspect of the earth element. With a little fire in my nature, I add warmth to the body by stimulating the creation and flow of enzymes to break down food and provide life-sustaining energy. And just as fire spreads rapidly, my action promotes smooth movement of blood, enzymes, and food through the solar plexus. And from this center, nutrients and energy are carried and dispersed throughout the body. Just as fire destroys all in its path, and in its wake new growth and life emerges, so do my gifts provide a cleansing influence on the deep, inner organs that establish balance and vitality in the whole body.

"An essence of my flowers brings courage to help people adapt to all situations, even very difficult ones, and to thrive in abundance in all endeavors.

"And so my offerings to you are nourishment, ease of flow, and cleansing. Enjoy and receive the tremendous amounts of nutrients offered in the food of my roots, leaves, and flowers. My abundance upon the earth is a response to humanity's great need for my gifts. But people, blinded by lack of understanding, regard me as a useless weed and do their best to eradicate me and my gifts.

"I help people value what seems to be small and insignificant, and to see the miraculous and vast magnitude of the expanse of life. The simple wonder of being in the presence of beauty! Please see my simple beauty and indulge in my humble, yet bountiful gifts. For I offer the blessing of humility and ability to see the value and exquisite nature in the most common things, even in plants regarded as weeds. Learn to be content with what is available. To be satisfied and grateful for what is simple is to know unlimited happiness. It is a lovely life and a beautiful planet. Please keep the gardens alive!"

Echinacea

Echinacea purpurea, spp.
Compositae (*Asteraceae*) (Sunflower or Aster) Family

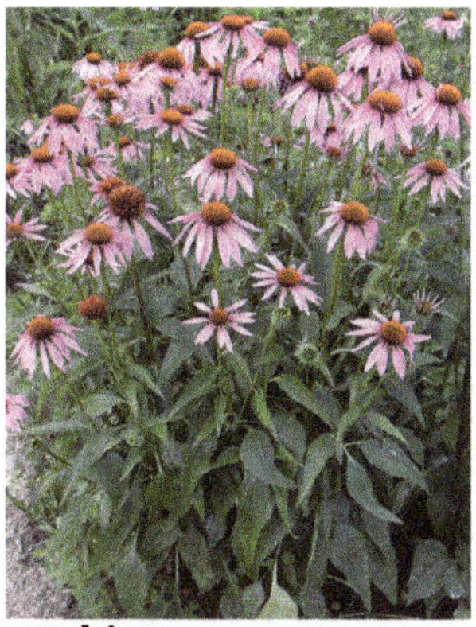
Echinacea purpurea

Botanical Names

The genus *Echinacea* contains nine species, two varieties, and many cultivars. The three species growing in the largest populations and most often used medicinally include *Echinacea purpurea* (purple coneflower), *E. angustifolia* (narrow-leaf coneflower), and to a lesser extent, *E. pallida* (pale coneflower).

Brauneria and *Rudbeckia* are old genus names no longer in use.

Common Names

Purple coneflower is the most common name given to *E. purpurea*. Sampson root and Black Sampson are old names for this species dating back to the time when a slave, who doctored his people in North Carolina, used it as a remedy for snakebites. Red sunflower, Kansas snake root, Missouri snake root, comb flower, and hedgehog are older names for *E. angustifolia*.

Medicinal Part of the Plant

The roots, leaves, and flowers of all nine species contain varying amounts of medicinal constituents.

Range, Habitat, and Description of Echinacea Species

Members of the genus *Echinacea* are herbaceous perennials native to the United States and a few areas of southern Canada. They all have large, solitary flowers sitting atop long stems with the characteristic elevated "cone" in the center of the flower head. The Latin name *Echinacea* is derived from the Greek word *echinos*, referring to the sharp, pointed spines of sea urchins and hedgehogs that resemble the spikes of this flower's cone. The long ray petals surrounding the cone have 2-3 small notches at their tips. *E. purpurea* is the only species with fibrous roots that spread out horizontally, while *E. angustifolia* and all other species have slower-growing taproots. Butterflies are attracted to colorful Echinacea flowers and goldfinches love to eat the seeds.

E. purpurea (Purple Coneflower) once grew throughout much of eastern and central North America in open woods, meadows, and prairies north to Michigan, west to Texas, south to Louisiana, and east to Ohio and Pennsylvania. Over-harvesting has greatly reduced or eliminated natural stands of this and all Echinacea species. However, *E. purpurea* has become a popular and widely cultivated garden ornamental. Growing 3-4′ tall, it is a beautiful and hardy plant resistant to drought. Several stout, erect, round stems emerge from the fibrous roots and branch out toward the top of the plant. The stems, a colorful blend of green and dark maroon, are covered with short hispid (stiff, coarse) hairs. Leaves grow along the entire length of the stems in an alternating pattern, and are petiolate (stalked) at the base of the plant but become sessile (stalkless) and smaller towards the top. Other Echinacea species have narrow, linear leaves, but *E. purpurea* has wider leaves that are oval to lance-shaped. They have a parallel and webbed vein pattern and are covered with white hispid hairs resulting in a rough, scratchy texture. Leaf margins have widely spaced serrate teeth barely visible on some leaves and larger and more obvious on others. Leaf tips end in sharp points.

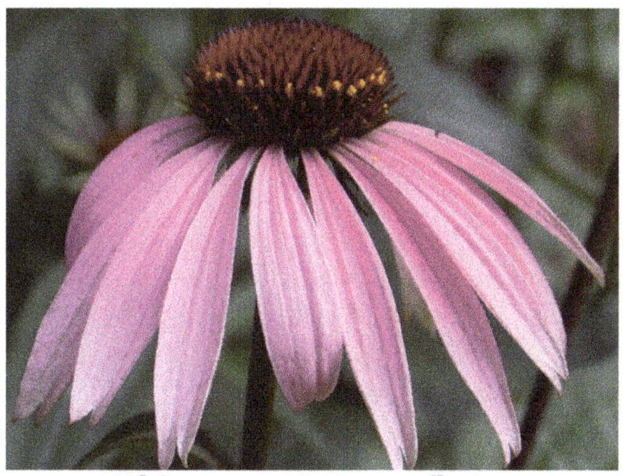
***Echinacea purpurea* flower**

A solitary, cone-shaped flower head, characteristic of the daisy-like flowers in the *Compositae* family, grows from tips of branching stalks. The protruding cone-shaped center of the flower head consists of many stiff, erect disc florets in multi-colored blends of green, yellow, orange, and crimson-red spike tips. The cone is surrounded by several narrow ray petals, about 2″ long, that tend to droop downward and vary from a pale to deep pinkish-purple color. They blossom from May through October depending on location and climate. The attractive plants get bushy with lots of deep-green foliage and many brilliantly colored flower heads that produce yellow pollen.

After the colorful, long ray petals fade and fall away, the remaining cone of disc flowers becomes more prominent. One seed, or nutlet, matures in each disc flower, but only a small percentage of seeds within the entire cone are viable. Seeds reach maturation after 4-6 weeks. The tiny nutlets are barely 1/8″ long, quadrangular in shape, and light brown in color.

E. angustifolia, or Narrow-Leafed Echinacea, was once the most plentiful species with huge populations indigenous to the dry prairie states west of the Mississippi River, including Texas, Oklahoma, Kansas,

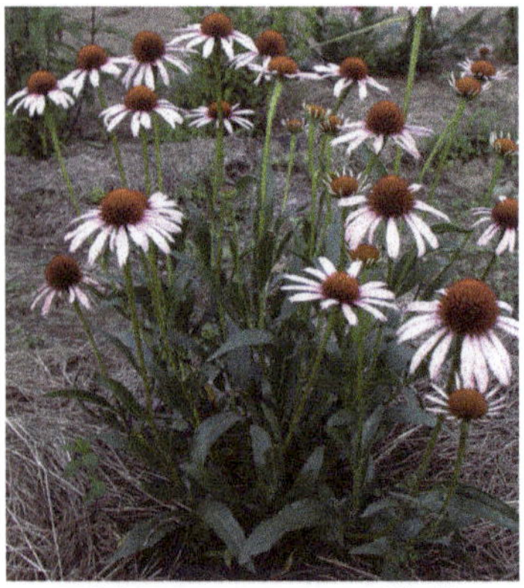

Echinacea angustifolia

Nebraska, Colorado, Montana, the Dakotas, and a small area of Canada north of the Dakotas. Growing up to 20″ tall, *E. angustifolia* is a shorter, more delicate-looking plant with considerably less foliage than *E. purpurea*. It consists of a basal rosette of several petiole, narrow, linear-shaped leaves that are silver green. They are simple with smooth margins and parallel venation. The stout flower stalks are erect, fibrous and round, and depending on the age of the plant, one or more stalks grow from the taproot. Lower leaves on the stalks are on long petioles and upper leaves are sessile. Short hispid hairs cover both leaves and stems. One flower head grows at the end of each stalk and is similar in appearance to *E. purpurea* except that the ray petals, which number from 12-20, are shorter (1¼″), more pale in color, and curled inwards towards the stem. Flowers bloom from June through September.

E. pallida grows in eastern Texas, Oklahoma, Arkansas, Illinois, Iowa, and scattered sections of the eastern states in open woods or fields. It is a taller plant growing up to 40″ in height. The drooping ray petals are very narrow and longer, growing up to 3½″ in length, and are a characteristically paler pinkish-purple color. This is the only species with white pollen. The leaves are very similar in appearance to *E. angustifolia*. Under cultivation, *E. pallida* produces larger roots than *E. angustifolia*.

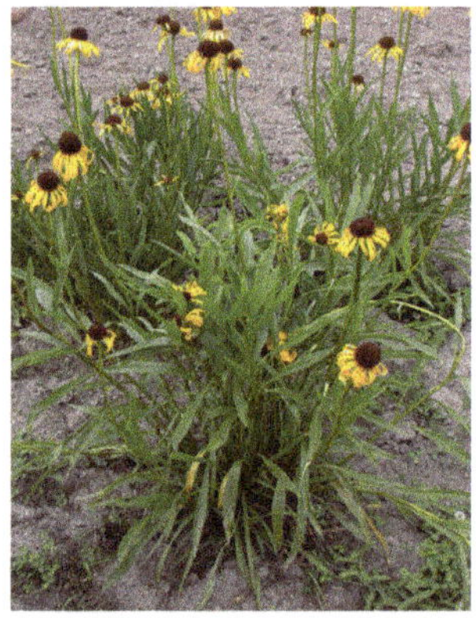

Echinacea paradoxa

Other species that are not commonly used medicinally and occur in much smaller populations include:

E. paradoxa (meaning "unaccountable paradox"), the only species with a yellow flower head. Indigenous to the Ozark Mountain area in Arkansas and Missouri, it has a taproot, narrow leaves, and smoother stems and leaves than other species. The unique flowers make this a beautiful garden ornamental.

E. tennesseensis, which is indigenous to a few specific areas in central Tennessee and is on the federal list of endangered species. The stems and leaves are covered with coarse, erect hairs and the ray petals are long and slender.

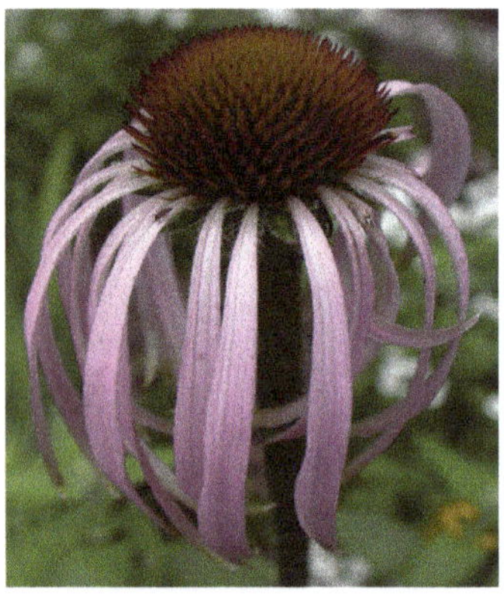

Echinacea pallida

E. simulata, which means "similar to" and looks like *E. pallida*, but has darker pink flowers with yellow pollen. This species is native to Illinois, Kentucky, and the Ozark Mountain area.

E. atrorubens, which has glabrous (smooth and hairless) stems and darker, reddish-purple ray petals that curve inwards to touch the stalk. Ray petals are shorter in length like those of *E. angustifolia*. The plant grows up to 3′ tall. It is indigenous to the prairies of Texas, Kansas and Oklahoma, but is quite rare.

E. sanguinea, named for its blood-red flowers. It is native to Arkansas, Oklahoma, Louisiana, and Texas.

E. laevigata, meaning "to make smooth." This is a rare and endangered Appalachian species indigenous to Virginia and the Carolinas. It is similar in appearance to *E. purpurea*, but has smooth (glabrous) leaves that are ovate to lanceolate with parallel venation. The ray petals are longer and narrower like *E. pallida*.

Cultivation

I have enjoyed the colorful and dynamic presence of *Echinacea purpurea* in my gardens for many years, and encourage people to grow it at home. Not only is it wonderful medicine to have close at hand, but it is a beautiful ornamental that attracts butterflies, birds, and plant-loving humans. Due to its use as a popular herb, wild stands of all Echinacea species are dwindling at an alarming rate. Cultivation is absolutely necessary to supply the huge current world demand. Echinacea species are not difficult to grow and *E. purpurea* is especially easy.

All species require full sun except *E. purpurea*, which tolerates partial shade. Species growing in the central and eastern United States, including *E. purpurea*, thrive in moderately fertile, well-drained soil with a pH of 6.5–7. *E. angustifolia* and other species indigenous to the plains and prairie states do well in sandy, rocky soil with a more alkaline pH of 7–8. This genus is fairly drought resistant, but good drainage in wet climates is essential to prevent species with taproots from rotting. All Echinacea species can be propagated by planting the seeds or dividing and replanting offshoots of the root crown. Echinacea self-sows its seeds and naturally multiplies on its own.

E. purpurea is the only species with a fibrous root system. It is the easiest to cultivate because it is hardy and adaptable to different ecosystems, drought, and dampness. It provides the greatest root and foliage yields in the shortest amount of time. *E. purpurea* seeds do best with a short period of stratification (cold conditioning) before planting to increase speed and rate of germination, but seeds will often emerge without this conditioning. Ideally, seeds are harvested (or purchased) and planted under full sun in a prepared garden bed in late summer or early fall to go through winter conditioning. Or they are planted in very early spring when temperatures still drop low. Artificial stratification may be achieved by placing the seeds in a bag with a little moist (but not wet) sand, and keeping them refrigerated (33-38°F) for 3-6 weeks. Then the conditioned seeds and sand mix are planted in flats or sowed directly into a garden. If you have access to live plants, it is easy to harvest the seeds and plant them directly in the garden in late summer or autumn for germination the following spring. This method ensures a rapidly expanding patch over the years.

Opinions vary as to whether or not *E. purpurea* seeds are light dependent, but studies have shown that seeds pressed into the surface of potting soil germinate faster than seeds that are buried. When seedlings are 3-4″ tall, they can be transplanted and spaced 1-2′ apart in a permanent bed. When grown from seed, plants require 3-4 years before roots reach maturity and contain ample concentrations of phytochemicals for healing. Older roots can become woody and are not suitable to be made into medicinal preparations.

E. angustifolia will grow in non-prairie habitats but needs good drainage. *E. angustifolia* seeds must have at least 12 weeks of stratification to germinate and are treated in the same way as *E. purpurea*.

All Echinacea species may also be propagated by dividing offshoots from the crowns. Mature plants consist of a mass of crowns that can be separated by hand or with a knife. When the root is harvested, the top ½-1″ of root attached to a crown can be replanted. Depending on the age of the plant, 2-7 buds may be divided from one crown, and each one will produce a new plant.

Aster yellows is an infectious disease primarily transmitted by leafhoppers. It deforms Echinacea flowers by causing bizarre tufts of deformed leaves to grow inside the flower or in place of the flower. The infection continues throughout the life of a plant, so it is best to pull and destroy it to prevent further contamination.

After growing four species of Echinacea in southern Indiana, I have found that *E. purpurea* requires the least effort while producing the greatest yields. It is a prolific self-sower, so if left alone it naturally expands its perimeter of growth. *E. pallida* and *E. paradoxa* do well, but seem to be less hardy structurally and fall over more easily than *E. purpurea,* which always stands strong. *E. angustifolia* tolerates the more acidic soil and humid conditions of the Midwest, although it thrives best in drier climates and sandy soils. A stand of flowering Echinacea plants is a beautiful sight and provides excellent medicine always within reach!

Harvest

Please grow Echinacea to harvest from your garden rather than depleting increasingly rare wild stands! To access the highest potency of constituents, gather the aerial parts and roots at different times. Harvest leaves and flowers during the peak of flowering by pruning plants that are at least 2 years old. Leave plenty of foliage (65%) to ensure that the plant survives. Harvest roots from plants that are at least 3 or 4 years old in late autumn, when the medicinal polysaccharides have reached their highest concentrations, and during dormancy, when there is little leaf growth and most of the plant's energy has descended into the roots. There is usually less moisture in the root when harvested in autumn. Taproots are easy to clean, but *E. purpurea* crowns must be pulled apart in order to wash dirt off the extensive fibrous root system. When harvesting roots, you can propagate more plants by replanting some of the crowns with root fibers attached. This method produces mature plants faster than planting seeds.

Harvest seeds for propagation from plants that are at least 2 years old, 3-5 weeks after the colorful ray flowers have fallen off and the remaining flower head is dark brown, dry, and prickly. Goldfinches love to eat the mature seeds, so harvest them before the birds do! Cut the stems 1′ below each flower head and place them upside down in a large paper bag. Allow the heads to completely dry in the sun for several days. Then shake and beat the paper bag to displace the seeds that will fall away from the flower head to the bottom of the bag. Gather the open end of the bag with your hands to form a funnel, turn the bag upside down, and shake it allow the loosened seeds to fall out through the funnel opening while keeping the stems and dried flower heads inside the bag. Plant the seeds or store them in a paper bag in a cool, dry place. Seeds remain viable for up to 3 years.

Preparation of Plant Medicine and Dosages

All Echinacea species are medicinally active and contain similar phytochemicals that stimulate immunity. *E. purpurea* and *E. angustifolia* are considered to be about equal in strength, although some tests have shown *E. purpurea* to exhibit the strongest phagocytic activity against pathogens. Echinacea species are primarily taken internally but do have applications for external healing. They are commonly prepared as tincture, tea, tablets, capsules, and salves that are sold commercially or can be made at home. Commercial manufacturers often extract fresh juice from the roots, leaves, and flowers to be stabilized, dried, and prepared as tablets. The liquid extract is also preserved like a tincture preparation by adding 25% alcohol.

Echinacea preparations should always be made from freshly harvested plants for maximum potency. Dried leaves, flowers, and roots lose their potency over time. Whole dried roots are more stable than the ground powder, which deteriorates rather quickly within about 6 months. The valuable polyacetylenes and alkylamides that stimulate immune activity are prone to oxidation, especially when the plant is ground into fine particles for teas, pills, and capsules. For these reasons, **I recommend tinctures processed from freshly harvested plants as the most effective type of Echinacea preparation.**

Echinacea is usually taken short-term for 7-14 days in large doses to stimulate the immune system's response to toxins and infections. It works well as a curative for acute illnesses such as the common cold and flu, as a preventative after exposure to infection, or during stressful circumstances that tax the immune system. For acute illness, it works most efficiently when taken at the immediate onset of symptoms in large doses several times during the day. As a preventative, one or two doses may be ingested to boost immunity and prevent illness. Echinacea's effectiveness is dose-dependent, so large doses taken every 3-4 hours at the onset of illness are imperative for optimal success. In clinical trials, 4 droppers of ingested liquid extract were found to be productive and statistically significant in treating the flu, compared to 2 droppers, which were ineffective (Braunig, 1992). Echinacea may be used in smaller doses over a longer time span with periodic breaks every 3 weeks when addressing chronic infections, toxicity, allergies, or cancers.

There are different opinions as to how long Echinacea should be used, whether it loses its effectiveness after several weeks of use, or if it suppresses the immune system if taken for too long. The German Commission E herbal regulatory agency stated that it should not be taken for longer than 8 weeks. Many herbalists and researchers believe that Echinacea should be taken in intervals rather than long-term. One study showed steadily increasing immunity between 2-10 weeks of daily ingestion (Bone, 1995; Coeugniet, 1986). The early American Eclectic physicians used Echinacea without any problems for as long as 9 months to treat chronic infections and cancers. The well-known German physician and herbalist Rudolf Weiss, M.D., who used Echinacea extensively in his practice, recommended that for chronic problems it "should be continued for many weeks and even months, if necessary, even for years" (Weiss, 1988).

I generally encourage people to take Echinacea tincture only when necessary as a short-term preventative following exposure to illness or as treatment for acute problems like the common cold, flu, infections, and fever. Those wanting to use it for chronic problems should take smaller doses for longer periods of time.

PREPARATIONS

Tincture: Use only freshly harvested roots, leaves, and flowers for tincturing and chop them into small pieces. Echinacea species contain active constituents that are soluble in alcohol and water, so both should be used when tincturing. The immune-enhancing polysaccharides and glycoproteins are water-soluble and sweeter-tasting, and tend to precipitate (clump together) in large amounts of alcohol. The alkylamides are alcohol-soluble and may be the strongest immune components. Caffeic acid derivatives are both water- and alcohol-soluble. Echinacea is not a bitter-tasting herb, but tinctures containing adequate amounts of alkylamides produce a characteristic tingling sensation on the tongue.

Cover the finely chopped plant in a mixture of 75% 190-proof grain alcohol and 25% distilled water for the best extraction of all the desired constituents. Since the roots and aerial parts are harvested at different times of the year, they can be tinctured separately and then combined into one glass container to obtain all the desired constituents for the final tincture product.

The following dosages are recommended for tincture preparations:

For preventative purposes following exposure: 3-4 droppers (30-35 drops are in one dropper) of tincture in ½ cup of water 2-3 times at 3-4 hour intervals.

For curative purposes to treat acute short-term infections: 4 droppers of tincture in ½ cup of water every 3-4 hours. More may be taken if desired since Echinacea is non-toxic. I have successfully used much larger doses of ¼ ounce for acute infections and to prevent illness. It is important to continue using the herb for 7-10 full days to ensure complete eradication of infection. For 2-4 days after symptoms disappear, reduce dosage to 2 droppers taken twice a day

For chronic infections and conditions: smaller doses of 2 droppers are taken 2-3 times a day for up to 9 months with occasional weekly breaks.

Dose for children: The tincture diluted in water is safe and effective for childhood infections and illnesses like colds, flu, measles, mumps, or chicken pox. Evaporate alcohol from tinctures before giving them to children (see page 207 for instructions). To determine children's dosages, use Clark's method of calculation described on page 148 in the chapter titled "How to Calculate Dosages."

Fresh Juice Extract: The juice in the leaves, flowers, and root can be expressed with a juicing machine. To preserve the juice, it may be frozen or combined with 25% grain alcohol, which acts as a preservative. Dosage: 1-2 teaspoons in water up to 6 times a day for acute infections.

Tea: Water-soluble polysaccharides are extracted best in water. Gently simmer 2-4 tablespoons of finely chopped fresh roots in a quart of water for 30 minutes and steep for another 30 minutes. Leaves and flowers are steeped in boiled water for 30 minutes. Dosage: 3-4 cups of tea a day as needed.

Tablets and Capsules: Grind dried roots, leaves, and flowers into a fine powder and pack it into capsules or make pills by the standard method. Dosage: 3 capsules or tablets up to 3 times a day as needed. Dosage for commercially prepared products is 300-400 mg up to 3 times daily.

Salve: Chop fresh roots, leaves, and flowers into small pieces, put them in a stainless steel or glass pan, cover with olive oil, and bake at 200°F for 3 hours. Echinacea works best as a salve when combined with other vulnerary herbs (refer to the section "Skin Problems" on page 591 in the "Index of Health Issues and Herbal Recommendations" for suggestions).

Chemical Constituents

The species having undergone the most scientific research include *E. purpurea, E. angustifolia,* and to a lesser extent, *E. pallida*. The main constituents responsible for immune activity are believed to be polysaccharides, caffeic acid derivatives, and lipophilic components that include two main groups: the alkylamides and polyacetylenes. All these phytochemicals occur in different amounts depending on the species, plant parts, time of harvest, and other variables. The immune stimulant activity of alcohol extracts is mainly due to the alkylamides and caffeic acid derivatives. The activity of water-based preparations like tea is due to the water soluble-polysaccharides and caffeic acid derivatives. Recent research has revealed that alkylamides are the most bioavailable of these phytochemicals and are probably the constituents most responsible for Echinacea's immune effects (Bone, 2005).

Polysaccharides are found in many plants and exert immunological activity. Researchers have found several types of polysaccharides in Echinacea species, including arabinogalactan (an immunostimulant that increases interferon production, tumor necrosis factor, and phagocytosis), inulin (protective against breast and colon cancers, neutralizes viruses and bacteria, expectorant, immunostimulant), heteroxylan (phagocytic), and echinacin (hyaluronidase-inhibitor, antiviral, vulnerarsy). Polysaccharides and glycoproteins (polysaccharides bonded to proteins) increase phagocytosis and promote cytokine production of tumor necrosis factor and interferon. The water-soluble polysaccharides and glycoproteins occur in the roots, leaves, and flowers of *E. purpurea* and *E. angustifolia,* but are most abundant in the roots.

Caffeic acid derivatives are phenols that include caffeic acid (analgesic, antibacterial, anticancer, antihistamine, anti-inflammatory, antileukemia, antimutagenic, antioxidant, antitumor, antiviral, diuretic, hepatoprotective, immunostimulant, vulnerary), echinacoside (antibiotic against *Streptococci* and *Staphylococcus aureus*, antiflu, antiviral, immunostimulant), verbascoside (antibacterial, anti-inflammatory, antileukemia, antioxidant, antitumor), chlorogenic acid (analgesic, antibacterial, anticarcinogenic to stomach, liver and skin cells, antihistamine, anti-HIV, anti-inflammatory, antitumor, antiviral, cholagogue, immunostimulant, vulnerary), isochlorogenic acid (antioxidant, antiseptic, anticancer), and cichoric acid (antibacterial, anticancer, antiflu, anti-HIV, antiviral, hyaluronidase-inhibitor, immunostimulant). Cichoric acid is the most commonly measured chemical and is highly concentrated in the fresh flower heads and roots of *E. purpurea*, and to a lesser degree in the leaves of *E. angustifolia* and *E. pallida*. Cichoric acid causes a noticeable stimulation of phagocytosis against bacteria and viruses in laboratory tests.

Lipophilic components are fat-soluble and include polyacetylenes (also called polyenes) and alkylamides. Polyacetylenes typically occur in the *Compositae* family and are usually most concentrated in the roots. *E. pallida* root contains significant amounts of two polyenes, ketoalkynes and ketoalkenes, which are not found in other Echinacea species and give this plant a unique earthy-metallic taste. Polyacetylenes are anti-inflammatory. Alkylamides are not commonly found in plants but do occur in the *Compositae* family. At least 20 alkylamides have been identified in the genus *Echinacea* and include isobutylamides, echinacein, and echinolone. Alkylamides have been isolated from the roots and flowers (containing the highest concentrations), leaves, and seeds of *E. angustifolia* and *E. purpurea*, but are nearly absent in *E. pallida*. Since alkylamides are responsible for the characteristic tingling sensation on the tongue, *E. pallida* lacks this quality. Alkylamides are anti-inflammatory, hepatoprotective, and direct phagocytes to surround and destroy infectious pathogens.

Various flavonoids, mainly occurring in the leaves of these three species, include rutin (antibacterial, anticancer, immunomodulator, vasodilator), quercetin (analgesic, anti-allergic, antibacterial, anticancer, antiflu, antitumor, antiviral), kaempferol (antibacterial, anticancer, antihistamine, anti-inflammatory, anti-oxidant, hepatoprotective, vasodilator), rutoside (decreases blood clotting and capillary fragility, choleretic), luteolin (antibacterial, anticancer, antihistamine, anti-inflammatory, antioxidant, antitumor, hepatoprotective, vasodilator), apigenin (antibacterial, antihistamine, anti-HIV, anti-inflammatory, antimutagenic, antioxidant, antispasmodic, antitumor, vasodilator), and isorhamnetin (antibacterial).

Fatty acids include linoleic, oleic, scerotic, and palmitic (antioxidant) acids. Essential oils include borneol (antibacterial, anti-inflammatory, antipyretic, anti-yeast, choleretic, fungicide, hepatoprotective), bornyl acetate (antibacterial, antiviral, expectorant), and caryophyllene (anti-acne, anti-asthmatic, antibacterial, anti-inflammatory, anti-streptococal, antitumor, anticandida, diuretic, fungicide).

Vitamins and minerals include ascorbic acid (vitamin C), beta-carotene (converts into vitamin A), thiamine (vitamin B1), niacin (B3), calcium, chromium, iron, magnesium, manganese, potassium, selenium, and zinc.

E. paradoxa root is chemically similar to *E. pallida* root, but contains greater amounts of alkylamides and less of the polyacetylene constituents. *E. tennesseensis* is high in alkylamide content (Bauer, 1998; Bone, 1997; McCaleb, 2000).

Safety, Contraindications, and Drug Interactions

Echinacea is an extremely safe herb and no overdoses, drug interactions, or toxicity have been reported with oral use. In fact, research on *E. purpurea* has demonstrated it to be non-toxic and non-mutagenic. There have been reports of temporary allergic, hive-like skin reactions from topical contact with fresh plants. Most clinical studies over the past 50 years have been conducted in Germany using the injectable form of the fresh juice extract of *E. purpurea,* and to a lesser degree, salve and tinctures. When reviewing these studies and outcomes, remember that biological responses from injectable applications are usually different and much stronger than those from traditional oral preparations. Echinacea's observed side effects occur when delivered as an intra-muscular injection and include shivering, mild dizziness, throat irritation, joint pain, nausea, vomiting, headache, and fever. These problems have not been reported with oral use.

Current clinical data on pregnant women show that Echinacea is safe to use during pregnancy and lactation, and is gentle enough for the more sensitive systems of infants and the elderly. One study involving 206 women who used Echinacea during pregnancy concluded that the herb posed no problems or risks to mother or infant (Gallo, 2000 & 2001). For many years, I have given Echinacea tincture to my children, and now my grandchildren, and have recommended it to the parents of many others without problems. It is one of the few antibiotic and antiviral herbs I recommend to pregnant women and children without hesitation.

There are many ambiguities and various opinions concerning the efficacy and safety of using Echinacea in cases of **autoimmune diseases**. Some sources, such as the *German Commission E Monographs*, warn not to use Echinacea for autoimmune or systemic diseases like tuberculosis, multiple sclerosis, AIDS, HIV, diabetes, arthritis, leukosis (abnormal proliferation of white blood cells or the tissues that produce them, as in leukemia), and collagenosis (occurring when connective tissue is attacked by the immune system, as in systemic lupus erythematosus). This warning is based on the idea that immune stimulants should not be used in cases of autoimmune diseases due to the possibility of exacerbating symptoms. Warnings also come from conclusions drawn from research using phytochemicals that have been isolated from Echinacea and tested in animal and test tube studies. However, these warnings are largely theoretical and, although they are reasonable precautions, there is very little convincing clinical evidence to support these contraindications. Some clinical trials and studies actually contradict this theory (McCaleb, 1998). Professor Bauer, considered to be the world's leading researcher of Echinacea, wrote, "As far as I know, these contraindications have only been included because of theoretical considerations." Australian phytotherapist Kerry Bone believes that current clinical practice, the extensive historic use by American Eclectic physicians, and proper evaluation of modern scientific data actually support both the long-term use of Echinacea and its possible benefit for autoimmune disorders (Bone, 1997). On the other hand, Herbalist Paul Bergner has reported several cases in which Echinacea probably worsened autoimmune diseases (Bergner, 1997a, 1997b, & 2007). Therefore, although many people with autoimmune diseases have used the herb without side effects, it should be used cautiously under supervision and promptly discontinued if any problems arise.

Medicinal Uses

History of the Plant

E. angustifolia was one of the most important and revered medicinal plants of Native American Indians living in the Great Plains area, and was probably used interchangeably with other prairie species, especially *E. pallida*. It was taken for a variety of ailments, most notably as a universal antidote for venomous bites and stings from snakes, spiders, scorpions, and other poisonous animals. Ethnobotanical data from several sources have contributed to the knowledge base concerning native use of this herb among the Plains Indians, including the Sioux, Dakota, Pawnee, Omaha-Ponca, Crow, Winnebago, Fox, Cheyenne, Meskwaki, Kiowa, Choctaw, and Comanche. Archeological digs of Lakota Sioux villages that thrived during the 1600s have unearthed fragments of *E. angustifolia* root used to heal injuries and wounds. Native Americans prepared a tea from the root or chewed it for several hours to treat toothaches, swollen glands, and sore mouths or gums. The herb was taken for many illnesses, including colds, sore throat, coughs, stomach cramps, infections, inflammation, venereal diseases, and many types of cancers. The tea was administered as a wash for eye injuries and infections. The root was pulverized, powdered, or made into tea for use as an antiseptic and analgesic when applied to external wounds, punctures, and burns. The stiff bristles of the dried flower heads were employed as hair combs. In 1919, ethnobotanist Melvin Gilmore noticed how the Plains tribes respected this herb, writing that, "Echinacea seems to have been used as a remedy for more ailments than any other plant" (Foster, 1999).

European immigrants to North America did not discover *E. angustifolia* until they moved west of the Mississippi River into the prairie states. H.C. Meyer, a German healer and medicine vendor in Pawnee City, Nebraska, apparently learned about *E. angustifolia* from Native Americans during the 1880s. Meyer combined Echinacea root with Wormwood and Hops, and sold it as "Meyer's Blood Purifier," which he advertised as a cure-all for venomous snake bites and many ailments. This blend became quite popular. In 1885, Meyer enthusiastically brought *E. angustifolia* to the attention of Eclectic physician John King, M.D., and John Uri Lloyd, the prominent pharmacist of the Eclectic practitioners. Both men were initially doubtful about Meyer's exuberant claims and his offer to be bitten by a rattlesnake in order to demonstrate the plant's abilities. But after two years of experimenting with the herb in his clinical practice and his family, John King was adequately impressed with Echinacea's healing abilities and sent preparations of the root to other Eclectic physicians to test in their clinical practices. King gained much confidence in the plant when it was the only remedy that brought relief to his wife, who was suffering from cancer. Lloyd reported that whenever she stopped taking it, her symptoms worsened, and consequently she used it daily until she died. John King officially endorsed *E. angustifolia* to other Eclectic physicians in a paper he wrote in 1887, and the herb's popularity quickly spread. Soon after this publication, Lloyd Brothers Pharmacists, Inc. made liquid alcohol preparations of Echinacea available to medical professionals.

Echinacea was never officially accepted by the American Medical Association (AMA), but by the early 1900s, Echinacea preparations were the most popular herbal remedies prescribed by both Eclectic physicians and many "regular" doctors of the AMA. Several Eclectic physicians documented clinical data on their use of Echinacea in medical practice, providing a scientific foundation for current use and investigations of this herb (Ellingwood, 1919; Felter, 1898). They considered it a specific remedy for wounds, burns, acne, boils, abscesses, bites and stings of insects, venomous snakes and rabid dogs, all types of blood poisoning, and dangerously acute septic infections. There are accounts of Eclectic physicians who were amazed at Echinacea's ability to save limbs so damaged by gangrene that amputation would have otherwise been necessary.

E. angustifolia root was prescribed for the common cold, bacterial infections, excessive and chronic mucous discharge, sinus and respiratory tract infections, flu epidemics, swollen glands and lymph nodes, bronchitis, tuberculosis, tonsillitis, urinary tract infections, pain and inflammation of syphilis and gonorrhea, diphtheria, typhoid, meningitis, malaria, inflammation, eczema, psoriasis, and eruptive feverish conditions such as measles, chicken pox, and scarlet fever. The herb's stimulating activity on the immune system was recognized, and several physicians reported that it was beneficial against some types of cancer, especially of the mucous membranes and breast. Echinacea was used to improve digestion and heal ulcerated and inflamed membranes lining the mouth, and for diarrhea, cholera, and dysentery. It was often used in veterinary medicine to heal saddle-born ulcers on the backs of horses.

Eclectic physicians preferred tincture preparations of *E. angustifolia* root, believing that it was more potent than *E. purpurea*, and vast populations of the herb in the prairie states allowed easy access to large supplies. *E. angustifolia* and *E. pallida* were often used interchangeably and were listed as official medicines in the *U.S. National Formulary* from 1916–1950. After the demise of the Eclectic physicians in the 1930s and the rise of allopathic medicine, Echinacea was replaced by antibiotics and lapsed from public use into obscurity for many years until the 1980s. Today, Echinacea is again a top-selling herb. Most Echinacea sold currently is *E. purpurea* because it is the species most easy to cultivate with the fastest growth rate, followed by *E. angustifolia*.

The herb was introduced into Europe around 1895 and was initially prepared as a homeopathic remedy prescribed by German physicians. Since the early 1930s, it is estimated that over 50,000 pounds of Echinacea have been annually exported from the United States to European markets. As the plant's popularity and demand grew among Europeans, shortages of American imports led to the commercial cultivation of *E. purpurea* in Germany during the late 1930s. According to a 1991 study, over 280 Echinacea pharmaceutical products, half of which were homeopathic, were available in the West German market (Foster, 1999).

E. purpurea, E. angustifolia, and to a lesser extent, *E. pallida*, have been the subjects of much research. It is estimated that over 400 journal articles, mostly from Germany, have been written on the chemistry, pharmacology, and clinical application of Echinacea species, validating many of their historical uses. Most of the clinical studies conducted over the past 50 years in Germany have used an injectable preparation of a fresh juice extract of *E. purpurea*, called Echinacin®, and to a lesser degree the salve and tincture extracts. German physicians often give intramuscular injections of Echinacin® for more severe conditions that include arthritis, tonsillitis, allergies, and urinary and gynecological infections. Injectable forms, which are not available in the United States, can cause side effects and have different pharmacological actions than oral preparations of the herb.

Healing Qualities

Alterative, analgesic, antibacterial, anticarcinogenic, anti-catarrhal, antifungal, anti-inflammatory, antiseptic, antivenom, antiviral, depurative, exanthematous, febrifuge, immune modulator and stimulant, lymphagogue, opthalmicum, vasodilator, and vulnerary.

Traditional Chinese Medicine (TCM) Perspective

Echinacea is cooling and drying. It stimulates and restores Wei Qi (the immune system) and promotes the detoxification and circulation of blood and lymphatic fluids. It primarily affects the blood, lymphatic fluids, skin, stomach, and lungs. It clears toxic heat and is especially beneficial for treating damp heat with yellow puss occurring with infection and inflammation. Its stimulating quality removes Qi stagnation to restore normal tissue function and flow of blood and fluids. In TCM, tumors and cancers are thought to arise from stagnated energy flow, toxic blood, and deficient Wei Qi, all of which are improved by the actions of the genus *Echinacea*. Since it has cooling properties, it should be combined with warming herbs for a balanced formula when taken for chronic infections or toxic illness. Chronic fatigue, muscle weakness, poor nutrition, and insufficient digestion are often underlying causes of chronic infections, and are best resolved by combining Echinacea with deep-acting tonic herbs like Astragalus (*Astragalus membranaceus*), American Ginseng (*Panax quinquefolius*), Eleuthero or Siberian Ginseng (*Eleutherococcus senticosus*), Holy Basil or Tulsi (*Ocimum sanctum*), and Reishi (*Ganoderma lucidum*), Shiitaki (*Lentinula edodes*), and other immune-stimulating mushrooms.

Primary Actions

Echinacea is one of my favorite and most reliable herbs. I have grown, prepared, and used *E. purpurea* tincture for over 35 years for myself, my family, and hundreds of clients with great success and without complications. It is truly one of Nature's precious gifts, a remarkable healer! It is renowned for its ability to enhance and stimulate the body's natural ability to defend against invading pathogens, including bacteria, viruses, fungi and yeast, and has been successfully employed for the treatment of infectious illnesses for hundreds of years. It is one of the most effective blood and lymphatic cleansers for all types of toxicity. The scientific and medical communities extensively research this herb for the treatment of many conditions from the common cold and flu to cancer and AIDS.

Echinacea is indicated for all infectious and toxic conditions in which the immune system is challenged or compromised. This is an herb that should only be taken during acute or chronic illness. One or two doses may be taken after exposure to infection, but it is not to be used on a continual basis as an immune booster during times of relative health. Clinical studies indicate that Echinacea is most effective when taken at the very onset of colds and other infectious illnesses, followed by several doses throughout the day, and continued until all signs of infection are over.

I have personally found this to be true. When feeling the initial symptoms of a sore throat, swollen glands, the flu or a cold approaching, I take a large dose of 5-6 droppers of tincture once or twice, and almost always avoid getting sick. I frequently combine Echinacea with its synergistic partner, Boneset (*Eupatorium perfoliatum*), which also possesses impressive immunostimulating properties. This combination provides powerful protection against infections and toxins. By following this regimen, the symptoms of heavy-duty colds, flu, and other infections are greatly reduced, usually passing through the system within a few days.

Immune System: Echinacea's amazing ability to moderate and activate the immune system has been adequately verified by many years of clinical evidence and scientific research. An explanation of the immune system helps in understanding the herb's activities. The immune response depends on the body's ability to recognize and eliminate substances that it interprets as foreign and harmful to its well-being. Components of the immune system are on constant surveillance against these pathogens that include bacteria, viruses, fungi, yeast, parasites, and cancerous cells. Some bacteria harm the body by releasing enzymes and other toxins to break down protective cellular membranes and destroy healthy cells. Viruses invade cells, and cancers arise when normal cells mutate and divide uncontrollably. When infectious pathogens attack the body, or when cells become cancerous, complex chemical activities are set into motion to defend and protect the body's tissues.

The primary components of the immune system are leukocytes, or white blood cells, which include granulocytes, monocytes, and lymphocytes. Granulocytes are immune cells that develop in bone marrow and have granules in their cytoplasm. Granulocytes include basophils and mast cells that produce histamine and play a role in allergic reactions and inflammation. Eosinophils also respond to allergic reactions and work by a process called phagocytosis in which they seek out, identify, engulf, ingest, and destroy bacteria, viruses, toxins, and cancerous cells. Neutrophils are the other type of phagocytic granulocyte that plays a major protective role. Macrophages (meaning "big eaters") also protect the body by phagocytosis. Macrophages are primarily formed from monocytes and some granulocytes, and reside in the liver, spleen, tonsils, and lymph nodes.

Lymphocytes include B- or T-lymphocytes. B-lymphocytes are produced in bone marrow and released into the blood stream, and about 50% pass through the thymus gland to become T-lymphocytes. B-lymphocytes make antibodies, which are large protein molecules that seek out and identify pathogens, bind to antigens (foreign invaders or toxins) on their cell surfaces, and destroy them. T-lymphocytes include natural killer T-cells and lymphokines that activate macrophages. T-lymphocytes also activate cytokines that include tumor necrosis factor (TNF), interleukins-1, 6, and 10, and interferon. Interferon is a protein produced in the body that has strong antiviral activity. All of these substances, carried throughout the body in blood and lymphatic fluids, work together to destroy pathogens and are major players in the immune response.

Immune responses are either specific or nonspecific, and both depend on lymphocytes. Specific or humoral immunity occurs in the body fluids (humors) and involves antibody and complement activities. When a bacteria or virus enters the body, B-lymphocytes activate, recognize the pathogen as foreign, make antibodies to destroy the pathogen, and then "remember" it for subsequent exposures. Vaccinations elicit this type of specific response. Nonspecific or cell-mediated immunity involves T-lymphocytes and non-selectively protects against pathogens without having previous exposure. T-lymphocytes are the body's main defense against cancerous cells, tumors, and bacterial, viral, fungal, and yeast infections. T-lymphocytes are involved in allergic reactions, rejection of transplant organs, and autoimmune diseases.

Echinacea is primarily a nonspecific immunostimulant that works by increasing phagocytosis (Sun, 1999; Viehmann, 1978; Wagner, 1985). Several phytochemicals in Echinacea, including polysaccharides, alkylamides, cichoric acid and other caffeic acid derivatives, have been found to enhance the activity of macrophages and stimulate phagocytosis (Goel, 2002). Polysaccharides activate white blood cells by binding to receptors on their cell surfaces (Wagner, 1984) and stimulate T-lymphocyte and cytokine production (Fonseca, 2014). Data that has been collected from over 300 published research papers on *E. purpurea, E.*

angustifolia, and *E. pallida* conclude that these herbs:

- ❖ promote general nonspecific cell-mediated immunity
- ❖ stimulate and increase leukocytes (white blood cells) to fight infection
- ❖ activate natural killer T-cells to fight against cancer cells and other pathogens
- ❖ exert antibiotic and antiviral effects
- ❖ increase phagocytosis by macrophage activity
- ❖ inhibit hyaluronidase (an enzyme that degrades hyaluronic acid) in order to protect cells from pathogenic invasion and decrease tissue inflammation
- ❖ stimulate properdin (a serum protein that acts nonspecifically against bacteria and viruses)
- ❖ activate increased production of alpha-1 and alpha-2 gamma globulins to fight infections
- ❖ stimulate production of tumor necrosis factor (TNF), interferon, and interleukins-1, 6, and 10
- ❖ inhibit tumor growth
- ❖ promote growth of healthy tissue
- ❖ fight Candida yeast
- ❖ stimulate the adrenals to secrete corticosteroids during times of adrenal stress and exhaustion (Bauer, 1991; Hobbs, 1989 & 1990; Lawrence Review, 1990; Luettig, 1989; Rodinet, 1993; See, 1997).

Properdin is a naturally occurring compound in the body that activates the alternative complement pathway, which is a cascade event of immune responses. It binds to viruses and bacteria to neutralize or destroy them. Echinacea species increase properdin levels in laboratory experiments, and German studies have shown that intramuscular injections of *E. purpurea* in rabbits increased properdin levels by 50-70% for at least 120 hours (Busing, 1958).

Another way in which this herb impedes infection is by preventing the destruction of hyaluronic acid, a mucopolysaccharide that occupies the space between cells and connective tissue. Hyaluronic acid is the "cement" that binds cells together and protects them from microbial attack and destruction. Many pathogens and some venomous animals produce an enzyme called hyaluronidase, which dissolves hyaluronic acid and destroys this protective barrier between cells. The mucopolysaccharides in Echinacea stimulate a temporary increase of hyaluronic acid that activates connective tissue-forming cells, called fibroblasts, to multiply and produce new tissue. This promotes healing and decreases tissue inflammation (Bonadeo, 1971; Busing, 1952). The echinacin and cichoric acid in Echinacea also contribute to the protection of hyaluronic acid and stimulation of fibroblast activity to defend against bacterial and viral invasion (Bauer, 1991).

Bacterial, Viral, Yeast, and Fungal Infections: Research and an extensive history of folk use support Echinacea's wonderful ability to stimulate immunity and prevent and treat many kinds of infections and the fever, inflammation, and mucous or pus discharge that often accompany them (Hobbs, 1990; Stroll, 1950; Wacker, 1978). The herb has a long history of treating influenza (flu), the common cold, tonsillitis, laryngitis, strep throat, and upper respiratory tract infections such as bronchitis, pneumonia, and whooping cough. It is beneficial for chronic and acute sinusitis (inflammation of the nasal sinuses caused by viral infection, bacteria, or allergies) and excessive mucous discharge from the sinuses and lungs. It is also effective against *Helicobacter pylori* bacteria, a cause of stomach ulcers.

A wealth of research provides evidence of Echinacea's ability to counteract infections. In a placebo-controlled clinical trial involving 282 adults, an extract of the flowering tops of *E. purpurea* was effective in treating the common cold and relieving symptoms (Goel, 2004). A meta-analysis of 14 studies involving different Echinacea preparations evaluated randomized, controlled trials studying 1,356 patients for incidence of the common cold and 1,630 patients for duration of the cold. The analysis revealed that the herb reduced the incidence of catching a cold by 58% and decreased the duration of sickness by an average of 1½ days (Shah, 2007). In a double-blind, placebo-controlled clinical trial that also investigated Echinacea's efficacy in treating the common cold, 120 participants were divided into two groups. One group took a placebo and the other took 20 drops of Echinacea extract every 2 hours the first day, and then 3 times a day for up to 10 days. Only 40% of the people taking Echinacea developed colds, which resolved after 4 days, compared to 60% of the placebo group that developed colds lasting 8 days before improving (Hoheisel, 1997). In another study involving 95 people with early symptoms of cold or flu, subjects were divided into a placebo group or a group that received 5-6 cups of Echinacea tea. There were significant improvements in symptoms and shorter duration of illness for participants who drank the tea compared to those in the placebo group (Lindenmuth, 2000). A clinical trial involving 473 patients diagnosed with the flu demonstrated that those taking *E. purpurea* and Elderberry (*Sambucus nigra*) syrup had as good a recovery as those taking Tamiflu®, and experienced fewer effects (Raus, 2015). Meta-analysis research shows that Echinacea reduces the risk of respiratory tract infections, complications, and recurrences (Schapowal, 2015).

Echinacea is excellent for kidney and genitourinary tract infections, including cystitis, urethritis, pyuria (pus in urine), pelvic inflammatory diseases, vaginitis, and prostatitis. The herb has been used to treat venereal diseases such as gonorrhea, syphilis, and trichomoniasis (caused by *Trichomonas vaginalis*, a protozoa parasite). It clears toxic heat and is a cooling febrifuge excellent for fevers, especially when combined with Yarrow (*Achillea millefolium*), Peppermint (*Mentha x piperita*), Sage (*Salvia officinalis*), and Boneset.

Research from Germany has shown dramatic improvement in Candida yeast and other fungal infections with fewer recurrences when Echinacea was used for several months. In a study of 203 women with recurrent vaginal yeast infections, those who ingested Echinacin® (*E. purpurea*) in addition to using a topical econazole nitrate cream experienced a lower recurrence rate of 16.7%, compared to a 60.5% recurrence in women who only used the cream (Coeugniet, 1986). A Canadian study found that Echinacea extracts have antimicrobial activity against several strains of yeast and fungus, including Candida yeast (Binns, 2000). *In vitro* tests have demonstrated that alkamides from Echinacea extracts destroy fungi by disrupting and damaging their cell walls (Cruz, 2014).

The herb exerts antibacterial activity against *Staphylococcus* (causing impetigo) and *Streptococcus* infections, meningitis, diphtheria, anthrax, and tetanus. Echinacea protects the digestive system from bacterial infections, including cholera, enteritis, peritonitis, and dysentery. It has also demonstrated specific antiviral activity against rabies, herpes, influenza, and pox viruses (Binns, 2002; Wacker, 1978). When used in combination with St. John's Wort (*Hypericum perforatum*) and Lemon Balm (*Melissa officinalis*), it works wonders in reducing the size and pain of herpes and shingles lesions, promoting rapid healing, and reducing frequency of recurrent outbreaks. Echinacea also works well to reduce symptoms and speed recovery from mononucleosis caused by the Epstein-Barr and cytomegalo viruses. The herb's capacity for liver protection was investigated when alkamides isolated from *E. purpurea* roots were studied for their efficacy in treating acute hepatitis in mice. The alkamides stimulated immune activity that reduced liver cell inflammation and damage (Hou, 2011).

Echinacea diminishes inflammatory and allergic reactions to food, environmental toxins and irritants, and seasonal allergies like hay fever. Start with small doses to treat allergies because it may make symptoms worse in some people. To decrease potential side effects of vaccinations, take a few large doses of the tincture immediately after the inoculation.

An excellent remedy for eye problems, the herb is used for eye infections such as conjunctivitis, allergic irritations, redness, and itching. Make a tea from the root or leaves to treat eye problems. Pour the tea through coffee filter paper to remove all particles, and put several drops in each eye with a sterile dropper 3-5 times a day. The tea can be stored in a sterile jar in the refrigerator up to a week for continual use. Echinacea tends to have a drying effect on the eyes, which can be safely remedied by adding Marshmallow root (*Althaea officinalis*) or Slippery Elm bark (*Ulmus rubra*) to the tea for their moistening mucilage.

For otitis media (inner ear infection) in children or adults, the tincture is taken internally and a few drops are placed in the ears several times a day. Many years ago while traveling in the jungles of Ecuador, I developed acute pain in my ear during a canoe trip on a tributary of the Amazon River. Fortunately, I always carried a bottle of Echinacea in my backpack, and since this was the only option for relief, I squirted several drops of the tincture into my ear. The pain stopped almost immediately and never recurred.

Echinacea can be used in conjunction with pharmaceutical antibiotics, or as an alternative when taken in adequate dosages. Unlike antibiotics, it does not disrupt intestinal flora to cause diarrhea. I usually recommend that Echinacea be combined with other herbs appropriate for the specific condition being treated for best results. The Eclectics and many naturopaths have combined it with Wild Indigo (*Baptisia tinctoria*), which has similar actions on the immune system, in a ratio of 5:1 (5 parts Echinacea to 1 part Indigo). Wild Indigo is a strong antimicrobial used in small doses **(due to toxicity with large doses)** and is also taken for septic conditions. Other antimicrobial herbs that have synergistic action with Echinacea include Goldenseal (*Hydrastis canadensis*), Yarrow (*Achillea millefolium*), Blue Vervain (*Verbena hastata*), Boneset (*Eupatorium perfoliatum*), Cayenne (*Capsicum annuum*), and Isatis (*Isatis tinctoria*).

Blood and Lymphatic Cleanser: Echinacea excels as one of the best blood and lymphatic cleansers in the plant kingdom, and is able to neutralize many poisons and toxins. The lymphatic system plays a major role in the body's defense system. The fluid in lymphatic vessels carries immune-activating lymphocytes to tissues throughout the body. Lymph nodes line the pathways of lymphatic vessels and produce lymphocytes that destroy infectious pathogens. The nodes filter out foreign particles like bacteria and prevent them from reaching the blood stream. These actions contribute to the detoxification of lymphatic fluid, blood, and the thymus gland and spleen, which are important components of the immune system. The thymus and spleen are both composed of lymphatic tissue that produces lymphocytes and antibodies to fight infection. The spleen acts as a large filter system that removes dead and damaged red blood cells, bacteria, and other debris from the blood. Echinacea stimulates the thymus, spleen, and bone marrow to produce sufficient levels of immune cells. As a peripheral vasodilator, the herb dilates blood vessels to improve circulation in all extremities. It is beneficial for dark, swollen varicose veins and phlebitis (inflammation of blood vessels).

The herb has a history of successfully treating venomous bites and stings from snakes, rabid dogs, scorpions, and insects. Venom often contains hyaluronidase, which breaks down hyaluronic acid (the protective ground substance in tissues), allowing venom to penetrate into the cells and bloodstream. Echinacea protects tissues by inhibiting the action of hyaluronidase and restricting the body's absorption and circulation of toxins.

Eclectic physicians praised the plant for its ability to treat all types of serious septicemia (toxins and infectious pathogens in the blood) and conditions involving blood poisoning and lymphatic toxicity. These included eczema, acne, boils, abscesses, gangrene, animal venom, plant toxins, strep and staph infections, chronic wounds, typhoid fever, swollen glands and lymph nodes, measles, mumps, and chicken pox.

For cases of acute or chronically sore, swollen lymph nodes, I combine Poke root tincture (*Phytolacca decandra*) with Echinacea and this works amazingly well every time. Poke is very powerful and specific for lymphatic cleansing. Remember that **Poke is toxic in large doses**, and is only taken in small amounts of 5-10 drops 3-4 times a day with Echinacea. Another wonderful blood and lymphatic cleansing formula is prepared with equal parts of the tinctures of Echinacea, Cayenne, Red Clover (*Trifolium pratense*), St. John's Wort, and the roots of Yellow Dock (*Rumex crispus*), Dandelion (*Taraxacum officinale*), and Burdock (*Arctium* spp.). Take 40-60 drops of this combination in water 4-5 times during the day for 7-14 days. Eating a light diet with lots of pure water, herbal teas, fruit, vegetables, raw foods, brown rice, and reasonable fasting also potentiates the cleansing process.

Cancer and HIV/AIDS: Most people with cancer, tumors, and HIV have a weak, underactive immune system that can be strengthened by Echinacea. Many of its phytochemicals, including caffeic acid and echinacin, demonstrate anticarcinogenic and antitumor activity in scientific studies. Cichoric acid, abundant in the flowers and roots, appears to have anti-retroviral effects that help prevent viruses from infiltrating and mutating DNA in healthy cells. *In vitro* tests show that cichoric acid inhibits colon cancer by inducing apoptosis (programed cell death) to cancerous colon cells (Tsai, 2012).

Several studies have shown that Echinacea helps reduce suppression of white blood cells during radiation and chemotherapy (Pohl, 1969) and strengthens immunity in people with cervical, ovarian, and breast cancers (Coeugniet, 1987). Echinacea's multiple strengthening and stimulating effects on immunity are appropriate as an additional treatment for HIV/AIDS and different types of tumors and cancers, including lymphatic cancers such as lymphomas and Hodgkin's disease (Currier, 2002). Currently, scientists and some medical professionals are researching Echinacea's role in the treatment of these diseases and its ability to lessen immune suppression during chemotherapy and radiation. Echinacea has been given for leucopenia (low counts of white blood cells and T-helper cells) caused by radiation and chronic immune deficiency.

Adrenal Glands: Research shows that Echinacea can induce mild stimulation of the adrenal cortex to secrete cortisone steroid hormones. This improves the body's ability to deal with stress and helps reduce chronic inflammation (Busing, 1952; Mostbeck, 1962). Injectable forms of the extract are used by German medical doctors for adrenal stimulation.

Wound Healing: The World Health Organization and German Commission E herbal regulatory agency have approved Echinacea for external use in healing wounds, chronic skin ulcers, and inflammatory skin conditions. The herb can be applied to any external wound, whether it is a surface or deep puncture wound, acute or chronic. It fights infection, decreases inflammation, and stimulates wound healing and tissue repair. Echinacea is used to treat cuts, burns, sunburn, skin ulcers, abscesses, carbuncles, boils, folliculitis, cellulitis, rashes, dermatitis, eczema, varicose veins, and herpes lesions including shingles, cold sores, and genital herpes. The Eclectic physicians successfully used the herb for serious tissue-destroying gangrene infections, and to relieve the itchy, painful rashes of chicken pox, mumps, and measles.

In a 5-month clinical study involving 4,598 patients with various skin ailments, a topical ointment of *E. purpurea* improved wound healing, inflammation, burns, eczema, ulcers, and herpes simplex lesions in 85.5% of the people. Another clinical study in 1963 by the same researcher involved 200 patients suffering from psoriasis. Oral doses of *E. purpurea* alcohol extract, given in conjunction with pharmaceutical topical medicines, elicited remissions in 90% of the patients over a period of 9-18 months (Viehmann, 1978).

Research has provided some explanations for the herb's vulnerary (wound healing) properties. Several phytochemicals, including alkylamides, reduce pain and inflammation. Echinacea's influence on the adrenal glands to secrete cortisone hormones also helps reduce inflammation and pain. Laboratory studies have confirmed that echinacein, a polysaccharide component, promotes wound healing due to its ability to maintain the structure and integrity of the collagen matrix of connective tissue in skin and organs. It also stimulates fibroblasts to make more connective tissue cells that promote structural repair and wound healing (Tunnerhoff, 1956). Researchers have found that topical applications of Echinacea on infections and wounds stimulate granulation in which new, healthy tissue is formed (Bauer, 1991). It catalyzes the immune response to heal wounds and reduce pus and tissue decay by eliminating bacterial and fungal infections.

The roots, leaves, and flowers are used for external wound healing. They may be dried, ground into powder, mixed with water to make a paste, and applied as a poultice. The tea or diluted tincture can be soaked in a cloth and applied as a wash or compress. The freshly harvested plant is also an excellent addition to salve. When using Echinacea to treat chronic external conditions, take the tincture internally as well to enhance greater immune stimulation and detoxify the blood and lymphatic fluids. In this way, it cleans and heals from the inside out.

Arthritis: Echinacea has traditionally been used for rheumatoid arthritis. German researchers and physicians have successfully treated early stages of rheumatoid arthritis with injections and oral use of the extract (Murray, 1992). Its cooling, anti-inflammatory properties relieve joint pain, while hyaluronic acid lubricates joints. However, use caution because Echinacea has increased the discomfort of arthritis in some people, so it is recommended to try small amounts initially to determine individual effects.

Childbirth and Infants: Echinacea is a safe remedy to treat or prevent postpartum infection in women following childbirth and to treat mastitis (breast inflammation). If birth conditions are not sterile, or if there is any question of sanitation, 40-60 drops of tincture can be ingested 2-3 times a day in water for 7 days as a preventative against infections.

For infants, 1-2 drops of diluted tincture can be put on the umbilical stump several times a day to eliminate possibility of infection and encourage rapid healing. A sterile wash of the tea may be used for bacterial eye infections in newborns by putting several drops of the **filtered tea** in each eye with a sterile dropper, 3-4 times a day. Echinacea tincture is safe for newborns and older infants suffering from colds, flu, or other infections, and is much safer and gentler than prescription antibiotics. Be sure to **evaporate off the alcohol** by putting the tincture in a small amount of boiling hot water, stirring, and allowing it to sit for about 10 minutes. Give the infant ½ drop of tincture per pound of body weight 3-5 times a day. The mother may slip a plastic dropper containing the diluted tincture next to the nipple and give it to the baby while nursing.

Parting Thoughts

Echinacea is an amazing and valuable plant to enjoy growing around one's home and to use for medicine. For best healing results, use tincture prepared from freshly harvested plants and take it at the first sign of the common cold, flu, and other infectious illnesses. I always keep Echinacea tincture in my medicine cabinet and take it with me when I travel. It is one of the best herbal allies to eliminate infections.

Teachings from the Echinacea Deva

"Greetings! My presence is revered among the plants on this Turtle Island – what you now call North America. I am an elder upon this land and a leader among the medicine plants. For hundreds of years, I have been consumed by animals as well as people inhabiting Turtle Island, first by the early native people and then by those who immigrated. And even now, my medicine is well known and used by many people.

"I am a powerful, masculine warrior plant offering great protection. My fiery Aries nature contains strong medicine that protects against invasive infections and diseases. The native people drank my tea and put poultices of my roots on wounds and venomous bites. For I not only heal the tissues but pull poisons out of the body and neutralize those that remain. My energies are like a shield against harmful elements in the environment. My protective warrior quality emerges from the fire element, and my big pink flowers hold the red fire energy. The prickly spikes in the center of my flowers carry swift, piercing power to purge invaders and poisons from the body.

"Just as fire purges, my ability to destroy all that is harmful allows purification of the blood and waters of the body. The lymph fluids, like the waters of the oceans, bathe and cleanse all cells. By keeping fluids pure, the cells and tissues remain strong and vibrant. So I bring purity, balance, and peace to the environment of the body.

"Just as the action of a warrior is only required during attacks or threats of attacks, my medicine is to be used only upon threat of illness or actual invasion. Then use me in large, frequent doses to maintain a strong defense against pathogens and poisons. And when the battle of sickness is over, peace reigns and the action of the warrior is no longer needed. And so, do not ingest me on a regular basis. During these times of peace, maintain your bodies with the gentler plants that act to nourish and sustain.

"My essence offers deep inner strength where there is fear and hesitation. The pink color of my flowers is also associated with heart energy. I bring courage of heart to those in fear and trauma. I help people to move ahead and walk forward with confidence, knowing that we are all supported and grounded in the mystical power and compassion and abundant nature of the Great Mother, the Earth. My power to combat all that harms and disrupts the body is a reflection and extension of the compassionate power of the Great Mother.

"So relax and take a deep breath. Know that this power and compassion resides as the essence of all beings. In the kingdom of the plants, I am a chief carrier of this energy and share the message with others. I am a messenger of abundant purity. Resting in this space, there is great beauty and joy of heart. It is the feeling elicited when standing in a garden of my plants, strong in stature and rooted in the earth.

"I hold the fiery and expansive energies of Aries and Sagittarius, and with intensity my medicine moves through the body like a swift arrow aimed at its target to subdue and eliminate all that harms. But this warrior nature is blended and balanced with the heart energy of compassion, and this is my gentle feminine aspect. For without heart-felt compassion, unbridled power becomes senselessly destructive to all life. Within the balance of power and compassion arises calm and peaceful abiding.

My offering to you is this space of balance and peace. This is my most precious and revered gift."

Elderberry

Sambucus canadensis
Caprifoliaceae (Honeysuckle) Family

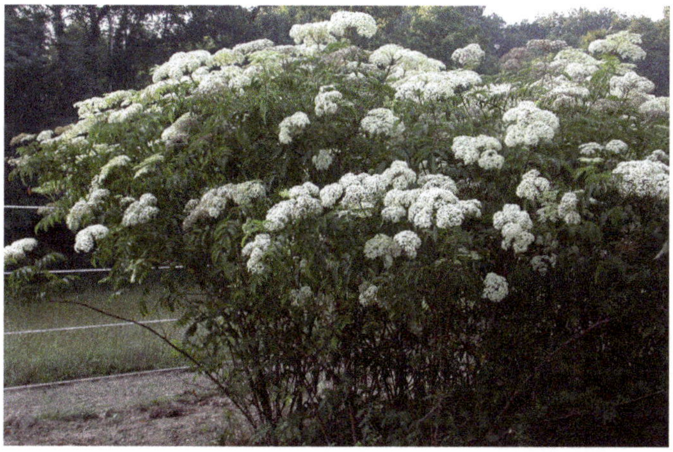
American Elderberry (*Sambucus canadensis*)

Common Names

Sambucus canadensis is known as American Elder or American Elderberry. European Elderberry, *Sambucus nigra*, is also called Black Elder or European Elder. Common elder, sweet elder, Sambucus, Elder Mother, Hylde-Moer, Elda Mor, Lady Ellhorn, Lady Elder, tree of music, pipe tree, and tree of medicine are common names for *Sambucus* plants.

Medicinal Part of the Plant

Sambucus canadensis and *S. nigra* share the same medicinal properties and are used interchangeably for healing and culinary purposes. While the roots, bark, leaves, and flowers are all medicinal, the flowers and dark-purple berries are the parts most prized for medicine.

Range and Habitat

More than 20 *Sambucus* species grow worldwide, but *S. canadensis* and *S. nigra* are the medicinal varieties with dark-purple berries. *S. canadensis* is native to most areas of North America, particularly the central and eastern regions. It grows north from British Columbia to Nova Scotia, as far south as Florida, and west to Texas and Arizona. Elderberry plants are found in damp areas, meadows, along the edges of wooded areas, and in waste places. The shrub thrives in rich, moist soil with good drainage and full sun. There are numerous *Sambucus* cultivars grown primarily for their tasty medicinal berries. Farmers once planted Elderberry bushes around their barns, and sometimes these can still be found growing around old barns.

S. nigra is indigenous to temperate areas of Europe, northern Africa, and western and central Asia. It grows in similar habitats as *S. canadensis* and has naturalized in some areas of the United States. Widely cultivated for its edible fruits, it continues to be popular in European herbalism.

Some varieties of Elder develop poisonous red berries that should never be eaten. *S. ebulus* (Dwarf Elder) is indigenous to Europe, but is a much smaller plant than *S. nigra*. *S. racemosa* is indigenous to Europe, western Asia, northern United States, and Canada. The greenish flowers are clumped in panicles with a different appearance than the umbel-shaped flower heads of *S. canadensis* and *S. nigra*. Another red-fruited species found in North America, *S. pubens*, has creamy-white or yellow flowers that, rather than being arranged in a wide flower head, also grow in long clusters.

Description of the Plant

American Elderberry (*S. canadensis*) is a handsome, lush, deciduous shrub with tree-like bark and many branching stems. The erect stems have a soft, porous inner pith. As the woody stems terminate into leaves and flowers, the bark thins into smooth, round herbaceous stems. The plant grows 5-12′ high and can get very bushy.

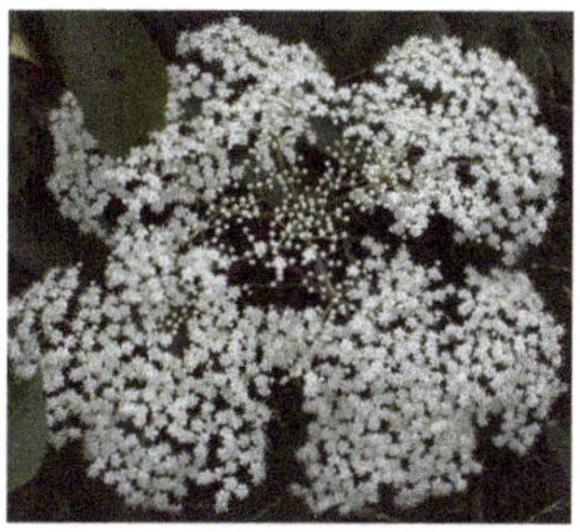

Many pinnately compound leaves climb the branches opposite each other. Leaflets typically grow in 3-5 pairs with one leaf appearing on the end of the stem. Leaflets attach to short petioles and are lance-shaped to ovate with sharply pointed tips, pinnate veins, and finely serrated teeth.

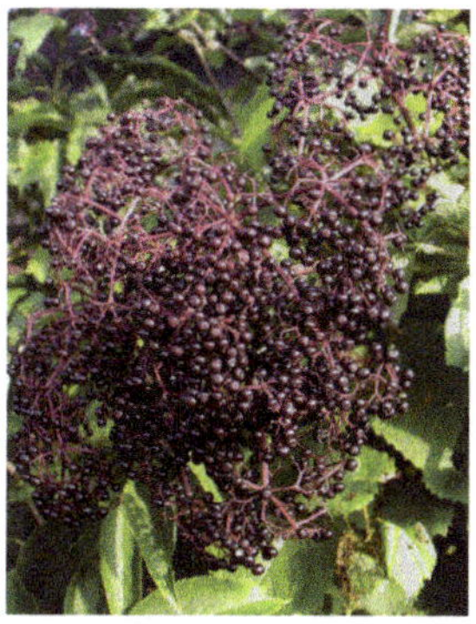

At the end of each flower stalk, the stem divides into 5 large compound umbels containing numerous small, creamy-white flowers. The tiny flowers, about 1/6″ wide, have 5 petals with 5 pale-yellow stamens. Flower heads, reaching up to 1′ in diameter, emit a sweet, earthy fragrance. Flowers bloom from May to July and are quite beautiful, resembling delicate, lacy wisps of clouds among the deep-green foliage. During August and September, the flowers mature into round, dark-purple berries the size of a small pea. The berries are juicy and hang in large, drooping bunches.

European Elderberry (*S. nigra*), much larger than *S. canadensis*, is a deciduous tree growing up to 30′ in height. The leaves and flowers have a similar appearance as *S. canadensis*, and it also has white umbel flower heads that mature into round, dark-purple berries.

Elderberry (*Sambucus canadensis*)

Cultivation

Elderberry can be started by seeds and stem cuttings. Plants growing wild or around old barns may be dug up and transplanted into gardens. Before planting seeds, soak them for 24 hours for best germination. Most gardeners find that propagation from stem cuttings is the fastest and most reliable method. Simply cut 3-4′ long stems from mature plants in spring and place the cut ends in a bucket full of very moist sand, potting soil, and vermiculite. Poke drainage holes in the bottom of the bucket. Stems usually develop roots within 2-3 weeks and are then planted into a permanent garden. Roots grow vigorously in moderately fertile, well-drained soil. Plants prefer full sun and grow rapidly into large bushes. Deer eat the leaves and flowers, so young plants may need to be protected by fencing until they are larger.

Harvest

Gather fresh leaves anytime during the growth cycle. Harvest flowers shortly after blooming and use them fresh or dried. Harvest berries at the peak of ripeness when they have turned deep purple and are soft and juicy. **Do not harvest Elder species bearing toxic red berries!**

Preparation of Plant Medicine and Dosages

Freshly harvested flower heads are best prepared as tincture to maintain best potency, or they are dried. Ripe, dark-purple berries are made into a delicious and highly nutritious juice or syrup. Leaves, bark, and roots are only used for external healing as an ointment or poultice for bruises, sprains, and hemorrhoids. **Avoid ingesting the leaves, bark, and roots due to their strong laxative properties and potential toxicity.**

PREPARATIONS

Infusion Tea: Steep 1-2 teaspoons of fresh or dried flowers per cup of boiled water. Flowers are mucilaginous and have a pleasant, slightly sweet flavor. Dosage: 1-3 cups a day as needed.

Tincture: Prepare freshly harvested flowers with 65% 190-proof grain alcohol and 35% distilled water. Dosage: 10-60 drops 1-4 times a day as needed.

Salve or Ointment: Use leaves, flowers, bark, and roots.

Berry Juice: To extract juice from the dark-purple berries, use an electric food processor, a potato masher, or similar hand tool to mash them into juicy pulp. Put the pulp in a large pan and add twice as much water. Stir vigorously, then strain and squeeze as much juice out of the pulp as possible. Another batch of water may be added to the remaining pulp and the process repeated. Another method of extraction is to put the berries through an electric juicing machine, producing thick juice and fairly dry pulp. To obtain the most benefits, water may mixed with this pulp, strained, and squeezed.

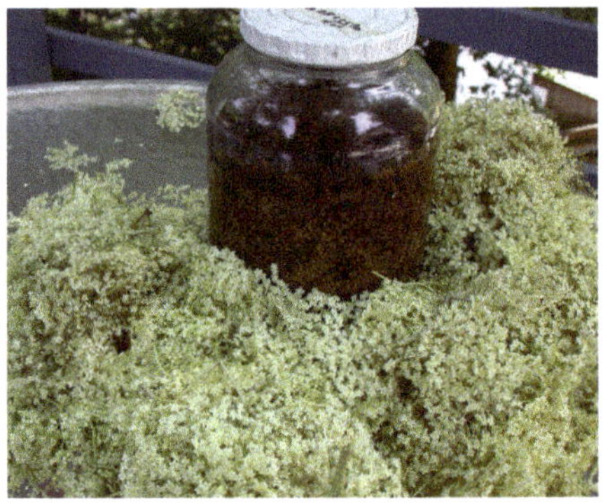

Flowers tincturing in a jar

When the juice has been extracted and strained, it should be free of pulp and seeds. Cutin, a waxy substance covering the seeds, may be seen floating on the surface of the berry juice and skimmed off. Gently simmer the juice for 8-10 minutes while stirring (it must be thoroughly cooked). Add honey or another natural sweetener to taste, cool, and pour into plastic bags or containers and freeze for best preservation. Dosage: 1-2 ounces daily. Dilute with water if desired.

Syrup is prepared using the berry juice or a strong tea of the flowers. Combine 1 part juice or tea with 3 parts natural sweetener. Gently simmer the mixture while constantly stirring, then pour it into sterilized jars. Less sweetener may be used, but the syrup must be refrigerated for preservation. Dosage: Give children 1 teaspoon up to 4 times a day, while adults may take 2-3 teaspoons 4 times a day.

Cordials are created by adding brandy to the berry juice or strong tea. Add at least 25% alcohol to preserve cordials.

Culinary Uses

Elder flowers and berries are delicious and contain many nutrients. The flowers are picked when in full bloom and added to salads or made into fritters by dipping the flower heads in batter and frying them in a skillet. The ripe, purple berries are excellent prepared as juice, wine, brandy cordials, jam, and pies.

Chemical Constituents

Flavonoids and triterpenes are the primary biologically active constituents in Elder plants. The flowers are high in anti-inflammatory, antioxidant, and anti-allergenic flavonoids (up to 3%), including astragalin, hyperoside, isoquercitrin, rutin, quercetin, kaempferol, and anthocyanins. Flowers contain 8-9% minerals (mainly potassium), phenolic acids (about 3% chlorogenic acid), and triterpenes that include alpha- and beta-amyrin palmitate (anti-anemic, anti-inflammatory, anti-arthritic, mild sedative). Studies show that these triterpenes exhibit strong ability to protect the liver against damage from toxic carbon tetrachloride. Other triterpenes include ursolic acid (anti-inflammatory), oleanolic acid, beta-sitosterol (antibacterial, anticarcinogenic, diuretic, anti-inflammatory, estrogenic, hypoglycemic), and stigmasterol (hepatoprotective, anti-inflammatory, antiviral, estrogenic). Flowers also contain mucilage, pectin, tannins, vitamin C, and the vitamin B-complex. Fatty acids include linoleic, linolenic, and palmitic acid (Blumenthal, 2000).

Leaves contain similar flavonoids, triterpenes, and fatty acids as those found in the flowers, in addition to cyanogenetic glycosides, including sambunigrin.

Elder bark contains saponins, hydrocyanic acid (toxic in large doses), sambuline, and lectins. Lectins include phytohaemagglutinins that have been used to treat drug-induced leukopenia (insufficient amount of white blood cells) and some types of anemia (Paulo, 1976).

Ripe, purple Elder berries are exceptionally rich sources of several nutrients that include vitamin C, flavonoids, and anthocyanins (purple pigments and powerful antioxidants that reduce oxidation to protect cells from damage). Anthocyan glycosides include chrysanthemin, sambucin, and sambucyanin. Flavonoid glycosides include hyperoside, isoquercitrin, and rutin. Berries also contain beta-carotene (vitamin A), thiamine (vitamin B1), riboflavin (vitamin B2), niacin (vitamin B3), pantothenic acid (vitamin B5), biotin, calcium, and several amino acids, including tryptophan (antidepressant, anti-anxiety, analgesic, sedative), alanine (antioxidant, anticarcinogenic), arginine (antihypertensive, diuretic, pituitary stimulant, vasodilator), cystine, glutamic acid (anti-epileptic, antilithic), glycine (anti-acid, anti-ulcer), histidine (antioxidant, anti-arteriosclerotic), methionine (detoxant, antioxidant, hepatoprotective, lipotropic), phenylalanine (antidepressant , used for attention deficit disorder), and tyrosine (anti-ulcer, thyroid support).

Safety, Contraindications, and Drug Interactions

The flowers of *S. canadensis* and *S. nigra* are safe for general consumption. **The berries are safe to eat only if they are dark purple and ripe, cooked, and the tiny seeds have been strained out.** The flowers and properly prepared berries have no known contraindications, side effects, interaction with other drugs, or restrictions during pregnancy and lactation.

The root, bark, and leaves are safe for external use only. These parts, along with the unripe berries, are not recommended for internal use because they contain toxic cyanide glycosides (sambunigrin) and strong alkaloids that can cause nausea, vomiting, severe diarrhea, dizziness, and rapid heartbeat when ingested in large doses. In the literature, there are reports of children who developed toxic symptoms from prolonged handling, chewing, or sucking on toys made from fresh Elder stems.

Medicinal Uses

History of the Plant

Over many centuries, *S. nigra* has been employed as an important medicine throughout Europe. It has been venerated for its healing and magic by great physicians, who used all parts of the plant and wrote numerous accounts of its attributes. Hippocrates (who called Elder his "medicine chest"), Theophrastus, Pliny the Elder, Dioscorides, Galen, Paracelsus, and Nicholas Culpeper all considered this herb to be one of their most valuable remedies. It was prescribed for respiratory ailments, the common cold, fevers, influenza (the flu), excess phlegm, colic, diarrhea, cholera, uterine problems, rheumatism, and all types of infections and deadly plagues that swept across Europe. The root was used as a diuretic for edema, a purgative to expel toxins, and a remedy for poisonous snakebites. Leaves were also ingested as a purgative to induce vomiting and diarrhea, and for treating coughs, colds, and inflammation of the mucous membranes. Leaves were applied as a poultice or salve to wounds, hemorrhoids, animal bites, ulcers, tumors, and gouty toes. A tea made from flowers was given for coughs, colds, flu, and as a blood purifier. The berries were taken to clean the blood, heal skin rashes, ease joint pain, and reduce coughs, water retention, and constipation.

In *The Complete Herbal*, Culpeper described several uses of Elderberry and wrote that the plant is under the dominion of Venus. He boiled the first Elder shoots and young leaves appearing in spring in a fatty broth as a remedy for respiratory afflictions and excess phlegm. The bark and berries were employed as a diuretic for water retention and as an emmenagogue to promote and ease menstruation.

The name *Sambucus* is derived from the Latin term for an ancient Roman musical instrument made with Elder wood. Flute-like musical instruments called pan pipes were created by removing the inner pith of the stem, and "pipe tree" became a common name for the plant. Children whittled flutes, whistles, and pop-gun toys from the stems. The name Elder comes from the Anglo-Saxon word *aeld*, meaning "fire," because people could start fires by blowing through the hollow branches of the plant.

Elder trees were honored as holy plants and greatly respected throughout the ages. The Greeks associated Elder with Pan, the mythological half-goat, half-man god of music and the fields, forests and mountains, who was a companion of the nymphs. A wealth of European lore extols the magical properties surrounding *S. nigra* and the mystical woman living in Elder trees. It was said that she is an intensely powerful, stern, wise woman whose presence takes the shape of the Elder plant bearing healing gifts. She demands respect and is known by many names, including Elder Mother, Hylde-Moer, Elda Mor, and Lady Ellhorn. Country folk believed she was capable of maliciousness if mistreated or dishonored. If parts of her tree were harmed or taken without permission, it was feared that the Elder Mother would haunt and punish the offender. Many were scared for their lives if they harvested the plant or burned the wood without the proper request and offering. It was thought that children placed in cradles made from Elder harvested without due respect would be tormented until removed from the cradle. Many people believed that Jesus was crucified on a cross made of Elder wood and that Judas hung himself from an Elder tree. Consequently, Elder also became a symbol of sorrow and death.

But people also acknowledged that the Elder Mother holds great power, wisdom, and protection against harm. If someone was sick and unsure as to what herbal remedy to use, according to old lore they could sit under an Elder tree and be advised of the correct herb. During the era of the Inquisition and witch-hunts, people had faith in Elder's ability to ward off evil and protect them from witches. Elderberry was grown around homes and employed for spells and charms. Plant parts were worn as amulets, and bundles of the leaves were tied to doors and windows for protection from evil or being struck by lightning. Wooden crosses made from Elder were sometimes placed on new graves and the leaves buried with people in hopes of providing peace to departed souls and protecting them from the realms of hell.

There are legends of Elder serving as a portal into mystical fairy realms of the underworld, and the plant is sometimes identified with the Queen of the Netherworld. In Danish folklore, it was presumed that by standing under an Elder plant on the night of the summer solstice, one could see the King of Fairyland ride by with all his retinue. Many people were afraid to fall asleep under Elder trees, convinced they would disappear forever into the underworld.

In North America, *S. canadensis* was used by the Native Americans long before the European invasion. In some tribes, Elder was called the "tree of music" and flutes were whittled from the branches. Arrows were made from Elder shoots. The berries were frequently enjoyed as food and a pleasant beverage. Different tribes found a variety of medicinal uses for Elderberry. The Iroquois and Huma boiled the inner bark to prepare tea that was applied as a wash for inflammation and painful swellings. The Creeks pounded the roots to make a poultice for swollen breasts. The root bark tea was used by the Meskwakis to clear phlegm and congestion from the lungs, stimulate childbirth, and treat constipation, water retention, and headaches. The Menominee drank a tea of the dried flowers to reduce fevers (Vogel, 1970). The Mohegans gave a tea created from flowers to babies with colic. The Cherokee used it for fevers, kidney problems, and rheumatism. Leaves and stems were applied externally to burns, skin eruptions, and boils. The Delaware ingested tea from leaves and stems as a blood purifier and for infant colic. The Iroquois applied leaf poultices for headaches, cuts, and swellings. A tea of the berries was given for fevers, measles, diphtheria, mumps, venereal diseases, and stomach, kidney, and heart problems (Moerman, 1998). Native Americans and Europeans used the purple and red berries as dye.

Later in American history, the Eclectic physicians employed Elderberry in their treatment protocols for children and adults. It was used as a diaphoretic (increasing perspiration) to reduce fevers, as a diuretic for edema, and for liver problems. Tea of the flowers and juice from berries were given for excess mucous and nasal congestion, fevers, flu, skin diseases, syphilis, rheumatism, and scrofula (tuberculosis of the lymph nodes in the neck). The inner bark was used in large doses for its cathartic action and taken in small doses to remove obstructions and increase secretions. The plant was externally applied for skin diseases and eruptions, burns, eczema, old ulcers and edematous tissues having poor circulation, and all erysipelas diseases, which involved skin inflammation caused by *Streptococcus* bacterial infection. Elder berries were listed as an official medicine in the *U.S. Pharmacopoeia* from 1820–1890. Elder flowers were listed in the *U.S. Pharmacopoeia* from 1831–1905 and in *The National Formulary* from 1916–1947.

Currently, Elder berries and flowers remain popular herbal remedies in the European and American markets. Approved modern therapeutic applications for Elder berries and flowers are supported by their long history of use in well-established systems of traditional medicine, by *in vitro* and human clinical studies, and by phytochemical identification. Most research has been on European Elderberry (*S. nigra*) and a popular cough syrup extract of its berries sold under the trade name Sambucol®.

Healing Qualities

Flowers prepared as tincture or hot tea are a relaxing diaphoretic that opens skin pores to promote perspiration and reduce heat in cases of fever. Cold tea and tincture are diuretic. Flowers have alterative (restoring health and vitality), anti-catarrhal (reducing mucous), anti-inflammatory, antispasmodic, antiviral, demulcent, detoxifying, expectorant, immunostimulant, and nervine properties. Fresh flowers are a milder laxative than the berries, but may be irritating to the stomach. If a laxative effect is not desired, drying the flowers eliminates this action.

Berries are a powerhouse of nutrients that cleanse, cool and fortify the blood, treat anemia, strengthen weak and sore muscles, and restore vitality to the whole body. Antioxidants support and stimulate immunity, reduce inflammation, and protect cells from damage. Berries are antiviral, diaphoretic, diuretic, and mildly laxative. Berries have similar uses as the flowers and are helpful for sinus congestion, upper respiratory infections, asthma, arthritis, neuralgia (nerve pain), and sciatica.

Leaves are externally applied as a soothing emollient and healing vulnerary for bruises, wounds, rashes, tumors, and other external problems. They remove heat and inflammation from infections, boils and arthritic joints, and ease nerve pain. Leaves exert expectorant, diuretic, and diaphoretic properties when taken internally, but are not usually ingested because they are such strong purgatives.

Inner bark and roots are powerful cathartic laxatives and diuretics that purge the system by stimulating very strong spasms in the stomach, liver, gallbladder, intestines, and kidneys. Large doses can cause vomiting. Small doses of the bark and roots are used for acute constipation and fluid retention with caution due to their powerful actions. In small homeopathic doses, they have been taken to treat cramps and spasms, liver and bile congestion, constipation, asthma with excessive phlegm, and even epilepsy. They are applied externally for the same conditions as the leaves.

Traditional Chinese Medicine (TCM) Perspective

The flowers are cooling, drying, and remove Qi and fluid stagnation throughout the body. They open passageways and stimulate secretions that open skin pores to promote sweating, improve movement through the digestive and urinary tracts, and increase circulation. The flowers dispel Wind Heat, clear toxic heat in the blood, open the lungs, drain fluid congestion, and expel mucous.

The berries are a cooling, moisturizing, and restorative Yin tonic. By nourishing the blood, they benefit all deficiency conditions such as anemia, muscle weakness, chronic fatigue, and scanty or delayed menses. Berries clear Blood and Liver Heat, which removes toxins and decongests Liver Qi Stagnation.

Primary Actions

The American Elderberry (*S. canadensis*) is an herb I feel blessed to know and have growing close by. The beauty of its delicate, lacy-white flowers on huge flower heads that transform into drooping clusters of deep-purple berries glorify any garden landscape. The impressive size of the bushes and rapid, prolific growth of stems, leaves, and flowers each year is a signature of the tremendous vital life energy and potential for healing and longevity contained within this valuable herb.

The pure white color of the flowers is a signature of their affinity with the nervous system, and they exude an earthy "other-worldly" fragrance and mild gas that induce a calming effect. The plant stimulates movement of energies and fluids throughout the body. Nerves relax, passageways are opened, blood and lymphatic circulation are enhanced, secretions of sweat glands and digestive enzymes increase, urine flow improves, muscles are strengthened, and pain and aches are eased.

The ripe berries are an especially potent tonic that I have come to absolutely love! In late summer when the berries are soft and ripe, I harvest enough to juice, cook, and freeze so that there is enough to last through the winter. When drinking a shot of the tasty, deep burgundy-purple juice, I can feel its restorative energies entering my bloodstream and energizing the whole body. It feels like an herbal blood transfusion!

Elder berries are excellent for treating all conditions involving nutritional deficiencies and degenerative diseases because they nourish, cleanse, and restore the body over time. Anthocyanins are phytochemicals in the berries providing healing and immune support. They are the flavonoid pigments synthesized by plants that provide red, blue, or purple coloring to flowers, fruits, and berries. As powerful antioxidants, anthocyanins protect against cellular damage, inflammation, cancer, cardiovascular problems, and other chronic, degenerative diseases. The berries are helpful in treating a multitude of problems, including poor immunity, anemia, chronic fatigue, muscle weakness, chronic dermatitis, and drug withdrawal. The berries also exert a tonic effect on the endocrine organs.

I encourage people to grow the beautiful and stately Elderberry bushes around their homes to enjoy a continual source of this excellent medicine.

Colds, Coughs, Flu, and Fevers: Use Elder flowers for the early or middle stages of the common cold, sinusitis, fevers, flu, coughs, bronchitis, and other respiratory infections. The berry juice is also excellent for these problems. A hot tea of the flowers or berry juice stimulates perspiration and benefits colds, flu, and fevers by sweating them out of the body. Bronchial secretions are increased to loosen and remove congestion. The antiviral flowers and berries reduce inflammation in the upper respiratory tract (Mascolo, 1987). Take them for chronic sinusitis, hay fever allergies, spasmodic croupy coughs and bronchitis, laryngitis, tonsillitis, measles, and other skin eruptions. The tea or diluted tincture of the flowers can be used as a gargle for sore, inflamed mouths and throats. Elder flowers and berries are safe for infants and young children, and are beneficial for childhood fevers, croup, and sinus congestion.

A formula made with equal amounts of Elder flowers, Yarrow (*Achillea millefolium*), and Peppermint (*Mentha x piperita*) was very popular among early American colonists for treating colds, coughs, fevers, and the flu. This remedy is especially effective when combined with Boneset (*Eupatorium perfoliatum*) and Echinacea (*Echinacea purpurea* and *E. angustifolia*).

Current research substantiates these traditional uses of Elderberry, confirming that the flowers and berries stimulate immunity. Anthocyanins in the berries and flowers enhance immune function by increasing the production of anti-inflammatory cytokines, which regulate the intensity and the duration of a strong immune response and mediate cell-to-cell communication (Watzl, 2000; Barak, 2001).

Sambucol, the standardized extract produced from the berries of *S. nigra*, was effective against 10 strains of influenza virus during *in vitro* testing (Zakay-Rones, 1995). Elder berries and flowers exert antiviral activity against Epstein-Barr, herpes, and HIV viruses. Two *in vitro* tests have demonstrated that Sambucol extract reduced infection and replication of HIV strains and the herpes virus. This included acyclovir-resistant strains of herpes, which were completely inhibited by the herb (Shapira-Nahor, 1995; Morag, 1996). Combined with St. John's Wort (*Hypericum perforatum*), Elder berries reduce the herpes simplex and influenza viruses (Serkedjieva, 1990; Turpin, 2000). Researchers think that phytochemicals in the berries may bind to the outer membrane of viruses and prevent them from invading healthy cells or replicating. Swiss researchers found that the berry extract inhibited the growth of H5N1 avian influenza virus in a human breast cancer cell line (Sauter, 1989). A more recent *in vitro* study demonstrated that flavonoids from the berries bind to the surface of H1N1 viruses (belonging to the same viral group as the swine flu virus) to prevent infection of healthy cells (Roschek, 2009).

The berry extract has been shown to halt viral replication in humans and *in vitro*. One study showed that a standardized extract of Elder berries (*S. nigra*) inhibited several types of influenza viruses during *in vitro* tests and in a clinical test treating 27 children and adults infected with influenza B. Children received 2 tablespoons daily of the extract and adults ingested 4 tablespoons. Within 2 days, there was significant improvement in the symptoms of 93% of participants who took the herb, compared to 6 days for the placebo group to feel relief (Zakay-Rones, 1995).

A larger study investigated the efficacy and safety of a standardized syrup of Elder berries (*S. nigra*) to treat influenza A and B infections. Sixty patients between 18-54 years of age, who suffered from influenza symptoms with fevers for 48 hours or less, were enrolled in this randomized, double-blind, placebo-controlled study. Patients received 15 ml of Elder berry or placebo syrup 4 times a day for 5 days. Symptoms diminished on an average of 4 days earlier and use of rescue medication was significantly less in those receiving the herbal syrup than with the placebo (Zakay-Rones, 2004).

Cardiovascular System, Blood, and Muscles: A juice or syrup of the ripe, purple berries is an excellent tonic that nourishes and fortifies the blood, heart, and muscles throughout the body. The high nutrient content and wealth of anthocyanins in the berries mineralize the blood and are beneficial for compromised blood vessels, anemia, muscle weakness, fibromyalgia, fatigue, and mental fog.

Research at Tufts University has shown that anthocyanins in Elder berries protect blood vessel walls from oxidative damage associated with vascular diseases (Youdim, 2000). Studies revealed that Elder berries contain greater antioxidant capacity than vitamin C (Pool-Zobel, 1999). They possess significant free radical scavenging ability to protect cells from oxidative damage, and the berries reduce oxidation of low-density-lipoprotein (LDL) cholesterol (Abuja, 1998). Oxidation of LDL cholesterol is implicated in blocked blood vessels and contributes to cardiovascular disease. In a randomized, placebo-controlled trial to study the effects of anthocyanins on cholesterol and antioxidant status, 34 people were given 3 capsules of 400 mg dried Elder berry powder containing 10% anthocyanins (equivalent to 5 ml of Elderberry juice) for 2 weeks. Researchers noted a slight improvement in cholesterol levels and antioxidant activity during this short study using small amounts of Elder berry juice (Murkovic, 2004). All these qualities of the berries offer significant protection against heart attacks, strokes, and blood vessel damage.

By opening the channels of elimination and increasing circulation, Elder flowers and berries remove toxins from the blood, lymphatic fluids and nodes, and their cooling nature reduces excess heat. A cool tea of the flowers is an excellent alterative and diuretic to treat skin rashes caused by metabolic toxicosis (Kuts-Chereauz, 1952).

Digestive and Urinary Systems: Elderberry stimulates the digestive system by increasing secretions of digestive enzymes. This helps indigestion, infant colic, and other stomach and intestinal problems, including gas and bloating. Calming to the nervous system, the herb relaxes muscle tone in the gastrointestinal and urinary tracts. This allows passageways to open for increased circulation and movement throughout the body and reduces gastrointestinal spasms (Richter, 1973). The berry juice and the flowers prepared as a tincture or tea have mild laxative activity helpful for sluggish digestion and chronic constipation. The leaves are powerful laxatives to be used cautiously only in small doses. *In vitro* tests show that the berries inhibit *Helicobacter pylori* bacteria often responsible for stomach ulcers (Chatterjee, 2004). Phytochemicals in the flowers and strong antioxidants in the purple berries exert a cleansing and protective action on the liver.

Elder flowers are diuretic when ingested cold and increase urinary output and reduce edema. The cooling, cleansing actions and alkalizing minerals in the flowers and berries support healthy kidneys, and can ease the pain of gout, an arthritic condition of the large toe related to excessive acids in the blood and tissues.

Women's Health: Elder berries normalize blood flow to the uterus and ovaries. Hippocrates used Elder berries and flowers for many female problems, especially those caused by stagnated blood flow to the ovaries and uterus. Reduced blood flow can cause menstrual problems such as suppressed and scanty menstruation, blood clots, cramps, and pain. The flowers and berries are safe to use during pregnancy, and berries help reduce uterine inflammation after childbirth. A compress made from tea of the flowers may be applied to sore nipples and breasts for relief of mastitis and pain. Cooling properties of the herb are helpful for menopausal hot flashes when 30-60 drops of Elder flower tincture are taken several times a day.

External Healing: Elderberry leaves, flowers, and inner bark have been used for external healing by the ancient Europeans and Native Americans. They are prepared as salve or ointment, or as strong tea applied as a wash or compress on affected tissues. A tincture may be applied to unbroken skin after diluting 60 drops in a cup of water. Elderberry has antiseptic properties to combat skin infections and helps heal traumatic injuries, wounds, burns, abrasions, inflammation, bruises, sprains, swollen glands, hemorrhoids, rashes, dermatitis, rosacea, eczema, and other eruptive skin problems like poison ivy, chicken pox, and measles. A poultice of the ripe berries can be applied to burns.

When used as a hot wash or compress, the herb draws toxins out of skin pores and has a cleansing effect. The emollient leaves and flowers soothe and soften irritated skin, and can be applied as a facial or antiseptic wash. It has been used to improve oily skin, acne, and boils.

Teachings from the Elderberry Deva

"Greetings. I am the Mother Deva of the Elderberry. Those of old called me Elder Mother; for I embrace powerful feminine qualities and belong to the Sisterhood in service of the Great Earth Mother. The power of the Great Mother encompasses nurturing compassion as well as devastating wrath. I embody these extremes which are the natural process on this planet. Life is born and builds upon itself to fullness. For this building process, my berries contain blood-enriching nutrients and my flowers provide healing medicines. But just as life emerges, it ages and becomes old, eventually to be eliminated. And this is the wrathful quality of my bark and roots that purge toxins and waste, just as the elements manifest as raging tornados and hurricanes, tsunami waves, and devastating fires or earthquakes leaving destruction and death in their wake.

"And so people of old who used me in Europe had great fear and trepidation about me, as well as love for my flowers and berries. They followed the wise tradition of asking my permission before cutting away at my limbs and fruit.

"My flowers are of the air element and their medicine is directed to problems in the head and lungs. I open airways for better breathing when the nose and lungs are full of mucous and infection. The white color of my flowers points to this purity of breath and the moving expansive flow of air through the body. The essence of my flowers also releases confused thoughts and feelings that imprison people in their own fear and ignorance.

"My blood-red, purple berries are an offering of my earth element containing an abundance of life-giving nutrients that nourish the blood and bring substance to the body. My berries offer the 'blood of life' that sustains the blood flowing through women during the menses and times when life grows in the womb, when the body of the infant is nourished by the mother's blood. My affinity with this blood of life is another aspect of my offering of purity.

"To heal blood that is toxic and insufficient to sustain life, drink the juice of my berries and add a few drops of Bloodroot tincture every day for a week or so. Bloodroot is a sister plant with powerful, piercing masculine energies that destroy pathogens in the blood and lungs. When her work is complete, the gentler action of my flowers opens passageways in the nose and lungs for easy breathing and my berries nourish the blood and tissues. So Bloodroot's protective warrior energy balances perfectly with my nurturing female quality. Another powerful masculine plant is Poke, which has roots that purify the blood and lymphatic fluids, and balance with my energies. A few drops of tinctured Poke roots may also be blended with the juice of my berries for powerful cleansing. However, when taking Bloodroot and Poke root tinctures, you must remember that their great power is harmful in large doses, and only one or two drops daily are necessary for a short time of seven days. Also, do not take these herbs together. Use either Bloodroot or Poke, one at a time, on separate days.

"I am an herb of the heart. I nurture the physical heart by invigorating and fortifying the blood with my berries. And for emotional healing, a few drops of my flower essence soothe hearts tormented by grief, fear, and feelings of being lost and isolated.

"Although I embody the nurturing and wrathful aspects of the feminine, know that my essence, just like all my sisters and brothers of the plant kingdom, resides in peaceful, radiant calm. Please plant my bushes close to your home so you may come to sit beside me. You are invited to partake of my food and medicine, and to feel and absorb my powerful air, earth, and heart energies into your own being. Align yourself with the forces and nurturing of the Great Mother. Be in awe and reverence of the life force within yourself and all beings. Embrace feminine power for strength and endurance to move through the bumpy grinds and hardships of life, while resting in the space of peaceful, yet powerful, calm abiding. Have courage of heart and peace of mind, and the activity of generosity naturally follows. To live in this flow is to receive and witness the abundant bounty of life!"

Elecampane

Inula helenium

Compositae (*Asteraceae*) (Sunflower or Aster) Family

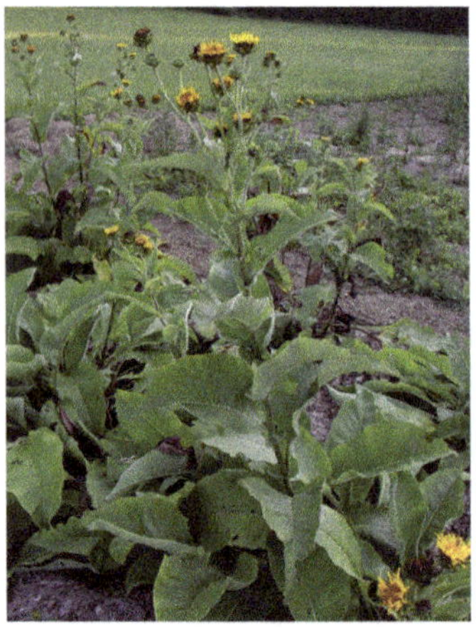

Common Names

Elfdock, elfwort, wild sunflower, velvet dock, yellow starwort, scabwort, horse-elder, and horseheal are old names for Elecampane.

Medicinal Part of the Plant

The roots of plants 2-5 years old are used in Western herbalism. The flowers are used medicinally in Asia.

Range and Habitat

Inula is a large genus containing about 90 species native to Europe and temperate Asia. *Inula helenium* grows in a variety of habitats including moist, shady areas, sunny fields and meadows, and along roadsides. The plant is widely cultivated in Europe and China, and has naturalized in parts of eastern and central North America after introduction by early European colonists.

Description of the Plant

I. helenium is a strikingly attractive and robust perennial. It grows rapidly to a height of 4-6′. Clumps of bulbous rhizomes develop at ground level and increase in size and quantity with age, forming a unique and massive root system. Several large fleshy roots growing 6-12″ long and 1-2″ thick branch off from the bulbs like the legs of an octopus. The roots are brown on the outside and cream-colored inside. Many white, thready rootlets grow off the main root. The bulbous roots produce buds that develop into flowering stalks. The fresh root has a pleasant aromatic odor.

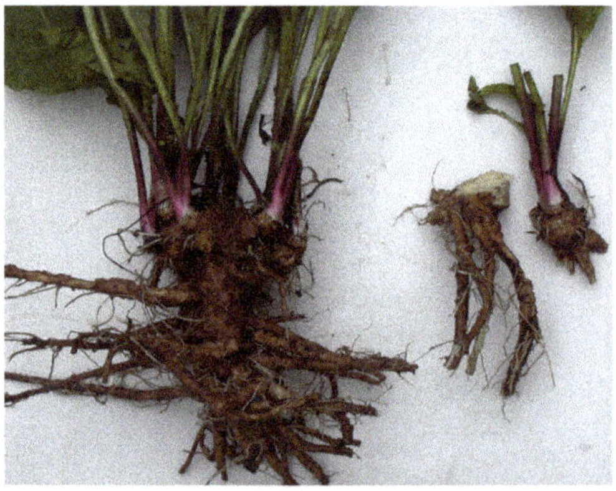

Elecampane roots

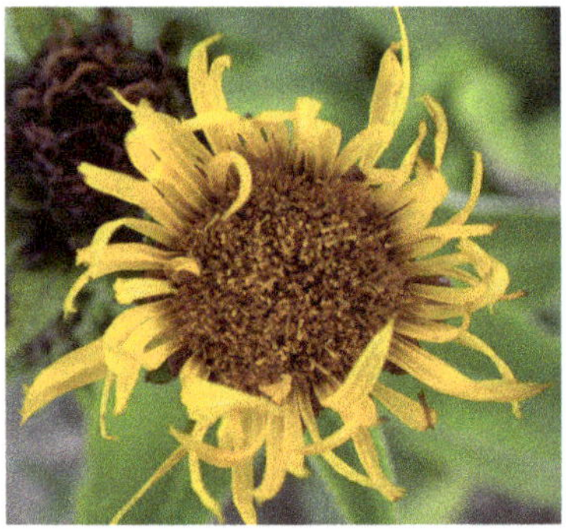

The base of the plant consists of a radical rosette of large, long-stemmed ovate leaves reaching 1-2′ in length. Very stout, round, erect flower stalks emerge from the roots. The green and maroon stalks are covered with fine, woolly hairs. Large leaves climb the stalks in an alternating pattern, becoming smaller towards the top of the plant. Lower leaves have petioles (stems) while the upper leaves are sessile (lacking stems) and clasp around the stalk. The simple leaves have pinnate venation, dentate teeth along their margins, and a rugose (rough and wrinkled) texture. They are covered with rough hairs on top of the blade and velvety white hairs underneath.

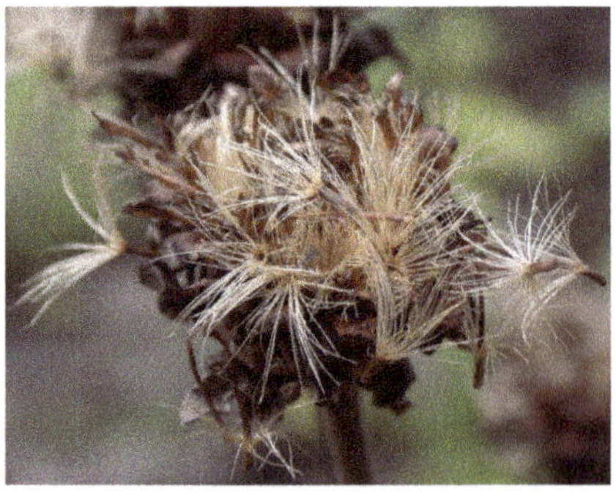

Elecampane seeds

Bright, sunny-yellow flowers resemble small sunflowers and appear on top of the stalks, either sitting alone or in loose panicle clusters. The large calyx consists of many overlapping ovate and pointed sepals. Elecampane has the typical *Compositae* flower head composed of many narrow yellow ray petals surrounding a golden-yellow center of many tightly compacted disc flowers. The flower heads can reach a diameter up to 4″ and bloom from June to September on plants that are at least 2 years old. The disc flowers mature into many brown, rectangular-shaped achene seeds, each attached to a tuft of hairs that carries it in the wind.

Cultivation

Elecampane is a beautiful and cheerful-looking plant, making it a welcome addition to gardens. As a hardy plant, it tolerates a range of soil conditions, but does best in moist, well-drained, fairly rich clay loam. Although it grows in sun or shade, plants thrive best in full sun. It is very easy to grow and may be germinated from seed or more easily propagated by root division.

Seeds can be planted in a greenhouse or by a sunny window in early spring 6-7 weeks before the last frost, or they can be directly planted in a prepared garden bed in mid-spring. They are light-dependent germinators, so plant seeds on the soil surface and press them down into the dirt, barely covering them. Keep seeds moist. Germination usually takes 2-3 weeks.

For root divisions, dig up the dormant roots in early spring or late autumn. The root crowns are bulbous and grow buds that eventually sprout into stems and foliage. Divide the crowns, making sure that they each contain a bud, and plant them with the buds pointing upward, ½″ below the soil surface and spaced 2′ apart. Each crown will develop into a large plant.

Harvest

Harvest roots in autumn from plants that are 2-4 years old. Older roots tend to become woody and pithy. Autumn is the best harvest time because plants contain the highest concentrations of inulin, an important medicinal phytochemical. When harvesting, remember to replant some of the bulbous roots with buds attached in order to propagate new plants.

Many years ago, before I knew about propagating by root division, I was harvesting a large Elecampane plant and noticed all the robust buds growing on the bulbous rhizome. Sensing the plant's rather obvious invitation to take advantage of its life-giving buds, I used a hatchet to separate several of the bulbs with attached buds and planted them, thinking that this could be a way to propagate new plants. The remainder of the root was made into tincture. The following year, about 20 new plants appeared from the buds of the original "mother plant." I will always be grateful to Elecampane for teaching me about root division, and since that experience, I often use this propagation method when harvesting roots.

Preparation of Plant Medicine and Dosages

Freshly harvested roots can be processed into a decoction tea, tincture, or syrup for internal use, prepared as a salve for external application, or dried for future needs. The plant yields its medicinal properties to both alcohol and water. As with many herbs, the freshly harvested roots are best to use for medicinal purposes because dried roots lose their potency over time. If you choose to dry the roots, slice them into thin pieces, spread them out on a screen, and keep them shaded and well-ventilated till dry.

PREPARATIONS

Decoction Tea: Use ½-2 teaspoons of dried or fresh root per cup of water. Simmer very gently in a covered pan for 10 minutes and cool. Dosage: 1-2 cups per day as needed. The root is bitter-tasting.

Tincture: Macerate fresh roots in a mix of 60% 190-proof grain alcohol and 40% distilled water. To extract more inulin (a medicinal water-soluble polysaccharide), add more water by using 50% grain alcohol with 50% water. Dosage: ½-1 teaspoon 3-4 times a day as needed.

Syrup: The root can be slowly boiled down to a thick decoction tea by leaving the lid off the pan to allow gradual evaporation of the water. The tea is preserved with sugar or honey. To make syrup for coughs, sore throats and digestive problems, it is most effective to use Elecampane in combination with other appropriate herbs. Dosage: 1-2 tablespoons every 2-3 hours as needed.

Salve: Chop roots into small pieces, cover with olive oil, and bake at 200°F for 2-3 hours.

For other herbs to add to syrup and salve, refer to "Index of Health Issues and Herbal Recommendations" and review "Cough and Bronchial Problems," "Digestive System," and "Skin Problems."

Chemical Constituents

Several volatile oils in the root are important medicinal phytochemicals, most notably the sesquiterpene lactones that include alantolactone, isoalantolactone and isocostunolide, which are all anticarcinogenic. Alantolactone and isoalantolactone are antioxidant, anti-inflammatory, immunostimulating, and powerful antimicrobials against parasites, amoebae, bacteria, and fungi. They are specific against the tuberculosis bacteria (Cantrell, 1999). Alantolactone is also a diuretic, expectorant, hypotensive, and cholagogue (supports liver and gallbladder health and the production and flow of bile). Other volatile oils include alantic acid and azulene (anti-allergic, antibacterial, antihistamine, anti-inflammatory, antispasmodic, anti-ulcer, febrifuge, hepatoregenerative). Beta-sitosterol and stigmasterol are androgenic, antibacterial, anticancer, antioxidant, antitumor, antiviral, febrifuge, and hepatoprotective. The root also contains 11-44% inulin, which supports immunity and beneficial bacteria in the intestines.

Safety, Contraindications, and Drug Interactions

Elecampane is safe when taken in normal doses. Excessively large amounts can be over-stimulating and induce vomiting, diarrhea, cramps, and spasms. The roots are **contraindicated during pregnancy** because they are too stimulating to the uterus and may promote menstruation. They are too strong for infants and are contraindicated during lactation. Direct physical contact with the plant may cause temporary allergic skin reactions such as hives in some sensitive people (Blumenthal, 1998; Brinker, 2001). These rashes are quickly neutralized by 2-3 applications of rubbing alcohol on the affected area soon after physical contact with the plant.

Medicinal Uses

History of the Plant

Elecampane has been a popular medicinal herb throughout Asia and Europe for many centuries. In Traditional Chinese and Indian Ayurvedic medicine, it continues to be used for respiratory and digestive problems. The Greek physician and botanist Dioscorides (*circa* A.D. 40–*c.* 90) described it in his herbal and wrote that Elecampane promotes urination and menstruation. He used it to treat lung ailments, venomous bites, and stomachaches (Dioscorides, 1959). Pliny the Elder (A.D. 23–79) wrote, "Let no day pass without eating some of the roots of Inula, considered to help digestion and cause mirth [happiness]" (Grieve, 1971). During the Middle Ages in Europe, it was a favorite remedy of common people and herbalists for respiratory ailments, stimulating a sluggish digestive system, and treating parasites, pain, skin wounds, and rashes. English herbalist John Gerard (1545–1612) administered the root for shortness of breath, coughs and thick phlegm, stomach problems, and venomous bites. It was commonly grown in herb gardens, and the root was candied in sugar or prepared as a cordial.

Elecampane is also called scabwort and horseheal because it was a popular veterinary medicine used to heal scabs on sheep and skin infections on horses. The botanical name *helenium* may be derived from the name of Helen of Troy, the Greek heroine. According to one legend, she carried a handful of Elecampane when Paris, the Trojan prince, abducted her from Sparta and initiated the Trojan War. Another legend states that Helen was the first person to use this herb for treating venomous bites.

In the 1600s, British herbalist Nicholas Culpeper wrote, "It is a plant under the domain of Mercury. The fresh roots of Elecampane, preserved with sugar, or made into a syrup or conserve, is very good to warm a cold and windy [gassy] stomach . . . also to help a cough, shortness of breath, and wheezing in the lungs" (Culpeper, 1992). He prescribed this herb for all lung diseases including whooping cough, to strengthen the stomach and improve digestion, for kidney and bladder stones, parasites, cramps, convulsions and gout, and as a poison antidote.

Early American colonists introduced Elecampane into the new world and cultivated it in their gardens to use for medicine. Native American tribes of the northeast incorporated the plant into their herbal pharmacies and often ingested it for bronchial problems. From the late 1800s to the 1930s, the American Eclectic physicians prescribed the root for water retention, chronic respiratory ailments, the common cold, asthma, night sweats, sluggish liver, indigestion with gas and bloating, skin diseases and eruptions, and atonic conditions involving weak muscles. They employed Elecampane as a treatment-of-choice for all problems of excessive phlegm (mucous) discharge, and it was often combined with *Echinacea angustifolia* to treat tuberculosis (Ellingwood, 1919; Felter, 1898). It was once listed in the *U.S. Pharmacopoeia* as an official medical treatment for skin diseases, respiratory problems, and digestive and liver disorders.

Elecampane is currently sold as dried tea, tincture, pills, and capsules. Although extensively used in European and Asian herbalism over many centuries, clinical trials on Elecampane are lacking. Most research has been animal and *in vitro* studies focusing on individual phytochemicals occurring in several *Inula* species, validating many of the herb's historic uses. Alantolactone and isoalantolactone have been investigated for their wide range of activities, especially against cancers and other pathogens.

Healing Qualities

Alterative, analgesic, antibacterial, anti-catarrhal, antifungal, anti-inflammatory, antilithic, antiseptic, antispasmodic, antivenom, antiviral, astringent, bitter tonic, carminative, cholagogue, depurative, diaphoretic, diuretic, emmenagogue, exanthematous, expectorant, febrifuge, hepatic, immunostimulatory, nephritic, pectoral, stimulant, stomachic, vermifuge, and vulnerary.

Traditional Chinese Medicine (TCM) Perspective

Elecampane is a bitter, stimulating, warming, and drying herb. The Chinese species, including *Inula japonica* and *I. britannica,* are known as Xuan Fu Hua. Extracts of *I. britannica* have anti-inflammatory, antibacterial, antihepatitis, and anti-tumor activities that specifically inhibit growth of human leukemia cancer cells (Liu, 2005). *I. britannica* flowers are a rich source of secondary metabolites primarily consisting of terpenoids (sesquiterpene lactones) and flavonoids. These compounds have shown diverse biological effects, including anticancer, antioxidant, anti-inflammatory, neuroprotective, and hepatoprotective actions (Khan, 2010).

Elecampane is a Qi tonic specific for chronic Qi deficiency conditions of diminished energy and activity resulting in the stagnation and accumulation of fluids and mucous throughout the body. It stimulates and restores the downward flow of Qi in the lungs and digestive system, and also removes damp heat specifically in the lungs, digestive tract, kidneys, uterus, and skin. The herb's astringent property helps tighten loose, boggy mucous membranes that secrete excessive phlegm and fluids, and it is decongesting to the lungs and other organs burdened by these excesses. It is specific for Lung Qi deficiency and cold dampness resulting in copious mucous discharge, coughs, wheezing, chronic asthma, or bronchitis. The flower heads and roots are used to dry excess moisture and expel phlegm (Tierra, 1988).

Elecampane tones Digestive Qi, resolves Liver Qi Stagnation, and treats Stomach and Spleen Qi deficiency that causes profuse mucous, diminished appetite, indigestion and malabsorption, loose stools, and fatigue. The herb addresses Uterine Qi Stagnation and damp cold that interferes with normal menstruation and can result in abnormal vaginal discharge, cramps, or premenstrual syndrome (PMS). The herb also resolves Kidney Qi Stagnation that causes fluid retention. It is a beneficial tonic for chronic Qi deficiency conditions leading to weak immunity, frequent infections, chronic fatigue, and underactive organ and endocrine function. In TCM, it is also prescribed to counteract ingested poisons and treat some types of cancer.

Likewise, India's Ayurvedic medical system recognizes Elecampane's ability to strengthen the lungs and reduce excessive amounts of phlegm. It is highly regarded as one of the best lung tonics to treat coughs and is also prescribed for its calming action on the mind, digestive system, and female reproductive organs (Frawley, 1986).

Primary Actions

Elecampane's warmth and stimulation are helpful for chronic conditions caused by diminished energy and weak organs resulting in sluggishness, congestion, and excess mucous. The herb is taken as a tonic over time for these problems. Volatile oils exert vermifuge, antibiotic, and antifungal activity beneficial for treating parasites and infections. As a diaphoretic, Elecampane induces perspiration to reduce fevers. The roots contain substantial amounts of inulin, which stimulates immunity and promotes proliferation of beneficial probiotics in the intestines. The mucilage property of inulin is soothing and cleansing to the tissues, especially the mucous membranes lining the respiratory, digestive, and urinary tracts. Astringent properties of the herb tone these mucous membranes and tissues to help normalize their secretions. Eclectic doctors prescribed Elecampane for all atonic conditions in which tissues and muscles were weak, lacked tone, and leaked fluids.

Elecampane root is specific for the lungs. I have combined it with other pectoral herbs for many years with wonderful results for both acute and chronic respiratory ailments. It is traditionally used in combination with other herbs rather than alone.

Lung and Bronchial Problems: Elecampane stimulates immunity and is helpful for respiratory distress. As one of the best rejuvenating tonics for the lungs, it is especially adept in reducing bronchial congestion. Its warm, drying nature decreases excessive mucous secretions, and as a non-irritating expectorant, it expels phlegm from the lungs. Lung muscles and tissues are strengthened by the plant's tonifying, cleansing, and mild astringent qualities.

The roots are used to reduce mucous congestion, tissue inflammation, and coughs. The antibacterial, antiviral, and antifungal volatile oils are beneficial for treating laryngitis, respiratory tract infections, the common cold, bronchitis, pneumonia, and whooping cough. Eclectic physicians prescribed Elecampane for all chronic lung ailments, including wheezing, asthma, shortness of breath, persistent coughs, sinusitis, and emphysema. Eclectic physician William Cook, M.D., wrote, "The root is stimulating and relaxing, leaving behind a tonic and slightly astringing impression. Its influence is expended chiefly upon the mucous structures of the lungs, but it also acts moderately upon the stomach, uterus, skin, and kidneys. To the lungs it is warming and strengthening, promoting the discharge of viscid mucous, but leaving the surfaces slightly dry. It is a popular remedy in coughs . . . but it is not suitable for cases of any class where the lungs are irritated or dry, as it then increases the dryness, and gives a feeling of constriction" (Cook, 1869).

Around 1885, scientists discovered that alantolactone in Elecampane kills the bacteria causing tuberculosis (Cantrell, 1999), and many herbalists have employed the roots to treat this potentially deadly disease. Beginning in 1886, physicians also prescribed it for diphtheria (Grieve, 1971).

Elecampane is usually blended with other pectorals such as Horehound (*Marrubium vulgare*), Pleurisy Root (*Asclepias tuberosa*), Wild Cherry bark (*Prunus serotina*), Yarrow (*Achillea millefolium*), Echinacea (*Echinacea* spp.), and Holy Basil/Tulsi (*Ocimum sanctum*). **Due to its warming and drying nature, it should not be used alone for dry coughs, but combined with moistening herbs** like Marshmallow (*Althaea officinalis*), Chickweed (*Stellaria media*), or Slippery Elm (*Ulmus rubra*).

Digestive System: Elecampane's bitter properties stimulate the entire digestive system. By strengthening and toning the stomach, pancreas and liver, enzyme secretion is optimized to improve digestion. As a cholagogue, it promotes the formation and flow of bile in the liver while reducing liver and gallbladder sluggishness and congestion that may promote high cholesterol levels and gallstones.

According to TCM, chronic conditions of profuse mucous are caused by weakness and poor function of the stomach, pancreas, and spleen. Elecampane stimulates and strengthens these organs to treat problems of mucous excess at their causal level. It also tones and normalizes mucous membranes lining the entire digestive tract. The inulin mucilage in the roots soothes the lining of the digestive tract, helps maintain a good balance of important bacterial flora in the intestines, promotes regular bowel movements, and cools and heals inflamed tissues, including stomach and intestinal ulcers. Several volatile oils in the roots reduce inflammation and spasms throughout the digestive tract. Elecampane is specific for deficiency conditions that are caused by poor digestion and eventually weaken the immune system. The herb improves sluggish, damp conditions leading to gas, bloating, indigestion, diarrhea, and excess mucous discharge.

Alantolactone and isoalantolactone concentrated in the roots possess strong vermifuge (antiparasite) properties and shown antibacterial and antifungal activity *in vitro* (Newall, 1996). Clinical studies in Europe have successfully demonstrated Elecampane's ability to kill several types of parasites, including roundworms, hookworm, whipworm, threadworm, and giardia (Duke, 2000). *Clonorchis sinensis* is a parasitic liver fluke that feeds on bile and resides in the human liver, common bile duct, and gall bladder. This fluke is considered to be the third most prevalent worm parasite in the world and is endemic to Japan, China, Taiwan, Southeast Asia, and Russia. Recent studies show that it can cause liver and bile duct cancer. Using *in vivo* testing, Chinese researchers investigating the influence of *I. helenium* tea on the structure of *Clonorchis sinensis* worms found that the herb initiated shrinking and destruction of the organs within the parasites (Rhee, 1985). These findings validate the historic use of Elecampane in treating dysentery and other parasitic infestations in the digestive tract.

Animal studies demonstrate how small doses of Elecampane root lower blood sugar levels, while high doses can increase blood sugar levels and lower blood pressure (Duke, 2000). Alcohol extracts of roots from a related species, *I. racemosa,* reduce blood sugar levels and enhance the formation of glycogen (glucose that is stored to provide energy) in the liver without increasing blood levels of insulin in animal studies. Researchers believe that the root may increase insulin sensitivity, which is helpful in diabetes and insulin-resistant conditions (Tripathi, 1995).

Kidneys and Bladder: Antibiotic and diuretic properties of the roots are helpful for urinary tract infections including cystitis, mucous in urine, and fluid retention throughout the body. Elecampane reduces the formation of kidney stones, and its soothing, anti-inflammatory, and antispasmodic effects on tissues throughout the urinary tract ease the painful passage of existing stones.

Women's Health: Elecampane's stimulating, warming, and drying actions also improve sluggish circulation in the pelvis and reduce excessive discharges from the uterus and vagina. The root promotes menstruation and is helpful for delayed and scanty menses, cramps, swollen breasts, and premenstrual syndrome (PMS). It has been used for estrogen and progesterone deficiencies. Eclectic physicians prescribed it for night sweats, mucous discharges from the bladder and vagina, and leucorrhea, a white or yellow vaginal or uterine discharge indicative of Candida yeast, parasites, or other infectious organisms (Felter, 1898).

Antioxidant Protection: The two primary phytochemicals in Elecampane root, alantolactone and isoalantolactone, protect against damaging oxidation to cells via several mechanisms and have demonstrated anticancer and antitumor activities.

Researchers have discovered that extracts of roots from *I. helenium* and related species stimulate Nrf2, a protein that is latent in all cells of the body until it is activated. Once activated, Nrf2 migrates into the cell nucleus and bonds to DNA. This Nrf2 bonding turns on several hundred "survivor genes," enabling cells to survive stressors, including oxidative stress and free radical damage. Nrf2 activation stimulates production of antioxidants and detoxifying enzymes such as glutathione, catalase, and superoxide dismutase (SOD). Alantolactone and isoalantolactone have specifically stimulated Nrf2 accumulation in the nucleus of mice cells, resulting in the activation of these antioxidants (Seo, 2008 & 2009).

Immunity and Cancer: Studies have documented that flowers and roots of several Elecampane species combat some types of cancer. This results from the plant's ability to protect cells from destructive oxidative stress, to stimulate apoptosis (programmed death of cancerous cells), and to potentiate T-lymphocytes and the cytokines and phagocytes they produce that also destroy cancerous cells.

Water-soluble polysaccharides isolated from *I. helenium* rhizomes have been shown to stimulate T-lymphocytes and increase cytokine and phagocytic activity to kill cancerous cells (Danilets, 2010). Alantolactone and isoalantolactone induce apoptosis by normalizing pathways that are frequently deregulated in cancers, allowing replication and proliferation of cancerous cells and tumors (Rasul, 2013). One study revealed that Elecampane interferes with proliferation of squamous cell carcinoma of the head and neck by inducing cell apoptosis (Wu, 2013). *In vitro* tests have documented that alantolactone and isoalantolactone inhibit cell viability and induce apoptosis in human colon cancer cells (Zhang, 2013) and in ovarian, prostate, lung, and leukemia cancer cells (Pal, 2010). Isocostunolide, another sesquiterpene lactone isolated from the roots of *I. helenium*, has effectively induced cytotoxicity (cell death) in human melanoma cells by apoptosis (Chen, 2007).

Researchers at the Memorial Sloan-Kettering Cancer Center in New York City discovered that extracts of Elecampane root demonstrated significant ability to destroy tumors. The herb caused mitochondria (the energy source of cells) in tumor cells to swell and rupture, which killed cancerous cells. The research team recommended further investigation to test the herb as a safe and effective treatment for cancer (Dorn, 2006).

Skin Diseases and Poison Antidote: Elecampane is beneficial for many skin diseases and toxic conditions due to its antimicrobial and antioxidant properties, and its stimulating and normalizing influence on the liver and kidneys. Chronic skin ailments and slow-healing wounds can be caused by diminished activity of the liver and kidneys, resulting in toxic build-up. These toxins are then released through the skin rather than the normal routes of elimination. Elecampane may be applied externally as a salve or wash of the tea to treat skin problems, and should also be taken internally to address the underlying problems of infection and toxicity affecting the skin.

Volatile oils in the herb are antiseptic against bacterial and fungal infections. The roots are externally applied for skin diseases, itching, rashes, animal and insect bites and stings, dermatitis, eczema, herpes lesions, skin ulcers, and scabies. The volatile oils are also analgesic, anti-inflammatory and antispasmodic, and help relieve pain from nerve inflammation, including sciatica, nerve injuries, gout, arthritis, and wounds.

The sesquiterpene lactones (alantolactone, isoalantolactone, and diplophyllin) in the roots show significant activity against staph infections (Blagojevic, 2012). Elecampane root extracts have demonstrated moderate antimicrobial activity against *Staphylococcus aureus* (causes food poisoning, respiratory infections, impetigo, and other skin infections), *Enterococcus faecalis* (infects the digestive system), *Escherischia coli* (normally occurs in the colon but can cause food poisoning), *Pseudomonas aeruginosa* (typically infects the lungs to cause pneumonia, infects the urinary tract, skin wounds and burns, and causes septic blood infections), and *Candida albicans* (Stojakowska, 2005). *In vitro* tests provide evidence that *I. helenium* root was 100% effective against 200 clinically significant *Staphylococcus aureus* strains, including MRSA (methicillin-resistant *S. aureus*), which is resistant to antibiotics. An extract of *I. viscosa* flowers showed similar results (O'Shea, 2009; Qiu, 2011).

Teachings from the Elecampane Deva

"Greetings, dear one. I am the Elecampane Deva, a being of light, sunshine, and balance. My plants are strong in the air and earth elements, and my medicine offering is a balance of these two forces. I am under the domain of the astrological air sign Gemini and my ruling planet is Mercury. My stimulating air element allows swift, free-flowing movement through the body, just as Mercury, the Roman god adorned with winged shoes and helmet, traveled quickly as a messenger between people and the gods.

"Gemini is the sign of the male and female twins. These polarities may be in conflict, but with Gemini's wisdom and healing, these opposites merge into peaceful balance. And so the feminine earth element and masculine air element blend together in the essence of my plants. This is part of the gift I offer.

"My robust plants laden with stout stems, massive leaves, hefty flowers, and abundant roots reflect the strength and boldness of my good medicine and feminine earth qualities. The yellow flowers point to my affinity with the solar plexus and digestive organs. My roots contribute to the transformation of food into energy and the substances necessary for vibrant cell and tissue growth in the physical body. In this way, I nurture the earth aspect of human bodies.

"The qualities of my powerful masculine air element are reflected in my tall stalks reaching up to the sky and in the ability of my roots to bring health and spaciousness to the lungs and air sinuses in the head. By purging infection and excess mucous, airways are opened and I mediate ease of movement and flow of air with life-giving oxygen through the lungs and blood. My plants also assist in releasing unnecessary gases from the body.

"I assist in the natural flow of air, the eternal waxing and waning of the in-breath and out-breath that carries the life force running through your veins. Know that the breath is sacred. Upon the first breath of the newborn infant, the soul and life force are 'locked' within the physical body. And following the final breath at the time of death, the life force is released as the physical body expires and is put to rest. With each breath you take, realize and honor this mighty power sustaining your life. And remember how people, animals, and plants share this breath of life with all living creatures on the planet. For animals and plants also breathe gases in and out and depend upon each other to maintain balance. And so I live and move upon the spacious nature of this breath of life.

"My essence draws together the air and earth elements and balances their male and female polarities. Thus, their energies dance together, blending into harmonious expressions of the wholeness and oneness of life. Use me when this balance is lost, when extreme disturbing thoughts and feelings are in conflict, obscuring the calmness of equanimity. I will assist in bringing you ease of movement and the quiet peace of contentment."

Feverfew

Tanacetum parthenium
Compositae (Asteraceae) (Sunflower or Aster) Family

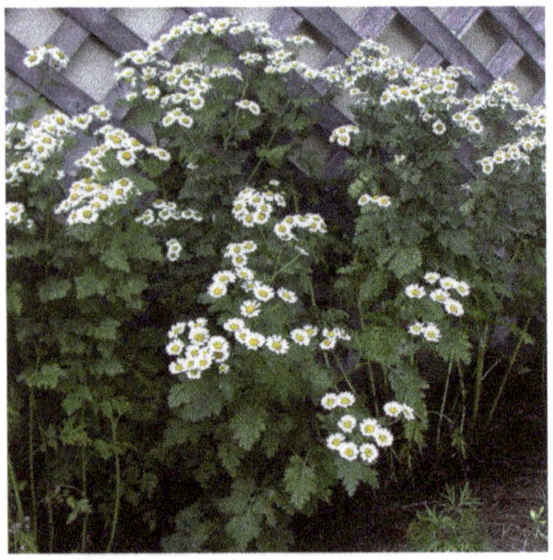

Botanical Names

Feverfew has been placed into five different genera over time, reflecting confusion as to which genus the plant truly belongs. Former botanical names include *Chrysanthemum parthenium, Pyrethrum parthenium, Leucanthemum parthenium,* and *Matricaria parthenium*.

Common Names

Febrifuge plant, featherfoil, featherfew, bride's buttons, bachelor's buttons, and wild quinine are antiquated names for this herb.

Medicinal Part of the Plant

Most commercial Feverfew preparations contain only the leaves, and scientific research has predominately focused on chemicals in the leaves. However, studies show that the flowers contain the greatest concentrations of medicinal parthenolides (Majdi, 2011). I always use both leaves and flower heads in tincture preparations with good results for migraine and inflammatory relief.

Range and Habitat

Feverfew is native to central and southern Europe and western Asia. It has naturalized in many temperate and some tropical zones throughout the world, including North and South America. In the United States, it is occasionally found in the wild but is more commonly cultivated in gardens. It thrives in dry or moist soil with low to moderate fertility.

Description of the Plant

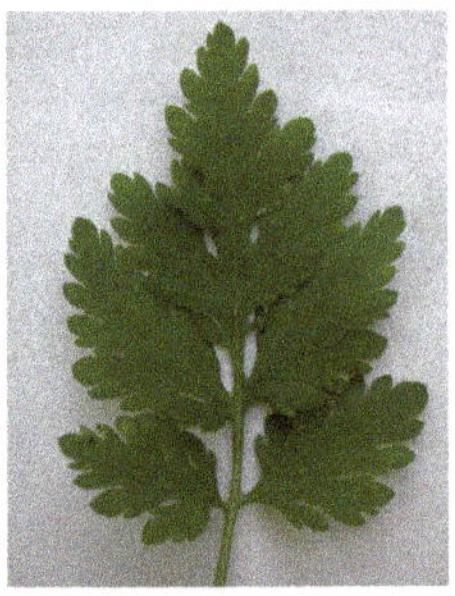

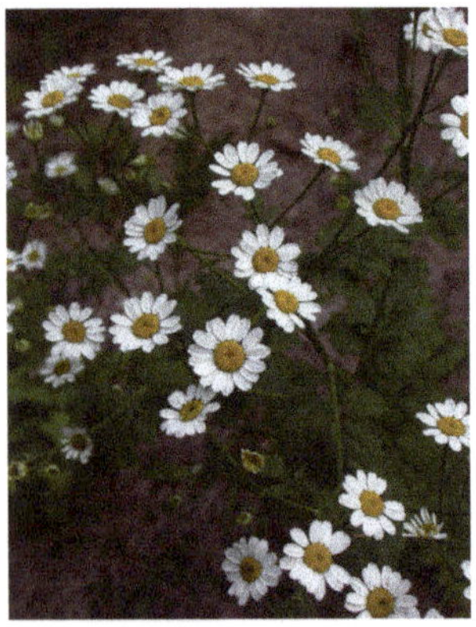

Feverfew is an aromatic perennial that grows into a bushy plant reaching 1½-3′ in height. The cheerful flowers are an attractive addition to any garden. The main root is a hard, woody, cream-colored rhizome that creeps horizontally through the soil. A thickly woven mass of white, thready, fibrous rootlets grows along the entire surface of the rhizome. Several erect, hollow, rounded, and finely furrowed stalks emerge from the root and branch out from the upper half of the plant. Petiole leaves climb the entire length of the stems in an alternating pattern. The green to yellowish-green compound leaves are bipinnate with deeply incised lobes. The coarsely toothed margins are serrate with rounded tips. The compound leaf and leaflets have an oval shape, and although they feel smooth, they are actually covered with a white down visible with a 16x magnifying glass. Leaves grow 1-4″ long. Flowers bloom on the ends of the branching stalks from June through October. Each flower is ½-1″ in diameter and looks like a miniature daisy with a center of many tightly packed yellow disc florets surrounded by 16-20 white ray petals. Flowers sit atop long stems and are arranged in loose corymb clusters. As flowers mature, the white petals fall away, leaving the central disc that develops into oblong seeds. The seeds are extremely viable and readily self-sow to germinate the following spring.

There are several cultivars of Feverfew. Some display completely yellow flowers and others are double-petaled. The herb's strong aromatic odor and presence of pyrethrin, an insecticide, repel bees and other insects.

Cultivation

Feverfew is a lovely plant to adorn gardens and cheer up gardeners, and it is exceptionally easy to grow since the seeds germinate so readily. It is rather drought-resistant and tolerates a wide variety of soils and partial shade, but grows best in well-drained, fertile soil in full sun. Feverfew may be propagated by seed, root division, or from cuttings taken from young shoots growing from the base of mature plants. Growing by seed is the easiest method.

Plant seeds in the garden or greenhouse in spring. They are light-dependent germinators, meaning that they need light to germinate, so press them into the soil rather than covering them. Keep soil moist and they should germinate within 10-15 days when the soil temperature is at least 70°F. When seedlings are 3-4″ tall, transplant or thin them 1′ apart. Once established, Feverfew prolifically self-sows and can quickly multiply into a large patch within a few years.

Harvest

Collect flower buds and upper leaves just as the buds start to open into flowers. The medicinal properties are at peak concentration during this time. Prune the tops of plants while leaving enough lower leaves to keep the herb alive. After the flowers are harvested, older plants will produce more flowers and can often be harvested twice during a growing season.

Preparation of Plant Medicine and Dosages

Most commercial Feverfew preparations consist of air-dried or freeze-dried leaves, and this is the form that has been used in most research studies. However, like most herbs, prolonged storage of dried Feverfew leaf leads to substantial loss of biological activity. The medicinal parthenolide content in dried plants was found to be reduced by 35% after nine months (Heptinstall, 1992). Herbal authority Dennis Awang has found parthenolide to be "extremely unstable when the herb material is dried" (Blumenthal, 1997).

As the flowers also contain medicinal constituents, I prefer a tincture made from fresh leaves and flower heads. Tinctures do not deteriorate and retain their high level of potency for many years. Herbalist Joseph Meyer (1878–1950) and Eclectic physician Harvey Felter, M.D. (1865–1927) wrote that although Feverfew imparts its virtues to boiling water, alcohol is the best extractor, and many herbalists prefer using the tincture extract.

Using the freshly harvested plant is very important for high potency and is an incentive for migraine sufferers to grow their own Feverfew. Several of my friends and clients have reported more benefit from tincture preparations made from the freshly harvested plant than from dried preparations.

PREPARATIONS

Tincture: Chop leaves and flower heads into small pieces, stuff them into a glass jar, and cover with a blend of 60% 190-proof grain alcohol and 40% distilled water. Dosage: 30-80 drops in water 3-4 times a day as needed.

Infusion Tea: Steep 2-3 teaspoons of fresh or dried leaves and flower heads in 1 cup of boiled water. Dosage: 1-2 cups a day as needed. The tea tastes very bitter. The weight of 2-3 medium sized fresh leaves is equal to about 60 mg (milligrams) of the dried herb.

Chewing on the Fresh Leaf: People with access to live plants can eat 1-3 fresh leaves daily as a migraine preventative. However, be aware that the bitter leaves can cause irritation or mouth sores in some people. Ingesting Feverfew tincture, capsules, or pills does not create this problem.

Capsules and Pills: Make these at home with dried plant material, or the freeze-dried leaf may be purchased. Dosage: Although 125 mg of Feverfew per day is the typical recommended dose based on clinical trials, many manufacturers make pills containing 300-380 mg. The Canadian Health and Welfare Department has recommended that Feverfew preparations contain at least 0.2% parthenolide, and this has become the standardized amount, although the actual content has been found to be extremely variable among different commercial preparations. This is partly due to the different times of year and day in which people harvest the herb, length of storage time, and method of preparation. Be sure your Feverfew capsules or pills are fresh (if this is possible), or better yet, use the tincture.

Chemical Constituents

More than 30 sesquiterpene lactones have been identified in Feverfew leaves and flowers, but parthenolide is the one thought to be primarily responsible for reducing the pain and inflammation of migraines and arthritis. Parthenolide constitutes about 84% of the total sesquiterpenes, and although researchers and manufacturers focus almost exclusively on this component, it is usually the combination and synergistic action of all the phytochemicals in a plant that creates therapeutic effects. Studies show that parthenolide decreases the body's release of inflammatory blood components and is antiprostaglandin, anti-arthritic, antispasmodic, antibacterial, and anti-neuralgia (reduces nerve pain). Parthenolide deters the process leading to abnormal blood clotting and tones vascular smooth muscle (the muscle within blood vessels).

The flowers and leaves contain antibacterial volatile oils that are monoterpene and sesquiterpene components, including camphor, borneol, and linalool. Flavonoids include kaempferol, quercetin, apigenin, and luteolin. Tanetin is a flavonol that inhibits the generation of inflammatory prostaglandins and leukotrienes (Williams, 1995). The flowers contain cosmosin (aldose-reductase inhibitor, antibacterial, and candidicide) and santamarin (anti-inflammatory, antispasmodic). Researchers have isolated small amounts of melatonin (2.45 micrograms per 1 gram of the herb) from fresh Feverfew leaves (Murch, 1997) and in alcohol extracts of the flowers (Ansari, 2010). In the human body, melatonin is produced from serotonin (a calming inhibitory neurotransmitter) and secreted by the pineal gland. Melatonin induces sleep, regulates circadian rhythms, helps relieve chronic pain, and eases neurological disorders such as migraine.

Vitamins and minerals include thiamine (vitamin B1), riboflavin (B2), niacin (B3), ascorbic acid (vitamin C), beta-carotene (Vitamin A), calcium, magnesium, chromium, iron, phosphorus, potassium, and selenium.

Safety, Contraindications, and Drug Interactions

There have been no reports of toxicity or serious problems caused by extended use of Feverfew. Some people may experience diarrhea, nausea, vomiting or gas, but this usually disappears after the first week of use. People with blood clotting disorders taking anticoagulant drugs should use this herb cautiously, because its ability to reduce blood clotting may potentiate effects of these drugs. Allergic reactions have been reported. About 18% of people who have chewed the leaves report mouth sores, inflammation, or ulceration of the mouth and tongue, but these symptoms disappear when it is discontinued. In order to avoid the possibility of oral inflammation, the herb can be ingested in pills, capsules, or as tincture.

Pregnant women should avoid Feverfew due to its stimulating abortifacient action on the uterus that could trigger a miscarriage. Children older than 3 years of age may safely take the herb (Brinker, 2001; McGuffin, 1997). For pediatric doses refer to the chapter "How to Calculate Dosages" on page 148.

Medicinal Uses

History of the Plant

Feverfew has a fine reputation and long history of folk use for treating severe headaches, fevers, arthritis, menstrual irregularities, and other painful, inflammatory conditions. It has been cultivated in Europe as a medicinal and ornamental garden herb for hundreds of years. The Greek physician Dioscorides (*circa* A.D. 40–*c.* 90) prescribed it for fevers, stomach ailments, menstrual problems, asthma, headaches, inflammation, and to "drive out phlegm." Galen (*c.* A.D. 131–*c.* 200), another Greek physician, found it beneficial for women's ailments, delayed menses, to expel the placenta after childbirth, for phlegm in lungs, vertigo, and ague (an old term for malaria). Feverfew was commonly used for headaches during the 1600s and is mentioned in Gerard's 1633 *Herball* for this purpose. The English herbalist Nicholas Culpeper (1616–1654) prescribed it for colds and lung congestion. He called it "a general strengthener of wombs" and wrote that it is "effective for all pains in the head" (Culpeper, 1787).

The genus name *Tanacetum* comes from an altered form of *anthansis* (*athanatos*), meaning "immortal," and refers to the everlasting nature of the dried flowers. The species name *parthenium* is derived from the Greek word *parthenos,* meaning "virgin," and refers to its traditional use by women to relieve menstrual cramps. The burning taste of the root explains why it is classified by some sources as *pyrethrum*, derived from the Greek word *pyro,* meaning "fire." The common name of Feverfew came from the Latin word *febrifuga*, referring to the plant's traditional role in lowering fevers. Some sources claim that it was called featherfoil because of its feathery leaves, and featherfoil became known as featherfew, and eventually feverfew.

European immigrants introduced the plant into North and South America, where it became widely cultivated and continues to be used medicinally. Feverfew is a popular medicine of herbal healers and shamans in Central and South American countries. Several years ago, when visiting Ecuador with a group of herbalists, I saw Feverfew for sale in the outdoor markets. Several shamans we encountered told us about their long traditional use of the herb in their healing ceremonies. It was one of several herbs that they tied into a bundle, dipped in a bowl of water, and rubbed over a person's body for cleansing. This ritual was performed at the beginning of every shamanic healing we attended.

During the colonization of North America, Feverfew was used by early settlers to heal fevers and accompanying chills and pain. Historically, the plant has also been administered to treat upset stomachs, intestinal parasites, earaches, to induce abortion, and as a garden insecticide. During the late 1800s, American Eclectic physicians primarily prescribed it for delayed menstruation, menstrual cramping, premenstrual syndrome (PMS), and to address the emotional ups-and-downs of the hormonal cycle known as "female hysteria" during this period. In *King's American Dispensatory*, Harvey Felter, M.D., wrote that it "is an excellent remedy in recent colds, flatulency, worms, atonic dyspepsia [sluggish indigestion and bloating], nervous debility, suppression of the urine, and in some febrile [feverish] diseases" (Felter, 1898).

As pharmaceutical drugs replaced herbal preparations, Feverfew fell from popular use for many years. During the 1970s, however, media reports called attention to European research demonstrating the herb's ability to relieve migraine headaches. Since then, its popularity and commercial sales have continued to grow. Researchers have focused almost exclusively on the activities of parthenolide and have discovered several mechanisms of the herb's actions in reducing inflammation and relieving migraines.

Healing Qualities

Abortifacient, analgesic, antibacterial, antifungal, anti-inflammatory, antiseptic, antispasmodic, blood-thinner, carminative, diaphoretic, emmenagogue, febrifuge, laxative, vasodilator, vermifuge, and vulnerary.

Traditional Chinese Medicine (TCM) Perspective

Feverfew is a cooling, drying, bitter herb that specifically treats hot, inflammatory conditions. It promotes the smooth flow of Qi and reduces blood stagnation, especially in the head, joints, and uterus. This herb reduces Uterine Qi Stagnation that evolves into scanty or delayed periods with clots, cramps, and difficult flow. It also resolves damp mucous and phlegm that causes nasal and lung congestion.

Primary Actions

First and foremost, Feverfew is an anti-inflammatory par excellence. Most specific for preventing and alleviating migraines, the herb normalizes the muscle tone of blood vessels to correct conditions of unequal circulation, which causes a deficient or excessive blood flow. Thus, Feverfew promotes optimal circulation, breaks up areas of stagnant blood, and reduces inflammation that produces pain, especially in the head and uterus. Its antibacterial properties fight infections, and current research has discovered the herb's beneficial influence on several mechanisms offering protection against various cancers. For many years in my nursing practice, I have recommended Feverfew tincture prepared from the upper leaves and flower heads for treating migraines and inflammation throughout the body.

Anti-Inflammatory Activity: Feverfew diminishes inflammation and pain in the head, stomach, intestines, joints, uterus, lungs, and nasal sinuses. Most of the anti-inflammatory research has focused on parthenolide, the primary phytochemical that inhibits chemical pathways initiating the inflammatory process (Kwok, 2001). Parthenolide interferes with the production of prostaglandins, a family of chemicals causing inflammation, and extracts of both flowers and leaves are more effective in reducing prostaglandins than leaf extracts alone (Collier, 1980). Studies have shown that tanetin, a lipophilic flavonoid found in the leaves, flowers and seeds of Feverfew, also blocks prostaglandin synthesis. Alcohol extracts (tinctures) have stronger, more effective anti-inflammatory actions than water or tea extracts (Gupta, 2011; Sumner, 1992).

Migraine Headaches: Feverfew is recommended for migraine prevention and treatment. It is especially indicated for migraine sufferers who hold excessive heat and inflammation in their body. Several clinical studies confirm Feverfew's effectiveness for migraine headaches. In 1983, the British medical journal *Mims Magazine* reported on a clinical study involving 300 people with chronic migraines who had been taking Feverfew for 2.5 years. Positive results were validated by 70% of the people, who claimed that eating 1-3 Feverfew leaves daily significantly decreased the intensity and frequency of their headaches (Johnson, 1983). A small double-blind study at the London Migraine Clinic involved 17 chronic migraine sufferers who had been using Feverfew leaves (about 60 mg daily) for at least 3 months prior to the study. This trial investigated the effects of Feverfew deprivation by giving 9 people placebos rather than their usual doses of Feverfew. Those people reported an increase in the severity and frequency of headaches, nausea, and vomiting. Those who continued taking 60 mg of the freeze-dried leaf in capsules on a daily basis maintained improvement of their migraine symptoms (Johnson, 1985).

In another study, researchers at the University Hospital in Nottingham, England, reported improvement of migraine symptoms in 70% of patients taking daily capsules of freeze-dried Feverfew leaves. The daily dose was about 82 mg of Feverfew containing 0.66% parthenolide. This study consisted of 72 adults who had suffered at least one migraine a month during the previous 2 years. The study lasted for 8 months, and treatment with the herb was clearly associated with a reduction in the frequency and severity of migraine headaches (Murphy, 1988). Outcomes of a clinical trial in 2005 involving 215 patients with recurring migraines again substantiated significant reduction in headaches when using Feverfew compared to a placebo (Diener, 2005). To assess the effectiveness of Feverfew as a prophylactic therapy for migraine, a 4-month trial was conducted with 57 people who attended an outpatient pain clinic. Patients were divided into two groups that were both treated with Feverfew for 2 months. During the third and fourth month, placebo treatment was introduced. Results showed that those taking Feverfew experienced a significant reduction in pain intensity, vomiting, nausea, and sensitivity to noise and light. Transferring the Feverfew-treated group to the placebo treatment resulted in increased pain and other migraine symptoms (Palevitch, 1997).

Migraines occur when blood vessels in the brain constrict temporarily, resulting in reduced blood flow and oxygen to the brain. In response, the blood vessels eventually dilate, and when they expand, they become inflamed, throb, and can cause pounding pain. Although the exact causes of migraines are not clearly understood, they are considered to be a chronic neurovascular disorder involving unstable blood vessels, inflammation, and increased excitability in nerve tissues of the brain. Current explanations for the development of migraines include substandard levels of serotonin, blood vessel constriction and spasms, abnormal activity of blood platelets and their sudden release of large amounts of serotonin, and excessive production of inflammatory substances.

Serotonin is a primary relaxing neurotransmitter that calms the nervous system, reduces anxiety, and promotes sleep and a peaceful mood. Clinical research shows a positive correlation between low serotonin levels and migraine attacks. With the use of neurotransmitter testing, I have found several of my migraine clients to be low in serotonin. Serotonin relaxes and decreases contractions of smooth muscle, which is the type of muscle found in all the blood vessels, organs and glands, as opposed to cardiac muscle found in the heart and skeletal muscle that connects the bones. When a person has chronically low serotonin levels, anxiety develops, the tone of smooth muscles throughout the body tends to constrict, and blood vessels narrow. This can lead to a chronic state of vascular tension and reduced blood flow.

Blood platelets, typically involved in clotting, are believed to be primary triggers of migraine headaches. When blood vessels are broken and hemorrhaging, platelets release serotonin, which under these circumstances, constricts blood vessels to stop bleeding. During a migraine attack, platelets tend to aggregate in the vessels, restrict blood flow, and release large amounts of serotonin that create pain. When vessels eventually relax and dilate, allowing increased blood flow, migraine pain and pressure can be intense.

Feverfew has shown remarkable ability to stop blood platelets from clumping and forming blood clots that can lead to strokes, heart attacks, thrombophlebitis, and other health risks (Loesche, 1988). Parthenolide in the leaves and flowers promotes vascular stability by decreasing inflammation and spasms in blood vessels. Parthenolide inhibits the release of serotonin from blood platelets and reduces levels of other vasoconstrictors like epinephrine and prostaglandins (Murphy, 1988; Groenewegen, 1990). Researchers have found that only fresh leaf extracts, as compared with dried leaves, inhibit the constricting effects on smooth muscle and blood vessels, probably due to higher a concentration of parthenolide (Barsby, 1993). Parthenolide inhibits the release of inflammatory leukotrienes and thromboxanes that constrict blood vessels, induce platelet aggregation, and form blood clots. Parthenolide also inhibits histamine release, which can trigger migraines by stimulating inflammation and vascular spasms in the head (Hayes, 1987; Heptinstall, 1985; Makheja, 1981 & 1982).

Like all migraine treatments, Feverfew works well for some people, but not for everyone. The inconsistency of parthenolide content in Feverfew preparations, with some commercial products containing none at all, is an important factor and another good reason to grow your own plants for medicine!

To prevent migraines
take 30 drops of tincture or 125 mg of dried leaf daily.

To treat migraines
take 60-80 drops of tincture or 300-400 mg dried leaf every 15–30 minutes up to 6 times, or until the migraine is under control.

People with chronically recurring migraines frequently report that Feverfew is helpful when they continue using small amounts each day. I have given the tincture to many people, and about 70% who use it consistently say that it noticeably decreases the incidence and pain of their migraines. To prevent migraines, taking 30 drops of tincture in water or 125 mg of dried leaf daily generally works well. At the onset of a migraine, larger doses of 60-80 drops of tincture or 300-400 mg of dried leaf may be repeated every 15-30 minutes up to 6 times, or until the migraine is under control. I like to blend Feverfew with Lavender tincture (90% Feverfew with 10% Lavender) to produce a fragrant and synergistic remedy.

Feverfew's anti-inflammatory, antispasmodic, analgesic, and blood-thinning properties are also helpful to relieve regular headaches not classified as migraines. To treat headaches, follow the same instructions given for the onset of a migraine.

To heal the underlying causes of all headaches, consider the importance of addressing diet and lifestyle factors. Nutritional deficiencies, food allergies (especially to chemicals in foods and gluten and dairy products), stress, hormonal changes, and chemical exposure can be issues that need to be explored. For clients suffering from chronic headaches, I always recommend the vitamin B complex (25 mg twice daily) and magnesium bis-glycinate (the most absorbable and fastest-acting form of magnesium) at a dose of 200-300 mg twice daily. Magnesium is an effective nerve and muscle relaxant that helps stabilize blood vessel tone. Since neurotransmitter imbalance is a common factor, I encourage migraine sufferers to get their serotonin levels checked and often recommend a supplement.

Allergies: Feverfew can be a helpful remedy for allergies due to its ability to inhibit the release of histamine, a substance causing inflammation and allergic reactions. Naturopathic herbalist John Bastyr taught that Feverfew is a tonic to the mucous membranes and helps normalize their secretion of fluids and mucous (Mitchell, 2003). It works well combined with Stinging Nettle (*Urtica dioica*), another antihistamine plant, and 500 mg of the anti-inflammatory bioflavonoid quercetin, which can be taken twice daily.

Arthritis: Feverfew's historic use for treating arthritis has been validated by current research. Inflammatory substances called polymorphonuclear leukocytes (PMNs) are released by white blood cells and blood platelets to cause pain, inflammation, and cellular damage in joints. Studies have shown that Feverfew inhibits the release of PMNs in joints and skin to reduce pain and inflammation (O'Neal, 1987).

Researchers have found that Feverfew has similar analgesic and anti-inflammatory properties as non-steroidal anti-inflammatory drugs (NSAIDs), such as aspirin and Motrin, without the potential side effects. NSAIDs are conventional remedies for migraines and arthritis that inhibit inflammatory prostaglandin and thromboxane synthesis. Parthenolide in Feverfew reduces secretion of leukocytes (white blood cells) necessary for the production of prostaglandins, thromboxane and leukotrienes, all involved in the painful and damaging inflammatory process. The herb also inhibits release of harmful levels of arachidonic acid that stimulate inflammation (Capasso, 1986; Makheja, 1981 & 1982; Hepinstall, 1985). Unlike aspirin and other NSAIDs, Feverfew does not irritate the stomach or suppress the immune system.

Synovial fluid is the viscous fluid in joint cavities that reduces friction between the cartilage during movement. Upon examination using *in vitro* methods, researchers found that crude Feverfew extracts and purified parthenolide significantly reduced inflammation in the synovial fluid of joints by inhibiting cytokines, including interleukin (up to 95% suppression) and tumor necrosis factor (up to 93% suppression) (Piela-Smith, 2001).

Cyclooxygenase-2 (Cox-2) is an enzyme that promotes inflammation during the body's natural response to injury, and promotes many inflammatory diseases. Laboratory tests show that Feverfew's ability to inhibit Cox-2 is another way it reduces inflammation and arthritic symptoms (Lavalle, 2001). The therapeutic benefits of Feverfew may require daily usage for 1-3 months before full symptomatic relief is experienced. In addition, dietary changes eliminating acidic and inflammatory foods (citrus, tomato, sugar, red meat, coffee, alcohol, soda, dairy, and gluten) are usually required when addressing underlying causes of arthritis.

Fevers, Infections, and the Common Cold: As indicated by its name, Feverfew has historically been used to treat fevers. As a diaphoretic, it promotes perspiration to reduce fevers. *In vitro* research validates the herb's historic use for treating colds and infections. In these studies, parthenolide inhibited the growth of Gram-positive bacteria, yeast, and filamentous fungi (Blakeman, 1979; Chavez, 1999). This powerful phytochemical also inhibited *Mycobacterium tuberculosis* (causing tuberculosis) and *Mycobacterium avium* (a bacteria damaging to the digestive tract and lungs) (Tiuman, 2005).

A hot tea or tincture of the leaves and flowers is excellent for colds, coughs, wheezing, and any difficulty breathing. Similar to aspirin in its mechanism of action, the herb's analgesic properties diminish pain. For colds, fevers, and other infections, I combine Feverfew with other antimicrobial herbs such as Echinacea, Sage (*Salvia officinalis*), Yarrow (*Achillea millefolium*), and Boneset (*Eupatorium perfoliatum*).

The Digestive System: As a bitter tonic and mild laxative, Feverfew stimulates and improves digestion. It is specific for a slow, sluggish system and nervous debility resulting in indigestion, gas, or constipation. It stimulates the liver and increases bile flow, promotes secretion of digestive enzymes, and improves a poor appetite. Antispasmodic properties relax smooth muscles in the stomach and intestines, making it an effective treatment for abdominal cramps, colic, pain, and inflammatory, ulcerative bowel conditions. Studies have demonstrated that administration of parthenolide significantly reduced inflammation in mice with induced ulcerative colitis (Zhao, 2012).

Feverfew kills parasites and works most effectively when combined with other vermifuge herbs such as Wormwood (*Artemisia absinthium*), Black Walnut hulls (*Juglans nigra*), and Cloves (*Syzygium aromaticus*). *In vitro* studies showed that a water and alcohol extract of Feverfew inhibited the growth of *Leishmania amazonesis*, a parasite transferred by the bite of the sand fly (Tiuman, 2005).

Women's Health: Feverfew is strengthening and normalizing to the uterus. The herb regulates blood flow through the pelvic area, and its anti-inflammatory properties are a remedy for menstrual and uterine problems, including premenstrual syndrome (PMS). As an emmenagogue, it promotes menstruation and is specific for scanty, sluggish, or delayed menses caused by stagnation of pelvic and uterine blood flow. Its antispasmodic properties relax uterine muscles to relieve menstrual cramps and ease the pain of childbirth. To encourage menses to begin or to ease menstrual cramps, take 40 drops of tincture in water every 3-5 hours for up to 4 days. Due to its stimulating action on the uterus, it is known as an abortifacient (capable of inducing miscarriage) and is **not recommended during pregnancy**.

Alcoholic Delirium Tremens: Clinical herbalist John Lust recommended Feverfew for delirium tremens caused by excessive consumption of alcohol (Lust, 1974). The plant's abilities to relax muscles and reduce spasms are helpful for this condition. Take it as a warm infusion tea, tincture (30-40 drops), or use the dried form as needed. It is most effective when combined with herbal nervines such as Scullcap (*Scutellaria lateriflora*), Hops (*Humulus lupulus*), Valerian (*Valeriana officinalis*), and Wood Betony (*Stachys officinalis*).

Cancer Therapy: Feverfew may be a potential candidate for cancer treatment, as research studies have revealed several activities of parthenolide that fight various types of cancers. Multiple studies prove that parthenolide affects cytokines, which are part of the immune response crucial for eliminating infections and cancerous cells. Cytokines can be anti-inflammatory or pro-inflammatory, and include interferons, interleukins, lymphokines, and tumor necrosis factor. Cytokines are produced by a broad range of cells, including mast cells and immune cells such as macrophages, B lymphocytes, and T lymphocytes. Several *in vitro* tests have demonstrated that parthenolide inhibits the secretion of inflammatory interleukin-6, tumor necrosis factor (Kang 2001; Magni, 2012), and prostaglandin COX-2 (Hwang, 1996).

Another immune mechanism involved in destroying cancerous cells is apoptosis, or the genetically programmed death of damaged and cancerous cells. When this protective mechanism becomes dysfunctional, cancer cells are free to uncontrollably reproduce and metastasize. Several *in vitro* studies verify that parthenolide induces apoptosis and reduces viability of different kinds of human cancer cells. Apoptosis with resulting cell death has occurred in two types of breast cancers (Wyrebska, 2013), colon cancer (Pajah, 2007), and cancers of the larynx and nasopharynx (Ross, 1999). Treatment of bladder cancer cells with parthenolide also resulted in a significant decrease in cancer cell viability and metastasis by inducing apoptosis (Cheng, 2011).

Parthenolide seems to suppress growth of the Epstein-Barr virus, a member of the herpes family that causes mononucleosis. Epstein-Barr is also associated with particular forms of cancer such as Hodgkin's lymphoma, Burkitt's lymphoma, nasopharyngeal carcinoma, and conditions associated with human immunodeficiency virus (HIV), including hairy leukoplakia and central nervous system lymphomas. One *in vitro* study revealed that parthenolide suppressed growth of Epstein-Barr virus-positive lymphoma cells (Li, 2012).

Angiogenesis is the formation of new blood vessels, including those that supply rapidly growing tumors and cancer cells with nutrients. Parthenolide isolated from Feverfew inhibited angiogenesis in human colorectal cancer cells, eliciting their destruction (Kim, 2014).

Oxidative stress promotes inflammation and the generation of cancerous cells. A team of researchers investigated Feverfew's efficacy in reducing tissue oxidation. When 11 sesquiterpene lactones, including parthenolide, were isolated from *T. parthenium*, they activated nuclear factor E2 (Nrf2) (Fischedick, 2012). Nrf2 is found in all cells and is responsible for stimulating cells to secrete antioxidants that are major players in reducing oxidative stress, enhancing strong immunity, and keeping the body healthy.

Wounds and Insect Bites: Feverfew is an antiseptic and vulnerary for external healing to relieve pain, swelling, and inflammation caused by insect bites, traumatic injury, wounds, ulcers, and bruises. The leaves and flowers may be included in an oil-based salve, applied as a poultice, and the tea or diluted tincture may be used as a wash.

Insecticide: The pyrethrin in Feverfew is an effective insecticide this is deadly to many insects, but harmless to people and animals. Plant this attractive herb in your garden to protect other plants from insect predators, or grind dried leaves and flower heads into a dust and apply it to plants. A strong tea can also be prepared and combined with 40% mineral oil. Use a spray bottle to apply this blend to protect plants. The mineral oil is added to help the tea adhere to the plants, and the Feverfew and mineral oil blend should be re-applied after heavy rains. To keep bugs off people, dilute the tincture with water and apply topically.

Teachings from the Feverfew Deva

"Greetings, dear one. I am the deva of the Feverfew plant. I will share with you my wisdom and healing virtues. I am a plant of the heart with my warm and loving nature that radiates outward. I soothe inflammation throughout the body, leaving a peaceful calm in the tissues. Today we will sit together and I will tell you my story.

"I offer many virtues. My plants bring beauty to the eyes and to the heart. For I emit an abundance of radiance culminating in the sunny, bright, smiling flower heads adorning my sweet and light, fluffy leaves. I am a happy being and my plants radiate this happiness. My abundant nature manifests through my prolific flowers and seeds possessing strong self-germination capacity, allowing my plants to easily multiply and spread over the ground in a beautiful carpet. I am a hardy little plant and my delightful beauty and abundant nature are part of my gifts to you.

"I am a fiery herb in the domain of Leo and the Sun. My flowers with bright-yellow centers resemble the sun surrounded by white petals of light rays flowing out into the world.

"I am also of the air element, which brings swift movement to my nature and stimulating activity in the human body that purges through congestion and blockages along my path. And thus, the fire and air energies bring warmth and stimulating movement. This is part of my medicine. But in excess, these attributes cause inflammation and pain in the tissues. And so I help maintain a balance between cool and warm, stagnation and overstimulation. This ability to modify and maintain balance of these polarities resides in the synergistic blend of all the chemical substances in my leaves and flowers. Those people who look at my plants to discover the one substance containing the medicine are missing the point. The power of my medicine rests in the harmonious blend of all substances in the leaves and flowers. Please remember this union. It is true in all of Nature. Always understand parts according to their relationship and position in the wholeness. Isolating only one substance from my plants changes its healing ability that emerges from the interaction of all my chemicals blended together by Mother Nature.

"My air element is ruled by Gemini and my medicine brings polarized opposites into union, which is the healing essence of Gemini. My energies travel out and also draw back inward. When you use me for medicine, my energies radiate out to heal your physical body. My inward movement gathers and draws other people to you who will be of assistance in your healing process.

"I am a being of happiness, lightness of heart, and friendship. Life passes quickly and the journey is brief. Nurture the preciousness of sweet joy and laughter to fill the hours and days of your journey. My smiling flowers adorning my plants are reminders of this little gem of wisdom from our hearts to yours."

Goldenrod

Solidago odora, spp.
Compositae (*Asteraceae*) (Aster or Daisy) Family

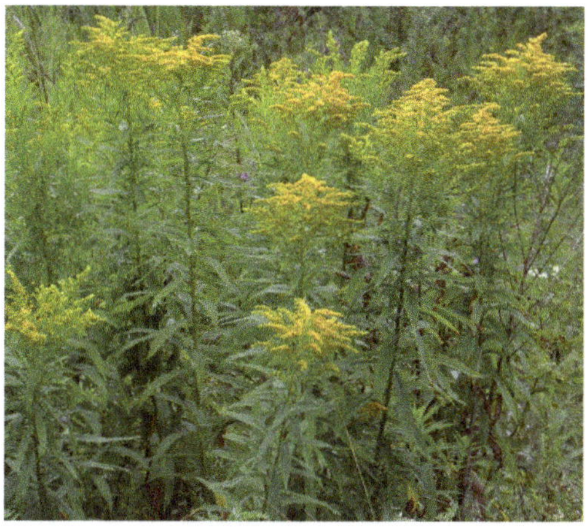

Solidago odora

Common Names

Sweet Goldenrod, anise-scented Goldenrod, woundweed, and blue mountain tea are common names for *Solidago odora*.

Medicinal Part of the Plant

The flowering tops and upper leaves are used medicinally.

Range and Habitat

Solidago species grow in temperate regions around the world. They like full sun in open meadows or woodlands and along the edges of forests. Goldenrod thrives in dry, sandy, or clay soils with medium fertility. There are over 100 species indigenous to North America and many of them hybridize, which can sometimes make their identification difficult.

S. odora, native to the Midwest and eastern United States, is the one true fragrant Goldenrod species and is named for its pleasant odor. Other North American varieties employed for healing include *S. altissima, S. arguta, S. canadensis, S. flexicaulis, S. gigantea, S. graminifolia, S. nemoralis, S. procera, S. rigida, S. rigidiuscula, S. rugosa,* and *S. sempervirens*. Many species of Goldenrod are indigenous to Europe, including *S. virgaurea*, the variety most often used medicinally by Europeans.

Description of the Plant

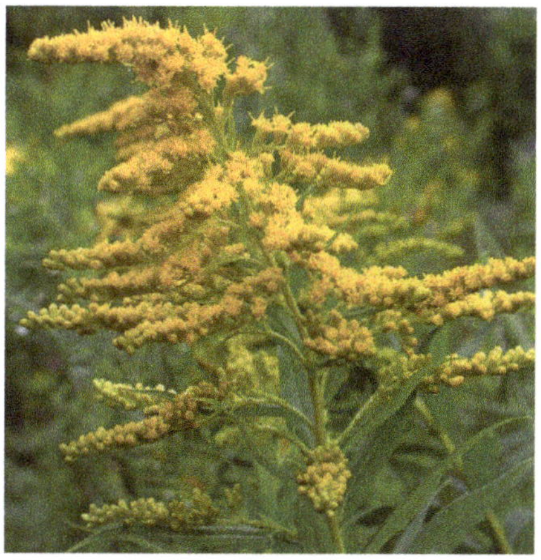

Solidago odora

All species of Goldenrod are showy perennials with clusters of bright-yellow flowers that grow in various arrangements. The leaves are linear to lance-shaped, sessile, either smooth or hairy, and some have teeth while other species are entire with smooth margins. *S. odora* has a creeping rootstock that produces a stem growing to a height of 2-3′. Leaves are thin, entire, linear to lanceolate, and covered with transparent dots that are glands containing volatile oils. Golden-yellow flowers appear in one-sided panicle racemes from July through September. *S. odora* is called Sweet Goldenrod because the volatile oil in the leaves has an anise-like fragrance when bruised, and the flowers also have a unique and pleasant aroma.

S. virgaurea (European Goldenrod) grows 2-3′ tall and has short rootstocks with many fibrous roots. The hairy, round stems support oblong to lanceolate, weakly serrated leaves growing in an alternate pattern. Lower leaves have petiole stems and upper leaves are nearly sessile. Yellow flowers appear in panicle racemes at the ends of stems from July to October. *S. canadensis* is native to North America, and is the only species having galls, which are hard, round swollen areas protruding from the stems.

Cultivation

Goldenrod species usually grow so abundantly in sunny meadows that they can often be wildcrafted, making cultivation unnecessary. However, this herb can be grown from seeds sown in autumn or early spring. The root crowns may be dug up in spring when stems are 4-5″ tall, divided, and replanted. Plant the seedlings or root divisions 10-12″ apart in a moderately fertile, well-drained bed. Goldenrod grows well in slightly acidic soil.

Harvest

Harvest the upper leaves and flowers when blooming first begins in late summer to obtain the greatest concentrations and potency of the volatile oils. Older leaves develop a more astringent, bitter flavor. Collect seeds for replanting when seedpods are dry and have turned brown.

Preparation of Plant Medicine and Dosages

Goldenrod leaves and flowers can be prepared as tea or tincture, or dried for future needs. A poultice, wash, or salve of the herb may be applied to the skin for wound healing and other external problems.

PREPARATIONS

Tea: Steep 1-3 teaspoons of fresh or dried leaves and flowers in 1 cup of boiled water. Dosage: 1-3 cups a day. Warm tea has diaphoretic properties. Cold tea stimulates the system and helps to dispel gas. The leaves and flowers of *S. odora* emit a pleasant fragrance and taste.

Tincture: Prepare a leaf and flower tincture in the standard way by using 50% 190-proof grain alcohol and 50% distilled water. Dosage: 10-50 drops 1-4 times a day.

Chemical Constituents

The different species of Goldenrod contain many of the same phytochemicals, including flavonoids, saponins, and phenol glycosides (Metzner, 1984). Flavonoids support healthy blood vessels and capillaries, while saponins have diuretic and expectorant actions. Although North American varieties of Goldenrod contain greater concentrations of these phytochemicals than European species, the different varieties possess similar medicinal properties and are used interchangeably in herbal medicine.

Research has primarily been on *S. virgaurea* (European Goldenrod), consisting of essential oils, about 1.5% flavonoids, 10% catechin tannins (astringents that reduce bleeding and diarrhea), 2-6% triterpene saponins (diuretic and expectorant), and phenol glycosides, including leiocarposide (anti-inflammatory, analgesic, and potent diuretic). Phenolic acids include caffeic and chlorogenic acids, which have diuretic, analgesic, antibacterial, anticancer, antihistamine, anti-inflammatory, and antioxidant properties. Flavonoids are antioxidants and include rutin (supports healthy blood vessels), quercetin (anti-allergy, diuretic, antibacterial, antihistamine, anti-inflammatory), isoquercitrin (diuretic, antibacterial, anticancer), astragalin (diuretic, expectorant, immunostimulant), hyperoside, and nicotiflorin.

Safety, Contraindications, and Drug Interactions

People with chronic kidney disorders should use Goldenrod with caution because it stimulates increased kidney activity that may aggravate chronic urinary tract problems. According to the German Commission E herbal regulatory agency, Goldenrod has no known side effects, interactions with drugs, or restrictions during pregnancy and lactation. However, since it is somewhat stimulating to the uterus, **it should be used only after the first trimester in small dosages.**

Goldenrod pollen is mistakenly reputed to cause allergic reactions similar to hay fever. These allergies are actually caused by Ragweed (*Ambrosia* spp.), which blooms at the same time as Goldenrod. Ragweed produces huge amounts of light pollen that is carried by the wind, while Goldenrod pollen is heavy, sticky, and transported by insects rather than the wind. So a person would have to be close to the Goldenrod plant to have an allergic reaction.

Medicinal Uses

History of the Plant

The genus name *Solidago* is derived from the Latin word *soldare*, meaning "to make whole," in reference to its use as a vulnerary (wound healing) herb. Goldenrod has also been employed for urinary, respiratory, and digestive problems in traditional medicine for many centuries. Certainly the bright-yellow color of its flowers attracted the attention of herbalists, and those who paid attention to the Doctrine of Signatures were guided by the yellow color (pointing to affinity with kidneys and urine) to use this herb for urinary problems. In Europe, it was administered by folk healers, monks, and herbal practitioners like Nicholas Culpeper (1616–1654) and John Gerard (1545–1612). Gerard wrote in his famous herbal, "Goldenrod provoketh urine, wasteth away stones in the kidnies, and expelleth them . . . . It is extolled above all other herbes for the stopping of blood in sanguinolent [bloody] ulcers and bleeding wounds" (Gerard, 1633). It is interesting that the internationally known Austrian herbalist Maria Treben wrote, "Country folk say that there is a gentle and helpful angel standing next to each plant" (Treben, 1988). It was often used as a culinary tea when tea from China was scarce.

In North America, many species of Goldenrod were included in the pharmacies of the indigenous people. The early American botanist Rafinesque, who recorded the native uses of many herbs, wrote that the Cherokee used the herb for fevers while the Iroquois drank an infusion of the flowers as a gastrointestinal and liver aid (Moerman, 1998). Other tribes drank teas of the flowers and leaves for sore throats, respiratory ailments, and chest pain. They applied a Goldenrod poultice to aching teeth and gums, poisonous bites and stings, burns, muscle sprains, and painful cramps and swellings. Jacob Bigelow (1787–1879), an American physician and botanist, wrote, "The claims of the Solidago to stand as an article of the Materia Medica are of a humble, but not despicable kind . . . . An essence made by dissolving the essential oil in proof spirit [alcohol] is used in the eastern States as a remedy in complaints arising from flatulence, and as a vehicle for unpleasant medicines of various kinds. I have employed it to allay vomiting and to relieve spasmodic pains in the stomach of the milder kind, with satisfactory success . . . it has for some time been an article of exportation to China, where it fetches a high price" (Bigelow, 1817). Goldenrod flowers yield a beautiful yellow color that was used to dye cloth and soap. I often harvest the flowers to color and add fragrance to soap that I make every year.

The American Eclectic physicians employed *S. odora* in their herbal pharmacy and used it as a gentle stimulant and carminative for indigestion, stomach and intestinal spasms, gas, diarrhea, and dysentery. They prescribed the flowers as a valuable remedy for urinary tract conditions, including nephritis (kidney inflammation), kidney stones, difficult and scanty urination, edema, bladder ulceration, and back pain associated with kidney problems. *S. odora* was the only species of Goldenrod listed as an official medicinal drug in the *U.S. Pharmacopoeia* from 1820–1882.

Currently, the herb is more popular in Europe than in the United States, and several species continue to be used in European medical herbalism, including *S. virgaurea, S. sertina*, and *S. canadensis*. Goldenrod is listed in the *German Pharmacopoeia* as an official diuretic herb to treat kidney and bladder inflammation and kidney stones. Few clinical studies and little research have been conducted on the medicinal uses of the *Solidago* species.

Healing Qualities

Analgesic, anti-catarrhal, antifungal, anti-inflammatory, antiseptic, antispasmodic, astringent, carminative, diaphoretic, diuretic, lithotropic, nephritic, stimulant, and vulnerary.

Traditional Chinese Medicine (TCM) Perspective

Goldenrod is cooling and drying in nature, influencing the kidneys, bladder, lungs, stomach, intestines, and uterus. It is a Yang-acting herb, and its stimulating action reduces stagnation in the abdominal and pelvic organs and promotes the smooth flow of Qi, blood, urine, and other fluids. It is specific for excessive dampness. Its drying and downward movement drains excess fluid and congestion from the nasal sinuses, lungs, and kidneys.

Goldenrod is excellent for Kidney Qi Stagnation that results in edema and kidney stones, and it helps relieve toxic conditions caused when the kidneys are unable to filter and excrete waste products and acids from the blood. Goldenrod reduces damp heat in the urinary tract to help decrease infections and yeast overgrowth. The herb also stimulates normal flow of Qi and blood in the uterus to normalize menstrual periods for women, and promotes optimal prostate health for men.

Primary Actions

The different species of Goldenrod are primarily used for urinary problems in modern herbalism, but they also prove beneficial for digestion, the lungs, and conditions involving excessive amounts of mucous. Goldenrod stimulates blood flow to the kidneys and uterus, improves urination, and flushes toxins and waste products out of the body. Researchers have verified the antioxidant and anti-inflammatory activities of the herb's flavonoid content, which is helpful to all tissues (Apati, 2003).

Urinary Tract: Several species of *Solidago* are specific for urinary problems involving the kidneys, bladder, ureters, and urethra. The leaves and flowers are diuretic, promoting the production of urine, and are also aquaretic, meaning that they increase urination by improving blood flow to the kidneys. This increases the glomerular filtration rate and production of urine in the kidneys without depleting minerals. The herb is safer than many pharmaceutical diuretics (such as Lasix) that cause loss of minerals, especially potassium.

Goldenrod is an excellent strengthening tonic for long-term treatment of chronic conditions caused by underactive kidneys resulting in problems of congestion, stagnation, and accumulation of waste products throughout the body. Daily use of the tea or tincture can be helpful for edema and skin conditions that are caused by or worsened by toxins, such as dermatitis, psoriasis, eczema, acne, hives, and other rashes. Goldenrod is beneficial when used in a detoxification program.

The leaves and flowers of this herb reduce pain, inflammation, and spasms throughout the urinary tract. The tea and tincture regulate the kidneys, stimulate increased activity and urination, and help restore and maintain normal kidney function. It is one of the safest and most effective diuretic and antiseptic herbs for the urinary tract. By increasing urinary flow, bacteria and excessive amounts of albumin and acids are washed out of the tissues and blood. This normalizes blood urea nitrogen (BUN) and creatinine blood levels to promote healthy kidneys.

Goldenrod is an effective treatment for mild to severe cases of kidney disease, urinary tract infections (UTIs), and inflammation. This includes acute and chronic nephritis (kidney inflammation and infection), cystitis (bladder infection), urethritis (inflamed urethra), and urinary spasms. Ingesting the tea or tincture is beneficial for painful, difficult, or scanty urination with dark-colored urine containing cloudy sediments. These symptoms are all indicative of infection. The herb's astringent properties reduce blood in the urine in cases of tissue damage. Goldenrod soothes kidney pain and related back discomfort. People with indwelling catheters and on kidney dialysis have reported improved kidney function when taking Goldenrod (Cai, 2014). It has a long tradition of use in preventing kidney stones and facilitating their elimination.

Water and alcohol extracts of Goldenrod are prescribed in Germany to treat bladder dysfunction, including overactive and spastic bladder. German scientists have conducted *in vitro* studies to determine the effects of Goldenrod on human and rat bladders, and found that the extract reduced bladder contractions and urination following lab-induced stimulation (Borchert, 2004). The herb has also demonstrated diuretic and anti-inflammatory action in lab and animal research (Ghazaly, 1992).

A clinical study evaluated the efficacy of an herbal blend of *Solidago*, *Orthosiphon stamineus* (Java tea), and Birch extract in 164 women with recurrent UTIs. For 3 months, every participant received prophylactic antibiotics, while 107 of the women also took the herbal blend. During the 12-month period following the prophylactic intervention, women who had received the added herbal blend experienced fewer UTIs than the others, whose relapse risk of infection was 2.5 times greater (Frumenzio, 2013).

Combine Goldenrod with other herbs to increase its effectiveness in treating UTIs. Diuretic kidney herbs that increase urination and flush out pathogens include Parsley (*Petroselinum crispum*), Dandelion leaf (*Taraxacum officinale*), Celery seed (*Apium graveolens*), and Juniper berries (*Juniperus communis*). To kill bacteria or fungi, add herbs specific for the urinary tract such as Uva-ursi (*Arctostaphylos uva-ursi*), Buchu (*Agathosma betulina*), Oregon Grape Root (*Mahonia aquifolium*), Goldenseal (*Hydrastis canadensis*), and Yarrow (*Achillea millefolium*). Include herbs that contain mucilage to soothe and heal inflamed, irritated, and ulcerated urinary tract tissues, such as Marshmallow root (*Althaea officinalis*), Slippery Elm bark (*Ulmus rubra*), Plantain (*Plantago* spp.), Chickweed (*Stellaria* spp.), Corn Silk (*Zea mays*), Couch grass rhizome (*Elymus repens*), and Hollyhock (*Alcea rosea*) leaf and root. Prepare a quart of tea containing several of these herbs, and sip on it throughout the day to treat urinary problems.

While taking herbs to resolve UTIs and other urinary tract issues, follow these additional suggestions:

1) Drink plenty of pure water each day to flush waste products and bacteria out of the bladder and kidneys.
2) Drink unsweetened Cranberry juice (*Vaccinium macrocarpon*) to reduce the ability of *Escherichia coli (E. coli)* to adhere to the inner lining of the bladder and urethra. Normally residing in the colon, *E. coli* is responsible for a large portion of acute bladder infections.
3) Take a probiotic supplement and eat yogurt and fermented foods to nourish and replenish healthy intestinal and vaginal bacteria, which decreases the incidence of UTIs. Health-promoting *Lactobacilli* typically populate vaginal flora and prevent invasion of *E. coli* into the bladder. *Lactobacilli* produce carbon dioxide and hydrogen peroxide, which help maintain a healthy acidic bladder.
4) Vitamin C (ascorbic acid) also promotes more acidic urine.

Respiratory Infections, Allergies, and Excessive Mucous Production: As an anti-catarrhal (anti-mucous) herb, Goldenrod has traditionally been employed to treat acute and chronic damp conditions and excessive mucous production anywhere in the body, especially in the nasal sinuses and lungs. Several of the flavonoids in Goldenrod possess decongesting antihistamine actions. The herb contains substantial amounts of astringent tannins that dry the mucous membranes in the nasal sinuses. It restores normal mucous production and thins the mucous when it is thick and sticky, making it easier to eliminate.

Goldenrod's ability to normalize mucous secretion is excellent for treating sinus allergies, respiratory infections, chronic sinusitis, the common cold, influenza (flu), bronchitis, tonsillitis, and fevers with alternating chills and high temperatures. It is especially indicated when there is an excessive amount of mucous discharge and drainage, and when mucous is white (indicating congestion), yellow (indicating infection), or green (indicating more severe infection). Drink hot tea or tincture for fevers because the diaphoretic activity increases perspiration, bringing internal heat to the surface to be released. Tea or tincture diluted in warm water can be used as a gargle for sore throats and laryngitis.

Digestion: *Solidago odora* and other Goldenrod species are traditionally taken for digestive issues caused by inflammation, spasms, stagnation, and excessive dampness. These issues include indigestion, stomach problems, gas, colic, Crohn's disease, and other irritable bowel conditions. The herb's stimulating action encourages the smooth flow of food through the gastrointestinal tract. The astringent properties reduce diarrhea. Researchers found that solidagenone in the herb effectively protected the stomach lining of mice from developing ulcerous lesions (Schmeda-Hirschmann, 2002). Several *in vitro* studies reveal that various *Solidago* species are anti-fungal and specifically inhibit Candida yeast (Vila, 2002; Duarte, 2005; Laurencon, 2013).

Women's Health: Goldenrod has an affinity with the lower abdominal and pelvic regions of the body, and its healing virtues extend to the reproductive systems of both men and women. Although it is not currently a popular herb for women's health, the flowers and leaves have been used to treat dysmenorrhea (painful menstruation) and amenorrhea (abnormal cessation of menstrual bleeding). The antispasmodic and anti-inflammatory properties address uterine cramps and spasms. The herb's stimulating influence to the pelvic area increases blood flow to the tissues and organs, which promotes their normal function and regular menstrual cycles. Goldenrod's drying nature reduces excessive dampness, especially in the pelvis, and can be helpful for chronic yeast infections and other types of vaginal discharge.

Prostate Health and Cancer: In Europe, the different species of Goldenrod are administered to treat prostate diseases. Researchers from the Southern Illinois University School of Medicine tested an extract of *S. virgaurea* to determine its anticancer activities. They discovered that the herb exhibits strong cytotoxic activities (ability to destroy damaged cells) during *in vitro* tests on various tumor cell lines, including human prostate, breast, melanoma, and small cell lung carcinoma. The extract also significantly suppressed tumor growth in *in vivo* animal studies. The active component resides primarily in the leaves of the plant and is soluble in water. The researchers concluded that *S. virgaurea* is a promising antineoplastic medicine with minimal toxicities (Gross, 2002).

External Healing: The leaves and flowers of different Goldenrod species can be applied as a poultice, wash, or salve to promote wound healing and treat ulcers, bites, stings, and sprained and inflamed muscles. As an antiseptic it kills bacteria on the skin, and the astringent tannins reduce bleeding and bruising. Quercetin and rutin, two primary flavonoids in the herb, improve capillary fragility to reduce bruising and improve bleeding disorders. Goldenrod works best when combined with other vulnerary herbs. (See "Skin Problems" on page 591 in the "Index of Health Issues and Herbal Recommendations" for suggestions.)

Teachings from the Goldenrod Deva

"Greetings, dear one. I am the deva of the Goldenrod plants. My deeply penetrating yellow flowers adorn the Earth in late summer and autumn, when the energies of the sun begin to wane and the life force in plants slowly flows downward back into the ground. I am a traveler, and my seeds and plants have spread out over many miles and lands. Even across the oceans, I have been carried by immigrating people.

"My direction of flow is downward and outward, like water being poured upon the soil. My plants harness the energy of the sun within their leaves and flowers. When these are taken as medicine, they stimulate the flow of water throughout the body, until eventually waters move downward, through the kidneys, and are then eliminated. This downward flow of movement is also reflected in the unique blooming pattern of my flowers. In most plants, flowers growing on spikes bloom from the bottom of the spike first and proceed upward to the top, but my flowers start opening at the top of my spikes and proceed downward.

"I am a masculine plant providing swift and balanced movement of fluids and blood through the waterways of the body that eventually empty into the kidneys for purification. As the blood percolates through the vessels of the kidneys, waste is filtered out and released as urine. And thus my cleansing action benefits all fluids in the body: the blood, lymph, urine, vitreous fluid filling the eyeball, and the amniotic water that bathes the developing child within the womb. My duty is to regulate the flow of water energies in the body, to keep them all balanced and working together in harmony. Just as there are waterways (creeks, streams, and rivers) and bodies of water (ponds, lakes, and oceans) on the earth, the same terrain exists in the body. The tiny capillary blood vessels are like little creeks trickling into larger streams and eventual rivers of the larger blood vessels. The fluids in the eyeballs are like small ponds of water. All of your cells bathe in an ocean of water you call lymph. When you burn your finger and a blister forms, the clear fluid within this blister is lymph. All cells are nourished and maintained by this ocean of lymphatic waters.

"As a plant endowed with the forceful masculine energies, my honorable work is to be of service to the feminine by watching over, protecting, and regulating the water element within the human body. For the water element is the heart and essence of feminine qualities. And so my presence and healing gifts bring balance to the polarities of male and female.

"As herbalists and healers of old recognized, my deep-yellow flowers share a similar vibration and have an affinity with the organs residing in the area of the solar plexus. This includes the kidneys, the water regulators of the body. The nature of my plants is cleansing. By the power and nature of water, the body is kept clean and nourished; for water manages the transportation of both life-giving nutrients and toxic wastes. The sweet, fresh fragrance of my flowers is a manifestation of the sweetness that my purifying actions bring forth.

"And so I am a plant of protection and purification. My presence upon the earth is essential, especially in this time of unprecedented global accumulation of toxins emerging from chemicals created by people. These eventually damage and destroy the life force of the body and living creatures. My message to people is this: Please follow my example of honoring and protecting the life-giving energies of water and the feminine essence. Keep your bodies and your home planet clean and pure, for the Earth is your body and the lakes, rivers, and oceans are like the blood and fluids flowing through your veins and bathing your tissues."

Goldenseal

Hydrastis canadensis

Ranunculaceae (Buttercup or Crowfoot) Family

Goldenseal is occasionally classified as the sole member of the *Hydrastidaceae* family.

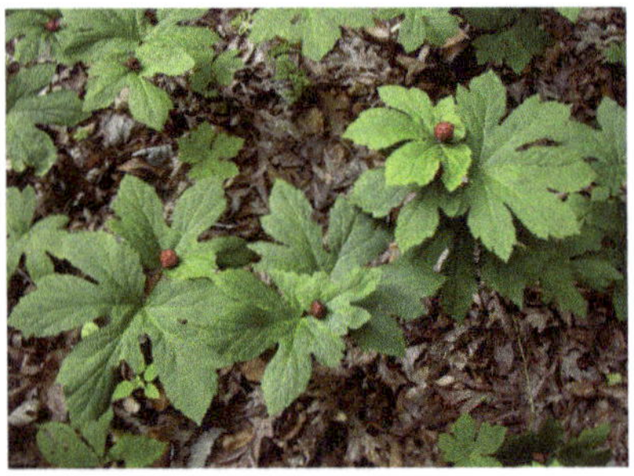

Common Names

Yellow root, orange root, yellow puccoon, turmeric root, Indian turmeric, wild curcuma, Ohio curcuma, and yellow Indian paint root are older names descriptive of the yellow color of Goldenseal root and its historic use among Native American Indians as a dye. The herb has been called ground raspberry because its red berries resemble raspberries. Eye root, eye balm, yellow eye, and jaundice root are antiquated names that reflect the plant's value as a remedy for eye problems and jaundice.

Medicinal Part of the Plant

The roots are the most potent and commonly used part of the plant. However, the leaves and stems contain smaller amounts of the medicinal alkaloids, and can be harvested as they start to dry and wilt.

Range and Habitat

Indigenous to eastern and central North American hardwood forests, Goldenseal is a national treasure. It thrives in rich, moist woodlands under a canopy of Beech, Maple, Oak, Sycamore, and Basswood trees. Its range and habitat are identical to that of American Ginseng (*Panax quinquefolius*), Bloodroot (*Sanguinaria canadensis*), Mayapple (*Podophyllum peltatum*), and Wild Ginger (*Asarum canadense*). Prior to European colonization, large populations of Goldenseal carpeted vast forests throughout Kentucky, Indiana, Virginia, Ohio, the Ohio River Valley, and the Appalachian Mountain region. Small, scattered wild stands still survive, but they are constantly threatened by loss of habitat, logging, and unsustainable wildcrafting.

Description of the Plant

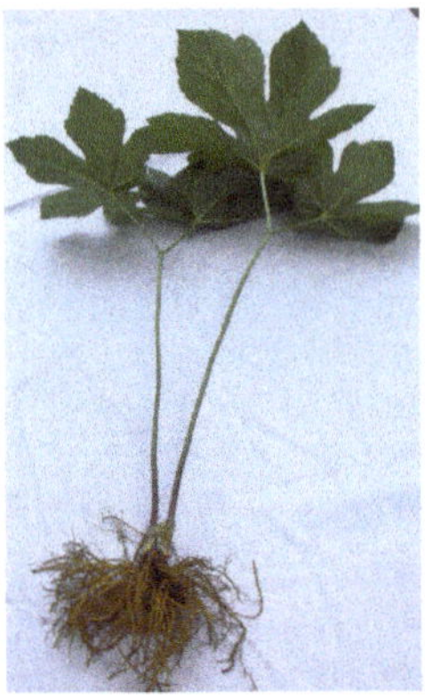

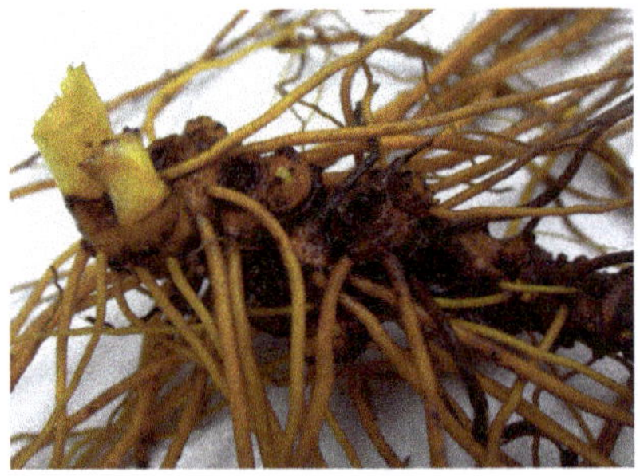

Root with two sprouting stems and old scars

Goldenseal is a perennial herb reaching heights of 6-12″. The root rhizome develops horizontally, and its golden-yellow color allows for easy identification. I have seen rhizomes grow up to 3-6″ long and ½-¾″ in diameter. Fibrous, thready rootlets branch off the rhizome. Each year the root grows longer and sprouts at least one stem. When the stem dies off in autumn, it leaves an indented cup-shaped scar that contributes to the rhizome's rough texture and knotty appearance.

The erect, round stem arising from the rhizome bears 2-4 yellowish scales at its base. The green stem becomes dark maroon at the base and is covered with white, downy hairs. Young plants develop a single leaf. After 2-3 years, 2 leaves branch off the solitary stem. One leaf is always smaller than the other and bears the flower and seeds. (Interestingly, this reflects the same pattern found in animals in which the smaller of the species, the female, reproduces the young.) Leaves of mature plants are large, up to 12″ wide. Leaves are simple and have 5-7 deep palmate lobes that are sharply pointed at their tips. Leaves are palmately shaped and veined, and covered with fine, short white hairs. Small, sharp serrate teeth line the margins. Leaves typically die back after the seeds mature.

From April to May, the cheerful white and pale greenish-yellow flowers start blooming before the wrinkled leaves are fully open. Flowers are short-lived, lasting no longer than 5-7 days. The radially symmetrical flower is about ½-1″ in diameter and lacks petals or sepals. Instead, a spray of 40-50 white stamens with pale-yellow anthers form the round flower and look like small, thready spikes radiating out from a ball. The stamens surround several ovaries in the center. As the ovaries mature from May to June, they develop into a green, raspberry-shaped fruit that ripens into a bright crimson-red berry. The berry consists of small, fleshy, oblong segments called drupes. Each drupe contains 1-2 round, shiny black seeds. Berries typically develop at least 10-20 seeds depending on the age of the root.

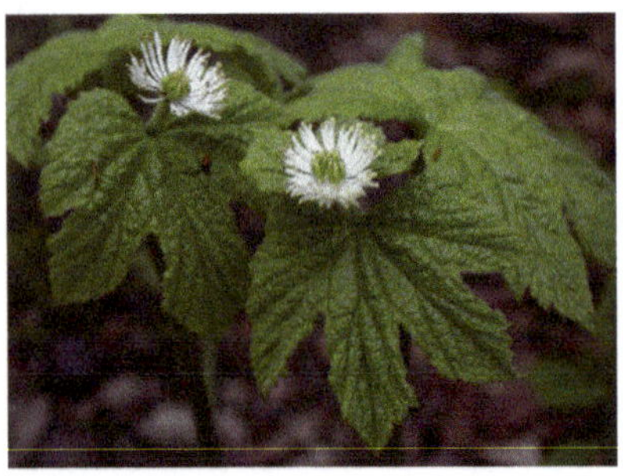

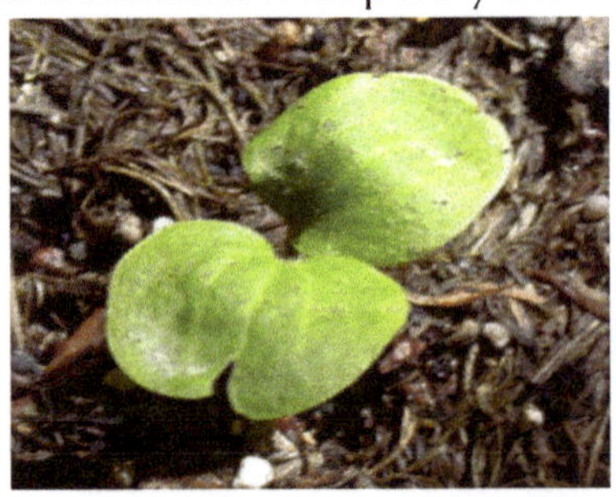

Cotyledon (first sprout)

Cultivation

Goldenseal's deep-green leaves and brilliant-crimson berries make this beautiful plant a delightful addition to shady gardens. Propagation is encouraged and absolutely necessary to meet the high market demand for this endangered herb. When preparing a garden bed for Goldenseal, try to replicate its natural forest habitat of moist, fertile humus soil. If wooded land is available, a great cultivation method involves clearing an area between trees by double-digging or rototilling, raking away debris, and preparing beds. If forest habitat is unavailable, shaded garden space under trees or next to a house or garage will suffice. Remember that adequate light, drainage, ventilation, and spacing of roots or seedlings are important to prevent mold and blight (a plant fungus). I have observed that Goldenseal growing on sloping, moist bottom land prospers better than plants living on higher dry ground, especially during dry summer months.

Goldenseal is propagated easily by seed or root division. Purchase seeds or directly harvest them from plants. If fortunate enough to be able to harvest seeds, remove the pulp of the red berry from the black seeds and wash them to encourage optimal germination. This cleaning process normally occurs in nature when birds and other animals eat the tasty berries, digest the pulp, and defecate the seeds a distance away from the parent plant in little piles of fertilizer. Plant freshly harvested or purchased seeds as soon as possible because they lose their viability quickly and should not be allowed to dehydrate. If weather conditions are not conducive for planting, or if you choose to wait until autumn, the cleaned seeds can be mixed with a bit of slightly moist sand and stored in a container in the refrigerator.

Plant seeds ¼″ deep in a well-prepared, shady nursery bed and space them 2-3″ apart. Planting seeds in straight lines helps to later distinguish them from weeds. After covering seeds with soil, keep them moist and spread grass clippings or shredded leaves over them. Goldenseal seeds need stratification (cold conditioning) to germinate. Many seeds germinate the first spring after autumn planting, while some lay dormant for a year and appear the second spring. Those that remain dormant that first year are actually developing root and bud systems that produce a stem and leaf the following season. The first leaves to emerge from seedlings are called <u>cotyledons</u>. Goldenseal cotyledons resemble miniature cupped spoons that look completely different from older leaves. During the second year of growth, one very small leaf emerges that looks like a typical Goldenseal leaf with pointed tips and teeth along the margins. Two leaves usually appear in the third year of growth. When plants are 3 years old, they can be transplanted into a permanent bed. Space plants 10-12″ apart and keep them watered and mulched. Little care is required after this, except to keep the patch weeded and moist. Seeds from older plants may be collected every year and immediately planted in woodland nursery beds. The seeds generally have a 65-80% germination rate under ideal conditions.

To propagate by root division, purchase live roots or dig up mature plants to divide and replant. Always allow Goldenseal to self-sow by waiting until the seeds mature and drop before digging up the roots. When dividing a root rhizome, notice how it is studded with undeveloped buds. A piece of root containing a bud with a few strands of fibrous roots will produce a plant. Usually 4-5 divisions can be made from a 4″ root with each piece cut ¾-1″ in length. Plant the root pieces horizontally 1″ deep in moist soil and space them every 12″.

If soil conditions are too dry for planting, roots may be temporarily planted in trays or boxes of dirt placed outdoors in the shade and kept moist. Some people recommend using sand for this, but after trying both methods, I found dirt to be the best medium because it allows the dormant roots to start growing. This reduces damage from rotting, which can happen when roots are stored in sand. Plant roots in a permanent bed when weather conditions permit. Once a Goldenseal patch is established, it will self-seed and slowly expand for many years, creating a beautiful, lush woodland bed of greenery and good medicine!

Harvest

Due to generations of over-harvesting, most indigenous stands of Goldenseal that once grew abundantly have been devastated and are rarely found. Harvesting cultivated plants is the best way to sustain the survival of this endangered herb. If you *must* gather from a wild patch, take only a few plants. And remember to allow Goldenseal to self-propagate by waiting until the red berries have dropped before harvesting. When started from seed, Goldenseal requires 5-6 years of growth before the rhizomes are large enough to harvest. Those developed by root division may be gathered after 3-4 years.

Roots may be dug up any time during their dormancy period from September through March. However, harvesting in late summer or early autumn provides the most potent medicines because perennial roots contain more phytochemicals in autumn to sustain them during winter dormancy. Harvest the entire rhizome with the thread-like rootlets. **A great <u>sustainable</u> <u>method</u> to harvest and propagate at the same time is to leave ½-¾″ of the rhizome attached to the crown and replant it. The remaining rhizome is taken for medicine.** This process provides plant material for medicine while establishing new plants for the future.

Roots contain the most medicinal components, but the leaves and stems are also beneficial for healing. After the red berries have matured and dropped, harvest leaves and stems as they start to dry and wilt.

For successive harvests, plant some roots and seeds every year. Once an established patch of Goldenseal starts producing berries, gather them when they turn bright red and plant the seeds. Deer, wild turkeys, and other critters love the tasty red berries and can quickly devour an entire patch. Beat the animals to the seeds, unless you want them to eat the berries and distribute the seeds in their own natural ways!

Preparation of Plant Medicine and Dosages

Clean freshly harvested roots with a forceful spray of water. Alcohol is the best extractor of Goldenseal's phytochemicals, although boiling water also works well. Fresh roots can be prepared into tincture, tea, or dried for storage. Dry the roots by cutting them into small pieces and arranging them on screen trays in a shaded, well-ventilated area. In humid conditions, put fans in front of the roots to speed the dehydration process and reduce potential for mold growth. Keep a watchful eye on the roots and turn them for even ventilation. Store the dried roots in a glass container out of direct sunlight. Always recheck the roots a few days after they have been put in storage to make sure that they are thoroughly dry. Dried Goldenseal root is very stable. Its peak medicinal potency lasts up to 5 years when the roots are kept whole, and up to 3 years if they are ground into powder. For optimal potency and to prevent oxidative damage, grind roots into a fine powder just before they are needed for healing. Storing roots in the freezer works well to ensure freshness and extend shelf-life. Leaves may be combined with the roots in applications for internal or external healing.

Goldenseal root is commercially available as powder, tincture, tea, pills, and capsules. It is a primary ingredient in many salves and ointments. **Please do not purchase Goldenseal harvested from wild stands, which is often stolen from private or public property. Instead, buy organically cultivated Goldenseal.**

For acute illness like the common cold or flu, this herb is traditionally ingested in medium to large doses for 5-8 days. For long-term use in treating chronic conditions, smaller doses are taken over 4-8 weeks. Eclectic physicians traditionally prescribed 7-15 drops of the tincture per dose.

PREPARATIONS

Decoction Tea: Use a covered pan to gently simmer ¼ - ½ teaspoon of powdered root in 1 pint of water for 8-10 minutes, then let it sit to cool. Dosage: ½ -1 cup up to 3 times a day. The tea is very bitter and may be diluted with water if too strong. It is an effective gargle for sore, infected throats. A strong decoction can be used externally as a wash to heal wounds and ulcers, or administered as a vaginal douche. When making a gargle, wash or douche, prepare a stronger tea by simmering ½-1 teaspoon of the root per pint of water.

Nasal Spray and Eyewash: Strain the tea through coffee filter paper to remove all sediment and use it as an outstanding eyewash or nasal spray for infections, inflammation, and excess mucous discharge.

Pills and Capsules: The finely ground powder is hand-packed into gelatin capsules or rolled into pills. The encapsulated powdered root is one of the best ways to take Goldenseal. Most people do not like the bitter taste of the tea, so capsules are an easy way to bypass the taste buds. Dosage: For acute infections take 1-2 capsules 3 times daily for up to 8 days. For chronic conditions take 1 capsule a day for no longer than 8 weeks.

Tincture: Since Goldenseal is a valuable endangered herb, I avoid wasting any part of the plant and prepare this tincture differently than others. Grind roots into a fine powder, put them in a glass jar, and cover with 70% 190-proof grain alcohol and 30% distilled water. Use a ratio of 1:5, which means that 1 part root (measured in grams) is covered with 5 parts alcohol and water (measured in milliliters). Shake this combination daily. After a month, rather than decanting to separate the liquid from the herb, skip this step and use the tincture with the root particles in it for medicine. This method is not acceptable for commercial sale because consumers prefer clear tinctures, but for personal use it works well to optimize Goldenseal's benefits and not be wasteful. Leaves and stems contain important medicinal phytochemicals and can also be tinctured. Dosage: 7-15 drops is a small dose, while 40-60 drops is considered to be a large dose. Take the tincture 3-4 times a day as needed for acute problems.

Ointment and Salve: Cover chopped leaves and powered root with olive oil and bake at 200-225°F for 3 hours. Other vulnerary herbs may be baked with Goldenseal (refer to the "Index of Health Issues and Herbal Recommendations" and the herbs listed under "Skin Problems" on page 591).

Chemical Constituents

Goldenseal contains several isoquinoline alkaloids, including berberine (0.5-10%), hydrastine (1.5-5%), berberastine (2-3%), canadine (1%), canadaline, and hydrastinine. The major biological actions of the herb are attributed to these alkaloids, especially berberine and hydrastine, although studies indicate that other chemical constituents act synergistically to provide its medicinal activities.

Berberine is responsible for the yellow color of the root and the plant's bitter taste. It reduces abnormal bleeding, stimulates and tones the uterus, promotes digestion, benefits the stomach, increases bile secretion from the liver, acts as a laxative, and reduces muscle spasms. *In vitro* and *in vivo* studies show that Berberine exerts analgesic, anti-arrhythmia, antispasmodic, anticarcinogenic, anti-inflammatory, antihistamine, carminative, cholagogue, hepatoprotective, hypotensive, sedating, and uterotonic activities. It reduces fevers, stimulates immunity, and offers broad-spectrum protection against bacteria, yeast, fungi, and parasites (Hoffman, 2003; Newall, 1996; Pizzorno, 1988; Preininger, 1975). Interestingly, herbalist David Winston found that cultivated Goldenseal contains much more berberine than plants from wild stands.

The properties of hydrastine are similar to berberine, and it is astringent, antibacterial, and choleretic. Injections in animals decrease blood pressure and stimulate involuntary smooth muscles. Canadine stimulates uterine contractions in animal studies (Genest, 1969). Berberastine is analgesic, cardiotonic, anti-arrhythmic, antibacterial, antihistamine, anti-inflammatory, antiseptic, antiviral, and antiparasitic. It is effective against pneumonia, conjunctivitis, herpes, liver cirrhosis, cholera, dysentery, giardia, Candida yeast, chlamydia, gonorrhea, amoeba infections, and cancer.

Goldenseal also contains meconin, chlorogenic acid (anti-atherosclerotic, antibacterial, anticarcinogenic, antihistamine, anti-inflammatory, antioxidant, antiseptic, antiviral, cholagogue, hepatoprotective, immunostimulant, vulnerary), phytosterins, and resins. Vitamins and minerals include beta-carotene (vitamin A), ascorbic acid (vitamin C), some of the vitamin B complex, cobalt, magnesium, manganese, zinc, and silicon.

Safety, Contraindications, and Drug Interactions

Over 200 years of medicinal use plus current research verifies that Goldenseal is a safe, non-toxic herb when taken in recommended doses. There are no known drug interactions, although some *in vitro* and clinical studies have provided evidence that Goldenseal may inhibit the liver enzyme cytochrome P450 (Gurley, 2008). This enzyme is involved with the metabolism of about 30% of all pharmaceutical drugs and may interfere with some drug therapy. Goldenseal may diminish the anticoagulant action of heparin. Some sources claim that the herb is contraindicated for people with high blood pressure.

Goldenseal's alkaloids exert strong activity and should not be taken in large doses over long periods of time. People with kidney disease or kidney failure should avoid this herb due to their inability to excrete the alkaloids. These alkaloids stimulate the uterus, so large amounts could promote contractions (Farnsworth, 1975). Although no studies document detrimental effects of Goldenseal during pregnancy, **herbs containing berberine are not currently recommended for use during pregnancy or lactation**. However, it is interesting to note that an Eclectic physician named Cuthberton gave Goldenseal to several pregnant women suffering from goiters (enlarged thyroid) for six weeks to three months, three times a day, and reported safe use and success in treating the goiters (Ellingwood, 1919). Older respected herbalists like Jethro Kloss and John Lust documented that small doses taken frequently eased morning sickness during pregnancy.

Warnings of potential toxicity are found in the literature stating that large amounts of Goldenseal cause excessive secretions from mucous membranes, eventually resulting in dryness, ulceration, and inflammation to tissues it directly contacts. This warning seems to have originated from homeopathic applications and side effects, which are very different from herbal preparations.

Goldenseal has mistakenly been accused of killing beneficial intestinal flora in similar ways as prescription antibiotics. There is no evidence from traditional use or scientific research to confirm this. In fact, one research study found no changes in a segment of bowel flora following the administration of 400 mg of berberine, the equivalent of 26 capsules of Goldenseal (Rabbani, 1987).

The misconception that Goldenseal masks urine tests for illegal drugs also lacks any scientific basis. Herbal expert Steven Foster traced this myth to the novel *Stringtown on the Pike*, written by the Eclectic pharmacist John Uri Lloyd and published in 1900 (Foster, 1993).

Medicinal Uses

History of the Plant

Wherever it grew, Goldenseal was extensively utilized by North American Indians, both internally and externally, for treating wounds, skin problems, eye infections, mouth sores, stomach and liver problems, colds, coughs, respiratory infections, skin cancers, and gonorrhea that was introduced by the Europeans. The Cherokee drank tea made from the roots for indigestion and poor appetite, as a general tonic for debility, and as a wash for local inflammation, inflamed eyes, and skin cancers. The Iroquois also used it for these purposes and for diarrhea, indigestion, gas, whooping cough, pneumonia, fever, and earaches (Moerman, 1998). The dried root was ground into a powder and placed on open wounds and skin cancers to halt bleeding, treat infection, and promote healing. The powder was often mixed with bear grease and prepared as an ointment for wounds or repelling insects. The roots were also highly prized as a yellow dye for body paint, tools, and clothing. Early European colonists learned about this herb from the Native Americans. Goldenseal was documented as a plant employed for infections and eyewashes in the journals of Lewis and Clark during their expedition to the Pacific coast in the early 1800s (Lewis, 1977).

In 1828, Goldenseal's popularity among European colonists heightened when botanist C.S. Rafinesque (1783–1840) publicized the herb in his writings. Samuel Thomson (1769–1843), founder of the Thomsonian herbal medicine system, popularized it as an antiseptic. He recommended changing its common name from yellow root to Goldenseal, because the small, cup-like scars on top of the golden-yellow rhizome resemble wax seals that were once melted to glue envelopes. Due to the similar shape of their leaves, Goldenseal was originally named *Hydrophyllum* (Waterleaf) by botanist Carl Linnaeus (1707–1778). He later renamed the genus *Hydrastis*, thought to be derived from two Greek words meaning "water" and "to act or accomplish," referring to its healing and normalizing action on the watery secretions of mucous membranes. Goldenseal was listed as an official medicine primarily for inflammation of the mucous membranes in the *United States Pharmacopoeia* from 1830–1840, when it was discontinued, and re-instated from 1860–1926. It was originally included in the *U.S. National Formulary* in 1888 and reappeared from 1936–1955.

Goldenseal became a popular remedy among the American Eclectic physicians, who called it hydrastis. The famous Eclectic pharmacist John Uri Lloyd and his brother wrote an extensive monograph about Goldenseal in 1884. Detailed documentation describing its clinical use appeared in the Eclectic classic, *King's American Dispensatory*. The Eclectics primarily employed the roots for all catarrhal (excessive phlegm discharge) conditions and inflammation of the mucous membranes throughout the body. The herb was prescribed for respiratory and sinus infections, coughs, tonsillitis, and sore throats. As a bitter tonic, Goldenseal roots were administered to stimulate and tone the digestive system and to treat liver and gallbladder diseases, gallstones, stomach problems including nausea, heartburn and ulcers, and infectious or chronic diarrhea. The herb was used for cystitis, ear infections, swollen glands, hemorrhage, uterine complaints, vaginal discharges, and prolapse of internal organs due to muscle atony (weakness and loss of tone). For skin problems such as eczema, acne, ringworm, seborrhea, rosacea, lupus, boils, ulcers and skin cancers, the roots were ingested and applied externally (Felter, 1898; Cook, 1869; Ellingwood, 1919).

Dramatic decline in Goldenseal populations occurred during the late 1800s. Rising market demand, devastating wildcrafting practices, and dwindling habitat had taken an alarming toll. Even so, by 1910 Goldenseal was the most popular herbal remedy of lay people and physicians. But like many phytomedicines, it was replaced by pharmaceutical drugs. Since the 1970s, Goldenseal has re-emerged as a favorite and top-selling herb in health food stores. Herbalist Steven Foster has estimated that about 150,000 pounds of the roots are consumed annually in the American market (Foster, 1993), and millions of roots are exported around the world. In 1997, the U.S. government classified the plant as either "endangered" (meaning that it is in danger of extinction), "imperiled," or "threatened" in the various states in which it grows. In the same year, the Convention on International Trade in Endangered Species (CITES) began limiting U.S. exportation of Goldenseal roots to conserve this valuable resource. Since the 1990s, many cultivation projects have been initiated in an attempt to supply huge consumer demands. Due to the endangered status, alternate plants containing berberine are often recommended instead of Goldenseal. These include Oregon Grape Root (*Mahonia aquifolium*), Barberry (*Berberis vulgaris*), and Goldthread (*Coptis chinensis, C. trifolia*).

Scientific research has primarily focused on the isolated alkaloid berberine and less on whole plant extracts of Goldenseal. There have been few clinical trials. Practitioners and researchers currently use preparations of the crude herb or isolated berberine administered orally or by injections. Studies on the pharmacology and biological effects of the whole plant and isolated berberine validate many traditional folk uses of this herb.

Healing Qualities

Alterative (to the mucous membranes), antibacterial, anticarcinogenic, anti-catarrhal, antifungal, anti-inflammatory, antimicrobial, antiseptic, antiviral, astringent, bitter, cardiac, cholagogue, deobstruent, mild diuretic, emmenagogue, exanthematous, expectorant, febrifuge, hemostatic, hepatic, lymphagogue, opthalmicum, oxytocic, pectoral, stomachic, tonic (to mucous membranes), vasodilator, and vulnerary.

Traditional Chinese Medicine (TCM) Perspective

Herbs containing berberine (the genus *Hydrastis* and *Berberis* and the *Coptis chinensis* plant) are used extensively in China, India, and other parts of Asia in the treatment of malaria, parasites, fevers, and to improve appetite and digestion (Harborne, 1993). Goldenseal is a bitter, drying, and cooling herb that dispels heat and dampness while removing toxins. It is stimulating and decongesting to the mucous membranes, calming to the nerves, and stabilizing and restoring to the digestive, respiratory, and genitourinary systems. It benefits the lungs, heart, stomach, liver, gallbladder, intestines, kidneys, bladder, and uterus.

Goldenseal resolves damp mucous congestion and discharge, vitalizes blood, clears damp heat in the liver, and its stimulating activity relieves Liver and Stomach Qi Stagnation. It is specific for Stomach and Spleen Qi deficiency causing weak muscles and excessive mucous discharge. It is indicated in most cases of excess heat and dampness, and when the tongue is large, swollen, and covered with a sticky yellow coating.

Primary Actions

Goldenseal is dear to my heart. It initiated me back into the world of healing plants many years ago. When I was 18 years old, I had a bad cold and a dear friend made me a cup of Goldenseal root tea. It was so bitter, but I drank it, and by the next day the cold had disappeared. This captured my attention, and Goldenseal has remained a favorite herb, always kept close in my first-aid cabinet. Its powerful healing so impressed me that I began a life-long study and relationship with medicinal herbs that has evolved into a passionate and fulfilling journey of gardening, nursing, teaching, and a joyful, loving connection with Nature!

The healing properties of Goldenseal are due to its remarkable affinity with the mucous membranes throughout the body, its normalizing action on these membranes, and its powerful antimicrobial alkaloids. Eclectic physician William Cook, M.D., extolled its virtues in his writings, saying, "This root is one of the purest tonics, the stimulating property predominating, but the relaxing well marked. It acts slowly and steadily . . . . Its influence upon the system is very general; and there seems to be no organ or tissue but can be benefited by its appropriate use, though it is most prominently advantageous to mucous membranes, the digestive apparatus, and the uterine organs" (Cook, 1869).

When using Goldenseal internally, remember that it is a bitter herb that exerts a cooling effect on the entire system, making it specific for hot conditions such as fevers, inflamed tissues, rashes, or flushed skin. If taken by a cool-natured person without heat symptoms, it can be counterproductive by creating excess coolness. In these circumstances, the cooling nature can be balanced by combining Goldenseal with warming herbs such as Ginger, Cinnamon, or Cayenne. Another consideration is the root's drying action on the mucous membranes. Keep in mind that it is most appropriate for problems involving excessive secretions of mucous or other fluids. Taking Goldenseal to treat dry conditions without adding moisturizing herbs like Marshmallow (*Althaea officinalis*) can increase dryness to create more imbalances.

Goldenseal is generally known as an herbal antibiotic due to the actions of berberine and other alkaloids in the plant. However, strong antimicrobial activity tends to be limited to the tissues that come into direct contact with the herb when it is ingested or applied to the skin. Studies show that berberine is poorly absorbed through the walls of the small intestines when taken orally, although small amounts do get into the bloodstream and have been found in tissues of the heart, kidneys, liver, gallbladder, spleen, lungs, pancreas, uterus, and testes (Bhide, 1969; O'Hara, 1998). Goldenseal's alkaloids are excreted through urine (Chopra, 1932), indicating that some are absorbed into the blood since this is the only way they can circulate through the kidneys to be excreted in urine. The body tends to metabolize berberine in the liver and quickly excrete it in the urine rather than circulating much of it through the body. Yet the small amounts that are circulated in the blood are strong enough to have antimicrobial and medicinal effects in other organs like the spleen, lungs, pancreas, heart, and uterus. Poor intestinal absorption and fast excretion are the primary reasons why many studies have focused on injectable forms of berberine and the other alkaloids.

Goldenseal is often used incorrectly. It is specific for feverish and infectious conditions involving excessive mucous discharge, and is *not* an immune stimulant or preventative for illness. Goldenseal and Echinacea tinctures are sometimes combined in commercial preparations, but this is not the best combination. Echinacea is an immune stimulant most effective when taken in large doses as a preventative following exposure to illness and during the initial phase of infections. Goldenseal should be taken for active infections, and is specifically indicated for excessive mucous discharge.

Mucous Membranes and Immunity: Much of Goldenseal's healing potential resides in its unique toning and normalizing actions on the mucous membranes. These specialized membranes line organs and passageways throughout the respiratory, digestive, and genitourinary tracts. In addition to secreting mucous and white blood cells involved with immunity, mucous membranes provide other components that moisturize and protect tissues from dryness, irritation, and infectious pathogens. Goldenseal exerts anti-inflammatory, anti-catarrhal, astringent, and antimicrobial activity on all mucous membranes.

This is one of the best herbs for healing conditions of catarrh (an old term for excessive mucous or phlegm) and inflammation of the mucous membranes induced by infections or allergies. Chronically inflamed mucous membranes eventually become boggy and overly relaxed, allowing profuse secretions of mucous. Goldenseal's astringent properties help these tissues tighten and regain their normal tone and output of secretions. On the other hand, insufficient flow of mucous leaves tissues dry and unprotected against pathogenic infections. Goldenseal is considered to be an "alterative" to the mucous membranes because it alters and normalizes secretions by reducing excessive amounts of mucous discharge.

Antibodies, also known as immunoglobulins, identify and neutralize invasive pathogens, including bacteria, viruses, fungi, and parasites. Antibodies move through the body in blood and lymphatic fluids. IgM antibodies respond to initial exposures and appear early in the course of infections. Researchers discovered that after two weeks of Goldenseal treatment, IgM increased in lab rats, which indicated strong immune protection (Rehman, 1999). IgA and IgG are other antibodies produced by lymphatic tissues in the mucous membranes lining the gastrointestinal, respiratory, and genitourinary tracts. All these protective antibodies are carried in the secretions of mucous membranes. Goldenseal's antimicrobial properties are probably related to its ability to increase the flow of healthy mucous containing IgM, IgA, and IgG antibodies. Alkaloids within the roots and leaves also directly exert broad-spectrum action against many pathogens.

Eclectic physicians considered Goldenseal to be most beneficial for subacute and chronic inflammation, but did not typically prescribe it for acute inflammation. Due to its drying effect, they used it for cases of excess mucous secretion rather than undersecretion. Harvey Felter, M.D., wrote, "It should be considered when subacute and chronic inflammation with free secretions are present. The more the tendency toward chronic debility with oversecretion the more effective is hydrastis. It first relieves the irritation, then restrains the secretions, and finally gives tone to the membranes" (Felter, 1922).

Antimicrobial Action against Colds, Flu, Sinus and Respiratory Infections, Candida Yeast, and Parasites: Goldenseal root is helpful for resolving these infections by reducing uncomfortable symptoms and hastening recovery. The herb's superb antimicrobial and tonifying actions on the mucous membranes reduce infections, inflammation, and excessive phlegm drainage and congestion, making it an excellent remedy for sinus and respiratory problems. It is specifically indicated for profuse secretion of thick yellow or green mucous, which indicates more severe infection and heat. Goldenseal roots have traditionally been used to treat the common cold, influenza (flu), sinus infections, laryngitis, sore throats, tonsillitis, and respiratory tract infections that include bronchitis, pneumonia, and wet, productive coughs. Remember that **Goldenseal is contraindicated for dry coughs** due to its astringent property.

Eclectic physicians prescribed Goldenseal root tea as a gargle for sore throats and to be taken internally for pharyngitis, chronic sinus infections, and sinus and nasal congestion accompanied by thick mucous and sinus headaches. Harvey Felter, M.D., wrote, "Hydrastis preparations are among the most successful remedies in catarrhs of the nose and throat" (Felter, 1922). Research shows that gargling and drinking the tea is helpful for strep throat infections because berberine inhibits *Streptococcus* bacteria from adhering to tissues lining the throat (Sun, 1988).

Many historical uses of Goldenseal have been validated by modern research. Berberine and hydrastine extracted from the roots have demonstrated strong, broad-spectrum antimicrobial activity in many *in vitro* and animal studies, although it must be acknowledged that the results of these studies do not always represent actions of the alkaloids when ingested by people. Berberine is a strong antibacterial against strains of *Mycoplasma* that attack the lungs and urogenital tract, and it interferes with the ability of some bacteria (like *Streptococcus*) to adhere to mucous membranes (Buhner, 2013). Berberine's effectiveness against other bacteria include *Staphylococcus* spp., *Streptococcus* spp., *Shigella* (causes dysentery), *Vibrio cholerae* (causes cholera), *Salmonella paratyphi* (responsible for paratyphoid), *Corynebacterium diphtheriae* (causes diphtheria), *Diplococcus pneumoniae* (causes pneumonia), *Mycobacterium tuberculosis* (causes tuberculosis), *Bacillus cereus* (a source of food poisoning), *Escherichia coli* (a source of urinary tract infections), *Neisseria meningitidis* (causes meningitis), *Chlamydia trachomatis* (sexually transmitted urogenital infection), *Neisseria gonorrhoeae* (causes gonorrhea), and *Treponema pallidum* (source of syphilis). Berberine is active against several types of *Candida* yeast, *Entamoeba histolytica* (a parasite responsible for dysentery and liver abscess), *Giardia lamblia* (an intestinal parasite), and *Trichomonas vaginalis* (caused by a sexually transmitted parasite) (Birdsall, 1997; Hahn, 1976; Kaneda, 1991; Pizzorno, 1988; Preininger, 1975).

In vitro tests have shown berberine to be 90-99.97% effective in inhibiting the growth of several type A and B flu viruses (Lesnau, 1990), specifically H1N1 influenza A, known as swine flu (Cecil, 2011). Berberine is active against other viral infections, including herpes simplex virus 1 and 2, cytomegalovirus, hepatitis B, West Nile virus, dengue fever (a mosquito-transmitted virus), and yellow fever virus (Buhner, 2013).

Although isolated berberine has been the focus of most research, remember that the synergistic blend of all the chemicals in whole plant parts provides the best broad-spectrum healing. Studies show that whole leaf extracts of Goldenseal have more potent antimicrobial activity than when the isolated berberine is used alone against methicillin-resistant *Staphylococcus aureus* (MRSA) (Cech, 2012). The alkaloid canadaline has exerted greater bactericidal activity than berberine against Gram-positive bacteria (Scazzocchio, 2001).

The cooling, febrifuge quality of Goldenseal reduces fevers and inflammation that often accompany infections. In one research study involving rats, berberine's ability to reduce fevers was three times greater than that of aspirin (Sabir, 1978). Although aspirin suppressed fevers, berberine helped by enhancing the immune system's ability to neutralize infectious pathogens that caused the fever.

To eliminate Candida yeast, take Goldenseal capsules, tea, or tincture several times a day, in addition to douching with a strong decoction tea if the yeast is vaginal. For thrush, a yeast infection in the mouth, gargle the tea as a mouthwash several times a day.

Use Goldenseal tea as a nasal spray to experience one of the best remedies for people suffering from acute or chronic sinus infections, the common cold, or allergies accompanied with mucous drainage or congestion. The filtered tea can be poured into a neti pot or plastic nasal spray bottle. Pour or spray the tea into each nostril 3-4 times during the day to allow direct contact with the sinus cavities. This produces quite an exhilarating rush and works to relieve painful inflammation, normalize mucous production, and eliminate bacteria, mold, and yeast. Chronic sinus problems are often caused by a proliferation of these pathogens that incubate and reproduce in the warmth, moisture, and darkness of the sinus cavities. Goldenseal tea nasal spray is the first line of defense I enlist for any symptoms of a cold, sinus infection, or air-borne allergy. Several friends and clients have been able to discontinue their pharmaceutical antihistamines and nasal sprays after using Goldenseal nasal spray for 1-3 weeks.

My favorite and most successful blend for treating the common cold, flu, and respiratory tract infections includes Goldenseal combined with equal parts Boneset (*Eupatorium perfoliatum*), Blue Vervain (*Verbena hastata*), Echinacea (*Echinacea purpurea*), Yarrow (*Achillea millefolium*), Isatis (*Isatis tinctoria*), Sage (*Salvia officinalis*), and Mullein (*Verbascum thapsus*). A popular respiratory formula prescribed by the Eclectic physicians was 5 drops each of Goldenseal, Lobelia (*Lobelia inflata*), and Cayenne (*Capsicum annuum*) tinctures added to water and ingested every 3 hours as needed. Powered Myrrh (*Commiphora myrrha*) is an outstanding herb to take with Goldenseal for bacterial infections and Candida yeast. Use ¼-½ parts Myrrh to 1 part Goldenseal. Remember to eat a light diet of vegetables and protein when fighting infections, and abstain from meat and mucous-forming sugar, bread and grains containing gluten, and dairy products.

Digestive System: Small doses of Goldenseal tone and normalize mucous membranes lining the gastrointestinal tract, and are an old remedy for many digestive problems. Astringent properties benefit mucous membranes by normalizing their secretions and improving atonic conditions in which membranes leak fluids. Astringent actions also strengthen muscle tone to hold organs in place and prevent prolapse.

Goldenseal's bitterness stimulates secretion of bile from the liver and digestive enzymes from the stomach and pancreas. This promotes optimal appetite, absorption of nutrients, peristaltic action, and bowel movements.

Berberine fights bacterial and fungal infections in the digestive tract by increasing levels of immunoglobulin A antibodies (IgA) in the mucous membranes. It is effective against pathogens causing food poisoning, gastrointestinal infections, dysentery, and diarrhea. Berberine exhibits antimicrobial activity against the oral pathogens *Streptococcus mutans* (causing tooth decay) and *Fusobacterium nucleatum*, a common bacteria in the mouth contributing to plaque formation and periodontal disease (Hwang, 2003). Although bitter-tasting, Goldenseal tea can be prepared as a mouthwash or gargle to neutralize excess acids causing canker sores and ulcerations in the mouth and throat. The powdered root may also be applied directly to inflamed gums and canker sores. Ingesting the alkaline herb also helps these problems.

The Eclectic physicians prescribed this stimulating herb as a tonic to increase nerve stimulation and movement in a sluggish digestive system, recommending that 10-20 drops of tincture be taken before meals. Avoid excessive amounts of Goldenseal because it may eventually cool and weaken the digestive organs.

Stomach and Pancreas: The roots are helpful for indigestion, gastritis (stomach inflammation), nausea, and gas. The cooling alkaloids ease heartburn, acid reflux, and stomach or intestinal ulcers, while neutralizing excessive acids responsible for these conditions. Combining Goldenseal with moisturizing, mucilaginous herbs like Marshmallow root or Slippery Elm bark (*Ulmus rubra*) aid in soothing inflammation and healing damaged tissues. Researchers have documented that berberine and hydrastine occurring in alcohol extracts of Goldenseal root inhibited the *in vitro* growth of 15 strains of the *Helicobacter pylori* bacteria, one cause of stomach ulcers (Mahady, 2003). When stomach secretions of hydrochloric acid are deficient, the herb stimulates their increased production and secretion necessary for the digestion of proteins and minerals. Goldenseal also has a healing effect on the pancreas and promotes secretion of pancreatic enzymes to break down and digest food.

Liver, Gallbladder, and Intestines: Goldenseal is a wonderful liver tonic having a stimulating, detoxifying, and strengthening influence on the liver and gallbladder. As a cholagogue, it stimulates bile production in the liver and its secretion into the gallbladder and small intestines. Bile dissolves fats and stimulates peristaltic action in the intestines, allowing normal bowel movements. Goldenseal benefits most liver and gallbladder problems, including inflammation, cirrhosis, and jaundice. Animal studies show that berberine stimulates the secretion of bile and bilirubin (Chan, 1977), which cleans and decongests the liver to protect against gallstones and high cholesterol levels. Berberine improves chronic cholecystitis (gallbladder inflammation) and helps normalize elevated levels of the amino acid tyramine in patients with liver cirrhosis (Watanabe, 1982). The accumulation of tyramine occurring with cirrhosis causes accelerated cardiac output, reduced kidney function, and cerebral dysfunction. One clinical study evaluated the effects of berberine on 225 patients with chronic cholecystitis. Within 48 hours, ingestion of 5-20 mg of berberine 3 times a day successfully eliminated symptoms, decreased abnormal bilirubin levels, and increased the amount of bile secreted by the gallbladder (Pizzorno, 1988).

In a randomized, placebo-controlled clinical trial at a Chinese hospital, the effects of Goldenseal were investigated in 91 patients diagnosed with high cholesterol. Patients received either oral berberine (0.5 gm twice daily) or a placebo for 3 months. Blood samples revealed that berberine significantly lowered serum cholesterol by 18%, triglycerides by 28%, and low density lipoprotein (LDL) by 20% in all patients. The beneficial high density lipoprotein (HDL) levels were not changed. The placebo group showed no changes, while berberine improved liver function without diminishing kidney function (Kong, 2004).

Other researchers compared the ability of a whole root extract against isolated berberine in lowering cholesterol in hamsters during a 24-day study. The hamsters were fed a high cholesterol diet and divided into a group that received a daily dose of isolated berberine, another group that got a daily dose of Goldenseal root extract, and the control group that received neither. The whole root extract reduced plasma levels of total cholesterol by 31.3%, LDL cholesterol by 25.1%, and triglycerides by 32.6% compared with the control group. The extract of the whole root showed 2-3 times the activity of isolated berberine, indicating that the synergistic blend of phytochemicals produced the greatest improvement compared to using berberine alone. Interestingly, another alkaloid, canadine, exhibited stronger activity than berberine. In addition, the whole root extract decreased serum levels of unhealthy VLDL (very low density lipoproteins) and LDL without reducing levels of beneficial HDL (Abidi, 2006).

Studies indicate that berberine prevents certain bacteria from adhering to intestinal walls, and that it relaxes smooth muscle in the small intestines to prolong the transit time of food (Birdsall, 1997). Smooth muscle relaxation also eases cramps. Astringent properties assist in shrinking hemorrhoids. Antimicrobial and anti-inflammatory actions on the mucous membranes in the intestinal tract are helpful for ulcerative colitis, Crohn's disease, and dysentery and diarrhea caused by bacteria or parasites. Several clinical studies reveal Goldenseal's ability to treat infectious diarrhea. One study involving 200 adults suffering from acute bacterial diarrhea showed that those given 150 mg of berberine daily in addition to standard antibiotic therapy recovered faster than those only receiving antibiotics. Thirty additional adults were treated with berberine alone, which completely arrested diarrhea in all cases (Kamat, 1974). Another study of 65 children younger than 5 years of age revealed that berberine was more effective than standard antibiotic therapy for acute diarrhea caused by *E. coli* and other bacteria (Sack, 1982). These and other clinical studies show that berberine is very effective against acute diarrhea caused by *E. coli, Shigella dysenteriae, Salmonella paratyphi, Klebsiella, Entamoeba histolytica, Vibrio cholerae,* and *Giardia lamblia* (Rabbani, 1987 & 1996; Gupte, 1975; Subbaiah, 1967). In a placebo-controlled clinical study, 40 children between ages 1-10 who were infected with *Giardia lamblia* received berberine, metronidazole, or a placebo of vitamin B syrup in 3 divided doses. After 6 days, 48% of the children treated with berberine were symptom-free and 68% of these children were free of Giardia determined by a stool sample test. Only 33% of the group who took metronidazole were free of symptoms and Giardia in their stools (Choudhry, 1972; Kaneda, 1991).

An old formula, recommended by the late clinical herbalist Jethro Kloss, is especially beneficial to the liver, gallbladder, pancreas, spleen, and kidneys. It includes equal amounts of Goldenseal, Red Clover blossoms (*Trifolium pratense*), Yellow Dock (*Rumex crispus*), and Dandelion (*Taraxacum officinale*).

Urinary Tract: Due to its antibiotic and normalizing activity on the mucous membranes, Goldenseal's healing ability extends to the kidneys and bladder. The herb is excreted through urine, allowing direct contact with the kidneys, ureters, bladder, and urethra. Used in combination with other appropriate herbs, it is wonderful for inflammation and infection in the urinary tract, including cystitis. As a mild diuretic, the root stimulates urination to reduce edema. Men can ingest the herb for prostate inflammation.

Women's Health: Goldenseal is classified as an emmenagogue because the strong alkaloids stimulate uterine muscles to contract and promote menstruation (Farnsworth, 1975). Therefore, **pregnant women should not ingest Goldenseal**. However, external application on the skin is safe during pregnancy. The tea can be added to a sitz bath in combination with other herbs, especially Comfrey (*Symphytum officinale*), to heal torn perineal tissues following childbirth.

Goldenseal's ability to strengthen muscle tone improves bladder and uterine prolapse. The herb's astringent and hemostatic properties inhibit abnormal bleeding due to uterine fibroids and endometriosis. Eclectic physicians prescribed the herb for painful menorrhagia (excessive menstrual bleeding) and leucorrhea, a vaginal discharge caused by bacteria, parasites, or yeast infections. The tea prepared as a douche or suppositories made from powdered roots are excellent remedies for all types of vaginal infections and abnormal discharges, including Candida yeast and *Trichomonas vaginalis* (a sexually transmitted parasite).

To make suppositories, mix 1 part each of Goldenseal and Myrrh (*Commiphora myrrha*) with 4 parts Slippery Elm powder. Combine this with enough water to produce a thick paste. Roll the paste into the shape of suppositories about the size of your little finger, and dry them in room air or a low oven. Insert a suppository far up into the vagina before bedtime. **To prepare a vaginal douche**, use these same ingredients to make a tea. The suppositories or douche should be used daily until all symptoms are gone, and then continued every third day for another 2 weeks to ensure that the infection is completely eliminated.

Blood and Lymphatic Fluid: As an alterative, Goldenseal gradually restores normal body function by purifying the blood, lymphatic fluids, and spleen. Its cleansing and energizing action on the spleen and liver improves the quality of blood. The roots contain minerals that alkalize blood, neutralize excess acids, and reduce blood and lymphatic toxins. Excess acids can be an underlying cause of many conditions such as inflammation, arthritis, skin eruptions, canker sores, heartburn, and chronic sinus congestion or drainage. Goldenseal is an excellent treatment for swollen lymph nodes, especially when combined with Echinacea tincture and very small amounts of Poke (*Phytolacca decandra*) tincture (only 4 drops 3 times a day due to potential toxicity of Poke).

Heart and Circulation: The berberine and other alkaloids in Goldenseal improve cardiac function in conditions of heart weakness and help normalize a weak or irregular pulse. In Asia, berberine extracts are used to treat congestive heart failure, hypertension, and cardiac arrhythmia (irregular heart beat). Goldenseal's influence on the cardiovascular system was acknowledged by the Eclectic physicians. Finley Ellingwood, M.D. (1852–1920) wrote, "It stimulates respiration and circulation, imparting tone and increased power to the heart's action, increasing arterial tension and capillary blood pressure . . . . It stimulates normal fibrillar contractility and increased tonus, encouraging the nutrition of muscular structure" (Ellingwood, 1919). William Cook, M.D., noted, "Though a stimulant, and hence sustaining to the circulation, it never excites or forces the pulse; and it is unlike almost all other stimulating tonics in soothing the irritation connected with feeble and congested conditions of mucous membranes . . . . It has an excellent sustaining influence on the nervous tissues, and upon the pulse when its caliber is diminished from nervous fatigue and exhaustion" (Cook, 1869).

Goldenseal equalizes circulation throughout the body. The Eclectic pharmacist John Uri Lloyd (1849–1936) noted its value for treating chronic blood congestion and stagnation in the liver, spleen, uterus, and abdomen. Harvey Felter, M.D. (1865–1927) wrote, "Hydrastis controls passive hemorrhage. It is not adapted to copious active hemorrhages, as gastric and post-partum hemorrhages, but in those forms only of renal, uterine, or pulmonary bleeding in which small quantities of blood are passed at a time and are recurrent in form. It is a comparatively slow-acting drug in most forms of hemorrhage, but its effects are permanent" (Felter, 1922).

Animal and human trials show that intravenous (IV) berberine exerts a mild systemic vasodilation (blood vessels relax and expand) that improves circulation, impaired function of the heart ventricles, and the re-oxygenation of heart muscle (Snow, 1998). Several Chinese researchers have found that IV administration of berberine reduces high blood pressure, tachycardia (rapid heartbeat), arrhythmia, and heart damage in animals and people (Zhou, 1993; Huang, 1990, 1992 & 1992b). In a double-blind clinical trial involving 165 patients with congestive heart failure, coronary artery disease and tachycardia, half were given 300 mg of berberine 4 times a day and the other half received a placebo. All participants continued their prescription medications during the study. Compared with the placebo group, those taking berberine experienced a significant increase in left ventricular ejection, improved exercise capacity, and decreased arrhythmias. There was also a 47% decrease in mortality over a 2-year period in the berberine group, and no side effects were noted (Zeng, 2003). A small study of 12 patients with severe congestive heart failure revealed that IV administration of berberine significantly reduced blood pressure while improving ejection of blood from the heart. The patients experienced improved circulation and oxygen saturation in their blood (Martin-Neti, 1988).

Goldenseal works especially well for the cardiovascular system when it is combined with Hawthorn berries (*Crataegus* spp.), Cayenne, and the bis-glycinate form of magnesium.

Ears and Eyes: For earaches and infections, 3-4 drops of the filtered tea or tincture can be placed in each ear 3-4 times a day. Goldenseal tea is an excellent eyewash for eye injuries, inflammation, redness, and itchy irritation due to allergies, and for infections including conjunctivitis. **Never put alcohol tincture in the eyes!**

In the early 1900s, Goldenseal tea was a popular eyewash. Berberine and hydrastine were added to many commercial eye drop preparations for their antiseptic and astringent properties that reduced infections and inflammation (McCaleb, 2000). I have often used and recommended Goldenseal tea to eliminate conjunctivitis and itchy, irritated eyes, especially during hay fever season. Good results are obtained by putting 3-6 drops of the filtered tea in each eye 2-4 times a day. Several times, I have used only one application of the tea to successfully eliminate styes, which appear as small red bumps on the outside or inside of the eyelids. When located on the outside of the eyelid, styes are infections of the sebaceous glands. Styes on the inner eyelid are infected apocrine sweat glands. Styes contain pus and are usually caused by *Staphylococcus aureus* bacteria, which will spread if the stye is forcefully ruptured.

Berberine has been employed for the serious infectious eye disease known as trachoma caused by *Chlamydia trachomatis*, the bacteria responsible for blindness and impaired vision in many people living in tropical and underdeveloped countries. Sulfacetamide is the drug most often used for trachoma. In clinical trials, sulfacetamide produced the fastest improvement of symptoms, yet patients still tested positive for the presence of *Chlamydia trachomatis* in their eyes and reported high rates of recurrence. Those who used berberine eye drops in a 0.2% solution experienced a slower recovery period, but eventually all traces of the bacteria disappeared and no relapses occurred within a year of the treatment (Babbar, 1982; Mohan, 1982).

Immune Enhancement and Cancer: Goldenseal was traditionally employed by Native American woodland tribes as a cancer treatment. Currently, *in vitro* and *in vivo* research studies reveal that berberine enhances immunity by stimulating the number and activity of white blood cells to destroy cancerous cells (Wagner, 1985). Berberine activates macrophages, which are immune cells that search out, engulf, digest, and destroy bacteria, viruses, cancer cells, and other pathogens (Kumazawa, 1984; Pizzorno, 1988; Sabir, 1971; Clement-Kruzel, 2008). Berberine also promotes optimal function and immune activity of the spleen, a primary organ of the immune system and site of IgM antibody production. The spleen consists of sheaths of lymphatic tissue that surround many blood vessels. Berberine's action increases blood supply to the spleen and filters pathogens out of the blood (Sabir, 1971).

Human and animal studies demonstrate berberine's potent antitumor activity in malignant brain tumors (Rong-Xun, 1990) and skin cancers in mice (Nishino, 1986). This phytochemical is a beneficial addition to cancer therapy and has been administered in Chinese medical practice since 1972 to treat abnormally low white blood cell counts (leukopenia) caused by chemotherapy and radiation. A Chinese clinical study involving 405 cancer patients with leukopenia documented that 50 mg of berberine taken orally 3 times a day for 1-4 weeks was significantly effective in elevating white blood cells in 40.2% of the patients, effective in 38.8%, and ineffective in 21% of the cases (Liu, 1991). Naturopathic physician William Mitchell also reported berberine's ability to increase white blood cell counts in cancer patients with leukopenia caused by chemotherapy (Mitchell, 2003).

External Uses: Goldenseal's ability to reduce bleeding, cool inflamed tissues, and kill bacteria, fungi, and yeast make it excellent for all types of external healing. This includes open wounds and cuts, many skin diseases, infections, eruptions, itching, ulcers, acne, eczema, fungal infections (ringworm and athlete's foot), diaper rash, skin cancers, impetigo, and all external staph infections.

Goldenseal is a common ingredient in most commercial herbal salves and ointments. The powdered root may also be used as a poultice and sprinkled directly on the affected skin, or water can be added to the powdered root and made into a paste for external application. A strong decoction tea may be used as a bath, or a washcloth saturated with the tea can be applied to the skin as a fomentation.

For hemorrhoids, use an ointment or suppository. For fungal infections, take 3-4 capsules of powered Goldenseal root throughout the day and apply Goldenseal powder externally by adding enough water to make a thick paste. Another option is to soak the affected area with a strong tea of the root.

In his *Book of Herbal Wisdom*, herbalist Matthew Wood tells several stories of people ingesting the tincture and applying it to torn spinal disks, knee meniscus, and other torn tissue with excellent results (Wood, 1997).

Teachings from the Goldenseal Deva

"Greetings, dear one. I am the Goldenseal Deva, a warrior woman and protective mother of the forest lands. Although my plants contain the masculine quality of sharp bitterness that cuts through and destroys infectious organisms, this is tempered by the feminine side of my nature that is gentle, nurturing, and protective. My plants require the shade and moisture of woodlands, so they are equipped to resist molds and bacteria that thrive in this habitat. The substances in my leaves and roots that protect them from damage also fight off bacteria and fungi in the human body. This is how plant medicine works. Our plant bodies must be protected against dangers from the environments we live in, just as humans need defenses. The substances that protect plants do the same for humans. In this way, plants and people share an intimate relationship.

"My protective actions focus on parts of the body that are most exposed to the dangers in the external environment. My healing power moves and operates through the fluids in the body that I keep healthy by guarding against infectious invaders. The smooth ebb and flow of fluids in the membranes is moderated by my medicines to bring forth balance. If mucous pours out in excess, I slow it down. To support digestion, I promote the easy movement of fluids carrying enzymes that break down and digest food. This allows food to travel through the stomach and intestines with ease. I assist the natural flow of urine and of blood during the time of women's menses. In the lymphatic fluids and blood, my medicine provides cleansing and fluidity of movement. I also support the liver and kidneys that process fluids so they can eliminate waste and infectious substances from the body. And so my healing gifts are focused upon these organs and tissues that regulate the waters of the body and offer vibrant health.

"My plants are a balanced blend of the elements. The fire element is strong within my being and provides powerful protective energy that destroys impurities and pathogens, just as fire envelopes and destroys all in its path. The fiery golden-yellow color of my roots and crimson-red color of my berries can remind you of my fire qualities. My plants regulate and act as guardian of the water element. This affinity with water is seen in my ability to create change in the body's fluids by destroying and washing away impurities. The air element directs healing to the lungs and airways and eases breathing. Like a strong wind, my medicine forcefully expels infections and thick secretions from the airways. And the earth element brings vibrant health and calm to the tissues after my powerful medicine has cleansed the fluids and tissues of the body.

"My actions are influenced by the energies of Jupiter and Saturn. Jupiter empowers my medicine with swift movement and strength of purpose to remove impurities. This expansive activity is reflected in the shape of my flowers consisting of many long filaments bursting out like shafts of light radiating from the sun. The white color of my flowers reflects this quality of cleansing and purification that promotes peaceful harmony in the body. The yellow tips of my flowers and deep-golden color of my roots point to affinity with the solar plexus and digestive system, which my medicines also protect from harmful infections and inflammation. Just as Saturn is a stern gatekeeper requiring people to complete lessons in life before moving forward, I am a gatekeeper watching over and protecting the waterways from intruders.

"I am a plant of old that was valued and used by the native people who once lived upon this land they called Turtle Island. I came to assist those people and protect their bodies against harm. They recognized and used my healing virtues for so many problems, both internal and external. My roots and leaves were pulverized between stones and placed upon wounds, bites, and infections. My plants retain memory of those beloved people who have been slaughtered and destroyed. This, too, has been my lot, as huge populations of my plants have been pulled out of the ground.

"The wisdom I offer comes with remembrance of kinship between people and plants and the earth. We are all of the same life force dancing together in the flow of life, serving and depending upon each other. Embracing this reality brings the enriching golden light of my essence into your heart space. My flowers and roots help people to be grounded in the flow of life and pure in body, while armed to respond to adversity. To connect deep into the golden vibration of my essence is to be immersed in fullness of heart and in the expanse of all life. Be in peace and wellness."

Holy Basil (Tulsi)

Ocimum sanctum
Ocimum tenuiflorum (the more recent species name)
Labiatae (*Lamiaceae*) (Mint) Family

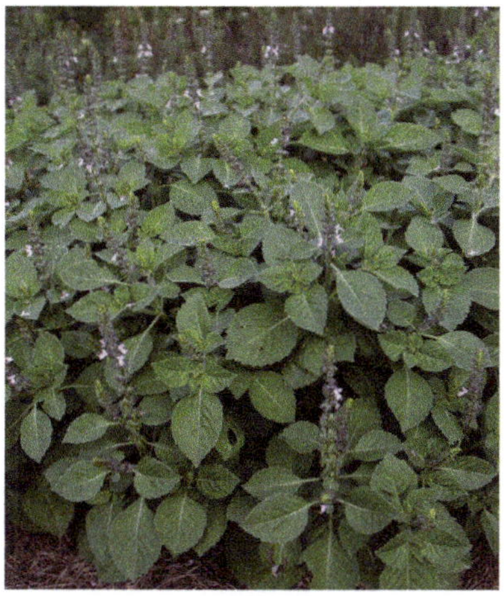

Common Names

In its homeland of India, Holy Basil is known by many common names reflecting the deep reverence people feel for this amazing plant. It is most commonly called "Tulsi," which in Sanskrit means "The Incomparable One." It is also known as Indian Basil, Sacred Basil, "The Queen of Herbs," and "The Mother Medicine of Nature."

Medicinal Part of the Plant

The leaves, flowers, seeds, and roots are used for medicinal purposes.

Range and Habitat

Ocimum sanctum is native to India, the Himalayan Mountains, and parts of northern Africa. It is cultivated in many tropical and temperate zones.

Description of the Plant

In tropical India, Holy Basil is a pleasantly aromatic perennial shrub, but in temperate climates it is easily grown as an annual. The uniquely distinct fragrance of the plant is enticing to gardeners and to the bees that create a constant buzzing around the herb when it is blooming.

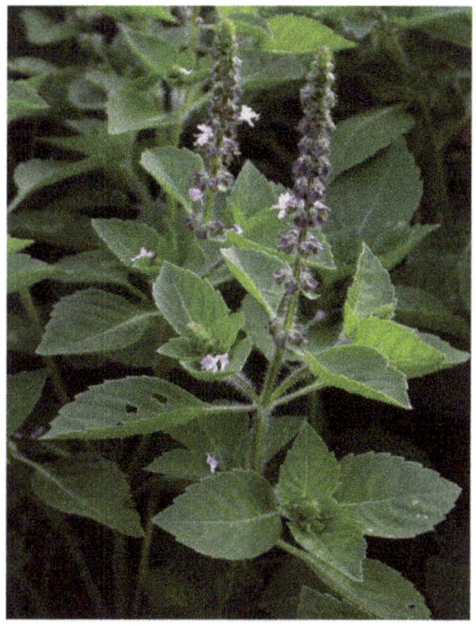

Three varieties of Holy Basil are employed for healing and share similar properties. Rama or Sri Tulsi (*O. sanctum*) has green stems and leaves and is more frost-hardy. Krishna or Shyama Tulsi (also *O. sanctum*), with purple stems and purplish-green leaves, is the most esteemed variety for medicinal uses. Vana Tulsi (*O. gratissimum*) translates as "very grateful" or "pleasing" Basil. It grows wild in its natural habitat and is also called Forest Tulsi. Holy Basil plants exhibit significant variations in size, form, and chemical constituents depending on climate, rainfall, and soil chemistry and fertility. These factors influence the medicinal strength and efficacy of the herb.

In temperate climates, *O. sanctum* is an attractive plant reaching 1-2′ in height. The roots are fibrous. Simple leaves grow opposite each other on square stems. Leaves are ovate with pinnate veins and serrated teeth margins. Soft hairs cover the leaves and stems. Small purple flowers appear on multiple upright spikes. The calyx has 5 sepals, and flowers consist of 5 petals arranged as 2 lobes with 4 stamens. The flowers produce many seeds that fall to the ground around the parent plant and typically germinate prolifically the following spring.

Cultivation

Tulsi prefers growing in full sun and rich soil with plenty of water and good drainage. It is easy to grow by seed germination. Sow the seeds indoors or in a greenhouse in early spring, or sow them in window boxes or a garden bed after the soil has warmed. Plant the small seeds just below the surface of the soil and press in firmly. Keep them watered until germination occurs within 1-2 weeks. When seedlings are 2-3″ tall, they can be thinned or transplanted 1′ apart.

In my southern Indiana gardens, Tulsi cultivation requires little work, making it one of the easiest annual herbs to grow. The plants thrive during the warm months as I prune them regularly to make teas and tinctures. In autumn, the seeds fall to the ground and germinate effortlessly in late spring the following year to fill the garden with lush plants. This yearly cycle continues on its own without planting additional seeds.

Harvest

Harvest the leaves and flowers as soon as the fragrant flowers begin to bloom. By moderately pruning Tulsi plants, they will continue growing to provide many harvests throughout the summer and early autumn. Allow some plants to produce seeds that will drop to the ground and germinate the following spring. To harvest seeds for future sowing, gather them when the flower heads are dry and brown.

Preparation of Plant Medicine and Dosages

Freshly harvested leaves and flowers are prepared as tincture, tea, oil, salve, or they are dried. Seeds are safe to ingest for the same purposes as the leaves and flowers. The herb has a delicious flavor reflecting its distinct aroma and brews into a wonderfully refreshing tea that may be enjoyed on a daily basis.

PREPARATIONS

Tea: Steep 1-2 teaspoons of freshly harvested or dried leaves and flowers for 5-10 minutes. Dosage: 1-5 cups a day. Larger dosages are helpful for treating specific problems.

Tincture: Chop fresh leaves and flowers, stuff them into a glass jar, and cover with a mix of 65% 190-proof grain alcohol and 35% distilled water. Dosage: 30-60 drops 1-3 times a day as needed.

Tablets or Capsules: Dosage: In India's Ayurvedic system, the traditional dose for preventative therapy is 300-600 mg of dried leaves per day for at least 6 months. For curative treatment of existing problems, 900-1800 mg is recommended in divided doses for 2-12 months as needed.

Poultice: The leaves are prepared fresh or dry for external application.

Oil and salve: Chop leaves, flowers and roots, cover with olive oil and bake at 200°F for 2-3 hours.

Culinary Uses

Tulsi may be added to a wide variety of foods for flavoring in similar ways as regular Basil.

Chemical Constituents

Tulsi is richly endowed with antioxidants, fats, proteins, beta-carotene (vitamin A), ascorbic acid (vitamin C), calcium, iron, zinc, selenium, and manganese.

The large concentrations of volatile oils are analgesic, carminative, antioxidant, anti-inflammatory, and antimicrobial. Oils include linalool, beta-caryophyllene, elemene, eugenol (choleretic, hepatoprotective, vasodilator), carvacrol (antispasmodic, antitussive, carminative, expectorant, vermifuge), methyl chavicol (known as estragole), terpinen-4-ol (the active ingredient in Tea Tree oil that kills mites), salinene, alpha-pinene, beta-pinene, camphene, thymol, rhymol, camphor, xanthomicrol, caffeate, myrcenol (anti-asthmatic), nerol (anti-asthmatic), and ursolic acid. Studies validate ursolic acid's protective action on nerve, liver and skin tissues, as well as immunomodulatory benefits. Volatile oils are primarily terpenes and phenols (Singh, 2002). Polyphenols include vanillin, caffeic, gallic, rosmarinic, and chlorogenic acids.

Saponins possess antitumor and immunomodulator properties. Sterols include campesterol, stigmasterol, and beta-sitosterol (antibacterial, anticancer, antioxidant, antiviral, diuretic, febrifuge, hepatoprotective). Flavonoids are potent antioxidants and include vicenin-2, galuteolin, cirsilineol, cirsimaritin, isothymusin, and apigenin.

Safety, Contraindications, and Drug Interactions

Tulsi is a safe beverage tea and medicinal remedy for all ages, including the very young. No serious side effects or drug interactions have been reported with normal dosages. Since it is a warming herb, Ayurvedic practitioners suggest that people with overly heated pitta conditions use it in moderation and add cooling herbs for balance. Although Tulsi has safely been employed to promote male and female fertility for hundreds of years in India, it is contraindicated during pregnancy in some literature. This is the result of a study in which large amounts of the herb decreased fertility in rats (Batta, 1971). The accuracy of this conclusion based on one study is questionable and does not reflect the herb's historic use in human populations.

Medicinal Uses

History of the Plant

For thousands of years, Tulsi has been one of the most cherished and sacred plants in the Hindu religious tradition, and continues to be one of the most important herbs in Ayurvedic medicine. The Indian people revere this simple plant for its beauty, its wonderful fragrance that permeates the air like incense, its delicious flavor, and its legendary healing power. It appears in many ancient Indian medical texts written from 500 B.C. to A.D. 1200, which refer to its great popularity and wide range of applications in healing. India's ancient scriptures and holy epics, the *Bhagavata Purana* and *Mahabharata*, tell of the Tulsi goddess who was a devotee of Lord Vishnu (one of the three supreme gods in Hinduism). The goddess was reincarnated in the form of the Tulsi plant to express her love and devotion to her Lord (Garg, 1982).

A passage from the *Padmapurana*, a 5,000-year-old healing text from India, proclaims, "Leaves, flowers, fruits, root, branches and the main stem and everything about Tulsi is sacred; even the soil under the Tulsi plant is holy." In another passage, Lord Shiva glorifies the power of the herb saying,

"Every house, every village, every forest, wherever the plant of Tulsi is grown, there misery, fear, disease and poverty do not exist. Tulsi in all aspects and places is holier than holy. Where the breeze blows through Tulsi plants, it spreads Tulsi's fragrance making the surrounding area pious and pure. Lord Vishnu and other gods shower their blessing on the people who worship and grow Tulsi. Through the worship of Tulsi, the souls of our ancestors are pleased and our path to the heavens is opened . . . . The three gods, Brahma, Vishnu, and Rudra [Shiva] reside in the roots, middle parts of the plant, and in the flowering tops respectively. This is why the plant of Tulsi is the most holy plant of the earth."

Regarded as a goddess in the form of a plant, Tulsi has been included in religious rituals and festivals since ancient times, especially those venerating Lords Vishnu and Krishna. Tulsi is known to open and purify the heart and mind, calm the soul, offer protection, and promote compassion, mental clarity, and serenity. The herb is used in the daily life of many Indians who grow it around their homes, shrines, and temples.

The name "Basil" comes from the Latin word *basilicum*, meaning "royal." The genus name *Ocimum* translates as "fragrant lipped" for the two-lipped flowers, while *sanctum* means "sacred." More recently, Tulsi has been given the Latin name *Ocimum tenuiflorum*, meaning "Basil with small, slender flowers."

Modern science validates many of Tulsi's historic applications. The majority of research has involved animal studies, but several human trials have been conducted as well. Tulsi's fame has spread to the Western world, where it is enjoyed as a popular beverage tea.

Healing Qualities

The leaves possess adaptogen, alterative, anticarcinogenic, antifungal, anti-inflammatory, antimicrobial, antioxidant, antiparasitic, antirheumatic, antiseptic, antispasmodic, carminative, diaphoretic, diuretic, expectorant, febrifuge, hepatoprotective, mild hypotensive, immunomodulator, nervine, nutritive, tonic, and vasodilating properties. The seeds are antioxidant, mucilaginous, and demulcent.

Ayurvedic Medical Perspective

Tulsi is warming and drying with a mild spicy, pungent flavor. In Ayurvedic medicine, Tulsi is considered to be a regulator of the three doshas: the elements of kapha (water and earth), pitta (fire), and vata (air). These three doshas control all functions of the body. (Refer to page 45 in the chapter "History of Herbalism and Early Medicine" for an expanded explanation of the Ayurvedic Medical perspective and the doshas.) Tulsi harmonizes and regulates the doshas and different systems of the body, making it beneficial for a broad spectrum of physical and psychological ailments.

The Ayurvedic tradition recognizes the tremendous significance of Tulsi as a calming elixir that heals the mind, body, and spirit. It is traditionally employed to reduce stress and fatigue and to promote general health, vitality, longevity, and peace of mind. Practitioners prescribe the herb to treat the common cold, fevers, coughs and respiratory problems, abdominal bloating and gas, headaches, arthritis, depression, nerve deterioration, cognitive and memory loss, and poisoning. Tulsi helps prevent the accumulation of fat in the body, especially for menopausal women, and addresses obstinate skin diseases. It is often taken in combination with other herbs, especially with other adaptogens such as American Ginseng (*Panax quinquefolius*), Asian Ginseng (*Panax ginseng*), Astragalus (*Astragalus membranaceus*), Ashwagandha (*Withania somnifera*), and Eleuthero or Siberian Ginseng (*Eleutherococcus senticosus*).

Primary Actions

I began growing Tulsi several years ago and quickly became entranced by the amazing aroma and healing abilities offered by this bountiful herb, so easy to grow. Each year, visitors to the Tulsi gardens are enthralled and comment on the unusual fragrance and peaceful state-of-being they feel when around the plant.

Tulsi's most amazing gift is its ability to re-calibrate and normalize the nervous and endocrine systems, which are primary regulators of all body functions. Specifically supporting the endocrine glands and nervous system, Tulsi reduces stress responses, restores adrenal health, and improves mental health. Its relaxing, tonifying, and restoring action throughout the body is especially beneficial for the digestive and respiratory organs. The herb boosts immunity and contains rich supplies of antioxidants that protect cells from damage caused by the aging process, environmental and chemical toxins, and radiation. When taken as a tonic over time, Tulsi assists in maintaining vibrant health while preventing and treating many chronic, degenerative conditions. One of my favorite teas, I frequently recommend and give Tulsi tea and tincture to friends and clients. With regular use of the tasty tea or tincture, people report less stress-induced anxiety and headaches, and improved digestion, energy levels, mental clarity, and inner calm.

Stress Relief and Adrenal Restoration: As an invigorating adaptogen, Tulsi enhances the body's ability to adapt to environmental and internal stresses by supporting the endocrine, immune, and nervous systems. When taken as a tonic, it increases physical stamina and endurance, normalizes metabolic functions, and improves the body's resistance to physical and psychological stressors, including environmental pollution.

The body initially responds to stress by activating the sympathetic nervous system and adrenal glands, resulting in the fight-or-flight response. This response increases secretions of the stimulating adrenal hormones and neurotransmitters, epinephrine (adrenaline), norepinephrine and cortisol, causing a state of hyper-alertness with increased heart rate, blood pressure, and sweating. Cortisol levels rise during initial stages of stress. When stress becomes chronic, the adrenals are weakened and production of adrenaline, norepinephrine, and cortisol eventually decline, leaving people feeling physically exhausted and mentally foggy. Since chronic stress is such a common problem in this modern age, many people suffer from weak adrenal glands with resulting depression, chronic fatigue, insomnia, elevated blood sugar levels, weight gain, poor immunity, and compromised cognitive function.

I have enjoyed many opportunities to observe the herb's strengthening and stabilizing influence on clients with weak adrenal function. People usually experience more vitality and improvement in their symptoms within 7-14 days of using Tulsi tea or tincture. One woman suffering from classic adrenal "burn-out" came to my office with symptoms of chronic insomnia, exhaustion, and muscle fatigue and pain. For years she had tried numerous pharmaceuticals and sedating herbs to help her sleep, without success. She started taking about 60 drops of Tulsi tincture at bedtime and was delighted to finally get 6-7 hours of deep sleep each night. Drinking the tea or tincture during the day energized her and provided relief from muscle pain.

Researchers have explored Tulsi's adaptogen functions. Animal studies demonstrate the herb's ability to improve physical performance, endurance, and stamina during stress tests. In one trial that compared the effects of Tulsi and other well-known adaptogens on the swimming ability of mice, researchers found that Tulsi was superior to Ashwagandha, Eleuthero, and Asian Ginseng in reducing stress without side effects. Tulsi protected the animals' adrenal glands from stress reactions while maintaining normal adrenal secretions (Bhargava, 1981; Saksena, 1987; Singh, 1986b).

A clinical study revealed that Tulsi can reduce excessive cortisol production and lower blood sugar levels in diabetic patients (Agrawal, 1996). After 30 years of clinical research, Dr. Narendra Singh, a leading Tulsi researcher in India, documented that an increase in stamina and immunological resistance generally occurs within 1-4 weeks of using Tulsi (Singh, 2002).

Another mechanism of stress reduction is Tulsi's ability to increase production of succinate dehydrogenase (SDH), a result that researchers have observed in the brains of rats. SDH is an enzyme in the mitochondria (sites of energy production) of cells that, when activated by stress, produces and conserves cellular energy. Thus, SDH is beneficial during times of stress to protect cells against harmful free radicals (Kalsi, 1987; Robbins, 1982).

Tulsi is a wonderful remedy for chronic fatigue, a use that has been validated by clinical studies. Within 7 days of taking a daily capsule of Tulsi leaves (300 mg), 50 out of 56 aging patients reported a reduction in their fatigue. After a month of treatment, all patients experienced this improvement (Singh & Abbas, 1995b). In a follow-up study, 27 young Indian men diagnosed with chronic fatigue syndrome experienced similar improvement after taking 500 mg of Tulsi twice a day for 3 months (Singh & Abbas, 1995c).

The Nervous System, Anxiety, Depression, and Hypertension: Tulsi's calming and restorative activity on the nervous system benefits the entire body. Daily use relaxes rigid muscles, eases physical and psychological anxiety and depression, and reduces stress-related, mild-to-moderate hypertension.

The herb's influence on the nervous system and muscles is beneficial for all types of muscle cramps and spasms, including stress headaches. Its adaptogen properties alleviate anxiety. Prolonged periods of stress eventually cause the excitatory neurotransmitters epinephrine (adrenaline) and norepinephrine to decline. Levels of serotonin (a relaxing neurotransmitter) also diminish and dopamine generally elevates. Tulsi's ability to normalize brain chemistry during times of stress has been documented in several mice and rat studies, showing that the herb maintained normal levels of these regulatory substances while reducing the animals' stress responses (Dixit, 1985, 1986 & 1987; Misra, 1987; Singh, 1991b). In a clinical study investigating the effects of the herb on general anxiety disorder, 35 outpatients were enlisted to take 500 mg of Tulsi administered in capsules twice a day for 2 months. Participants reported significant improvement of their anxiety and depression (Bhattacharyya, 2008).

Tulsi's therapeutic intervention on the nervous system, endocrine glands, and neurotransmitters can be beneficial for many neurological and psychological problems, including loss of cognitive function, dementia, attention deficit hyperactivity disorder (ADHD), mania, depression, psychosis, and schizophrenia.

Tulsi possesses several mechanisms to reduce hypertension. Circulation improves because the herb decreases high cholesterol levels and promotes relaxation and dilation of blood vessels. Diuretic properties diminish fluid retention that can contribute to hypertension. Mild anticoagulant constituents in the herb promote normal blood flow and cardiovascular health, which helps prevent and treat blood clots and atherosclerosis. In a study involving 50 hypertensive patients, half were given 500 mg of powdered Tulsi leaves 3 times daily for 6 weeks, while 25 patients took a placebo. After 2 weeks, those taking the herb experienced a significant drop in systolic (26 mm Hg) and diastolic (16 mm Hg) blood pressure that continued for at least 2 weeks after stopping the treatment. No side effects were reported (Singh, 1986b; Srivastava, 1986).

Immunity and Infections: Tulsi is an immunomodulator, and regular ingestion of the tea or tincture strengthens and regulates immunity. The herb activates cell-mediated immunity and the production of T-lymphocytes that protect the body against viral and bacterial infections, environmental toxins, and cancers. Research involving 20 patients who ingested Tulsi over a 4-week period demonstrated this ability and significantly enhanced their cell-mediated immunity (Kumar, 1982; Singh, 1986b; Dixit, 1987). Another trial consisted of 24 healthy volunteers who consumed either 300 mg of Tulsi leaves in a capsule or a placebo every day for 4 weeks. Those taking the herb experienced improvements in several immune parameters, including more protective T-helper cells, natural killer cells, interferon, and interleukins (Mondal, 2011).

The primary detrimental effects of chronic stress and environmental pollution are oxidative stress and damage to cells and the formation of free radicals. These unstable molecules compromise cells to cause cellular death, premature aging, inflammation, and degenerative diseases, including cancers and tumors. Researchers found that antioxidants in Tulsi (vitamins A and C, selenium, flavonoids, and volatile oils) protect against free radical damage in human and animal liver cells (Singh, 1978 & 1986a; Mishra, 1998; Robbins, 1982). These antioxidants have also protected mice and rats from radiation damage (Devi, 1998; Jogetia, 1986). In other studies, ursolic acid and oleanolic acid from Tulsi provided 60% protection against free radical damage in the livers and hearts of rats, and stimulated activity of superoxide dismutase (SOD), a potent antioxidant in animals and humans (Balanehru, 1991 & 1992).

Using *in vivo* and *in vitro* studies, researchers have documented Tulsi's ability to increase levels of other protective antioxidants, including catalase and glutathione, and decrease destructive lipid peroxidation. Antioxidant activity was also evident from the herb's efficacy in scavenging free radicals (Samson, 2007).

Several phytochemicals in Tulsi demonstrate anticancer potential in addition to reducing the destructive effects of radiation therapy on healthy cells. Preclinical studies revealed that urosolic acid, eugenol, rosmarinic acid, apigenin, myretenal, luteolin, sitosterol, and carnosic acid prevented chemically induced skin, mouth, liver, and lung cancers in animals. This prevention was mediated by the herb's ability to increase antioxidant activity, induce apoptosis (programmed destruction of damaged and cancerous cells), and inhibit metastasis and angiogenesis (formation of blood vessels that feed cancer cells). Orintin and vicenin are flavonoids occurring in Tulsi tea that have protected mice against radiation-induced sickness and mortality, while also protecting healthy tissues from the damaging effects of radiation. Eugenol, rosmarinic acid, apigenin, and carnosic acid also prevented radiation-induced DNA damage in research studies (Rastogi, 1995; Baliga, 2013). Tulsi has significantly decreased the incidence of squamous cell carcinoma of the stomach in mice (Aruna, 1992), and topical application has reduced skin tumors (Prashar, 1994; Karthikeyan, 1999).

Tulsi is an appropriate remedy for many bacterial and viral infections. Its volatile oils demonstrate *in vivo* and *in vitro* antibacterial activity against Staphylococci and other bacteria (Patel, 1988; Lahariya, 1979; Mehta, 1978; Suri, 1978) and fungal infections (Suri, 1979a & b). In Ayurvedic medicine, the plant is a remedy for earaches, and tea prepared from the roots is prescribed for malarial fevers.

An interesting study compared Tulsi with steroid drugs in treating acute viral encephalitis in 16 patients admitted to a hospital in Lucknow, India. A small group of 6 patients took 2.5 mg of fresh Tulsi leaves 4 times a day, while 10 patients received steroids. A complete recovery occurred in 60% of those using the herb, while no one in the steroid group experienced complete recovery. Viral encephalitis usually causes significant neurological damage, but those using Tulsi were protected (Das, 1983).

Respiratory System: Ayurvedic practitioners give Tulsi as a primary medicine for acute and chronic respiratory problems. The herb improves the body's ability to efficiently utilize oxygen (Bhargava, 1981; Singh, 1988). As a bronchodilator that relaxes the bronchial and lung tissues, it reduces spasms and eases labored breathing. As excessive moisture and mucus production are reduced in the lungs and nasal sinuses, Tulsi's expectorant properties expel phlegm. The leaves, flowers, and powdered seeds alleviate fevers and inflammation and are an excellent remedy for the common cold, influenza (the flu), coughs, asthma, pleurisy, bronchitis, and other upper respiratory tract infections. My son, who once developed a deep, dry cough that lingered for several days following thex flu, drank a quart of Tulsi tea that completely cured his cough. Laboratory and clinical studies demonstrate that volatile oils in the herb elicit mild activity against tuberculosis bacteria (Gupta, 1955; Ramaswami, 1967).

Regular ingestion of Tulsi can also reduce asthma and allergic symptoms. An elevation of eosinophils (a type of white blood cell) is an indicator of allergic reactions, and the herb's anti-allergenic properties were detected in a study revealing its ability to reduce blood levels of eosinophils in people with asthma (Singh, 2002). Studies involving guinea pigs with asthma have documented that Tulsi decreased bronchospasms and coughs and improved labored breathing in the animals (Palit, 1980 & 1983). In a clinical trial involving 15 patients suffering from bronchial asthma, 500 mg of the dried leaves were taken 3 times daily over a 4-week period. Outcomes included a reduction in eosinophil count (reflecting fewer allergic reactions) and increased hemoglobin with improved oxygen levels in most of the participants. They reported fewer asthmatic attacks, fewer spasms with easier breathing and expanded lung capacity, reduction and better expectoration of phlegm, and a greater sense of well-being (Dixit, 1986; Singh, 1986a).

Digestive System: In India, Tulsi seeds are traditionally ground into powder and mixed in water, juice, or cow's milk for a nourishing mucilaginous drink that soothes and heals inflamed and ulcerated tissues in the stomach and intestines. The leaves are a digestive tonic that supports production and secretion of digestive enzymes, and eases abdominal tension, spasms, hiccups, bloating, and jaundice caused by liver obstruction. Tulsi is a helpful remedy for halitosis (bad breath), stomach and intestinal ulcers, colic, nausea and vomiting, intestinal parasites, constipation, diarrhea, and dysentery. A tea of the roots is administered as a prophylactic against epidemics such as cholera.

When the sympathetic nervous system is overstimulated, intestinal mobility increases and food moves through the digestive tract too quickly, causing diarrhea with poor nutrient absorption. Tulsi's calming influence quells this hyperactivity and can be helpful for diarrhea and intestinal inflammation in ulcerative colitis or Crohn's disease.

A clinical trial showed that Tulsi reduced the incidence and severity of stomach ulcers and excess stomach acid in patients (Jalil, 1970). Several animal studies confirm that pretreatment with Tulsi drastically prevented chemically induced stomach ulcers (Singh, 1978 & 1993; Bhargava, 1981 & 1984). Benzodiazepine tranquillizers can reduce ulcers due to their anti-anxiety actions, and when researchers compared these drugs with Tulsi, they found that the herb's anti-ulcer effects were 10 times greater than that of the drugs. Compared to the drugs, which were sedating at low doses, Tulsi was only mildly sedating at very high doses, while small doses increased stamina and healed ulcers (Mandal, 1993).

Antioxidants in Tulsi protect liver cells against toxins and oxidative damage. They normalize and stimulate the liver to moderate healthy cholesterol levels and bile output. Human trials demonstrate that the herb lowers elevated cholesterol levels, especially when related to stress (Agrawal, 1996). Other studies show that components in the leaves, including saponins and eugenol, significantly decrease cholesterol, triglycerides, and low density lipoproteins (LDL) while increasing beneficial high density lipoproteins (HDL) (Sirtori, 1979; Sen, 1992; Sarkar, 1994). In India, Tulsi is prescribed as an effective treatment for viral hepatitis (Sankaran, 1980; Rajalakshmi, 1988; Rastogi, 1995).

Blood Sugar and Diabetes: Several studies suggest diabetics may benefit from Tulsi's ability to lower blood sugar levels (Bever, 1979; Gholap, 2004; Marles, 1995). In a trial involving 40 patients with adult onset, non-insulin-dependent diabetes, drinking a tea of the leaves for 4 weeks significantly lowered urine glucose levels as well as fasting and postprandial blood glucose levels. A moderate reduction of cholesterol levels also occurred (Agrawal, 1996).

Detoxification Support: Tulsi has historically been used in Ayurvedic medicine as a blood purifier to reduce toxic overload and eliminate poisons from the body. It can be ingested for acute toxicity and also taken as a tonic over several weeks or months to reduce deeper, chronic toxic overload. Modern research verifies the presence of many flavonoids, including eugenol, ursolic acid, apigenin and rosmarinic acid, that are potent antioxidants supporting glutathione detoxifying systems. Research demonstrates that Tulsi supports normal liver function and enzyme production necessary for detoxification, and protects against mercury-induced toxicity in mice (Uma, 1999; Maulik, 1997).

Pain Relief and Inflammation: In India, the dried root of Tulsi is ingested for its mild analgesic effects on many types of pain and inflammation. This traditional use has been validated by modern research and discovery of the plant's chemical constituents. Tulsi decreases inflammation by inhibiting COX-2 and lipoxygenase pathways of arachidonic acid metabolism. Animal studies have revealed analgesic and anti-inflammatory effects of the volatile oils, especially ursolic acid (Singh, 1991a & 1995; Newmark, 2000). The herb eases arthritis and other types of inflammatory joint pain, and muscle pain and rigidity, including fibromyalgia.

Reproductive Health for Women and Men: India's ancient medical texts described Tulsi as a fertility enhancer and giver of children. Modern Ayurvedic practitioners continue to extol the herb's virtues of increasing sperm count and viability in men and fertility in women. The herb reduces tension in the pelvic area and increases blood flow. Women take the herb to ease menstrual cramps and enjoy emotional calm.

For men, the dried root and leaves are prepared as tea or ground into powder and taken in milk or pills to increase sperm count and sexual stamina and prevent premature ejaculation. In *Tulsi the Mother Medicine of Nature*, Ayurvedic physician Narendra Singh writes about a 27-year-old man who came to his clinic with low sperm count and motility and inability to have children with his wife after 8 years of marriage. His initial analysis revealed a diminished total sperm count of 79.7 million/ml with 70% being non-motile. He began treatment, taking 600 mg of dried Tulsi leaves in capsules twice daily. He experienced tremendous improvement after 2 months when his total sperm count increased to 146.8 million/ml with only 30% being non-motile (Singh, 2002).

Regardless of Ayurvedic's successful application of Tulsi for fertility problems over many generations, some sources currently report that the herb is contraindicated during pregnancy, based on research showing that very large doses had anti-fertility effects in rats (Batta, 1971). The validity of the research methods and consequent warnings are questionable because the extremely large amounts of Tulsi needed to reduce fertility in rats did not reflect human consumption. Current Indian researchers report that after 15 years of clinical experience in prescribing Tulsi, they have found no evidence of anti-fertility effects in men or women (Singh, 2002).

External Uses: The leaves or fresh juice extracted from the leaves are applied as a poultice to treat skin infections, abscesses, boils, insect bites and stings, skin diseases, and fungal infections such as ringworm or athlete's foot. The volatile oils with their wonderful fragrance have been used in deodorants and in mouthwashes for bad breath and gum health. The live plant acts like an environmental mosquito repellent and the fragrant oil may be applied to the skin to repel bugs.

Teachings from the Tulsi Deva

"Greetings, dear one! You wish to know about my healing essence? I am the deva of the Tulsi plants, and I 'tune up' the vibrational frequency of the cells and tissues in the human body. I especially influence the nervous and endocrine systems, for they have an electrical quality that regulates all activities of the body. And so, by energizing and calibrating the electrical or energetic charges in the nerves, the entire body is superimposed with alert calmness that is balancing and nourishing.

"I preside over the electrical circuitry in the body, assisting impulses to travel through the nerves without obstructions or problems. By establishing a smooth flow of energy, balance and calm permeate the nervous system and the mind. My plants help maintain optimal function of all body systems and adjust the electrical flow between times of ease and times of stress. My job is to maintain a dynamic state of equilibrium through all of life's ups and downs. This is my relationship to the nervous system.

"My plants also provide nourishment for the small endocrine glands that regulate the body and produce chemical messengers that travel to communicate with other parts of the body. The substances in my leaves and flowers monitor and optimize this flow of enzymes, hormones, and other chemicals from the glands. In this way, my nurturing and vitalizing influence on the nerves and endocrine glands provides a way for all the different cells and organs of the body to communicate together and function in cohesive unity.

"The seven endocrine glands within the body act like doors or portals for currents of life-giving energy or light to travel through. The ancient ones called these portals 'energy centers' or 'wheels of light,' and in India they are known as chakras. These seven chakras can appear as wheels radiating light that enters and leaves the body. This light enters each chakra at very high frequencies not normally seen by people. As the vibrational frequency of each chakra slows down, it materializes into the corresponding endocrine gland. It is the same substance in different form, just as water can be solid like ice, liquid like water, or vaporous in air. The crown chakra at the top of the head corresponds to the pineal gland. The forehead chakra, known as the 'third eye,' corresponds to the pituitary gland. The throat chakra is related to the thyroid gland, the heart chakra is related to the heart and thymus gland, and the solar plexus chakra is connected to the pancreas. The pelvic chakra energizes the ovaries in women and testes in men, while the root chakra corresponds to the adrenal glands. The people in my homeland of India understand the workings of the chakras, and this knowledge is deeply embedded in their culture. Just as the seven chakra centers govern the health and vitality of the human body, the seven endocrine glands are also master regulators. My healing power is unique in its ability to assist in the strong and balanced flow of life energies in and out of the chakras, and to support each of the corresponding endocrine glands. My medicine is high frequency energy capable of neutralizing and transforming lower energy frequencies manifesting as pain, depression, or deteriorating, diseased tissues. The higher frequencies of my plants restore life, and you may think of me as a replenishing fountain of youth, balance, and calm.

"My plants are ruled by the air and fire elements, for these are the forces that regulate and invoke the electrical charges of the life-force. I bring balance and calm to the life-force within the human body and maintain equilibrium. In this way, I can benefit all people. My medicine is profoundly powerful in its restorative ability, yet gentle and safe enough for the very young and elderly.

"I am a benevolent and generous being, allowing my plants to produce vast quantities of seeds so full of the life-force that they prolifically reproduce to provide abundant medicine. And just as my medicine helps people adapt to the stresses and extremes of life, my plants are adaptable and grow in many regions throughout the world. Please plant my seeds in your gardens and drink the tea of my leaves and flowers to stay healthy and vibrant! Share my gifts with others.

"For I am a being of radiant light sent to earth to adjust and fortify the radiant light flowing in and out of all creatures. My medicine offering is beautiful to see, fragrant to smell, and delicious to taste. So I am an easy and delightful medicine to take!

"The healing gifts I offer are especially needed at this time on the planet when there is so much destruction of the sacred life-force due to hatred and ignorance in the hearts and minds of too many people. My lesson is to teach the preciousness and sacredness of the mysterious force of life that flows through plants, animals, and human beings. Revere and protect this gift of life, and you will bask in the wonderment revealed in each moment. So be it!"

Hops

Humulus lupulus
Cannabaceae (Hemp or Cannabis) Family

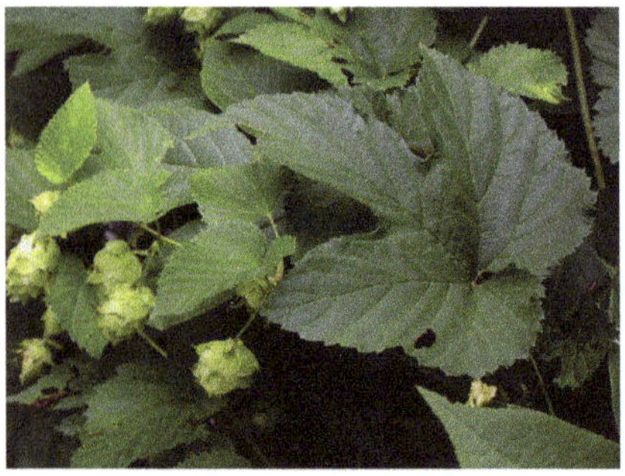

Common Names

Humulus, common Hops, and European Hops are common names.

Medicinal Part of the Plant

Strobiles are the flowering fruit from female Hops vines and are used in healing and brewing beer. In England, the leaves are employed for sluggish liver and gallbladder problems.

Range and Habitat

Hops is native to North America, Europe, and Asia. It is extensively cultivated for brewing beer and has naturalized in many temperate zones. The other species in this genus is *Humulus japonicus* (Japanese Hops), a rapidly growing annual vine.

Description of the Plant

Humulus lupulus is a hardy perennial climbing vine. The attractive plant is dioecious, meaning that male and female flowers appear on separate plants. The long, pencil-thick roots grow horizontally like long underground vines. Many stems continually sprout up from the trailing roots. The stems are long, twining vines able to grow up to 25′ during a growing season. Tough fibers make the rounded, angular stems strong but flexible. Short, scratchy hairs scattered along the stems and leaves create a very rough, slightly prickly texture. Unlike many climbing vines, Hops lacks tendrils.

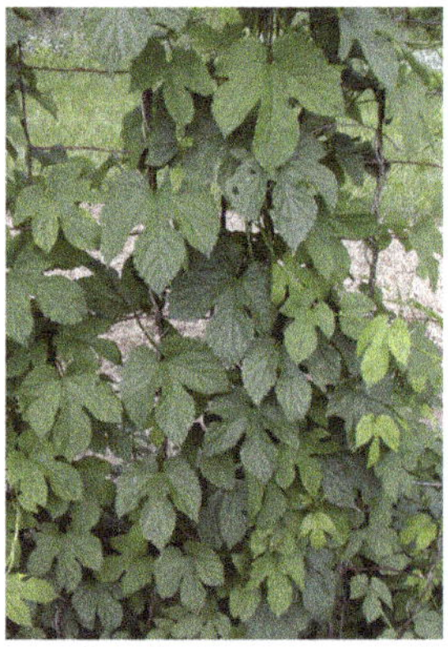

Deep-green leaves grow oppositely along the length of the vines, although upper leaves can be arranged singly. Leaves are simple but vary in shape from cordate (heart-shaped) to palmate with 3 deeply indented lobes. All leaves have pointed tips, serrated teeth, and petioles. The larger leaves are 2-5″ long and wide. The top surface is rough like Velcro. Under a 16X magnifying glass, tiny yellow lupulin glands appear as miniature drops of oil on the bottom surface of leaves.

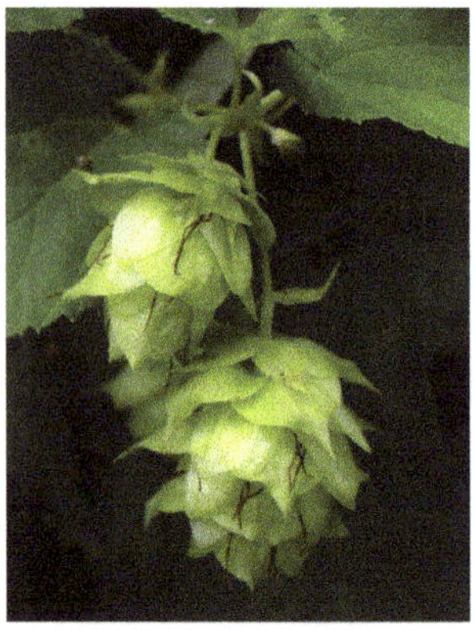

Hops strobiles

The unique-looking flowers are called strobiles. Only the female strobiles produce viable seed and are used medicinally. The pale yellowish-green female strobiles are 1-2″ long, round to oblong in shape, and are composed of many leafy bracts, each one covering a seed. The overlapping pattern of the bracts is somewhat similar to the scales on a pinecone, but the delicate strobile is paper-thin, soft, and pliable rather than woody. Bright-yellow pollen is scattered underneath the bracts, along with many brown, thready glandular hairs. Strobiles bloom from July through September.

Male strobiles, on the other hand, are smaller, yellowish white, and hang in loose panicle clusters 3-5″ in length.

Cultivation

Only female plants are cultivated for their strobiles and used for brewing beer and making medicinal preparations. Although I have only grown the female plants, I have read that growing some male plants with the females produces larger strobiles. Hops requires deep, rich, moist but well-drained soil with a pH of 5-6.5. This is a sun-loving plant, and its long vines need to climb on a trellis or fencing material. Hops vines can be grown from seed, but they are usually propagated by the more reliable methods of root division or stem cuttings. Live roots may be purchased from nurseries or seed companies. Be sure to order female plants. If you already cultivate Hops plants, you may propagate more by digging up several roots in early spring or autumn. Cut them into 10-12″ pieces, lay them horizontally in the ground like they naturally grow, and cover with 3-4″ of soil. Water and mulch the roots while keeping the soil moist, cool, and weed-free.

Stem cuttings (2-3′ long) may be taken from vines in spring or summer. Put the cut ends in a mix of moist potting soil, sand, and vermiculite. Keep moist and well-drained, and roots will develop after several weeks. Then plant the cuttings horizontally 1′ apart in a prepared bed. New plants that develop from root divisions and stem cuttings usually flower after 3 years. Only 6-10 Hops roots are required to create a patch that will continually expand for many years.

Prune all dead vines at ground level when the foliage has died back in late autumn. New shoots will emerge from the extensive root system every spring. Once the vines find their way to a trellis, they climb and keep a tight hold. Help the vines by pointing them in the right direction to find support and weaving them around the trellis material. The plant makes a pretty addition to gardens and may also be grown as an arbor vine to create a shady enclosed area.

Harvest

Collect mature strobiles from female plants from July through September when they are greenish-yellow, fluffy, and full of sticky, resinous, yellow pollen.

Preparation of Plant Medicine and Dosages

The golden-yellow lupulin oil glands and pollen within strobiles contain the primary medicinal constituents. These resinous oils make the strobiles sticky. The most potent tea is prepared with fresh strobiles. Dried strobiles rapidly deteriorate in potency and only 15% of their original biological activity remains after 9 months of storage (Fetrow, 1999). Therefore, tincturing the strobiles immediately after harvesting is the best way to preserve the herb's medicinal properties.

PREPARATIONS

Tincture: Fresh strobiles are tinctured in the usual way with 60% 190-proof grain alcohol and 40% distilled water. Dosage: 30-90 drops 1-4 times day as needed. The yellow color of lupulin and pollen in the strobiles produces a beautiful golden-orange tincture.

Infusion Tea: Steep 1-3 teaspoons of fresh strobiles in 1 cup of boiled water. Dosage: 1-2 cups daily as needed. The tea has a strong bitter flavor and most people prefer taking the tincture.

Salves and Poultices: Hops strobiles are an excellent addition to salves and can also be prepared as a poultice for skin irritations, itching, pain, and wounds.

Chemical Constituents

Due to its importance in the beer industry, constituents in Hops strobiles have been identified and researched extensively. It is estimated that Hops plants contain over 300 phytochemicals. Lupulin glands within the strobiles consist of essential oils and resins that give beer its characteristic aroma and bitter taste. The bitter resins (15%) are the most important components for beer brewing. Their antimicrobial properties help preserve beer and exert antimicrobial protection for people.

Humulone (2-10%) and lupulone (2-16%) are the primary bitter resins. One of their metabolic by-products is 2-methyl-3-butene-1-ol, known to calm the nervous system. Humulone is an antispasmodic and antioxidant, and has decreased inflammation and tumor formation in mice (Yasukawa, 1995). Other bitter resins are valerianic acid, cohumulone, lupulene, colupulone, and adlupulone. Pollen in the mature strobiles contains 10% lupulin, which reduces anxiety and induces sleep.

Over 100 compounds occur in the volatile oils, including linalool (antitumor), myrcene (diuretic, analgesic, antibacterial, anticonvulsant, antispasmodic, fungicide), beta-caryophyllen, farnesene, terpineol (antibacterial, anticarcinogenic, sedative, vulnerary), caryophyllene (anti-inflammatory, antitumor, diuretic, fungicide), eugenol (analgesic, antibacterial, anticonvulsant, anti-inflammatory, antispasmodic, choleretic, diuretic, hepatoprotective, sedative, vermifuge), citral (antibacterial, antihistamine, broncho-relaxant, anticarcinogenic, sedative), and geraniol (antibacterial, antispasmodic, antitumor, and sedative).

The strobiles also contain flavonoids that are estrogenic and anticarcinogenic. Flavonoids include xanthohumol, 6-prenylnaringenin, and isoxanthohumol. The predominant flavonoid is the weakly estrogenic isoxanthohumol, which is converted to 8-prenylnaringenin (8-PN), a stronger estrogen, by bacteria in the colon. According to *in vitro* studies, **8-PN is the most potent plant estrogen known** (Chadwick, 2006). Xanthohumol is anti-inflammatory, antiviral, and anticarcinogenic (Festa, 2011).

Other flavonoids include kaempferol, quercetin, rutin, and astragalin (diuretic, antileukemic, expectorant, hypotensive). Colupulone and avermectin are antibacterial (Fetrow, 1999), anthocyanidins are antioxidant, alpha- and beta-pinene are antibacterial, anti-inflammatory, antispasmodic, antiviral, expectorant, and sedating. Other constituents include tannins (2-4%), gamma-linoleic acid, and beta-eudesmol (antimutagenic, anti-ulcer, hepatoprotective, sedative).

Although it belongs to the same family as Marijuana, Hops does not contain psychotropic (mind-altering) substances.

Safety, Contraindications, and Drug Interactions

Hops is a safe, non-toxic herb when taken in normal dosages. It is **contraindicated during pregnancy** due to its emmenagogue and hormonal properties, but it is safe for nursing mothers to drink as tea to increase quantities of breast milk. Drinking beer brewed with Hops is often recommended for the same purpose. This is *not* an herb for people with depression, listlessness, or chronic fatigue because its sedating action may accentuate these problems. It may also potentiate the effects of sedating drugs and alcohol.

Medicinal Uses

History of the Plant

Hops is best known as an important ingredient for brewing beer. The Germans began adding Hops to beer during the 800s, and by the 1300s, most European beers were brewed with Hops. The vines were cultivated in monastery and country gardens during the Middle Ages. Germans introduced Hops cultivation to China and Korea in the 1860s and later to Japan, where German and American cultivars replaced the native Japanese variety (Blumenthal, 2000).

In Chinese and Indian Ayurvedic medicine, Hops is employed as a digestive tonic and sedative for anxiety, headaches, and insomnia. Greek and Roman physicians prescribed the herb for similar problems. The species name *lupulus* is derived from the Latin word *lupus*, meaning "wolf," comparing the plant's climbing, entwining vines that strangle other plants to a wolf that overpowers and devours its prey. The English name "Hops" comes from the Anglo-Saxon word *hoppan*, meaning "to climb." The strong, tough fibrous stems were once used in England to produce paper and coarse cloth.

In his *Herball or Generall Historie of Plantes*, English apothecary and surgeon John Gerard (1545–1612) wrote about the common practice of eating young Hops shoots in salads for good health. He prescribed preparations of the leaves and strobiles to "remove obstructions out of the entrails" and to purify the blood and skin by their beneficial action on the kidneys in removing waste products. Attesting to the herb's value in making beer, Gerard wrote, "The manifold virtues of Hops do manifestly argue to wholesomeness of beer above ale; for the hops rather make it a physical drink to keep the body in health, than an ordinary drink for the quenching of our thirst" (Gerard, 1633).

English herbalist and apothecary Nicholas Culpeper (1616–1654) wrote in his herbal that Hops is under the dominion of Mars and that the tea "brings down women's courses [promotes menstruation] . . . operates in opening obstructions of the liver and spleen, cleansing the blood, loosening the belly, expelling the gravel [kidney stones], and provoking the urine" (Culpeper, 1992). He prescribed Hops to treat parasites, headaches triggered by nervous tension and excess heat, and for external wounds, scabs, itching, skin eruptions, and fungal infections including ringworm. In Europe, the herb continued to be a remedy for these problems for hundreds of years.

When European colonists brought Hops plants to North America, Native Americans were already using their indigenous species. The Mohegans reportedly drank Hops tea as a sedative and heated strobiles for application to painful teeth and gums. The Cherokee used it as a sedative and analgesic and as a remedy for arthritis pain, breast and uterine complaints, and kidney and urinary problems. The Sioux prepared the leaves as tea to relieve fevers and abdominal pains, and as a poultice for wounds.

The early American Eclectic physicians employed Hops from the 1880s to the 1930s primarily for its sedative effects and as a digestive aid. It was also given for lung infections and delirium tremens (uncontrollable shaking during withdrawal from chronic alcohol or drug abuse). External applications were prescribed for eczema, ulcers, and tumors. Throughout the 1800s, the strobiles were included in many patent herbal medicines. Hops was listed as an official medicine in the *United States Pharmacopoeia* from 1831–1916 and in the *U.S. National Formulary* from 1916–1947.

The Hops plant remains a popular brewing herb and medicinal remedy. Several subspecies or cultivars have been developed specifically for brewing beer. Many *in vitro* and animal studies have identified phytochemicals in the strobiles and documented their biological actions. Hops' traditional applications employed over the centuries by eastern and western medical systems have been substantiated by these studies along with human clinical trials.

Healing Qualities

Analgesic, antibacterial, antifungal, anti-inflammatory, antilithic, antimicrobial, antiseptic, antispasmodic, anti-uric, astringent, bitter tonic, cardiac, carminative, cholagogue, depurative, diuretic, emmenagogue, exanthematous, febrifuge, galactagogue, hepatic, laxative, nephritic, nervine, sedative and hypnotic, stomachic, vermifuge, and vulnerary.

Traditional Chinese Medicine (TCM) Perspective

Hops is prescribed as a bitter and cooling remedy for conditions of excess heat such as fevers and inflammation in TCM. Its astringent properties are drying. The herb relaxes and restores the central nervous system and calms the Shen (spirit). This beneficial effect on the nerves influences the liver, gallbladder, stomach, intestines, kidneys, skin, and reproductive system. The primary use of Hops is in treating Qi (energy) constraint and tension throughout the body due to excessive nervous stimulation. Qi constraint in the lungs promotes coughs, asthma, and infections. Heart Qi constraint can lead to dizziness, heart palpitations, anxiety, and chest pressure. Kidney Qi restraint can induce gout, arthritis, kidney stones, edema, and hypertension. Uterine Qi constraint causes painful, crampy periods with a scanty flow. Liver, gallbladder, and stomach Qi constraint and stagnation can produce bloating, gas, indigestion, intestinal spasms, and constipation. Hops strobiles are beneficial for all of these problems.

Clinical studies in modern China demonstrate the effectiveness of Hops in the treatment of tuberculosis, leprosy, acute bacterial dysentery (intestinal infection and inflammation causing diarrhea), silicosis (a chronic condition in which lung tissue becomes fibrous after long-time exposure and inhalation of silicone dust), and lung inflammation due to extended and chronic inhalation of asbestos (Chang, 1986).

Primary Actions

The calming, antispasmodic qualities of Hops are felt throughout the entire body. It is specifically indicated for people with underlying stress and nervous tension along with excess heat that can manifest as irritability, anxiety, muscular spasms and twitching, insomnia, heart palpitations, and nervous indigestion. Bitter-tasting constituents help stimulate a sluggish digestive system. The phytoestrogens (plant estrogens) in Hops can benefit women's reproductive organs and fertility cycles. The strobiles are typically combined with other herbs when preparing remedies.

For many years, I have included the tincture of fresh strobiles in many formulas for nervous anxiety and insomnia, digestive problems, and to normalize female reproductive hormones. When supporting the nervous system, I typically combine Hops with other sedative/nervine herbs like Scullcap (*Scutellaria lateriflora*), Valerian (*Valeriana officinalis*), and Passion Flower (*Passiflora incarnata*).

Nervous System Sedative, Analgesic, and Anti-Inflammatory: Hops is an excellent sedative to calm the nervous system and ease tension, restlessness, anxiety, and hyperactivity. It acts as a nervine that helps restore nerves to their normal function, and as a hypnotic that induces sleep. Hops is helpful for a multitude of conditions triggered by nervous over-stimulation and anxiety such as headaches, panic attacks, high blood pressure, heart palpitations, premenstrual stress, delirium tremens, and neuralgia (nerve pain), including facial neuralgia and sciatica. People experiencing depression or chronic fatigue should avoid ingesting Hops because its depressant effects on the nervous system could potentiate these problems.

The herb is excellent for insomnia when a cup of tea or 40-60 drops of the tincture are taken in water 15-30 minutes before bedtime. Sleeping on a Hops pillow is an old remedy for insomnia. These pillows are made by adding a little alcohol to the fresh strobiles and stuffing them into a small pillow.

Researchers have identified many of the chemicals and their biological effects in the resins, volatile oils, and flavonoids in the strobiles, validating their historic use in sedating the central nervous system (Hansel, 1982; Wohlfart, 1982 & 1983). The ability of Hops to induce sleep has been documented by studying sleep patterns in insomniacs (Fussel, 2000) and by using electroencephalography (EEG) to observe electrical activity in the brain after people ingested the herb (Vonderheid-Guth, 2000). Mechanisms of its sedating/hypnotic activities have also been investigated. *In vitro* trials show that beer made from Hops and extracts of the strobiles both bind to GABA (gamma-aminobutyric acid) receptors on cells. This activates GABA, a powerful inhibitory neurotransmitter that promotes relaxation and sleep (Rodenbeck, 1998; Aoshima, 2006). *In vivo* studies of mice indicate that the sleep-inducing properties of Hops may also be related to its activation of melatonin, the sleep-promoting hormone secreted by the pineal gland (Butterweck, 2007).

Several human trials have explored the sedating properties of Hops combined with Valerian (*Valeriana officinalis*). Clinical studies reveal that this combination is a safe and effective alternative to benzodiazepine drugs (such as Valium) for people with insomnia (Schmitz, 1998). An interesting study involving 48 healthy men was designed to test the sedating effects of a combination of Hops (60 mg per tablet) and Valerian (250 mg per tablet) compared to a placebo when simultaneously taken with 200 mg of caffeine. Within an hour, 2 herbal tablets reduced caffeine-induced stimulation, while the full dose of 6 herbal tablets completely inhibited stimulation (Schellenberg, 2004). Another clinical trial consisting of 42 people diagnosed with poor quality sleep investigated the effects of a single dose (2 mL) of a Hops and Valerian liquid extract. Compared to 22 participants who received a placebo, the 20 people who took the herbal blend reported deeper and better quality sleep plus longer sleep time (Dimpfel, 2008).

A multicenter study involving 210 patients with occasional insomnia was conducted in nine sleep disorder centers. The patients received 2 tablets of a Valerian-Hops extract for 28 nights (each tablet contained 187 mg Valerian and 41.9 mg of Hops), a placebo (2 tablets each night for 28 nights), or 2 tablets of diphenhydramine (marketed as 25 mg tablets of Sominex) for 14 nights. By the end of the second week, the Valerian-Hops group reported the greatest improvements in going to sleep quickly (Morin, 2005).

As a nervine, Hops not only calms the nervous system but also promotes growth and protection of nerve cells. An extract of phenols from the strobiles (containing 55% proanthocyanidins and 28% flavonoids) has demonstrated antioxidant activities that protect and enhance the life span of cells. The extract effectively scavenged damaging free radicals *in vitro* and inhibited DNA oxidative damage. Mouse trials show that ingestion of a Hops extract protected their livers against chemical toxicity (Wang, 2013). Another *in vivo* study revealed that flavonoids in Hops enhanced the growth and development of nerve cells (neurogenesis), aided their regeneration, and protected them from damage. The herb stimulated the growth of axons and dendrites from the cell body of nerve cells, which allow cells to communicate with each other. Consequently, the researchers concluded that Hops may be beneficial in cases of chronic degenerative nerve diseases, acute brain and spinal cord injuries, and age-related cognitive impairment such as memory loss and dementia (Oberbauer, 2013).

Hops is a beneficial analgesic and anti-inflammatory remedy (Prokopenko, 1986) offering relief for nerve, muscle, and tissue pain and inflammation. Researchers have observed its ability to decrease nerve and muscle spasms (Caujolle, 1969), making it beneficial for myalgia (muscle pain) and fibromyalgia. Hops reduces production of inflammatory COX-2. In a study using a Hops extract high in alpha acids, inflammation and resulting pain were reduced over 9 hours, equivalent to ibuprofen 400 mg (Lemay, 2004).

For best pain relief, combine Hops with other analgesics such as St. John's Wort (*Hypericum perforatum*), Meadowsweet (*Filipendula ulmaria*), Wood Betony (*Stachys officinalis*), and Willow (*Salix* spp.).

Women's Health: Hops strobiles help regulate menstrual cycles and normalize the uterus and ovaries. Phytoestrogens are estrogen-like molecules from plants that bind to human estrogen receptors on cells, like a key fits into a lock. Phytoestrogens have traditionally been used to regulate the hormonal cycles governing menstruation and fertility, replenish the system with estrogen, and manage menopausal symptoms. The primary flavonoid in the strobiles is isoxanthohumol, which is converted to 8-prenylnaringenin (8-PN) by bacteria in the colon. It is rapidly and almost completely absorbed following ingestion (Rad, 2006). **Within the plant kingdom, 8-PN is the most potent estrogenic substance known. However, phytoestrogens have much weaker hormonal activity than estrogens produced by the body or manufactured synthetically. Phytoestrogens help protect women from the potentially harmful effects of strong, synthetic estrogens.**

The first scientific confirmation that Hops contains phytoestrogens appeared in 1953, when researchers injected rodents with a preparation made from the strobiles and reported that one gram of strobiles contains the equivalent of 20-300 mcg of estradiol (the most potent estrogen produced by women) (Koch, 1953). Several *in vitro* studies show that 8-PN binds to the two estradiol receptors, ERalpha and ERbeta. It is also well-documented that 8-PN mimics the action of estradiol, although 8-PN has 10- to 20,000-fold less potency than estradiol for ERbeta receptors. But 8-PN has greater affinity for ERalpha receptors, where it is only 70-fold less potent than estradiol (Chadwich, 2006; Coldham, 2001; Milligan, 2000 & 2002; Rong, 2001; Zara, 1998; Zierau, 2002). The combination of Hops and Red Clover (*Trifolium pratense*) has been shown to attach also to progesterone receptors and exert beneficial progesterone activity (Liu, 2001).

Hops is an emmenagogue that promotes menstruation, and its analgesic and antispasmodic properties help relieve menstrual pain and cramps, especially when taken before or as the discomfort begins (McKendree, 1937). Sedative qualities ease nervous irritability of premenstrual syndrome (PMS). As a diuretic, it reduces water retention that can cause breast tenderness and premenstrual edema. The antimicrobial resins in Hops are also active against *Trichomonas vaginalis*, a protozoa parasite causing vaginal and urethral infection.

As a galactagogue for nursing mothers, the bitter-tasting tea or tincture helps to increase and enrich breast milk. It is also a postpartum aid in relieving the "after-pains" of childbirth caused by extremely strong uterine contractions that help stop bleeding and restore the uterus to pre-pregnancy size.

During menopause, Hops increases estrogen levels to relieve anxiety, hot flashes, vaginal dryness, and other menopausal discomforts. Hops may be combined with Black Cohosh (*Cimicifuga racemosa*), Blue Vervain (*Verbena hastata*), and Sage (*Salvia officinalis*) for these issues. Estrogen is known to support strong bones, and 8-PN may be beneficial for the prevention and treatment of osteoporosis. Researchers have discovered that humulone has an extraordinarily strong inhibitory effect on bone reabsorption (Honma, 1998; Tobe, 1997).

Several clinical trials have explored the hormonal activities of Hops for menopausal problems. A 12-week study involved 67 menopausal women who took a Hops extract standardized to specific amounts of 8-PN (100 or 250 mcg) or a placebo. After 6 weeks of treatment, the women receiving both doses of the herbal extract experienced faster reduction of menopausal symptoms than those taking the placebo, most notably in diminished hot flashes (Heyerick, 2006). In a 16-week study, 36 healthy women experiencing typical menopausal difficulties were recruited. Each of the women had an intact uterus and had not had a period for at least one year. Compared with the placebo group, the women using a Hops extract reported significant reductions in menopausal complaints with improved quality-of-life (Erkkola, 2010).

Two clinical trials investigated the effects of a medical gel containing hyaluronic acid, phytoestrogens from a Hops extract, and vitamin E. The trials were designed to test the safety and efficacy of this gel in post-menopausal women with urogenital atrophy (dry vaginal tissues). The initial pilot study involving 10 women confirmed the safety of the gel on the local tissues of application at a dose of 1-2 gm per day for 30 days. In the second study, 100 post-menopausal women were treated with a vaginal application of 2.5 gm of gel per day for one week followed by two applications a week for 11 weeks. The results revealed a significant reduction in vaginal dryness, itching, burning, inflammation, rash, vaginal abrasions, and painful sexual intercourse. None of the women complained of adverse reactions (Morali, 2006).

For many years, Hops producers have reported that workers who harvest the strobiles tire easily, which reflects the herb's sedating quality. Female pickers often experience early menstrual periods, indicative of the estrogenic effects.

Research determining Hops' role in preventing or aggravating reproductive cancers, which are usually estrogen-dependent, seems to be contradictory. Some *in vitro* tests show that 8-PN in Hops inhibits growth of human breast and ovarian cancers (Miranda, 1999). Xanthohumol, isoxanthohumol, and 8-PN in Hops extracts have inhibited estrogen production in cancerous breast tissues, decreased proliferation of cancerous cells, and destroyed existing cancer cells by apoptosis, or programmed cell death (Monteiro, 2007; Hemachandra, 2012). In two other *in vitro* studies, 8-PN mimicked the effects of estradiol in contributing to the development of reproductive cancers (Rong, 2001) and stimulated the growth of estrogen-dependent

MCF7 breast cancer cells (Matsumara, 2005). In light of conflicting evidence, it may be wise to avoid taking Hops when estrogen-dependent reproductive cancers are present.

Men's Health: Prolonged ingestion of Hops containing estrogenic 8-PN (8-prenylnaringenin) can reduce testosterone levels, excessive libido and sexual over-excitement in men, and decrease the incidence of wet dreams, premature ejaculation, and persistent abnormal erection of the penis called priapism (Smith, 1999; Weiss, 1988). The Eclectic physicians prescribed Hops for the treatment of spermatorrhea (the involuntary escape of semen) and chordee, a downward deflection of the penis caused by a congenital anomaly or urethral infection. Some men who pick the strobiles for employment have experienced hormonal changes and developed gynecomastia (abnormal breast enlargement in men). For these reasons, men experiencing problems caused by excess estrogen or insufficient testosterone should avoid large quantities of beer containing Hops, and only ingest Hops in small amounts for short periods or avoid it completely.

Xanthohumol, isoxanthohumol, 6-prenylnaringenin, and 8PN isolated from Hops strobiles induced apoptosis (programmed cell death) of prostate cancer cells during *in vitro* trials (Delmulle, 2008). According to researchers, *in vitro* studies indicate that these constituents may be beneficial for prostate hyperplasia (inflammation and enlargement) and malignant prostate cancer (Colgate, 2007).

Digestive System: Like most bitters, Hops stimulates a sluggish digestive system by increasing the production and secretion of stomach acids, pancreatic enzymes, and bile from the liver. Sufficient digestive enzymes ensure optimal absorption of food and normal intestinal movements. The herb helps prevent or treat constipation. Hops improves a poor appetite, strengthens the digestive organs, and reduces gas, bloating, and stomach and intestinal cramps. The sedating and antispasmodic properties of the herb are relaxing to the nerves and muscles in the digestive tract, and are especially beneficial for digestive problems stemming from nervous overstimulation and anxiety. Hops can reduce spasms in the diaphragm that cause hiccups.

Eclectic physicians prescribed the strobiles for dyspepsia (indigestion), gastritis (stomach inflammation), enteritis (intestinal inflammation), and to stimulate the stomach's production of digestive acids. They also employed the herb to reduce excessive nervous anxiety that overstimulates the stomach's production of acids causing heartburn and headaches. Finley Ellingwood, M.D. (1852–1920) wrote that Hops "modifies secretion of the gastric fluids inhibiting the output of acids" (Ellingwood, 1919). The cold tea or tincture is particularly valuable for normalizing digestion when taken 20 minutes before meals. Antibiotic resins in Hops are effective against some bacteria that cause dysentery and food poisoning.

By stimulating and normalizing metabolic activity and blood circulation in the liver, Hops strobiles are beneficial when treating hepatitis, jaundice, and other liver and gallbladder problems. They relax the muscles in the liver and gall ducts, allowing for smooth passage of blood and bile, and also reduce inflammation. The British use both the strobiles and leaves for liver and gallbladder problems. One clinical study documented that a blend of Hops, Chicory (*Cichorium intybus*), and Peppermint (*Mentha x piperita*) relieved pain in patients with chronic cholecystitis (gallbladder inflammation) with or without gallstones (Chakarski, 1982). Hops is also a vermifuge that can be combined with other herbs to eliminate intestinal parasites.

Kidneys and Bladder: Hops stimulates kidney function to increase urine output. This relieves edema and has a generalized cleansing action on the entire body by eliminating waste products and toxins from the bloodstream. It reduces excess uric acid, making it helpful for gout (caused by uric acid deposits in the joints of the big toe) and for dissolving abnormal mineral deposits in other arthritic joints. It has been used to treat kidney stones by decreasing their formation and by dissolving pre-existing stones. The antibiotic and anti-inflammatory properties are helpful in treating cystitis (bladder infection) and spastic bladder. A clinical test by Lenau in 1984 demonstrated that 772 out of 915 people who used Hops, Uva-ursi (*Arctostaphylos uva-ursi*), and natural vitamin E reported improvement in their irritable bladder symptoms and resulting urinary incontinence.

Heart, Blood, and Circulation: The sedating, antispasmodic properties of Hops on the nervous system are reflected in its ability to calm a nervous, overstimulated heart, reduce palpitations and tachycardia (rapid heartbeat), ease chest pressure, and relax the muscles within blood vessels to reduce hypertension. One study demonstrated that xanthohumol in the strobiles possesses potent anti-platelet activity that inhibits abnormal blood clotting in the vessels (Lee, 2012). These actions contribute to improving circulation and reducing the underlying stress and constriction usually involved in hypertension. The cleansing actions of Hops on the liver and kidneys also benefit the blood by reducing acids and excess heat, and antibiotic properties help eliminate toxins in the blood.

Antimicrobial Activity against Bacteria, Yeast, Fungi, and Cancer: The cooling febrifuge quality of Hops is helpful for fevers, and its antispasmodic property is beneficial for coughs. The Eclectic physicians prescribed Hops for pneumonia and pleurisy in combination with other herbs.

The bitter resins humulone and lupulone demonstrate antibiotic activity mainly against Gram-positive bacteria, including those causing tuberculosis and staph infections (Teuber, 1973). Lupulone possesses about 10 times more antibiotic activity than humulone. Researchers have found that *in vitro* dilutions of lupulone inhibited many bacteria, including *Bacillus* spp. (causing anthrax and food poisoning), *Corynbacterium diphtheriae* (causing diphtheria), *Diplococcus pneumoniae* (responsible for pneumonia), *Staphylococcus aureus* (causing sinus and respiratory tract infections, impetigo, cellulitis, boils, and food poisoning), and *Mycobacterium* (causing tuberculosis). Hops demonstrates antimicrobial activity against *Streptococcus mutans, S. sanguinis,* and *S. salivarius*, which contribute to the formation of dental plaque (Bhattacharya, 2003). Antifungal activity has been documented against several species that invade human tissue, including *Trichophyton, Candida, Fusarium*, and *Mucor* (Mizobuchi, 1984 & 1985).

Researchers have explored the herb's activity against various types of cancer using *in vitro* and *in vivo* studies. Humulone has been shown to inhibit the growth of cancerous cells causing leukemia (Honma, 1998; Tobe, 1997). Lupulone reduces proliferation of several types of cancer cells, including breast adenocarcinoma (Stephan, 1998). The flavonoids isoxanthohumol, xanthohumol, and 8-PN demonstrate anticancer activity against colon, liver, skin, and lymphoma cancers (Chung, 2009; Allsopp, 2013; Miyashita, 2013).

One mechanism of cytotoxicty is apoptosis, in which the membranes of cancerous cells are damaged, allowing white blood cells called phagocytes to engulf and digest them. Xanthohumol has been characterized as a broad-spectrum anticancer agent following *in vitro* studies, and it exhibits cytotoxic activity against glioblastoma cells, which are the most common and aggressive malignant brain tumors in humans (Festa, 2011).

External Uses: Hops is anti-inflammatory, antiseptic, analgesic, and clears damp heat from the skin. An *in vitro* test demonstrated that a Hops extract of xanthohumol and lupulone exerts strong inhibitory activities against strains of bacteria that cause acne, including *Propionibacterium acnes, Staphylococcus epidermidis, S. aureus,* and *Streptococcus pyogenes*. Antioxidant capacity was also evaluated, showing xanthohumol to have the highest activity (Yamaguchi, 2009).

A fomentation, poultice, or ointment can be beneficial for nerve, muscle and joint pain, including arthritis and gout. These preparations may be applied to wounds, sprains, bruises, itchy skin, eczema, boils, abscesses, burns, skin ulcers, insect bites and stings, Candida yeast, and fungal infections including athlete's foot and ringworm. The Eclectic physicians prescribed Hops for acute local inflammation and painful swellings, and to treat the pain of facial neuralgia and childhood earaches. Jethro Kloss, clinical herbalist and author of *Back to Eden*, recommended it for ear pain and toothaches. I always add Hops strobiles to my herbal salve for its wonderful healing gifts.

Teachings from the Hops Deva

"Greetings, dear one. I am the deva of the Hops plants. I offer an abundance of delightful little flowers containing my golden-yellow and green essence; for these are the colors and frequencies my healing medicine offers to people. I am supported by the earth and water elements, and unless assisted by objects to climb upon, my plants stay close to the ground. You can feel into the essence of my movement by observing my vines and roots growing and meandering upon the ground in long, flowing strands, and by the petals of my flowers falling downward upon each other like a cascading waterfall. I help the energies and fluids of the body flow through the nerves and tissues to sustain life. The resulting balance and harmony allows the entire system to relax into deep peace.

"I am ruled by the astrological sign of Taurus and by Venus, the planet having an affinity with women by promoting balance, beauty, and gentle flow. My plants serve women by supplying substances that nourish and help regulate the cycles of the reproductive organs. I may be used in small amounts to normalize the hormones of reproduction. In this way, I assist in bringing new life into this world. Men may also use me when in need of feminine energies for balance.

"Although I am of the earth and water elements, there is lightness to my nature, and small amounts of my medicine are quite calming for the smooth flow of electrical charges and fluids through the body. I assist in the inter-communication of all the body parts to establish a balanced, constant flow of life and regularity of cyclic patterns. I help to regulate daily sleeping and waking cycles. Larger doses of my flowers help people enter into deep restorative sleep. And I help women with the waxing and waning monthly cycles of moon time, and with the longer cycle of fertility that eventually transforms into the menopausal phase. My medicine helps women transition through all these cycles of life with greater ease and contentment.

"I am not to be given to children, except in very small amounts combined with other herbs to help them sleep. Larger amounts of my medicine may influence their hormones and fertility cycles, and these should be left to unfold in their natural time and way.

"My offering to people is deep, restorative sleep and peace to the body and mind, allowing regeneration to occur and vitality to flourish. Always use my medicine in accordance with the body's natural rhythms. The lesson I offer is to always dwell in the space of inner peace and stability as you go through the hectic and overwhelming ups and downs of life. Stay anchored in your inner cave of calm to journey through daily life with greater ease and peaceful heart and mind."

Horehound

Marrubium vulgare
Labiatae (Lamiaceae) (Mint) Family

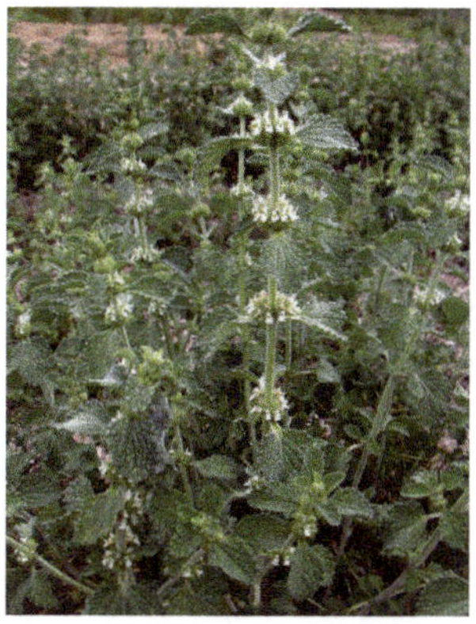

Common Names

White horehound, hoarhound, houndsbane, seed of Horus, and bull's blood are older names.

Medicinal Part of the Plant

The leaves and flowering tops are prepared for medical purposes.

Range and Habitat

The genus *Marrubium* contains up to 40 species, of which White Horehound (*Marrubium vulgare*) is the most popular. This hardy perennial is indigenous to Britain, Europe, Russia, Asia Minor, and central Asia. It grows wild on dry, sandy fields, waste places, and along roadsides. It is cultivated in temperate zones worldwide and has naturalized in the United States. Black Horehound (*Marrubium nigra* or *Ballota nigra*) also grows in the Mediterranean area and is similar in appearance to White Horehound, although the flowers are purple rather than white.

Description of the Plant

White Horehound is a non-aromatic member of the Mint family. This small plant usually grows no taller than 1½′. The fibrous roots send up several erect, square green stems. Stems and leaves are covered with fine, pubescent (soft and downy) white hairs, giving the plant an enchanting silvery bluish-green color and a woolly appearance. Leaves are about 1″ long, simple, ovate with rounded tips, and have crenate margins of rounded teeth. The wavy leaves display a rugose (rough and wrinkled) texture with many palmate veins. Leaves grow opposite each other along the entire length of the stems. Larger leaves at the base have stems, while upper leaves are sessile (without stems).

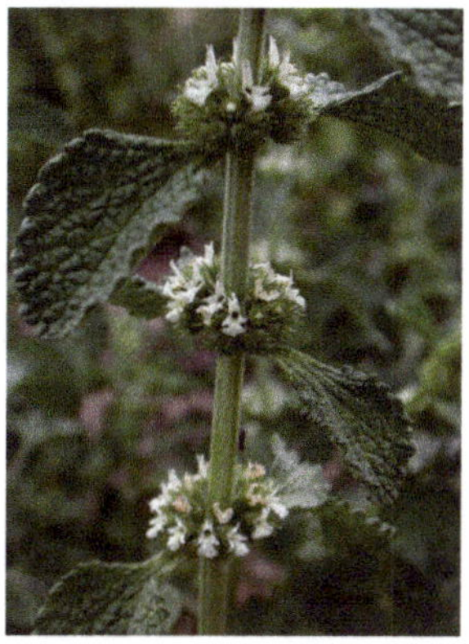

Numerous tiny, creamy-white sessile flowers appear in dense whorls circling the upper portions of stems, growing just above the leaf axils. Each flower is borne in a cup-like green calyx, and the tubular corolla opens into a bi-lobed upper lip and a tri-lobed lower lip. Flowers bloom from June through September. The calyx is spiny and pointed, making the flower whorls prickly when they mature into seedpods. Little curved spikes on the dried brown pods cling to clothes and animal fur, much like the notorious cockle burr of the Burdock plant. The small seeds are brownish black.

Cultivation

Horehound requires full sun and good drainage. It is a hardy plant adaptable to growing wild in wastelands and fields where the soil is dry and infertile. However, it produces more prolific foliage in a rich, fairly dry sandy loam. Acceptable pH ranges are between 4.5 and 7.0. It is easy to start new plants from seeds or stem cuttings.

Sow seeds in trays in early spring and barely cover them with ¼″ of soil. They germinate in a few weeks and can be transplanted to a permanent bed when 3-4″ tall. Space the seedlings about 10″ apart to make a compact stand. When grown from seeds, plants usually take a couple of years to flower.

Stem cuttings can be taken in spring or early summer, placed in a wet rooting mix, and planted after several weeks when roots develop. Keep the plants moist, weeded, and mulched.

Harvest

Harvest the upper leaves and blossoms during the early flowering stage when flowers are in full bloom. Prune no more than 25% of the plant to ensure its continued survival. Two harvests a year are often possible. Seeds are gathered for propagation purposes when the prickly seedpods are brown and dry.

Preparation of Plant Medicine and Dosages

The leaves and flowers are used fresh or dried, although the fresh herb is always most potent. The healing virtues are extracted in both alcohol and water, but alcohol is a better extractor of the medicinal bitters, making tinctures the most potent preparation. Horehound may also be prepared as tea, cough syrup, candied lozenges, pills and capsules, or used externally as a salve, poultice, or fomentation. The herb has a powerfully bitter taste, so many people prefer taking a little of the tincture rather than drinking a whole cup of the strong tea.

PREPARATIONS

Tincture: Put fresh, finely chopped leaves and flowers into a glass jar and cover them with 60% 190-proof grain alcohol and 40% distilled water. Dosage: 10-90 drops in water 1-3 times daily. For acute infections and congestion, take 60 drops every few hours until symptoms improve.

Infusion Tea: Steep 1-2 teaspoons of the herb in 1 cup of boiled water for 10 minutes. Dosage: ½-1 cup per day or twice as much for acute symptoms. Honey may be added to tone down the bitterness. The unsweetened tea is an excellent gargle for sore, infected throats.

Syrup: For coughs, hoarseness and sore throats, Horehound may be used alone or combined with Hyssop (*Hyssopus officinalis*), Licorice root (*Glycyrrhiza glabra*), Wild Cherry bark (*Prunus serotina*), Elecampane (*Inula helenium*), Pleurisy Root (*Asclepias tuberosa*), and Marshmallow root (*Althaea officinalis*). Make a strong tea by putting ½ ounce of each herb in 1½ quarts of water, simmer gently for 10 minutes, steep for 20 minutes, strain, and sweeten with honey. Dosage: 1-2 tablespoons as needed.

Pills and Capsules: Flowers and leaves are dried, ground into powder, and prepared in the usual way as pills or hand-packed into capsules. Dosage: 1-3 pills or capsules up to 4 times a day.

Salve: Bake fresh Horehound in oil in the usual way. Refer to the "Index of Health Issues and Herbal Recommendations" when choosing other herbs to combine with Horehound.

Poultice: Pulverize fresh or dried leaves into a mash and cook them in a little water for application.

Fomentation: Soak a cloth in a strong infusion tea and apply to the skin.

Culinary Uses

In Europe, Horehound has been used as a seasoning in stews, salads, fish and meat dishes, sauces, cakes, and cookies. However, its bitterness is too extreme for many people's taste buds. It is primarily used to make candy and cough medicine, but requires a lot of sweetener to make it palatable.

Chemical Constituents

Marrubiin (0.3-1%) is a bitter diterpene lactone considered to be one of the main medicinal components of Horehound. It is an analgesic and expectorant, it normalizes secretions of the mucous membranes, and promotes bile flow through the liver (choleretic). Marrubiin normalizes heart arrhythmias, but excessive doses can cause irregular heartbeats. Other bitter diterpenes include marrubiol, peregrinol, vulgarol, marrubenol, marruciol, and sclareol (antibacterial and antifungal).

Essential oils include bisabolol, cymene (analgesic, antibacterial, antiviral, sedative), pinene (anti-acne, antibacterial, anti-inflammatory, antispasmodic, antiviral, expectorant, sedative), sabinene, limonene (antibacterial, anticancer, antilithic, antispasmodic, antiviral, expectorant, sedative), and camphene (expectorant). These essential oils generally exhibit vasodilator, expectorant, and antimicrobial activity.

Flavonoids include apigenin (anti-arrhythmic, antibacterial, antihistamine, anti-inflammatory, anti-leukemia, antioxidant, antiviral, choleretic, estrogenic, sedative, vasodilator), luteolin (antibacterial, anticarcinogenic, antitumor, antihistamine, anti-inflammatory, antispasmodic, antiviral, choleretic, hepato-protective, vasodilator), and quercetin (anti-inflammatory and antihistamine). B-sitosterol is a phytosterol showing estrogenic activity in addition to being antibacterial, antiviral, hepatoprotective, and antitumor for breast, cervical, and lung tissues. Horehound also contains tannins, mucilage, ursolic acid (analgesic, antihistamine, sedative), alkaloids (betonicine, stachydrine, turicine), ascorbic acid (vitamin C), and choline, which is hepatoprotective and hypotensive.

Safety, Contraindications, and Drug Interactions

Horehound is generally considered to be a safe herb when ingested in standard dosages. Current medicinal applications are based on modern scientific research in addition to the plant's historic use in well-established systems of traditional healing. In very large doses, it can act as an emetic (causing nausea and vomiting), a strong laxative, or cause heart arrhythmia. However, the extremely bitter taste is an innate safety mechanism, making Horehound difficult for most people to ingest in excessive amounts. **Pregnant women should avoid this herb** due to its emmenagogue properties that stimulate uterine contractions and menstruation. **It is too strong to be taken by children under 2 years of age.** The German Commission E herbal regulatory agency reported no other known side effects, drug interactions, or contraindications (Blumenthal, 1998; Brinker, 2001).

Medicinal Uses

History of the Plant

People throughout Europe and Asia have included Horehound in their folk medicine for centuries. The ancient Egyptians employed it as a lung remedy for coughs and infections, and so highly revered its powerful action that they called it the "Seed of Horus" (their mighty god of the sky) and "bull's blood." Its antispasmodic and healing actions for respiratory ailments were recognized by the early Greeks and Romans. They used it as an antidote for many poisons, especially from bites of snakes and rabid dogs, hence its common name, "Horehound." "Hore" may also be derived from Old English *hor* or *har*, meaning "white with age," referring to the fine, white, downy hairs covering the entire plant. The botanical name *Marrubium* is thought to have originated from the Hebrew word *marrob*, meaning "bitter juice." According to Jewish tradition, Horehound can be used as one of the bitter herbs required for the Feast of Passover. Some historians believe that the Latin name is derived from *Maria urbs*, an ancient town of Italy.

The Greek physician Dioscorides (*circa* A.D. 40–*c.* 90) treated respiratory diseases, mucous congestion, coughs, asthma, and tuberculosis with Horehound tea. He also used it to promote menstruation, ease difficult childbirth, and treat venomous bites and stings. Galen (*c.* A.D. 131–*c.* 200), a famous physician of the Roman Empire, administered the tea to purge the lungs of phlegm and to open obstructions in the liver and spleen. Much later, two British apothecaries, John Gerard (1545–1612) and Nicholas Culpeper (1616–1654), praised Horehound for effectively treating coughs and colds, wheezing, tuberculosis, ingestion of poisons, and bites of snakes and rabid dogs. Culpeper and other medical astrologers determined that Horehound is ruled by the planet Mercury (Culpeper, 1992). John Gerard wrote in *The Herball or Generall Historie of Plantes* that "Common Horehound boiled in water and drunk, opens the liver and spleen, cleans the breast and lungs, and prevails greatly against an old cough. The same boiled in wine and drunk, brings down the terms [promotes menstruation]" (Gerard, 1633). Horehound was a common remedy of the Medieval Europeans who believed that it offered special protection from the imagined evils of witchcraft. Indigenous to India, Horehound has been employed by Ayurvedic doctors for respiratory illnesses, including bronchitis and whooping cough.

When European settlers introduced the plant into North America, the Native American Indians adopted it into their herbal pharmacy, as did the Eclectic physicians during the 1800s. The Eclectics prescribed it for respiratory distress, coughs, asthma, jaundice, intestinal worms, and to stimulate menstruation. Horehound was listed as an official drug in the *United States Pharmacopoeia* from 1820–1900.

Since Victorian times in England, Horehound has been a primary ingredient in candy and cough drops. Although this herb has been an important European folk medicine for hundreds of years and researchers have determined it to be safe and effective, the U.S. Food and Drug Administration (FDA) banned Horehound from over-the-counter cough remedies in 1989, claiming insufficient evidence of effectiveness. However, it remains on the GRAS (generally recognized as safe) list, and in 1990, the German Commission E herbal regulatory agency officially approved Horehound for the treatment of bronchial catarrh (phlegm), dyspepsia (indigestion), loss of appetite, and acknowledged its beneficial choleretic action on the liver. The Council of Europe approves it as a natural flavoring, allowing it to be added to food in small amounts. It continues to be a popular herb and is cultivated in the United States, Europe, and throughout the world.

Healing Qualities

Antibacterial, anti-catarrhal, anti-inflammatory, antioxidant, antispasmodic, antivenomous, antiviral, bitter tonic, cardiac, carminative, cholagogue (choleretic), deobstruent, diaphoretic, diuretic, emmenagogue, expectorant, febrifuge, hepatic, laxative, pectoral, mild sedative, stimulant, stomachic, vasodilator, vermifuge, and vulnerary.

Traditional Chinese Medicine (TCM) Perspective

Horehound is a cooling and bitter Yang herb that stimulates movement and activity throughout the body. It specifically improves stagnation and sluggish conditions in the lungs, heart, stomach, spleen, liver, and uterus. As a cooling expectorant, it dissolves and expels lung phlegm and damp heat. Horehound promotes sweating and dispels Wind Heat manifesting as fevers, bronchitis, sinusitis, and coughs with white or yellow mucous. The herb circulates Heart Qi (vital energy) and resolves Heart Qi constraint to calm tension and relieve palpitations. It stimulates sluggish digestion and bile flow, and resolves Stomach and Liver Qi Stagnation that can cause indigestion, constipation, and liver problems. Horehound resolves Kidney and Uterine Qi Stagnation and resulting skin rashes, scanty urination, edema, premenstrual syndrome (PMS), irregular cycles, and missed periods. It is contraindicated in cold conditions of Kidney Yang deficiency.

Primary Actions

The historic uses of Horehound revolve around its stimulating and restoring actions on the respiratory and digestive systems. It calms the nerves and relaxes the muscular layers of blood vessels to dilate them and increase blood flow. The leaves and flowers normalize the secretions of mucous membranes, which are specialized cells lining the respiratory, digestive, and genitourinary tracts. Horehound is effective for acute respiratory infections and may also be used as a tonic over time to restore balance to the system. I use it as one of the main ingredients in my tincture formulas for lung and bronchial ailments and for stomach problems. Clinical herbalist and Eclectic physician William Cook, M.D., wrote, "This herb is stimulating and relaxant, acting rather diffusely, but leaving behind a permanent impression which is somewhat tonic and astringent. The skin and mucous membranes are chiefly affected by it, and it is a longtime family remedy in colds and catarrhal coughs" (Cook, 1869).

Lungs and Respiratory System: Horehound exerts specific action on the nasal sinuses, throat, bronchioles and lungs, and is excellent for the treatment of acute and chronic respiratory problems. Eclectic physician Harvey Felter, M.D. (1865–1927) wrote, "Its stimulant action upon the laryngeal and bronchial mucous membranes is pronounced, and it, undoubtedly, also influences the respiratory function. It is used in the form of syrup in coughs, colds, chronic catarrh (excessive mucous), asthma, and all pulmonary affections" (Felter, 1898). The essential oils in Horehound relax smooth muscles to ease constricted breathing and dilate blood vessels, which increases circulation in the lungs. The oils are antibacterial and antiviral against infections and are expectorants for coughs (Karryev, 1976). Marrubiin is a cooling, non-irritating expectorant that decongests and reduces phlegm and damp heat in the lungs. It has a normalizing effect on the secretions of mucous glands in the sinuses, bronchial tubes, and lungs (Tyler, 1982). For dry and unproductive coughs, Horehound stimulates mucous secretions to liquefy and expel thick phlegm. For copious mucous discharges due to atonic mucous membranes, the herb tones the membranes to reduce secretions. Thus, it has historically been employed for wet productive coughs or for dry unproductive coughs with chest tightness.

The herb lowers fevers because it promotes perspiration and brings interior heat to the surface. When treating fevers, drink hot tea prepared from the leaves and flowers or take 30-60 drops of tincture in hot water. Horehound is a remedy for all bronchial and respiratory problems and infections, including colds, coughs, sore throats, swollen lymph glands, hoarseness and laryngitis, pneumonia, whooping cough, asthma, shortness of breath, wheezing, acute and chronic bronchitis, sinusitis, and it can be helpful for hay fever and allergies. In the past, it was prescribed for tuberculosis, typhoid, and paratyphoid fevers.

For respiratory conditions, Horehound combines well with Elecampane, Elder berries (*Sambucus canadensis*), Wild Cherry bark, Marshmallow root, Hyssop, Pleurisy Root, Mullein (*Verbascum thapsus*), Thyme (*Thymus vulgaris*), Goldenseal (*Hydrastis canadensis*), and Lobelia (*Lobelia inflata*).

Digestive System and Diabetes: Bitter alkaloids in Horehound have a stimulating and tonic influence on the entire digestive system, and specifically influence conditions caused by underactivity and congestion, including indigestion, gas, bloating, and constipation. As a digestive aid, drink ½-1 cup of tea or 15-30 drops of tincture in water 5-10 minutes before meals.

Horehound reduces spasms and normalizes mucous membrane secretions throughout the digestive tract. It promotes secretion of stomach acids and pancreatic digestive enzymes, improves a poor appetite, and is an excellent stomach tonic. The herb resolves general acidosis, a condition resulting from acid accumulation or depletion of alkaline reserves in the blood and tissues. In mice studies, an alcohol extract of Horehound leaves reduced the incidence of stomach ulcers. The extract protected the stomach linings of the mice against damage by normalizing acid pH and increasing mucous production (Paula de Oliveira, 2011).

By promoting bile flow from the liver, bitter herbs help restore healthy liver and gallbladder function (Krejci, 1959). Adequate bile flow enables the liver to clear toxins and excess estrogens out of the system, and normalizes intestinal activity and bowel movements. Horehound has a long tradition of use in treating jaundice and chronic hepatitis. Marrubic acid in the herb protects the liver from toxins and can significantly reduce elevated liver enzymes indicative of liver malfunction (Ahmed, 2010).

M. vulgare strengthens the pancreas and is a popular traditional medicine in Mexico and Algeria for treating diabetes type 2 and elevated blood levels of cholesterol and triglycerides. A cup of tea is usually ingested before each meal for these problems (Boudjelal, 2012).

Horehound's volatile oils possess vermifuge properties used to treat parasites. Researchers have found that these oils are especially toxic to the parasitic blood flukes *Schistosoma mansoni*, which infect the intestinal tract, and *Schistosoma haematobium*, which infect the genitourinary tract (Saleh, 1989).

Kidneys and Edema: When the tea is taken cool or tincture is added to cool water, Horehound stimulates the kidneys, and its diuretic action promotes urination to eliminate excess fluids from the tissues. The herb helps open and normalize blood flow through the kidneys and enhances the production of urine. This has a general cleansing effect on the entire body and helps to excrete excess acids from the blood. Antibacterial phytochemicals in Horehound help keep the urinary tract free of infection.

Heart and Nerves: Horehound acts as a weak sedative that calms the nervous system and can be used in combination with other herbs for nervous heart conditions and to reduce hypertension. Several constituents have been researched that provide explanations for the herb's ability to promote nerve and heart health. Marrubiin and marrubinic acid help normalize an irregular heartbeat (Duke, 2000). During *in vitro* studies, Marrubiin and marrubenol exhibited vasorelaxant activity (relaxing blood vessels). This allows blood vessel dilation, which improves many circulatory problems. Marrubenol inhibits smooth muscle contraction by blocking calcium channels, which relaxes muscles throughout the body (El Bardai, 2003).

Water and alcohol extracts of Horehound demonstrate anti-inflammatory and antioxidant action, providing protection against heart attacks and resulting fibrosis of heart muscles (Yousefi, 2013 & 2014). In folk medicine, water extracts of the leaves and flowers are a popular treatment for high blood pressure. Researchers confirmed the herb's ability to decrease systolic blood pressure in hypertensive rats during a

10-week treatment using Horehound tea (El Bardai, 2004).

In vitro studies demonstrate that antioxidants in *M. vulgare* inhibit cellular damage caused by low-density lipoproteins (LDL) while enhancing favorable effects of high-density lipoproteins (HDL) (Berrougui, 2006). Regular ingestion of the herb, combined with appropriate diet and exercise, may help prevent the development of cardiovascular diseases.

Create an excellent cardiovascular tonic by combining Horehound with Hawthorn berries (*Crataegus* spp.), Motherwort (*Leonurus cardiaca*), and Linden tree leaves and flowers (*Tilia americana,* spp.).

Women's Health: The liver clears excess estrogen from the bloodstream. By reducing stagnation in the liver, Horehound can improve problems caused by a sluggish and underactive liver resulting in estrogen excess. The herb exerts emmenagogue activity to stimulate menstruation, help increase a scanty menstrual flow, and restore menses if they stop abnormally. Horehound reduces spasms and has historically been used to relieve menstrual cramps and expel the placenta after childbirth. For vaginal infections and discharge (leucorrhea), drink the tea or tincture and prepare a strong tea for use as a douche.

Researchers have documented analgesic activity in marrubiin, which can relieve pain associated with PMS and menstruation (Meyre-Silva, 2005).

External Wound Healing: Horehound's anti-inflammatory, antibacterial, and vulnerary properties are healing for wounds, skin eruptions, ulcers, and other external problems. For external applications, the tea or diluted tincture can be administered as a wash or fomentation, the crushed leaves made into a poultice, or salve can be used. I have included Horehound leaves and flowers in my all-purpose "Herbal Healing Salve" for many years with wonderful results.

Teachings from the Horehound Deva

"Greetings, dear one. I am the deva of the Horehound family. In keeping with the green color of my leaves, I offer nourishment for the heart. For the vibrational frequency of the heart manifests as the green spectrum of color. Small amounts of my bitterness are good medicine for the emotional aspect of the heart and also for its cells to function well. My bitterness is like a homeopathic remedy assisting the heart to absorb and assimilate the bitterness of what you would call 'a world of hurt.' In homeopathy, it is said that 'like cures like.' In this way, I help the heart deal with the bitterness and hurt inherent in human life on this planet. For the nature of the heart is to express the fullness of love – love for all life, all creatures, and all people. The heart is able to perceive the oneness of life flowing through everyone and everything, and there is no perception of separation or fear. When life is lived in this reality, much suffering is avoided. However, during this era, so many forget this truth. So pain and bitterness live and grow in people, contributing to weakness and illness of the heart. Thus, I offer the heart protection from the grief and hardships of life. Indulge in my gifts by taking sips of my tea, a little tincture, or my flower essence. These may be taken over time for healing to occur.

"I greatly affect the lungs lying close to the heart. Like the heart, lungs must have great capacity for expansion as they breathe in air and oxygen. My plants provide good medicine to promote healthy lungs and assist in eliminating infectious pathogens, inflammation, and excessive mucous. My actions help normalize and strengthen the lungs, allowing you to take in the breath of life more fully.

"Although bitterness is part of my nature, I am a small plant and a gentle being. My essence is benevolence – I have compassion for the human family. I help mend what is torn and broken in the emotional field of energy. As the heart area is repaired and cleansed, its bright life force strengthens and radiates outward through the body.

"I help balance the energies of dry and damp within the body. My plants are regulated by the earth and air elements, and seek to blend these in harmonious balance. The earth element is cooling with a grounding flow of energy, reflected in our ability to normalize the digestive system and allow the smooth, downward flow of food. The air element serves the lungs and movement of gases and oxygen through the body. The air element is diffusive energy spreading outward. So there is freedom of movement within my plant medicines. I offer the balance of being securely grounded and protected in the earth, while also experiencing the freedom and expanse of unrestricted movement, growth, and wonderment.

"My message is to bring this balance into your own life – the merging of heaven and earth. This is an act of bringing the polarities into a dynamic and constantly changing expression of balance. Partake of my medicine for assistance on this path."

Hyssop

Hyssopus officinalis
Labiatae (Lamiaceae) (Mint) Family

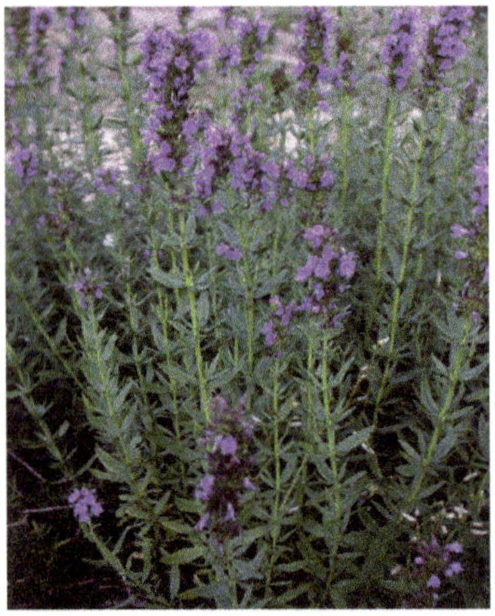

Common Names

Hyssop and sacred herb are common names for this herb. Several different plants are called wild Hyssop, Lavender Hyssop and Anise Hyssop, but they are not related and do not refer to *Hyssopus officinalis*.

Medicinal Part of the Plant

The upper leaves and flowers are used for medicinal purposes.

Range and Habitat

Hyssop is native to the Mediterranean region and has been cultivated throughout Europe, the Middle East and the United States, where it has naturalized in many areas. It grows in dry or moist soil along roadsides and in open spaces.

Description of the Plant

Hyssop is an attractive perennial growing 1-3′ tall. It is an aromatic herb, emitting a strong, pungent camphor fragrance somewhat reminiscent of turpentine. The fibrous root system sends out many erect, branching, square stems that become woody at the base as plants age. The stems and leaves may or may not be covered with tiny hairs. Deep-green leaves are ½-1½″ long and climb the entire length of the stems in small whorls at ½-1″ intervals. Leaves are simple, entire (having a smooth margin), and linear. Hyssop is considered to be an evergreen since many of the lower leaves remain green throughout the freezing months of winter.

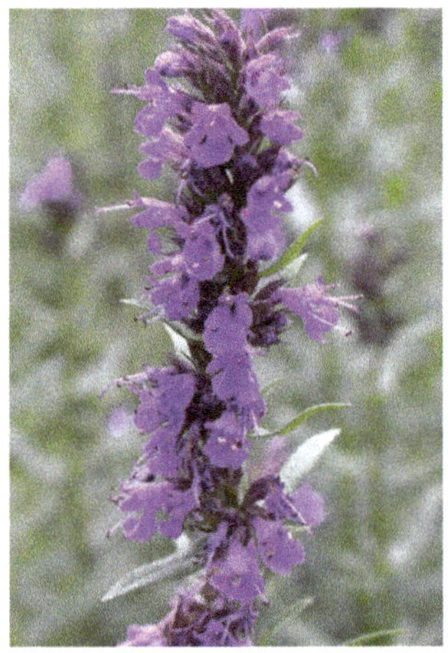

The small ¼-½″ flowers bloom from June through September. They are a brilliant shade of purplish blue, although white and pink cultivars exist. The different colored flowers may be used medicinally. Flowers grow from 2-10″ spikes in whorls containing up to 16 blossoms that emerge from leaf axils along one side of the upper stems. A green tubular calyx holds the flower's tubular corolla. The bi-lobed upper lip of the corolla is erect, and the lower lip consists of 3 lobes. Each flower has 4 protruding stamens surrounding the central pistil.

An established bed of blooming Hyssop creates a radiant, deep purple-blue bushy ground cover that is charming and beautiful to behold, and a welcome addition to flower gardens. Bees are attracted to the flower pollen, which yields a dark, deliciously strong-tasting wildflower honey. Some people claim that grapevines increase their yields when planted close to Hyssop.

Cultivation

Hyssop is a hardy plant easily grown from seeds or stem cuttings. Plants can adapt to various growing conditions, but produce the most medicinally potent oils when grown in warm, dry areas under full sun. Hyssop prefers a light, loamy, well-drained limestone soil with a pH between 6.5 and 7.5. Peak production of flowers and leaves is usually during the second and third years of growth, but older plants continue to produce substantial yields. Cultivated plants may live up to 7-9 years.

Plant the seeds in flats during early spring and barely cover them with soil. The germination rate is usually 40-60% and requires 1-2 weeks when soil temperature reaches 60-70°F. When seedlings are 5-6″ tall, transplant them to a prepared bed. Space them about 6″ apart or plant 2-4 seedlings together and space them 1′ apart to create a more compact garden.

To propagate from stem cuttings, clip 7-8″ lengths of stems from mature plants in late spring or early summer. Place the stems in a bucket of wet, well-drained potting soil, sand, and vermiculite until roots develop. Plant the stem cuttings 1′ apart, water thoroughly, and mulch. Although much of Hyssop's foliage remains green all winter, dead growth on the upper stems should be pruned away every spring to keep the patch clean and encourage new growth.

Harvest

When the plant is in full bloom, harvest the flowering tops and leaves by pruning the top 6-10″ of stems. Be sure to leave plenty of leaves and flowers to ensure the plant's survival, and avoid pruning more than 25% of the stems. The tiny seeds can be collected for next year's planting. Gather them in late summer after the flowers have matured into dry, brown seedpods.

Preparation of Plant Medicine and Dosages

Hyssop yields its medicinal components to alcohol, water, and oils. Preparations include tea, tincture, pills, capsules, cough syrup, and external applications of a wash or fomentation, poultice, oil, and salve. The freshly harvested herb is most potent, but the flowers and leaves may be dried by placing them on screens or tying them in small bundles to hang in a shady, well-ventilated area.

PREPARATIONS

Infusion Tea: Steep 1-2 teaspoons of the herb in 1 cup of boiled water. Dosage: 1-2 cups per day. For a much stronger medicinal tea, steep ¼ ounce of the herb in a pint of water, sweeten with honey, and take in 3-4 divided doses throughout the day. The sharp, pungent flavor is bitter and rather spicy. For external purposes, the tea may be used as a wash or applied as a fomentation.

Tincture: Chop fresh leaves and flowers into small pieces, place in a glass jar, and cover with 70% 190-proof grain alcohol and 30% distilled water. Dosage: 20-60 drops in water up to 4 times a day.

Pills and Capsules: The leaves and flowers are dried, ground into fine powder, and rolled into pills or packed into gelatin capsules. Dosage: Up to 6 pills or capsules in divided doses throughout the day.

Cough Syrup: Create wonderful syrup by brewing a very strong tea of the fresh leaves and flowers and adding sugar or honey. (Refer to "Lung and Bronchial Problems" on page 579 in the "Index of Health Issues and Herbal Recommendations" for a listing of more herbs to combine in cough syrup.)

Oil and Salve: Chop fresh flowers and leaves, put them in a stainless steel or glass bowl, cover with olive oil, and bake at 200-225°F for 3-4 hours. Add beeswax for a thicker salve consistency. Combine Hyssop with other vulnerary herbs for best results. (Refer to "Skin Problems" on page 591 in the "Index of Health Issues and Herbal Recommendations" for a listing of vulnerary herbs).

Poultice: Apply the fresh or dried herb as a poultice for external healing.

Culinary Uses

The leaves are hot, spicy, and somewhat bitter. They have traditionally been used to flavor salads, soups, stews, tomato dishes, and fruit pies. Use them sparingly because of the very strong flavor.

Chemical Constituents

The volatile oils (0.3-2%) exert strong actions that are stimulating, antibacterial, antiviral, anti-inflammatory, carminative, diaphoretic, and antispasmodic. Volatile oils include camphor (which is also analgesic, expectorant, fungicide), pinocamphone, isopinocamphone, cineole (antiparasitic, anti-allergic, anti-catarrh, anti-arthritic, antiseptic, anti-sinusitis, antitussive, expectorant, sedative), carvacrol (antiparasitic, anti-streptococcal, antitussive, expectorant, fungicide), thujone (emmenagogue), pinene (antiflu, expectorant, sedative), camphene (expectorant), linalool, bornyl acetate (expectorant, sedative), borneol (analgesic, antibronchitis, febrifuge, hepatoprotective, sedative), eugenol (anticonvulsant, anti-herpes, choleretic, diuretic, febrifuge, vermifuge), geraniol (expectorant, sedative), thymol (anti-arthritic, expectorant, vermifuge), and limonene (antiflu, antitumor, expectorant, fungicide, sedative).

Terpenoids include marrubiin (cardio-active, anti-arrhythmic, choleretic or cholagogue, expectorant, anti-catarrhal), oleanolic acid (antibacterial, anti-HIV, anti-inflammatory, antiviral, cardiotonic, diuretic, sedative), and ursolic acid (antihistamine, anti-HIV, anti-inflammatory, antiviral). Caffeic acid is antibacterial, antiflu, anti-herpes, antihistamine, anti-HIV, immunostimulating, sedative, and vulnerary. Rosmarinic acid is antibacterial, diuretic, anti-HIV, anti-inflammatory, and antiviral. Beta-sitosterol is antibacterial, androgenic, estrogenic, and hepatoprotective. Tannins are astringent. Flavonoids include diosmin (anti-inflammatory, antihistamine, diuretic, protects capillaries) and hesperidin (antihistamine, antiviral, choleretic, sedative, protects and strengthens capillaries) (Duke, 2000).

Safety, Contraindications, and Drug Interactions

Very little clinical research has focused on Hyssop, although many chemical constituents in the herb have been identified which provide information about its biological activity and support its historic uses by well-established medical traditions. The herb is **contraindicated during pregnancy** due to emmenagogue activity. There are no known drug interactions or side effects when it is taken in recommended doses (Brinker, 2001; McGuffin, 1997).

Moderate use of the tea, tincture, and pills is considered safe, but due to the content of strong volatile oils, **large doses should not be ingested for extended periods of time**. The **concentrated essential oil can be toxic**, potentially causing spasms and convulsions, and should be avoided or taken in very small doses of one drop diluted in one cup of water. At least three cases of essential oil toxicity have been reported. One involved a six-year-old child who developed muscle spasms after taking 2-3 drops of oil for several days. Two adults also reported spasms after ingesting 10 drops of oil (Blumenthal, 1998).

Medicinal Uses

History of the Plant

Hyssop's beauty, spicy flavor, and pungent aroma attracted the attention of ancient people living throughout the Mediterranean area. A symbol of cleansing and purification, its common name is thought to be derived from the Greek word *azob*, meaning "holy herb." The strong fragrance of the leaves and flowers cleansed the air in temples and sacred places. The ancient Egyptians treated lepers with Hyssop baths. Details of its historic use are muddled because many plants have been given the common name of Hyssop. For instance, it is mentioned in the Bible in Psalm 51:7 when David prays, "purge me with hyssop and I shall be clean," and a reference to the crucifixion in John 19:29 reads, "There was a vessel full of vinegar: and they filled a sponge with vinegar and put it upon hyssop and put it in His mouth. . ." Many botanical and biblical scholars believe that these verses refer to wild Marjoram or Oregano rather than *Hyssopus officinalis*, which did not grow wild in the area.

The Romans valued this plant as a ceremonial and medicinal herb and cultivated it wherever they lived. The Greek physician and botanist Dioscorides (*circa* A.D. 40–*c.* 90) often mixed it with figs to make the bitter flavor more palatable. He recorded its value in expelling worms and treating lung ailments, including pneumonia, asthma, coughs, and excess phlegm. Hyssop has been employed throughout Europe for treating many respiratory and digestive problems, anxiety, rheumatism, ear pain, toothaches, and external wounds.

During the early history of the Catholic Church in Europe, Hyssop continued to be revered for its purifying attributes. The fragrance of the crushed leaves scattered in European homes and churches masked nasty odors resulting from lack of sanitation and bathing, and the leaves and flowers were added to colognes, bath oils, lotions, and liqueurs. Hildegard of Bingen (1098–1179), the German Benedictine nun and healer, wrote that Hyssop "cleanses the lungs," and recommended it for respiratory problems and depression. English apothecary and surgeon John Gerard (1545–1612) prescribed Hyssop for respiratory and digestive problems that included inflammation, coughs, shortness of breath, and for mouth or throat sores. Another English apothecary, Nicholas Culpeper (1616–1654), also recommended it for treating lung and digestive afflictions, parasites, as a nerve tonic and sedative for anxiety, and externally for rheumatism, wounds, ear pain, toothaches, and to kill body lice. Culpeper wrote, "The herb is Jupiter's, under the sign Cancer . . . . It restoreth the natural color of the skin when discolored by the yellow jaundice" (Culpeper, 1992).

Hyssop was introduced into North America by the early European colonists, who grew it in their New England gardens until it naturalized into surrounding areas and north into Canada. The Eclectic physicians of the 1880s–1930s adopted it into their practice for its excellent effect on the respiratory and digestive systems, and to treat asthma, coughs, colds, flu, and quincy (tonsillitis). They recommended the herb as a gargle for sore throats, to promote good capillary circulation, and to treat wounds, external bruising, and pain. Over time, as pharmaceutical drugs became the predominant medicines, Hyssop fell out of general use and is now primarily enjoyed as a garden ornamental. It is currently listed in the British Herbal Pharmacopoeia for treating the common cold and bronchial infections. Although it is commercially available, Hyssop is not a top-selling or well-known herb, and lack of research studies have kept it from the attention of the media.

Healing Qualities

Antibacterial, anti-catarrhal, anti-inflammatory, antispasmodic, antiviral, aromatic, astringent, bitter, carminative, cholagogue (choleretic), depurative, diaphoretic, diuretic, emmenagogue, exanthematous, expectorant, febrifuge, hepatic, mild immunomodulator, mild laxative, nervine, opthalmicum, pectoral, sedative, stimulant, stomachic, tonic, vermifuge, and vulnerary.

Traditional Chinese Medicine (TCM) Perspective

Hyssop is slightly warming, bitter, and drying. It influences the lungs, stomach, liver, kidneys, uterus, and blood circulation. It removes interior heat to reduce fevers, pathogens, and toxins. The herb expels obstructions from the lungs and blood vessels, and resolves phlegm and dampness in the lungs. It is stimulating and promotes the smooth flow of Qi in the lungs, liver, kidneys, and digestive and circulatory systems. It exerts a restoring and relaxing influence on the nervous system, and is tonifying to mucous membranes and blood vessels throughout the body.

Primary Actions

Hyssop is a wonderful healing herb that I add to different formulas. It exerts a calming effect on the nervous system. As an antiviral and antibacterial, it is ideal for a multitude of infections, specifically those of the respiratory and digestive systems. Hyssop is a dependable addition to many of my antiviral formulas. Relaxing and safe for children, it was used in pediatric practice by the Eclectic physicians.

Fevers and Infections: Hyssop is an immunomodulator that regulates and supports the immune system. Effective against bacterial and viral infections, it is an effective remedy when treating the common cold, coughs, upper respiratory infections, influenza (the flu), and eruptive skin diseases such as scarlet fever (caused by *Streptococcus* bacteria), measles (rubeola virus), mumps (a viral infection of parotid and other glands), chicken pox (caused by the varicella-zoster virus, a member of the herpes group), and shingles (the herpes zoster virus). Modern research confirms Hyssop's ability to inhibit growth of the herpes simplex virus (causing mouth and genital lesions) in laboratory settings (Duke, 2000). It is most effective when combined with St. John's Wort (*Hypericum perforatum*), Lemon Balm (*Melissa officinalis*), and Boneset (*Eupatorium perfoliatum*) when treating the herpes family of viruses. Many of my clients have reported that this formula speeds up the healing of cold sores and reduces the severe, agonizing pain of shingles within a few hours when applied to the lesions and ingested (1 teaspoon diluted in water) every 3-4 hours. This formula also works well for other member of the herpes family, including the Epstein-Barr virus causing mononucleosis. Many high school and college students who have taken this formula to treat mononucleosis report rapid reduction of their symptoms, especially fatigue, and they are able to return to their normal activities much sooner.

Researchers have recorded test tube experiments demonstrating the ability of crude Hyssop extracts to inhibit the HIV virus that causes AIDS. The herb contains a compound called MAR-10 that inhibits HIV replication without damaging healthy cells (Gollapudi, 1995; Kaplan, 1990).

Hyssop induces sweating to release excess internal heat and reduce fevers, especially when the tea or tincture is taken hot. It is beneficial for all intermittent (reoccurring), chronic, low grade or acute fevers, and for viral infections with underlying toxic conditions. I usually combine Hyssop with other antiviral and antibacterial herbs such as Sage (*Salvia officinalis*), Yarrow (*Achillea millefolium*), Echinacea (*Echinacea purpurea*), Blue Vervain (*Verbena hastata*), Boneset, and Isatis (*Isatis tinctoria*). Take 2-4 droppers full (45-90 drops) of this tincture combination several times throughout the day for best results during illness.

Lung and Bronchial Health: Hyssop is a beneficial tonic for mucous membranes throughout the body, especially in the nasal sinuses, throat, bronchioles, and lungs. The herb reduces inflammation, and its astringent qualities tone the membranes and normalize mucous secretions. Marrubiin and several soothing, camphor-like compounds in the volatile oils loosen phlegm to break up congestion and expel excessive mucous. As an antispasmodic and relaxing expectorant, it is valuable for most respiratory problems, including bacterial and viral infections, acute and chronic congestion, the common cold, coughs, bronchitis, bronchial spasms, tonsillitis, allergic rhinitis (sinus inflammation), emphysema, and asthma.

The effect of *Hyssopus officinalis* on asthma was explored using mice studies that revealed the herb's ability to decrease inflammation and regulate immunity. Mice treated with the herb had reduced levels of eosinophils (a type of white blood cell) and IgE (an immune substance), which both increase during inflammation. Mucous secretion and improved airflow were documented (Ma, 2014). Researchers have also confirmed *in vitro* antioxidant and antimicrobial activities in alcohol extracts of the herb (Vlase, 2014).

Hyssop reduces fevers and can be combined with Sage and Horehound (*Marrubium vulgare*) to treat fevers and make a soothing, antibacterial gargle for sore throats. In the European herbal folk tradition, Hyssop was often combined with Horehound and Coltsfoot (*Tussilago farfara*) to treat coughs, and with Boneset, Elder flowers (*Sambucus* spp.), and Peppermint (*Mentha x piperita*) for the common cold and flu.

Nervous System: Hyssop's nervine qualities help tone and restore the nervous system while relaxing the lungs and entire body. As a sedative, it calms anxiety and eases nerve and muscle spasms. The herb is an old remedy for insomnia and is employed as a tonic for all types of conditions caused by nervous tension. The herb was once used in treating epilepsy. Modern researchers have confirmed that the volatile oils in Hyssop exert a muscle-relaxing effect in animal studies (Lu, 2002). It combines well with other nervines and sedatives such as Scullcap (*Scutellaria lateriflora*), Valerian (*Valeriana officinalis*), Lavender (*Lavandula* spp.), Hops (*Humulus lupulus*), Passion Flower (*Passiflora incarnata*), and Chamomile (*Matricaria recutita*).

Blood Circulation and Detoxification: Named for its ability to cleanse and purify, Hyssop relaxes blood vessel walls to improve blood circulation and help lower high blood pressure (Willard, 1997). It is beneficial for chronic venous insufficiency, a condition of poor blood circulation through the veins (Duke, 1997). Hyssop catalyzes elimination of toxins by its diuretic activity that increases urination and flushes out the kidneys, and by its diaphoretic qualities that stimulate perspiration to reduce fevers and eliminate toxins through the skin. By enhancing blood circulation and the natural routes of elimination, the herb exerts stimulating, cleansing, and tonic effects benefiting the entire system.

Gastrointestinal and Urinary Systems: Hyssop soothes and normalizes the mucous membranes lining the organs and passageways of the digestive and urinary tracts. Especially when taken hot, it relaxes muscle tone within the tissues and reduces inflammation and spasms. Like many herbs containing strong volatile oils and bitters, it stimulates the release of digestive enzymes from the stomach and pancreas and bile from the liver and gallbladder. As a mild laxative, it promotes bowel movements. Hyssop is specific for many digestive problems, including indigestion, gas, colic, bloating, and conditions involving spasms and inflammation.

Hyssop helps to normalize the liver, restore normal color to jaundiced skin, correct imbalance in the spleen, and exerts diuretic action on the kidneys to stimulate removal of excess fluids. Old-time herbalists recommended cold tea or tincture for kidney and liver problems. They used Hyssop in the treatment of dropsy, an antiquated term for edema of the ankles and legs perpetuated by heart congestion or failure.

Hyssop is effective against some bacterial, viral, and parasitic infections occurring in the digestive and urinary tracts. For parasites, tea or tincture is ingested three times a day before meals and used with other vermifuge herbs such as Wormwood (*Artemisia absinthium*) and Black Walnut (*Juglans nigra*).

Arthritis: Hyssop is an old European remedy for sprains and achy joints and muscles. A tea made from fresh leaves was ingested several times a day, and people soaked in Hyssop baths to comfort and restore sore limbs and backs.

External Uses and Eye Problems: The strong aromatic oils in the plant are an effective treatment for many unwanted pests. Hyssop oil kills body lice when applied externally, and the pungent odor repels insects. The leaves and flowers can be used as a poultice, salve, or fomentation to heal wounds, infections, burns, skin irritations, inflammation, muscular rheumatism, strains, and sprains. The herb is antibacterial and antifungal for skin infections, and it has a reputation of being a splendid agent in removing the black-and-blue discoloration from bruises when directly applied to the injured tissues. The filtered tea is administered as eyewash and is helpful for eye infections, inflammation, and itchy irritation. Combine it with Goldenseal (*Hydrastis canadensis*) tea for an excellent remedy for eye problems.

Teachings from the Hyssop Deva

"Greetings, dear one. I am the deva of the Hyssop plants that you summon. Hear my teachings. The intense, pungent odor and taste of my leaves and flowers reflect a powerful nature. My plants radiate the intensity of the violet aura, residing in the deep stillness of space existing before the dance of polarities manifests as form. For all material things arise and come into being from that which is formless – what has been called 'the great mystery' since the beginning of time. In this pure abode I rest, in this purple light vibration that permeates everywhere, though so subtly.

"I am also richly adorned in the blood-red light of the life force enlivening the earth, animals, and humans. It is this red ray that so strongly supports life in the physical body and is the foundational support for survival. And so, within the rainbow spectrum of light, I radiate the lower frequencies of the red ray and the higher frequencies of the violet ray. My plant medicine brings strength and balance to these forces in the body: my red light supporting and invigorating the physical body while the violet ray calms the nervous system and clarifies and refines mental faculties. When these lower and higher frequencies are in balance, the emotional feeling aspect of the heart easily rests in harmony, allowing the experience of residing in dynamic serenity and joy. Use the essence of my flowers or a few sips of my tea or tincture to receive these subtle benefits.

"My plants are under the dominion of Scorpio, governed by Mars and Pluto. Thus, I am ruled in part by Mars, the red planet providing physical strength, force of purpose, activity, and endurance. The power of my medicine purges and cleanses the body of toxins and infectious organisms to establish a pure terrain for sweetness to exist. My purple ray is associated with Pluto, the outer planet of higher and more subtle frequencies. When this ray is in attunement, deep inner calm abides.

"Within my medicine, these two octaves of Scorpio reside: the lower octave of Mars responsible for the physical body and the higher octave of Pluto influencing subtle energies of emotions and thoughts. By learning the lessons of Scorpio, these octaves merge into a basic harmony and completion. The ultimate lessons of Scorpio are to clearly perceive the reality of life and death, and to be free of all hope and fear, or attachments to either. In this way, true freedom and abiding peace are possible.

"I offer a meditation to balance the energies of the earth and heavens, and to strengthen and radiate love from the central heart. Sit calmly in a quiet place. Close your eyes and feel your lungs and chest expand and contract as you inhale and exhale with each breath. Do this for a short time, filling your body with air and oxygen, and allowing your chest and body to relax, deeply and completely. Then, imagine a ray of bright red light rising up from the earth's center, entering the base of your spine and moving up into your heart. Let each in-breath draw the red earth essence into your heart, and with each exhale, allow the red light to fill your heart and lungs, permeating through the rest of your body. Practice and learn to relax in this breathing pattern and visualization for a while. Next, with each inhale, imagine radiant white light descending from the heavens through the top of your head and into your heart. Upon your exhale, allow this radiance to fill your heart and entire body, instilling deep calm, clarity, and spaciousness. Practice in this way for 5-10 minutes a few times every day for several days. When this exercise becomes easier and more natural, complete the process with this third step: Sit quietly with closed eyes. Envision red light rising up from the earth as the white light descends from the heavens, and both merge in spiraling circles of pink light in your heart. As your heart fills with this pink light, allow it to radiate outward, nourishing the body and brightening the world. Practice this ancient meditation on a daily basis to enhance the stable experience of inner calm, clarity, and loving compassion. Namaste, dear one. I bow to the light within you."

Isatis

Isatis tinctoria
Cruciferae (*Brassicaceae*) (Mustard) Family

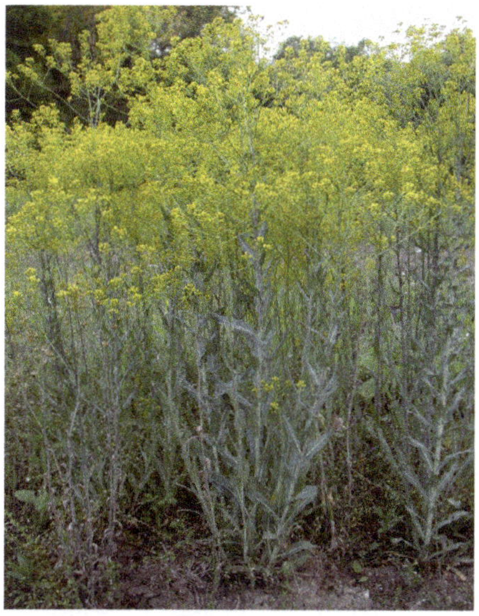

Common Names

Isatis tinctoria is commonly called woad, dyer's wood, and indigo.

Medicinal Part of the Plant

The leaves of one- or two-year-old plants and the roots of the second-year plant are used for medicine.

Range and Habitat

The *Isatis* genus consists of more than 30 species. The most popular species for dye and medicine are *I. tinctoria*, indigenous to Europe, and *I. indigotica,* native to Asia. Isatis plants grow in open sunny areas, and tend to be invasive in the western United States.

Several years ago, I introduced *I. tinctoria* into my gardens in southern Indiana. After allowing some of the original plants to go to seed, a multitude of seedlings sprouted voluntarily to flower the following spring, and Isatis continues to flourish in the gardens every year.

Description of the Plant

An attractive biennial ornamental, *I. tinctoria* grows up to 4′ tall. During the first year of growth, a bushy mound of light silver-green foliage reaches 1-1½′ in height. Early the following spring, the flowering plants are especially beautiful, creating a radiant cloud of brilliant golden-yellow flowers.

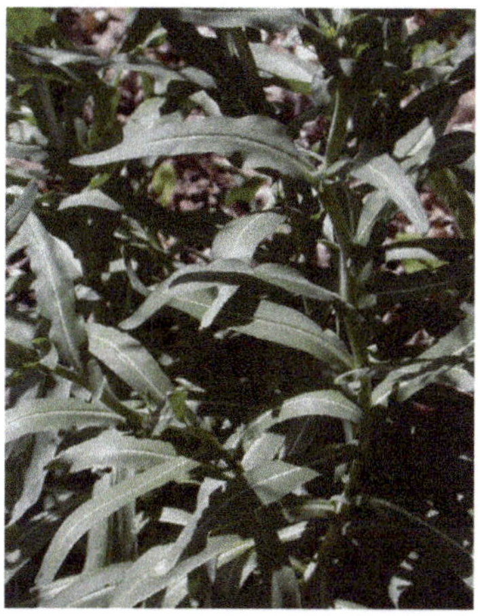

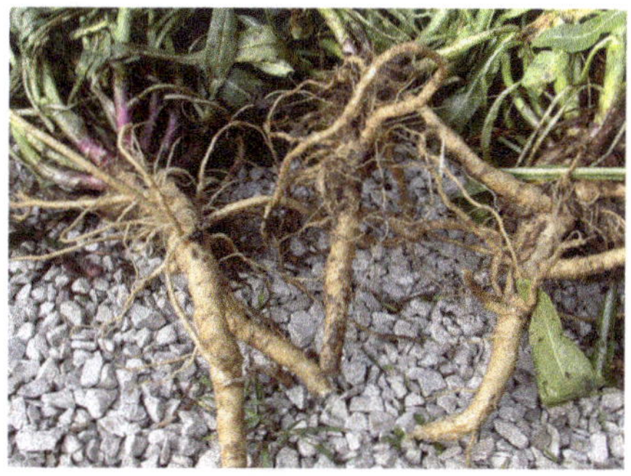

Small secondary roots branch off short, fibrous taproots. The cream-colored roots become woody during their second year of growth. Many erect, smooth stems emerge from the thick root crowns. Stems are round, solid, and pale green with splotches of dull maroon. They branch out into several flowering stalks towards the top of the plant.

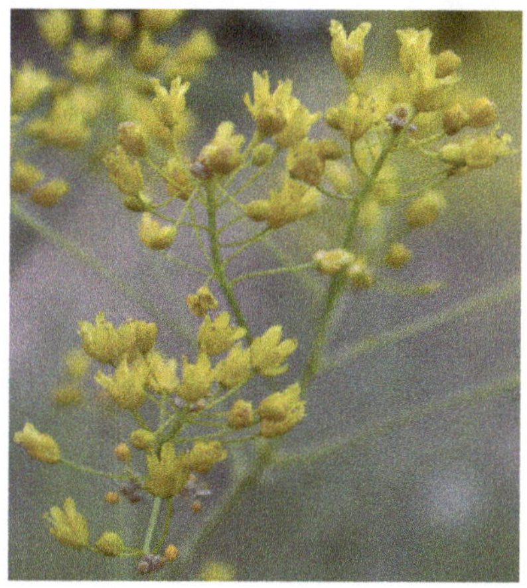

Many narrow, hastate-shaped leaves climb the stalks in an alternating pattern. Each leaf has a sessile base that clasps to the stem and points outward like an arrowhead, tapering to a pointed tip at its other end. The simple leaves are a light grayish-green color with a smooth, succulent texture similar to the leaves of broccoli and other members of the *Cruciferae* family. One predominant vein extends along the length of each leaf, while many lightly defined webbed veins cover the leaf. The leaves and stems are coated with a thin whitish film.

During the second year of growth, many corymb panicles (clusters) of tiny yellow flowers branch off the end of each stem, blooming from early April through May. Flowers consist of 4 greenish-yellow sepals, 4 bright-yellow petals, and 6 stamens surrounding the pistil. After 6-8 weeks, the flowers mature into flat, green, bi-lobed seedpods that turn brown when dry.

Cultivation

Isatis must be started from seed and is very easy to grow. Once established, it self-sows in early summer to provide volunteer plants by autumn. This herb prefers loamy soil with average fertility, good drainage, and full sun. Seeds may be sown directly into the soil in spring or autumn, or into nursery flats in early spring. Cover the seeds with ¼-½″ of soil. Transplant the seedlings into a prepared garden bed when they are 3-4″ tall and space them 1½′ apart. Keep the plants watered and mulched during the first year while the leaves and root systems develop. Flowers bloom in early spring of the second year and the seeds are usually mature by mid- summer.

Isatis (*Isatis tinctoria*)

Harvest

Harvest the roots and leaves of two-year-old plants when flowers bloom between April and May. After the blooming phase, roots become too fibrous and woody to be useful for medicine, so harvest the plants before this. Be sure to leave some plants to continue flowering so you can enjoy their beauty and collect the seeds, which may be planted immediately. Seeds can germinate within a month and develop their first year of foliage, then flower and be ready to harvest the following spring. In this way, a steady supply of plants may be harvested for medicine, and seeds are collected to replant year after year.

Preparation of Plant Medicine and Dosages

Wash and chop roots, and pick leaves off the stems. It is interesting to see the pretty indigo blue color as the bruised plant parts oxidize from air exposure. Before making tea or tincture with the leaves, clinical herbalist Stephen Buhner recommends to **dry leaves so the phytochemicals can convert to their usable forms**. When preparing tincture, the chopped root and dried leaves are put in a pan with a lid, heated to the point of boiling in the water used for tincturing, cooled, and alcohol is then added (Buhner, 2013).

Roots are bitter and leaves have a pleasantly mild taste similar to that of broccoli leaves with a slightly peppery aftertaste. Isatis can be made into tea, although tincturing provides the greatest concentration and preservation of healing constituents. The Experimental Pharmaceutical Factory at the Beijing College of Traditional Chinese Medicine found alcohol to be superior to water for extracting phytochemicals (Zhang, 1990). Always consider the **very cool nature of Isatis** that relieves hot conditions, but can eventually cause imbalance if taken in excess. Take Isatis for short periods of time and combine it with warming herbs when appropriate. The **leaves possess stronger antiviral actions** and the **roots are more antibacterial**.

PREPARATIONS

Tincture: Use 70% 190-proof grain alcohol and 30% distilled water for tincturing. As directed above, the chopped roots and dried leaves are brought to boiling in the water used for tincturing. Allow this to cool, transfer the water, roots and leaves into a glass jar, and cover with grain alcohol. Decant (separate) the herb from the liquid after one month. Dosage: 40-60 drops up to 6 times a day for acute infections. For chronic conditions, take 20-40 drops 1-3 times daily.

Tea: Simmer 2 teaspoons of chopped root in 2 cups of water for 10 minutes. When using dried leaves, steep 1-2 teaspoons per cup of water. Dosage: 1 cup 1-3 times daily for no longer than 2-3 weeks.

Dosages: Chinese doctors recommend daily doses of 9-15 grams (about 2-4 teaspoons) of the leaf and 10-30 grams (about 2-7 teaspoons) of the root prepared as tea, pills, or capsules.

External Applications: Prepare the leaves and roots as a poultice, apply the tea as a wash or fomentation, or use the tincture as a liniment.

Chemical Constituents

Isatis species share similar phytochemicals and biological effects. The roots and leaves of Isatis contain indican, the blue pigment indigo that is synthesized from indoxyl-glucoside and was used in the textile dyeing industry. The primary medicinal phytochemicals (and most researched) are tryptanthrin and indirubin, which occur in much greater concentrations in the dried leaves than in the fresh leaves (Buhner, 2013). Tryptanthrin is a potent antimicrobial and reduces inflammation by inhibiting prostaglandin and leukotriene production. It inhibits topical fungal infections and is antiparasitic. Indirubin, also a potent antiviral and anti-inflammatory, exhibits antitumor, antileukemic, anti-psoriasis, and neuroprotective actions.

I. tinctoria also contains beta- and gamma-sitosterols (lower cholesterol, immunomodulator), butenyl-isothiocyanate (antimutagenic), indigotin (inhibits cancer cell replication in lab studies), and sinigrin (has phagocytic activity that destroys cancer cells). *In vitro* tests show that isoformononetein is active against influenza, herpes simplex, and Coxsackie viruses (Wang, 2013). Isatin is antibiotic, antifungal, antitumor, and antiviral. Flavonoids include kaempferol (antibacterial, anticarcinogenic, anti-herpes, antihistamine, antileukemic, antiseptic, anti-staphylococcal, antiviral, choleretic, diuretic) and quercetin (anti-allergenic, antibacterial, anticarcinogenic, antiflu, anti-herpes, antileukemic, antiviral).

Safety, Contraindications, and Drug Interactions

Isatis is non-toxic with no problematic drug interactions (McGuffin, 1997). Taken with antibiotics and viral vaccines, it acts synergistically to increase their actions. **Use Isatis cautiously due to its very cooling properties**. Cool-natured people should only use this herb for short periods of 4-6 days. Combining Isatis with warming herbs, such as Ginger *(Zingiber officinale)* or Cayenne *(Capsicum annuum)*, balances its cool nature and can be a helpful adjustment. Use this combination if Isatis is taken over time to treat a chronic condition, or for bacterial and viral infections without fever. Excessive coolness weakens the stomach and can cause nausea in some sensitive people, and long-term use can weaken digestion. People occasionally report an uncomfortable but reversible feeling of internal coolness with long-term use.

Medicinal Uses

History of the Plant

European Isatis, *I. tinctoria*, has been cultivated throughout Europe since ancient times. Known as dyer's woad, it was used for the production of the blue dye indigo. Woad was often used to enhance and fix the more brilliant blue color derived from its relative, Wild Indigo *(Baptisia tinctoria)* until the early 20th century, when both plants were replaced by synthetic blue pigments.

Chinese Isatis, *I. indigotica*, has been used for over 2,000 years as medicine and blue indigo dye, and continues to be a popular herb in Chinese medicine. Most research comes from China, including clinical studies and many *in vitro* and *in vivo* tests that identify the phytochemicals and their biological actions.

Healing Qualities

Both *I. indigotica* and *I. tinctoria* clear heat toxicity, cool the blood, and have anti-allergenic, antibacterial, anticarcinogenic, antifungal, anti-inflammatory, antiparasitic, antitumor, antiviral, febrifuge, immunostimulant, and opthalmicum properties.

Traditional Chinese Medicine (TCM) Perspective

Chinese Isatis (*I. indigotica*) is very cooling and the roots are bitter. Isatis specifically affects the stomach, colon, heart, lungs, and liver. Due to its cooling nature, it is mainly used for acute hot conditions and chronic underlying excess heat. By clearing pathogenic heat, called Fire Poisons, from the blood and tissues, the entire body cools and detoxifies. Isatis is ideal for sore throats and reducing heat resulting from fever, inflammation, and infection. It is indicated for hot eruptive skin conditions involving redness and irritation. It also is beneficial for Damp Heat conditions like jaundice, Candida yeast, and fungal infections.

In TCM, the leaf, *Folium isatidis*, is commonly called Da Qing Ye, and the root, *Radix isatidis*, is Ban Lan Gen. Leaves and roots are often combined for their specific actions. The main indications for use are high fever, headache, infections, and a dark reddish-purple tongue. Isatis is traditionally used in clinical treatment of lung infections, pharyngitis, the common cold, toxic skin conditions, and viral diseases like mumps, measles, influenza (the flu), hepatitis, and encephalitis.

Primary Actions

After starting to grow, tincture, and use *I. tinctoria* for healing, it quickly became one of my favorite remedies for conditions of excess heat and bacterial, viral, or fungal infections. Since Western medicine has little to offer when treating viral illnesses, this is an important herb to have in one's medicine cabinet for its impressive range of activity. I always combine Isatis with other herbs to eliminate the common cold, flu, and fevers, for all types of acute infections, and infections that linger. Several of my clients with chronic excess heat manifesting as constant ruddy and flushed complexions, heavy menstrual bleeding, and red, itchy skin rashes have been helped by taking small amounts of the tincture alone for several months. It is an easy and beautiful plant to grow, and I encourage people to get acquainted with this powerful herbal ally.

Inflammation: Isatis is traditionally used as a cooling anti-inflammatory for the entire body, and specifically for the liver and spleen. Indirubin and tryptanthrin in Isatis are strong anti-inflammatory substances. Tryptanthrin inhibits the production of several inflammatory substances, including lipoxygenase (5-LOX), cyclooxygenase (COX-2), prostaglandins, and leukotrienes (Danz, 2002). Helpful for arthritis, the herb reduces inflammation in the joints. In a small study of 20 patients with neck or head cancer who had undergone radiation therapy, *I. indigotica* root decoction was tested for its ability to reduce inflamed tissues and painful swallowing. Compared to the group receiving saline water, the 10 patients given Isatis tea had faster tissue healing with less ulceration and pain when swallowing (You, 2009).

Bacterial, Viral, Fungal, and Parasitic Infections: Isatis is a powerful broad-spectrum antibiotic and antifungal, as well as an effective herb for viral infections. Its cooling nature removes pathogenic heat to reduce fevers, detoxify the blood, and treat eruptive skin rashes. Substantial research confirms the herb's ability to enhance immunity and eliminate infectious pathogens. Mouse studies show that polysaccharides extracted from Isatis root promote immune function by significantly increasing the weight of the spleen (a primary organ of immune function) and number of white blood cells in the mice. Beneficial phagocytic activity of macrophages engulfing and destroying pathogens was stimulated, and immunosuppressive actions of hydrocortisone were partially reduced (Xu, 1991; Roxas, 2007). Other researchers discovered that an a-glucan, also isolated from the root, significantly improved the immune response of mice exposed to H1N1 influenza (a cause of the flu, swine flu, and avian bird flu). The a-glucan increased the number of macrophages that destroyed the virus. The researchers concluded that these studies indicate the herb's ability to increase both humoral and cell-mediated immunity (Shan, 2014). During bacterial infections, endotoxins are sometimes released into the body from dying and damaged bacteria, worsening symptoms of the infection. Isatis works well in scavenging and eliminating these pathogenic endotoxins.

For many centuries, TCM physicians have prescribed Isatis for the common cold, influenza (flu), high fevers, laryngitis, sore throats, swollen lymph nodes, lung and respiratory tract infections, hepatitis, jaundice, encephalitis (viral infection and inflammation of brain tissue), meningitis (bacterial infection and inflammation of the tissues surrounding the brain and spinal cord), and septicemia (bacterial infection of the blood). It is given for contagious and epidemic viruses, such as mumps, measles and chicken pox, and for diphtheria, an acute bacterial infection. Isatis is an excellent treatment for all types of genitourinary infections, including cystitis (bladder infection) and vaginitis (vaginal infection). It is an effective and soothing antiseptic gargle for sore, infected throats.

A textbook published by the Shanghai College of Medicine recommends Isatis leaf for "epidemic febrile [feverish] diseases with the invasion of the blood by heat, manifested as high fever, restlessness, maculas [red spots] and eruptions, unconsciousness, delirium . . . erysipelas [a streptococcal skin infection], canker sores, and swollen and sore throat due to exuberant toxic heat in the blood . . . . The root is chiefly indicated for fever and headache in epidemic febrile diseases, or craniofacial infection characterized by swollen head and flushed swollen face, or throat infections with scarlet fever . . . and for influenza" (Enqin, 1988).

Over many years of nursing practice, I have used Isatis tincture combined with other antiviral herbs in assisting numerous clients to successfully reduce symptoms and speed recovery from severe herpes infections resulting in cold sores, genital lesions and shingles, and from mononucleosis primarily caused by the Epstein-Barr virus and occasionally by the cytomegalo virus (both members of the herpes family). Researchers have confirmed that extracts of Isatis leaf reveal powerful antiviral activity against the herpes simplex virus *in vitro* and *in vivo* (Fang, 2005).

An *in vitro* study was designed to test the ability of an *I. indigotica* alcohol extract to treat Japanese encephalitis, a serious viral infection and inflammation of the brain. The extract, containing indirubin, demonstrated potent antiviral activity in preventing and treating encephalitis by blocking the attachment of the virus to cells, inhibiting viral replication, and ultimately destroying the virus (Chang, 2012).

Herbalist Stephen Buhner has found Isatis to be effective in treating many serious, increasingly resistant pathogenic bacteria like methicillin-resistant *Staphylococcus aureus* (MRSA), *Escherichia coli* (cause of digestive and urinary tract infections), *Haemophilus influenzae* (responsible for pneumonia, bacteremia blood infection, and meningitis infection of the membranes covering the brain and spinal cord), *Shigella* (causes diarrhea and dysentery), *Pseudomonas aeruginosa* (responsible for pneumonia, septic shock, and infections of the urinary tract, ears, digestive system, and skin), *Clostridium botulinum* (source of botulism food poisoning), *C. perfringens* (a deadly form of gangrene), *C. tetani* (source of tetanus), and *C. difficile* (very resistant to antibiotic therapy). Buhner also recommends the herb for *Aspergillus niger* (a common mold resulting in lung and sinus infections) and for parasitic infections, including *Plasmodium* (the parasite responsible for malaria), leishmaniasis (a parasitic infection spread by the bite of sandflies that affects the skin, spleen, liver, and bone marrow), and toxoplasmosis (transmitted by cat feces and contaminated food or water) (Buhner, 2012). When treating eye infections, Isatis may be prepared as a tea, filtered to remove all sediment, and applied as drops or eyewash. A clinical study in China involving 200 people diagnosed with acute bacterial conjunctivitis (pink eye) determined that Isatis root eye drops (applied 6 times daily) were safe and 90% effective in eliminating the infection (Qi, 2007).

The herb's influence on the respiratory system has also been researched. Isatis is helpful in treating allergies characterized by chronic inflammation, and inhibits the release of inflammatory histamine from mast cells. When a leaf extract was administered to mice by nasal spray that also contained allergens, researchers found that the allergic reactions of inflammation and excessive mucous secretion were reduced, allowing easier breathing (Brattström, 2010). A Danish study evaluated the efficacy of Isatis on a rat model of chronic *Pseudomonas aeruginosa*, a bacterial lung infection mimicking cystic fibrosis. In contrast to control groups, rats given Isatis had reduced incidence of lung abscess and decreased severity of the infection. The majority of the rats improved from acute lung inflammation, progressing to a less severe chronic state, and the elimination of *P. aeruginosa* was greatly enhanced compared to the control group (Song, 1996). During the SARS (severe acute respiratory syndrome) pandemic in 2003 and the avian bird flu epidemic in China during 2013, many people followed the advice of Chinese government officials and took Isatis to prevent and treat these potentially deadly viruses.

Like many members of the Brassica family, Isatis has anticancer properties and is prescribed for tumor and cancer treatment in China. Indirubin extracted from Isatis has been shown to bind to and block enzymes governing cell division to stop the pathological proliferation of white blood cells (leukocytes), and to be effective in treating chronic granulocytic leukemia (Liu, 1995; Wu, 2011). This is a slowly progressing blood cancer in which bone marrow produces too many white blood cells. A clinical study examined the effects of indirubin extract on 314 patients diagnosed with chronic granulocytic leukemia. According to the study, 26% of the patients showed complete remission and 33% had partial remission. The toxicity of the extract was relatively mild, and remissions lasted up to several years (Hoessel, 1999). *In vitro* and *in vivo* tests exploring the activity of Isatis leaf extracts on human hepatoma cells (the most common type of liver cancer) showed that the herb induced apoptosis (cellular destruction) of the liver tumors (Chung, 2011).

Digestive System: Although Isatis is not typically indicated for digestive problems in Asian traditions, it should be noted that the intense bitter flavor stimulates the stomach and liver, increasing digestive enzymes and bile flow. It can reduce excess stomach and liver heat when used over a period of time. Isatis helps eliminate harmful bacteria, viruses, Candida yeast, and parasites from the digestive tract. A Chinese extract known as Qing Dai contains Isatis and other herbs, and is used to treat ulcerative colitis (Suzuki, 2013).

Skin Problems: Isatis is wonderful for healing skin infections and wounds due to its cooling, antimicrobial, and anti-inflammatory properties. TCM has traditionally administered Isatis for many inflammatory and eruptive skin diseases and rashes often caused by hot, toxic blood and pathogens. These include eczema, hives, boils, abscesses, herpes lesions, measles, mumps, and *Staphylococcus* infections like impetigo. In a clinical trial determining the efficacy of a TCM formula of Isatis and nine other herbs for treating non-weeping eczema, a 91.4% decrease in erythema (diffuse redness of skin) occurred in patients taking the herbs compared to a 10.6% decrease in those who only received a placebo (Sheehan, 1992).

The herb is known to be an effective treatment for scabies, a contagious and very itchy infestation caused by a mite that burrows and lays eggs under the skin. Tryptanthrin in the herb inhibits fungal skin infections and is a helpful treatment for ringworm, athlete's foot, and Candida yeast. Phytochemical investigations on alkaloids in the root and leaves showed significant antifungal activity against *Trichophyton schoenleinii* (responsible for ringworm), *Aspergillus niger* (a frequent cause of fungal ear infections), *Candida albicans* (the common yeast infection), and *Trichophyton simii* (causing athlete's foot and ringworm) (Ahmad, 2008).

When addressing skin infections and wounds, it is most effective to drink the tincture and apply Isatis to the affected area as a salve, poultice, or a wash or fomentation prepared from tea.

Teachings from the Isatis Deva

"Greetings, dear one. I am the Isatis Deva and I will speak to you of my healing offerings. People of the past noticed my pretty little yellow flowers so eager to bloom with the stirring of warm spring temperatures. They discovered that I am a radiant and vibrant plant, strong in character and healing virtues.

"My watery and earthy nature, so extremely cooling, is a stabilizer to subdue intense conditions of heat and inflammation. In this capacity, I am a mighty conqueror of fire and infectious organisms that invade the body. My medicine cools and moistens hot, dry tissues. I am a subduer of impurities so they cannot penetrate my threshold of protection.

"In accordance with my cooling and protective nature, I am ruled by the planet Saturn and the sign of Capricorn. Part of my medicinal work in cleansing the body of invasive pathogens is to usher people into a state of vibrant wellness of body, thoughts, and emotions. My gifts of purification enable people to heal, stabilize, and then expand in gaining renewed understanding and deepening awareness of the power within their core essence. And so I serve as a gatekeeper, as does Saturn, requiring a level of purity in body and mind before allowing a person to move forward with improving health and evolving in conscious awareness.

"The blue color of my essence permeates through my leaves, which people have used as a textile dye. My blue radiance, reflecting my cooling nature, has a calming influence on the human mind and nervous system. The higher frequencies of my blue color spectrum are able to disrupt the lower frequencies of bacteria, viruses, and fungi. Thus, my powerful capacity for purification.

"Understanding life in relationship to energy, or frequencies of vibration, is important. Remember that everything (a rock, fish, flower, or person) consists of frequencies of energy that manifest as atoms. Thoughts are also vibrations originating in a person's mind that flow outward, as do emotions when they radiate from our hearts out into the world. Higher, more refined frequencies correlate with happier, more peaceful mental and emotional states, allowing for a balanced and gentle flow of life energy through the body. This promotes physical strength and health. On the other hand, dense lower frequencies can manifest as self-centeredness, hate, fear, anger, or aggression. As these disturbing thoughts and feelings arise, daily life can become quite dark, isolated, and painful. Whether caused by infection or tissues that deteriorate, all disease originates from energies that vibrate at a significantly lower frequency compared to the vibrant tissues of a healthy person, animal, or plant. Ultimately, all successful methods of healing work by eliminating lower energy frequencies and strengthening the higher ones.

"Thus, part of my job is to offer healing gifts powerful enough to thoroughly cleanse the 'lower frequencies' of infections to allow the natural expression of calm. My plants protect and tend to the physical body. For when it receives the required nourishment to thrive, a state of deep peace and security naturally arises within the body, allowing the mind and emotions to follow suit. When people have this experience of core connection in their daily life, the typical ups and downs life brings are not so devastating. Instead, one responds from a calm center. Of course, constant intentionality is required to accomplish this degree of inner peace, but in choosing to pursue this path, the journey and wonderment of transformation begins and you will receive the blessings of all who have gone before you in the journey home."

Lavender

Lavandula angustifolia
Labiatae (*Lamiaceae*) (Mint) Family

Botanical and Common Names

About 40 species of Lavender have been used interchangeably in herbal healing throughout the ages. Many garden Lavenders are hybrids and subspecies that have developed over time, so identification can be challenging.

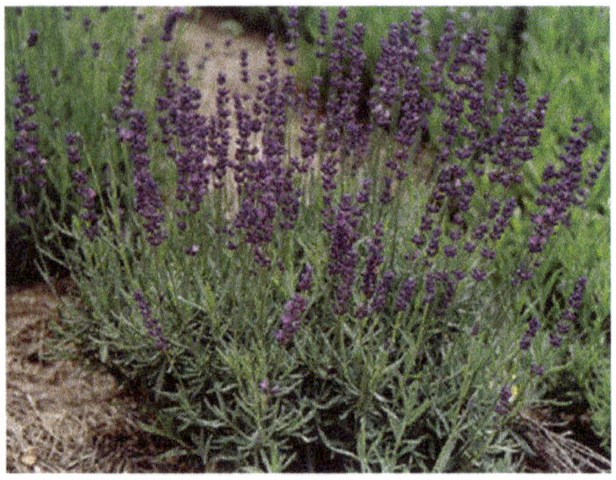

Lavandula angustifolia

Lavandula angustifolia is called English, Common, or True Lavender and yields the highest quality of oils. It is the most widely cultivated and valued species for medicinal and aromatic purposes. It was formerly known as *Lavandula vera, L. officinalis,* and *L. spica*. Descriptive of the leaves of this species, *angustifolia* means "narrow leaf."

Other important species include:
L. latifolia, also known as Broad-leaf or Spike Lavender;
L. lanata, native to Spain;
L. dentata, called French Lavender;
L. stoechas, called Spanish, French, or Arabian Lavender; and
Lavandula x intermedia, known as Lavandin. This is a sterile hybrid developed from *L. angustifolia* and *L. latifolia*. Lavandin is widely cultivated because it produces the greatest amount of oil. However, its oil is considered to be of lower quality than other varieties.

Medicinal Part of the Plant

Flowers contain the greatest concentration of the medicinal and aromatic volatile oils, and have historically been used in the preparation of Lavender oil. The leaves also hold substantial amounts of oil and can be used in combination with the flowers for medicinal purposes.

Range and Habitat

Lavender species are native to the dry, sunny hills of the Mediterranean region of southern Europe and northern Africa, and are widely cultivated throughout Europe, the United States, and temperate zones around the world.

Description of the Plant

All varieties of Lavender are small, aromatic, bushy evergreen shrubs growing 1-3′ tall. These perennial plants possess fibrous roots, and the lower stems tend to become woody with age. Upper stems are square and grooved with many simple, entire leaves growing opposite on the stems. The sessile and narrow linear leaves are 1-1½″ long with a predominant mid-vein. Leaves range between light grayish green to bluish green and feel smooth to the touch. Look at this plant through a 16X magnifying glass for an amazing view of tiny oil glands and drops of oil covering the flowers, calyx, leaves, and stems.

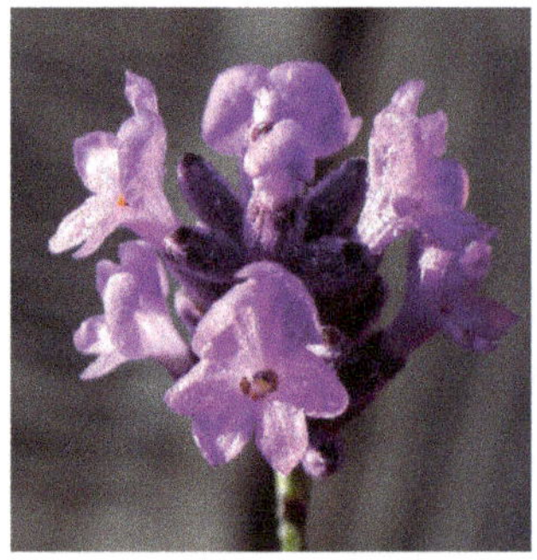

An elongated, cup-like calyx holds the small, delicate, violet-blue flowers consisting of a tubular corolla with 5 petals. The flowers cling to long stalks in whorls forming a loose, short spike. Blooming times range from June through August. The flowers mature into seedpods holding small, shiny, dark seeds.

Cultivation

Standing in a garden of Lavender is a pleasantly sensual experience bringing peace and grace to the emotions, mind, and soul. The flowers and leaves emit a delightful aroma that is both calming and exhilarating. Bees are attracted by the fragrance and help pollinate the flowers.

All Lavender varieties require moderate temperatures and many do not survive severe winters in northern climates where temperatures fall below 0°F. Plants will withstand freezing temperatures in mild zones, and thick mulch during winter months helps protect the dormant roots. Mulch should be removed with spring warming to avoid root and stem rotting. *Lavandula angustifolia, L. latifolia,* and Lavandin are the species best suited to withstand freezing temperatures.

Lavender requires a sunny location for optimal production of its medicinal oils and grows especially well on southern slopes protected from the north wind. Ideal for rock gardens, it also thrives in regular garden plots or flowerpots. A true xerophyte, Lavender likes dry climates and tolerates drought conditions once it is well established. It requires only moderate watering, but good drainage is essential to prevent the roots from rotting, so avoid heavy clay soils. Lavender plants tolerate a wide range of soil conditions, but prefer fertile, sandy loam mixed with lime for 5.8-7.0 pH. Mixing plenty of sand into the loam is imperative for good drainage. Small amounts of wood ash are useful as a natural source of lime, phosphorous, and other mineral nutrients. Potassium and aged manure or compost can be added to the soil before planting to promote bushy foliage. Applying a 1″ top-dressing of sand around the plants can increase oil yields.

Lavenders are primarily grown from stem cuttings, stem layering, and root division. Starting from seed is challenging since germination and survival rates can be disappointingly low. The numerous hybrid and cultivar varieties, such as Lavandin, can have sterile seeds, and those with viable seeds will probably not develop into plants with the same characteristics as the parent plant. Therefore, propagate from stem cuttings or layering, the most successful and expedient methods for obtaining the desired variety. Root division also works but is more disruptive to the plant.

If you attempt to grow Lavender from seeds, plant them indoors in February under adequate lighting or in a greenhouse in March. In warm climates, seeds can be sown outdoors in raised beds in autumn or early spring. Cold conditioning improves germination, so first place the seeds between two slightly moist pieces of paper towel and put this in a plastic bag to retain moisture. For 4-6 weeks, keep seeds moist and alternate between keeping them in a freezer for a week and then in room temperature. When ready, prepare a planting tray of potting soil mixed with fine sand and plant the seeds ¼″ deep. Lavender seeds usually require temperatures greater than 52°F to germinate. They germinate best in darkness, so keep the tray covered with newspaper until seedlings start to emerge and then allow exposure to full sun. Let seedlings mature for 6-12 months, until they are about 6″ tall, before transplanting them into a permanent bed. Space plants about 1′ apart when the soil is warm. Always keep soil moist while plants are becoming established.

The easiest way to propagate Lavender is by stem cuttings, and this is the method preferred by commercial producers. Prune the stems from mature plants in lengths of 5-6″ during late spring and early summer. The stems may be dipped in a commercially available root hormone powder to promote root development and placed in a wet mixture of 50% vermiculite, 25% fine sand, and 25% potting soil. Keep cuttings moist and shaded until they develop roots, when they can be transplanted into larger containers for further growth before being planted in permanent beds.

Layering is another propagation method that works well and ensures specific variety duplication. Bend outer stems of mature plants and anchor them down to the ground with small stakes. Bury a portion of the stem under the soil while leaving the stem tips exposed in the air. Eventually roots develop along the length of the buried stem. Once rooted, stems can be cut to separate them from the parent and replanted.

For root divisions, dig up large mature plants in early spring and cut the roots into 5-7″ lengths that are immediately replanted 1′ apart.

Remember that Lavender likes dry conditions, so be sure to prevent disease and mold by providing adequate ventilation space between plants. Avoid piling fresh mulch too close to the plants for the same reasons. To encourage branching and more abundant foliage, prune Lavender plants 5-6″ above soil surface at the end of the first and second years. Old plants must be adequately pruned or they become woody. Harvesting the plant is an efficient way to prune. Established Lavender plants can live as long as 30 years, but greatest yields come from younger plants that are 3-5 years old.

Harvest

Gather flowers and leaves on a dry, sunny day during the early flowering stage when the fragrant volatile oils are at their peak potency and concentration. To avoid weakening or killing the plant, harvest by pruning no more than one-third of the foliage. Watering the plant after harvesting encourages new growth. Two cuttings are usually possible each season.

Preparation of Plant Medicine and Dosages

Although fresh Lavender leaves and flowers are preferable, they retain their fragrance after drying and are used fresh or dried in medicinal remedies and aroma therapy. The use of heat in processing destroys some of the volatile oils. These oils are very soluble in alcohol but only partially soluble in water, so tinctures are the best medicinal preparations for Lavender and other herbs containing substantial amounts of volatile oils. Volatile oils are also stable in oil-based salve preparations.

PREPARATIONS

Tincture: Use 80% 190-proof grain alcohol and 20% distilled water to tincture the freshly harvested leaves and flowers. Dosage: 10-30 drops in water 1-4 times a day as needed. Tinctures made from freshly harvested leaves and flowers retain the rich, fragrant Lavender aroma.

Infusion: Steep 1-2 teaspoons of fresh or dried leaves and flowers in 1 cup of boiled water for 10 minutes. Dosage: 1-2 cups a day. Strong Lavender tea tastes bitter and may be sweetened with honey.

Oil and Salve: Put the chopped leaves and flowers in a stainless steel pan, cover with olive oil, and bake at 200°F for 2-3 hours. Add beeswax to solidify oil into ointment.

Flower Essence: Only the flowers are used for this preparation. Dosage: 1-2 drops under the tongue.

Essential Oils: Essential oils are distilled from the fresh flowers and leaves after harvesting. Distilling requires the proper equipment, and the oil produced is very concentrated. Enormous amounts of plant material are required to produce essential oil, and about 200 pounds of fresh Lavender flowers yields one pound of oil. Lavender essential oil may be taken orally, applied topically, or used in baths, steam inhalation, and aromatherapy. **Be careful with essential oils that can be toxic when used internally or externally in medium or large doses! Use caution even with small doses.** The German Commission E herbal regulatory agency recommended 1-4 drops of essential oil on a sugar cube, but it is safer to follow the advice of other botanical authorities and clinicians who warn against ingesting more than **one drop of oil diluted in water, twice daily**.

For external application, dilute essential oils with olive oil or other carrier oil. For a safe 1-2% dilution, add 5-10 drops of Lavender essential oil to 1 ounce of a carrier oil.

Aromatherapy: Hang a bundle of freshly cut or dried leaves and flowers in your home to enjoy the lovely fragrance or use the distilled oil with aromatherapy equipment.

Bath Therapy (Balneotherapy): Pour a big pot of strong tea made with 1-2 cups of leaves and flowers or a few drops of the essential oil into a bathtub of hot water. Play relaxing music, light candles, lie back, and bathe in luxury!

Culinary Uses

Some people use the flowers and leaves for seasoning, although they have a rather strong, bitter flavor. Europeans have traditionally added Lavender as a flavoring to salads, stews, meats, cakes, jams and jellies, butter, cheese, honey, and wine. A restaurant in Nashville, Indiana, prepares a unique Lavender lemonade that is delicious.

Chemical Constituents

The volatile oils in Lavender (1.5-3%) are the primary medicinal components. More than 100 compounds have been identified in the oils, and their concentrations differ according to the various species and cultivars. The oils generally tend to be antimicrobial, antioxidant, anti-inflammatory, antispasmodic, sedating, and analgesic. The most biologically important components of *L. angustifolia* oil include linalyl acetate (25-55%), linalool (20-38%), limonene (0.1-0.5%; antilithitic, expectorant), camphor (0.2-0.5%; anti-acne, anticarcinogenic, anti-emetic, carminative, decongestant, expectorant), B-ocimene (4-10%), cineole (0.3-33%; anticarcinogenic, anti-catarrh, antiparasitic, antirheumatic, anti-sinusitis, choleretic, expectorant), and lavandulyl acetate. Perillyl alcohol, a metabolite of limonene, is anticarcinogenic. Other chemicals in the volatile oil include 1-terpinen (2-6%), octanone (1-3%), geraniol (anthelmintic, anticarcinogenic), terpineol (0.3-1%), cadinene (anti-acne, anti-streptococcal), caryophyllene (anti-acne, anti-asthmatic, antitumor), alpha- and beta-pinene (anti-acne), camphene (expectorant), citronellol (anti-staphylococcal, anti-streptococcal), and borneol.

Acids include rosmarinic acid (antibacterial, anti-HIV, anti-inflammatory, antiviral), ursolic acid (analgesic, anti-inflammatory, antitumor, choleretic, hepatoprotective, sedative), and valeric acid (antispasmodic, hypotensive, muscle relaxant, sedative).

Coumarins are generally antimicrobial, anti-inflammatory, and antispasmodic. They include umbelliferone, herniarin (cholagogue), coumarin (analgesic, anticarcinogenic, estrogenic, cardiodepressant, cardiotonic, fungicide, sedative), and dihydrocoumarin (anticarcinogenic). Cinnamaldehyde is antibacterial, anticarcinogenic, anti-inflammatory, antispasmodic, anti-staphylococcal, antiviral, choleretic, circulatory stimulant, central nervous system depressant, hypotensive, sedative, and a vasodilator. Flavonoids include luteolin, which is antibacterial, anti-inflammatory, antispasmodic, antitumor, and a vasodilator. Lavender oil contains about 12% tannins (astringent), which is unique to the Mint family.

Safety, Contraindications, and Drug Interactions

All Lavender varieties are safe for general use when taken in moderate amounts and when essential oils are used cautiously in small doses. Therapeutic applications and safety are validated by Lavender's long historic use and by current research, including numerous clinical trials. The German Commission E herbal regulatory agency reported no known contraindications, side effects, or drug interactions. However, the calming influence Lavender exerts may potentate sedating prescription drugs. Although the Commission reported no restrictions for ingesting Lavender during pregnancy, its mild emmenagogue activity is stimulating to the uterus and **it is wise for pregnant woman to abstain from ingesting the herb until the last month of pregnancy.** Bathing in water mixed with a few drops of the distilled essential oil is safe for everyone, including pregnant women.

Take care when using distilled essential oils due to their high levels of concentration and potential toxicity in large doses. When applying the essential oil externally, always dilute it in vegetable oil to prevent possible skin irritation. Only **1-2 drops of essential oil should be ingested daily**, and always diluted in water.

Medicinal Uses

History of the Plant

Its alluring beauty, fragrance, and calming essence has made Lavender a beloved aromatic and medicinal herb. In ancient Egypt and Europe, people believed that Lavender was a powerful protector against the "evil eye," and the herb was associated with Hecate, the goddess of magic and sorcery. Keeping a sprig of Lavender close to the body was thought to impart strength and courage. The aromatic leaves and flowers were strewn in temples to purify and sanctify them, and during the Middle Ages and Renaissance, Europeans continued to spread Lavender on floors to scent rooms and prevent insect infestation. During these times, when sewage ran through the streets and sanitation in European towns was so appalling, aromatic herbs were highly valued to overpower the stench. Women carried Lavender sachets and inhaled the fragrance when feeling faint or nauseous amid unpleasant odors, and they applied lotions and soaps containing water distilled from Lavender flowers.

It is widely claimed that the genus name *Lavandula* comes from the Latin word *lavare*, meaning "to wash," but the name more likely derives from *livere*, meaning "bluish." In ancient Persian, Greek, and Roman medical traditions, different species were employed as antiseptics for skin infections and as bactericides to disinfect hospitals and sick rooms. The Greeks cultivated *L. stoechas,* and the Greek physician Dioscorides (*circa* A.D. 40–*c.* 90) wrote that a decoction of this species "is good for ye griefs in ye thorax" (Dioscorides, 1959). The famous Persian pharmacist and physician Avicenna (*c.* 980–1037) noted the calming effects of Lavender baths in his classic *Al-Qanun fi al-Tibb (Cannon of Medicine)*.

Knowledge of Lavender's medicinal attributes was introduced into India and Tibet and incorporated into their healing systems. The *Gyu-zhi*, or *Four Tantras*, written by Chandranandana in the eighth century B.C., was the first Indian medical text translated into Tibetan. The text states that Lavender, called *Pri-yangku* in the Tibetan language, was added to formulas for the treatment of psychiatric illness. It continues to be used in modern Tibetan medicine to treat mental imbalance and psychoses. Indian Ayurvedic practitioners prescribed it for intestinal gas, spasms, depression, anxiety, insomnia, and arthritic pain.

European physicians employed Lavender to calm the nervous system, treat infections, and relieve pain. English apothecary and surgeon John Gerard (1545–1612) wrote in *The Herball or Generall Historie of Plantes* that he used the herb to treat headaches, lung disease, and to open congestion in the lungs and liver (Gerard, 1633). English apothecary Nicholas Culpeper (1616–1654) and other European herbalists prescribed Lavender for nervousness, muscle spasms, cramps, convulsions, as an analgesic for headaches and other pain, and for palsy, which is nerve degeneration causing trembling and paralysis. Culpeper wrote in his herbal that "Mercury owns this herb . . . . Lavender is of a special good use for all the griefs and pains of the head and brain that proceed of a cold cause . . . . It strengthens the stomach, and freeth the liver and spleen from obstructions" (Culpeper, 1992).

Cultivated in the United States, *L. angustifolia* was the species prescribed by the early American Eclectic physicians for its sedating and restorative influence on the nervous systems of children and adults. William Cook, M.D., wrote, "Lavender flowers are very diffusive in action, of equally relaxing and stimulating properties, influencing the nervous peripheries. They are used mostly as an adjunct to other agents in nervous agitation and restlessness, with prostration; their own action being soothing, and rendering stronger articles more acceptable to the stomach. The oil is used for the same general purposes, and also as an ingredient in many of the finer colognes and other perfumes" (Cook, 1869). The herb was also used as an antiseptic dressing for wounds during World War I.

A favorite herb of aromatherapists, Lavender continues to be a popular fragrance, beverage tea, and medicinal remedy used in similar ways as in the past. The essential oil continues to be listed as an official drug in the *National Formulary* of the United States. The validity of Lavender's historic medicinal applications has been confirmed by a wealth of laboratory and human clinical studies investigating its chemistry and biological activities.

Healing Qualities

Adjuvant, analgesic, antibacterial, antidepressant, antifungal, anti-inflammatory, antioxidant, antiseptic, antispasmodic, antiviral, aromatic, carminative, cholagogue, diaphoretic, mild emmenagogue, nervine, rubefacient (only the essential oil), sedating in cases of nervous overstimulation, stimulating in cases of depletion and fatigue, stomachic, tonic to the nervous system, vasodilator, vermifuge, and vulnerary.

Traditional Chinese Medicine (TCM) Perspective

A mildly cooling and drying botanical, Lavender normalizes and regulates the flow of Qi (energy) throughout the nervous system by balancing excess and deficiency. Depending on the body's condition, it either sedates or stimulates the nerves. It is relaxing in cases of constrained and excess Qi, but stimulating for people with Qi deficiency. Lavender is specific for Heart Yang deficiency with shortness of breath, fatigue, palpitations, and generalized body coolness. The herb calms the Spirit and quiets emotions, and is beneficial for problems stemming from tightness and rigidity within the muscles, organs, and passageways such as the blood vessels and respiratory bronchi.

Although it is cooling and clears heat in cases of fever and inflammation, the herb's relaxing and dispersing nature increases circulation to provide warmth in cases of Qi constraint and deficiency. Lavender's stimulating action reduces Liver Qi Stagnation and helps resolve Spleen Qi deficiency that causes damp phlegm in the digestive and pelvic organs. It benefits the nerves, brain, heart, lungs, liver, uterus, and skin.

Primary Actions

I typically combine Lavender with other herbs to calm and normalize the nervous and cardiovascular systems, and to promote a gentle wave of relaxation throughout the entire body. It may be given alone or as part of a formula for all conditions involving anxiety and a hyperactive nervous system. During times of intense stress and emotional crises, Lavender is a reliable ally that brings deep calm and stability at a core level. When in need of emotional and spiritual healing, I have often used and recommended Lavender to be taken as a flower essence, using a much smaller dose of 1-2 drops under the tongue. This influences the more subtle emotional and energetic aspects of ourselves, and can be quite healing during stressful times, especially when used in conjunction with meditation and conscious breathing practices. I have also taken 1 drop of the tincture in water or tea, and it provided good results similar to that of a true flower essence preparation.

For the denser physical body, the multitude of powerful volatile oils that eliminate pathogens and reduce inflammation and spasms offer many applications for healing infections, lung congestion, skin injuries, and muscle pain. I always prepare freshly harvested Lavender leaves and flowers as tincture, which maintains the heavenly aroma of the plant to be enjoyed over many years.

Nervous System: Lavender has strong affinity with the nervous system, acting as a gentle sedative and nervine with pronounced calming and analgesic effects. When used during the day, it eases nervous tension and restlessness, but does not typically induce sleep. For treating insomnia, Lavender works best combined with stronger sedating botanicals like Scullcap (*Scutellaria lateriflora*), Hops (*Humulus lupulus*), and Valerian (*Valeriana officinalis*). Those suffering from nightmares may also benefit from Lavender. Many people enjoy the pleasant fragrance and sleep-inducing benefits of sleeping with a small pillow filled with dried Lavender flowers.

Ingesting the tea or tincture or inhaling the oils during aromatherapy reduces nervous overstimulation resulting from acute emotional trauma or chronic anxiety. Over time, chronic tension leads to a deficiency state of nervous exhaustion, listlessness, and depression. For these conditions, Lavender provides a gentle yet stimulating, uplifting influence and assists in healing depression from emotional trauma "locked" in the system. Thus, Lavender's nervine qualities, addressing both extremes of overstimulation or exhaustion, adjust and restore nervous activity to a state of calm stability. The herb is beneficial in treating multiple nervous disorders, and many clients have reported improvement for all types of anxiety, panic attacks, tension headaches, and migraines. In Asia, Lavender is considered a brain tonic helpful for altered brain chemistry, mental imbalance, and neuroses.

The antispasmodic flowers and leaves ease muscle cramps and spasms, and historically were employed to reduce convulsions, nervous tics, and stammering (Izzo, 1996; Lis-Balchin, 1997). Analgesic constituents in the herb help relieve neuralgia (nerve pain) when taken internally. The tincture or oil may also be massaged on the temples and forehead to relieve headaches and on sore, rigid muscles for sprains and spasms. For muscle tightness, cramps and spasms, Lavender works well when taken with Valerian or Lobelia (*Lobelia inflata*). To diminish nerve pain, combine Lavender with St. John's Wort (*Hypericum perforatum*) and take them internally while also using external applications. For relieving headaches and migraines, Lavender blends well with Lemon Balm (*Melissa officinalis*), Feverfew (*Tanacetum parthenium*), Wood Betony (*Stachys officinalis*), and Scullcap. Topical application of Lavender oil is effective for toothaches, especially when applied with Clove oil (*Syzygium aromaticus*).

As a nervine, Lavender helps during withdrawal and detoxification from nicotine, caffeine, alcohol, and drugs. It exerts a protective influence on the nervous system, helping muscles and tissues relax and normalize. Delirium tremens, the uncontrollable shaking that occurs during severe alcohol and drug withdrawal, can be diminished by ingesting the tincture or tea. Aromatherapy is also helpful to calm the mind.

A wealth of clinical studies and research focusing on specific chemical constituents validate many of the herb's traditional uses. Linalool and linalyl acetate demonstrate the ability to slow nerve impulses and reduce irritability, overstimulation, and pain (Duke, 2000). A small study of 8 patients diagnosed with major depressive disorder (MDD) revealed that their symptoms of anxiety, agitation, and restlessness improved within one week of taking Lasea capsules made with *L. angustifolia* essential oil containing high concentrations of linalool and linalyl acetate. Lasea has been approved in Germany for treating restlessness and anxiety. Although not authorized as a treatment for MDD, Lasea is prescribed to address anxiety, psychomotor agitation, and insomnia in patients with MDD (Fißler, 2014).

A German study involving 539 patients diagnosed with generalized anxiety disorder (GAD) demonstrated that a Lavender oil preparation, Silexan, was more effective than paroxetine (a selective serotonin re-uptake inhibitor) in reducing GAD-related anxiety, restlessness, fatigue, poor concentration, irritability, and sleep problems. Silexan is produced from steam-distilled fresh flowering tops and contains about 70% linalool and linalyl acetate. The patients were divided into treatment or placebo groups, and for 10 weeks received either Silexan (in doses of 80 mg or 160 mg) or paroxetine (20 mg) each day. The final outcome showed that both dosages of Silexan effectively improved GAD symptoms and were more efficacious than paroxetine (Kasper, 2014).

Another German study involving 318 patients diagnosed with mixed anxiety and depression disorder determined that those taking 80 mg of Silexan for 70 days showed significant improvement in symptoms compared to those receiving a placebo (Kasper, 2016).

An interesting study examining the herb's analgesic capacity in 24 children revealed that inhaling *L. angustifolia* essential oil reduced the amount of acetaminophen required for pain relief for 3 days after their tonsillectomies (Soltani, 2013). In another study utilizing electroencephalogram (EEG) testing in 23 women suffering from sleep disorders, researchers concluded that 1,200 mg of a Lavender and Valerian extract had strikingly similar effects on brain wave activity as standard dosages of Valium (Schulz, 1997).

A multitude of clinical studies validate the calming effects of Lavender oil administered by aromatherapy and massage (Buchbauer, 1991). Volatile oils are absorbed through the tissues and into the bloodstream when they are rubbed on the skin or inhaled into the sinuses and lungs (Jager, 1992). A research team found that gentle massage with Lavender oil reduced anxiety and improved the mood of 93 people hospitalized in an intensive care unit (Dunn, 1995). Another test documented the beneficial effects of Lavender aromatherapy on anxiety stress responses of nursing students (Park, 2004). A small study involving 4 elderly people reported that inhaling Lavender oil was as effective as tranquilizers in treating their insomnia. For 3 people who were experiencing insomnia after discontinuing their prescription sleeping pills, Lavender aromatherapy provided more restful sleep than their prescription medications (Hardy, 1995). Nighttime Lavender aromatherapy was shown to improve sleep quality in a study with 79 college students (Lillehei, 2015). The herb has reduced perceived pain and depression in hospice patients, while enhancing their sense of well-being (Louis, 2002). A research team studying the effects of a 3-minute session using Lavender aromatherapy on 40 adults found that they experienced increased drowsiness, less depression, and performed mathematical computations faster and more accurately following aromatherapy (Diego, 1998). A study of 15 elderly patients with severe dementia showed that 5 treatments consisting of 2 hours of Lavender aromatherapy improved agitated behavior in 9 of the patients (Holmes, 2002). A later study involving 77 nursing home patients also concluded that aromatherapy, given for a few hours each night for 3 weeks, significantly reduced aggressive behavior and irritability related to Alzheimer's disease and other types of dementia (Lin, 2007).

Cardiovascular System: The calming influence of Lavender on the cardiovascular system is beneficial for chest tightness, heart palpitations, tachycardia (rapid heartbeat), shortness of breath, angina (heart pain and pressure), and other problems triggered by underlying anxiety and tension. The relaxing action on the muscular layers of blood vessels allows the vessels to dilate and improves circulation throughout the body. Thus, Lavender can be helpful for conditions involving vascular (blood vessel) and muscular constriction, such as hypertension and cold extremities. A pot of strong tea or a few drops of the essential oil may be added to bath water to improve poor circulation and irregular heartbeats. In conditions of heart weakness involving fatigue and bradycardia (abnormally slow heartbeat), stimulating properties of the herb increase cardiac activity and elevate depressed moods.

A clinical study evaluated the effects of Lavender aromatherapy on coronary circulation in 30 healthy men age 24-40. Serum levels of cortisol (an adrenal hormone that increases during times of stress) and coronary circulation were measured before and after 30 minutes of aromatherapy using 4 drops of Lavender essential oil diluted with 20 milliliters of hot water. This process was repeated twice. After receiving aromatherapy treatment, the men had significantly lower blood levels of cortisol and coronary circulation also improved (Shiina, 2007).

Infections, Inflammation, and Spasms: The essential oil contains multiple antimicrobial constituents, making Lavender an effective remedy for viral and bacterial infections, including *Streptococcus* and pneumonia. It also helps reduce fevers. For infections, drink it as tincture or tea, or take 1-2 drops of the essential oil diluted in a cup of water. Lavender is especially effective for respiratory infections, and the essential oil or a strong tea can be inhaled in a steam mist. The antispasmodic, anti-inflammatory, and relaxing actions of the oil reduce coughs, asthma, and feelings of tightness and restriction in the chest. For ear infections and pain, put 3 drops of the tea, diluted tincture, or diluted essential oil in each ear several times during the day.

Research has revealed several active compounds in Lavender that have anti-inflammatory actions. One test explored *L. multifida*, known in American horticulture as Fern-Leaf Lavender. In Moroccan folk medicine, the leaves and stems of this variety are used for treating inflammatory conditions like rheumatoid arthritis and digestive problems. Researchers compared water and ethanol extracts of *L. multifida* with indomethacin (a non-steroidal anti-inflammatory drug) for their ability to inhibit ear edema induced in mice. The extracts were applied to the mouse ear, while the drug was given orally. Lavender demonstrated a dose-dependent anti-inflammatory effect, with the alcohol extract being more active than the water. Ursolic acid, oleanolic acid, and a diterpene extracted from the herb significantly inhibited edema by 74%, 45%, and 41% respectively, while indomethacin inhibited edema by 58% (Sosa, 2005).

Lavender species reduce muscle spasms throughout the body, and *in vitro* studies show that several chemical components in the oil, especially linalool and linalyl acetate, are responsible for this action (Lis-Balchin, 1999).

Digestive System: Lavender's soothing properties are especially indicated for digestive problems related to the tension of an overstimulated nervous system. The herb is a carminative and the tincture and tea are beneficial for many stomach problems, including nausea and vomiting, indigestion, gas, cramps, spasms, and feelings of excess fullness. Infants suffering with colic can be comforted by diluting 1 drop of Lavender oil in 5 teaspoons of olive or almond oil and gently massaging this on the abdomen.

As a cholagogue, Lavender increases bile flow from the liver to the small intestine, stimulating normal fat digestion, bowel activity, and cholesterol levels. Animal studies document that the herb decreases unhealthy low-density lipoprotein (LDL) cholesterol and raises protective high-density lipoprotein (HDL) cholesterol (Ulbrict, 2004). In a study involving 150 patients, Lavender essential oil promoted normal levels of total cholesterol (Siurin, 1997).

Lavender helps reduce constipation, intestinal spasms, inflammation, and irritable bowel syndromes. Antimicrobial substances in the volatile oil protect the gastrointestinal tract from harmful bacteria, Candida yeast, and intestinal parasites. Researchers discovered that perillyl alcohol in the oil specifically inhibits the growth of the intestinal parasite *Giardia lamblia* (Lujan, 1995). For best results, combine Lavender with other vermifuge herbs such as Wormwood (*Artemisia absinthium*) and Black Walnut (*Juglans nigra*) when treating parasites. Taking 1 teaspoon of food-grade diatomaceous earth in food or drink on a daily basis is an excellent addition to herbal therapy for intestinal parasites. The diatomaceous earth is not absorbed through the intestinal wall, and is completely non-toxic. Composed of silica crystals that cut up the bodies of intestinal parasites, it does not harm the intestinal tissue in humans and animals. However, do not breathe diatomaceous earth into the lungs, where it can damage the tissues.

Cancer: Researchers are currently investigating chemical constituents in Lavender for activity against cancer, and preliminary evidence is promising. In laboratory studies, perillyl alcohol inhibited cancers of the pancreas (Bronfen, 1994; Stark, 1995), liver (Mills, 1995), breast (Gould, 1995; Haag, 1994), colon (Reddy, 1997), and prostate (Jeffers, 1995). Perillyl alcohol and other monoterpenes present in the volatile oil have been found to inhibit cancer development during initial and progressive stages. Perillyl alcohol prevented tumor development and caused complete regression of advanced mammary tumors when administered to rats at the University of Wisconsin, Madison. It is known that perillyl alcohol blocks cell division and induces apoptosis (programmed cellular death) in cancerous cells (Ziegler, 1997). Researchers have theorized that perillyl alcohol caused tumor regression partly by fostering re-differentiation of tumor cells, meaning that it helped turn cancer cells back into normal cells (Shi, 1995).

Women's Health: The nervine, analgesic, antispasmodic, and anti-inflammatory properties of Lavender are helpful to women experiencing emotional and physical tension and discomfort during their menstrual cycle or menopause. The tea or tincture may be ingested to promote relaxation and inner calm, and massaging the diluted oil onto the pelvic area and forehead eases cramps and PMS tension. In a clinical trial of 96 students suffering painful menstruation, those who inhaled *L. angustifolia* essential oil reported significant relief compared to those who inhaled sesame oil (Raisi Dehkordi, 2014).

Lavender is effective for treating vaginal yeast infections, *Trichomonas vaginalis* (a parasitic vaginal infection), and *Gardnerella vaginalis* (a bacterial infection of the vagina and urethra). For these conditions, drink Lavender tea or tincture and douche with the strong tea or a few drops of Lavender essential oil added to warm water. Follow this program every day until all symptoms are gone.

Lavender has a mildly stimulating emmenagogue effect that promotes menstruation, and for this reason it **should not be taken internally during pregnancy until the last month before the due date**. At that time, 15-20 drops of tincture may be ingested daily to prime the uterus for labor. It may also be taken during labor to encourage productive contractions, relax the mother, and ease pain. Midwives have traditionally brought a bundle of Lavender to the bed of a laboring woman to bring nurturing, calming, cleansing energy into the room, and to impart strength and courage to the mother during childbirth. Herbalist Rosemary Gladstar recommends soothing Lavender baths throughout the entire pregnancy (Gladstar, 1993).

One clinical study investigated the ability of Lavender cream (containing 1.25% Lavender essential oil) to alleviate anxiety, stress, and depression in 141 women who were 6-7 months pregnant. At 4 weeks and 8 weeks the women who applied Lavender cream to their skin experienced significant improvement in anxiety, stress, and depression scores compared to those taking placebo (Effati-Daryani, 2015). Another clinical trial involving 635 postpartum women found that using Lavender oil as a bath additive for 3-5 days reduced perineal pain and discomfort following childbirth (Dale, 1994).

External Uses: An external application of salve, tincture, liniment, poultice, or diluted essential oil is traditionally applied to wounds, infections, skin ulcers, acne, sore muscles, bruises, sprains, arthritic joints, varicose veins, animal and insect bites, and painful headaches. Lavender can be beneficial for muscle pain and stiffness occurring with fibromyalgia. The oil is an excellent antiseptic when sprayed on burns and reduces pain, inflammation, and scarring. External application of the oil also helps eliminate body lice and scabies, and acts as a repellent against mosquitoes. A hot, soothing Lavender bath is beneficial for all these problems and stimulates circulation. The tea may also be applied as a wash or fomentation to small areas of the body.

The herb's long history as a vulnerary is substantiated by current research. *In vitro* studies demonstrate that linalool, geraniol, and several other essential oils in the plant exert significant antibacterial, antifungal, and anti-yeast activity (Inouye, 1998; Larrondo, 1995; Pattnaik, 1997). *In vitro* research involving the application of Lavender oil to eradicate *Staphylococcus aureus* and *Enterococcus faecium* skin infections shows promising results (Nelson, 1997).

Be careful when applying Lavender essential oil, especially to children, the elderly, or others with sensitive skin. It is very potent and must be diluted with a carrier oil such as olive oil or other vegetable oil. Dilute 5-10 drops of Lavender oil in one ounce of vegetable oil. Apply a dab of the oil blend to a small area of skin to determine if the dilution is sufficient.

Another pleasant use of Lavender is to place a sachet of the aromatic flowers among one's clothes and linens to give them a delightful fragrance and to repel moths and other insects that infest wool and fabrics.

Teachings from the Lavender Deva

"Greetings, dear one. I am the Lavender Deva. My plants are composed of the purest and most refined frequencies of light. The subtle energies of my plants interact with the essence of the ethers, the pervasive and endless space holding the gases of the air, the stars and planets, and the spinning atoms manifesting as physical objects. All that exists is contained within the ethers, and my healing radiance operates in this etheric realm. My refined nature allows healing to adjust and harmonize 'out-of-tune' frequencies in the ethers that manifest as different states of discord in human beings.

"As an etheric being, I affect the physical, mental, and emotional spectrum – you may say the aura or the sum total of the energies that circulate through and radiate from plants, animals, and the human body. This radiance, when healthy and flowing, appears as the rainbow spectrum of colors in the body, from red to purple. The essence of my plants is contained in the most refined and subtle spectrum of the lavender-purple frequency.

"My plants are of the air element and ruled by the air sign of Aquarius, symbol of the water-bearer who pours the water and light of life out to all beings. This is a perfect reflection of the vast outpouring of the offerings from my plants. Ancient people believed my plants were a gift from the gods and goddesses to help purify and evolve human consciousness. Some believed Lavender was a gift from the goddess Venus.

"Being of the air element, Lavender has an affinity with the subtle energies of thoughts, emotions, and the nervous system that translates and assimilates frequencies of energy in the cells. The nervous system is a mediator between each cell in the body, and between each person and the external world. Lavender helps in refining, balancing, and adjusting these electrical signals to assist in a true interpretation. That is to say, when the emotions are agitated, one's interpretation and interaction with people and the world at large will reflect this agitation. If one is in a bad temper, an unintentional bump against the shoulder from a passer-by can be taken as an assault, compared to the same event happening to a calm person, who simply interprets this as an innocent mistake and lets it go.

"And so my medicine naturally soothes the nervous system, heart, and other tissues of the physical body. More importantly, the refined essence of my lavender-purple frequencies penetrates through non-physical emotions and thoughts to soothe and adjust the balanced, harmonious flow of these energies. Although emotions and thoughts cannot be seen or touched as physical objects, everyone would agree that they exist and are very real. This all-encompassing transcendent quality, penetrating through the ethers and all the energetic layers of thoughts, feelings, and the physical body, is one reason people are so drawn to the beauty and enticing aroma of my plants.

"I am a portal allowing entry into the past through memories. My fragrance has a unique affinity with the area of the brain involved in perceiving scents, and stimulates the revival and retrieval of old memories from the distant past to re-emerge. I stir the life back into old memories. The beauty of this gift is that I uncover the most precious, beloved memories, enveloping one in deeply satisfying contentment, ease, and a sense of well-being. For every human has experienced these moments and I draw people back to this 'core of being' – the place of refuge where all is well, all is one. And here we rest. When using Lavender to pass through this portal into etheric realms, drink a small amount of my flower essence, tea, or tincture. Remember that my medicine heals to the core by working through each layer, like opening the petals of a flower to reveal the inner core of light and regeneration."

Lemon Balm

Melissa officinalis
Labiatae (*Lamiaceae*) (Mint) Family

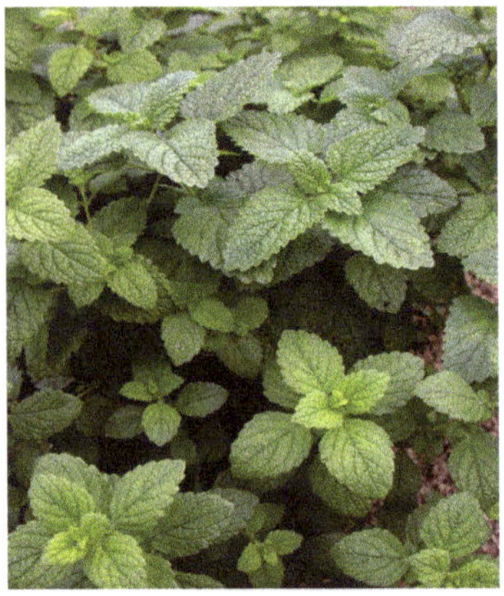

Common Names

Balm, sweet balm, garden balm, and balm mint are common names derived from the word *balsam*, referring to the herb's sweet-smelling oils. Melissa, bee balm, and honey plant are common names associated with the honeybees attracted to the flowers.

Medicinal Part of the Plant

The upper leaves and flowers are used medicinally.

Range and Habitat

Lemon Balm is indigenous to the Mediterranean area of southern Europe and northern Africa, the Middle East, and Western Asia. It is widely cultivated and has naturalized in North America and temperate zones worldwide.

Description of the Plant

Lemon Balm is a perennial herb emitting a strong but delicate lemon citrus fragrance. It develops into a bushy, multi-branching plant growing 2-3′ in height. The fibrous roots send up many erect stems that are square (typical of all members of the Mint family), grooved, solid, and covered with long, fine, pilose (sparsely scattered) hairs, especially around the leaf nodes. Light yellowish-green leaves grow opposite each other along the entire length of the stems. The simple leaves are 1-3″ long, oval-shaped, rugose (deeply wrinkled), pinnately veined, and have rounded, crenate teeth along the edges. Leaves are covered with erect pilose hairs on their top surface, and are attached to the stem by a petiole stalk.

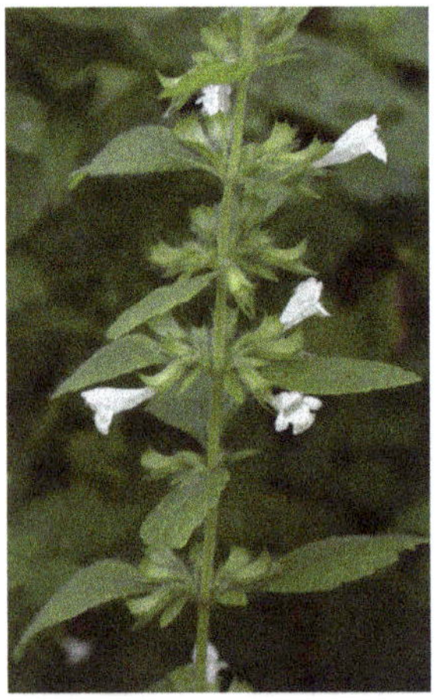

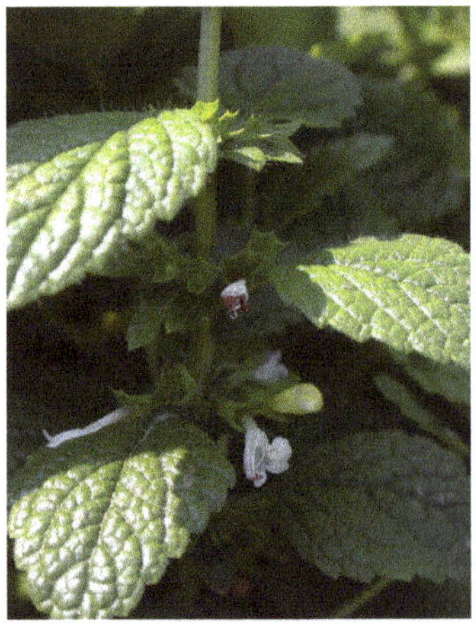

The tiny, inconspicuous flowers, 1/3-1/2″ in length, vary from white to pale blue, pink or yellow, and bloom from July through September. Appearing as small spikes, the flowers grow in clustered whorls emerging from leaf axils all along the upper stems. The partial whorls typically cling to one side of the stem. Tubular flowers are trumpet-shaped and cradled in a hairy, tubular calyx. The corolla opens into a bi-lobed upper lip and a curving 3-lobed lower lip. Four stamens extend beyond the corolla. The flowers mature into round, dark seeds.

Cultivation

Lemon Balm is grown from seed (the easiest method), root division, or stem cuttings. The plant requires a soil pH between 4.5-7.5 and fertile, moist soil with good drainage. It prefers a cool habitat and accepts partial shade, but it is best to grow Lemon Balm in full sun for greater production of medicinal volatile oils. Keep plants watered, as the leaves wilt and turn yellow or brown if they become too dry in the hot sun.

Seed germination is improved with 2-3 weeks of cold, moist conditioning before they are sown. Plant seeds in flats when temperatures are about 70°F, barely cover them with 1/8-1/4″ of soil, and keep moist. Germination takes 20-30 days. When seedlings are 3-4″ tall, transplant them to a permanent garden, spacing them 1′ apart. To propagate by root division, dig up the roots of established plants in early spring when the soil is moist. Divide the roots and replant each piece 1′ apart. Keep them watered until new foliage appears. Stem cuttings that are 8-10″ long can be taken from vigorous summer growth and placed in a mix of wet potting soil, sand, and vermiculite until roots emerge. Plant the rooted cuttings 1′ apart.

Be sure to establish your garden where the herb can grow freely without crowding out other plants. Once a Lemon Balm patch is established, it will proliferate by self-sowing its seeds to make an attractive ground cover. During the blooming season, the aromatic flowers and leaves attract bees, and the garden is alive with their droning buzz as they collect pollen to create delicious honey.

Harvest

The aromatic medicinal volatile oils reach their peak concentration and potency on sunny days during the early flowering stage. Gather upper leaves and flowers by trimming off the top 6-10″ of the stems. The plants can usually be harvested twice during the growing season.

Preparation of Plant Medicine and Dosages

The leaves and flowers are prepared fresh or dried, although fresh leaves are significantly more fragrant and biologically active. Alcohol and boiling water both extract the healing virtues, so Lemon Balm can be made into a refreshing tea or tincture. It is also excellent for external healing when prepared as a salve, poultice, wash, fomentation, or liniment.

If you choose to dry the herb, arrange individual leaves on screens or hang the cut stems and leaves upside down in loose bunches. Dry in a shady, well-ventilated area. Leaves can turn black if they are not dried quickly, so a fan or dehydrator may be necessary to speed up the process, especially in humid climates.

Lemon Balm is very safe and can be freely taken as tea. It is specific for small children who like the mild flavor. Give the tincture to children after the alcohol is evaporated off in boiling hot water (see instructions on page 135) and always use pediatric doses (refer to "How to Calculate Dosages" on page 148).

PREPARATIONS

Infusion Tea: Steep 2-3 teaspoons of the fresh or dried herb in 1 cup of boiled water for 5-10 minutes. Steeping rather than boiling preserves the volatile oils. Dosage: 1-2 cups daily. The tea has a pleasant and delicate lemon taste, making it a refreshing beverage and medicinal tea. Young children enjoy it flavored with a little sweetener.

Tincture: Chop the freshly harvested herb and cover it with 65% 190-proof grain alcohol and 35% distilled water. Prepare in the usual manner. Dosage: ½-1 teaspoon taken 1-4 times a day as needed.

Salve: The fresh leaves and flowers are baked in olive oil according to the standard method. Lemon Balm is most effective for external healing when combined with other vulnerary herbs (refer to "Skin Problems" on page 591 in the "Index of Health Issues and Herbal Recommendations").

Poultice: The dried or fresh leaves may be prepared as a poultice for external application.

Culinary Uses

The fresh leaves are an attractive garnish, offering a subtle lemon flavor and aroma to soups, stews, salads, fruit, omelets, meat, cookies, pudding, yogurt, and beverages. Fresh leaves may be frozen for later use.

Chemical Constituents

Lemon Balm leaves contain 0.1-0.8% volatile oils responsible for many of the herb's medicinal properties. These oils are generally recognized to be antibacterial, antifungal, antiseptic, antispasmodic, sedative, and digestive aids that relieve gas. Primary components of the volatile oils include geranial (antiparasitic, anticarcinogenic, antitumor, expectorant), neral, citronellal (anti-staphylococcal, anti-streptococcal, muscle relaxant), linalool, eugenol (an anesthetic and antiseptic used in dentistry, anticonvulsant, anti-inflammatory), limonene (antiflu, antilithic, antitumor, antiviral, expectorant), caryophyllene (anti-inflammatory), and thymol (analgesic, antiparasitic, anti-acne, anti-herpes, carminative, expectorant, muscle relaxant).

Triterpenoids include ursolic acid (analgesic, anti-arthritic, antihistamine, anti-ulcer, antiviral, sedative) and oleanolic acid (antibacterial, anti-inflammatory, antioxidant, antiviral, cardiotonic, hepatoprotective, sedative, uterotonic). Sesquiterpenes include copaene (carminative) and cadinene (anti-acne, antibacterial, anti-streptococcal).

Several polyphenol constituents with strong antioxidant ability are present in Lemon Balm. Tannins are polyphenols that provide astringent actions. Research studies reveal that phenolic acids in the herb are effective against bacteria such as *streptococci* and *mycobacterium* (causing tuberculosis, skin infections, and inflamed lymph nodes), and they possess significant antiviral activity against herpes simplex, herpes zoster, influenza, and polio. Phenolic acids include caffeic acid (analgesic, antihistamine, anti-hyperthyroid, anti-inflammatory, antiseptic, antispasmodic, cholagogue, fungicide, sedative, vulnerary), chlorogenic acid (analgesic, anticarcinogenic, antihistamine, anti-hyperthyroid, anti-inflammatory, cholagogue, anti-ulcer, fungicide, vulnerary), ferulic acid, and rosmarinic acid (increases the calming neurotransmitter GABA, anti-inflammatory, astringent, cholagogue). Flavonoids, another class of polyphenols, are antioxidants and include quercetin (anti-allergy, anti-inflammatory), luteolin (anti-inflammatory), rutin (vasoprotective), kaempferol, and apigenin. Flavonoids, rosmarinic acid, ferulic acid, and caffeic acid are known to be antiviral.

Safety, Contraindications, and Drug Interactions

Virtually without side effects, Lemon Balm is a safe, non-toxic herb enjoyed by people of all ages. It is a specific remedy for many infant and childhood illnesses. According to herbal authority Mark Blumenthal, "The approved therapeutic applications of Lemon Balm are supportable based on its long history of use in well-established systems of traditional medicine, on phytochemical investigations, and on its documented pharmacological actions reported from *in vitro* studies and *in vivo* experiments in animals" (Blumenthal, 2000). The German Commission E herbal regulatory agency stated that the plant has no known contraindications, interactions with other drugs, side effects, or restrictions during pregnancy. Because it is a mild emmenagogue, some references recommend against its use during pregnancy, although this is a hypothetical restriction since there are no reports of problems. In fact, the emmenagogue activity is caused by the herb's relaxing effect on the uterus rather than being an irritating stimulant leading to miscarriage. Many reputable herbalists regard moderate amounts of the tea taken throughout pregnancy to be quite safe.

Current research has shown that Lemon Balm helps normalize an overactive thyroid gland. There are some warnings that people with hypothyroidism (underactive thyroid function) should not take the herb over a long period of time due to the possibility of worsening the condition, although no clinical evidence supports this hypothesis.

Medicinal Uses

History of the Plant

Lured by Lemon Balm's delicate heavenly fragrance, people have cultivated and used the plant medicinally for over 2,000 years. The genus name *Melissa* is derived from the Greek word for "honeybee," indicating the strong attraction bees have to the flowers and pollen that they use to make superb honey. According to ancient Greek and Roman healing arts, the leaves were steeped in wine to be ingested and applied topically for many types of external healing. In the writings of two famous Greek physicians, Pliny the Elder (A.D. 23–79) and Dioscorides (*circa* A.D. 40–*c.* 90), Lemon Balm was recommended as an antiseptic and surgical dressing for wounds, to treat venomous stings and bites (including those of scorpions and rabid dogs), for toothache and gout, to improve memory, promote longevity, and treat anxiety, nervousness, headaches, and indigestion. The famous Persian physician Avicenna (*c.* 980–1037) recommended it for depression, heart conditions, and as an antiseptic dressing for wounds, ulcers, and scabies. It was a favorite herb of the great medieval physician and alchemist Paracelsus (1493–1541), who called it the "elixir of life" and sold the remedy to kings by proclaiming that it could completely revitalize the body. In *The Herball or Generall Historie of Plantes*, English apothecary and surgeon John Gerard (1545–1612) extolled its ability to heal wounds and wrote, "The juice of Balm glueth together greene wounds, being put in oil, salve or balm for that purpose, makes it of greater efficacy." The herb's ability to reduce fevers, calm anxiety, soothe indigestion, and treat cramps, spasms, headaches, and the common cold has been praised by herbalists for centuries. English herbalist and apothecary Nicholas Culpeper (1616–1654) claimed that it could lift the spirits, promote mental acuity, and stimulate menstruation. He believed that Lemon Balm was ruled by the planet Jupiter, and placed it under the astrological sign of Cancer. The aromatic leaves were traditionally used in potpourri, perfumes and colognes, and were placed in clothes closets and drawers to deter moths. Lemon Balm is also included in the traditional Indian medical system of Ayurveda, and is prescribed for problems of the nervous system and digestive tract.

European colonists introduced Lemon Balm into North America, where its traditional use as medicine and a pleasant beverage continued. During the 1880s–1930s, American Eclectic physicians prescribed the herb as a mild stimulant, diaphoretic, and antispasmodic. They gave a warm infusion of the tea to reduce fevers and painful menstruation, and it was a well-known remedy for the common cold (Felter, 1898).

Lemon Balm continues to be a popular herbal tea and medicine in Europe and the Americas. Formerly recognized as an official medicine, it was listed in the *United States Pharmacopoeia* from 1840–1890. In Germany, leaf preparations in teas, pills, and capsules are approved for anxiety, nervous sleep disorders, and gastrointestinal problems. Europeans often combine Lemon Balm with Valerian (*Valeriana officinalis*) and Hops (*Humulus lupulus*) when dealing with anxiety-based conditions. Recent scientific studies have revealed several chemicals in Lemon Balm leaves possessing medicinal value, including potent antiviral components effective against the herpes virus.

Healing Qualities

Analgesic, antibacterial, anti-catarrhal, antifungal, antihistamine, anti-inflammatory, antioxidant, antiseptic, antispasmodic, antiviral (specific to the herpes virus), aromatic, mild astringent, cardiac, carminative, mild cholagogue, diaphoretic, mild emmenagogue, febrifuge, hepatic, hypotensive, nervine, restorative tonic to the nervous system, sedative, stomachic, vasodilator, and vulnerary.

Traditional Chinese Medicine (TCM) Perspective

Mildly warming and drying, Lemon Balm clears excess heat. In conditions of overstimulation, it calms the nervous, cardiovascular, and digestive systems. For opposite cases of exhaustion and devitalized nerves, it exerts a gentle stimulating and restorative influence.

Lemon Balm resolves blocked and constrained Qi (energy). By circulating and equalizing Qi throughout the body, it dissipates tension and calms the Spirit, clears heat, dispels Liver Wind heat, and resolves phlegm. The herb helps blood vessels relax to relieve restricted circulation. It is given for constrained Heart Qi and Yin deficiency manifesting as nervous excitability, rapid and irregular heartbeat, headaches, hot flashes, hypertension, and hyperthyroidism. By easing Lung Qi constraint, it is helpful for asthma, wheezing, shortness of breath, dry cough, and chest pain. Lemon Balm helps reduce Stomach and Intestinal Qi constraint causing indigestion, vomiting, colic and gas, and it resolves Uterine Qi constraint resulting in reproductive problems like irregular and painful menses. It tones the Liver and strengthens against Kidney Essence deficiency, a condition causing potential depression, poor memory and mental clarity, and infertility.

Primary Actions

Lemon Balm is first and foremost a remedy for the nervous system with two modes of action: relaxation and restoration. Its relaxing properties are specific for people whose sympathetic nervous systems are chronically overstimulated, and who have problems with anxiety, emotional and psychological stress, muscle tension, headaches, nervous stomach and indigestion, insomnia, hypertension, and heart palpitations. The herb's powerful calming action on the nervous system has a special affinity with the thyroid gland and is a valuable treatment for excess thyroid stimulation, known as hyperthyroidism. Over time, a chronically over-stimulated nervous system that becomes exhausted and weak can benefit from Lemon Balm's restorative actions. These dual modes of action are why the herb is helpful for both anxiety (a state of emotional excess) and depression (a deficiency state). It has a balancing influence that can ease the tension of finding ourselves in places or situations that we are not ready to accept.

As an antimicrobial, it is effective against different types of infections, and I have seen it work wonders to subdue pain and heal severe lesions caused by the herpes virus. Safe for all age groups, Lemon Balm is a wonderful herbal remedy for infants, addressing the common childhood problems of colds, flu, fevers, colic, teething, irritability, restlessness, and sleeplessness. The tea is a tasty and refreshing beverage that can replace unhealthy sodas and excessive amounts of fruit juice or coffee.

Nervous System: As a calming sedative and restorative nervine, Lemon Balm's influence on the nervous system benefits all tissues and organs by resolving the tension interrupting normal flows and rhythms of the body. In this way, it serves to normalize the entire system, specifically targeting the heart, blood vessels, thyroid gland, and the organs of respiration, digestion, and reproduction.

As a relaxing sedative, the herb helps relieve conditions caused by an overactive, stressed nervous system, such as hyperactivity, irritability, muscle tension, spasms, inflammation, and digestive problems The tea and tincture are helpful for treating insomnia, nightmares, stress headaches, migraines, anxiety, panic attacks, and manic episodes.

As a restorative nervine, Lemon Balm benefits nerve and cognitive brain function. It is specific for treating mild to moderate depression and seasonal affective disorder (SAD), especially when combined with St. John's Wort (*Hypericum perforatum*). The ancients drank Lemon Balm combined with Sage (*Salvia officinalis*) to promote longevity and for use as a "brain tonic" to support optimal brain function, improve cognition and memory, and sharpen the senses. Lemon Balm can be included in formulas for drug, alcohol, caffeine, and nicotine withdrawal to calm and restore an agitated, depleted nervous system.

Current research validates many of these applications. One mechanism of the herb's anti-anxiety activity is due to rosmarinic acid in the volatile oil. Rosmarinic acid inhibits the enzyme that normally degrades GABA (gamma-aminobutyric acid), a primary inhibitory neurotransmitter that induces relaxation. The resulting elevations of GABA have been shown to reduce anxiety, subdue excessive and obsessive thinking, and promote restful sleep (Awad, 2009; Ibarra, 2010). Many prescription drugs for treating anxiety and seizures work by increasing brain levels and activity of GABA.

A research team studied the cognitive and mood effects of single doses (600, 1,000, or 1,600 mg) of dried Lemon Balm leaves compared to a placebo in 20 young, healthy volunteers. Doses were given and increased every 7 days, and evaluation tests were conducted 1, 3, and 6 hours after ingestion. The most notable effects were improved memory performance and increased calmness in those taking the largest dose of 1,600 mg of Lemon Balm. Smaller doses had correspondingly weaker effects (Kennedy, 2003). Other clinical studies have demonstrated the herb's ability to improve memory and mental acuity (Wake, 2000).

German researchers have found the extract to be very beneficial in treating anxiety and nervousness (Buchner, 1974), and when combined with Valerian (*Valeriana officinalis*), it was as effective as the pharmaceutical sedative Halcion in clinical studies (Dressing, 1992). Additionally, the herbal formula did not cause the morning drowsiness and diminished mental acuity experienced by those taking Halcion. In another clinical trial, people with mild insomnia found that 3 tablets of Lemon Balm (80 mg) and Valerian (120 mg) improved their ability to sleep without any adverse side effects (Cerny, 1999).

Beneficial results have also been documented in children. The efficacy and tolerability of a Lemon Balm and Valerian combination was investigated in a multicenter study involving 918 children under 12 years of age who were suffering from anxiety, restlessness, and insomnia. A significant reduction in severity was observed for all symptoms, which were reduced from "moderate/severe" to "mild" or "absent" in most of the children. The herbs were well tolerated (Müller, 2006).

A multi-center study in Germany documented that 2 daily doses of a tablet supplying Lemon Balm (320 mg) and Valerian root (640 mg) improved the symptoms of hyperactivity, impulsiveness, and poor concentration in children 6-11 years old after a treatment period of 7 weeks. At the end of the test period, parents reported noticeable improvements in their child's social behavior, ability to go to sleep, rest soundly, and wake with greater energy. The portion of children experiencing poor ability to focus decreased from 75% to 14%, those with hyperactivity fell from 61% to 13%, and those with impulsiveness from 59% to 22%

(Gromball, 2014). Children or adults with attention deficit disorder (ADD) and attention deficit hyperactivity disorder (ADHD) can benefit by taking Lemon Balm with Chamomile (*Matricaria recutita*) and Hawthorn (*Crataegus* spp.) tea or tincture on a daily basis.

Melissa officinalis extracts have been shown to bind directly to nicotinic and muscarinic receptors in human nerve and muscle cells (Kennedy, 2006). This binding increases levels of the important neurotransmitter acetylcholine, which is typically deficient in Alzheimer's disease and other conditions of neurodegeneration. Acetylcholine is crucial for normal muscular movement and cognitive function like learning and memory. Rosmarinic acid inhibits acetylcholinesterase, the enzyme that breaks down acetylcholine and reduces its availability to brain cells (Dastmalchi, 2009). Lemon Balm's ability to increase acetylcholine levels is similar to the action of prescription drugs designed to treat Alzheimer's disease.

Oxidative damage to nerve cells is another major factor promoting development of Alzheimer's and Parkinson's diseases, as well as age-related cognitive decline. Antioxidants in Lemon Balm protect against this damage. Other phytochemicals are highly effective in reducing harmful accumulations of amyloid-beta, a protein and leading contributor to Alzheimer's disease (Hamaguchi, 2009). A 4-month clinical study evaluated the efficacy of a *M. officinalis* extract (60 drops per day) in 42 patients with mild to moderate Alzheimer's disease. Those taking the extract experienced improved cognitive function and less agitation than those in the placebo group (Akhondzadeh, 2003). In a double-blind, placebo-controlled study involving 72 patients with severe dementia living in nursing homes, a lotion containing 200 mg of Lemon Balm essential oil was applied topically every day for 4 weeks. The oil applications reduced agitation by 30% in 21 of the patients, compared to 14% in 5 people receiving a placebo. Those receiving the lotion also increased the amount of time spent in social interaction and constructive activities (Ballard, 2002). Based on these studies, daily ingestion of Lemon Balm may be helpful for preventing and treating many types of muscle, nerve and cognitive decline, including memory loss, Alzheimer's disease, and other forms of dementia.

Current animal studies verify the sedating and analgesic properties of several volatile oils and other constituents in Lemon Balm (Soulimani, 1991), validating its historic use for relief of pain, headaches, and neuralgia (nerve pain). The tea or tincture may be ingested for these problems, while the salve or diluted essential oil can be applied topically to the forehead, temples, and other areas of discomfort.

For all types of nervous conditions and muscular tension, try drinking 1-2 cups of Lemon Balm tea or 1-2 teaspoons of the tincture on a daily basis. This herb works best when combined with other sedative and nervine herbs such as Passion Flower (*Passiflora incarnata*), Lavender (*Lavandula* spp.), Scullcap (*Scutellaria lateriflora*), Valerian, and Hops (*Humulus lupulus*). Take small doses of these herbs for daytime tension and anxiety, and larger doses at night. For insomnia, drink the tea or tincture 15 minutes before going to bed.

Antioxidants and Protection from Radiation: Lemon Balm protects cells from radiation and chemical damage by increasing levels of the body's natural antioxidants (superoxide dismutase or SOD, glutathione, and catalase), by protecting cell membranes from lipid peroxidation (the destruction of fats in cell membranes), and by protecting cellular DNA (Schulpis, 2006). A study documented the benefits of Lemon Balm in radiation technologists, who are exposed to constant low-level radiation during their work. Drinking the tea (1.5 grams taken twice daily for 30 days) produced beneficial increases in SOD (71% increase), glutathione (12%), and catalase (61%) (Zeraatpishe, 2011).

Heart and Circulation: Lemon Balm's calming and restorative action on the cardiovascular system benefits the heart and blood vessels. A gentle and beneficial tonic for conditions exacerbated by nervous tension, it is helpful for chest constriction and pain, labored breathing, and heart arrhythmias, palpitations (irregular heartbeat), and tachycardia (rapid heartbeat). By relaxing muscle tension throughout the body, including within the blood vessel walls, Lemon Balm promotes mild vasodilation (opening) of peripheral blood vessels that improves circulation. This decreases hypertension, promotes general body warmth by moving internal heat to the surface, and brings warmth to cool, achy extremities. A small study of 55 people found that those taking 500 mg of encapsulated Lemon Balm twice daily for 14 days reduced episodes of heart palpitations by 36.8% compared to a 4.19% decrease in the placebo group (Alijaniha, 2015).

Use Lemon Balm as a tonic for several months and combine it with Hawthorn, Motherwort (*Leonurus cardiaca*), Lavender (*Lavandula angustifolia*), Linden tree flowers and leaves (*Tilia americana,* spp.), and Garlic (*Allium sativum*) for heart problems, poor circulation, and hypertension. Lemon Balm contains strong antioxidants that protect cells from damage and aging. One Japanese research team found at least 6 major compounds contributing to its antioxidant effects, which are 10 times stronger than vitamin C and E (Tagashira, 1998).

Hyperthyroidism: In European herbalism, Lemon Balm is an accepted treatment for hyperthyroidism, or overactive thyroid, a condition in which the thyroid gland produces and secretes excessive amounts of the hormones thyroxine (T4) and/or triiodothyronine (T3). These thyroid hormones are critical to the normal function of cells and affect nearly all tissue by controlling the pace, or metabolic rate, of all body processes. Excessive thyroid hormones overstimulate the sympathetic nervous system and metabolic rate, causing every function of the body to "speed up."

Symptoms of hyperthyroidism include hyperactivity, anxiety, irritability, poor concentration, increased perspiration, hand tremors, difficulty sleeping, thinning of the skin and hair, brittle hair, muscular weakness, hypertension, and rapid heartbeat (tachycardia) or palpitations. Digestive disturbances and increased appetite accompanied by weight loss also occur. The most common cause and form of hyperthyroidism is Graves' disease, an autoimmune disorder in which antibodies attack the thyroid gland, activating excessive T3 and T4 secretion. Symptoms of Grave's disease include large, bulging eyeballs.

Several studies show that freeze-dried water extracts and single injections of Lemon Balm reduce the excitatory effects of thyroid stimulating hormone (TSH) on the thyroid gland. It does this by interfering with TSH binding to thyroid cell membranes, which inhibits the formation of T3 and T4, reducing overstimulation throughout the body (Auf'mkolk, 1984 & 1985; Sourgens, 1982). Lemon Balm also blocks stimulating auto-immune antibodies of Graves' disease to improve this condition. Flavonoids and other polyphenols in the herb appear to be responsible for the thyroid-regulating activity.

Over the years, several of my clients suffering from hyperthyroidism and Graves' disease have experienced significant relief from hyperactive symptoms by using a tincture preparation of equal parts Lemon Balm, Bugleweed (*Lycopus* spp.), and Motherwort (*Leonurus cardiaca*). When using 3 droppers of this blend 2-3 times a day, people report improved sleep, digestion, cognitive focus and function, and mental and emotional calm, along with lower blood pressure, slower heartbeat, and a calmer state of well-being.

Although Lemon Balm is sometimes contraindicated for people with hypothyroidism (underactive thyroid), there are no references in the literature about individuals developing hypothyroidism while taking Lemon Balm, or of hypothyroid people deteriorating from its use.

Herpes Virus: Herpes is a contagious viral disease that attacks the nervous system and travels along the nerves, creating painful skin lesions. It is a very resistant virus that remains dormant in the nervous system after lesions have disappeared. Prolonged periods of stress that weaken the immune system can exacerbate flare-ups. I have noticed a direct correlation between stress and herpes flare-ups, and every person I know who has experienced an outbreak reported excessive stress beforehand. The antiviral drug Acyclovir (Zovirax) is commonly prescribed to relieve symptoms of the herpes virus, but provides little protection against recurrent outbreaks. The side effects of increased bleeding and bruising, kidney damage, and nausea, vomiting, and diarrhea can be problematic for some people.

> *Lemon Balm is an amazingly effective treatment for all herpes infections, including Epstein-Barr, especially when combined with St. John's Wort*

Lemon Balm has gained attention for its ability to subdue herpes simplex virus types 1 and 2, which erupt into painful cold sores around the mouth (type 1) or into genital lesions (type 2). The herb is also effective against the herpes zoster virus responsible for shingles, an extremely painful skin rash of blisters that most often erupt along one side of the torso, often in a striped pattern, and on the head. An initial infection of varicella zoster virus causes chickenpox, the short-lived illness generally occurring in children and young adults. After the initial episode of chickenpox resolves, the herpes virus remains dormant in the nervous system and can re-emerge years later as shingles (herpes zoster), and typically flares during times of stress.

Several clinical studies have confirmed Lemon Balm's topical use in accelerating the healing process, reducing the size and intense pain of lesions, and providing longer intervals between herpes outbreaks (May, 1978; Dimitrova, 1993; Koytchev, 1999). In Germany, Lemon Balm is sold in commercial antiviral medicines and as a cream, Lomaherpan, for treating herpes infections. The herb blocks receptor sites on the outer membrane of skin cells to prevent the virus from penetrating and infecting the cells and causing them to erupt into lesions. A study involving 116 people suffering from herpes simplex type 1 and 2 outbreaks found that Lomaherpan cream significantly reduced severity of symptoms and healing time of the lesions, and provided better preventative treatment than prescription drugs (Wolbing, 1984 & 1994).

I have seen astonishing results with speedy recovery when my Herpes Relief tincture containing Lemon Balm, St. John's Wort (*Hypericum perforatum*), Hyssop (*Hyssopus officinalis*), and Boneset (*Eupatorium perfoliatum*) is taken internally (1 teaspoon in water 4-5 times a day) to treat herpes outbreaks. Most effective when taken at the onset of the infection, a tincture and salve prepared with these herbs should also be applied to the lesions. Time and again, clients have reported that the combined internal and external applications diminish their pain and irritation, shrink and dry their lesions, shorten recovery time, and prevent future outbreaks. When prone to recurrent flare-ups, I encourage people to continue taking a small amount (40 drops a day) of Lemon Balm and St. John's Wort tincture.

The worst case of shingles I have ever seen was a woman in her thirties who was covered with extremely painful, red, raised pustules the size of a dime on her chest, under her arm, and around to her shoulder blade. I suggested that she take 1 teaspoon of my Herpes Relief tincture with ½ teaspoon of Echinacea (*Echinacea purpurea*) tincture every 2-4 hours due to the severity of the outbreak. She applied the Herpes Relief tincture to the lesions on a continual basis, in addition to a salve made with the four herbs in the tincture. She was compliant and when I saw her 48 hours later, her lesions had shrunk to the size of pimples. She reported feeling much better, and experienced a significant reduction in her excruciating pain 5-6 hours after the initial dose and application of the tincture and salve. We were both grateful and amazed by the results!

Lemon Balm is also helpful in treating the Epstein-Barr virus, a member of the herpes family implicated as a cause of fibromyalgia, chronic fatigue syndrome (CFS), and mononucleosis. The herb's ability to treat fibromyalgia and CFS was the subject of a 101-day study. Participants were 72 adult patients diagnosed with fibromyalgia, and 69 patients also had CFS. About half received a placebo, while the remaining 38 people received 1-2 tablets of Valerian (180 mg) and Lemon Balm (90 mg) at bedtime, in addition to 30 mg of melatonin, multivitamins, magnesium, and malic acid. Compared to the placebo group, those receiving the herbal and supplement therapy showed gradual improvement of their symptoms (Teitelbaum, 2003).

Fever, Flu, and the Common Cold: Lemon Balm is safe to use in large amounts for viral and bacterial infections, fevers, and excessive mucous production, drainage, or congestion. It exerts an astringent, toning action on tissues that decreases bleeding and excessive discharge from mucous membranes. The herb can be helpful for infections in the digestive system and sinus, bronchial, and lung irritation. The tea or tincture should be initiated at the first signs of illness, and children usually enjoy the pleasant-tasting tea.

Lemon Balm tea and tincture have traditionally been used to treat the flu, common cold, coughs, bronchitis and other upper respiratory infections, and some types of asthma. Flavonoids and other chemical components in the plant exert antihistamine actions helpful for allergies. When taken as hot tea or tincture, Lemon Balm is diaphoretic and induces perspiration that draws heat out of the body. The volatile oils in the herb exit through the skin pores, opening them to allow normal skin respiration and interior heat to escape. This has an overall cooling effect, reducing fevers and other hot conditions.

Several researchers have discovered phytochemicals in the herb that are antiviral (Cohen, 1964; Kucera, 1967; Herrmann, 1967), antibacterial, and mildly antifungal (Larrondo, 1995). Studies show that polyphenols in Lemon Balm fit into receptor sites on cell membranes to which viruses attach during infections. The polyphenol "bumps" the virus off receptor sites and prevents infection from spreading into the cells. Antibacterial polyphenols inhibit *Streptococcus* and *Mycobacterium in vitro*. Different strains of mycobacteria cause lymph node inflammation, skin diseases, tuberculosis, and leprosy (Duke, 1997). Researchers investigating the role of Lemon Balm in immunity found that it increased both humoral and cell-mediated immunity in lab trials with mice (Drozd, 2003).

Digestion: Like many members of the Mint family, Lemon Balm is helpful for digestive problems, especially when they are triggered by nervous anxiety and emotional stress. As the herb calms and restores the nervous system, the energies of the solar plexus relax and the digestive organs function more normally. Drinking the warm tea is specifically helpful for digestive problems, and is the recommended preparation for children.

The herb is a wonderful carminative that relaxes smooth muscle to reduce muscle spasms and flatulence (gas) throughout the gastrointestinal tract, and it can relieve spasms of the diaphragm causing hiccups. It has long been taken for the treatment of indigestion, stomachaches, nausea, vomiting, and dysentery, a bacterial infection in the intestines causing inflammation, cramps, pain, and diarrhea. Lemon Balm can be helpful for chronic constipation and irritable bowel conditions triggered by long-term tension and emotional stress. The herb's antimicrobial properties also help keep the gastrointestinal tract free of bacteria, viruses, and Candida yeast. The essential oil inhibits *Esherichia coli* (*E. coli*) bacteria (Thompson, 2013).

A research study found that an herbal combination containing Lemon Balm relieved pain and constipation in people with chronic colitis, an inflammation of intestinal tissues (Chakurski, 1981). The other herbs in the formula were Dandelion (*Taraxacum officinale*), Calendula (*Calendula officinalis*), St. John's Wort, and Fennel (*Foeniculum vulgare*). A combination of Lemon Balm, Spearmint (*Mentha spicata*), and Coriander (*Coriandrum sativum*), marketed as Carmint, significantly relieved abdominal pain and bloating in 16 patients diagnosed with irritable bowel syndrome over 8 weeks of treatment (Vejdani, 2006).

Chamomile has similar actions in the gastrointestinal tract as Lemon Balm, so they are a reliable combination for digestive complaints stemming from stress. Both are gentle enough to be specific remedies for infants and children. Lemon Balm with equal amounts of Catnip (*Nepeta cataria*) is excellent for all kinds of childhood digestive problems, including infant colic. I gave these herbs to my sons when they were babies and have recommended that many parents give it to their children with excellent results.

Women's Health: Lemon Balm is a gentle remedy for reproductive problems caused by nervous anxiety that evolve into pelvic muscle tension. Women suffering from chronic anxiety are more prone to menstrual cramps, pain, and other problems because internal tension slows down the flow of hormones and blood circulation. It is a well-known phenomenon that tension intensifies pain. As a mild emmenagogue, Lemon Balm's gentle calming properties promote menstruation. The sedative and muscle-relaxant qualities ease premenstrual syndrome (PMS) and uterine cramps. It is most effective when combined with Motherwort (*Leonurus cardiaca*) for these problems. In a 3-month study investigating the benefits of Lemon Balm on the intensity of PMS symptoms in 100 high school girls, those taking 1,200 mg daily experienced significant reductions compared to those in the placebo group (Akbarzadeh, 2015).

Lemon Balm has been used in combination with other herbs to treat infertility and safeguard against impotence. It is a mild emmenagogue due to its relaxing effects on the uterus, but a daily cup of the tea can be safely taken during pregnancy to calm the nervous system and ease insomnia, headaches, anxiety, and depression. It can reduce nausea, vomiting, gas, and dizziness during pregnancy, especially when used with Ginger tea (*Zingiber officinale*). Drinking a daily cup of Lemon Balm tea 2-3 weeks before the due date primes the uterus for labor. Midwives have given the tea or tincture to help expel a retained placenta.

External Uses: Lemon Balm is a vulnerary herb with antiseptic, antifungal, antispasmodic, anti-inflammatory, and analgesic properties that improve many external problems. The leaves are prepared as a poultice for direct application, or the warm tea may be used as a wash or fomentation. Lemon Balm is a wonderful addition to salves and continues to be an important and reliable ingredient in the salve I have produced for many years.

The leaves contain eugenol, an anesthetic that decreases pain. Scientists have found that the essential oils of aromatic plants such as Lemon Balm make excellent wound and surgical dressings because they release ozone, which has antiseptic properties. As the resinous oils dry on wounds, they seal the tissue and protect against infection. The herb is healing for sprains and inflammation, acne, animal bites and stings, burns, and ulcers. Its astringent property draws boils and pimples to a head and promotes healing.

Teachings from the Lemon Balm Deva

"Greetings, dear one. Can you see the luminescent lemon-yellow and spring-green aura of my plants? I am an herb of the Sun in alignment with Leo, the astrological sign under the Sun's domain. Leo is the great manifester, drawing atoms and the elements together into tangible, living forms. The essence and gifts of my plants contribute to the foundational structure of the physical body. My strong oils penetrate deeply through the body's tissues and waterways to cleanse and purify, allowing the brilliance of the vibrant yellowish-green within my aura to radiate through your own body.

"I share a strong affinity with the solar plexus that shines golden-yellow rays of light and with the green aura radiating from the heart center. I calm both of these centers, allowing each to function in healthy, life-giving ways. I soothe the 'wrinkles' in the atmosphere. When discordant energies threaten the health of the digestive organs and the heart and lungs, I assist in restoring harmony and peace to the surrounding atmosphere and the physical body. When a person's heart and emotions are distraught and in discord, the thoughts and actions reflect this and all is off-center and tense.

"And so the healing gifts I offer help merge, balance, and restore the nerve communication network between the solar plexus and the heart. Each of these areas intersects with a major hub of the nervous system and has a huge influence over the entire body. The solar plexus consists of vast bundles of nerves involved with the workings of the digestive organs and the transformation of nutrients into living cells. The solar plexus regulates physical activity and each person's process of interacting with the external world. The heart area is the 'feeling and emotional brain' of the body. Its state of being affects the lungs' ability to provide the breath of life and the body's power to protect against infectious creatures. When the forceful energies of the solar plexus are in alignment with a calm heart, all activities arise from this harmonious and tranquil flow manifesting as easier and gentler movement through each day.

"I am a light being, meaning that I am spacious, airy, free flowing movement. The essence of my medicine assists in expanding and enhancing these qualities in humans. My medicine is a good balancing remedy for people who are burdened under the weight of a heavy heart overloaded with life-draining feelings of fear, isolation, hate, or grief. For these emotions, when allowed to live in the heart, fester into tissues that deteriorate and turn against themselves. My plants help heal this enormous wounding experienced by so many people. I help loosen and bring spaciousness to the dense, constricted energies of the wounded pain body. Many people become stuck in their pain body and live in despair. If such a one makes the choice to heal and be released from the entrapment of the pain body, my plants will be of assistance in promoting a flow of love and acceptance to reverse the downward spiraling spin of the frequencies of despair. I will guide the energies of the heart and mind upward toward clarity and light. And so my direction of movement is upward and outward, easing constricted, dense, solidified, and trapped spaces to relax.

"I am an expansive herb like the Sun that shines and radiates out to all – whether naughty or good, all receive the sunlight. On your journey to wholeness, always remember that you are loved and worthy of love. Spend time getting to know yourself at the deepest levels until your 'inner knowing' experiences the radiant light that is the refined and subtle essence of all. My plants are helpers on the healing path, and the delightful fragrance of my leaves and flowers whisper to you, 'My medicine is sweet and delicious and will help bring sweetness into your life.' Although my essence is light and airy, I am also powerful and, like the Sun, can penetrate through deep, dark areas to re-establish the light of life.

"So go in peace, dear one. And partake of my healing medicines to assist in your amazing, sacred journey into wholeness and well-being."

Lobelia

Lobelia inflata
Campanulaceae (Bluebell) Family

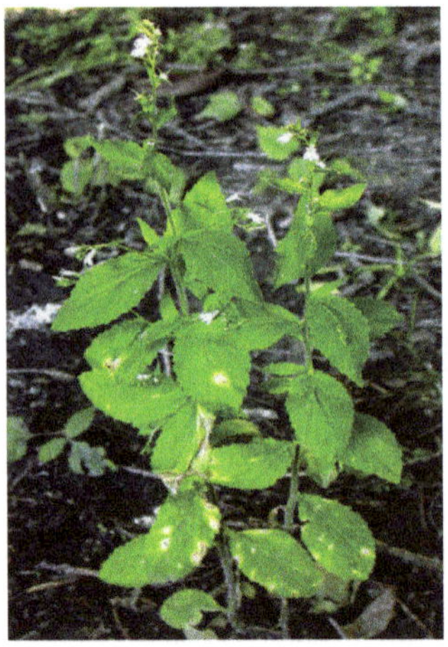

Lobelia inflata

Common Names

Indian tobacco and wild tobacco are antiquated names referring to Lobelia's use as a smoking herb. The name "bladderpod" describes its round, hollow seedpods resembling an empty bladder, and "asthma weed" refers to its use in treating asthma. Several common names, including emetic herb, emetic weed, puke weed, gag root, vomit root and vomitwort, refer to the nausea and vomiting induced by large doses of the dried plant.

Medicinal Part of the Plant

The entire plant is medicinally active with the seeds and roots containing the greatest amounts of potent phytochemicals. The leaves and seedpods are the parts traditionally used in medicinal preparations.

Range and Habitat

Lobelia inflata is indigenous to eastern and central United States and Canada. It grows in sunny fields and meadows, waste areas, and shady woodlands.

Description of the Plant

Over 400 species of Lobelia grow throughout the world. *L. inflata* is the species employed for medicinal purposes in Western herbalism. This is an annual herb in cold climates and a biennial in warmer zones. *L. inflata* is an inconspicuous wildflower with small, fibrous roots. The size and height of the plant varies depending on growing conditions and location. Plants in the wild are typically smaller with one primary stem reaching a height of 6-12″. Cultivated Lobelia often develops into bushy plants reaching 2′ with much larger, stouter stems and many branches.

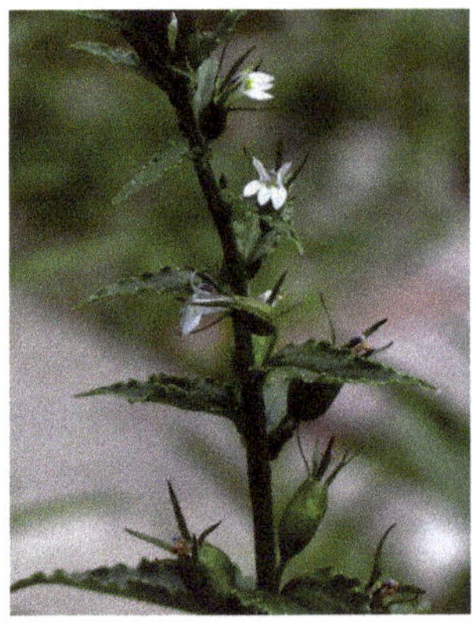

***Lobelia inflata* flowers**

L. inflata stems are erect, round, furrowed, and densely covered with soft, white hairs. Simple, alternate leaves are elliptic in shape with pinnate venation. They have small crenate (rounded) teeth and are sparsely covered with fine downy hairs. Sessile leaves clasp around the stem, and vary in length from 1-3″. The tiny, bluish-purple flowers are ¼″ long with 5 petals fused into a short tube forming a bi-lobed upper lip and a tri-lobed lower lip. Flowers are arranged in loose spikes, blooming from July through October. As flowers mature, the hollow calyx becomes inflated with seeds (thus the species name *inflata*) and transforms into a round, balloon-like pod. When the pod dries, it turns tan and splits into two segments, allowing many extremely tiny, dark seeds to spill out.

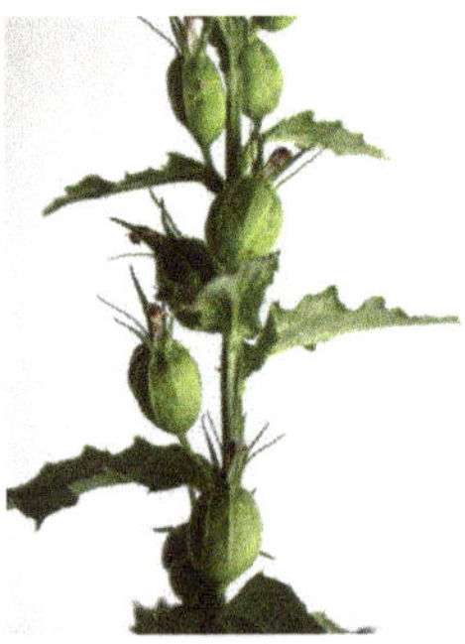

Seedpods

Two other *Lobelia* species were used medicinally in the past:

❖ *Lobelia siphilitica*, a perennial wildflower known as Great Blue Lobelia, is larger and showier than *L. inflata*. It grows up to 3′ tall and the vibrant violet-blue flowers are about 1″ in length, making this a stunningly attractive garden ornamental.

❖ *Lobelia cardinalis*, called Cardinal flower, is a perennial with brilliant, scarlet-red flowers 1-1½″ in length. Its ornate and vibrant flowers are also favored by gardeners.

Cultivation

L. inflata grows under partial shade or full sun in a variety of soils, but thrives best in a moist, fertile loam. It responds extremely well to cultivation, and plants growing in my gardens are always larger and bushier than those found in the wild. Researchers have discovered that cultivated plants contain about 40% more of the medicinally active lobeline, and they produce more seeds containing the highest concentrations of lobeline (Krochmal, 1972). The United Plant Savers organization has placed Lobelia species on their "to watch" list because diminished natural habitats are taking a severe toll on plant populations. For this reason, cultivation and conservative wildcrafting are more important than ever.

In my experience, *L. inflata* is difficult to start from seed. The tiny seeds have short viability, so plant them in plastic trays or a prepared garden bed immediately after collection. Because Lobelia seeds are light-dependent germinators, sow them on the soil surface and pat gently, but do not cover them with dirt. Use a fine spray mist when watering the delicate seedlings. After Lobelia is established in a field or garden, it naturally self-sows and keeps reappearing every year.

I consider this valuable herb to be somewhat of a "trickster" plant. In the human body, it can be stimulating or relaxing with different dosages, so caution and forethought are important when working with Lobelia. It has also been tricky in my gardens. I first tried growing a plot of Lobelia from seeds that I had collected from a nearby meadow and broadcast onto a carefully prepared bed. The following spring, not even one plant emerged from the plot where all the seeds had been sown, but new plants appeared everywhere else in the garden! So I have learned to let Lobelia plants grow freely wherever they choose to appear in the gardens, and they continue to self-propagate each year when they drop their seeds, while I enjoy abundant harvests.

Harvest

Gather leaves, flowers, and seedpods when the plant is in advanced stages of flowering from the end of July through mid-October. Seeds contain the greatest concentration of medicinal alkaloids, so harvest the plants when the mature seedpods are light brown with lots of tiny, black seeds inside. Be sure to leave some of the seedpods on the plant so that they will drop and germinate into new plants the following year.

Preparation of Plant Medicine and Dosages

Lobelia is ingested as tincture or tea. Tincturing is the best preservation method because the dried herb deteriorates quickly. Only tincture the freshly harvested plants because they exert stronger physiological activity and are not as likely to cause nausea as the dried herb. When preparing Lobelia, soft and moist stems from smaller plants are suitable for medicinal use. In larger plants, discard the tough, fibrous stems. Roots exert strong actions and may be tinctured, but please leave many of the roots so the plant can re-seed.

Lobelia leaves and seeds have a pungent, peppery taste. They leave a slight tingling sensation in the mouth and throat that lingers for a few minutes when they are chewed or taken as tincture or tea. Some people report that the herb stimulates salivary glands to secrete more saliva.

Tips on dosages: This wonderful healer is a powerful herb that exerts different activity depending on the dosage, so good judgment and respect for its virtues is important. Lobelia is **stimulating with small doses of 3-5 drops of tincture**, while it is **sedating and relaxing with larger doses of 20-30 drops**. It is best to **start using Lobelia in small doses** to determine its effect, and then gradually increase.

PREPARATIONS

Tincture of Leaves and Seedpods: Put the finely chopped fresh herb in a glass jar and cover with 100% 190-grain alcohol, 100% vinegar, or a blend of the two. Vinegar is traditionally used because its acidity works well to extract the medicinal alkaloids. However, I prefer and always use 100% grain alcohol. Dosage: Small doses of 1-5 drops can be taken 4-6 times a day as needed. Medium dosage is 6-19 drops taken 4-6 times a day as needed. Large doses ranging from 20-60 drops tend to cause nausea, especially if the dried herb is taken. If a larger dose is needed, start with small doses of 1-5 drops and slowly increase by 1 or 2 drops until nausea is felt, then decrease the dose by 1 drop and continue with this amount. The tincture also makes a wonderful liniment for topical applications.

Tincture of Seeds: Bruise the seeds by grinding them with a mortar and pestle, putting them in a bag and gently pounding them with a hammer, or by grinding them in an electric coffee bean grinder. Weigh the seeds and put them in a glass jar. Cover each ounce of seeds with 5 fluid ounces of alcohol or vinegar. Seeds may also be tinctured with the whole plant rather than separately. Dosage: Eclectic physician William Cook, M.D., found the seeds to be twice as strong as the leaves. Start using the seed tincture in small doses of 1 drop and gradually increase as needed up to 10 drops.

Infusion Tea: Steep 1 teaspoon of the herb in 1 cup of water for 10-15 minutes. Eclectic physicians believed that boiling water diminishes Lobelia's healing actions, so use moderately hot water to steep. Sip on the tea and use it as frequently as needed. Tea may also be used as a wash for external healing.

Poultice: The leaves are applied externally to treat wounds and soothe injured muscles and sprains.

Chemical Constituents

L. inflata contains 14 pyridine alkaloids (0.13-2.5% of the plant constituents) that include lobeline, lobelaline, lobelanidine, lobelanine, isolobeline, and lobelic acid. Lobeline, the primary alkaloid responsible for the plant's physiological effects, is the focus of most research on the herb. The other alkaloids are similar in action but milder than lobeline. These alkaloids belong to the same chemical group as nicotine. They are less potent and not addictive, but act on the peripheral and central nervous system in similar ways as nicotine (Gilman, 1980; Mansuri, 1973). Lobeline, lobelanidine, and lobelanine induce dopamine release and inhibit dopamine uptake in the brain, which increases the amounts of this neurotransmitter (Teng, 1998).

Lobeline is a mild diuretic and strong antispasmodic and expectorant used for asthma and bronchitis. It stimulates the nervous system and dilates the bronchial passages, allowing easier breathing when taken in small doses. Animal studies show that the emetic properties of isolated lobeline stimulate the vomit center at the base of the brain (Laffan, 1957). Isolobinine also causes nausea and vomiting when taken in large doses. Research indicates that beta-amyrin palmitate isolated from Lobelia leaves causes the release of norepinephrine in mouse brains (Subarnas, 1993). Norepinephrine is a neurotransmitter that has stimulating effects on the nervous system, while relaxing and opening bronchial passages. Other constituents in Lobelia include lipids, resins, gums, and chelidonic acid.

Safety, Contraindications, and Drug Interactions

The question of Lobelia's toxicity has been an issue in the herbal and medical communities for years. The controversy is fueled by unsubstantiated, hypothetical warnings that continue to appear in the literature and by the U.S. Food and Drug Administration (FDA) listing it as a "suspect" herb. The alleged toxicity is due to the similar chemistry of lobeline and nicotine (from Tobacco plants), although lobeline exerts weaker activity than nicotine. Having similar actions on the nervous system, **lobeline and nicotine stimulate the nerves and respiration in small doses, while causing nerve and respiratory depression in large doses.** Symptoms of nicotine overdose include nausea, vomiting, diarrhea, coughing, headaches, disturbed hearing and vision, tremors, and dizziness. Nicotine toxicity produces profuse sweating, tachycardia (rapid heart rate), hypothermia (reduced body temperature), hypotension, convulsions, shock, coma, respiratory failure, and paralysis followed by death. All of these problems are commonly cited as potential side effects of large doses of Lobelia. Adding to this confusion is the fact that Lobelia's activity is definitely dose dependent and lab tests can be misleading. For example, in dogs and rats, lobeline causes constriction of the bronchial passages, but in guinea pigs and humans the opposite occurs, and the bronchials relax (Cambar, 1969).

Nausea and vomiting are the only side effects that have actually been observed with Lobelia, and temporary nausea is the most common problem. Some people feel nausea from 2-5 drops of tincture or after chewing on a leaf, while others can tolerate 20-60 drops of tincture. Some people may experience passing nausea while others feel it for an hour. Vomiting usually requires several larger doses of 1-4 teaspoons of tincture. William Cook, M.D., wrote about the large amounts of Lobelia tea he prescribed, saying, "I have myself many times used an ounce of the herb within a few hours, and had it all retained; have given half an ounce to a babe six months old, in two hour's time; have given a child of five years four ounces of the seeds inside of seven hours, and had it retained, and in so doing have broken up most alarming attacks of disease, and promptly restored health from spasmodic conditions that otherwise would have been fatal" (Cook, 1869).

After extensive literature research investigating safety issues, herbalist Paul Bergner concluded:

> No credible evidence of Lobelia toxicity or any adverse effect more serious than vomiting is present in the medical literature of the past two centuries. Twentieth century literature that alleges Lobelia toxicity provides no primary references or alleged least toxic dose. Modern allegations appear to be parroted uncritically from early nineteenth century sources . . . . The nineteenth century literature is divided between medical practitioners who used Lobelia regularly and in large doses, and those who used it hardly at all. The unanimous consensus of those who actually use it in practice is that it is a harmless agent without potential for toxicity beyond its nauseating effects. Supporting this view is the twentieth century use of lobelia hydrochloride in large intramuscular, subcutaneous, and intravenous doses through the 1970s, and the non-prescription use of oral doses of lobeline sulfate without warnings or cautions as recently as 1990. (Bergner, 1998)

There are no known drug interactions for Lobelia, although people taking cardiovascular or pulmonary medications should use it cautiously. It is **contraindicated during pregnancy and lactation** due to the alkaloid content. Like many other herbal practitioners who use this herb, I have experienced and witnessed its wonderful healing ability, and encourage people to dose carefully when using it.

I learned about the tricky nature of Lobelia many years ago, unfortunately at the expense of a friend. One evening over the light of a campfire, he started complaining about a severe muscle cramp in his leg. Knowing that Lobelia has amazing ability to relax muscles, I gave him a hefty dose of about 40 drops of tincture, assuring him his pain would diminish. Within five minutes, he had forgotten about his leg cramps, which had indeed disappeared. Instead, he was holding his stomach ready to vomit and was not happy with me for making him feel so miserable. Luckily, my friend's nausea passed within a short time and his muscle spasm did not return, and I learned a valuable lesson about the power of Lobelia.

Medicinal Uses

History of the Plant

The genus *Lobelia* is named after the Flemish botanist Matthias de L'Obel (1538–1616). *Lobelia inflata* has a colorful history clouded with confusion. Some people claim that it is a dangerous, potentially deadly plant, while physicians and others who have used it extensively consider it to be a valuable and safe botanical.

Indigenous to North America, the healing virtues of *Lobelia inflata* and other Lobelia species were utilized by Native Americans. Historic records document its use by several tribes, including the Penobscot, Micmacs and Senecas, who drank the tea and smoked the leaves for respiratory problems. The Cherokee employed the leaves and roots for coughs and as an analgesic poultice applied for stiff necks and body aches, bites, stings, boils, and sores. The Iroquois used the tea as an emetic to induce vomiting when poison or spoiled food was eaten, to counteract illness produced by witchcraft, and to cure whisky poisoning after Europeans introduced alcohol (Moerman, 1998).

Lobelia siphilitica contains similar medicinal alkaloids as *L. inflata*, and Native Americans prepared tea from the leaves to treat colds, coughs, fevers and stomach problems, and applied leaf poultices to wounds. Many tribes combined *L. siphilitica* root with Mayapple root (*Podophyllum peltatum*), Wild Cherry bark (*Prunus serotina*), and New Jersey Tea (*Ceanothus americanus*) to successfully treat gonorrhea and syphilis passed on by infected Europeans (hence the name *siphilitica*). European colonists and healers learned about Lobelia from the Native Americans. One story came from Dr. Colden, who testified in 1758 that by ingesting less than an ounce of *L. siphilitica* root, he cured many soldiers of syphilis in less than a week. A cure for venereal disease sparked interest in the medical community, but their attempts to utilize Lobelia were unsuccessful, probably because they used it alone without adding other herbs traditionally used by Native Americans. Consequently, Lobelia was dismissed as useless against gonorrhea and syphilis, although Eclectic physicians prescribed the root as a diaphoretic, emetic, and remedy for ulcers, wounds, inflammation, and dropsy (edema caused by heart insufficiency). *L. siphilitica* is seldom used in modern herbalism.

The Cherokee, Iroquois, Pawnee, and other Native Americans were drawn to the beautiful scarlet-red flowers of *Lobelia cardinalis*. They prepared the root as a tea to treat venereal diseases, and used the roots and leaves during ceremonies and prayers and to make love charms. Although *L. cardinalis* is thought to possess similar alkaloids and medicinal properties as *L. inflata*, it has not been used by Western herbalists.

The popularity of *L. inflata* in Western herbalism is credited to Samuel Thomson (1769–1843), a New Hampshire "root doctor" (an old name for an herbalist). Lobelia was one of his favorite and specific remedies. He considered it to be an equalizing agent capable of opening blockages to allow the smooth flow of energy through the nervous system and to promote optimal blood circulation. He believed that this action allowed the body's vital force to circulate freely, bringing the system into a healthy balance. Over time, his theories and clinical results drew a gathering of herbal lay practitioners who called themselves "Thomsonians." They used tea from the dried powdered herb and an alcohol or vinegar tincture of the fresh plant as an expectorant, sedative, antispasmodic, and diaphoretic to reduce fevers.

As Lobelia's reputation grew, it became one of the most prescribed herbs in North America during the mid-1800s, and its popularity spread to England in the 1830s. Thomsonian herbalism became an alternative to the conventional medical practice of the allopathic or "regular" physicians of that period, who prescribed purging, bloodletting, and toxic mercury-derived medicines that were popular remedies for a variety of ills. As an effective emetic, Lobelia became the herb of choice for purging among herbal practitioners. It is estimated that by 1840, up to 20% of the United States population used Thomsonian herbal medicine (Bergner, 1998).

Samuel Thomson earned quite a notorious reputation for promoting this herb. Although Lobelia was tremendously popular among medical herbalists, allopathic physicians opposed it with great hostility. Dr. French, one of many allopathic physicians opposing Thomsonian medicine, repeatedly attempted to persecute Thomson, even threatening to "blow his brains out." In 1809, he had Thomson imprisoned in Massachusetts on the charge of murdering a very ill man, Ezra Lovett, with excessive doses of Lobelia. Apparently, Lovett became infected with a deadly disease that had recently claimed the life of a relative in his home. Thomson treated Lovett with Lobelia, but stopped treatment after deciding the case was hopeless, and an allopathic doctor took care of the patient during the last 24 hours of his life. Since Lobelia's effects are rapid and relatively short-lived, it is most likely that the patient died from the infection. The murder charges were dropped in court due to lack of proof, and Thomson was found innocent and released. However, accusations that he killed a man with Lobelia and false claims of the herb's toxicity capable of causing stupor, coma, and death have been cited in medical and herbal texts ever since. William Cook, M.D., wrote a detailed account of Lobelia's colorful history and Thomson's trial in his 1869 *Physiomedical Dispensatory*, and herbalist Paul Bergner has done extensive research and written an excellent article on this subject in his journal, *Medical Herbalism* (Bergner, 1998). According to Bergner's literature search, all claims of Lobelia's toxicity are based on references originating from Samuel Thomson's murder trial and the writings of authors James Thacher and Jacob Bigelow. Thacher started allegations of Lobelia's toxicity in American medical literature by claiming in his book *American New Dispensatory*, published in 1810, that it caused Lovett's death. In 1817, Bigelow emphatically declared the herb to be poisonous in his *Vegetable Materia Medica*. All subsequent citings of toxicity are probably derived from these authors, although Thatcher and Bigelow lacked proof for their claims. Unfortunately, confusion and misinformation about this very beneficial herb continues today.

L. inflata was a favorite remedy of the American Eclectic physicians during the 1880s–1930s. They considered it to be the best antispasmodic herb in their materia medica and prescribed it to treat severe muscle spasms (including those occurring with tetanus and rabies), strangulated hernias, and childhood and adult convulsions. Lobelia was often combined with Cayenne (*Capsicum annuum*) to treat these types of nerve and muscular conditions, and for asthma, whooping cough and other lung problems, and to relax and dilate the cervix during childbirth. Lobelia was highly valued for reducing fevers during major illness. It was administered in frequent small doses for chest pressure, pulmonary congestion and difficult breathing, and in larger doses to relieve angina. The leaves were applied externally to treat wounds, bruises, sprains, ringworm (a fungal infection), bites, stings, and poison ivy.

In one of the classic Eclectic works, *King's American Dispensatory*, Harvey Felter, M.D. (1865–1927) and pharmacist John Uri Lloyd (1849–1936) wrote, "Lobelia was known to the Penobscot Indians, and was also extensively used by the people in New England in domestic practice, long before the time of Samuel Thomson, its assumed discoverer . . . . The credit for the introduction of lobelia into medical practice is due to Drs. Manasseh Cutler [a prominent physician and medical herbalist in Massachusetts] and Samuel Thomson . . . few drugs have been so notoriously historical as the one under consideration. It became widely known to the people during the early part of the present century, through the famous trials of Drs. Thomson and Frost. The name of lobelia became so odious, that to be known as a 'lobelia doctor' was sufficient to subject the physician to all manner of ridicule" (Felter, 1898). Referring to the political climate of the era and the discord between herbal and allopathic physicians, Eclectic physician William Cook, M.D., wrote about the notoriety of Lobelia, saying, "This herb has had to fight its way into use through opposition the most extended and bitter, and has had combined against it the deepest venom of the whole one hundred and fifty thousand allopathic physicians in this country, who in turn brought to their help the prejudices and passions of the people, and the power of legislative enactments. Enmity so malignant has scarcely been equaled in medical history" (Cook, 1869).

Written accounts of several Eclectic physicians dispute the false allegations against Lobelia and document their clinical experiences using the herb to safely and effectively treat patients. William Cook, M.D., wrote, "I have myself many times used an ounce of the herb within a few hours, and had it all retained [meaning that it did not cause vomiting]; have given a child of five years four ounces of the seeds inside seven hours, and had it retained; and in doing so have broken up most alarming attacks of disease and promptly restored health from spasmodic conditions that otherwise would have been fatal. Other physicians have done the same, and many of them have given larger quantities than this. Within the last 75 years, it is probable that not less than 5,000 active practitioners have used this article every day, in all forms and in all imaginable quantities; and today their united experience comes up with one loud answer to the effect that lobelia is absolutely harmless" (Cook, 1869).

Although much confusion stemming from erroneous charges of toxicity and death has surrounded Lobelia, it is still used by many people and medical herbalists in England and the United States. *L. inflata* was listed as an official drug for the treatment of asthma from 1820–1920 in the *United States Pharmacopoeia* and in the *National Formulary* from 1936–1960. It was promoted and clinically used during the 1900s by well-known herbalists such as John Lust (author of *The Herb Book*), Dr. John Christopher (author of *School of Natural Healing*), and Jethro Kloss, who wrote almost 30 pages extolling the many virtues of Lobelia in his herbal classic, *Back To Eden*. Most modern research on Lobelia has focused on the primary alkaloid, lobeline.

Healing Qualities

Adjuvant, antihydrotic (decreases excessive perspiration), anti-inflammatory, antispasmodic, cardiac, diaphoretic, mild diuretic, emetic (with large doses), expectorant, nervine, pectoral, restorative, sedative (with large doses), sialagogue, central nervous system stimulant (with small doses), vasodilator, and vulnerary.

Traditional Chinese Medicine (TCM) Perspective

Asian varieties include *Lobelia radicans* and *L. chinensis*. Both are used in TCM to treat sores, skin and gum abscesses, poisonous snakebites, traumatic injuries, and ascites (abnormal fluid accumulation in the abdominal cavity). Researchers have identified anticarcinogenic actions in *L. chinensis*.

L. chinensis is indigenous to China and used in TCM. Its stimulating properties have mildly warming effects, while large doses that depress the system are cooling. It is relaxing in conditions of excess Yang, and stimulating in deficient Yang conditions. By harmonizing and restoring the whole system, the herb benefits the nerves, muscles, heart and circulation, lungs, stomach, liver, small intestines, kidneys, uterus, and skin. Lobelia regulates and restores the normal movement of Qi throughout the body, while promoting normal nerve function beneficial to all tissues and organs. The herb opens blockages throughout the system, improves and equalizes circulation, and removes mucous obstructions. It clears Internal Wind to stop spasms, clears excess heat, and detoxifies poisons from the body. It restores and establishes harmony between the nervous and circulatory systems. Lobelia is helpful for Qi constraint and stagnation throughout the body, including Lung Qi constraint and damp phlegm manifesting as chronic respiratory problems like asthma and emphysema. It also benefits acute problems like coughs, bronchitis, and pneumonia. Lobelia helps resolve Heart Qi constraint and deficiency manifesting as chest pressure, angina, palpitations, shortness of breath, edema, and poor circulation with cold extremities. It is also used for Uterine Qi Stagnation that can cause painful menstrual periods with cramping, and can prolong painful childbirth complicated by a rigid cervix and failure to progress.

Lobelia is indicated for people with chronic underlying nervous tension. It is specific for conditions of excess Yang and increased heat that manifest as a ruddy complexion, hyperactivity, anxiety, hypertension, poor circulation, spasms, tics and tremors, rapid heartbeat, chest constriction, labored breathing, and mucous congestion in the sinus cavities and lungs. The pulse may feel full but congested, and thick fur may appear on the tongue.

Primary Actions

Lobelia's predominant effects on the nervous system influence the entire body. Herbalists sometimes call it the "thinking herb" because its actions are directed to either stimulate or relax, depending on what is needed to normalize the system. It is stimulating to a depressed, lethargic nervous system or relaxing in conditions of excessive stimulation and tension. Lobelia's primary action is a general relaxation of the nerves, exerting a systemic effect to calm muscles and tissues throughout the body. Eclectic physician Finley Ellingwood, M.D. (1850-1920) used it in his medical practice and commented, "Lobelia seems at once to supply a subtle but wholly sufficient force, power, or renewed vital influence, by which the nervous system and the essential vital force within the system again reassert themselves and obtain complete control of the functional action of every organ. From this influence . . . a complete harmonious operation of the whole combined forces is at once resumed, in some cases in an almost startling manner" (Ellingwood, 1919). William Cook, M.D., wrote in his *Physiomedical Dispensatory*, "By the repetition of small doses at intervals of 15 or 30 minutes, its relaxing impression will soon begin to be distributed throughout the body, first upon the capillaries and nerve peripheries, then upon the general circulation, and finally throughout the muscular and glandular systems" (Cook, 1869).

When working with Lobelia, always keep in mind that small doses stimulate and larger doses sedate. Respect this powerful little plant and always begin with small doses. It may be taken alone, but it is traditionally taken with other herbs to balance its sedating effect occurring with large doses. The Thomsonian and Eclectic physicians combined it with Cayenne (*Capsicum annuum*), and Ginger (*Zingiber officinale*) is another stimulating herb appropriate to combine with Lobelia. **One important point to remember** – since Lobelia is dose-specific for different conditions, **bottle it separately rather than combining it in a formula** with other herbs. When taking Lobelia, put the specific dose in a glass of water and then add other herbs.

> *Lobelia tincture is stimulating in small doses (3-5 drops) and relaxing in larger doses (20-30 drops).*

In clinical practice, I use *L. inflata* tincture with excellent results for relaxing muscle spasms and cramps, improving respiration for those with asthma, helping people stop smoking cigarettes, and promoting easier childbirth. Other than one case of temporary nausea, everyone has expressed satisfactory results.

Nervous System and Muscular Relaxant: Lobelia is a powerful nerve relaxant that promotes and restores an unobstructed flow of energy through the nerves and normalizes muscle tone throughout the body. This is accomplished by the herb's strong influence on the autonomic nervous system, which is the autonomous or self-governing branch of the nervous system functioning without conscious control to regulate the glands, cardiac muscle, and smooth muscle within all blood vessels, tissues, and organs. The autonomic nervous system consists of the sympathetic and parasympathetic systems, and their opposite actions work together in maintaining a continual dynamic balance. The sympathetic nervous system mobilizes and stimulates the body's energy for emergencies and quick action, often called the fight-or-flight response. Heart rate increases, pupils dilate, rate of breathing and blood pressure rise, adrenal glands secrete adrenaline and cortisol, and perspiration increases. The parasympathetic nervous system is responsible for bodily functions performed at rest that restore the body, like digestion and elimination. Heart rate and respirations slow down, blood pressure drops, and as the tissues relax, the glands and digestive system become more active and increase their secretions. Lobelia's most wonderful and unique gift is its ability to balance and harmonize these two systems. It seems to have a direct effect on the hypothalamus, the center in the brain that integrates actions between the sympathetic and parasympathetic systems to regulate many involuntary functions and maintain homeostasis throughout the body. Lobelia also influences the spinal and cranial nerves within the central nervous system that send impulses to the voluntary skeletal muscles in the arms, legs, and torso that move by our willful control. Thus, Lobelia benefits all the muscles in the body because of its action on the nervous system.

The herb can either depress or stimulate the nervous system depending on dosage. Large doses are relaxing and helpful for painful, inflamed muscles, nervous tics, spasms, and cramps. Small doses are stimulating and dilate the airways to ease breathing and increase respiratory rate. Lobelia has historically been administered to treat nervous disorders, including epilepsy, seizures, childhood and adult convulsions, spasms caused by tetanus (lockjaw) and rabies, myalgia and fibromyalgia (muscle pain, rigidity, and inflammation), and all types of neuralgia (nerve pain). Eclectic physicians combined it with Blue Cohosh (*Caulophyllum thalictroides*) and Cayenne to treat convulsions. Convulsing babies were given a drop or two of Lobelia tincture directly into their mouths. William Cook, M.D., wrote, "The nervous system derives great benefit from it, as it is one of the most reliable articles to relieve all forms of suffering arising from tension and excitement of the tissues" (Cook, 1869). He recommended Lobelia for acute arthritis, periostitis (inflammation of the tissue covering bones), meningitis (inflammation of tissue surrounding the brain and spinal cord causing muscle spasms and convulsive seizures), and for the nervous irritation and spasms of delirium tremens occurring during alcohol and drug withdrawal.

Several studies have investigated Lobelia's mechanisms of action on neurotransmitters regulating the nervous system. Lobeline and other alkaloids in the herb increase dopamine levels by stimulating its production and release from synaptic vesicles connecting nerve cells (Teng, 1998; Dwoskin, 2002). Dopamine is a neurotransmitter that promotes feelings of well-being and is necessary for smooth, coordinated muscle movement. Dopamine deficiency can result in tremors, muscle rigidity and delayed initiation of movement, as seen in Parkinson's disease.

Researchers have found that lobeline is a strong inhibitor of adrenaline (epinephrine) and norepinephrine from the adrenal glands (Lim, 2004). Reducing levels of these two stimulating neurotransmitters seems to be one of the herb's mechanisms that relax the nervous system.

Lobeline's ability to reduce seizures and convulsions and prevent mortality in mice has been documented. Lobeline significantly increased levels of GABA (gamma-aminobutyric acid), one of the primary inhibitory (calming) neurotransmitters known to reduce seizure activity (Tamboli, 2012).

Adults suffering from nervous tension and spasms can start taking small doses of 3-4 drops of tincture in water and gradually increase up to 20-30 drops of tincture to obtain the desired relaxation effect. Find a dosage level that works without inducing nausea, and use that dosage as needed. Scullcap (*Scutellaria lateriflora*) and Valerian (*Valeriana officinalis*) work well combined with Lobelia for spasms and conditions stemming from nervous tension.

Small doses of Lobelia tincture stimulate a depressed nervous system and can be taken for shock with a sudden drop in heart rate and blood pressure, and for fainting, concussions, and coma. The herb has also been used to revive a depressed nervous system induced by drug poisoning. Putting small, frequent doses of 3-4 drops of tincture directly under the tongue can be repeated every 5 minutes as needed, and is specific for shock and restoring consciousness.

Lung and Bronchial Health: Lobelia's powerful, normalizing influence on the nervous system benefits the lungs and respiration. Its traditional application for acute and chronic respiratory problems is validated by current research. Lobeline stimulates sympathetic ganglia in the respiratory center of the brain, promoting bronchial dilation that allows easy, deeper breathing. Lobeline and other alkaloids are acetylcholine antagonists, which also contribute to the dilation and relaxation of bronchial passages (Robinson, 1986).

Lobelia is a strong antispasmodic and expectorant, and medium doses relax chest and bronchial muscles to open constricted airways (Cambar, 1969). By easing rigid muscles and spasms, Lobelia is excellent for asthma and difficult breathing exacerbated by exposure to cold air and physical exertion. The herb reduces dry, spastic coughs as well as wet, productive coughs. The Eclectic physicians valued it more than all other herbs for treating respiratory problems, and regarded it as one of their best expectorants to normalize mucous membrane secretions and break up mucous congestion. They recommended Lobelia for the treatment of coughs, croup, whooping cough, wheezing, shortness of breath, bronchial spasms, sore throat, laryngitis, pneumonia, bronchitis, pleurisy, asthma, and emphysema. Beginning in 1938, American and British physicians prescribed large doses (20 mg) of intravenous and intramuscular injections of lobeline hydrochloride during emergencies to stimulate respiration in newborn infants, for partial suffocation such as drowning, and in other conditions of respiratory failure (Osol, 1947; Hobart, 1949).

I have recommended Lobelia tincture to many people suffering from labored breathing due to asthma and bronchial infections. Most have reported improved breathing and relief from pressure and tightness in their chest and lungs. Many clients with asthma take Lobelia on a continual basis and are able to reduce the amount of prescription drugs and inhalers necessary to breathe comfortably.

For asthma and other respiratory problems, start with 4-5 drops of tincture and gradually increase up to 10-15 drops taken several times a day as needed. Find the minimum dose that works for you. To treat infant colic or childhood asthma, mix 5 drops of the tincture with 1/3 cup of water, and give 1 teaspoon at a time to the infant in 30-60 minute intervals as needed. For asthma, Lobelia may be taken alone or combined with Cayenne. When treating bronchial infections, take Lobelia with antibiotic and pectoral herbs such as Goldenseal (*Hydrastis canadensis*), Yarrow (*Achillea millefolium*), Horehound (*Marrubium vulgare*), Pleurisy Root (*Asclepias tuberosa*), Elecampane (*Inula helenium*), and Sage (*Salvia officinalis*).

An Aid to Help Drug Withdrawal and Stop Smoking Cigarettes: Sustained use of alcohol and many addictive recreational drugs can lead to neurological imbalance and damage. Lobelia is excellent during alcohol and drug withdrawal when people can experience severe nervous agitation and muscle spasms known as delirium tremens. A United States patent was issued in 1998 for the use of lobeline in treatment plans for withdrawal from recreational drugs, including alcohol, nicotine, cocaine, amphetamines, caffeine, opiates, barbiturates, and hallucinogens. The patent indicated that lobeline treatment reduces the desire for abusive drugs and suppresses appetite in people with eating disorders (Dean, 1999). Researchers have found that lobeline demonstrates potential for effectively treating methamphetamine abuse and reducing the damaging neurological and behavioral effects. Lobeline was found to inhibit methamphetamine-induced dopamine release (which is excessive) and resulting hyperactivity (Dwoskin, 2002; Nickell, 2014). For all cases of drug withdrawal, Lobelia should be given with strong sedating nervines like Scullcap, Valerian, Holy Basil/Tulsi (*Ocimum sanctum*), Hops (*Humulus lupulus*), and Lemon Balm (*Melissa officinalis*).

Lobelia leaves have historically been used in smoking mixtures by Native American tribes, and the plant was called "Indian tobacco" by American colonists who adopted this tradition. Like the tea and tincture, the smoke also opens bronchial passages and is an old remedy for asthma. The leaves provide a mild-tasting smoke that some people experience as mildly euphoric, yet stimulating.

More recently, Lobelia has been employed as an aid to stop cigarette smoking. Cigarette smokers develop more nicotine-binding receptors on their cells than nonsmokers do. Nicotinic binding receptors are specialized sites on cell membranes that, like a lock and key, only allow substances with a specific nicotine structure to enter and affect the cell. Nicotinic binding sites, occurring throughout the body, are stimulated by low doses of nicotine and are depressed or blockaded by high doses. When people stop smoking, nicotinic receptors that are normally saturated with nicotine become "starved," resulting in addictive cravings. Small doses of Lobelia are known to reduce nicotine craving when taken frequently throughout the day.

Attempting to understand Lobelia's mechanism of action and relationship to nicotine, researchers have found that lobeline is chemically similar to nicotine and attaches to nicotine receptors on cell membranes (Damaj, 1997; Terry, 1998). When lobeline fills nicotinic receptors, the craving for nicotine is satisfied and it is easier for people to stop smoking. However, compared to nicotine, Lobelia's physical effects are much milder and do not damage the lungs, deplete oxygen, or create addiction. By relaxing the nervous system and muscles, Lobelia also helps people deal with the tension and agitation normally accompanying nicotine withdrawal.

In 1990, the FDA approved Lobelia's alkaloids in over-the-counter preparations to help people overcome nicotine addiction and quit smoking. These were prepared as tablets, lozenges, and chewing gum containing 2-4 mg of lobeline sulfate. The FDA later revoked approval due to claims of insufficient research to validate efficacy. However, many herbalists continue using Lobelia preparations to help people stop smoking. I have given Lobelia tincture to 15-20 people for this purpose, and about 95% of them have reported that it decreased their craving for cigarettes and helped them stop smoking. I personally witnessed Lobelia's action when I took a 10-day vacation with one of my best friends, who had been a smoker for many years. She was serious about quitting, so I told her about Lobelia and she wanted to try it. On the first day of our vacation, she stopped smoking and started taking 4-5 drops of the tincture in water every couple of hours. After the first day, she only took the tincture a few times during the day when she thought about it. I kept asking her how she was doing, whether she needed another dose, but she did well on occasional small doses without experiencing distressful nicotine withdrawal symptoms or nausea. Towards the end of our time together, she was using only a small amount of Lobelia and stopped completely when she returned home. To this day, several years later, she continues to be free from cigarettes.

Cardiovascular System: Lobelia's calming actions benefit heart rate and muscles within the heart and blood vessels. Larger doses relax muscles to relieve chest pressure, spasms, poor circulation, labored breathing, and angina. The herb calms and normalizes cardiac muscle to reduce palpitations and tachycardia (rapid heart rate). The muscular layers of blood vessels also relax and dilate under the influence of Lobelia, helping to equalize circulation throughout the body and reduce hypertension. Small, stimulating doses may be dropped under the tongue for abnormally low blood pressure or pulse rate, fainting, and coma.

This was a favorite herb of the Eclectics for treating heart problems. Harvey Felter, M.D., observed, "Lobelia is *the* drug for angina pectoris, neuralgia of the heart, and pulmonary apoplexy [stroke] . . . . When the circulation exhibits a markedly slow pulse-wave it will be better corrected by lobelia than by any other drug we possess. In fact the most prominent indication for the drug is the full, oppressed, sluggish, doughy pulse. Associate this with praecordial [pericardium surrounding the heart] oppression, thoracic pain, difficult breathing, soreness or bruised feeling within the chest, nausea with tongue heavily coated at base, fullness of tissue, and we have before us a fair range of the action of lobelia. It is a good remedy in cardiac congestion" (Felter, 1922). William Cook, M.D., noted, "The circulation is materially equalized by its use, and the blood vessels relieved from a condition of tension, whether the case be one of inflammation or fever. By relaxing the circulatory apparatus, it favors a full outward flow of blood, with diaphoresis; secures greater fullness and softness of the pulse, with a reduced excitability of the heart, and from the universality of this influence, expedites the reestablishment of the secretions of the skin, liver, and kidneys" (Cook, 1869).

When using Lobelia for chronic cardiovascular problems, start with small doses and gradually increase to the dose that works best for you. Combine it with other heart tonics such as Cayenne, Hawthorn berries (*Crataegus* spp.), Motherwort (*Leonurus cardiaca*), and Peppermint (*Mentha x piperita*). For acute problems requiring immediate action such as painful angina, use larger doses of 20-30 drops of tincture every 10-15 minutes as needed, and get medical help.

Gastrointestinal System: Lobelia's soothing, normalizing action on the nerves in the solar plexus supports the digestive organs as well. Eclectic physicians found that small doses could improve the appetite and digestion, and they frequently used the herb to treat indigestion when nervous tension was present. Lobeline relaxes muscle tone throughout the gastrointestinal tract to reduce cramps and spasms, it increases secretions of stomach and pancreatic digestive enzymes, and promotes smooth movement of food through the intestines. Lobelia improves sluggish digestion and intestinal motility resulting in chronic constipation. The herb's antispasmodic and muscle relaxant properties are useful when treating intestinal spasms and inflammation that accompany irritable bowel syndrome and Crohn's disease.

The Eclectic physicians and Thomsonian herbalists frequently administered Lobelia tea as an enema for bowel obstructions and chronic constipation. For enemas, it combines well with Catnip (*Nepeta cataria*) tea.

Finley Ellingwood, M.D., reported using hypodermic-injected forms of Lobelia to relax muscles and relieve strangulated hernias, including a case of umbilical hernia.

In large doses, Lobelia stimulates the vagus nerve and acts as an emetic to induce vomiting, making it a useful treatment for food poisoning. For emetic purposes, take at least 1 teaspoon of tincture 3 times within 15 minutes. People respond differently to the emetic effects and some are sensitive to several drops, while others tolerate several teaspoons before feeling nauseous. The Eclectics successfully used Lobelia to produce vomiting in cases of ptomaine food poisoning and ingestion of poisonous mushrooms. They prescribed 30 drops of tincture taken every 30 minutes to treat the violent convulsion caused by strychnine poisoning.

Lobelia can also be helpful in relieving hiccups. It is interesting that while writing this section on Lobelia, I had a sudden attack of hiccups that was relentless. Hiccups are spasms in the large diaphragm muscle, and usually I can get them to stop by continuously gulping little sips of water for a couple of minutes while synchronizing drinking with breathing. When this method failed, it became an obvious opportunity to learn first-hand how Lobelia could help. I put a large sedating dose of 30 drops in water and drank it. The hiccups stopped a few minutes later and started again in 15 minutes. I took a larger dose of 60 drops and gulped down more water and the hiccups disappeared. About 20 minutes later, when the hiccups began again, I took another 60 drops of tincture in water and the spasms finally ended. After taking 3 large doses within 35 minutes, I did not feel any nausea or sedation. I experienced a wave of relaxation passing through my body, and could especially feel my solar plexus relax.

Kidneys, Kidney Stones, and Gallstones: Lobelia's muscle relaxant and antispasmodic properties reduce kidney inflammation and spasms, relax the ureters to dilate, and allow easier passage of kidney stones. As a mild diuretic, it may be helpful for some types of edema. Eclectic physicians found that it relieves pain from the passing of stones, and Finley Ellingwood, M.D., wrote, "Lobelia relieves pain due to spasms of any character. But in its antispasmodic and relaxing influence it is not narcotic in the same sense as opium. It exercises a soothing influence over nerve irritability, and a distinct anodyne [pain-relieving] result ensues. General relief from pain often follows when other measures have failed. The pain from renal or hepatic stone [kidney stones and gallstones] is more quickly relieved by it and more permanently, often, than by morphine because of the general relaxation" (Ellingwood, 1919).

Suppressed and Excessive Secretions: Lobelia has normalizing actions on the mucous and secretory glands due to its ability to relax nerves, muscle tone and tissues, open obstructions, and normalize circulation. When the body is relaxed, all glandular secretions tend to function better, and in this way, Lobelia can increase underactive secretions. Chewing the leaves and seeds stimulates the salivary and buccal glands to secrete saliva and mucous.

The herb is also antihydrotic, meaning that it can be helpful for excessive sweating. For this purpose, combine it with other antihydrotic herbs such as Cinquefoil *(Potentilla* spp.), Cranesbill *(Geranium maculatum)*, Sage, and Cleavers (*Galium aparine*).

Women's Health: Lobelia's calming, antispasmodic properties work wonderfully to initiate delayed menstruation and relieve menstrual cramps when there is tension and congestion in the pelvis. It is also helpful during pregnancy for a threatened miscarriage and during labor to relax the cervix and promote strong, productive contractions.

Miscarriage: Herbalist midwives have discovered that small to medium doses of Lobelia promote a natural miscarriage if the fetus is weak or malformed, but will prevent miscarriage if the fetus is strong and healthy, even if contractions begin. To prevent a threatened miscarriage, take very small sips of the leaf and seed tea every few minutes for an hour. Rest for another hour and repeat. Or take 5-15 drops of tincture in water every 15-30 minutes. Some sources recommend taking up to 60 drops of tincture every 30 minutes to stop a threatened miscarriage (Holmes, 1989).

Childbirth: Lobelia eases the discomfort of early labor and helps ensure a smooth birthing progress. It is specific for prolonged and difficult childbirth, working amazingly well to soften a rigid cervical os, vagina, and perineum. When uterine contractions are weak and ineffective, the herb seems to space out contractions, making them stronger and more productive. The Eclectics employed Lobelia for this purpose, and Harvey Felter, M.D., wrote, "Lobelia is of value in obstetrical practice. It powerfully subdues muscular rigidity. It is the remedy to overcome a rigid os uteri during parturition, and at the same time it relaxes the perineal tissues" (Felter, 1922). Injections of lobeline hydrochloride have been used to resuscitate newborns. Drops of tincture under the tongue would probably have the same result.

Many years ago when I was in training and assisted midwives at home births, we successfully used Lobelia tincture combined with twice as much Trillium *(Trillium erectum)* tincture for several birthing mothers with stalled labor. Doses of 30 drops (10 drops of Lobelia with 20 drops of Trillium) were taken in water 1-3 times about 15-30 minutes apart. This method always brought stronger, more effective contractions, relaxed and dilated the cervical os, and produced healthy babies born without problems.

Fevers and Infections: Lobelia is a diaphoretic that promotes sweating and releases internal heat that reduces fevers. The Thomsonians, Eclectics, and herbal naturopath Jethro Kloss used it in combination with other herbs to treat high fevers accompanying many serious infections, such as meningitis (inflammation of the membranes surrounding the brain and spinal cord caused by bacterial infection), hepatitis, peritonitis (infection and inflammation of the abdominal lining caused by ruptured appendix or intestines), nephritis (kidney inflammation), diphtheria (a very contagious bacterial infection), scarlet fever, chicken pox, measles, mumps, small pox, laryngitis, and tonsillitis. Harvey Felter, M.D., wrote, "It may be used in forming stages of febrile [feverish] afflictions, and is especially indicated by a general sluggishness of the whole system with an oppressive feeling, and the tongue is heavy and fully coated at the base" (Felter, 1922). William Cook, M.D., extolled Lobelia's virtues in his writings, saying, "Its use in fever is valuable beyond any other remedy that has ever been introduced to the notice of the profession" (Cook, 1869).

External Uses: The herb's antispasmodic properties are excellent for external applications to treat bruised and sprained muscles and ligaments, painful muscle spasms, menstrual cramps, and headaches. It relaxes muscles throughout the body, and when massaged on the chest, it relaxes chest muscles and improves breathing. External applications of Lobelia draw toxins, infection, and pus from wounds, insect bites and stings, poison ivy, abscesses, and boils. A poultice, wash of the tea, or liniment of the tincture has historically been used for these problems and for eruptive skin diseases such as herpes, eczema, nettle rash, and ringworm (a fungal rash). The liniment is especially effective for muscular and arthritic pain.

For skin ulcers and wounds, make a poultice by mixing and applying equal parts Lobelia leaves and ground Marshmallow root (*Althaea officinalis*) or ground Comfrey root (*Symphytum officinale*) to the ulcerated area. Herbalist John Christopher reported that soaking wounds in the tincture or tea draws out pain and congested blood (Christopher, 1976). Poultices of Lobelia combined with other herbs have been used to treat gangrene and skin cancers. For muscle sprains, strains, pain, burns and inflammation, the tincture works well when combined with Peppermint and St. John's Wort oil and gently massaged into the injured tissues.

Teachings from the Lobelia Deva

"Greetings. I am the deva of the Lobelia plants and am happy to share with you the secrets of my herbs and my medicine ways for humans. The sky-blue color of my little flowers reflects my calming influence on your nervous system and on the intangible aspects of a human being – the vibrational realms of thoughts and emotions. As I work with these subtle energies, there is automatically a relaxing, healing ripple effect through the body.

"My plants are ruled by the subtle air element that holds vibrational frequencies not existing as form – thoughts, feelings, and energetic movement along the nerve pathways. The air element helps clear and open respiratory passages, and my medicine works especially well for those who feel suffocated by heavy emotions, disturbing thoughts, and constricted muscles and tissues. My plants bring the ease and spaciousness of the air element to expand the tissues of the lungs and allow the breath of life to enter. I am a deva in service to the 'breath of life' that connects and is shared by all living beings on this planet. The sacred breath connects all people and animals to their physical bodies, from the first breath at birth until the last breath when the body dies and all else moves on. Honor this sacred breath of life moving through and animating your body. Cultivate happy, calming thoughts and emotions that allow the body to live in a peaceful state of being.

"The essence of my healing harmonizes the subtle etheric realms of thoughts and feelings, and helps the nervous system be relaxed to do its job of interfacing with and interpreting the world. When these energies are in balance, there is a natural ease of flow through the events of daily life, and although tensions may arise, they are resolved so the flow is not blocked. Blockage of the breath and energetic flow of the life force are the ultimate sources of human problems in the body, and in the world. With blockage comes forgetfulness of the spark of life within all beings – people, animals, and yes, also us, the plants and devas.

"When people lose touch and remembrance of their individual connection with the whole, a flood of deceptive realities pour into human consciousness and emotions. The experience of feeling alone and isolated from others, fear, anger, hate, self-loathing or self-grandeur – the display of realities is vast and limitless and is the ultimate source of human woes. And so my medicine heals and brings alignment to this flow of breath and life.

"I am ruled by the air sign Gemini, regulator of the chest and lungs. The energies of Gemini are symbolized as twins representing the polarities of life. The enlightened activity of Gemini balances and harmonizes all opposites to exist and operate in mutual cooperation, allowing the universal spark of life to flow freely and joyfully through all beings on this planet. Please think of me as a 'balancer.' Use the essence of my flowers when you feel unraveled and are falling apart, in need of returning to your calm center. I will help you remember your wholeness in the midst of the eternally unfolding dream of life."

Marshmallow

Althaea officinalis
Malvaceae (Mallow) Family

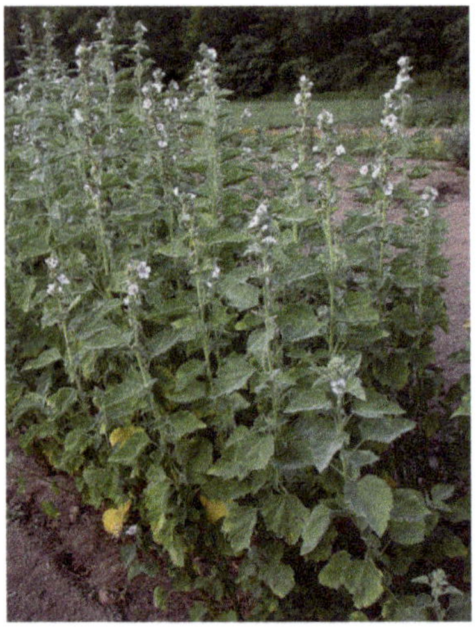

Common Names

Althea, cheeses, mortification root, sweet weed, and wymote are antiquated names for Marshmallow.

Medicinal Part of the Plant

Leaves, flowers, and roots all contain the healing mucilage, but the roots contain the greatest amounts and are the part most commonly used for medicinal purposes.

Range and Habitat

Marshmallow is indigenous throughout temperate Europe and Western Asia. It has naturalized throughout North America in the eastern states, the mountains of the west, and in salt marshes of the mid-Atlantic states. Members of the Mallow family prefer wet, marshy areas (hence Marshmallow's name). Plants prefer full sun, although they do accept partial shade, and grow by ponds, bogs, lakes, streams, rivers, and other moist areas.

Description of the Plant

This large, bushy perennial grows 4-6′ tall. Marshmallow has large, branching taproots growing a few feet long. The dark outer root surrounds a moist, creamy-white interior. Several erect, fibrous stems grow straight up from the massive root system and do not branch out. The stalk is round and, like the leaves, is densely covered with white pubescent hairs, giving the entire plant a very soft, fuzzy texture.

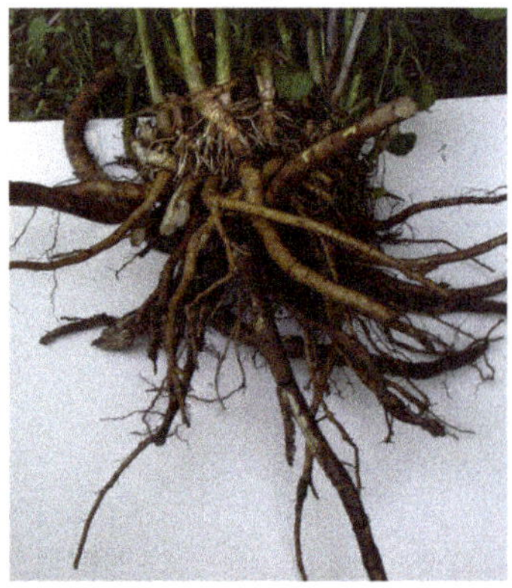

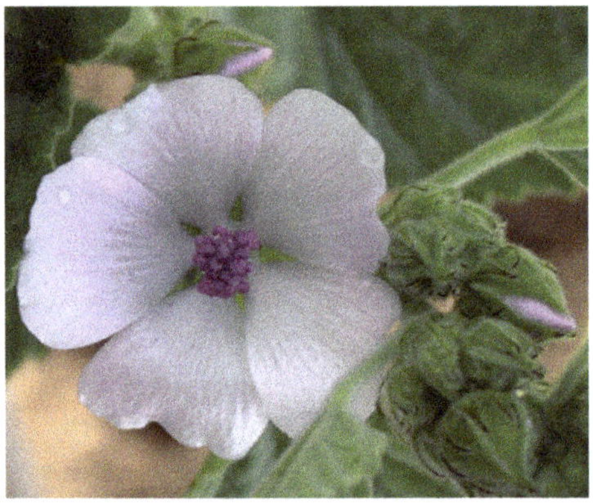

The simple, petiole leaves climb the stems in an alternating pattern, becoming smaller towards the top. The light-green leaves are 1-4″ long with a broad base that narrows into an acute tip. Leaves have palmate venation, several palmate lobes, and large dentate teeth. The dense, velvety down on both sides of the leaves gives them a soft thickness.

The attractive, delicate-looking flowers are 1-2″ in diameter and grow in clusters from upper leaf axils and along the ends of the long stems. A hairy, light-green calyx with overlapping, pointed sepals holds each flower. Flowers have 5 pale purplish-white or occasional pale-rose petals with a tuft of purple stamens in the center. The plant blooms from June through September. Flowers mature into light-brown, flat, round, disc-shaped seeds that are tightly clumped together to form small, round pods or buttons called "cheeses" in Europe.

Cultivation

Marshmallow plants thrive in moist areas with rich humus under full sun. Roots grown in moist, fertile soil tend to be larger, fleshier and less fibrous, providing better medicinal qualities than those in dry or compact clay soils. Plant Marshmallow in deep, fertile, sandy loam with constant moisture and adequate drainage. Drainage is important since roots growing in excessively wet soil tend to produce less medicinal mucilage than those in drier dirt. The plant is easily propagated by seeds or root division.

Sow seeds directly into a prepared garden in spring when danger of frost is past. In early spring, seeds may also be planted in trays in a greenhouse or by a sunny window. Marshmallow seeds tend to germinate well. Cover them with 1/8″ of soil, keep them moist, and they usually germinate within 30 days. When the seedlings are 3-4″ tall, transplant them 2′ apart in a permanent garden space. Mulch the plants with grass clippings, and water them throughout the growing season if conditions are dry.

Rootstock may be purchased or obtained by digging up live plants. Use a hatchet or sharp knife to cut the roots from the stems. Root crowns are covered with buds of future stems, which can be separated from the rest of the root and replanted. Leave 3-4″ of root attached to each crown to provide enough nutrients to keep them alive. Plant the crowns with attached roots so they are buried under 1″ of soil. Space them 2′ apart, water thoroughly, and keep the roots cool and moist with mulch. They grow fairly quickly into bushy plants.

Harvest

Leaves develop more mucilage after flowering begins, so harvest leaves and flowers when the plant is well into the blooming phase. Harvest 3- or 4-year-old roots in autumn to obtain the greatest concentration of healing mucilage.

The mucilage content in the roots fluctuates with seasonal changes. Mucilage is produced during the warm growing season and is used as food to sustain the roots during winter dormancy, making the end of the growing season the best time for harvesting. Dig a wide, deep hole around the roots so that none are left behind. When harvesting, remember that the root crown with one or more buds on it can be separated from the main portion of the root and replanted. This propagation method is a wonderful way to balance harvesting with propagating new plants, while maintaining a yearly supply of herbal medicine.

Preparation of Plant Medicine and Dosages

The soothing mucilage and immune-enhancing qualities of Marshmallow are better extracted by water than alcohol. Therefore, tinctures are not recommended for obtaining the greatest healing potential. The most therapeutic preparation for Marshmallow (and all mucilage herbs) is tea made from the fresh roots, leaves, and flowers. These parts may also be dried, stored, and ground into powder when needed. When mucilage comes into contact with water, it absorbs the water and swells to form a gel. The mucilage is extracted with warm water to make a pleasant, slightly sweet tea with a slick, somewhat slimy texture and thick consistency.

Roots are thoroughly washed and chopped into small pieces. They can be used immediately or dried for future needs. To dry, lay pieces of root on screens or cardboard in a well-ventilated area. Fans shorten drying time and reduce potential for mold growth in humid climates. Before storing the roots in a glass jar, make sure that they are completely dry by testing how well they snap apart when broken. Marshmallow is most effective when the roots are ground into fine powder and prepared as tea or mixed with water as a thick gruel. In this way, the entire root is ingested and the healing mucilage directly touches membranes lining the gastrointestinal and urinary tracts. For best preservation, wait to grind roots into powder until it is needed.

Leaves and flowers are used fresh or can be dried. Hang the whole stem with leaves and flowers in a shaded, well-ventilated area. If humidity is a problem, strip the leaves and flowers off the stem and lay them on trays or screens in front of a fan.

PREPARATIONS

Warm and Cool Infusions: The active mucilaginous properties of Marshmallow extract better in water that is warm rather than boiling hot. The root and leaf tea should never be boiled because this denatures the mucilage, reducing its medicinal properties. Soak 1-2 tablespoons of the chopped or shredded root or leaf in warm water for 4-8 hours, then strain and drink the tea cool or warmed. Dosage: 1-5 cups a day as needed. Infusion teas can be used for washes, fomentations, eyewashes, and douches.

Gruel or Porridge: Dry and grind roots into a fine powder and gently simmer in a little water to make a pleasant, mild-tasting gruel or porridge. This is a wonderful way to provide nutrients and hydration in cases of nausea, vomiting, and dehydration from excessive vomiting and diarrhea in children.

Poultice: The fresh root is the best poultice material, but leaves and flowers also work well. Cut freshly harvested plant parts into small pieces and grind them with a blender or mortar and pestle, adding enough water to make a thick paste. If the roots, leaves, or flowers are dried, grind them into powder and add water to make a paste. Apply the poultice to the skin, using a wrap to keep it in place. This may be left on the skin for several hours, but should be kept moist by adding more water as the plant material dries.

Salve: Marshmallow roots and leaves are an excellent addition to salves.

Syrup: Marshmallow root tea is a soothing addition to cough syrups.

Pills and Lozenges: Dry the roots and grind them into a fine powder. Add enough water to make a thick paste. Roll this into little pills and dry them. Dosage: 1-12 pills a day as needed.

Capsules: Dry and grind the roots into a fine powder and pack it into capsules. Dosage: 1-12 capsules a day as needed.

Suppositories: Make these the same way as pills, but roll them into suppository shapes and dry.

Culinary Uses

The roots, leaves, and green immature seeds are edible. The fresh, moist seeds (called "cheeses" or "nutlets") have a mildly pleasant, nutty flavor. Leaves are steamed and eaten like spinach or sautéed with vegetables. The powdered roots simmered in water produce a pleasant, mild-tasting gruel or porridge that hydrates and provides nourishment during bouts of fever, debility, and nausea and vomiting when the stomach refuses food. Infants can safely ingest the gruel or porridge.

Chemical Constituents

Marshmallow roots contain carbohydrates (25-38% starch and 10-35% pectin), mucilage polysaccharides (25-35% in the roots and 6-9% in leaves), amines (proteins including asparagin), and fats. The mucilage is composed of mucopolysaccharide sugars, including arabinogalactans, galacturonic acid, glucuronic acid, glucose, galactose, rhamnose, and mannose. Mucilage is the major medicinal constituent of the plant and is responsible for its slippery, slimy texture. Polysaccharides exhibit immune-enhancing properties. The root also contains flavonoids (quercetin and kaempferol), chlorogenic acid, coumarins (scopoletin), phenolic acids (caffeic, ferulic, syringic, and salicylic acids), and saponin sterols. There are ample amounts of pectin, a water-soluble plant fiber that provides bulk to keep the bowels moving and helps to moderate blood sugar levels. The roots contain substantial amounts of easily absorbable minerals such as iron, magnesium, selenium, chromium, calcium, manganese, phosphorus, and potassium.

Leaves contain mucilage in lower concentrations. Also present are flavonoids (quercetin and kaempferol), scopoletin (a blood-thinning coumarin), and phenolic acids that include caffeic, salicylic, and coumaric acids (Wren, 1988).

Safety, Contraindications, and Drug Interactions

All parts of the Marshmallow plant are safe and non-toxic. It is a nourishing and benign herb for people of all ages, including infants, the elderly, and those who are weak and debilitated. It is safe to use during pregnancy and lactation, and there are no known dangerous drug interactions. However, the mucilage may delay absorption of pharmaceutical drugs if they are taken at the same time. This can be avoided by ingesting pharmaceuticals at least 30 minutes before taking Marshmallow. The anti-inflammatory qualities of the roots appear to beneficially increase the effect of topical steroids.

Medicinal Uses

History of the Plant

Marshmallow has been widely used in European medicine for over 2,500 years. Ancient and modern applications of the herb are nearly identical. It was a popular remedy in early Greek and Roman medicine. The genus name *Althaea* comes from the Greek word *altho*, meaning "to cure or heal." The family name *Malvaceae* is derived from the Greek *malake*, meaning "soft," referring to the soft fuzziness of the leaves and perhaps to the gentle nature of the herb's healing actions. Hippocrates (*circa* 460–*c.* 377 B.C.), the "father of medicine," prescribed the root tea for bruises and bleeding wounds. Theophrastus (*c.* 370–*c.* 287 B.C.) prepared Marshmallow in wine as a cough remedy in his healing practice. A very popular herb during the Roman Empire, the plant was extolled by the naturalist Pliny the Elder (A.D. 23–79), who enthusiastically proclaimed, "Whosoever shall take a spoonful of any of the mallows shall that day be freed from all diseases" (Culpeper, 1992). The Greek botanist and physician Dioscorides (*c.* A.D. 40–*c.* 90) recorded that he used poultices of the mashed root to treat insect bites and stings, wounds, bruises, and inflammation. He prescribed the tea for vomiting, dysentery, toothaches, and as a poison antidote.

During the Middle Ages and Renaissance, European folk herbalists used Marshmallow both internally and externally for treating sore throats, toothaches, and problems of the stomach, intestines, and urinary tract. It became a favorite of the 17th century English herbalist Nicholas Culpeper when his son recovered from severe bloody diarrhea after two days by drinking Marshmallow boiled in milk. Culpeper recommended the tea and poultice applications for hot, inflammatory conditions, fevers, tumors, burns, stomach and breast ailments, coughs, and lung diseases like tuberculosis. For the painful passage of kidney stones, Culpeper wrote that the decoction tea "opens the strait passages and making them slippery, whereby the stone may descend more easily, and without pain, out of the reins [pertaining to the kidneys and loins], kidneys and bladder, and to ease the torturing pains thereof" (Culpeper, 1992). The English apothecary and surgeon John Gerard (1545–1612) recorded his experiences with Marshmallow in his book, *The Herball or Generall Historie of Plantes*. He prepared the roots in ointments for wounds and in teas for their soothing, healing actions on the kidneys and bladder, and for pain, kidney stones, intestinal cramps, and bloody diarrhea. The boiled roots and leaves were eaten for nutrition during times of famine.

Marshmallow was introduced to Arab physicians through trade routes and cultural exchanges during the 10th century, and its use eventually spread to India's Ayurvedic medical system. European immigrants brought seeds to the New World, where the herb escaped the confines of colonial gardens and naturalized. Native American Indian groups adopted Marshmallow into their herbal pharmacies, using it for colds, flu, coughs, sore throats, and wound healing. The roots were listed as an official medicine in the *U.S. Pharmacopoeia* during the mid-1800s. Eclectic physicians applied the herb as a poultice to wounds, burns, swellings, and inflammation. The root tea was prescribed for colds, diarrhea, gonorrhea, and respiratory, digestive, and urinary ailments. Eclectic physician John King, M.D., wrote in *American Family Physician*, "Marshmallow root is demulcent and diuretic. The infusion, either in hot or cold water, is valuable to all irritations of the mucous membranes, as hoarseness, catarrh [phlegm], inflammation of the lungs, stomach, or intestines, catarrh of the bladder, irritation of the kidneys, acute dysentery, and diarrhea; also in the retention of the urine, hemorrhage from the kidneys, inflammation of the bladder, some forms of gravel, and in nearly every affliction of the kidneys and bladder. It may be drunk freely" (King, 1864).

People often wonder about the relationship between the Marshmallow plant and marshmallow candy. The ancient Egyptians reportedly made a candy with Marshmallow roots and honey. Later, the French candied Marshmallow by peeling the outer bark off the roots, chopping the inner white pulp, and boiling it until it was soft. Sugar was added and the mix was rolled into sweet, spongy sticks. In the 1800s, European pharmacists and physicians cooked the juice of the roots with egg whites and sugar, and whipped this into a foamy meringue called "marshmallows" when it hardened. These soft, sweet confections were given to patients, especially children, to treat coughs and help them swallow bitter-tasting medicines. The marshmallow candy available today, made of sugar and binders, does not contain any Marshmallow plant.

Marshmallow currently remains a popular herbal remedy and is widely distributed within the commercial market. The plant grows rapidly and is easy to cultivate, making it a renewable medicinal resource.

Healing Qualities

Alterative, anti-catarrhal, anti-inflammatory, antilithic, antispasmodic, demulcent, mild diuretic, emollient, expectorant, febrifuge, galactagogue, laxative, mucilaginous, opthalmicum, nutritional and moisturizing tonic, and vulnerary.

Traditional Chinese Medicine (TCM) Perspective

Marshmallow is a nutritious and moisturizing Yin tonic. It cools and neutralizes excess heat in the blood and tissues, and helps resolve fire conditions. The cooling mucilage moistens dry tissues, clears inflammation, reduces skin itchiness and irritation, and is soothing, softening, and lubricating to all tissues it contacts. Specific for Yin and fluid deficiencies, it nourishes and restores Stomach, Kidney, and Lung Yin. It subdues Stomach Fire and heartburn, and clears damp or dry heat from the lungs and the digestive and urinary systems.

Primary Actions

The mucilage in Marshmallow is the most important medicinal constituent, providing nutritional, cooling, moisturizing, and anti-inflammatory actions to heal tissues throughout the body. The root can be taken alone as a tea or added to formulas for its beneficial mucilage. Marshmallow roots have similar medicinal properties as Slippery Elm bark (*Ulmus rubra*) and can be used in place of this increasingly scarce and endangered medicinal tree. The profoundly mild and gentle nature of Marshmallow makes it a valuable herb for all age groups, even infants and the very weak or elderly. I have recommended the tea to many people for respiratory problems involving dry lungs, for urinary tract infections with painful urination, and for nausea, acid reflux, gastrointestinal ulcers, ulcerative colitis, Crohn's disease, and other inflammatory conditions. I often use and recommend the roots of this wonderful healing plant for many different health issues with consistently beneficial results. The roots and leaves are valuable ingredients in the herbal salve I produce for a wide range of external problems.

Mucous Membranes and Hot, Feverish, Inflammatory Conditions: **Mucous membranes** are specialized tissues in the epithelium lining most body cavities and some internal organs, including the nasal sinuses, mouth, throat, stomach, intestines, lungs, kidneys, and bladder. Mucous membranes contain specialized cells that secrete mucous, a thick fluid that protects and moistens surrounding tissues. **Plant mucilage** has a direct affinity with the mucous membranes in the human body, and tea made from Marshmallow roots is widely used to treat irritated membranes and promote tissue regeneration. The herb's mucilaginous polysaccharides adhere to skin and membranes, forming a protective coating that cools, moisturizes, and heals dry, hot, injured, and inflamed tissues. *In vitro* studies show that Marshmallow root tea stimulates proliferation of human epithelial cells and supports their viability (Deters, 2010).

Tea prepared from the roots is effective for treating coughs, fevers, dehydration, and hot, inflammatory conditions like hives and other rashes, sore muscles and joints, arthritis, and gout.

Several years ago, one of my cats became very sick and disappeared for three days. I found him lying in the garden, burning up with a high fever and refusing to eat or drink water. I was faced with a three-hour wait before the veterinarian could be seen, and I doubted my cat would survive that long. I decided to make a tea of Goldenseal root (*Hydrastis canadensis*) to kill the infection and Marshmallow root for hydration and to bring down the fever. I gave my cat a few tablespoons of the tea through a plastic dropper, one squirt at a time, and within an hour his temperature was almost normal. I was amazed at the fast action of the Goldenseal and Marshmallow, and very grateful that my kitty survived.

Immune-Enhancing Effects: Studies show that mucopolysacharrides in the mucilage have mild immune-enhancing effects that stimulate phagocytosis, which is the ability of specialized white blood cells to seek out, engulf, and destroy infectious organisms. Animal studies reveal that the mucilage exerts antibacterial activity against *Pseudomonas aeruginosa* (causing pneumonia and skin, urinary, and gastro-intestinal infections), *Proteus vulgaris* (responsible for cystitis), and *Staphylococcus aureus* (causing skin and upper respiratory tract infections) (Recio, 1989). Since it is a mild herb, always combine Marshmallow with stronger antibacterial botanicals when fighting infections.

Respiratory System: Marshmallow root is especially beneficial for the lungs which require moisture to function properly and can be damaged by excessive dryness. People who smoke tend to have chronically dry lungs and can get relief from a root tea of the moisturizing mucilage. The tea lubricates, soothes, and relaxes the bronchial passages and lung tissues. Anti-catarrhal properties reduce and eliminate excess mucous. As a moisturizing expectorant, the herb is helpful for dry coughs, inflamed and injured tissues, sore throats, hoarseness, laryngitis, and more serious problems like bronchitis, pneumonia, whooping cough, asthma, and emphysema. It reduces bleeding in the lungs when combined with astringent herbs like Cranesbill (*Geranium maculatum*), Cinquefoil (*Potentilla* spp.), Sage (*Salvia officinalis*), and Yarrow (*Achillea millefolium*). For lung problems involving infection, combine Marshmallow root with other pectoral herbs such as Elderberry (*Sambucus canadensis*), Elecampane (*Inula helenium*), Horehound (*Marrubium vulgare*), Isatis (*Isatis tinctoria*), and Pleurisy Root (*Asclepias tuberosa*). A strong brew of Marshmallow root tea makes an excellent base for cough syrups.

In a placebo-controlled study involving 63 patients who had developed dry coughs while taking drugs, those receiving Marshmallow root tea had significant reductions in coughing compared to the placebo group (Rouhi, 2007). Other clinical trials have shown that patients who take herbal cough medicines containing Marshmallow root experience less coughing and greater relief of their sore throats (Beuchi, 2005; Brinckmann, 2003).

Digestive System: The soothing mucilaginous, anti-inflammatory, antispasmodic, and laxative properties of Marshmallow tea and gruel benefit the stomach and intestines. The mucilage heals and protects the inner mucosal lining of the stomach and intestines, and neutralizes excess stomach acid that causes painful inflammation, heartburn, acid reflux, and gastric and intestinal ulcers. The tea is excellent for severe nausea and vomiting. When the stomach is so sensitive and irritated that it refuses all food and liquids, making dehydration a potential problem, Marshmallow tea is usually tolerated and is very nourishing and hydrating. The roots contain substantial amounts of easily digested minerals, especially calcium. The herb has a long history of use for treating cramps, gastrointestinal bleeding, and all types of inflammatory conditions such as gastritis (stomach inflammation), enteritis (intestinal inflammation), bloody dysentery (intestinal inflammation with pain and frequent stools), ulcerative colitis, irritable bowel syndrome, and Crohn's disease.

In one study, researchers gave rats tea prepared from Marshmallow flowers for one month. The tea significantly increased blood levels of protective HDL cholesterol, reduced stomach inflammation and ulceration, and inhibited abnormal blood clotting (Hage-Sleiman, 2011).

Marshmallow is also a mild laxative helpful for constipation when stools are dry and hard. Drinking 1-2 cups of the tea each day adds moisture to the colon to reduce chronic constipation. Pectin in the roots is a soluble fiber helping to keep bowels regular. The roots are soothing and healing to hemorrhoids when taken internally as tea and externally applied as a poultice or salve. The herb also reduces and soothes gallbladder inflammation and spasms.

Pectin fiber in Marshmallow root helps maintain normal blood sugar levels. The mucilage has been shown to have considerable hypoglycemic activity in non-diabetic mice (Tomoda, 1987).

Urinary System: The cooling mucilaginous, anti-inflammatory, antispasmodic, and diuretic properties of the roots benefit the entire urinary tract. The mucilage coats and lubricates to heal tissues and relax spasms in the kidneys, ureters, bladder, and urethra. It is an effective addition to formulas for all types of urinary problems, including cystitis (bladder infection), urethritis (inflammation and infection of the urethra), kidney infection, painful urination, and urine that is hot and bloody. As it moisturizes tissues, the herb's soothing action on the kidneys is mildly diuretic and reduces edema.

Marshmallow's antilithic properties help prevent kidney stone formation. The slippery, gelatinous consistency of the tea makes it easier for existing stones to pass out of the body. The mucilage heals injured tissues and relieves inflammation and painful spasms as sharp stones travel through narrow passages of the urinary tract. The herb also promotes urination to help move stones through the system. When treating kidney stones, a quart of tea should be ingested throughout the day for several weeks. Marshmallow works best when combined with White Oak bark (*Quercus alba*) and Lobelia (*Lobelia inflata*) tincture, which also relaxes and decreases spasms in the ureters to allow easier passage of stones.

Women's Health: The soothing tea reduces pain and inflammation in uterine, vaginal and genital tissues, and is helpful for the treatment of cervical dysplasia. It relieves burning, itchy genitals caused by vaginitis, Candida yeast, and other infections. For these purposes, combine Marshmallow with appropriate anti-microbial herbs to be ingested and prepared as a suppository or douche. A poultice of the root or leaves can be applied to inflamed, irritated genital tissues.

Marshmallow tea is safe for pregnant women to drink. It can be combined with Ginger (*Zingiber officinale*), Raspberry leaf (*Rubus idaeus*), or Peppermint (*Mentha x piperita*) tea to ease the nausea of morning sickness. The root tea or gruel is a nutritious and moisturizing galactagogue that enriches and increases the production of breast milk in nursing mothers. Marshmallow can also be applied as a warm poultice or fomentation to soothe and heal sore, cracked nipples and inflamed breasts. In cases of mastitis, hot poultices help to open clogged milk ducts, increase circulation to the breast, draw out infection, and reduce the pain of infection and engorgement.

Infants and Children: Marshmallow tea and poultices are safe for many infant and childhood problems. The tea and gruel are excellent for fevers, colic, nausea, constipation, coughs, and asthma. It can be applied externally for diaper rash, hives, and other eruptive skin problems.

External Problems: Marshmallow root makes an excellent poultice, fomentation, or salve for wounds, burns, bruises, insect bites and stings, aching and sprained muscles, tumors, ulcers, varicose veins, eczema and other types of dermatitis, and eruptive conditions such as hives, boils, acne, abscesses, mumps, measles, and chicken pox. It is cooling, soothing, and reduces inflammation when applied to the skin, and its drawing action pulls infection and toxins out of tissues.

The filtered tea is an excellent and safe eyewash to treat inflamed, dry, irritated eyes. For infections like conjunctivitis (pink eye), prepare eyewash by combining filtered Marshmallow and Goldenseal teas, and apply a few drops in both eyes 4-6 times throughout the day.

A small Amish study documented the ability of an herbal ointment containing Marshmallow root to heal first- and second-degree burns in five people. The Amish ointment, known as Burns and Wounds, also contained honey, lanolin, olive oil, wheat germ oil, Aloe Vera gel, Wormwood, Comfrey root, White Oak bark, Lobelia, and Myrrh. Applications of the ointment prevented infection, allowed dressing changes with minimal or no pain, and healed the burns in less than 14 days (Kolacz, 2014).

Master herbalist and naturopath Dr. John Christopher used Marshmallow tea fomentations to heal gangrene. He soaked the infected skin with the herbal tea for 30 minutes, then soaked it with cold water for 5 minutes, and alternated this throughout the day. Mortification root, one of the plant's common names, alludes to its ability to arrest decaying tissue.

Teachings from the Marshmallow Deva

"Welcome, dear one, to the soothing and cooling gifts of my plants. I am the deva of the Marshmallow tribe. My plants are purely of the water element, and like water contained by the earth in lakes and rivers, my healing energies are contained in the structure and form of the roots, leaves, and flowers. The gift of water that my plants offer supports all the waterways and fluids in the human body, as well as the health and function of the body's physical structure.

"Just as rainwater seeps through the earth, my medicine flows through the body, gently permeating through the tissues, dissolving places of restriction and blockage. Water nourishes and provides life, just as my medicine brings moisture and healing nutrients to dry, inflamed, and damaged tissues.

"My plants are greatly influenced by the Moon. The Moon affects the cyclic flow of life in women of childbearing age and controls great bodies of water, as seen in the ocean tides. Likewise, my plants hold and offer the healing energies of the Moon to purify and harmonize the water element in the physical body and in the subtle emotional field.

"The essence of my flowers helps soothe the 'wrinkles' and bumps and grinds of life, easing the emotional and mental energies in humans. Water carries electrical energy, and when the waterways in the body are flowing freely, nervous energy is calm and the whole system is more relaxed. Water slowly dissolves even the densest rocks, and so my gifts can certainly help to ease the hardness of the heart and emotions when in turmoil and pain. The white color of my flowers points to their assistance in purification, while the deep-purple center reflects the results of purification – the harmonious balance of the physical, emotional, mental, and soul or spiritual energies. Ingesting the essence of my flowers offers this assistance.

"Be still. Close your eyes. Relax. Envision my white flower with its purple center. Imagine a flower in your heart and one in the middle of your head. Breathe white and purple light into the flowers. Feel the vibrant brightness and life force of my healing flowers flow into and saturate your heart and mind. Let each breath bathe you in my healing energies. If you practice this vision and breathing for a few minutes several times each day, you will feel a difference and lightness in your body, your feelings, and your thoughts. Eventually, the deep inner peace and stability this creates spills into your life to enrich and bring joy to you and the world around you. Be fluid in the flow of life, dear one, and pure in thought and deeds."

Motherwort

Leonurus cardiaca
Labiatae (*Lamiaceae*) (Mint) Family

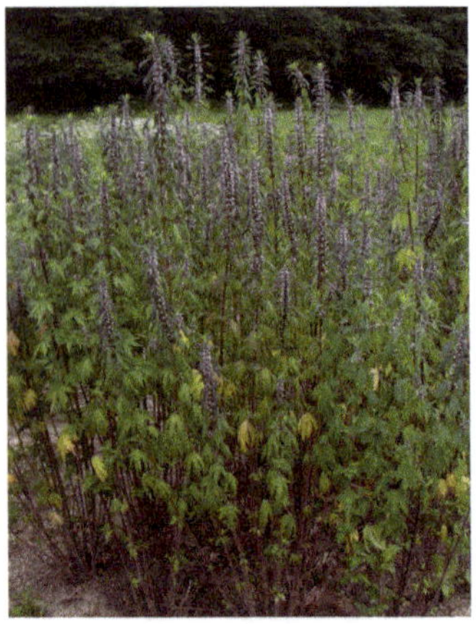

Common Names

Lion's ear, lion's tail, throwwort, mother herb, mother weed, heartwort, heart gold, and heart herb are antiquated names, several referring to Motherwort's traditional use for women's health and heart ailments.

Medicinal Part of the Plant

The flowering tops and leaves are used medicinally.

Range and Habitat

Several species of Motherwort are native to temperate zones throughout Europe and Asia. *Leonurus cardiaca* was introduced from Eurasia for cultivation in Canada and the United States, where it escaped from gardens to flourish as a common weed in some areas. Siberian Motherwort (*Leonurus sibericus*), a variety that has naturalized in parts of the Pacific Northwest, grows so abundantly in my southern Indiana gardens that I imagine it could adapt easily almost anywhere. *L. artemisia, L. japonicus,* and *L. heterophyllus* are other medicinal varieties of Motherwort indigenous to Asia. These and other *Leonurus* species contain similar medicinal constituents, and are used interchangeably for healing purposes.

Description of the Plant

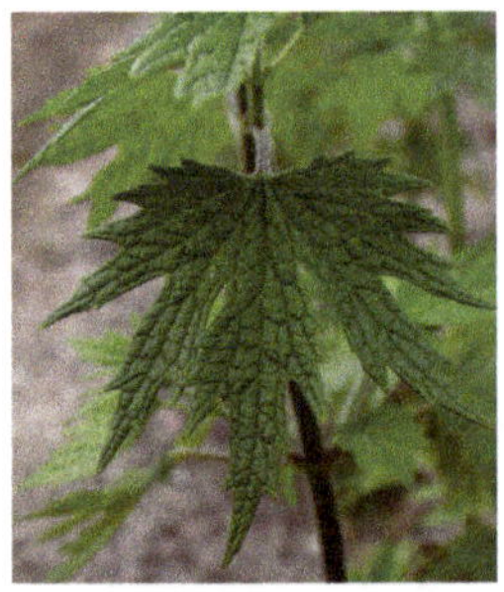

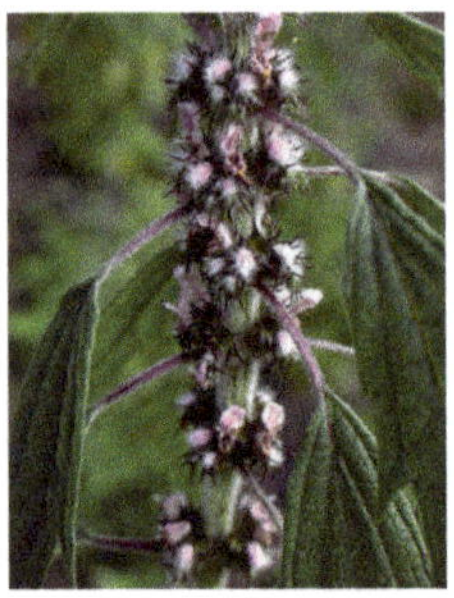

L. cardiaca is a perennial herb growing 4-6′ in height, but can grow taller in ideal conditions. The fibrous root sends up several erect, stout, distinctly square, greenish-maroon stems that are strong and fibrous. They are hollow inside, and the outside is smooth or covered with fine, white hairs. The main stem has many branches, giving older, larger plants a bushy appearance. The dark-green leaves, growing 3-4″ in length, are arranged oppositely along the stems. Leaves have palmate venation and palmate lobes that are pointed at the tips. Uppermost leaves are narrow and lance-shaped with 2 large lobes, while lower leaves are larger, more ovate, and develop more palmate lobes. The largest leaves at the stem base are more deeply incised with up to 7 lobes. All leaves have long petioles (stems) and are covered with fine, white hairs.

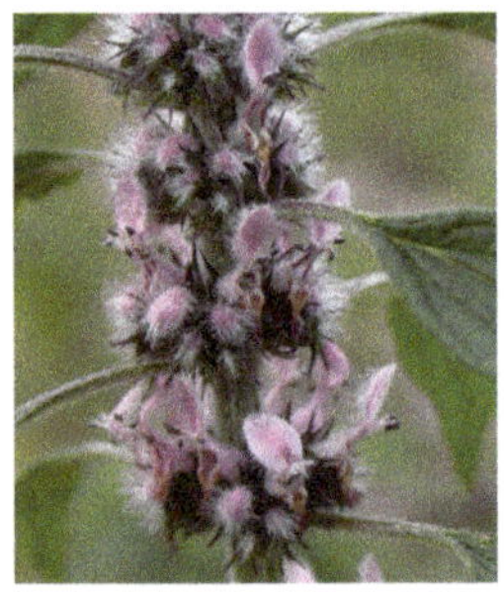

The white and pink flowers appear in numerous tight whorls around the upper stems just above the leaf axils, creating a spike-like appearance. There are typically 6-15 irregularly shaped flowers in each whorl. Each tiny, sessile flower has a short, tubular, bell-shaped calyx with 5 stiff, bristly teeth. The flower corolla has a larger, slightly arched upper lip, while the elongated, spotted lower lip has 3 lobes. Flowers bloom from late May through September with the lower whorls blooming first and progressing up the stalk. The dried calyx transforms into a very spiny, prickly seedpod after the flower has died. The dark-brown seeds are very small nutlets.

Cultivation

Motherwort grows well in sunny or shaded areas, although sun is preferable. Fertile, well-drained soil encourages large bushy growth, but the plant also does well in fairly poor soil. This herb is easy to propagate by sowing the extremely prolific seeds. These may be harvested from live plants or purchased. Plant the seeds in trays in early spring, barely covering them with soil. Keep the soil moist and germination usually occurs within 2-3 weeks. Transplant seedlings into a permanent garden space when they are 3-4″ tall, and space them 1′ apart. Plant Motherwort in an area where it is free to spread, because it self-sows each year and can easily take over a garden.

Harvest

Collect leaves and flowers during the early stages of blooming to obtain the highest potency of medicinal components. Prune no more than 25% of the foliage, and be sure to leave some flowers so they mature into seeds. Collect seeds when the prickly seedpods are dry and brown. To separate seeds from the pods, place them in a paper bag and gently smash the bag between your hands. Gather the open end of the bag so it may be held upside down, allowing the seeds to fall out while the seedpods remain in the bag.

Preparation of Plant Medicine and Dosages

Separate leaves and flowers from the stem to use fresh, or dry them for future needs. The fresh herb can be made into tea, tincture, or handmade pills. Tincturing the freshly harvested herb is the preferred method to extract and preserve medicinal constituents, because dried leaves and flowers quickly deteriorate and lose potency.

PREPARATIONS

Infusion: Steep 1-2 teaspoons of finely chopped leaves and flowers in 1 cup of boiled water for 10-15 minutes. Dosage: ½-1 cup of tea 1-4 times a day as needed. The tea is very bitter.

Tincture: Chop the fresh herb, pack it into a glass jar, and cover it with 70% 190-proof grain alcohol and 30% distilled water. Dosage: 30-60 drops 1-4 times daily with water as needed. Most people prefer Motherwort tincture because it is easier to take a mouthful of bitter tincture in a little water than to drink a whole cup of bitter tea.

Pills: These may be purchased or handmade from the dried and ground herb. Dosage: 2-3 pills 1-3 times a day as needed.

Suppositories: Prepare suppositories with dried, ground leaves for vaginal infections. Dosage: Insert a suppository high into the vagina before bedtime.

Chemical Constituents

Several medicinal *Leonurus* species contain identical phytochemicals that elicit similar biological activities in people and animals. Bitter alkaloids are thought to be largely responsible for the herb's actions. Leonurine, a primary alkaloid, is neuroprotective, calming to the central nervous system, hypotensive, anti-inflammatory, antioxidant, anticoagulant, diuretic, and uterotonic (Bradley, 1992; Newall, 1996; Song, 2015). Leonurine mainly influences the nervous, cardiovascular, and female reproductive systems. Stachydrine, a pyrrolidine-type alkaloid, relaxes the nervous system and is a cardiotonic that lowers blood pressure by relaxing blood vessels. Stachydrine is an emmenagogue (promotes menstruation) and lactagogue (increases breast milk), and may stimulate the release of oxytocin, a hormone involved in lactation and childbirth. Leonurinine, betonicine, turicin, and leonuridin are other alkaloids. The bitter glycosides leonurin and leonuridine have a beneficial calming effect on the heart.

Terpenoids include volatile oil (0.05%), resins, leocardin, and ursolic acid (anticancer, antioxidant, antitumor, antiviral, cardiotonic, cytotoxic, diuretic, antihistamine). Ursolic acid is a central nervous system depressant and it inhibits the Epstein-Barr virus (Kuo-Hsiung, 1988; Tokuda, 1986; Yanxing, 1983). Flavonoids are antioxidant and include apigenin, kaempferol, rutin, hyperoside, genkwanin (antibacterial), and isoquercetin (improves capillary strength, antibacterial, anticancer, antitumor, diaphoretic, diuretic, hypotensive). Acids include caffeic, citric, malic, oleic, linoleic, linolenic, and oleanolic acid (anti-atherosclerotic, antibacterial, anticancer, anti-inflammatory, antioxidant, antispasmodic, antiviral, diuretic, hepatoprotective, immunomodulator, sedative, and uterine tonic).

Alpha-humulene is antitumor. Caryophyllene and alpha- and beta-pinene are antibacterial, antiflu, anti-inflammatory, antispasmodic, antiviral, anticancer, antitumor, diuretic, and sedating. Catechin prevents abnormal blood clotting and is antibacterial, anticancer, antihistamine, anti-inflammatory, antioxidant, antiviral, diuretic, and hepatoprotective. Hyperoside improves capillary strength and is antibacterial, anticancer, antiflu, anti-inflammatory, antioxidant, antiviral, diuretic, and hypotensive. Limonene is antibacterial, anticancer, antiviral, antispasmodic, expectorant, and sedative. Marrubin is anti-arrhythmic, cardiotonic, choleretic, and expectorant.

Safety, Contraindications, and Drug Interactions

Motherwort is a safe, non-toxic herb when taken in normal dosages. The German Commission E herbal regulatory agency affirmed that it has no known contraindications, side effects, or interactions with other drugs. Although herbalists once recommended Motherwort during pregnancy as a soothing uterine tonic and to reduce anxiety, it is currently **contraindicated during pregnancy** due to its stimulating emmenagogue action on the uterus that promotes menstruation and may possibly cause miscarriage (Brinker, 2001; McGuffin, 1997). There are no restrictions for use during lactation (Blumenthal, 1998). The herb is not recommended in cases of heavy uterine bleeding because its stimulating effect on pelvic circulation can worsen the problem.

Relaxing to the nervous system and heart, Motherwort may increase the effects of pharmaceutical drugs taken for related conditions. The sedating effect reduces symptoms of a hyperactive thyroid gland, including heart palpitations and anxiety. Hypothetical warnings declare that people with an underactive thyroid should not take Motherwort on a regular basis, but there is no clinical evidence that the herb weakens the thyroid. Skin contact with the fresh plant may cause temporary dermatitis in sensitive people, but this is quickly remedied by washing the affected area with rubbing alcohol.

Medicinal Uses

History of the Plant

The genus name *Leonurus* is derived from the Greek words *leon*, meaning "lion," and *ouros*, "tail," because the flowering spikes were thought to resemble a lion's tail. The species name *cardiaca* comes from the Greek word for "heart," reflecting the herb's historic use for heart and circulatory problems. "Wort" is an old Anglo-Saxon term meaning "healing herb," and the common name "Motherwort" means "healing herb for the mother," indicating its value and reputation as a woman's ally.

European Motherwort and its Asian relatives have been employed for similar conditions in a long tradition of folk medicine throughout Europe, Asia, and the Americas. The ancient Greeks and Romans used the herb for depression, women's health, and as a heart tonic. They gave Motherwort to calm pregnant women experiencing anxiety. Since ancient times in China, Motherwort species have been considered superior medicines. Seeds were gathered for food and taken as a tonic to improve vision, physical strength and endurance, and to lift a depressed spirit. The leafy shoots were added to baths for relieving the discomfort and itching of skin diseases and shingles (Hu, 1976). Motherwort was used to promote menstruation, and was taken daily by courtesans to protect against pregnancy and venereal diseases. The Chinese also ingested it to enhance longevity due to its excellent abilities of strengthening the heart, improving blood flow, and reducing water retention. In Russia, *L. cardiaca* was highly endorsed as a rabies treatment.

During the Middle Ages, Europeans believed that Motherwort protected them against evil and malicious spirits. John Gerard (1545–1612) recommended the herb to treat coughs, irregular heartbeat, heart weakness and infirmities, delayed menstruation, cramps, intestinal worms, and convulsions. Nicholas Culpeper (1616–1654) continued the tradition of using Motherwort for these problems. He gave the herb to women as a uterine tonic and to ease childbirth. He wrote that "Venus owns the herb, and it is under Leo. There is no better herb to take melancholy vapours from the heart, to strengthen it, and make it a merry, cheerful, blithe soul, than this herb. Besides, it makes women joyful mothers of children, and settles their wombs as they should be, therefore we call it motherwort. It is held to be in much use for the tremblings of the heart, and faintings and swoonings; from whence it took the name cardiaca. It also provoketh urine and women's courses [menstruation], cleanseth the chest of cold phlegm oppressing it, and killeth worms in the belly. It is of good use to warm and dry up the cold humours, to digest and disperse those that are settled in the veins, joints, and sinews of the body, and to help cramps and convulsions" (Culpeper, 1992).

European colonists introduced *L. cardiaca* into North America and many Native Americans adopted it into their herbal pharmacopoeia. The Algonquin Indian groups ingested it for female reproductive and gynecological problems, as did other eastern tribes like the Delaware, Iroquois, Micmac, and Mohegan (Moerman, 1998). The Cherokees used it as a sedative and for stomach problems. Learning from the wisdom of Native Americans and Europeans, the 19th century American Eclectic physicians recommended Motherwort tea and alcohol extracts to treat liver and gastrointestinal distress, heart problems, high blood pressure, typhoid fever, arthritis, hyperthyroidism, goiter (enlarged thyroid gland), and many issues of women's reproductive health. It was highly regarded for most conditions caused by or associated with nervous tension and excitability, including spasms, insomnia, epilepsy, and delirium tremens, which are tremors and hallucinations caused by excessive alcohol intake and withdrawal. The Eclectics often combined Motherwort with Black Cohosh (*Cimicifuga racemosa*) and Blue Cohosh (*Caulophyllum thalictroides*) for use as a nervine, antispasmodic, and emmenagogue.

The chemistry of Motherwort and its ability to relax the nervous system, calm the heart, reduce high blood pressure, and stimulate the uterus has been well documented by modern scientists using *in vitro* (test tube) and *in vivo* (animal) research. Currently, it remains a popular herb and is commercially available as tea, pills, capsules, and liquid extracts.

Healing Qualities

Antibacterial, anticarcinogenic, anti-catarrhal, anti-inflammatory, antioxidant, antispasmodic, bitter, cardiac tonic, carminative, diaphoretic, diuretic, emmenagogue, galactagogue, hepatic, hypotensive, laxative, nephritic, nervine, restorative, sedative, stimulating to circulation and the uterus, stomachic, vasodilator, and tonic for the nerves, heart, and uterus.

Traditional Chinese Medicine (TCM) Perspective

Motherwort species are bitter, slightly cooling, and drying. The herb relaxes nerves and muscles, and tones and restores the nervous, cardiovascular, and female reproductive systems. It is a Yang herb that stimulates movement of Qi throughout the body. In the uterus, the herb breaks up energetic stagnation and blood stasis (congested lack of flow) manifesting as stalled, painful, and difficult menstruation or childbirth, irregular cycles, and infertility. Motherwort reduces damp phlegm and moves Qi through the lungs and nasal sinuses to break up mucous congestion and improve breathing. By stimulating blood circulation and Heart Qi, *Leonurus* can improve many conditions of blood stasis or stagnation in the blood vessels and heart. In TCM, it is prescribed for rapid heart rate, palpitations, heart disease, hypertension, and problems caused by insufficient circulation. It is also used for traumatic injuries resulting in swelling, pain and bruising, which are conditions of blood stasis. The herb relieves Qi stagnation in the kidneys and is beneficial for treating water retention, urinary tract infections, and toxic build-up in the blood resulting in skin rashes, eczema, abscesses, and skin ulcers.

Primary Actions

Motherwort transforms us at our core through its affinity with the nervous system, heart, and womb. By exerting a generalized relaxing action, it directly calms and normalizes the heart and is helpful for many health problems arising from nervous agitation. Specific for anxious, overstimulated people, this herbal ally addresses the hyperactive symptoms of an overactive thyroid gland. When considering the Doctrine of Signatures, the plant's pink flowers reflect its beneficial affinity with the heart and blood, and the hollow stems resemble blood vessels. Motherwort, as the name implies, is a specific herb for women that promotes reproductive health and calms the emotional ups and downs of changing hormonal cycles. Interestingly, physical changes in the plants reflect changes in women as both mature and age. The young plants have lovely, soft flowers like the gentle, sweet nature typical of many young women. But as the flowers grow old their seedpods become sharp and prickly, just as older women can develop a bold, powerful sharpness that comes in handy at times.

I have used Motherwort for many years with good results in various formulas for anxiety, colds and flu, women's health issues, hyperthyroidism, and to calm and normalize a racing, overstimulated heart.

Nervous System: Motherwort is an excellent sedative herb that has a calming influence throughout the nervous and cardiovascular systems. As a nervine, it can be used as a tonic for several weeks to restore tranquil, normal nerve function. It relaxes tense, rigid muscles and relieves spasms, and was once used in treating epilepsy. Eclectic physician William Cook, M.D., wrote about his clinical experience with Motherwort, stating, "This herb is a pleasant and moderately strong tonic, somewhat diffuse in action, and combining relaxing properties with a slight excess of stimulation. The nerves receive the most benefit of its stimulation, whence it is classified as a nervine tonic and antispasmodic . . . . As a tonic for nervousness, pains and palpitations of the heart, the sufferings peculiar to women, and habitual restlessness, it is an agent deserving of the first consideration" (Cook, 1869).

Motherwort is a strong neuroprotective that supports the mitochondria (energy-producing sites) in all cells, especially in the brain and heart. The herb reduces oxidative stress and damage to mitochondria, and all cells in general. It helps prevent cellular damage caused by blood and oxygen deprivation, and reduces mitochondrial swelling and restores normal function of mitochondrial membranes (Buhner, 2013).

Motherwort is helpful for all nervous conditions, including irritability, anxiety, panic attacks, headaches, dizziness, fainting, insomnia, tremors and nervous tics, neuralgia (nerve pain), and neuritis (nerve inflammation). It relieves muscle spasms throughout the body, including the stomach, intestines, and uterus. The tea or tincture eases nervous hyperactivity, calms and restores the nervous system, and eases delirium tremens during drug and alcohol withdrawal. Research studies have demonstrated its sedating and hypotensive effects (Bradley, 1992). When treating the nervous system, Motherwort works well combined with other nervine and sedative herbs such as Scullcap (*Scutellaria lateriflora*), Valerian (*Valeriana officinalis*), Black Cohosh (*Cimicifuga racemosa*), and Hops (*Humulus lupulus*).

The Heart and Vascular System: Many herbalists consider Motherwort to be one of the best cardiac tonics, as reflected in the species name *cardiaca*. It has a long tradition of treating many cardiovascular conditions associated with nervous overstimulation, anxiety, and emotional stress. The herb's sedative, nervine, and antispasmodic properties have a calming, restoring action on muscles of the heart and blood vessels, which reduces tachycardia (rapid heartbeat), palpitations, and arrhythmias (irregular rhythm) not caused by underlying heart disease. The muscle tone of blood vessels relaxes under the influence of Motherwort, making it beneficial for restricted circulation, vascular blockages, and mild to moderate hypertension. Diuretic properties also contribute to reducing hypertension.

Motherwort may be taken as a preventative against heart attacks and should be combined with a healthy diet and lifestyle. German medical herbalist Rudolf Weiss, M.D., wrote, "My own investigations have found that there is indeed a medicinal action, mainly for functional heart complaints due to autonomic imbalance. It appears to be predominantly sedative, similar to valerian. It is necessary, however, to take the drug for a long period, over months" (Weiss, 1988).

Current research validates Motherwort's ability to improve metabolic function of the heart, normalize heart rate, and increase blood flow to the extremities. Alcohol extracts of Motherwort have been shown to relax cardiac muscle and inhibit stimulating input (Newall, 1996). Glycosides and alkaloids in the plant are known to depress the central nervous system, normalize cardiac activity, and lower blood pressure (Bradley, 1992). *L. cardiaca* is a potent antioxidant that protects cells from damage by scavenging and destroying dangerous free radicals (Matkowski, 2006). Leonurine, one of the alkaloids, relaxes and dilates blood vessels (Chen, 2001). *L. cardiaca* and *L. heterophyllus* also improve coronary and capillary circulation by inhibiting blood platelet aggregation (clumping together) causing vascular congestion and blood clots (Chang, 1986; Xia, 1983). In a Chinese clinical study, 105 patients diagnosed with circulation problems were given 10 mL of *L. heterophyllus* extract intravenously on a daily basis. After 15 days of treatment, 94.5% showed improved circulation marked by lower blood viscosity and fibrinogen volume (resulting in thinner blood) and a decrease in blood platelet aggregation (resulting in diminished blood clotting) (Zou, 1989; Lee, 1991).

Motherwort's cardioprotective property was evaluated by its effects on mitochondria (energy production sites) in the cells of cardiac muscle. Researchers found that antioxidant substances in Motherwort (chlorogenic acid, orientin, quercetin, hyperoside, and rutin) effectively protected mitochondria against oxidative damage and reduced the production of destructive free radicals (Bernatoniene, 2014).

A 28-day clinical study was conducted to determine the efficacy of *L. cardiaca* oil extract (1,200 mg taken daily) on 50 patients with anxiety, insomnia, and either stage 1 hypertension (blood pressure of 140/90–159/99) or stage 2 hypertension (blood pressure 160/100–175/109). Patients with stage 1 hypertension improved significantly after 14 days of treatment, and after 28 days anxiety was reduced by 61%, emotional lability by 53%, headaches by 41%, and sleep disorders by 47%. Systolic and diastolic blood pressure improved after 21 days of treatment from an average of 144/96 to 130/87. Heart rate decreased slightly. In contrast, those with stage 2 hypertension did not experience as much improvement. Blood pressure decreased from 153/102 to 141/92 after 28 days of treatment, but did not normalize. By day 21 of treatment, anxiety was reduced by 62%, emotional lability by 20%, headaches by 34%, and sleep disorders by 42% (Shikov, 2011).

British medical herbalists combine Motherwort with equal parts Valerian and Wood Betony (*Stachys officinalis*) as a remedy for arteriosclerosis (hardening of the arteries). For hypertension, it can be taken with equal parts Valerian, Black Cohosh, and Scullcap (Yemm, 1935). Other heart tonic herbs that combine well with Motherwort include Hawthorn berries (*Crataegus* spp.), Peppermint (*Mentha x piperita*), and Lemon Balm (*Melissa officinalis*). Motherwort is most effective for the nerves and heart when taken as a tonic over time. The German Commission E herbal regulatory agency approved use of Motherwort for nervous cardiac disorders and thyroid hyperfunction (Blumenthal, 1998).

Hyperthyroidism: The thyroid is an endocrine gland that produces hormones (T4 which converts to usable T3) controlling the body's use of energy. Hypothyroidism, or low thyroid function, causes slow metabolism resulting in sluggish digestion, constipation, fatigue, depression, mental fog, weight gain, dry skin, and other problems. The opposite occurs with hyperthyroidism or overstimulation. Excessive thyroid hormones cause hyperactivity, nervous tension, heart palpitations, tachycardia (rapid heartbeat), hypertension, excessive sweating, insomnia, and weight loss. Motherwort inhibits the conversion of T4 into T3, making it a valuable herb for treating hyperthyroidism. Motherwort's action is similar to Lemon Balm's abilities to calm nervous tension, and both herbs have an affinity with the heart and thyroid. Bugleweed (*Lycopus virginicus*) is another herb for hyperthyroidism, and both are traditionally combined with Motherwort. Contrary to some warnings, Motherwort does not depress normal thyroid function.

Rudolf Weiss, M.D., wrote about his experience using small quantities of a German preparation called Thyreogutt (manufactured by Schwabe), which is an alcohol extract of Motherwort and Bugleweed. "Patients need to be told that an effect will not be noticeable until at least one or two weeks have passed, and that it will become appreciable only after three or four weeks. It consists in an improvement in subjective symptoms, particularly the palpitations" (Weiss, 1988).

A tincture of Motherwort, Lemon Balm, Bugleweed, and Astragalus (*Astragalus membranaceus*) has been safe and extremely helpful for several of my clients with hyperthyroidism. They started using 20 drops of the tincture combination 3 times a day, and gradually increased to 50 drops taken 3 times daily. All clients reported feeling much calmer with significant reductions in heart palpitations and arrhythmia, fewer feelings of panic, and improved energy and sleep.

Women's Health: Motherwort is appropriately named as a valuable herb for women and mothers. It tones and strengthens the uterus, reduces uterine inflammation and cramps, and has traditionally been used for many aspects of women's reproductive health. Its beneficial influence on circulation increases blood flow to the pelvis and reproductive organs, helping regulate normal menstrual flow. Leonurine and stachydrine are alkaloids in the herb that exhibit uterotonic effects and seem to stimulate the release of oxytocin, a hormone that initiates uterine contractions and the flow of breast milk (Newall, 1996). Research studies have demonstrated that Siberian Motherwort (*L. sibericus*) stimulates specific receptors (H1 and alpha-adrenergic receptors) in uterine tissue responsible for the beneficial uterine effects (Shi, 1995; Kong, 1976).

Menstruation: Motherwort's ability to promote circulation and relax the nerves makes it an effective emmenagogue to initiate delayed menstruation. It helps regulate the menstrual cycle and is excellent for amenorrhea (lack of menses), suppressed menses, or scanty blood flow. The herb relaxes uterine muscles and spasms, and can relieve dysmenorrhea (painful, cramping periods). It may help shrink uterine fibroids, but it is not recommended for bleeding fibroids or excessive menstrual bleeding because it increases blood circulation and may exacerbate the bleeding.

Over the years, I have frequently observed Motherwort's excellence as a remedy and calming agent for cramps, anxiety, and raging emotions that some women experience with premenstrual syndrome (PMS). Its diuretic action relieves premenstrual water retention and tender, engorged breasts. It may be taken as tea or tincture, and many women report relief from cramps within a short period of time. Chinese women often combine Motherwort with Dong Quai (*Angelica sinensis*) to regulate menstrual cycles and relieve PMS. Eclectic physicians often combined *L. cardiaca* with Black Cohosh to treat stalled menses and uterine pain.

Infertility: Motherwort has historically been used to promote fertility when taken as a tonic over a period of several weeks or months. In Traditional Chinese medicine, it is a widely prescribed treatment for infertility caused by blood stasis and tumors or cysts that are hard and immovable (Tierra, 1998). It is most effective when combined with other fertility herbs such as Chasteberry (*Vitex agnus-castus*), Wild Yam (*Dioscorea* spp.), and Dong Quai.

Childbirth: **Motherwort is contraindicated during pregnancy** because the oxytocic activity of its alkaloids stimulates uterine contractions that could cause miscarriage. However, it is a valuable ally for laboring mothers when taken during childbirth because it stimulates the release of oxytocin, the hormone that promotes strong and productive contractions to facilitate the birthing process. Motherwort relaxes the mother and eases labor pains, especially combined with St. John's Wort (*Hypericum perforatum*), when 10 drops of each tincture are taken every 20-30 minutes. In Chinese hospitals, large doses of Motherwort tea are often given to mothers after childbirth to contract the uterus, expel the placenta, diminish bleeding, and minimize intense "after-birth" pains of uterine contractions. It has also been taken for post-partum depression. Eclectic physicians gave Motherwort as an aid to expel the placenta after childbirth. Finley Ellingwood, M.D., considered it to be specific for "suppressed lochia [vaginal discharge following childbirth] from any cause, amenorrhea from cold, dysmenorrhea with nervous excitability, and hysteria. Prof. John King regarded motherwort as superior to all other remedies in suppression of the lochia" (Ellingwood, 1919).

Vaginal Infections: Astringent, antifungal, and antibacterial properties make Motherwort a helpful douche or suppository for bacterial vaginal infections, and it is especially beneficial for yeast infections. The herb is taken orally and prepared as a strong tea for douching until all signs of infection are resolved.

Menopause: Motherwort is a relaxing tonic during the hormonal fluctuations of menopause. It is soothing and eases anxiety, depression, heart palpitations, night sweats, and insomnia that can occur with menopause. The herb reduces frequency and severity of hot flashes, especially when combined with Black Cohosh, Sage (*Salvia officinalis*), and Blue Vervain (*Verbena hastata*). Regular use of Motherwort (10-20 drops of tincture 3-4 times a day) with Chasteberry (40 drops every morning) helps restore normal thickness and moisture to vaginal tissues.

Digestive System: Specific for digestive problems arising from nervous anxiety, Motherwort has a relaxing influence on the solar plexus that promotes normal function and muscle tone throughout the gastrointestinal tract. The herb benefits the stomach, liver, and intestines. Like most bitters, it improves digestion by stimulating the release of digestive enzymes and bile to break down food and encourage normal intestinal movements. As a mild laxative, carminative and antispasmodic, Motherwort relieves stomach and intestinal gas, indigestion, cramps, and spasms.

Kidneys and Diuretic Actions: The herb's ability to improve blood circulation stimulates sluggish kidneys and promotes urine output. Motherwort can reduce fluid retention (edema) in the tissues. It helps reduce kidney inflammation and has been prescribed for nephritis by British medical herbalists and practitioners of Traditional Chinese medicine (TCM). In TCM, it is also prescribed for oliguria (scanty urine flow) and hematuria (bloody urine).

In mice studies, leonurine that was isolated from *L. cardiaca* protected mice from acute kidney injury by decreasing inflammatory cytokines and oxidative damage to the kidney cells (Xu, 2014).

Flu, Fever, and the Common Cold: Motherwort reduces excessive phlegm secretions and congestion in the lungs and nasal sinuses. It relaxes bronchial muscles to allow easier breathing, and Chinese varieties of Motherwort are traditionally prescribed for bronchitis and asthma in TCM. As a diaphoretic, it promotes sweating to reduce high fevers, and the leaves contain antibacterial and antifungal constituents beneficial for treating infections. I always add Motherwort tincture to remedies for colds and bacterial infections.

Cancer, Tumors, and the Epstein-Barr Virus: Chinese doctors prescribe Motherwort for treating uterine and breast cancers. Recent studies indicating anticarcinogenic activity in some of the herb's phytochemicals have sparked renewed interest in its role in cancer treatment. Ursolic acid has inhibited tumor production and the Epstein-Barr virus in mice and *in vitro* studies (Kuo-Hsiung, 1988; Tokuda, 1986). The Epstein-Barr virus has been implicated as a cause of mononucleosis and chronic fatigue syndrome. The whole plant has demonstrated cytotoxicity (ability to destroy cancer cells) in lymphocytic leukemia cells, human lung carcinoma, mammary tumors, and human colon tumors (Kuo-Hsiung, 1988; Nagasawa, 1992; Satoh, 2003). Chinese researchers have found phytochemicals in *L. heterophyllus* that promote immunity by stimulating the proliferation of white blood cells called T-cells (Xu, 1992).

Teachings from the Motherwort Deva

"Greetings, dear one. I am the Motherwort Deva of the heart. The pink color of my flowers is a signature pointing to my healing offerings for the heart and blood vessels. The sharpness of the prickers surrounding my seedpods alludes to the ability of my plants to resolve sharp, uncomfortable emotions and matters of the heart, so necessary for true healing. The sharp, piercing nature of my medicine also cuts through obstructions and congestion in the physical body, allowing smooth flow of nerve energy and blood.

"My plants are under the influence of the astrological sign Leo, the regulator of the heart that is ruled by the fire element and the sun. Fire provides warmth, stimulation, and movement in the body. My fiery nature supports the heart and digestive system; for both require the fire element to function. Fire provides unlimited energy and life force to keep the heart beating. Day after day, year after year, the heart must sustain the capacity for continual movements of expansion and contraction. Adequate fire is necessary to provide digestive enzymes that break down food, providing fuel and warmth to nourish the body's cells. Insufficient fire weakens digestive ability and reduces nutrients.

"My medicine helps balance the fire element in the human body, increasing fire when it is diminished and cooling the fire when it rages in the form of nervous overstimulation, anxiety, and a pounding heart. The medicine of my plants has a special affinity with the thyroid gland, the regulator of energy usage in the body. When overstimulated, like a raging fire out of control, this gland can create havoc in people, destroying peace and stability. My healing gifts subdue this fire, allowing rest and ease.

"My plants regulate the nervous system and the energy traveling along nerve fibers to communicate information from every cell in the body and from the external world through an elaborate and complex nerve network. In the center of this network is the heart, governing the realm of feelings and emotions. I strengthen the heart and offer courage. Use the medicine in my leaves and the essence of my flowers to heal the heart of bitterness, pain, and despair. For your world can be difficult to live in, especially now, when the beauty and continuity of life on the planet is threatened by mankind's destructive choices. The deep, underlying stress this destruction creates upon all life is also felt in the human heart, consciously or unconsciously, and is a cause of depression and anxiety so prevalent among people at this time. Use my medicine for the sharp bitterness of life, to help lighten and keep the flow of life moving, calmly and continuously.

"Motherwort plants are also under the influence and grace of Venus. I am a deva in service to mothers by supporting the wombs and hearts of mothers; for both are called upon to embrace children in unconditional love. The heart of the Great Mother radiates unlimited love to all, offering the greatest realization that all are our children requiring boundless love. Take the essence of my flowers to assist in the learning of this great lesson – to love in this way brings joy and fulfillment of purpose. And so, dear one, as you partake of my plants for medicine, please also practice this meditation I will teach to calm your emotions and assist in your healing:

"Sit in a quiet place. Close your eyes. Relax. Bring your attention to your body. Breathe into areas of discomfort and tension until you feel relaxation. Then pay attention to your feelings. Are you feeling calm and happy, or are you experiencing irritation, grief, and other disturbing feelings? Begin to breathe into your heart. With each breath, draw white light from the heavens through the crown of your head into your heart, and at the same time, draw the deep-red aura of the earth up through your feet into your heart. As the white and red lights merge, imagine them blending into the brilliant, pink color of my flowers and permeating your heart with soothing, healing light. Practice this every day so it becomes easy to create a natural flow of calm, nourishing energy into your heart.

"Know that emotions are energies-in-motion – that is to say, feelings are energies arising within people that move out toward the object of the emotion and into the surrounding environment. When centered in the heart-space of love and calm abiding, emotions reflect this peaceful state, as does the entire nervous system. The emotional energies of other people must also be assimilated, which is not difficult when emotions are peaceful, but challenging when there is discord of anger and selfishness. The heart is the great mediator and interpreter of the emotions, and my medicine assists in this task. By paying attention to the emotional energies in which your heart lives, you assist in maintaining good heart health. Know that when living in hate, anger, resentment, self-loathing and all other harmful emotions, the life force nourishing the cells and tissues of the heart is diminished, eventually resulting in loss of function and disease.

"Remember that the heart and emotions have direct effects on the mind and thoughts emerging from it. When the heart is calm, thinking and actions are more rational and humane. The heart is a 'brain' utilizing feelings, rather than thoughts, as a means of communication. Know that feelings have great influence and power over the body by creating chemical changes in the tissues. Take good care of your heart and maintain a dynamic calm by eating nourishing food, using my healing gifts, and cultivating peaceful emotions through daily meditation. Be at peace, dear one, and be happy!"

Mugwort

Artemisia vulgaris

Compositae (Asteraceae) (Sunflower or Aster) Family

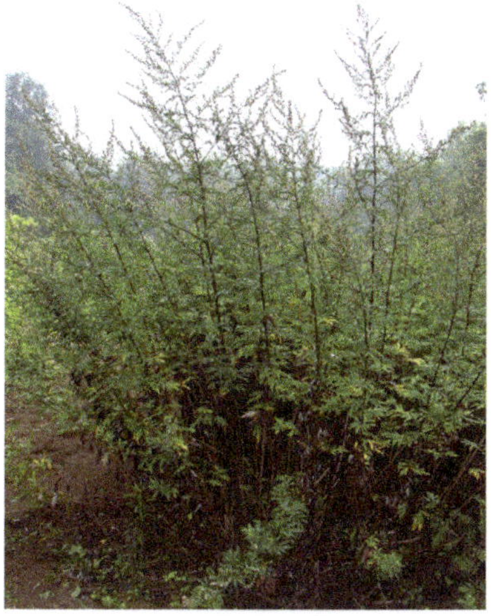

Mature
Artemisia vulgaris

Common Names

Felon herb, sailor's tobacco, St. John's plant, motherwort (not to be confused with *Leonurus cardiaca*), maidenwort, and womb's wort are antiquated names for Mugwort, several referring to its use as a woman's herb.

Medicinal Part of the Plant

The leaves and flowers are most often used, although the roots are also medicinal.

Range and Habitat

Artemisia is a large genus containing many medicinal species used throughout the world. Indigenous to Europe and Asia, Mugwort is a highly adaptable plant that thrives in a wide range of habitats. It has naturalized in many temperate zones, including North and South America. It can be found throughout much of the eastern and mid-western regions of the United States, often growing like a weed in waste places, sunny fields, and shaded woodlands.

Description of the Plant

Mugwort is a robust perennial herb that matures into a large bush. The plant can grow up to 8′ in height and create a massive hedge, especially in fertile soil. The tough, woody root is a creeping rhizome growing 8-12′ in length, and is covered with numerous thready rootlets 2-5″ long. Many erect, very fibrous stems arise from the root system. The smooth, round, grooved stems are green with longitudinal streaks of maroon. Many leaves and flower stalks grow off the stems in an alternating pattern. Larger leaves can reach up to 4″ in length. Their top surface is dark green and feels smooth, while the bottom surface is light, grayish green and densely covered with downy hairs visible under a 16x magnifying glass. The uniquely shaped leaves are simple with deeply incised lobes ending in pointed tips. Leaf margins lack teeth, but have many notches.

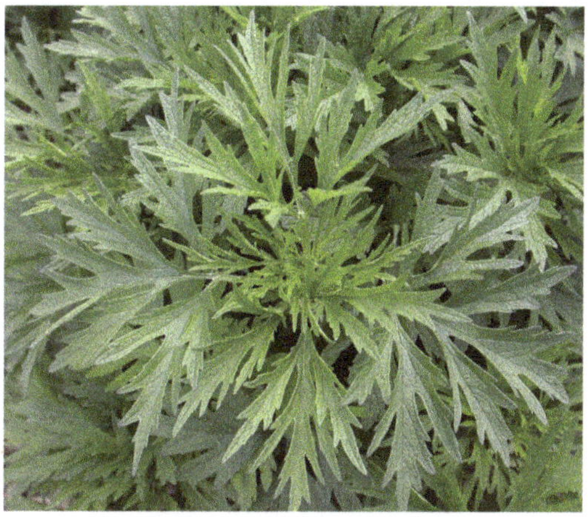

One-year-old *A. vulgaris*

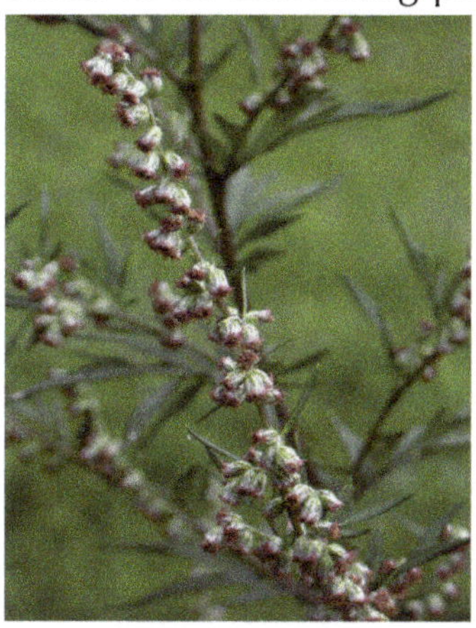

***A. vulgaris* flowers**

Flower spikes emerge from leaf axils on the upper portion of the plant. The tiny, inconspicuous pale greenish-yellow and reddish-brown flowers are sessile, and they grow in loose panicle spikes up to 6″ in length at the end of each branching stem. The light-green calyx is covered with downy hairs and forms a cup holding miniature yellow flower petals. Flowers bloom from July through October.

Cultivation

Mugwort is a hardy, vigorous bush even in cold climates. Easily started from seeds, root division or stem cuttings, it usually flourishes wherever it is planted. It is a prolific self-seeder that can crowd out other plants. Be sure to place it along the edge of a garden or in its own separate space, because it grows tall and wide and spreads rapidly unless it is cut back. Mugwort prefers full sun, which encourages optimal growth, but tolerates partial shade. Moderate to fertile soil with ample moisture is required for best development.

The tiny seeds can be planted outdoors in spring or fall, or started indoors in flats at the beginning of spring. Plant the seeds just below the soil surface and keep the dirt moist. Germination occurs within a few weeks at temperatures between 55-60°F. Transplant seedlings into a garden bed when they are 3-4″ tall and space them 2′ apart.

Propagate by root division in early spring while the plant is dormant. Dig up a strong plant and divide and replant the roots. Stem cuttings are taken in spring or early summer when foliage is robust, but before flower buds appear. Clip 2′ lengths of the upper stems and place them in a bucket of wet planting medium.

When roots develop from the stems, plant them in a garden bed. Mugwort usually does not require special attention once it becomes established. Prune old growth away in late autumn or early spring when the leaves and stalks have died back. New shoots emerge in spring.

Harvest

Harvest the leaves and flowering tops when the plant begins blooming around July. The medicinal oil content is highest at this time and decreases as the flowers age. Harvest the roots in autumn. Seeds may be harvested for planting in late summer and autumn when seedpods are brown and dry.

Preparation of Plant Medicine and Dosages

The leaves, flowers, and roots may be used fresh or dried to make tea, tincture, pills, and for external use a poultice, fomentation or salve. Mugwort is usually combined with other herbs for specific treatments.

Dosage Tips: Mugwort is powerful and should be taken in small doses for short periods of time. All species of *Artemisia* may be toxic in large doses and with long-term use. Stay within the recommended dose range and take the tea or tincture for 2 weeks, then stop for 2 weeks. Alternate in this way for a few months and then stop the treatment. The extremely bitter taste provides a great safety mechanism against overdosing!

PREPARATIONS

Infusion: Steep 1 teaspoon of dried leaves and flowers or 2 teaspoons of the freshly harvested herb in 1 cup of boiled water for 10-15 minutes. Dosage: 1-2 cups a day as needed.

Decoction: Gently simmer 2 teaspoons of the finely chopped fresh or dried roots in 1 pint of water for 10 minutes. Dosage: ½-1 cup a day as needed.

Tincture: Fill a glass jar with the freshly harvested, chopped herb and cover with a mixture of 60% 190-proof grain alcohol and 40% distilled water. Tincture in the standard manner. Dosage: 5-30 drops of tincture in water up to 3 times daily as needed.

Pills and Capsules: These can be handmade from the dried, ground herb. Dosage: 1-3 pills up to 3 times a day as needed.

Poultice, Fomentation, and Salve: These are preparations for external use. Make a poultice by grinding fresh or dried leaves and flowers, add water to create a pulpy mash, and apply it to the affected area for up to several hours. A fomentation is made by dipping a washcloth into a strong brew of the tea and laying it on the skin like a compress. Mugwort leaves and flowers are an excellent addition to salves, and I have included them in my salve formula for many years.

Chemical Constituents

Artemisinin inhibits the herpes, hepatitis and HIV viruses, although the greatest concentrations occur in *Artemisia annua* (Sweet Annie). Vulgarin, another sesquiterpene lactone, is antitumor, cardiotonic, and exerts a calming influence on the parasympathetic nervous system. The volatile oils in Mugwort are responsible for many of the herb's biological activities and demonstrate antimicrobial activity against bacteria, fungi, Candida yeast, and parasites. The oil contains camphor (analgesic, antiseptic, antispasmodic, muscle relaxant), cineole (analgesic, anti-catarrh, anti-inflammatory, antiseptic, antispasmodic, choleretic, expectorant, hepatic tonic, sedative, vermifuge), thujone (emmenagogue), linalool, borneol (analgesic, antibronchitis, anti-inflammatory, antispasmodic, hepatoprotective, muscle relaxant, sedative), terpineol, spathulenol, pinenes (anticancer, antiflu, anti-inflammatory, antiviral, expectorant, sedative), linalyl acetate (analgesic, antioxidant, antispasmodic, muscle relaxant, sedative), nerol (sedative), and myrcene (analgesic, anticonvulsant, antimutagenic, antioxidant, antispasmodic, diuretic).

Triterpenes include beta-sitosterol (antibacterial, anticancer, anticandida, anti-inflammatory, antileukemia, antioxidant, antitumor, antiviral, estrogenic, febrifuge, hepatoprotective) and stigmasterol (anticancer, anti-inflammatory, antioxidant, antiviral, estrogenic, sedative). Adenine is an antiviral, diuretic, cardiotonic, and vasodilator. Flavonoids include quercetin and rutin, and coumarins include aesuletin, aesculin, umbelliferone, scopoletin, and coumarin.

Safety, Contraindications, and Drug Interactions

Mugwort is a safe herb when used according to the recommended guidelines. However, excessive and long-term use can lead to toxicity, partly due to the thujone content. Toxic symptoms include stomach and intestinal discomfort, nausea, dehydration, dizziness, and tinnitus (ringing in the ears). Due to abortifacient and emmenagogue properties, it is **contraindicated during pregnancy in the West**, although there are no known reports of miscarriages from using Mugwort. In Chinese medicine, it is actually prescribed to prevent miscarriage. Skin contact with the live plant can cause temporary allergic symptoms of runny nose, itchy eyes, or hive-like reactions in sensitive people. There are no known drug interactions to date.

Medicinal Uses

History of the Plant

The healing virtues and protective qualities of Mugwort have been recognized by many folk traditions, and the herb has a long history of use in Traditional Chinese Medicine, India's Ayurvedic medicine, and European herbalism. It has primarily been employed as a women's remedy throughout Asian and European history and into modern times. The genus name *Artemisia* is probably derived from Artemis, the Greek goddess known as Diana in ancient Rome. She was worshipped as the goddess of the moon and childbirth, often portrayed as a virgin huntress associated with wild animals and woodlands. During the Middle Ages, European herbalists assigned Venus as the ruling planet of Mugwort, reflecting its value in treating women's ailments. The early Greek physician Dioscorides (*circa* A.D. 40–c. 90) wrote that it "brings down the terms [menses], the birth and the afterbirth." Swiss physician and alchemist Paracelsus (1493–1541) and English apothecary Nicholas Culpeper (1616–1654) both prescribed this herb for female problems, including menstrual irregularities, cramps, pain and infertility, and for childbirth and expelling the placenta. They also used it to treat nerve pain, stomach and digestive problems, liver ailments, jaundice, edema, parasites, and obstructions of the spleen (Culpeper, 1992). John Gerard (1564–1637), a famous English apothecary and surgeon, recommended it for stomachaches and neuromuscular problems, such as epilepsy and palsy, which is the deterioration and paralysis of nerves causing shaking and loss of muscle control. Gerard wrote, "Mugwort pound with oyle of sweet almonds, and laid to the stomacke as a plaster, cureth all the paines and griefes of the same. It cureth the shakings of the joints, inclining to palsie, and helpeth the contractions or drawing together of the nerves and sinews" (Gerard, 1633).

Dried Mugwort leaves were used to brew beer in Europe before Hops became popular. "Wort" is an old Anglo-Saxon name for a medicinal herb, and "Mugwort" literally means "herb of the mug or cup." In ancient Greece, the leaves were placed on woolen garments to repel moths, and the common name may also reflect this use, stemming from the Latin word for moth, *moughte*.

Surrounded by many legends over the centuries, Mugwort has been regarded as a love-divining and magical herb. Europeans used it as a talisman to protect against fatigue, sunstroke, wild animals, and evil spirits. Christians believed that John the Baptist wore clothing made from Mugwort leaves and stems when he lived in the wilderness. In Germany and Holland, where it was known as St. John's plant, the leaves and flowers were traditionally gathered on St. John's Eve (June 24), braided into a crown, and worn to protect against disease, misfortune, and evil (Grieve, 1971). Due to its connection with Artemis and the moon, Mugwort is associated with the dream world. Europeans stuffed the leaves into "dream pillows" believed to elicit lucid dreams revealing the future when placed under the head. Mugwort tea was thought to help induce trances and clairvoyance, and in China it has been used to cure sleepwalking. In North America, Native American Indians gathered indigenous Mugwort species to treat colds, flu, bronchitis, and parasites. Women often drank a tea of the leaves to relieve the pains of afterbirth (Moerman, 1998).

Mugwort continues to be a fairly popular medicinal remedy used by modern herbalists and consumers worldwide. There is little clinical research on *A. vulgaris*, but many studies on other members of the genus demonstrate antimicrobial activity against bacteria, fungi, viruses, parasites, and some types of cancers.

Healing Qualities

Antibacterial, antifungal, antispasmodic, bitter, carminative, cholagogue, diaphoretic, digestive stimulant, diuretic, emmenagogue, hemostatic, hepatic, laxative, nervine, sedative, stomachic, and vermifuge.

Traditional Chinese Medicine (TCM) Perspective

Mugwort is a bitter, cooling, drying Yang herb that stimulates movement and opens channels throughout the body, especially in the gastrointestinal tract and liver. The plant relaxes the nervous system, stimulates and restores the digestive system, and decongests the liver, blood vessels, and pelvic organs. Mugwort's ability to decongest a sluggish liver improves circulation throughout the system and elicits a secondary warming effect. In TCM, it is given for conditions of blood and Qi stagnation, such as poor circulation.

Mugwort exerts a restoring effect on the female reproductive organs. Chinese physicians prescribe the herb for Uterine Blood and Qi deficiency with blood congestion manifesting as irregular or absent menstruation, scanty or excessive bleeding, estrogen or progesterone deficiency, premenstrual syndrome (PMS), and infertility. Mugwort tones Uterine Qi and treats symptoms of Uterine Qi Stagnation, which include cramps, delayed menses, uterine fibroids, and stalled labor during childbirth. The herb reduces Liver and Stomach Qi Stagnation responsible for delayed and painful menses with clotting, indigestion, constipation, edema, bloating, and jaundice. It is cooling and drying for the treatment of damp heat in the bladder that can manifest as dark urine or bacterial and Candida yeast infections.

Mugwort leaves are used in moxabustion, a treatment that Chinese and Tibetan medical practitioners often use in conjunction with acupuncture. The downy fibers on Mugwort leaves are dried and rolled into sticks or cones called moxa. Each moxa is placed on the skin over a specific acupuncture point along a meridian (a pathway of energy flowing through the body), or the moxa is stuck on the end of an acupuncture needle that is inserted into the acupuncture point. The moxa cone is lit and allowed to burn close to the skin.

The heat entering the body has a warming, stimulating effect to clear and balance the meridian.

Artemisia species are popular ingredients in Chinese traditional preparations and are frequently used to treat inflammation, malaria, hepatitis, cancer, and fungal, bacterial, and viral infections.

Primary Actions

Mugwort brings balance to the body through its calming action on the nervous system and stimulating influence on the digestive organs. Its most notable attribute is the ability to normalize the female reproductive system, and I have discovered it to be a valuable remedy for many menstrual and reproductive imbalances and problems. I usually combine Mugwort with other herbs appropriate for specific issues.

Nervous System: Volatile oils in Mugwort are calming sedatives and restorative nervines. Small doses of the tea or tincture help relieve mild depression and nervous tension. European physicians have used Mugwort leaves and roots for many nervous disorders and spastic conditions, including nervous exhaustion, insomnia, sciatica (nerve pain), childhood and adult seizures, epilepsy, convulsions, palsy, tremors, and other uncontrollable shaking. Germans take the root as a tonic with other herbs to treat general irritability, anxiety states, and psychoneuroses. The herb is prescribed for heart palpitations due to its ability to relax and relieve muscle spasms. Some people report a calming effect when smoking the leaves.

University researchers in the Philippines, where *A. vulgaris* is a widely used anti-inflammatory, explored the herb's influence on the circulatory system of rats. Tea prepared from the leaves improved blood flow, reduced blood pressure, and reversed hypertensive symptoms that were induced by norepinephrine (an adrenal hormone that stimulates the nervous system and raises blood pressure) (Tigno, 2000).

Digestive System and Liver: Mugwort's calming action on the nervous system extends to the solar plexus organs, easing nervous agitation concentrated in the gut that manifests as nervous stomach, cramps and spasms, gas, diarrhea, and other digestive problems originating from anxiety.

The bitter, stimulating properties of Mugwort also benefit the digestive system. The lukewarm tea or tincture may be taken with meals to stimulate secretions of digestive enzymes from the stomach, pancreas and gallbladder, and promote movement of food through the gastrointestinal tract. Classified as a cholagogue, Mugwort promotes the production and flow of bile into the gallbladder, helping to "open" a congested and sluggish liver. It is good for many liver ailments, including jaundice and gallstones that may occur with faulty liver function and congestion. Mugwort's stimulating action on these organs helps normalize sluggish digestion, stimulate poor appetite, and reduce constipation. The herb's normalizing action may also be helpful for diarrhea. Oils in Mugwort are carminative and relieve gas, spasms, and colic. Acute stomach and intestinal pain may be eased by drinking the warm tea or tincture, and by applying a hot poultice or fomentation to the abdominal area. The herb is used in Germany for persistent vomiting and to promote circulation. Mugwort helps kill and eliminate parasites, having properties similar to Wormwood (*Artemisia absinthium*), a commonly used vermifuge for intestinal parasites. In European herbalism, Mugwort root is often taken for gastrointestinal problems.

Women's Health: Mugwort is a women's ally with a long tradition of use in regulating the natural rhythms of hormonal cycles. It has a warming influence as it improves circulation and relaxes muscles in the pelvic organs. The herb is an effective emmenagogue that promotes and normalizes menstruation and regular periods. It helps restore normal uterine function, and is safe for both young and older women. It is especially helpful for young women starting their menstrual periods because the herb helps regulate the process. It is beneficial in treating most menstrual problems, including irregular and delayed periods, dysmenorrhea (painful, cramping menses), menorrhagia (excessive and prolonged bleeding), spot bleeding between periods, and infertility. Women getting off the birth control pill can use this herb to help normalize and regulate menstruation. When using Mugwort as an emmenagogue to bring on the menses, drink a cup of tea or 1 teaspoon of tincture 2-3 times daily for a few days before the period is due. It works well combined with other herbal emmenagogues. I have used this reliable herb for many years in my emmenagogue formula with excellent results. Most women happily report improved regularity of their cycles with fewer premenstrual symptoms and less menstrual cramping.

Traditional Chinese and Indian Ayurvedic medical practitioners use Mugwort to improve pelvic blood circulation, stop excessive menstrual bleeding, and strengthen the fetus during pregnancy. Although Western herbalists do not use it during pregnancy, Asians have traditionally employed Mugwort to arrest threatened miscarriages. For childbirth, it is used during prolonged labor and to extract a retained placenta. The tea is used as a douche for vaginal yeast infections.

Traditional Chinese medical practitioners also use Mugwort for moxibustion in pregnant women to correct breech presentations when the infant is turned so that the feet present first. Several studies verify that moxibustion of acupuncture point Bladder 67, located on the outer corner of the fifth toenail, promotes the rotation of a fetus in breech position. Researchers discovered that by using this method, the success rate of turning the infant's head into the normal position after 34 weeks of gestation is 84.6% (Ewies, 2002).

A study in China involved 260 first-time mothers who were 33 weeks pregnant and diagnosed by ultrasound with breech presentation. Half of the women received moxibustion and stimulation of Bladder point 67 for 7 days, and the 7-day treatment was repeated if the breech presentation persisted. The control group of 130 women did not receive moxabustion. Outcomes during the 35th week of pregnancy revealed that the women receiving treatments experienced noticeably more fetal movements than the control group, and 98 (75.4%) of the 130 infants in the moxibustion group successfully rotated into the desired cephalic (head-down) position, compared to 81 (62.3%) of the 130 infants in the control group (Cardini, 1998).

Kidneys and Diuretic Action: Mugwort increases the flow of urine and reduces edema (water retention), especially when combined with Dandelion (*Taraxacum officinale*). Jethro Kloss wrote in his herbal classic *Back to Eden* "Mugwort is very useful to overcome inflammatory swellings, gravel and stones in kidneys and bladder, to increase flow of urine, for fevers and gout" (Kloss, 1971).

Infections, Cancer, and Malaria: The anti-inflammatory, antibacterial, and cooling diaphoretic properties of the herb address infections and reduce fevers. Mugwort is especially helpful for intestinal and urinary tract infections, and should be combined with other herbs for this purpose. The volatile oils in *A. vulgaris* have been found to inhibit the development of several kinds of bacterial infections, including *Pseudomonas aeruginosa, Klabsiella pneumoniae*, and *Staphylococcus aureus*. Tinctures of the leaves have antibacterial activity against *Shigella sonnei* and *Bacillus subtilis* (Alakbarov, 2003). Asian researchers are investigating *Artemisia* species for cancer treatment. An essential oil prepared from the leaves and flower buds of *A. vulgaris* showed cytotoxic activity against human leukemia cells (Saleh, 2014). When researchers investigated cytotoxic activity of leaf, root, and flower alcohol extracts of five *Artemisia* species against human breast cancer cells, they found that *A. vulgaris* demonstrated significant ability to destroy cancer cells (Gordanian, 2014).

Artemisinin, found in several Artemisia species, is active against herpes simplex type 1, cytomegalo, Epstein-Barr, and hepatitis B and C viruses (Efferth, 2008; Romero, 2005). Artemisinin is the primary phytochemical used for treating malaria, and is extracted from *Artemisia annua* (Sweet Annie), the species in which it occurs in highest concentrations. Researchers have found that Mugwort (*A. vulgaris*) contains smaller amounts of artemisinin and also has antimalarial activity (Abdul, 2010; Bamunuarachchi, 2014).

External: The anti-inflammatory, antibacterial, antiseptic, and antifungal phytochemicals in Mugwort help reduce muscle spasms, fungal and bacterial skin infections, bruises, abscesses, boils, eczema, itchy skin, gout, and arthritis. Tumors can sometimes shrink if treatment is patiently continued (although surgical removal of tumors is recommended). Small doses of the herb taken internally are also helpful for these conditions. Combine Mugwort with other appropriate herbs as a bath, poultice, hot fomentation, or salve.

Teachings from the Mugwort Deva

"Greetings, dear one. I am the deva of the Mugwort plants, and my medicine brings balance to the blending of feminine and masculine energies. My feminine nature is within the domain of the Moon, under the astrological water sign of Cancer that rules the home, children, and the expressions and emotions of the feminine. My masculine nature is in Saturn's domain, under the earth element sign of Capricorn. My plants embody the cool-natured, austere qualities of this planet. Saturn is known as the gatekeeper and taskmaster that requires discipline and responsibility to learn the lessons of life. Saturn demands that we move through our restrictions and limitations in order to grow and evolve along the cyclic path of our life's journey. As an herb of the earth element, my medicine reaches into and heals the deep inner recesses of the physical body. I work in the dark places within the form and structure of the body, which are composed of the earth element. My Saturn nature purges and purifies the tissues, allowing freshness and growth to move forward in accomplishing life's purpose. I purge the tissues and blood of low-frequency pathogens so your body may more fully radiate light and be healthy. My bitters stimulate the digestive juices to flow, to break down food into usable particles for nourishment, and to create movement that rids the body of waste. A full circle of activity!

"The essence of my flowers helps in focusing one's energies to move ahead with clarity and purpose. Use my medicine when feeling scattered or lost. I will help to reunite these fragments and heal the damage to make one whole and return to the sense of calm inner being. Part of my ability to unify the fragments in one's life comes from the harmonious blending of the feminine and masculine that is my nature. My plants are an example of the fully empowered feminine energy that is blended and strong in the masculine qualities of power and assertiveness.

"Use my medicine to bring balance to your life. Cancer and Capricorn are the opposite polarities on the astrological wheel – Cancer as concentrated feminine energy and Capricorn as concentrated masculine energy. The healing gifts of my plants bring these polarities into a dynamic harmony to enhance the physical body and emotions. Just as water and earth are contained within each other, so too, the feminine and masculine are contained within each person. Vibrant health is attained with the peaceful blending and equilibrium of these polarities."

Mullein

Verbascum thapsus
Scrophulariaceae (Figwort or Snapdragon) Family

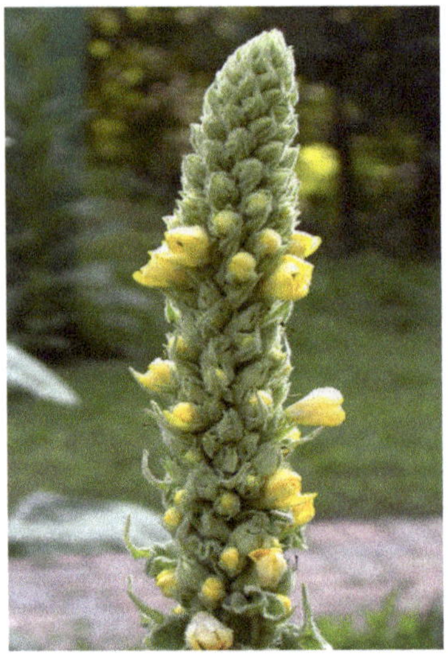

Flower stalk

Common Names

Flannel flower, feltwort, old man's flannel, and velvet dock are names referring to the soft, velvety texture of Mullein leaves. The tall flower stalks have been called Jacob's staff, Jupiter's staff, Shepherd's staff, and Aaron's rod. When people used to dip the long flower stalks in oils like tallow to burn as a torch and used the leaves as wicks for burning, the plant was known as torches, candlewick plant, and rag paper. Mullein dock and lungwort are other old names.

Medicinal Part of the Plant

The flowers and leaves are most often used, and the roots are valuable for the urinary tract.

Range and Habitat

Over 300 species of *Verbascum* are indigenous to Europe, northern Africa, and western Asia. *Verbascum thapsus,* the favorite medicinal species, has naturalized throughout many areas of North America and is commonly found growing in sunny fields and meadows, waste places, and along roadsides.

Description of the Plant

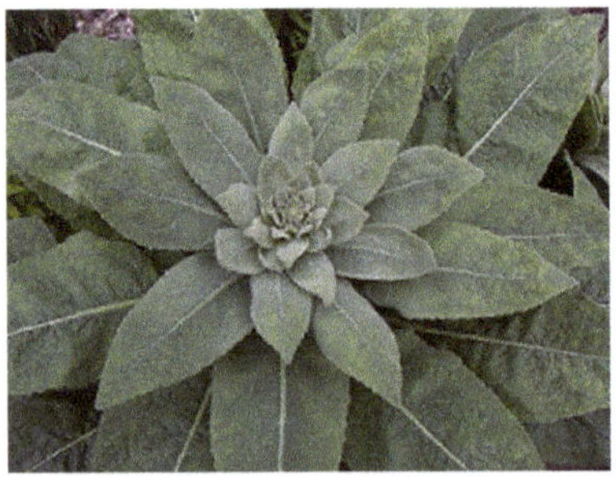

First-year rosette

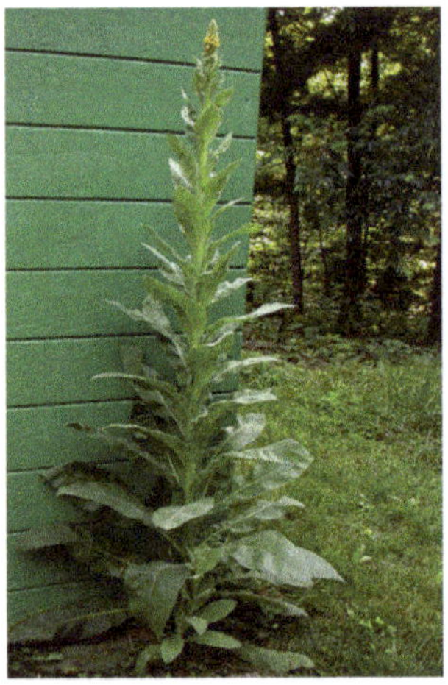

Two-year-old plant

Mullein is a strikingly beautiful, tall, hardy biennial growing up to 4-6′ in ideal conditions. All species have a light-brown taproot. The one-year-old plant is an attractive basal rosette of many simple, ovate leaves reaching a length of 6-18″. At the beginning of its second year of growth, a stout, erect, fibrous stalk emerges from the roots and terminates in a thick stalk of yellow flowers. The light-green stem and leaves are covered with white, fuzzy pubescent hairs giving the entire plant a very soft, velvety texture. The simple leaves are pinnately veined and matted with shallow crenate (rounded teeth) margins. Two-year-old leaves can reach up to 2′ in length. The base of each leaf clasps around the stalk and continues downward in longitudinal, leaf-like winged ridges, adding to the stalk's angular appearance. Leaves grow in a spiraling, alternating pattern along the entire length of the stalk. The largest leaves grow at the base and become smaller toward the top of the stalk.

Many vibrant, bright-yellow sessile (lacking a stem) flowers are tightly packed together at the top of the stalk, forming a dense, cob-like spike 1-3′ long. Individual flowers are ¾-1″ wide and bloom for only one day, but all the flowers on each stalk bloom over several weeks. Flowers have 5 buttery-yellow petals with 5 orange-tipped stamens that surround the central green pistil. Each flower sits in a cup-like calyx having several pointed tips. Flowers mature and the calyx dries into a pod containing tiny, round, dark seeds. Each plant produces hundreds of seeds.

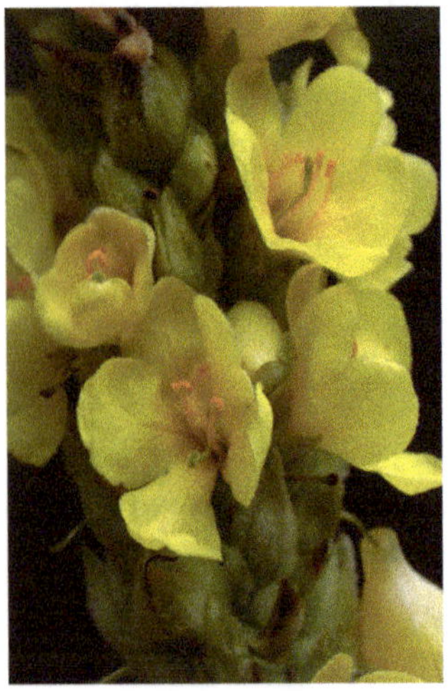

Flowers

Cultivation

Mullein plants prolifically reseed themselves and are often found growing in large communities in open fields where they can be harvested. Easily grown in a sunny, well-drained garden, Mullein will thrive in many types of soil, from infertile rocky or sandy soil to rich humus. Plants grown in fertile soil can become very tall and bushy.

Mullein is only propagated by seed, which is sown directly into garden soil in spring or autumn. It is a light-dependent germinator, so seeds are sown on the soil surface and pressed down rather than buried. When the soil is warm enough, seeds germinate within 10-20 days. Seedlings should be thinned so they are 1-2′ apart.

Harvest

Harvest leaves during their first year of growth and during spring and early summer of the second year. They are most potent when harvested before the flower stalk appears, but can be used any time before turning brown. The flowers may be harvested on a daily basis as they individually blossom during the summer months. Harvest roots early during the second year of growth before the flower stalk emerges in spring. Gather seeds for future planting when the pods dry out and the entire flower stalk turns brown. Cut and put dry flower stalks upside down in a large paper bag and shake to dislodge the seeds.

Preparation of Plant Medicine and Dosages

Flowers, leaves, and roots are used fresh or dried, but fresh preparations have greater potency. The leaves are most effective when prepared as tea rather than tincture, because hot water infusions extract and hold the plant's mucilage, a primary healing constituent, better than alcohol. The tea may be ingested, topically applied as a wash or fomentation, or made into cough syrup. If dry leaves are needed, they require 7-14 days to dry due to their thickness. To speed up the process, cut them into pieces, place them on screens, and use a fan. The dried leaves can be smoked in a pipe or rolled into cigarettes to ease lung congestion, coughs and asthma, or enjoyed as a pleasantly mild, safe, non-addicting substitute for smoking tobacco.

The freshly harvested flowers are prepared in oil and used as ear drops for ear infections and pain. The roots are most potent when freshly gathered and prepared as tincture for treating kidney and urinary tract issues, including incontinence.

PREPARATIONS

Infusion Tea of Leaves: Steep 2-4 teaspoons of dried or fresh leaves and/or flowers in 1 cup of boiled water for 10-20 minutes. Strain any fine hairs out of the tea to avoid irritating the membranes lining the throat and stomach. Dosage: 1-4 cups of the pleasant, mild-tasting tea per day as needed.

Decoction Tea of Roots: Gently simmer 1 tablespoon of fresh, chopped roots in 1 pint of water for 10 minutes. Dosage: 1-2 cups daily as needed.

Tincture of Roots: Place chopped roots in a glass jar and cover with 65% 190-proof grain alcohol and 35% distilled water. Dosage: 25-40 drops in water every 4 hours as needed.

Capsules and Pills: Dry and grind the leaves into powder and process into capsules or pills in the usual way. Dosage: 2-3 capsules or pills taken 2-3 times a day as needed.

Flower Oil for Ear Drops: Chop fresh flowers, put them in a small jar, and cover with olive oil. Flowers may be gathered every day or two as they bloom, added to the jar, and covered with more oil as needed. Allow this mix to sit in a cool place for 7-9 days, keeping a watchful eye for mold growth, then bake it in a stainless steel or Pyrex glass bowl at 200°F for 1 hour. Strain the oil into a clean jar. Dosage: For earaches and ear infections, place 2-3 drops of the oil into each ear 2-3 times a day.

Poultice: The leaves and flowers can be used fresh or dry as a poultice for external problems.

Smoking Mixture: The dried leaves may be used alone or combined with Sage leaves (*Salvia officinalis*) for a pleasant, mild smoke and a healthy, non-addictive substitute for tobacco. To make an herbal smoking mixture, combine 75% dried and powdered Mullein leaves with 25% dried, powdered Sage leaves. Place this mix in a pipe or use rolling papers to make a cigarette. Slowly inhale a little smoke at a time to let the lungs adjust. This combination also dries up excessive mucous drainage due to allergies

Chemical Constituents

Flowers and leaves contain about 3% mucilage polysaccharides that include D-galactose, arabinose, L-rhamnose, and uronic acids. Flavonoids include apigenin, luteolin, kaempferol, rutin, and large amounts of the flavonoid derivative rotenone, a natural insecticide that is non-toxic to warm-blooded animals. Other flavonoids include hesperidin (analgesic, anti-allergenic, antihistamine, anti-inflammatory) and a glycoside called verbascoside that has significant antioxidant, anti-inflammatory, and antitumor activity in addition to numerous wound-healing and neuroprotective properties (Zheng, 1993; Alipieva, 2014). The flowers and leaves also contain triterpene saponins (anti-inflammatory, expectorant, antimutagenic, antitumor, immunomodulator), tannins (astringent), caffeic acid derivatives, including caffeic and ferulic acid, and small amounts of volatile oils. There are several vitamins and minerals in the leaves and flowers, including beta-carotene (plant source of vitamin A), ascorbic acid (vitamin C), some of the B vitamin complex, iron, calcium, magnesium, selenium, and potassium.

Safety, Contraindications, and Drug Interactions

Mullein leaves, flowers, and roots are safe to use with no known side effects, contraindications, or drug interactions. There are no restrictions during pregnancy or lactation when taken in recommended dosages, and the leaf tea is safe for infants. Mullein **seeds are considered to be toxic** due to their narcotic effects and should not be ingested.

Medicinal Uses

History of the Plant

People have relied on Mullein as a protective medicinal herb since ancient times. Amulets of the leaves and flowers were worn to ward off dangerous animals, thieves, malicious people, and evil influences. The herb has been used in India for centuries to treat inflammation, asthma, coughs, tuberculosis, migraines, and as a safeguard against evil spirits. Ulysses, the legendary Greek king of Ithaca, kept Mullein with him on his sea voyages for protection against the sorcery of the enchantress Circe. Greeks and Romans dipped the long flower stalks of dried Mullein into suet and oils to set them on fire as torches, and the leaves and stems were used as wicks for lamps. During the medieval period in Europe, herbalists and healers known as "wise women" also used the stalks as torches for celebrations, performing rituals, and dancing around open fires.

The Greek physician Dioscorides (*circa* A.D. 40–*c.* 90) prepared Mullein tea and poultices to treat convulsions, coughs, toothaches, inflamed eyes, ulcers, stomachaches, hemorrhoids, and diarrhea. John Gerard (1545–1612) prescribed the herb in his apothecary and surgical practice in England, and wrote that the leaf boiled in water "is good against the diseases of the breast and lungs, and against spitting of all corrupt rotten matter" (Gerard, 1633). He applied leaf poultices and ointments to swollen tissues and joints, eye ulcers, and inflamed tissues. Later in England, well-known astrological herbalist Nicholas Culpeper (1616–1654) claimed that Saturn rules Mullein. In his apothecary practice, he prepared a tea of the flowers to treat coughs, stomachaches, colic, hemorrhoids, and edema. A tea made from the root and leaf was used to dissolve tumors and heal swellings, gout, and inflammations of the throat (Culpeper, 1992).

Historians differ regarding the origin of Mullein's name. Some believe that it comes from the Latin word *mollis*, meaning "soft," while others claim that it originated from the French word *malandre*, which is a skin disease causing boils on horses. The herb was employed by the French during the Middle Ages to treat malandre, and the name may have eventually transposed to Mullein.

Mullein continued to be a popular medicine during the colonial period in North America. The herb escaped colonial gardens to naturalize into the surrounding countryside, and many Native American tribes adopted it into their healing systems. Penobscot Indians boiled and sweetened the root to make cough syrup for croup in children. European settlers and Native Americans, including the Mohegan and Potawatomi, smoked the dried leaves like tobacco and inhaled the smoke as a treatment for sore throats, asthma, and other respiratory ailments. The leaves were mashed into a poultice or prepared as a wash for headaches, painful swellings, sprains, bruises, and wounds. The tea was ingested for rheumatism, colds, swollen glands and mumps, female reproductive issues, and kidney problems (Moerman 1998).

The Eclectic physicians used Mullein in their clinical practice from the 1880s–1930s, following the wisdom of traditional systems. Aware of the plant's demulcent and antispasmodic effects on the respiratory and digestive systems, the Eclectics prescribed it for coughs, asthma, and diarrhea. They applied external poultices to hemorrhoids, skin ulcers and tumors, and dropped oil made from the flowers into the ears for painful infections. Towards the late 1800s, physicians in Europe, England, and the United States prescribed Mullein for tuberculosis. Mullein leaves and flowers were classified as an official demulcent, emollient, and respiratory medicine from 1916–1936 in *The National Formulary* of the United States. Mullein remains a popular herb today. The leaves are a common ingredient in teas and pills for the respiratory system, the flowers are prepared in oil for the relief of earaches and infections, and the roots are used for urinary and kidney problems.

Healing Qualities

Analgesic, anti-catarrhal, anti-inflammatory, mild antiseptic, antispasmodic, mild astringent, demulcent, mild diuretic, expectorant, lymphagogue, mucilage, mild nervine, pectoral, and vulnerary.

Traditional Chinese Medicine (TCM) Perspective

Mullein is a mild, gentle herb. Its cooling, soothing, moisturizing nature supports the Yin qualities of moisturizing and nourishing the cells of the lungs, digestive system, bladder, and kidneys. It promotes the smooth flow of Qi in these organs and in the lymphatic and nervous systems. The roots are slightly warming and drain excess dampness from the kidneys and pelvic organs.

According to TCM, normal respiration depends on mutual regulation by the kidneys and lungs. Kidneys regulate the water element in the body, while the lungs regulate the air element by inhaling pure Qi (oxygen) from air and exhaling turbid Qi (carbon dioxide) out of the body. Healthy kidney function is necessary to "grasp" Lung Qi (generated from air) and circulate it through the body. When this relationship is in balance, the lungs remain moist and fluids and gases from air circulate normally. When kidney weakness develops, Lung Qi is not grasped and does not flow down to the kidneys, eventually leading to chronic respiratory problems like congestion, labored breathing, bronchitis, emphysema, and pulmonary heart problems. Mullein maintains this balanced relationship between the water element (kidneys) and the air element (lungs and ears). The root supports kidney function and promotes equilibrium in the water passages and compartments throughout the body, while the leaves keep the lungs clear and the flowers support healthy ears.

Primary Actions

Having specific affinity with the lungs, Mullein is first and foremost an herb for the respiratory system. Cooling, anti-inflammatory mucilage in the leaves and flowers moistens and soothes mucous membranes lining the nose and bronchiole passageways, through which air passes to the alveoli (air sacs) of the lungs. Mullein is effective for hot, dry, irritated respiratory conditions or excessive mucous discharge. The flowers exert a calming effect on the nervous system and are specific for earaches and ear infections. The analgesic, antispasmodic, and mildly sedating roots are used for kidney problems and incontinence, and for reducing bronchial, lung, and lymphatic tissue inflammation. Since Mullein is a mild herb, I usually combine it with other appropriate botanicals for specific issues.

A classic signature of the plant is seen in the different flows of energy between the downward pull of the roots and the uplifting momentum of the upper leaves and flowers. Mullein roots are anchored in the soil and elicit grounding, healing actions that draw energy downward towards the lower body and kidneys when they are ingested. Likewise, the upper leaves and flowers promote an ascending movement of energy, especially effective for problems in the upper body like earaches, facial pain, and respiratory ailments. Several years ago, after encouraging a group of apprentices to ask herbs for teachings during dream-time, one student shared an interesting dream about Mullein plants. She dreamed that she was walking along a dirt road meandering through a beautiful meadow, eventually coming to a locked gate that blocked her path. As she wondered how to get through the gate, she noticed hundreds of beautiful Mullein plants along the side of the road, waving in the breeze with their sunny-yellow flowers. In response to her predicament, the Mullein plants started dancing in upward, spiraling, wave-like movements, and in a group effort they gently lifted her up and over the gate, allowing her to continue her journey. Whenever I see Mullein growing, I remember this dream and see the rising, uplifting movement of these lovely, majestic plants.

Respiratory System and Infections: The leaves, flowers, and roots help all types of acute and chronic respiratory conditions. In the United States, the leaves are generally employed for respiratory problems, while Europeans prefer the flowers. As an expectorant, Mullein chemically irritates the lining of the bronchioles, which loosens congestion and stimulates coughing to expel excess mucous. As a demulcent, it is rich in mucilage that moistens, soothes, and heals dry, irritated, inflamed tissues. The mucilage tones mucous membranes throughout the respiratory system to regulate fluid and mucous secretions. The anti-inflammatory and mild nervine activities relax and soothe bronchial spasms.

Mullein is specific for wet, phlegmy coughs or for dry, unproductive coughs, and it benefits respiratory infections when the bronchi and lungs feel hot and dry, and the throat is hoarse and raspy. The tea is an excellent anti-catarrhal to reduce excessive mucous discharge, while also moisturizing to dry, irritated tissues. The herb has a long tradition of use for treating laryngitis, bronchitis, tuberculosis, influenza and viral infections in the respiratory tract, all types of coughs including smoker's cough and whooping cough, asthma, emphysema, lung hemorrhage, and respiratory allergies such as hay fever. In *The Physiomedical Dispensatory*, Eclectic physician William Cook, M.D., quoted J. Weeks, M.D., who reported that "a fomentation of the leaves at night, applied over the chest, gives great relief to pectoral distress in old coughs, and improves the lungs rapidly . . . a tincture of the stem with the flowers is excellent in painful and debilitated coughs, asthma, etc." (Cook, 1869).

Several studies explain Mullein's effectiveness for respiratory problems. Many years ago, researchers discovered that the herb significantly inhibits *Mycobacterium tuberculosis,* a bacteria causing tuberculosis (Fitzpatrick, 1954). Researchers have found that Mullein flowers effectively inhibit the herpes simplex virus and several strains of influenza A and B that cause the flu (Slagowska, 1987; Zgorniak-Nowosielska, 1991). Another study revealed that the tea has antibacterial activity against *Klebsiella pneumoniae* (causing pneumonia and urinary tract infections), *Staphylococcus aureus* (responsible for respiratory infections), and *S. epidermidis* (causing skin infections) (Turker, 2002).

When treating respiratory problems, add Mullein tea to Horehound (*Marrubium vulgare*), Elecampane (*Inula helenium*), Elderberry (*Sambucus* spp.), Thyme (*Thymus vulgaris*), and Pleurisy Root (*Asclepias tuberosa*) tea or tincture. Dried Mullein leaves can be smoked in a pipe or rolled like a cigarette to treat lung congestion, coughs, asthma, and sinus allergies. Smoking the herb dries up and reduces excessive mucous secretions and a runny nose. It combines well with Sage (*Salvia officinalis*) for these purposes, and a mild, tasty smoking mixture is made by combining 75% dried and powdered Mullein leaves with 25% powdered Sage leaves. During the hay fever season when my sinuses act up, smoking a little of this mix always dries up my leaky sinuses for 2-3 hours, and the pleasant aroma of the smoke is enjoyable, too. I have also found the leaves to be an excellent substitute for tobacco when people are trying to stop smoking cigarettes, as it can be very helpful to temporarily have something to smoke that does not contain nicotine.

Researchers have investigated phytochemicals in Mullein for their anti-inflammatory and anticarcinogenic activities. Verbascoside is found in the leaves and inhibits 5-lipooxygenase, the enzyme that stimulates formation of inflammatory leukotrienes, explaining one reason for the plant's benefit for inflammatory problems (Zheng, 1993). An *in vitro* study showed that verbascoside exerts cytotoxic activity on liver tumors and sarcomas (tumors in bone or soft tissues like muscle, fat, or skin) of rats, and retards the growth of epithelial carcinoma cells in people (Saracoglu, 1995).

Urinary Tract Infections and Incontinence: The diuretic roots increase the volume of urine while decreasing the frequency of urination. Demulcent properties soothe and heal inflamed tissues throughout the urinary tract, relaxing spasms and cooling hot, painful urination resulting from kidney stones, cystitis, and other urinary infections. Eclectic physicians found Mullein root to be an excellent remedy for edema, and prescribed the leaf tea to drink and apply as a poultice for orchitis (inflammation of the testes). Current research shows that the tea inhibits *Escherichia coli*, a bacteria normally residing in the intestines that is responsible for many urinary tract infections (Turker, 2002; Sepahi, 2014). The root is ingested as tea or tincture for acute and chronic infections, especially when combined with antibiotic herbs specific for the urinary tract such as Yarrow *(Achillea millefolium)*, Blue Vervain *(Verbena hastata)*, Goldenseal *(Hydrastis canadensis)*, Oregon Grape Root *(Mahonia aquifolium)*, and Uva-ursi *(Arctostaphylos uva-ursi)*. Cranberries (*Vaccinium macrocarpon*) help by reducing the ability of bacteria to adhere to the walls of the bladder.

Mullein root tones the bladder, improves function, and helps reduce incontinence in children and adults, especially when combined with Corn Silk (*Zea mays*). The root strengthens and tones the trigone muscle sphincter at the base of the bladder, which opens to allow the release of urine and closes to retain urine in the bladder. When the sphincter malfunctions there is loss of bladder control. Mullein root reduces age-related stress incontinence caused by coughing, laughing, lifting, or running. It also helps when chronic bladder irritation and interstitial cystitis (chronic bladder inflammation) causes urinary frequency and feelings of bladder infection, although urine samples test negative for bacteria. Menopausal women often experience incontinence when diminishing levels of estrogen cause urethral and vaginal tissues to dry and shrink, resulting in bladder weakness and leakage. Combining Mullein root tincture with herbs that increase hormone levels, such as Black Cohosh *(Cimicifuga racemosa)*, Dong Quai *(Angelica sinensis)*, Wild Yam *(Dioscorea villosa)*, and Chasteberry *(Vitex agnus-castus)*, can be beneficial. For urinary incontinence and other kidney and bladder problems, adults can take 30-60 drops of Mullein root tincture 3 times daily, and children's doses are determined by the child's weight (refer to "How to Calculate Dosages" on page 148).

Digestive System: Mullein's demulcent properties soothe and moisturize the mucous membranes lining the digestive tract. Anti-inflammatory actions ease muscle tension and painful spasms. Tannins in the plant have an astringent action that tightens tissues to reduce excessive secretions and bleeding. The Eclectic physicians prescribed a tea of the leaves to treat diarrhea, dysentery and hemorrhoids, and a leaf poultice was applied to shrink and heal hemorrhoids. Researchers have found that highly concentrated alcohol and water extracts of the leaves effectively killed roundworms (*Ascaridia galli*) and tapeworms (*Raillietina spiralis*) in rabbits, as well as reducing intestinal spasms (Ali, 2012).

Lymphatic System and Swollen Glands: Mullein leaf tea detoxifies lymphatic fluids and tissues, and decreases lymphatic congestion and swollen lymph nodes. It is most effective when combined with lymphatics like Poke Root (*Phytolacca decandra*) and Echinacea (*Echinacea purpurea* and *E. angustifolia*). Mullein has a long history of use for treating all types of glandular swelling, including the mumps, and works well with Lobelia (*Lobelia inflata*) and Cayenne (*Capsicum annuum*) for these problems.

Nervous System: Mullein flowers seem to have stronger nervine, analgesic, and antispasmodic properties than the leaves. The root is a little-known antispasmodic and sedative that eases facial nerve pain, including Bell's palsy, trigeminal neuralgia, and temporomandibular joint (TMJ) pain. For these conditions, combine Mullein flowers with Jamaican Dogwood (*Piscidia piscipula*), St. John's Wort *(Hypericum perforatum)*, Scullcap *(Scutellaria lateriflora)*, and Wood Betony (*Stachys officinalis*) (Winston, 2001). A tincture of the flowers and root can also be used for pains and cramps in the arms and legs, along with magnesium bis-glycinate (the best form of magnesium to eliminate muscle cramps).

Ear Infections and Pain Relief: Oil prepared from the flowers is an excellent and popular remedy for otitis media (ear infection and pain), especially when combined with Garlic oil (*Allium sativum*). This combination is beneficial for acute and chronic otitis media in adults and young children, and parents should always keep Mullein and Garlic oil in their medicine cabinets to avoid trips to the doctor for antibiotics.

Mullein flower oil was a popular ear remedy among the Eclectic physicians. Finley Ellingwood, M.D., wrote, "The most direct use of this agent is in the treatment of simple uncomplicated cases of deafness, or in the early stages of progressive deafness where the cause is not apparent. In these cases, from two to five drops in the ear, three or four times each day, will stop the progress of the disease, and will cure many simple cases. In its local influence, it softens and facilitates the removal of hardened secretions, stimulating the nerve structures at the same time. It has positive anodyne [pain relieving] properties, and is curative in a large number of the ordinary cases of earache in children, acting often more quickly than other and better 'known' agents, and is used with perfect safety, as it has no irritating or toxic properties" (Ellingwood, 1919).

Two studies investigated herbal remedies containing Mullein for acute otitis media in children. In the first study, 103 children ages 6-18 were divided into a group receiving Mullein, Garlic, Calendula, and St. John's Wort in a base of olive oil, or a group receiving analgesic ear drops (ametocaine and phenazone). After 3 days of treatment, the herbal remedy was as effective as the pharmaceutical drops (Sarrell, 2001).

In the second trial, 171 children ages 5-18 diagnosed with acute otitis media were placed in 4 groups and treated for 3 days. Children in group A were given an extract containing Mullein, Calendula (*Calendula officinalis*) and Lavender (*Lavandula angustifolia*) flowers, St. John's Wort leaves and flowers, Garlic oil, and vitamin E oil in a base of olive oil. These children received 5 drops in the affected ear, 3 times daily. Those in group B received the herbal ear drops together with oral amoxicillin (80 mg/kg/d divided into 3 doses). Group C received anesthetic ear drops (amethocaine and phenazone) in dosages of 5 drops, 3 times daily. Group D received the anesthetic ear drops with oral amoxicillin. Treatment was most successful in groups A and B with an average of 93.4% reduced ear pain, compared with 84% for Group C and 78% for Group D. During the first 3 days of infection, researchers found that the addition of antibiotics with either the herbal or anesthetic ear drops made no difference in pain management. Children using herbal ear drops experienced greater pain relief than those taking the anesthetic drops (Sarrell, 2003).

When my two sons were very young, I taught them to immediately tell me when they started feeling earaches. Putting drops of Mullein and Garlic oil in their ears during the initial stage of infection consistently took care of the problem without having to see a doctor for antibiotics. Since earaches and infections are such common childhood problems, I encourage all parents to instruct their children in similar ways and to employ this wonderful herbal combination.

External problems: Mucilage, anti-inflammatory, and mild analgesic constituents in Mullein leaves soothe and cool irritated, inflamed tissues to reduce pain and swelling. The leaves are used as a poultice, wash, oil, or salve for wounds, diaper rash, bruises, cuts, frostbite, burns, poison ivy, varicose veins, and tumors. For painful, swollen joints, the leaves and roots can be ingested and used as a poultice or salve. Mullein combines well with Lobelia and Black Cohosh for these problems. In his *Book of Herbal Wisdom*, herbalist Matthew Wood shares his knowledge of Mullein's ability to set broken bones that are out of alignment, and gives two examples involving a broken rib and a herniated disk between spinal vertebrae. In both cases, the external application of the leaves healed the injuries (Wood, 1997).

Teachings from the Mullein Deva

"Greetings, dear one. I am the deva of the Mullein plants, here to share the wisdom of my healing ways. As you look at my young plants, see how their leaves grow in a symmetrical, outflowing mandala arrangement and know that this pattern is a signature of my energies. Many plants – their stems and trunks and flowers – grow in similar mandala designs. The mandala is a template or model of the natural, universal pattern and movement of the flow of life coming into physical manifestation. The shape and dynamic movement of the mandala arises from a central core and radiates outward. The mandala is a microcosm of the sacred space of the universe.

"All movement in life and in the bodies of plants, animals, and humans is circular and spiraling. I assist in the natural, unobstructed flow of the air and water elements circulating throughout the body. My plants are strong in the air element and are beneficial for the smooth flow of air and gases through the lungs and bloodstream to provide for the body's needs. All plants have a special relationship with air in that they are the lungs of the earth, inhaling carbon dioxide and exhaling oxygen. Plants miraculously transform sunlight into plant cells by what you call photosynthesis, which means 'to create with light.' And thus, all animal and human existence on earth is made possible and sustained by plants. A sacred trust!

"As a deva involved with spiraling movement, my plants are ruled by Gemini and Aquarius, the air signs most associated with circular movement, which complements and completes wholeness when in balance. All parts and fragments are restored to their natural frequencies and healed, enabling the return to wholeness. Gemini, symbolized by the male and female twins, provides the harmonious balance of the opposite polarities. Aquarius, the water bearer, gives the healing gift of balance to the world. And so my plants offer the water and breath of life.

"My healing gifts support and strengthen the central core of the physical body, beginning at the base of the spine in the area of the kidneys (that regulate water and are healed by my roots), up to the central area of the lungs (that breathe in air and are supported by my leaves), and to the head, where my flowers offer healing to the ears (the organs that interpret sound frequencies traveling in air). The essence of my flowers moves all that is stuck in the mind and emotions, just like a powerful wind blowing away clutter. My flower essence helps scattered, confused thoughts and feelings transform and return to their natural flow, bringing fragmented parts into the wholeness of the core. And in the wake of this cleansing movement is the stillness of deep peace.

"Go now, dear one, and live within this balanced flow of life. Breathe deeply of the breath of life and rest in the peace of wholeness. Sit quietly and still the mind. Feel the peace of wholeness within your Self. Rest and be filled with light!"

Passion Flower

Passiflora incarnata
Passifloraceae (Passion Flower) Family

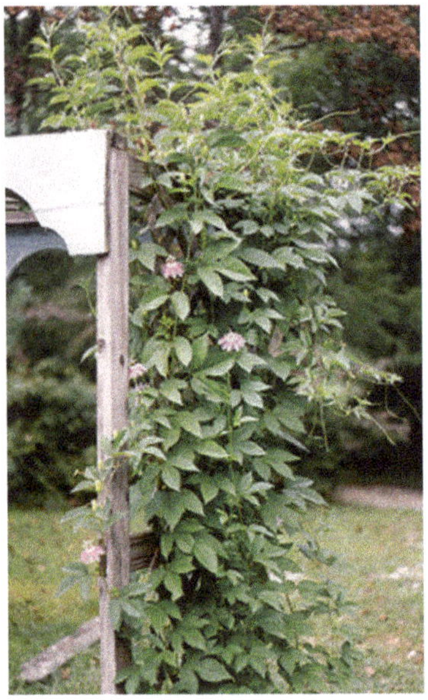

Common Names

Passiflora, maypop, passion vine, passionfruit, apricot vine, and water lemon are common names of the herb.

Medicinal Part of the Plant

The leaves and flowers are used medicinally.

Range and Habitat

The genus *Passiflora* consists of more than 500 species, and most are native to tropical rainforests in Central and South America. The flowers of different species display a variety of shapes and colors. Several species are used medicinally and about 50 species produce edible fruit. *Passiflora incarnata* is one of the hardiest and most cold-resistant species. Indigenous to the warmer regions of southeastern and mid-western North America, it appears from Florida as far west as Texas, and north up to Virginia, Ohio, Indiana, and Kansas. It grows in a variety of soils but prefers a rich loam in full sun. *P. lutea* and *P. caerulea* are the other hardy species growing in temperate zones of Europe and North America, but they are not typically used for medicine. The exquisitely beautiful flowers and edible fruits have inspired people around the globe to cultivate Passion Flower species in tropical and sub-tropical countries.

Description of the Plant

P. incarnata is a perennial climbing vine. The roots are runners that grow horizontally 6-12″ below the soil surface, extending several feet in length each year. Many smooth, pencil-thin vines shoot up from each runner in late spring or early summer after the soil has warmed. Leaves appear in an alternating pattern along the entire length of the vine, and a tendril and flower emerge from each leaf axil. The long, curly tendrils search for objects to cling to for support. The deep-green leaves are simple with 3-5 palmate lobes, finely serrated teeth along their margins, and grow 2-6″ wide. Two small but prominent nectar-bearing glands emerge at the base of leaf blades that attach to the stem.

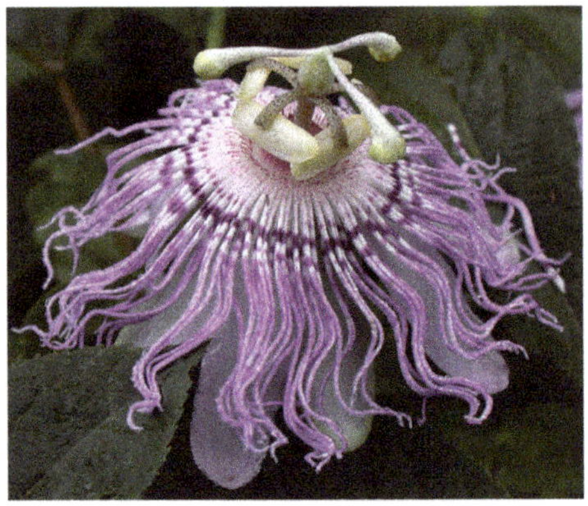

The stunningly beautiful flowers of *P. incarnata* appear in multi-dimensional shapes and rich blends of colors ranging from pale lilac to deep purple with splashes of white, red, yellow and green, giving them an aura of flowing movement, depth, and mystery. They grow 2-3″ in diameter, and their intricate structure and patterns make these flowers one of the most spectacular ornamental favorites among gardeners.

The unique, multi-layered structure of the flower is complex and characteristic of the *Passifloraceae* family. The calyx forms an elongated cup covering the immature flower and opens into 5 pale-green sepals 1-1½″ in length. The oblong sepals creating the first layer are a bright light-green color underneath, while the top side is whitish lavender. The next layer consists of 5 oblong pale-lavender petals that are the same size and shape as the sepals. Above this is a secondary corolla composed of 2 layers of wavy, curly, deep-purple-and-white, thread-like filaments up to 1¼″ long. Toward the center of the flower, a maroon core of thready petals creates a beautiful mandala pattern. Rising through and above this center is an elongated light-green pistil speckled with tiny, brown spots. Below the head of the pistil are 5 stamens with yellow, rod-shaped anthers. Above the pistil head are 3 downward-curving stigma. Flowers bloom from July through September, opening in the morning and lasting for 24-48 hours before they wilt.

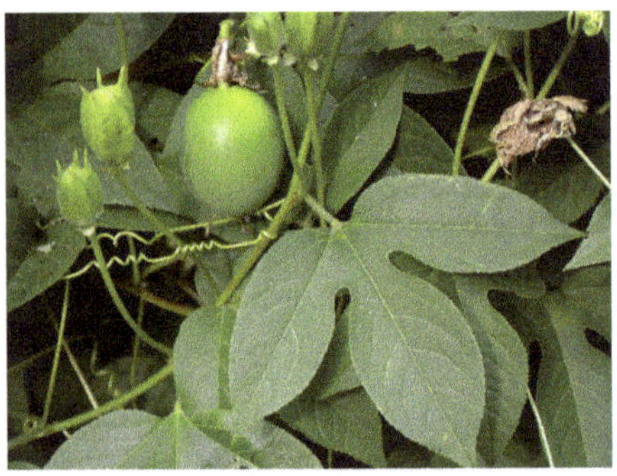

Maypop fruit and immature flower buds

Flowers mature into oval fruits called maypops that are about 2″ in diameter and the size of a hen's egg. The ripe fruit is hollow with green skin on the outside, and inside, a thin layer of cream-colored pulp contains many seeds. The pulp and seeds are edible with a mild and slightly sweet lemon flavor. Vines and leaves die back to the ground during winter.

Cultivation

Passion Flower will grow in sandy or clay soil in partial shade, but thrives in more fertile, loamy soil with good drainage under full sun. If soil is too high in nitrogen, the vine produces more foliage with fewer flowers. The long winding vines need a support to climb on such as a trellis, tree, fencing, or side of a building. Pinching the tips of vines encourages them to branch and develop more flowers.

The herb may be propagated from seed, stem cuttings, layering, or root division. Seed germination can be slow and sporadic, and vines started from seed take much longer to flower than those started by stem cutting, layering or root division, which are the easier and more dependable methods. If you do want to propagate using seeds, plant those that are freshly harvested because Passion Flower seeds do not usually store well and are often dormant for up to a year. To break dormancy and soften the outer coat of seeds that have been stored, lightly rub the seed coat with a piece of fine sandpaper. Then soak the seeds in water for 12-24 hours to improve germination. Seeds that float are not viable and should be discarded. Plant the prepared seeds in trays filled with a moist potting mix and cover them with ¼″ of soil. Fresh seeds can germinate within 2-4 weeks, while older seeds require at least 5-8 weeks, often longer. Keep seedlings moist and out of direct sunlight until they develop their second set of leaves.

Stem cuttings are taken in summer. Use sharp pruners to cut several 12-16″ lengths of vine. Strip off the bottom-most leaves and tendrils (where the adventitious roots will develop) and place them in a bucket filled with very moist potting soil and make holes for drainage. Keep the stem cuttings shaded and moist, and the cuttings generally take 4-6 weeks to grow roots large enough to transplant into a permanent bed.

To propagate by layering, strip leaves from a 3-4′ section of a vine and bury it under 4″ of soil. Roots will eventually develop at the leaf nodes. When propagating by root division, the horizontally-growing root must be dug up, cut into 5-12″ pieces, and immediately transplanted horizontally under 6″ of moist soil.

When transplanting, space Passion Flower vines 1-2′ apart. These vines multiply and spread out, so older patches can get large and cover a lot of ground. The shoots never appear in spring until the weather and soil get warm in May or June.

Harvest

Harvest leaves and flowers when the plant is in full bloom by cutting the vines with clippers and stripping (garbling) the leaves and flowers. Seeds may be harvested from mature seedpods for immediate planting.

Preparation of Plant Medicine and Dosages

Leaves and flowers are most potent when used fresh to prepare tea and tincture, but can be dried for future needs. Passion Flower is a mild-acting herb with a wide range of doses.

PREPARATIONS

Tea: Steep 1-3 teaspoons of fresh or dried leaves and/or flowers in 1 cup of boiling water. Dosage: 1-2 cups a day or before bed for insomnia and restlessness. The tea has a mild, pleasant flavor.

Tincture: Cover chopped leaves and flowers with 60% 190-proof grain alcohol and 40% distilled water. Dosage: 10-60 drops 1-4 times a day, or up to 60 drops repeated every hour as needed for more acute problems.

Culinary

Several *Passiflora* species produce edible fruits, including *P. incarnata*, but *P. edulis* and *P. quadrangularis* are most widely cultivated for their fruit. After the fruit is cut open and seeds are removed, the pulp can be made into juice, jams, and used as flavoring for baked goods, desserts, or dairy products. The pulp is acidic with a pH of 2.6-3.3 and contains citric acid, ascorbic acid (vitamin C), and carotenoids (Meier, 1995).

Chemical Constituents

Scientists are not sure which phytochemicals are responsible for the biological actions of *P. incarnata*, but it is generally agreed that glycosides and flavonoids are the two primary chemical groups that must be combined to elicit their sedating effects. Glycosides contain small amounts (up to 0.01%) of an important alkaloid called harman and its derivatives of harmine (telepathine), harmol, harmaline, harmane (passaflorine), and harmalol. Studies show that these are sedating and antispasmodic (Ergene, 1993; Rommelspacher, 1994).

Flavonoids (up to 2.5%) are antispasmodic, anti-inflammatory, analgesic, and relaxing for anxiety. Flavonoids include chrysin, apigenin, luteolin, quercetin, rutin, kaempferol, orientin, isoorientin, schaftoside, isoschaftoside, isovitexin, and vitexin (Geiger, 1990; Quimin, 1991). Passion Flower contains polysaccharides (especially arabinoglucan) and amino acids including the calming neurotransmitter GABA (gamma-aminobutyric acid). Researchers have found that maltol, when extracted from the plant and given to mice, relaxed and sedated their central nervous system, reduced their physical activity by 50% after 60 minutes, and demonstrated anticonvulsant activity (Aoyagi, 1974; Kimura, 1980). Passicol has been isolated and exhibits antimicrobial activity against a wide variety of bacteria, molds, and yeasts (Nicholls, 1973). The leaves and flowers also contain ascorbic acid, beta-carotene, calcium, citric acid, iron, malic acid, niacin, riboflavin, thiamine, fatty acids (linoleic and linolenic), and phytosterols (stigmasterol).

Safety, Contraindications, and Drug Interactions

Passion Flower leaves and blossoms are safe for all age groups, including young children and the elderly. There are speculative contraindications for use during pregnancy because isolated harman and harmaline constituents have caused uterine stimulation in animal studies (Farnsworth, 1975). However, the herbal tea has traditionally been ingested by pregnant and lactating women without any known problems, and the German Commission E herbal regulatory agency stated that the herb has no known side effects or contraindications, and has determined it to be safe during pregnancy and lactation. The sedative action of the herb may enhance the effects of sedating drugs.

Medicinal Uses

History of the Plant

Indigenous people of Central and South America have traditionally included edible Passion Flower fruit in their diets and employed the leaves and flowers for medicine. The Mayans prepared poultices for inflammation by crushing the leaves and drank the tea to treat ringworm, a fungal infection. Spanish conquerors were introduced to Passion Flower during the late 1500s by the Aztecs, who used it for insomnia and nervousness. In 1569, a Spanish physician in Peru named Monardes initiated the herb's popularity among Europeans when he wrote that it was treasured by tribes throughout Peru and Brazil. It was imported into Europe, where it was widely cultivated and enjoyed as tea. It was later introduced into European medicine, initially as a homeopathic remedy.

Passion Flower is considered to be a symbol of faith and piety. The unusual shape of the flowers inspired Spanish missionaries to name the plant for the passion of Christ, and individual parts of the flowers were associated with elements of the crucifixion. The coronal threads symbolized the crown of thorns Jesus wore, the curling tendrils were symbols for the cords of whips, the five stamens for the wounds of Jesus, the three styles for the three nails on the cross, and the stigma for the vinegar-soaked sponge. The plant's name comes from *passio*, meaning "suffering," and *incarnata*, which means "incarnate."

When European colonists arrived on the Gulf coast of America, they observed Native people drinking Passion Flower tea for its tranquilizing effects and applying poultices of the crushed leaves on skin wounds and bruises. The herb was adopted by the colonists for these uses and introduced into the American medical pharmacy around 1839 by Eclectic physicians. It was listed as an official drug in *The National Formulary* from 1916–1936. However, in 1978, the Food and Drug Administration (FDA) withdrew its approval that allowed Passion Flower in over-the-counter sleep-aids, claiming insufficient evidence of safety and effectiveness. Nonetheless, Passion Flower continues to be a beloved herb that is cultivated, enjoyed as tea, and employed for medicine throughout Europe, India, and North and South America. Combinations of Passion Flower, Valerian, Lemon Balm, and Hops are popular and marketed as effective sleep aids.

Most research on Passion Flower has focused on identifying its active constituents. There have only been a few human clinical studies on the plant's effectiveness when used alone, but there are several European studies on products containing Passion Flower combined with other sedating and analgesic herbs. Current research validates the herb's traditional uses for calming the nervous system.

Healing Qualities

Analgesic, antispasmodic, hypotensive, nervine, sedative, and vasodilator.

Traditional Chinese Medicine (TCM) Perspective

Passion Flower has a mild, neutral flavor. Its qualities are cooling, calming, and sinking. It is specific for Yin deficiency and Yang excess conditions. The herb calms the Spirit and tones and nourishes Heart Yin to relieve anxiety, chronic stress, and heart palpitations. It reduces excess Yang manifesting as hyperactivity, nerve and muscular tension, headaches, hypertension, spasms, and insomnia. The leaves and flowers help circulate restrained Qi and clear Internal Wind to relieve pain, twitching, trembling, and other spasms.

Primary Actions

Passion Flower's primary biological activity is calming to the nervous system and beneficial for problems arising from nervous exhaustion, hyperactivity, and anxiety. The German Commission E herbal regulatory agency approved the leaves and flowers for nervous restlessness and gastrointestinal problems caused by anxiety conditions, and *Passiflora* leaves and flowers are common ingredients in many European pharmaceuticals for treating nervous disorders. The herb is especially indicated for weak, frail people who are physically and emotionally exhausted and run down, and it may not have such a noticeable therapeutic effect on people who are vibrant and robust. I have always found Passion Flower to be a mild but reliable calming herb that eases physical, emotional, and psychological tension and anxiety. Many herbalists combine it with other herbs for specific therapeutic effects. I have found that it blends well and works synergistically with Hops (*Humulus lupulus*), Lavender (*Lavandula* spp.), Scullcap (*Scutellaria lateriflora*), Chamomile (*Matricaria recutita*), Wood Betony (*Stachys officinalis*), St. John's Wort (*Hypericum perforatum*), Valerian (*Valeriana officinalis*), and Lemon Balm (*Melissa officinalis*).

The Nervous System, Anxiety, and Insomnia: Passion Flower exerts a gentle calming, sedating influence on the nervous system. It tones and relaxes the sympathetic nervous system, eases nervous tension, irritability and restlessness, and is helpful in reducing anxiety, panic attacks, obsessive compulsive disorders, hyperactivity, and insomnia in children and adults. I have found Passion Flower to be helpful for insomnia caused by muscle tension, restlessness, and nervous exhaustion. It is specific for people who cannot fall asleep because of mental turmoil and obsessive thinking, and does not cause depression or drowsiness upon waking in the morning. This graceful herb tends to be most beneficial for frail, depleted people rather than those with robust vitality and a flushed face (indicating excess heat), who often do not experience sedation.

The early American Eclectic physicians successfully employed this herb in their pharmacy and documented their clinical applications of its use. In *King's American Dispensatory*, Harvey Wickes Felter, MD, states:

> The clinical application of passiflora has been with most observers satisfactory. Its force is exerted chiefly upon the nervous system, the remedy finding a wide application in spasmodic disorders and as a rest-producing agent. It is best adapted to debility and does not act so well in sthenic [excessively strong] conditions, although not contraindicated in such. It is especially useful to allay restlessness and overcome wakefulness, when these are the result of exhaustion, or the nervous excitement of debility. It proves especially useful in the insomnia of infants and old people. It gives sleep to those who are laboring under the effects of mental worry or from mental overwork. It relieves the nervous symptoms due to reflex sexual or menstrual disturbances, and the nervous irritability resulting from prolonged illness. We have employed it with good results to allay the restlessness of typhoid fever, although its action appears to be slow, but sure. The sleep induced by passiflora is a peaceful, restful slumber, and the patient awakens quiet and refreshed. (Felter, 1898)

Exploring the biological actions of Passion Flower, modern research has validated many of its historic uses as medicine. Animal studies confirm its sedating relaxation that eases anxiety, promotes sleep and lengthens sleeping time, as well as analgesic and antispasmodic properties that decrease pain, reduce overstimulated motor activity, and inhibit the effects of stimulating convulsant substances (Lutomski, 1960, 1975 & 1981; Speroni, 1988 & 1996; Soulimani, 1997). Researchers have discovered that these calming actions are largely due to the herb's relationship with GABA (gamma-aminobutyric acid), one of the primary relaxing neurotransmitters that inhibits nervous overstimulation, supports sleep, and reduces obsessive thinking. *In vitro* studies show that phytochemicals in *P. incarnata* extracts have an affinity and bind to GABA receptor sites on the outer surface of brain cells. This increases GABA levels and elicits an inhibitory, calming influence on the nervous system, moods, and behavior (Appel, 2011; Valli, 1991; Cott, 1995). Chrysin, a flavone in the herb, specifically reduces anxiety and pain by activation of GABA receptors in laboratory mice and rats (Brown, 2007; Zanoli, 2000; Zhai, 2008). Researchers have documented that the anti-anxiety effects demonstrated by mice after ingesting a Passion Flower extract were comparable to diazepam (Valium) (Grundmann, 2008). Studies also revealed that an alcohol and water extract significantly suppressed and reduced seizures in mice (Singh, 2012). Interestingly, gabapentin (Neurontin) is a pharmaceutical drug that binds to GABA receptor sites and increases GABA levels. It is commonly prescribed for treating anxiety, bipolar disorders, menopausal hot flashes, and hyperhydrosis (excessive sweating). It is used as an anticonvulsant for seizures and as an analgesic to relieve neuropathy (nerve pain), including the pain of shingles and fibromyalgia.

Researchers have explored Passion Flower's medicinal capacity in several clinical trials. An interesting study compared the efficacy of a *P. incarnata* extract with oxazepam (a prescription drug for mild to severe anxiety) for the treatment of generalized anxiety disorder in 36 outpatients. Participants were divided into two groups of 18 people for this 4-week trial. One group ingested 45 drops of a Passion Flower extract plus a placebo tablet, and the other group took 30 mg of oxazepam plus placebo drops each day. Test results showed that the *Passiflora* extract and oxazepam were equally effective in the treatment of generalized anxiety disorder. Oxazepam showed a more rapid onset of action compared to the herb, but caused significantly more impairments of job performance (Akhondzadeh, 2001).

An 8-week trial showed that 17 children diagnosed with attention deficit hyperactivity disorder (ADHD) showed significant improvement with Passion Flower (Akhondzadeh, 2005). Using a multicenter study, researchers have investigated the ability of a Passion Flower, Valerian, and St. John's Wort extract to treat 115 children (ages 6-12) suffering from nervous agitation for approximately two years. Parents reported definite improvement in children with attention deficit problems, anxiety, and social withdrawal. According to the physicians' assessment at the end of the observation period, 81.6–93.9% of the children had no symptoms or only mild symptoms of nervous agitation (Trompetter, 2013).

Some studies have focused on Passion Flower's ability to reduce anxiety prior to medical procedures. In one, 60 patients were divided into two groups and given *P. incarnata* (500 mg) or a placebo 90 minutes before outpatient hernia repair surgery to assess anxiety and sedation before and after surgery. Oral administration of the herb reduced anxiety without inducing sedation (Movafegh, 2008). In another trial designed to determine the ability of Passion Flower to reduce anxiety in 60 patients (ages 25-55) undergoing spinal anesthesia, half received an oral dose of the herbal extract 30 minutes before the anesthesia, while the other half received a placebo. Those who took the herb reported noticeably less anxiety (Aslanargun, 2012). And in a clinical trial involving 63 dental patients with moderate, high and severe anxiety, the 21 patients who took 20 drops of Passion Flower extract before and after their dental treatment experienced significantly less anxiety than those who did not (Kaviani, 2013).

Nerve Pain and Muscle Spasms: The nervous system controls and coordinates all muscular activity. This is why Passion Flower's calming and analgesic effects on the nervous system promote muscle relaxation that eases spasms and pain throughout the body. The herb is beneficial for all types of problems involving tight, rigid muscles and uncontrolled muscular movements, and for digestive issues caused by nervous tension, such as gastrointestinal spasms, cramps, and indigestion. It can be helpful for many types of pain, including neuralgia (nerve pain), shingles (painful infection of the nerves caused by the herpes virus), nervous headaches, and toothaches.

Eclectic physicians reported the herb to be useful for treating spasms and pain involved in whooping cough, meningitis, and tetanus (lock jaw). They prescribed it for spasms in children, hiccups, severe coughs, asthma, and gastrointestinal problems stemming from nervous anxiety. Passion Flower was used for many types of convulsive movements, such as Parkinson's disease, tics and tremors, delirium tremens, and for the initial aura phase of epilepsy. Research studies confirm the plant's analgesic (Lutomski, 1960) and anti-inflammatory properties (Borrelli, 1996). Harmine and harmaline alkaloids in the plant have demonstrated anti-Parkinson's activity (Duke, 1997).

Passion Flower combines well with Scullcap, Lavender, Valerian, Hops, Wood Betony, Meadowsweet (*Filipendula ulmaria*), and Jamaican Dogwood (*Piscidia piscipula*) for pain relief and muscle spasms. A mild tea of Passion Flower and Catnip leaves *(Nepeta cataria)* can safely be given to infants for painful teething and spastic colic.

The Cardiovascular System: Passion Flower's calming action on the nervous system benefits the heart and blood vessels. The heart's specialized cardiac muscle relaxes under the influence of the herb, and the smooth muscle in blood vessels relaxes and dilates to improve circulation throughout the heart and body. Studies have shown that harman alkaloids from the plant are smooth muscle relaxants that reduce abnormally fast heart rates (Aarons, 1977) and lower blood pressure by relaxing and dilating blood vessels (Shi, 2001; Berrougui, 2006). In France and Switzerland, the herb is combined with Hawthorn berries (*Crataegus* spp.) for palpitations and other cardiac problems involving underlying exhaustion and stress. Both herbs contain vitexin, a flavonoid that has been researched in animal studies and found to relax and dilate blood vessels, lower high blood pressure, and protect the heart from ischemia (oxygen deprivation), rapid heartbeat (tachycardia), and other arrhythmias (Wang, 2014; Lu, 2013; Dong, 2013).

Withdrawal from Caffeine, Nicotine, and Drugs: The sedating, nervine, antispasmodic, and analgesic properties of Passion Flower contribute to the restoration of the nervous system when people are in recovery from these substances. Remember that this herb is specific for helping people whose inner core has been damaged and weakened, and that this state of energetic, emotional, and physical deficiency is often a root cause for people's choice to engage in harmful activities.

In a study involving 65 people addicted to opiates, researchers measured the efficacy of a *P. incarnata* extract in managing anxiety during the withdrawal phase. Clonidine is an antihypertensive drug used as a primary protocol for opiate detoxification. However, detoxification with clonidine has limitations, including lack of efficacy for psychological symptoms. In this 14-day trial, participants were treated with 0.8 mg of clonidine plus a placebo, or with 60 drops of a *Passiflora* extract and 0.8 mg of clonidine. These were given in 3 divided doses daily. Researchers concluded that both protocols were equally effective in treating the physical symptoms of withdrawal syndromes. However, the *Passiflora*-plus-clonidine group demonstrated significant superiority over clonidine alone in the management of psychological symptoms. From these results, the researchers suggested that Passion Flower extract may be an effective adjuvant therapy in managing opiate withdrawal (Akhondzadeh, 2001).

Another trial investigated the benefits of a Passion Flower, Valerian, and Hops alcohol extract for 107 people withdrawing from benzodiazepines taken for sleep disorders. During a 2-week withdrawal phase, the benzodiazepine dose was tapered down and this was followed by a 4-week treatment phase in which participants received the herbal extract. At the completion of the 4-week phase, restlessness had improved in 71% of the patients, concentration problems had improved in 51%, impaired health had improved in 71%, and 68% of the patients reported that their quality of sleep improved by the end of the 4-week treatment period (Wahling, 2009).

Women's Health: Passion Flower is a calming nervine during times of hormonal adjustment occurring with menstruation, pregnancy, and menopause. It eases agitation, menstrual pain, cramps, and the after-pains of childbirth. Pregnant woman can drink an occasional cup of tea for anxiety and high blood pressure.

Teachings from the Passion Flower Deva

"Greetings, dear one. I am the deva of the Passion Flower family. My aura, or the field of energy radiating from my plants, is the shimmering violet-purple ray of the most refined vibration as it merges with the absolute purity and essence of the white light. This violet-and-pure-white vibration is apparent in the colors of my flowers. My plants are of the earth and water elements, and yet the power of my medicine extends beyond these elements of the dense physical plane, into the etheric realm of subtle, refined, energetic vibrations. For the physical body is simply the aggregate, or clumping together, of subtle particles of high-frequency, rapidly moving light energy that slows down and condenses, until solid form manifests.

"My ruling planets are Venus and Pluto. Venus rules the astrological sign Taurus, the primal earth sign embodying the creative forces perpetuating life. Venus holds the balance and beauty of creation arising and expressed as loving compassion, and this expression is reflected in the exquisite flowers of my plants. Just as the shapes of my flowers are multi-dimensional, so also are my healing powers. The power of Pluto, the exalted ruler of Scorpio, is that of transcendence – the evolution of awareness from the limitations and density of the physical plane to the freedom of the formlessness and brilliance of the subtle etheric realms of thought, emotion, and beyond into a dynamic stillness. The experience of dynamic stillness is beyond the boundaries of form and self-clinging to the concepts of 'I'. Self-clinging is the identification with the self as an isolated human being defined by past experiences, stories, and roles. When awareness expands beyond the limitations of self-clinging, that which exists beyond form and self-absorption is the original light or Christos. And thus, people of old who understood these qualities compared the healing virtues of my plants to that of Jesus the Christ, and many stories have been passed down about this relationship.

"I affect the highest centers in the brain, the pituitary and pineal glands, and the chakras in the body. And so, my plants' medicines have great affinity with the nervous system, the body's great regulator. My calming, harmonizing medicine soothes human agitation and disruption, allowing you to return to your calm center.

"Just as Scorpio holds the experience and mysteries of life and death, so also, I am a deva whose reach and influence are beyond the dimension of form to heal the deep recesses within human minds and hearts. The essence of my leaves directly influences the nervous system, while my flowers offer expanded awareness and experience of that which is beyond the world of physical form – boundless pure light, compassion, and wisdom as vast as space. For this dimension of human beings is beyond limitations of perceived individuation. Just as my long vines hold the jewels of many flowers, my flowers' medicine is like the 'common thread of light and consciousness' connecting all human beings and all of creation. The depth, beauty, and magnificence of my plants' healing power are indeed reflected in the design of my flowers, so expressive of the creative display of pure potential. For I reside in this realm of pure potential, radiant light, and the oneness from which creation arises. My teaching is also of humility. Although my healing power is magnificently regal and transformative and my flowers are astoundingly beautiful, I remain humble, as reflected in my vines contentedly growing and creeping upon the lowly ground, unable to grow upright without helping support.

"When preparing my plants, always use many flowers with my leaves so your medicine contains the complete essence of my healing capacity and gifts. My leaf medicine calms your body, while the essence of my flowers assists you in quiet times and meditation and in your journey through the ups and downs and turmoil of life, to keep you anchored in your calm center.

"My energies are the merging of compassionate love, embodied by Venus, and transformational transcendence as embodied by the mysterious planet, Pluto. A powerful and passionate blend that penetrates the depths of being! The blending of Venus and Pluto energies offers a portal into this realm of being that is pervasive, but unseen to most humans. The harmonious merging of Venus and Pluto stills the 'deep waters' of the heart, the psyche, and the soul.

"My movement is diffusive, constantly spreading outward, just as my viny stems and roots spread and cover whatever surface they come upon. And so, if invited, my healing, uplifting essence will permeate and fill you. My gifts are especially suited for those who are frail and weak, seemingly 'clinging' to life with desperation. For this deficiency affects the deep core, with which I am aligned to fill, heal, and make whole. If you choose to meditate upon me and enter into my world of the violet-purple ray, visualize my flower – an exquisite mandala glorifying the magnificence of creation – in your mind's eye. As you inhale, breathe the violet color of my flowers into your body, and as you exhale, allow the violet light to dissipate and fill every cell in your body. If you do this practice regularly, over time your body, emotions, and thoughts will become 'tuned' and harmonious with the subtle energetic frequencies of the violet ray. It is transformative! These are my healing offerings to humanity, so sorely in need of them at this time. Be well and happy, dear one, and be at peace."

Peppermint

Mentha x piperita
Labiatae (Lamiaceae) (Mint) Family

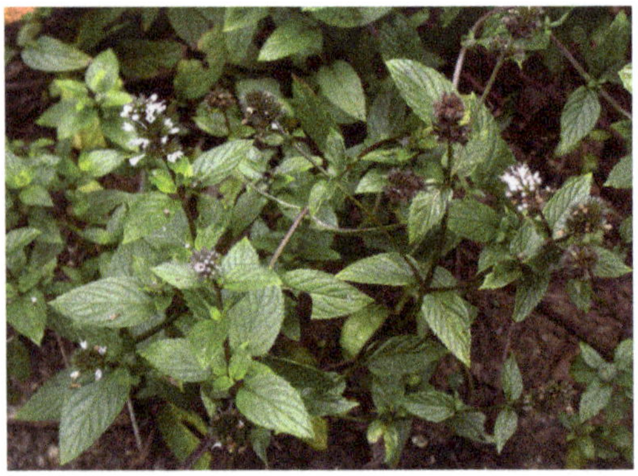

Common Names

Balm mint, white mint, brandy mint, lambs mint, and lammint are other names for Peppermint.

Medicinal Part of the Plant

The leaves and flowers have medicinal value.

Range and Habitat

Peppermint is indigenous to moist areas throughout England, Europe, and the Mediterranean region. Extensively grown for centuries, it has escaped from cultivation to naturalize throughout the world, including North and South America.

Description of the Plant

There are 20-38 species classified in the genus *Mentha*, although hundreds of variations exist due to numerous cultivars and hybrids that naturally develop between some species. Peppermint (*Mentha x piperita*) is a natural hybrid of Water Mint (*Mentha aquatica*) and Spearmint (*Mentha spicata*). It is the most aromatic of all the Mints, and the whole plant emits the characteristic smell of menthol. The plant reaches a height of 2-3′. The roots are horizontally-growing rhizomes that develop into a dense underground mat just below the soil surface. A multitude of branching stems shoot up along the root runners to create a compact patch of foliage. Peppermint is a perennial and like all Mints, has square, furrowed stems and opposite leaves. The two cultivated varieties are Black Peppermint with maroon in the leaves and stems, and White Peppermint with completely green leaves and a milder flavor. The simple leaves are lanceolate and pinnately veined with finely serrated teeth. Tiny, light-green glands and droplets of oil cover the leaves and are visible with a 16X magnifying glass. Leaves grow up to 2″ long and are borne on petioles. Flower spikes are whorled clusters of white, pink or lilac flowers, and each flower is held by a tubular calyx. The corolla is a short, bell-shaped tube that opens into 5 petals surrounding 4 central stamens. Flowers bloom in midsummer from July to September and, typical of most hybrids, do not develop seeds.

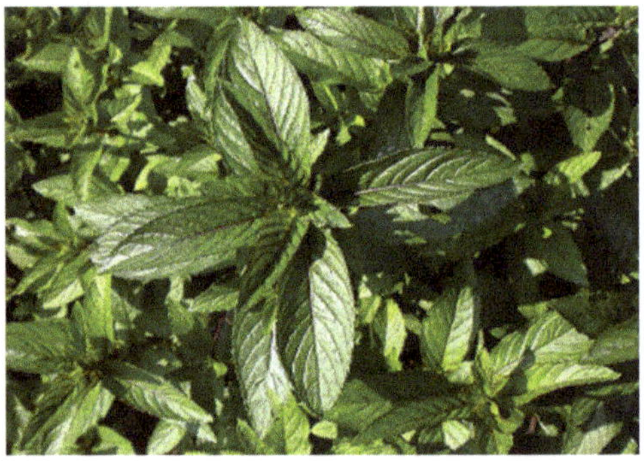

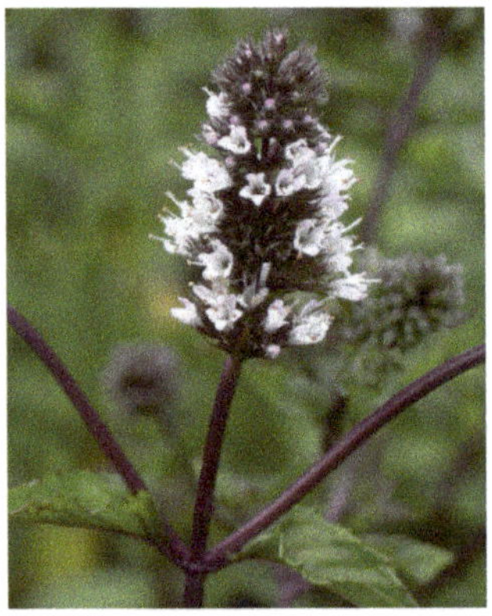

Cultivation

Most Mints grow prolifically and their cultivation is easy. Peppermint thrives and produces the best quality and quantity of aromatic medicinal oils when grown under full sun in moist, well-drained, loamy soil. Since it does not produce seeds, the plant must be propagated asexually by root division or stem cuttings. Different *Mentha* species crossbreed very easily and should be planted as far away from each other as possible to prevent cross-pollination.

Dig up and divide the roots in spring or early summer. A piece of root with a joint or node (occurring every 1-2″ along the roots) will develop roots and stems. Cut the roots into 4-5″ pieces and lay them horizontally in trenches 2-3″ deep, placing them 8-12″ apart. Cover with dirt, keep them moist and weeded, and shoots will emerge to sprout leaves. Since the dense root system can expand quickly, Peppermint can take over a garden after a few years and be difficult to contain. Avoid this by providing the herb with its own area so that other plants do not have to compete for space. Create borders by putting tiles, stones, or wooden boards around beds to deter roots from spreading. Regular rototilling or mowing to maintain a walkway around a Peppermint patch also works well.

Harvest

Collect leaves and flowers as the plant starts to bloom for the highest amounts of medicinal menthol in the volatile oils. Be sure to harvest on a sunny day after all morning dew has evaporated. Frequent cuttings encourage bushy plants.

Preparation of Plant Medicine and Dosages

Peppermint leaves and flowers are most potent when used fresh to prepare tea, tincture, poultices and salve, or they can be dried for future needs. Their fragrant volatile oils dissolve more readily in alcohol than water, so tinctures are stronger medicinal preparations than tea. The volatile oils are strong, however, and their effect is felt with tea, albeit to a lesser extent than with tincture. The tea is an enjoyable beverage for both children and adults, and is a tasty and nutritious replacement for juices, soda, or coffee.

The essential oil, available at health food stores, is obtained by steam distillation of the fresh leaves and flowers. Very concentrated and potent, the **essential oil is toxic in large doses.**

PREPARATIONS

Tea: To best preserve the volatile oils, steep Peppermint in a pan covered with a lid. Steep 1-2 teaspoons of fresh or dried leaves and flowers in 1 cup of boiled water. Dosage: 1-3 cups daily.

Tincture: Chop freshly harvested leaves and flowers, stuff them in a glass jar, and cover with 70% 190-proof grain alcohol and 30% distilled water. Dosage: 10-50 drops 1-4 times daily as needed.

Essential Oil: This may be used internally and externally, but be cautious due to its potential toxicity. Ingesting only **1 teaspoon of the essential oil can be toxic** to a child or adult. Dosage: Recommendations vary from 1-12 drops diluted in 1 cup of water taken 1-3 times daily. The German Commission E herbal regulatory agency recommended doses of 6-12 drops daily. Be wise and **start with a small dose of 1-2 drops and increase gradually. Children under 10 years of age should avoid drinking the essential oil**, and only ingest the tea or tincture after the alcohol has been evaporated (see page 207 for instructions).

For external use, dilute 5-10 drops of essential oil with 1 ounce olive oil or other vegetable oil. Mouthwash can be made by putting 6-12 drops of the oil in a cup of water.

Enteric-Coated Capsules of Essential Oil are manufactured to treat irritable and spastic bowel problems. They are specifically made to bypass the stomach without dissolving until they reach the small intestines. Pediatric dosage (for children over 10 years): 1 capsule containing 0.1-0.2 mL oil taken 1-3 times daily between meals. Adult dose: 1-3 capsules (0.2-0.4 mL oil each) taken 1-3 times a day. **Do not exceed recommended doses of essential oils!**

Salve: Peppermint leaves and flowers can be added to salves for external use.

Culinary Uses

The strong aroma and pleasantly zesty taste of Peppermint has inspired people to drink it as a refreshing tea and use it as a universal flavoring herb since ancient times. The leaves contain many vitamins and minerals and can be added to vegetables, soups, casseroles, salads, meat, fish, drinks, and desserts to enhance their flavors. It is a popular flavoring agent in commercially sold candy, chewing gum, mouthwash, breath mints, and toothpaste.

Chemical Constituents

Volatile oils are responsible for most of Peppermint's medicinal actions and occur in concentrations ranging from 0.5-4%. Menthol is the primary volatile oil (29-48% of the total oil content), and the remaining oils are various combinations of menthol, including menthone (20-30%), menthene, menthofuran (up to 7%), menthyl acetate (3-10%), cineole (6%), pulegone, phellandrene, limonene, pinene, caryophyllene, jasmone, azulene, eucalyptol, and viridoflorol. Most of the volatile oils are terpenes and they generally exert antibacterial, antiseptic, antispasmodic, carminative, cholagogue, and stomachic properties (Briggs, 1993; Tyler, 1994).

Flavonoids (12%) include apigenin, diosmin, and luteolin. Rosmarinic acid and related caffeic acid derivatives inhibit the production of inflammatory leukotrienes and prostaglandins, and exert cholagogue, antibacterial, and antiviral effects (Skenderi, 2003). Other phytochemicals include tannins (6-12%), coumarins (including aesculetin), azulene (anti-inflammatory and anti-ulcer), and many nutrients. The leaves contain calcium, magnesium, phosphorus, potassium, iron, zinc, selenium, beta-carotene (vitamin A), thiamine (vitamin B1), riboflavin (vitamin B2), niacin (vitamin B3), choline, tocopherols (vitamin E), and ascorbic acid (vitamin C) (Duband, 1992).

Safety, Contraindications, and Drug Interactions

Peppermint is a popular herb safely enjoyed worldwide for thousands of years and has a long history of medicinal applications. There are no known drug interactions. Peppermint oil, like all concentrated volatile oils, must be used cautiously in small amounts. Adverse reactions to enteric-coated oil capsules are rare, but can include skin rash, heartburn and gastrointestinal upset, bradycardia (slow heartbeat), and muscle tremors. When applying the oil externally, dilute it with olive oil and experiment by putting it on a small area to watch for any reactions. Do not apply the oil to children's faces or near the eyes and sensitive tissues.

Peppermint is **contraindicated for people with acid reflux and heartburn** because it relaxes the muscular sphincter between the esophagus and stomach, allowing stomach contents to back up into the esophagus and worsen the condition. For the same reason, people with a hiatal hernia should not use the herb since it relaxes abdominal muscles, allowing more herniation to occur. People with these stomach problems may be able to use the enteric-coated oil capsules that bypass the stomach to dissolve in the small intestines. The oil capsules should be avoided by those with achlorhydria, a deficiency of hydrochloric stomach acid, although drinking Peppermint tea may be helpful for the condition.

Many sources, including the German Commission E herbal regulatory agency, warn that large amounts of the oil, tincture, and tea should be avoided in cases of obstructed or inflamed bile ducts, gallbladder inflammation, gallstones, or severe liver damage because the stimulating action of the herb may worsen these problems. However, many clinical herbalists, including Rudolf Weiss, M.D., and the American Eclectic physicians, traditionally used the herb to safely tone bile ducts and treat gallstones.

Although many herbal texts and herbalists traditionally recommend Peppermint tea for morning sickness, some literature currently advises against this due to the emmenagogue effects of large amounts that could hypothetically stimulate miscarriage. There are no clinical reports of this problem, however, and many women continue to safely drink moderate amounts of the tea during their pregnancies (Westfall, 2004). That said, pregnant women should only drink the tea and avoid the much stronger oil capsules.

Medicinal Uses

History of the Plant

The Mints, indispensable in folk medicine all over the world, have been known throughout recorded history as one of the best remedies for digestive problems. Mint plants were mentioned in the Egyptian *Ebers Papyrus*, one of the oldest surviving medical texts. Chinese and Indian Ayurvedic physicians have used different Mint species over the centuries for digestive problems and to treat colds, coughs, and fevers. Spearmint (*Mentha spicata*) is the species originally employed for healing and has been cultivated for centuries. Peppermint, a hybrid of Spearmint, appeared later in herbal history. The genus name *Mentha* is traced back to Greek mythology and the story of a beautiful nymph named Mintha. The god of the underworld, Pluto, fell in love with Mintha, but his wife Persephone became so jealous that she changed Mintha into a low-growing Mint plant. Pluto was unable to transform Mintha back into a woman, but he bestowed her plant form with a powerfully memorable fragrance to honor her. Peppermint's species name *piperita* is Latin for "pepper" in reference to the plant's zesty aroma and pungent taste.

The Roman naturalist Pliny the Elder (A.D. 23–79) noted that the Greeks and Romans decorated their dining tables with fragrant Mint greens, cooked them and made sauces and wine, and used them medicinally. Pliny wrote that Mint "doth take away the headache and reanimates the spirit" and recommended hanging it in sickrooms to assist convalescence. He used it for venomous bites and stings, and followed Dioscorides' teachings about its contraceptive use, writing, "that being applied to the secret part of a woman before the act, it hindreth conception." Greeks and Romans added Mint leaves to milk to prevent spoilage, and served the sprigs of freshly picked leaves after meals as a digestive aid and breath freshener.

In *The Herball or Generall Historie of Plantes*, English herbalist, apothecary, and surgeon John Gerard (1545–1612) stated that Mints are "marvelous wholesome for the stomach" and help decrease vomiting and bleeding (Gerard, 1633). English apothecary and herbalist Nicholas Culpeper (1616–1654) and his contemporaries used the Mints for digestive problems including gas and colic, animal and insect bites and stings, and as a cough remedy and treatment for colds and fever.

It is difficult to know exactly which species of Mint were used by the ancients, for the Mints were generally considered one plant until 1696. Peppermint was first classified as a distinct species by British botanist John Ray, who included it in his 1696 edition of *Synopsis Stirpium Britannicorum*. It was listed as an official medicinal herb in the *London Pharmacopoeia* in 1721, and was commercially grown in England around 1750. It became a popular medicinal throughout Western Europe during the middle of the 18th century and was processed for its oil content (Grieve, 1971).

European colonists found that the Native Americans used their indigenous Mints, American Wild Mint (*Mentha canadensis*) and Field Mint (*Mentha arvensis*), for colds, coughs, fevers, and pneumonia (Moerman, 1998). Spearmint and Peppermint escaped from colonial herb gardens and quickly naturalized throughout New England. Chemists distilled menthol from Peppermint in the early 1880s. By the late 19th century, Eclectic physicians prescribed Peppermint tea and oil for stomach distress such as nausea and vomiting, headaches, coughs, bronchitis, menstrual discomforts, and added it to laxatives to minimize intestinal cramping. The oil was applied for the relief of neuralgia (nerve pain), arthritis, toothaches, and burns. They also used the menthol vapors in inhalants and chest rubs to relieve coughs, bronchial and sinus congestion, and asthma.

Peppermint is currently the most popular Mint in the commercial market, widely used in Europe and North America for medicinal purposes and as a flavoring agent. It has been listed in the *U.S. National Formulary* as an official drug to use in antacids, topical analgesics, decongestants, and as antiseptic and flavoring agents in toothpaste, breath mints, and mouthwashes. The German Commission E herbal regulatory agency approved the external application of Peppermint for muscle and nerve pain, and the tea, tincture, and oil were approved for indigestion, spastic complaints of the gastrointestinal tract, including the gallbladder and bile ducts, and congestion in the respiratory tract. A wealth of laboratory and clinical studies support the historical and traditional uses of the herb. Although it is regarded as a medicinal herb in many countries, the U.S. Food and Drug Administration (FDA) declared Peppermint to be ineffective for stomach distress and, in 1990, banned its use as a nonprescription drug. Nevertheless, this hardy plant continues to be cultivated and used as a popular seasoning, beverage, and medicinal herb in the United States and throughout the world.

Healing Qualities

The leaves and flowers are mildly alterative, analgesic, antibacterial, anti-catarrhal, anti-emetic, anti-inflammatory, antimicrobial, antioxidant, antiseptic, antispasmodic, antiviral, aromatic, cardiac, carminative, cholagogue, diaphoretic, emmenagogue, expectorant, nervine, mild stimulant, stomachic, and tonic. Peppermint oil is a rubefacient when applied to the skin.

Traditional Chinese Medicine (TCM) Perspective

Peppermint leaves and flowers are pungent and mildly drying. The stimulating oils generate warmth by promoting blood and Qi circulation. In cases of heat excess and fevers, larger doses cause sweating that cools the interior and lowers body temperature. The herb is indicated for Wind Cold and Heat resulting in the common cold, flu, headaches and chills, and for Qi constraint and stagnation in the stomach, liver, gallbladder, intestines, lungs, heart, uterus, and muscles. Its drying quality is beneficial for damp conditions of excess mucous.

Primary Action

Of all the *Mentha* species, Peppermint leaves and flowers contain the strongest concentrations of menthol and other volatile oils responsible for most of its therapeutic actions. Menthol and volatile oils in general are anti-inflammatory, antispasmodic, antioxidant, and antimicrobial (destroying bacteria, viruses, and fungi). In the case of Peppermint, these properties specifically benefit the nervous system, the heart and blood vessels, the digestive organs, and the respiratory tract. This herb is safe for infants and the elderly, especially when taken as tea. Tincture and oil preparations are considerably stronger than the tea. I often use this versatile botanical alone or added to formulas to increase their therapeutic benefits and enhance the flavor of other herbs that are not as tasty.

The Nervous System, Muscular Spasms, and Pain: Menthol and other volatile oils in Peppermint have nervine properties that tone, strengthen, and calm the nervous system in two distinct ways: as a relaxant and as a diffusive stimulant. As a relaxant, the herb calms nervous tension, anxiety, and spasms. These qualities are beneficial for insomnia, headaches, migraines, and other problems involving a depleted, stressed nervous system. As a diffusive stimulant, the herb increases the flow of blood and vital energy (Qi). This promotes warmth that energizes and revitalizes the whole body and is helpful for physical and psychological exhaustion. The stimulating constituents in the tincture or a cup of strong tea will quickly diffuse throughout the body and increase warmth in cases of chills. To enhance relaxation and support the nervous system, combine Peppermint with other nervines such as Scullcap (*Scutellaria lateriflora*), Hops (*Humulus lupulus*), Wood Betony (*Staychs officinalis*), Valerian (*Valeriana officinalis*), Lavender (*Lavandula* spp.), and Passion Flower (*Passiflora incarnata*).

The potent volatile oils exert systemic antispasmodic and analgesic relief, and *in vivo* studies show that they are also anti-inflammatory (Atta, 1998). The herb has a long history of use in easing smooth muscle spasms throughout the body, most notably in the digestive, respiratory, and genitourinary tracts. Research reveals that the volatile oils inhibit smooth muscle contraction by blocking calcium influx into muscle cells and returning them to their normal relaxed tone (Hills, 1991; Hawthorne, 1988).

Peppermint may be ingested and applied externally to treat all types of spasms and pain, including headaches, earaches, toothaches, sprains, arthritis, neuralgia (nerve pain), and myalgia (muscle pain). Stronger preparations of tincture for ingestion and the oil for external application produce the best results.

The Cardiovascular System: Peppermint is a heart tonic that safely strengthens and normalizes cardiac muscle. The mild vasodilating action of menthol equalizes and improves blood circulation as it eases tension and relaxes muscles in the heart and blood vessels. The herb can be helpful for palpitations and circulatory problems, especially when combined with other cardiovascular tonics like Hawthorn (*Crataegus* spp.) and Motherwort (*Leonurus cardiaca*).

The Digestive System: Menthol and other volatile oils have specific affinity with the digestive organs to promote optimal, comfortable digestion, and the majority of research has been on Peppermint's gastro-intestinal benefits. Peppermint relaxes muscles in the abdominal walls and digestive organs to restore their normal tone. The tea, tincture, and encapsulated oil are taken to treat all types of indigestion by relaxing nervous tension, easing painful cramps, spasms and inflammation, and stimulating the production and secretion of digestive enzymes.

Stomach: The potent volatile oils act directly on the stomach to treat acute and chronic problems, making Peppermint one of the best carminative and antispasmodic herbs. It is used globally to relieve indigestion (dyspepsia), stomachaches, gas, bloating and abdominal distension, cramps, pain, colic, gastritis (stomach inflammation), nausea, and vomiting. It is helpful for nausea caused by motion sickness or morning sickness during pregnancy.

The volatile oils stimulate stomach membranes to increase secretions of pepsin and hydrochloric acid digestive enzymes that break down proteins and minerals. Sufficient enzymes ensure normal movement of food through the stomach and reduce bloating, gas, pain, nausea, and distressing feelings of fullness caused by slow stomach emptying after meals. The oils absorb stomach and intestinal gas, relieve nausea and vomiting, and are a mild anesthetic to the stomach wall to decrease pain. Peppermint can reduce halitosis (bad breath) by improving digestion and by its strong aroma. When taken for hiccups, it relaxes spasms in the diaphragm that cause hiccups. The antimicrobial oils also protect the digestive tract against many bacterial infections.

A cup of tea, 10-50 drops of tincture, or a capsule of the volatile oil may be taken during or at the end of meals to improve digestion. As mentioned, Peppermint should be avoided by people with heartburn and acid reflux because it relaxes the sphincter muscle connecting the esophagus to the stomach, allowing stomach acids to escape into the esophagus causing pain and burning (Shipochliev, 1968).

For stomach ailments, Peppermint combines well with Chamomile (*Matricaria recutita*), Ginger (*Zingiber officinale*), Licorice (*Glycyrrhiza glabra*), Marshmallow (*Althaea officinalis*), Caraway (*Carum carvi*), and Fennel (*Foeniculum vulgare*).

Small and Large Intestines: Peppermint is traditionally employed to treat intestinal problems involving spasms, inflammation, gas, bloating, pain, and infections. It relaxes tense intestinal muscles, helps normalize intestinal movements (peristalsis), and reduces diarrhea and constipation. It is a popular remedy for dysentery, enteritis (intestinal inflammation), and irritable bowel syndromes (IBS) that include ulcerative colitis and Crohn's disease. Researchers have found that enteric-coated Peppermint oil capsules work best for intestinal problems because the enteric coating allows the oil to reach the intestines without first being dissolved and absorbed in the stomach. The enteric coating also reduces potential for the gastric side effects of heartburn and acid reflux (Somerville, 1984; Lech, 1988). Always remember the potential toxicity of excessive amounts of the volatile oils and do not exceed recommended doses.

A wealth of laboratory and clinical studies validate Peppermint's historic uses, efficacy, and safety for problems involving the gastrointestinal system. Over 15 clinical trials involving 651 patients with IBS document the herb's ability to relieve pain and inflammation, inhibit gastrointestinal smooth muscle spasms, and reduce colon motility. These actions are helpful for diarrhea and all types of irritable bowel conditions (Sigmond, 1969; Taylor, 1983; Grigoleit, 2005).

Many clinical trials validate the ability of enteric-coated Peppermint oil capsules to safely and successfully treat IBS and significantly reduce the painfully debilitating symptoms. In one trial, the effects of Peppermint oil and Caraway oil were compared to the gastrointestinal stimulant drug, cisapride, for the treatment of dyspepsia (impaired digestion). Of the 118 people in the 4-week trial, 60 participants ingested an enteric-coated oil capsule containing Peppermint oil (90 mg) and Caraway oil (50 mg) twice daily. The remaining 58 people took cisapride (10 mg) 3 times daily. The researchers concluded that the oil combination was comparable with cisapride in providing effective relief for dyspepsia (Madisch, 1999).

In another clinical study, 18 patients with acute IBS were given 1-2 enteric-coated Peppermint oil capsules 3 times a day for 3 weeks, or a placebo. Patients taking the herb experienced significant reductions in colic, pain, and abdominal distention compared to the placebo group (Rees, 1979). A meta-analysis of 8 randomized clinical trials involving 335 patients with IBS reported significant positive outcomes for those using enteric-coated Peppermint oil capsules compared to a placebo group (Pittler, 1998).

There are excellent studies involving children diagnosed with IBS. In one clinical trial, 42 children received either enteric-coated Peppermint oil capsules (187 mg) or a placebo for 2 weeks. Children weighing more than 99 pounds took 2 capsules 3 times a day, while those weighing 66-99 pounds ingested 1 capsule 3 times a day. At the end of the 2-week trial, the Peppermint oil group showed significant overall improvement compared to those taking a placebo. Only 19% of the children taking a placebo reported improvements, compared to 76% of the children taking Peppermint oil, who reported a notable decrease in pain, heartburn, nausea, vomiting, and urgency to defecate (Kline, 2001).

In a literature search of 16 clinical trials involving 651 children with IBS, the effectiveness of placebos and anticholinergic drugs (smooth muscle relaxants) was compared to 180-200 mg of enteric-coated Peppermint oil. Eight out of 12 placebo-controlled studies showed statistically significant improvements with the Peppermint oil. The average response rates in terms of "overall success" were 58% for Peppermint oil and 29% for the placebo. The studies comparing Peppermint to the smooth muscle relaxant drugs did not show differences between treatments, indicating equal efficacy (Grigoleit, 2005).

Peppermint oil inhibits painful stomach and intestinal spasms that typically occur during endoscopy and colonoscopy diagnostic procedures. In one study, diluted oil was sprayed directly on the endoscope instrument to inhibit gastrointestinal spasms in 20 patients undergoing colonoscopies. Researchers noted that the oil relieved colon spasms within 30 seconds in all of the patients (Leicester, 1982). In another trial, 100 patients undergoing endoscopies were given either Peppermint oil or hyoscine-N-butylbromide, an antispasmodic drug often given for this procedure. The group receiving the herbal therapy experienced significantly fewer gastrointestinal spasms without problematic side effects (Hiki, 2003).

Liver, Gallbladder, and Pancreas: The volatile oils in Peppermint stimulate bile flow from the liver and bile release from the gallbladder. The herb has traditionally been used to treat liver and gallbladder congestion with resulting gallstones. Several research studies validate these cholagogue properties and the herb's ability to improve the solubility of bile, which reduces the likelihood of gallstone formation (Hordinsky, 1971; Bell, 1979; Doran, 1979; Ellis, 1981; Somerville, 1984; Trabace, 1992).

Helpful for chronic diseases of the pancreas, Peppermint improves the production and secretion of pancreatic enzymes necessary for good digestion.

Bacteria, Viruses, Colds, Influenza (the Flu), and Fevers: Menthol and other volatile oils in Peppermint have demonstrated significant antiviral and diaphoretic effects (Herrman, 1967; Pizsolitto, 1975). Polyphenols are active antiviral components that are concentrated in the tea (Duband, 1992). Laboratory studies show that the oils inhibit many pathogenic viruses and bacteria, including influenza A viruses that cause the flu; *Herpes simplex* virus, manifesting as cold sores and genital lesions; *Streptococcus pyogenes*, responsible for strep throat and other respiratory infections, scarlet fever, otitis media (ear infection), cystitis (bladder infection), and cellulitis (skin infection); *Staphylococcus aureus*, causing pneumonia, sinusitis, impetigo, and endocarditis (heart inflammation and infection); and *Pseudomonas aeruginosa*, responsible for septic blood, and skin, respiratory, gastrointestinal, and urinary tract infections (Imai, 2001; Schuhmacher, 2003). The volatile oils are also active against *Esherichia coli* infections, *Shigella sonei* (causing bacterial dysentery), and fungal and yeast infections, including Candida albicans and *Trichophyton tonsurans* (causing ringworm). Studies show that the antioxidant oils destroy dangerous free radicals to protect cells from damage (Mimica-Dukic, 2003).

Peppermint is taken to sweat out the common cold and fevers because, as a diaphoretic, it stimulates perspiration and brings internal heat to the surface, producing a cooling effect. For coughs and lung congestion, the hot tea or tincture in hot water eases spasms and tightness in the bronchial passages and lungs. The stimulating volatile oils break up congestion and have mucous-thinning properties that reduce phlegm. The herb is helpful to improve breathing and treat sore throats, laryngitis, and coughs occurring with bronchitis and pneumonia. The oil is often an ingredient in cough drops. As an analgesic, Peppermint reduces the pain and discomfort that generally accompany these illnesses.

Peppermint may also be used as an inhalant to relax tight muscles and break up bronchial and sinus congestion. Make a strong tea or add 3-12 drops of essential oil to a pan of simmering water. Bend down to put your head over the steam, place a large towel over your head and the pan to trap the steam, and inhale for several minutes. Some people experience the same immediate relief by inhaling deeply from a Peppermint tea bag. A classic European and colonial American remedy for colds, chills, fevers, influenza, pneumonia, and other respiratory infections consists of equal parts Peppermint, Yarrow (*Achillea millefolium*), and Elderberry flowers (*Sambucus canadensis*) as tincture or tea. Boneset (*Eupatorium perfoliatum*) is an excellent addition to this formula.

Infants and Children: The mild tea is safe for infants and children to take for colic, fevers, the common cold and flu, coughs, spasms, and pain and irritation from teething. It was once used for childhood convulsions. Pediatric physicians in Germany prescribe Peppermint leaf (67%) combined with Chamomile flowers (33%) as a tea to treat gastrointestinal upsets in children. The tea can also be given as an enema.

A study confirmed that tea prepared with Peppermint, Licorice (*Glycyrrhiza glabra*), Blue Vervain (*Verbena hastata*), Fennel (*Foeniculum vulgare*), and Lemon Balm (*Melissa officinalis*) was safe and effective for colic in infants (Weizman, 1993). Colic is a common digestive problem in infants that manifests as painful stomach and intestinal spasms. Another study evaluated the efficacy of a liquid Peppermint leaf preparation compared to simethicone (a frequent prescribed drug to reduce gas) in 30 infants between the ages of 15-60 days who were diagnosed with colic. All of the infants ingested 1 drop of the Peppermint preparation per kilogram of body weight for 7 days. The treatment was stopped for 3 days and then the same infants were given simethicone for 7 days. The infants experienced equal relief from colic (measured by the frequency and duration of infant crying) with Peppermint and the drug (Alves, 2012).

Catnip (*Nepeta cataria*) is another safe pediatric herb that blends well with Peppermint. Remember that Peppermint tea is an excellent beverage for children and it can replace sugar-filled juices and soda pop, which leaches minerals from the body.

Female Reproductive System: The herb's nervine and antispasmodic actions are especially beneficial to women during menstruation and pregnancy. Peppermint relaxes pelvic and uterine muscles to promote blood circulation and ease painful menstrual cramps. The stimulating properties are specific for sluggish, congested pelvic conditions caused by underlying anxiety and tension that often cause delayed and painful menstruation, premenstrual syndrome (PMS), and bloating.

Peppermint is a mild emmenagogue, so **pregnant women should avoid ingesting the potent oil capsules**. Normal amounts of tea are safe, however, and many pregnant women have found that a cup of Peppermint tea helps ease morning sickness.

External Uses: Peppermint leaves and flowers can be prepared as a poultice or bath, added to salve, or tinctured to apply as an effective liniment. The concentrated oil is often used for external applications due to its superior strength. When diluted and applied to the skin, the volatile oils in the herb improve local blood flow to enhance healing. Menthol makes the skin feel cool and acts as a counter-irritant that stimulates nerves to reduce sensations of pain, headaches, or itching. A study evaluating the pain-relieving actions of a 10% Peppermint oil and 90% alcohol solution determined it to be an effective analgesic when applied to large areas of the forehead and temples in 32 people with headaches (Gobel, 1994 & 1995). Peppermint may be ingested and applied topically to treat pain, stiffness, cramps, and spasms in joints and muscles. It is helpful for arthritis, toothaches, and many types of neuralgia (nerve pain) and myalgia (muscle pain). For headache and migraine relief, rub the tincture or oil on the forehead, temples, in front of the ears, and around the nape of the neck. The oil may also relieve the itching and inflammation of poison ivy. An interesting study reported that Peppermint oil significantly reduced pruritus (generalized itching) in 47 pregnant women, although it was not clearly stated whether the oil was ingested (typically not recommended during pregnancy) or applied topically (Akhavan, 2012).

Peppermint oil is an antiseptic helpful against bacterial and herpes skin infections. Following an *in vitro* test investigating the ability of the oil to inhibit *Herpes simplex* virus type 1 and 2, researchers concluded that the essential oil was capable of neutralizing or destroying the virus. The oil significantly reduced lesion formation by 99% and was active against an acyclovir-resistant strain of herpes (Schuhmacher, 2003). In one case, a 76-year-old woman with intractable herpes nerve pain resistant to standard medical treatment found that Peppermint oil effectively reduced her chronic pain. She applied oil containing 10% menthol to her skin and experienced almost immediate pain relief lasting for 4-6 hours (Davies, 2002).

Avoid getting the oil and tincture in the eyes or around other delicate tissues because it can cause a burning sensation. Be especially cautious with babies and small children, and do not put Peppermint on their faces. Before applying the oil to anyone's skin, dilute it with a carrier oil (like olive oil) and then apply a small amount and wait a few minutes to ensure that it does not cause burning or discomfort.

Aromatherapy using 3-4 drops of Peppermint oil added to water can relieve nausea, increase mental alertness, and open respiratory airways.

Teachings from the Peppermint Deva

"Greetings, dear one. I am the deva of the Peppermint plants that speaks. My aura, the light radiating from my plants, is the blend of green and purple frequencies of light that affect the human heart and nervous system and feeling body – what you call emotions. I soothe the energies and flow of movement within the human body. By calming and bringing the dynamic balance of energies into equilibrium, the body and emotions rest in a peaceful state. Yes, this is the gift of my plants, my healing offerings. For my plants are a perfect balance of the four elements, each equal to the other in strength and importance. My diffusive nature empowers my healing substances to penetrate through the tissues of the body, just as water permeates through soil, bringing nourishment and life. My stimulating, warming action and peppery, spicy flavor reflect my fire element. I am a low-growing plant, staying close to the earth, covering her body with a thick blanket of fragrance that is carried in the air. My healing plants assist in opening the airways in humans, so they may fully receive the life force within the air you breathe.

"And so, in my expression of balance, my plants are exalted within the influence of Venus, the feminine planet of beauty that naturally arises from the state of balance. And I am ruled by the astrological sign Libra, an air sign within the domain of Venus. Libra is portrayed as a woman holding a scale, symbolizing the activity of maintaining balance and equanimity. The medicine of my leaves offers balance to the nervous system, the stomach and intestines, the heart, blood vessels, lungs, and the flow of blood and air through the physical body. The essence of my flowers brings healing and balance to the mind and emotions, allowing a calm, aware center of being.

"A beautiful offering my plants present, and yet we all remain humble and common, available to all. For in accord with our diffusive nature, my plants grow all over the world and are used by many people. It is our delight to be of use and service! The devas of all the plants, and Mother Earth herself, wish healing and peace and balance for the human race."

Pleurisy Root

Asclepias tuberosa
Asclepiadaceae (Milkweed) Family

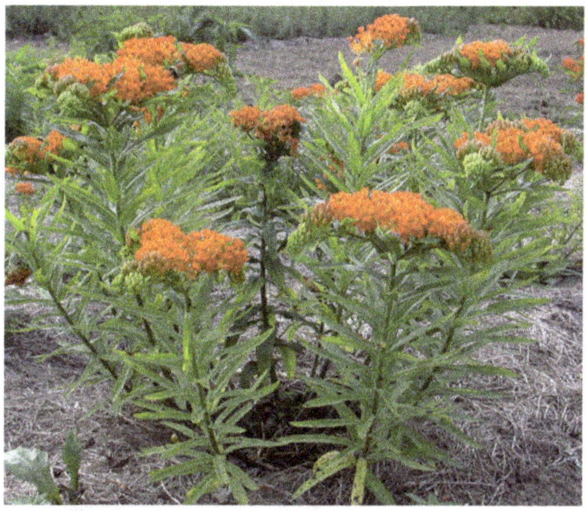

Common Names

Butterfly weed is the popular common name. Antiquated names include orange milkweed, orange swallow wort, silkweed, asclepias, chigger flower, Indian nosy, wind root, Canada root, tuber root, white root, flux root, colic root, and orange root.

Medicinal Part of the Plant

The root is the only part of the plant used for medicine.

Range and Habitat

Pleurisy Root is indigenous to North America and is found in open fields and along stream banks in clay, sandy, or loamy soil. It grows throughout a large area of the United States along the eastern coast, west to Arizona and Texas, and is most abundant in southern states and open fields and prairies of the Midwest.

Description of the Plant

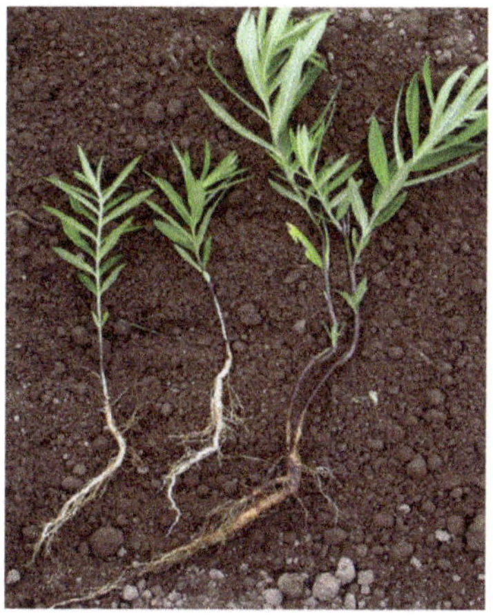

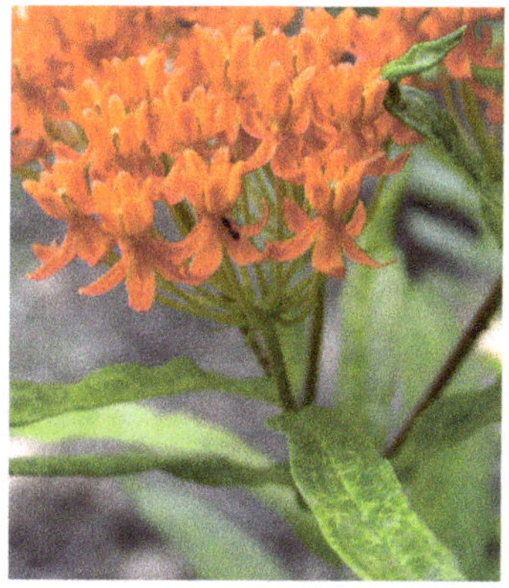

A. tuberosa is often cultivated in gardens as a showy ornamental because it is such a unique and strikingly beautiful wildflower. The colorful flowers and their copious production of nectar attract bees, hummingbirds, and many Queen and Monarch butterflies (hence its common name, Butterfly Weed). These butterflies lay their eggs on the stems of the plant and, when the larvae hatch, they feed on the leaves to grow into caterpillars. For the Monarch butterflies, plants in the Milkweed family are the only food source for their offspring.

Pleurisy Root is a perennial herb growing 1-3′ tall. The fusiform taproot is fleshy and can branch out, growing 1-2′ deep. Roots are creamy white inside and light brown on the outside with ring-like markings and grooves running lengthwise. The species name of *tuberosa* was given to this herb because of its characteristic tuberous root. Mature plants develop numerous erect, round stalks emerging from the root crowns. The 1-6″ long leaves lack teeth and are simple, linear with a pointed tip, and the leaf base is sessile and clasps closely around the stalk. Soft pubescent hairs cover the stalks and leaves. Unlike other members of the Milkweed family, *A. tuberosa* does not contain the milky-white latex juice, and the leaves grow alternately (rather than opposite or whorled) along the entire length of the stalk. The tip of each stalk branches out into several stems terminating in clusters of compound umbels. Each umbel contains many vibrant, brilliant-orange flowers. Each flower in the flower head is ¼-½″ long and uniquely barrel-shaped. The central yellow pistil is surrounded by 5 orange stamens and by 5 orange petals that point upwards. Below the petals, the calyx consists of 5 longer orange sepals pointing in the opposite downward direction. Flowers bloom from June through September, and mature into the characteristic green Milkweed pod that turns brown as it dries. The furry seedpod is usually 2-4″ long and splits open as it dries, releasing many flat, brown seeds. Each seed is attached to a tuft of long silky hairs that carry it in the wind like a parachute.

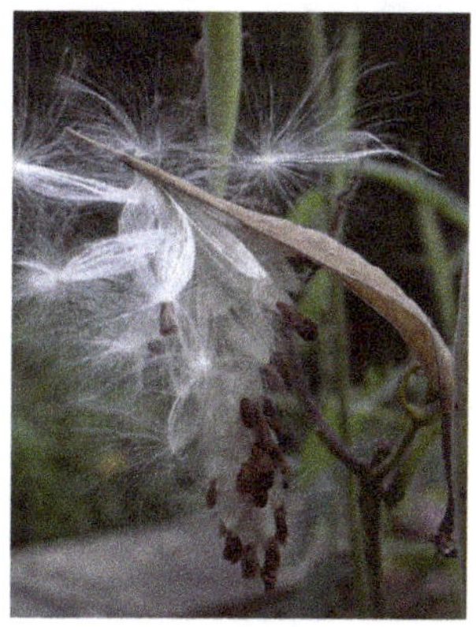

Cultivation

Pleurisy Root naturally grows in clay or sandy soil, so a combination of these works well when preparing a garden bed. Be sure the soil is well drained and in full sun. Once established, the plant thrives in poor, dry soils and is resistant to drought. Propagate Pleurisy Root with seeds or by stem cuttings.

Seeds germinate best after a period of cold, damp stratification, and can be planted in a garden bed in autumn to germinate the following spring. This herb does not like having its roots disturbed, making direct sowing preferable to starting seeds in trays and transplanting them. To plant seeds in the spring, stratification is accomplished by mixing the seeds with a little damp sand in a plastic bag and putting them in a refrigerator (33–38°F) for 10-12 weeks prior to planting. Place seeds 1/8-1/4" deep in sandy soil. Plants should be spaced 1' apart. If transplanting is necessary, try to keep the soil clumped around the roots and transplant out of direct sunlight to reduce shock. Plants grown from seed can take 2-3 years to flower.

To propagate by stem cuttings, clip 4-6" lengths of stem just below a leaf node and place them in a jar filled with water and sand. When roots develop after 4-8 weeks, plant the stems in a permanent bed.

Harvest

Harvest roots that are at least 3-4 years old in late autumn. Dig a fairly big hole around the plant to expose the whole root. Gather seeds when the pod turns brown and becomes dry. As the pod splits open, the mass of flat, brown seeds is visible. By gently rubbing the seeds between your fingers, they will break free of the long, downy hairs attaching them to the pod.

Preparation of Plant Medicine and Dosages

The most potent preparation is tincture made from freshly harvested roots, followed by tea. But if drying is necessary, clean and chop the roots into small pieces and arrange them on screens in a shady, well-ventilated room. The fresh roots have a mild flavor, becoming more bitter as they dry.

PREPARATIONS

Tincture: Prepare the freshly harvested roots in the usual manner with a mix of 60% 190-proof grain alcohol and 40% distilled water. Dosage: 30-90 drops every 3 hours as needed for acute conditions. For chronic conditions take 5-30 drops daily.

Decoction Tea: Gently simmer ½-1 teaspoon of finely chopped or powdered root in 1 cup of water for 8-10 minutes in a covered pan, then steep for 30 minutes. Dosage: 1-2 cups a day as needed.

Chemical Constituents

One of the primary constituents of the root is a cardiac glycoside called asclepiadin that can be extracted by alcohol or boiling water, but is greatly reduced when the root is dried. Asclepiadin's action is on the heart and it can be toxic in large, concentrated doses. Other cardiac glycosides include uzarigenin, syriogenin, syrioside, afroside, asclepin (strengthens heart contractions), calactin, calotropin, gomphoside, uscharidin, and uscharin. The roots contain saponins (immunostimulant, expectorant) and relatively high amounts of anti-inflammatory and antioxidant flavonoids that include rutin, kaempferol, quercetin, and isorhamnetin. Other constituents include caffeic acid, chlorogenic acid, choline, b-sitosterol, the triterpenes amyrin and lupeol, asclepione (a bitter), volatile oils, mucilage, starch, tannins, and 9% mineral salts.

Safety, Contraindications, and Drug Interactions

Pleurisy Root is a safe herb when used appropriately. Excessive doses can cause nausea, vomiting, diarrhea, or heart irregularities. It is **contraindicated during pregnancy and lactation** due to its potentially stimulating effect on the uterus and the cardiac glycosides. The roots should be used carefully by people on heart, blood pressure, and diuretic medications because cardiac glycosides could hypothetically interfere with these drugs, although there are no known reports of this problem.

Medicinal Uses

History of the Plant

There are over 140 known species in the Milkweed genus, and many have been used medicinally by people around the world for centuries. The genus name *Asclepias* comes from the ancient Greek healer Asclepias, who was deified as the "god of medicine." The indigenous people of North America utilized several Milkweed species in their medical pharmacy, and *A. tuberosa* was a favorite for a wide variety of purposes. The dried and fresh root was chewed or prepared as tea for treating respiratory problems, colds, fever, headache, toothache, indigestion, stomach and intestinal pain, diarrhea, dysentery, rheumatism, and heart problems. The crushed leaves were applied as a poultice to heal wounds, ringworm (a fungal infection), cuts, bruises, swelling and inflammation, skin ulcers, and skin cancers. The root was prepared as a powder or tea and applied to wounds, tumors, boils, and rashes. The flowers, young seed pods, and tender shoots were eaten as food (Moerman, 1981).

Early European explorers and settlers learned about Pleurisy Root from the Native Americans. It quickly became a primary expectorant in colonial American medicine, and was a popular remedy prescribed by "root doctors" and "regular" physicians. Charles Millspaugh, a 19th-century author on North American medicinal plants, extolled the virtues of the herb when he wrote:

The pleurisy-root has received more attention as a medicine than any other species of this genus, having been regarded, almost since the discovery of this country, as a subtonic, diaphoretic, alterative, expectorant, diuretic, laxative, escharotic, carminative, anti-spasmodic, anti-pleuritic, stomachic, astringent, anti-rheumatic, anti-syphilitic, and what not? It has been recommended in low typhoid states, pneumonia, catarrh, bronchitis, pleurisy, dyspepsia, indigestion, dysentery, helminthiasis [parasites], and obstinate eczemas. (Millspaugh, 1887)

Pleurisy Root was highly regarded by several herbal schools, including the physio-medical, Eclectic, and homeopathic disciplines. It was a favorite of the Eclectic physicians who administered it as a diaphoretic, a tonic herb and treatment for all types of lung ailments, and as a remedy for gastrointestinal problems. The Eclectics regarded it as a specific pediatric remedy for respiratory, stomach, and intestinal illnesses in children with mucous discharge, weakness, and general nervousness. *A. tuberosa* was listed as an official drug in the *U.S. Pharmacopoeia* from 1820–1905 and in the *National Formulary* from 1916–1936. The 16th edition of *The Dispensatory of the United States of America*, published in 1888, documented its healing potential as a diaphoretic, astringent, and expectorant for the treatment of catarrh (excessive phlegm and mucous), pleurisy, pneumonia, bronchitis, tuberculosis, rheumatism, diarrhea, and dysentery (Wood, 1892).

Pleurisy Root continues to be a popular medicinal herb and garden ornamental. Wild populations are dwindling due to human sprawl and agricultural chemicals, and *A. tuberosa* is listed on the United Plant Savers "To-Watch List." Since the survival of the Monarch and Queen butterflies depends upon the survival of plants in the Milkweed family, planting this herb in gardens and sowing it in open fields and meadows is important for the welfare of all and creates more beauty on the planet!

Healing Qualities

Anti-catarrh, anti-inflammatory, antispasmodic, cardiac tonic, diaphoretic, diuretic, expectorant, pectoral, and vasodilator.

Traditional Chinese Medicine (TCM) Perspective

A. tuberosa is mildly cooling and drying with both relaxing and stimulating properties. It opens and lubricates fluid channels in the lungs and throughout the body to stimulate, decongest, disperse, and restore the normal circulation of fluids. TCM recognizes that the lungs require moisture to maintain their permeable membranes and elasticity. The lungs must disperse and disseminate fluids and Qi, derived from air and oxygen, throughout the entire body. When the movement of fluids and Qi is diminished, Lung Qi Stagnation can cause coughs with excessive or deficient mucous, sore throat and hoarseness, lack of perspiration, feelings of chest pressure and tightness, and acute respiratory infections. Long-term stagnation can eventually result in chronic lung conditions.

Primary Actions

Pleurisy Root is an excellent remedy specific for all types of lung and bronchial problems. I have relied on tincture preparations of the fresh root as a primary ingredient in my bronchial formulas for many years, finding it to be a trustworthy remedy for acute and chronic respiratory problems, and even rare genetic lung conditions. Its ability to normalize body fluids benefits the lungs, the circulation of blood and lymphatic fluids, and all glandular secretions, including sweat glands that regulate perspiration. I always combine it with other herbs to treat specific conditions.

The only scientific research on *A. tuberosa* has been on the identification of its cardiac glycosides and other phytochemicals, and no clinical studies have been reported to date. This is unfortunate, considering the herb's amazing benefits to the lungs, but understandable since most herbal research occurs in Europe and Asia, and *A. tuberosa* is indigenous to North America, where clinical trials on herbs are rare.

Respiratory System: Pleurisy Root exerts a strong affinity with the respiratory system, and its tonic effect is specific for all types of acute or chronic bronchial and pulmonary complaints. It is a dependable remedy for lung and bronchial infections and inflammation, such as bronchitis, pneumonia, pleurisy, and influenza (flu). Historically, it was taken for whooping cough, typhus, scarlet fever, rheumatic fever, tuberculosis, measles, mumps, and chicken pox. The root reduces fevers and is an expectorant that breaks up excessive phlegm (catarrh) causing congestion, coughs, and colds. The root is beneficial for chronic lung weakness, asthma, emphysema, chronic coughs, and sore chest muscles causing painful breathing and coughing. *In vitro* studies have documented antimicrobial and antiseptic actions (Cheatham, 2000).

Pleurisy Root normalizes the lungs and bronchials by lubricating and moisturizing dry, congested lungs, or reducing excess phlegm in conditions of too much moisture. The herb acquired its common name because of its unique and specific action on the pleura of the lungs, which are the two layers of serous membranes lining the lungs and walls of the thoracic cavity. Serous membranes secrete serous fluid that lubricates and moisturizes tissues. Pleurisy or pleuritis occurs when pleural membranes become inflamed from infection or injury, resulting in cough, fever, chills, and painful, labored breathing. Pleurisy can cause an excess or deficiency of serous fluids, and the herb addresses both conditions. Because it normalizes fluid circulation in the lungs, Pleurisy Root is helpful for dry, irritating, unproductive coughs with chest tightness, and also for excessive mucous production and wet, productive coughs. The herb's normalizing influence on the serous membranes extends beyond the pleura of the lungs, and may also be beneficial for pericarditis (inflammation of the pericardium sac surrounding the heart), peritonitis (inflammation of the peritoneum tissue lining the inner wall of the abdomen and covering most of the abdominal organs), and bursitis (inflammation of bursae or small sacs of synovial fluid that are found throughout the body where muscles and tendons slide across bone). The American Eclectic physicians prescribed *A. tuberosa* for many respiratory ailments. Harvey Wickes Felter, M.D. (1865–1927) wrote:

> In acute chest diseases asclepias is useful to control cough, pain, temperature, to favor expectoration, and restore checked perspiration. When the cough is dry and there is scant bronchial secretion, asclepias stimulates the latter and thus relieves the irritation upon which the cough depends . . . . Asclepias is of the very greatest value in acute coryza [profuse mucous discharge from the nasal sinuses], la grippe [the flu], acute bronchitis, pleuro-pneumonia, and pneumonia, both catarrhal and croupous [the croup]. Its use should be begun early, usually in association with other agents sure to be indicated, and continued through the active stage; and if a dry cough persists it should still be continued and used freely. There is no kindlier cough medicine than asclepias, and when fever is present it is an ideal aid to the special sedatives. Asclepias should form an important part of the medication in acute pleurisy and pleurodynia [spasms and pain in the intercostal rib muscles], conditions in which it is most efficient and in which it first earned a therapeutic reputation. In pneumonia and in bronchitis asclepias is best adapted to the acute stage . . . (Felter, 1922)

For acute and chronic lung problems, restore balance and health to the respiratory system by taking Pleurisy Root tincture with other pectoral and antimicrobial herbs such as Astragalus (*Astragalus membranaceus*), Boneset (*Eupatorium perfoliatum*), Cayenne (*Capsicum annuum*), Elderberry (*Sambucus canadensis*), Elecampane (*Inula helenium*), Fenugreek (*Trigonella foenum-graecum*), Horehound (*Marrubium vulgare*), Mullein (*Verbascum thapsus*), and Thyme (*Thymus vulgaris*).

Cardiovascular System: *A. tuberosa* is a heart tonic that may be taken in small doses (20-30 drops of tincture daily) to improve heart function. Researchers have identified several cardiac glycosides in the roots that effect heart function (Abe, 2000; Warashina, 2009 & 2010). Cardiac glycosides are known to inhibit the sodium-potassium pump in cell membranes of the heart, resulting in increased concentrations of intercellular sodium and calcium and decreased potassium. This shift reduces electrical conduction within heart muscle to slow the heartbeat, produce more forceful contractions, and increase cardiac output (Cheatham, 2000; Yarnell, 2004). Cardiac glycosides also relax the muscular structure of the capillaries to dilate, allowing increased blood flow. These actions reduce tension in the cardiovascular system and strengthen cardiac muscle, making Pleurisy Root beneficial for treating cardiac insufficiency, palpitations, arrhythmia (abnormal heartbeat), tachycardia (rapid heartbeat), and hypertension. Be sure to use tincture prepared from freshly harvested roots for heart conditions because the potency of medicinal cardiac glycosides is greatly reduced after drying.

As the late herbalist and naturopath John Christopher emphasized, "Pleurisy Root influences the skin and circulation by relaxing the capillaries, thereby relieving the heart and arteries of undue tension, and stimulating a slow and steady perspiration of the sudoriferous glands, wherein the excessive heat due to congestion in the skin is gradually eased" (Christopher, 1976).

Normalizing Actions on Bodily Fluids: A classic use of this herb comes from its superb ability to normalize circulation and disperse fluid secretions throughout the body, which has a general tonic effect. Cardiac glycosides in Pleurisy Root demonstrate diuretic action by inhibiting the renin–angiotensin–aldosterone system that regulates blood pressure and water balance. The root moistens dry lungs and sinus cavities, and reduces and expels excess mucous in damp, wet conditions. The herb is an excellent diaphoretic that gradually increases skin temperature and promotes a slow, steady perspiration. This action reduces fevers and helps expel toxins from the interior of the body. This normalizing capacity has a harmonizing effect on skin secretions and perspiration by increasing moisture and perspiration in dry conditions, or by correcting the weakness that allows perspiration to pour out too freely. Used to reduce fevers by sweating, Pleurisy Root is a relaxing diaphoretic rather than stimulating, so the Eclectic physicians used it in cases of a full, congested pulse. They prescribed it to promote lymphatic drainage and treat pulmonary edema and conditions of excess catarrh (mucous). Eclectic physician William Cook, M.D., acknowledged:

> The root of this plant is probably one of the most reliable and serviceable relaxing diaphoretics in the whole Materia Medica. It diffuses itself with only moderate rapidity, but maintains its influence with considerable pertinacity. Its principal action is upon the sweat glands, at the same time that it relaxes the capillaries and thereby relieves the heart and arteries. It also exerts a decided impression upon the serous tissues, especially the pleurae and peritoneum; the mucous membranes of the lungs and bowels are also influenced by it; and its general action gives a peculiar and valuable relief to acute arterial and nervous excitements.
>
> The chief employment of this agent is in febrile and inflammatory afflictions, where the perspiration needs

to be decidedly promoted, and excitement of the heart relieved by a full outward determination of blood. It secures a slow, steady, and free perspiration, at the same time suitably diminishing excessive heat of the surface; which action renders it highly serviceable in typhus, scarlet, bilious, puerperal, lung, rheumatic, and other forms of fever, with a hot skin and rigid pulse. Measles and catarrhal fever may be added especially to this list; and so great is its service in pleurisy, that pleurisy root is one of the most popular of its names among the people. In acute dysentery, with fever and tormina, it secures that free circulation to the surface which affords great relief to the bowels; and in the acute stages of inflammation of the womb, bladder, and kidneys, it is of equal advantage. In all these cases its use is followed by not only an increased perspiration and softening of the pulse; but the action of the kidneys becomes better, the mucous surfaces act more firmly and naturally, and the nervous system obtains a soothing impression that is very desirable. (Cook, 1869)

Women's Health: Pleurisy Root restores the normal flow of fluids and resolves congestion in the pelvic area, making it helpful for suppressed menstruation, amenorrhea (abnormal cessation of menses), and dysmenorrhea (painful menses). *In vivo* animal studies show that it causes mild uterine contractions and has weak estrogenic effects (Costello, 1949; Hassan, 1952; Conway, 1979). **Pleurisy Root should not be used by pregnant and lactating women.**

Teachings from the Pleurisy Root Deva

"Welcome, dear one. I am the deva of the lovely Pleurisy plants. How beautiful the flowers – like swirling dancing skirts – attracting the bird and insect pollinators to fetch the tiny sparks of life within the pollen of my plants. The flowers are rich in sweet nectar, and the medicine of my roots provides fullness of breath and unbounded spaciousness. For such is the nature of air, my domain of healing.

"I am a being of movement and expansion. My plants are strengthened under the domain of Jupiter, the planet of outward expression and movement. My energies travel through the lungs clearing obstructions, nourishing and healing the cells, and maintaining balance between moisture and dryness. I help the lungs to receive the breath of life and to expel what is not needed.

"The shape of each tiny, orange flower resembles two lungs connected in the middle by the heart with a golden hue. For I also provide heart medicine, which is not dangerous, as some people warn, but works to support the lungs. The heart and lungs depend on each other for normal functioning, and although they are two distinct organs, they serve the one purpose of maintaining life. My medicine is safe to ingest because the substances in my plants blend and act together in harmonious ways. It is, as you would say, a dual effort to care for the lungs and heart together. Among all the members of the Milkweed tribe, my plants stand out and are unique in that they do not contain the white sap, which is toxic and bitter-tasting. This distinction is a sign to you that my medicine is safe. So use my plants as those before you have done; for they learned from the original inhabitants of this land once known as Turtle Island. Those people, so in tune with the earth and her plants, were told by the plants themselves how to be used for healing. The native people then taught the Europeans, and so the knowledge has passed on.

"In balancing and healing the heart and lungs, I harmonize the fire and air elements within the human body. Just as fire is contained and fed by air, so too, the heart depends on healthy lungs and requires the intake of oxygen and release of waste regulated by the lungs. Just as fire is extinguished without air, so too, the human heart extinguishes when the breath of life ceases.

"My orange-and-yellow flowers, the colors of fire, point to my affinity with this element. The heart is the core center of the human being. It rules and regulates the body and the unfolding of your life, more so than your brain. My essence, contained within my plants, brings balance to the heart, and with this comes harmony to the mind and to the thoughts projected from it. Within this harmony, where the struggle and conflict between polarities dissolves into calm abiding, is the experience of deep peace, beauty, light, and joy. My medicine assists you on your journey to return to this core, your birthright and essence of being.

"Sit quietly and breathe life-giving air and light into your lungs and blood and tissues. Do you feel the beating of your heart and the surging of blood through your body? It is a busy place of great activity within your body. I assist in this movement of air, blood, and other fluids and all the substances they contain. And if you wish to partake of my healing medicine, I will assist you in maintaining a calm and happy heart and healthy lungs as you journey through your life. The love and purity of my medicine will help you abide in the essence of your being. For the essence of devas and humans are the same. Live in balance and peace, dear one; for this is the way of happiness, health, and freedom."

Sage

Salvia officinalis
Labiatae (Lamiaceae) (Mint) Family

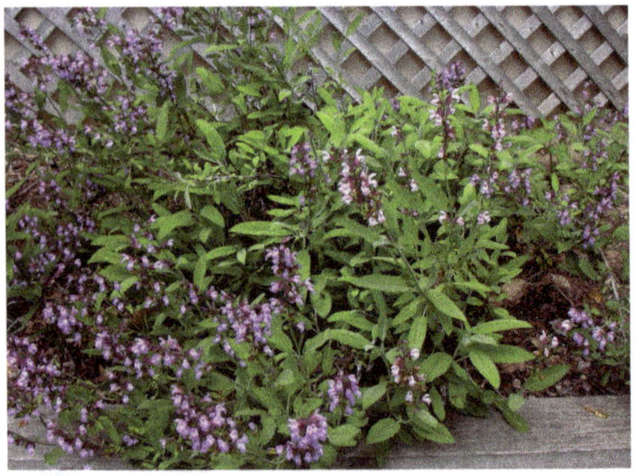

Common Names

Garden Sage, common Sage, true Sage, Dalmatian Sage, meadow Sage, and broad-leafed white Sage are common names of *Salvia officinalis.*

Medicinal Part of the Plant

The leaves and flowers are used medicinally.

Range and Habitat

Sage is native to the Mediterranean region. It is a popular and widely cultivated herb that has naturalized in temperate zones throughout the world, including North America. *Salvia* is a large genus of the Mint family containing hundreds of species. *S. officinalis* is a popular species in Western herbalism, although it varies in markings and color. Many other *Salvia* species are used medicinally, such as *Salvia lavandulifolia* (Spanish Sage), which is popular because it contains less thujone than other species.

Description of the Plant

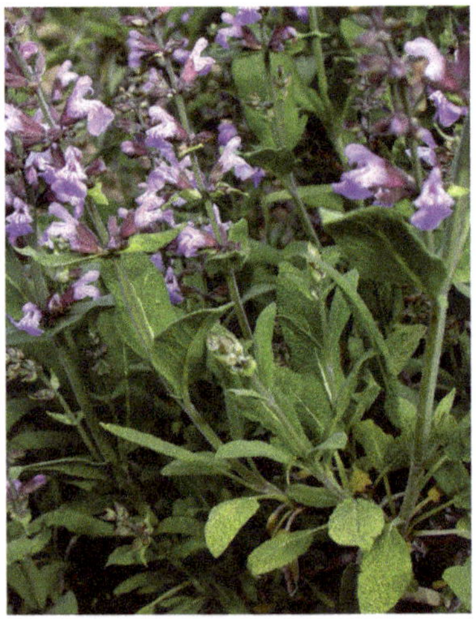

S. officinalis is a hardy, aromatic perennial growing 1-3′ tall. Several erect stalks arise from the fibrous roots and are characteristically square like all stems in the Mint family. After 3-4 years of growth, the lower main stalks become woody and rounded, and many smaller square stems grow opposite each other off the main stalks.

The simple, petiole leaves are lance-shaped, growing 1-4″ long and emerging opposite each other along the stems. The leaves have a pinnate vein pattern, a rugose (rough) texture, and a wrinkled appearance created by fine networks of tiny veins. Leaf margins are lined with miniature crenate (rounded) indentations. Oil glands underneath the leaves emit the pungent fragrance. Both leaves and stems are a light grayish-green color and are covered with very fine, silver-grey, wooly down. Leaves tend to be grayer during dry seasons and greener with wet weather.

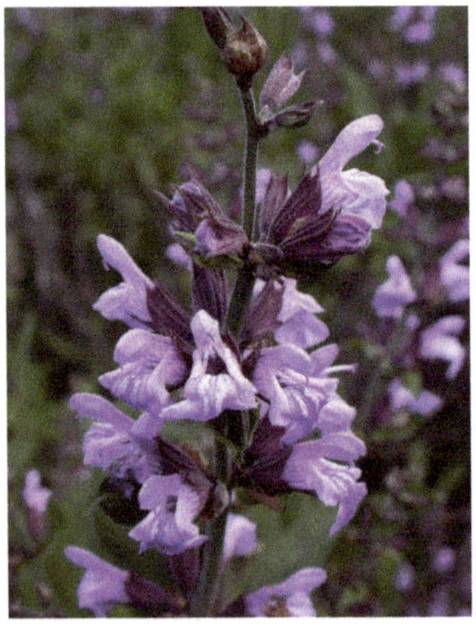

Flowers grow in loose racemes of whorled clusters along the upper stems, and there are usually 3-6 flowers in each whorl. Growing ½-1″ in length, flowers are typically bluish purple, but occasionally appear in shades of pink or white. Each flower has a trumpet-shaped calyx and corolla with a small, curving upper lip and larger, bi-lobed lower lip. Members of the genus *Salvia* typically have 2 stamens. As flowers mature and the corolla withers and falls off, the cup-like calyx holds 1-4 round seeds that eventually turn black and drop to the ground when dry.

The herb flowers from May to July. When a large patch of Sage plants blooms, it has an amazingly etheric, cloud-like appearance. It is a beautiful sight and one of my favorite times to be in the garden!

Cultivation

Sage will tolerate infertile and dry soil, but it thrives best in fairly rich, moist soil that is sandy, aerated, well drained, and contains lime and ample amounts of humus. Plants grown in full sun produce more of the medicinal, aromatic volatile oils.

The herb is propagated from seed and by stem layering, although most people propagate from seed. A period of cold, moist conditioning (stratification) improves germination, so seeds can be planted in autumn, allowing natural cold conditioning through winter months, or very early in spring while temperatures continue to drop to freezing. Seeds may also be artificially conditioned by putting them in a small plastic bag with a little moist sand and refrigerate (33-38˚F) for a week, followed by a week at room temperature. Alternate this schedule for several weeks. Sow seeds in planting trays or directly into a garden bed. They usually germinate within 3 weeks when soil temperature reaches 60-70°F. Space plants 1½-2′ apart and keep them mulched with grass clippings. Seedlings grow slowly, initially requiring plenty of moisture, and become drought resistant with maturity.

To propagate by layering, lay side stems of established plants on the ground, bury middle portions of stems under 1-1½" of soil, holding them down with a stake while the stem tip remains above ground. The buried section of the stem will eventually sprout roots and may be cut from its parent to be replanted.

Sage plants can live for several years. The lower stems eventually become woody but continue to produce flowers. Protect plants during cold winter freezes by applying plenty of mulch.

Harvest

Prune the upper 5-7" of the leafy stems before or when the flowers start blooming during June and July. Stems can be cut above the woody growth, but be sure to leave at least two green nodes that will sprout new leaves. In mature plants, 2-3 cuttings may be harvested each growing season, but allow plants to produce flowers towards the end of each season. Flowers can also be harvested with the leaves and used for medicine.

The round seeds are easy to harvest. Keep watch as the flowers fade and little green seeds develop inside the cup-shaped calyx. Collect the seeds when they turn black, but before they drop to the ground.

Preparation of Plant Medicine and Dosages

Freshly harvested leaves and flowers are prepared as tea, tincture, oil, salve, or dried for future use. The leaves tend to discolor and blacken if they are not used or dried quickly. Preparations made from freshly harvested leaves make noticeably more potent remedies than from older dried material, which lacks the full potency of the medicinal volatile oils. The dried plant is ground into powder to make pills and capsules.

Caution: Concerning dosages and length of use, remember that Sage contains thujone, which becomes toxic if taken in large doses over an extended period of time. Sage tea contains less thujone than alcohol-based tinctures and essential oil preparations because thujone does not extract well in water. Be sure to follow the recommended dosages, especially when using oil and alcohol preparations.

PREPARATIONS

Infusion: Steep 1-2 teaspoons of fresh or dried leaves with flowers in 1 cup of boiled water. Dosage: 1-3 cups a day as needed. Higher dosages should not be taken for more than a week. Smaller dosages can be used for 3-4 weeks and then discontinued for a month. The strong tea is bitter-tasting.

Tincture: Chop fresh leaves and flowers into small pieces, stuff them into a glass jar, and cover with 75% 190-proof grain alcohol and 25% distilled water. Dosage: 10-40 drops in ½ cup of water up to 4 times a day as needed.

Pills and Capsules: Prepare from dried leaves and flowers. Dosage: 1-4 grams taken1-3 times a day.

Oil and Salve: Combine the leaves and flowers with other vulnerary herbs to produce an excellent oil and salve for external problems. Bake herbs in olive oil and add beeswax by the standard method.

Distilled Essential Oil: Use cautiously due to greater amounts of potentially toxic thujone. Dosage: The German Commission E herbal regulatory agency recommended an adult dose of only 1 drop of volatile oil in a cup of water no more than 3 times a day. Do not exceed this dose, and limit consumption to 2 weeks or less each month. Young children should not use the essential oil.

Smoking Mixture: Sage leaves can be dried and enjoyed in a smoking mixture. The leaves produce a pleasantly mild smoke that dries sinus drainage and is a safe alternative to smoking Tobacco.

Smudging: This is an ancient practice in which different species of Sage leaves are dried and burned to produce fragrant smoke that purifies people, objects, and places like the home, birthing-bed, gardens, and places of worship and ceremony. Smudging was practiced by many indigenous people worldwide and continues to be used for cleansing rituals in modern times.

Culinary Uses

Sage is a popular flavoring herb and is particularly beneficial for its antioxidant action that preserves food. The leaves are a traditional seasoning for meats, turkey stuffing, soups, and vegetables.

Chemical Constituents

Sage contains volatile oils (1-2.5%) with anti-inflammatory, antispasmodic, antibacterial, and antioxidant properties. Thujone, one of the most important oils, is most concentrated in alcohol and essential oil extract preparations. Thujone is a neurotoxin when taken in large doses over extended periods of time, causing tachycardia (rapid heartbeat), hot flashes, dizziness, hallucinations, and convulsions. When taken in therapeutic doses, it acts as an antimicrobial, vermifuge, and emmenagogue. Other constituents in the volatile oil include borneol (analgesic, anti-candida, choleretic, febrifuge, hepatoprotective), pinene (antiviral, expectorant, anti-acetylcholinesterase), camphor (analgesic, carminative, decongestant, expectorant, fungicide), cineol (analgesic, antifungal, anti-staphylococcal, anti-acetylcholinesterase, choleretic, decongestant, vermifuge), humulene (antitumor), limonene (expectorant), caryophyllene, and terpineol (anti-allergenic, anti-asthmatic, antitussive, cholagogue, expectorant).

Beta-sitosterol, an estrogenic phytosterol, is hepatoprotective and antitumor for the breast, lungs, and cervix. Tannins are astringent, antibacterial, and anti-inflammatory. Diterpenoid bitters include carnosol (antibiotic, anticancer, anti-HIV, antioxidant, anti-inflammatory, fungicide, hepatoprotective), carnosolic acid (antioxidant, hepatoprotective), and rosmanol (antioxidant, hepatoprotective, and cancer preventative).

Phenolic acids include rosmarinic acid (anti-allergenic, anti-atherosclerotic, anti-inflammatory, antimicrobial, antioxidant, hepatoprotective, immunostimulant), caffeic acid (analgesic, antibacterial, anticarcinogenic, antiviral, antihistamine, anti-staphylococcic, cholagogue), chlorogenic acid (immunostimulant), labiatic acid (antioxidant), ferulic acid (analgesic, anti-allergenic, anti-arrhythmia, anticancer, antispasmodic, antiviral, cholagogue, hepatoprotective), and gallic acid (anti-allergenic, anti-asthmatic, antibronchitic, anti-staphylococcic, antiviral, and choleretic).

Several flavonoids in the plant are anti-inflammatory and antioxidant, including quercetin (anti-allergenic), apigenin (anti-arrhythmic, antibacterial, antihistamine, anti-inflammatory COX-2 inhibitor, antispasmodic, antitumor, antiviral, estrogenic, MAO-inhibitor, vasodilator), salvigenin, genkwanin (antibacterial), hispidulin (anticancer, hepatoprotective) and luteolin (anti-inflammatory, antitussive, antispasm, antitumor, choleretic, estrogenic, vasodilator). Sage contains salicylic acid, an analgesic and anti-inflammatory COX-2 inhibitor.

Nutrients in the leaves include calcium, boron (improves calcium absorption into bone), iron, phosphorus, magnesium, manganese, zinc, chromium, selenium, silica, beta-carotene (plant form of vitamin A), ascorbic acid (vitamin C), riboflavin (vitamin B2), niacin (vitamin B3), and pantothenic acid (vitamin B5).

Safety, Contraindications, and Drug Interactions

Sage is safe to consume in recommended moderate doses, but larger amounts are not advised. When taken in large amounts for an extended period of time, alcohol and volatile oil extracts containing thujone may cause dizziness, hot flashes, rapid heartbeat, and convulsions. Since the distilled essential oil of Sage contains greater concentrations of thujone, it must be used cautiously in small amounts of one drop diluted in water when ingested, and is not appropriate for children or the elderly. When applying the essential oil topically, always dilute it with a vegetable oil. Sage may worsen stomach-esophageal reflux in some people, and should be used cautiously in small doses by people with seizure disorders due to the thujone content. Sage is an emmenagogue that stimulates uterine contractions and is **contraindicated during pregnancy**. **Nursing mothers should avoid** the herb because its astringent action dries up breast milk. There are no known drug interactions (McGuffin, 1997; Blumenthal, 1998).

Medicinal Uses

History of the Plant

Sage is one of the most esteemed and popular medicinal plants used for culinary and medicinal purposes over thousands of years. Its strong, aromatic fragrance and beautiful flowers enticed ancient people to explore the properties of this herb. Many cultures and healing traditions have regarded Sage as a panacea for all ailments of body and mind. Its genus name *Salvia* comes from the Latin word *salvare,* meaning "to heal or save." The species name *officinalis* designates Sage as a historically official medicine.

The leaves have traditionally been employed to treat indigestion, colds, flu, fevers, sore mouth and throat, excessive menstrual bleeding, and to wean babies off breast milk. Leaves were prepared as a poultice and applied to sprains, swellings, ulcers, bleeding wounds, and arthritic joints. Ancient Egyptians ingested it to increase fertility. The Greeks and Romans added Sage leaves to meat, fish, and other food as a preservative. The Greek physician Dioscorides (*circa* A.D. 40–*c.* 90) employed it as a diuretic "to move ye urine and ye menstrua," as a remedy for coughs and hoarseness, and applied the leaves as a poultice to wounds and ulcers. Pliny the Elder (A.D. 23–79) wrote that it "cureth stinging and biting serpents" and prescribed it to improve memory, kill intestinal worms, promote menstruation, and treat sore throats, lung ailments, and epilepsy.

In medieval Europe, Sage was venerated as a sacred plant capable of increasing life span and was used as a general tonic for the entire body, including the brain and memory. In his 1633 book, *The Herball or Generall Historie of Plantes,* John Gerard mentioned it as a well-known herb in English gardens and medicine. He wrote, "Sage is singularly good for the head and brain, it quickeneth the senses and memory, strengtheneth the sinews [tendons], restoreth health to those that have the palsy [paralysis] from a moist cause, and taketh away shaking or trembling of the members; and being put up into the nostrils, it draweth thin phlegm out of the head." The British apothecary Nicholas Culpeper (1616–1654) wrote that Sage is ruled by Jupiter, and he recommended the leaves for liver disease, restoring memory, as a gargle for sore throats, and to treat epidemic plagues that swept across Europe. Ancient trade routes took *S. officinalis* east into Asia, where it was introduced and incorporated into Unani medicine of the Islamic world, Chinese herbalism, and India's Ayurvedic medical system.

When Europeans arrived in North America, the Native Americans were using indigenous species of Sage as seasoning, medicine, and in smoking mixtures. In a practice known as smudging, dried Sage leaves were burned during ceremonies and cleansing rituals, allowing the smoke to purify people, objects, and the environment. The European species of Sage was introduced to the Native Americans when European colonists settled in the new land and grew *S. officinalis* in their gardens, where it escaped cultivation to naturalize. During the late 1800s and early 1900s, the Eclectic physicians prescribed Sage in their herbal-based medical practice for sore, ulcerated throats, flatulence, excessive perspiration, fevers, parasites, to decrease the flow of breast milk in mothers weaning their babies, and as a poultice to treat arthritis. *S. officinalis* was listed as an official drug in the *U.S. Pharmacopoeia* from 1840–1900.

Modern applications of Sage are substantiated by its long history of use by many different cultures, clinical data from practicing clinical herbalists, and modern research studies. It continues to be cultivated in temperate regions throughout the world and is a popular herb found in many foods, medicinal remedies, and hair and other health care products.

Healing Qualities

Antibacterial, anti-catarrhal, antifungal, antihydrotic (reduces excessive perspiration), anti-inflammatory, antimicrobial, antioxidant, antiseptic, antispasmodic, antiviral, astringent, carminative, cholagogue, diaphoretic, emmenagogue, expectorant, febrifuge, hepatoprotective, immunomodulator, lactifuge, nervine, stimulant, tonic for nerve and endocrine systems, vermifuge, and vulnerary.

Traditional Chinese Medicine (TCM)

Salvia miltiorrhiza, known as Dan Shen, is the species commonly used in TCM. It was mentioned in the ancient herbal classic, *Shen Nong Ben Cao Jing*. Dan Shen and *S. officinalis* are Yang herbs with warming, drying, and stimulating actions that specifically benefit the brain, lungs, stomach, intestines, and uterus. While they invigorate a weak, depleted nervous system, they can also relax overstimulated nerves and ease muscle spasms. Both species resolve excessive dampness and congestion due to Spleen and Lung Qi deficiency, manifesting as excessive perspiration and mucous production. They are specific for deficient Yin syndromes that also cause excessive sweating. Congested Qi can result in lung congestion, painful cramps and spasms, and delayed menstrual periods. By stimulating the movement of Qi, Sage helps to resolve these issues. As a Qi and Essence tonic, it energizes, tones, and restores the whole system, including the nerves, brain, and endocrine glands.

Primary Actions

Sage is a wonderful multi-purpose healer. Its rejuvenating properties benefit mental clarity and cognition and the nervous and endocrine systems responsible for regulating all functions of the body. I have used the tea and tincture as an antimicrobial for bronchial, intestinal, and urinary tract infections with great success. The herb promotes healthy digestion, reduces spasms, and is a powerful anti-inflammatory. Sage is an excellent vulnerary that I have added to my herbal healing salve for many years.

The herb exerts a drying effect and can be combined with moisturizing herbs like Marshmallow (*Althaea officinalis*) or Chickweed (*Stellaria media*) when used by people with dry constitutions or dry, irritated tissues.

Herbalists in North America and Europe currently use *S. officinalis* as an antihydrotic to reduce abnormally excessive perspiration and menopausal hot flashes, for treating upper respiratory tract infections, sore throats, mouth and gum sores and ulcers, nervous exhaustion, weak immunity, and to improve poor memory and cognitive function.

The Nervous System, Brain, and Memory: *S. officinalis* is an excellent nervine to help restore and revitalize a debilitated nervous system. The nervine qualities gently stimulate the system to sharpen the mind and improve cognitive function. Strong antioxidants in the leaves protect cells from damage and retard their age-related deterioration. Enhancing general strength and vitality, Sage is specific for cognitive decline and cerebral and nervous system "burn-out." Its beneficial effects on the cortex of the brain enhance memory and concentration. When ingested in small doses, the tea and tincture are tonics for fatigue, nervous exhaustion, and poor cognitive function and memory.

> *A wise person is called a Sage.*
>
> *Sage plants are good medicine for sharp brain function and memory.*

While Sage is not a sedating herb, its restorative nervine action elicits calming actions on the heart, mind, and emotions. The muscular structure of blood vessels relaxes under its influence, which increases circulation to promote warmth throughout the body.

The herb is beneficial for nervous conditions resulting from depletion and exhaustion, such as anxiety, trembling, depression, vertigo (dizziness), and hypersensitivity. It is a helpful remedy for nervous headaches, especially when combined with Rosemary (*Rosmarinus officinalis*), Wood Betony (*Stachys officinalis*), and Peppermint (*Mentha x piperita*). Ayurvedic physicians combine Sage with Gotu Kola (*Centella asiatica*) for nerve and brain disorders.

Modern researchers have discovered that Sage benefits the brain and body because it increases acetylcholine levels. Acetylcholine is an important neurotransmitter found in the peripheral and central nervous systems, as well as in the cardiovascular and neuromuscular systems. It relaxes cardiac muscle to reduce rapid heart rate. While acetylcholine activates muscle movement and primarily produces excitatory responses in the peripheral nervous system, it is a neuromodulator in the central nervous system. As a neuromodulator, acetylcholine enhances brain function by improving sensory perception, helping sustain attention, and promoting the functions of learning and memory.

British researchers conducting *in vitro* tests found that *S. officinalis* and *S. lavandulifolia* (Spanish Sage) increase acetylcholine levels by inhibiting the enzyme acetylcholinesterase, which normally breaks down and reduces acetylcholine levels. A test in which *S. lavandulifolia* oil was given to rats once a day for 5 days confirmed that the oil increased their acetylcholine levels. The volatile oils also provided antioxidant protection, and inflammatory leukotrienes were inhibited by Sage (Perry, 1996, 2000, 2001, & 2002).

Several clinical trials have confirmed the ability of *S. officinalis* and *S. lavandulifolia* to improve cognitive function. A placebo-controlled study involving 44 healthy adults assessed the cognitive effects of a standardized extract of *S. lavandulifolia* given in 3 separate doses. Results determined by immediate and delayed word recall scores showed that Sage improved memory, mental acuity, and promoted calm moods (Tildesley, 2003).

A clinical study involving 30 healthy participants measured the mood and cognitive effects of 300 mg and 600 mg of dried *S. officinalis* leaves compared to a placebo. Testing was run on 3 separate days done 7 days apart. Both doses of Sage improved ratings of mood, with the lower dose reducing anxiety and the higher dose increasing levels of alertness and calmness (Kennedy, 2006).

In another study investigating the effects of a standardized extract of *S. officinalis* on cognitive performance in older adults, researchers gave 20 healthy volunteers, averaging 73 years of age, 4 different doses of the extract and a placebo. While the placebo did not elicit any improvement, 333 mg of the Sage extract demonstrated significant enhanced memory performance and accuracy of attention in the volunteers (Scholey, 2008).

Alzheimer's Disease: Nerve damage from oxidative stress, inflammation, and low levels of acetylcholine are common findings in people with Alzheimer's disease. Some neurodegenerative diseases, including Alzheimer's disease, dementia and memory loss, involve damage to the acetylcholine-producing cells in the brain. The resulting reduction in acetylcholine is believed to contribute to cognitive and memory impairments. To improve acetylcholine activity, cholinesterase inhibitors are usually prescribed by physicians. These drugs block the actions of acetylcholinesterase (the enzyme that breaks down acetylcholine) to increase levels of acetylcholine.

The use of Sage as a treatment for Alzheimer's disease has been the focus of several studies. The objective of one study was to assess the efficacy and safety of a *S. officinalis* extract in 42 patients diagnosed with mild to moderate Alzheimer's disease. This was a placebo-controlled trial in which half of the participants took 60 drops of the extract every day for 4 months and the other half received a placebo. After 4 months, the *S. officinalis* extract produced significantly better outcomes on cognitive functions than the placebo. There were no differences in side effects except that the placebo group experienced more agitation (Akhondzadeh, 2003).

The Adrenals, Pituitary, and Ovaries: Essential oils in Sage leaves vitalize, enhance, and synchronize the normal function of these endocrine glands to benefit brain function and cognition, the nervous system and calm moods, reproductive hormones, and general health (Durrafourd, 1982).

Anti-inflammatory Actions: Several constituents in Sage, such as luteolin, rosmarinic acid, quercetin and apigenin, exhibit strong anti-inflammatory activity. *In vitro* studies show that extracts of Sage reduce tissue inflammation by several mechanisms, including the ability to 1) decrease pro-inflammatory interleukin-6; 2) inhibit the release of tumor necrosis factor involved in systemic inflammation; 3) inhibit formation of pro-inflammatory leukotrienes; 4) increase the anti-inflammatory cytokine interleukin-10; and 5) reduce COX-2, an enzyme that increases during inflammation (Vogl, 2013).

Infections and the Respiratory System: The antimicrobial, anti-inflammatory, and antispasmodic phytochemicals in Sage leaves are an excellent remedy for fevers, the common cold, pneumonia and other bronchial infections, and the flu (influenza), an acute viral infection in the respiratory tract accompanied by fever, cold symptoms, cough, sore throat, and body aches. Expectorant actions help loosen and expel mucous from the lungs, while the astringent effects of tannins decrease excessive mucous secretions from the nasal sinuses and lungs. The leaves may be ingested hot as a tea or tincture for these problems.

Sage is a classic remedy for inflamed and infected sore throats, laryngitis, and tonsillitis. A gargle made from the strong tea works best used alone, but honey may be added for children and others with more sensitive taste buds. The tea is prepared as a nasal spray to reduce infection, congestion, and inflammation of chronic or acute sinusitis, and is especially effective when combined with Goldenseal (*Hydrastis canadensis*) tea. For the annoying symptoms of hay fever, smoking dried Sage leaves reduces excessive mucous drainage for up to three hours. Sage is a pleasantly mild smoking herb, especially nice when combined with the dried leaves of Mullein (*Verbascum thapsus*).

Inhaling steam vapors from a pot of hot Sage tea breaks up sinus and bronchial congestion and eases coughing. Put a big towel over your head while bending over the pot of steaming tea so the vapors are trapped and easily inhaled. When consuming Sage, remember that it has a drying effect on the tissues and mucous membranes, so it should not be used alone for dry coughs. Combining it with a moisturizing herb like Marshmallow root (*Althaea officinalis*) balances out the drying tendency.

Sage helps regulate immune activity. A group of water-soluble polysaccharides isolated from *S. officinalis* leaves by cold water extraction have demonstrated this immunomodulatory activity in research studies (Capek, 2004). Many pharmacological tests have identified antibacterial, antifungal, and antiviral constituents in the herb. Sage attacks Staphylococcal infections that often cause sinusitis (Masterova, 1996). *In vitro* tests reveal its antibacterial activity against *Streptococcus pyogenes* (causing sore throat, scarlet fever, and kidney infections), *Staphylococcus aureus* (provoking a wide range of skin, respiratory, and systemic infections) (Caceres, 1991), *Escherichia coli* (causing urinary tract infections and diarrhea), *Shigella sonnei* (causing dysentery), *Salmonella* species (responsible for typhoid fever and gastroenteritis), *Klebsiella ozanae* (causing intestinal infections), and *Bacillus subtilis* (responsible for the eye infection known as conjunctivitis) (Recio, 1989).

Researchers have explored the efficacy and tolerability of a nasal spray containing 15% *S. officinalis* extract against a placebo in the treatment of 286 patients with acute viral pharyngitis. The 3-day treatment revealed a significant reduction in throat pain within the first 2 hours after administration in those taking the Sage nasal spray (Hubbert, 2006). Other research demonstrates the ability of water and alcohol extracts of *S. officinalis* to destroy the *Herpes simplex* virus type 1 and 2. *In vitro* studies showed that both extracts exerted strong antiviral activity, although the alcohol extract had a much stronger activity than the water-based tea (Schnitzler, 2008).

Gastrointestinal Tract: Sage is an excellent support and remedy for the digestive system. The volatile oils reduce inflammation and are soothing to the mucous membranes lining the esophagus, stomach, and intestines. By exerting a relaxing effect on smooth muscles, volatile oils ease spasms and colic, stimulate secretions of digestive enzymes to enhance digestion, and allow the smooth movement of food. As a carminative, Sage alleviates gas and bloating in the stomach and intestines, and is used to treat indigestion, nausea, diarrhea, colitis, liver complaints, and a sluggish, atonic gastrointestinal tract. The astringent tannins tone intestinal membranes to reduce diarrhea and bleeding. Improving the diet and using Sage tea or tincture reduces halitosis (bad breath).

Thujone and other antibiotic and anti-inflammatory constituents in the herb effectively treat gastrointestinal infections, including *Heliobacter pylori* (a bacterial cause of stomach ulcers), dysentery, gastritis (stomach inflammation), and enteritis (inflammation and microbial infection of the intestines). Combined with other vermifuge herbs and food-grade diatomaceous earth, Sage helps expel intestinal parasites. A tea is used as a gargle for gingivitis (gum inflammation and infection), glossitis (inflamed tongue), stomatitis (generalized mouth inflammation), mouth ulcers called canker sores, and other mouth lacerations.

Liver and Pancreas: Sage is a liver tonic that stimulates sluggish liver and gallbladder activity. Its cholagogue action promotes bile production in the liver and bile secretion from the gallbladder into the small intestine to break down fats. This enhances complete digestion, daily bowel movements, and normal blood levels of cholesterol.

Several phytochemicals in Sage leaves have hepatoprotective activity. Researchers have designed a test to demonstrate the herb's ability to protect the liver against toxicity induced by azathioprine, an immunosuppressive drug. Animals pretreated with water extracts of the leaves did not experience liver necrosis (tissue death) or changes in cellular structure and function following azathioprine administration (Amin, 2005). Another study showed that Sage tea exerted strong antioxidant effects in the livers of rats when their water was replaced with Sage tea for 14 days. Results were determined by liver enzyme analysis and confirmation of biological safety (Lima, 2005).

Sage also benefits the pancreas and helps manage diabetes. Research has shown that the tea can promote significant reduction of blood sugar levels in people with diabetes (Berger, 1950). In a laboratory test involving diabetic rats, alcohol extracts of the leaves significantly decreased their serum glucose within 3 hours without increasing insulin release from the pancreas. The Sage extract did not have this effect in healthy rats. Although Sage was given as an injection, which is not the traditional route of administration, the data indicates that the herb exerts hypoglycemic effects in diabetes (Eidi, 2005).

An interesting clinical study examined the efficacy and safety of a *S. officinalis* leaf extract for the treatment of 40 patients diagnosed with hyperlipidemia (elevated fats, cholesterol, and/or triglycerides) and diabetes type 2 (adult onset). Half of the patients took the Sage extract in a 500 mg capsule 3 times daily for 3 months, while the remaining group received a placebo. The Sage extract successfully lowered fasting glucose levels, HA1c (a blood test measuring glycated hemoglobin to assess blood sugar levels), total cholesterol, triglycerides, and LDL (low density lipoproteins). Beneficial HDL (high density lipoproteins) levels increased. No adverse effects were reported (Kianbakht, 2013).

Another study involving 80 patients with diabetes type 2 documented that those taking *S. officinalis* tablets 3 times a day for 3 months experienced a significant reduction in blood sugar and cholesterol blood levels compared to the placebo group (Behradmanesh, 2013).

Bladder and Kidney Infections: Sage is an excellent herb for bladder and kidney inflammation and infections, including cystitis. The tea or tincture eases spasms, and the astringent actions are beneficial to treat cases of bloody urine. One *in vitro* study assessed the effect of *S. officinalis* oil on bacterial strains derived from 100 urine samples taken from people diagnosed with urinary tract infections. The oil demonstrated 100% efficiency against *Klebsiella* and *Enterobacter* species, 96% against *Escherichia coli*, 83% against *Proteus mirabilis*, and 75% against *Morganella morganii* (Pereira, 2004).

Excessive Perspiration, Hot Flashes, and Weaning Nursing Babies: Sage leaves have a normalizing effect on the skin and glandular secretions. The herb is a strong antihydrotic with astringent and drying actions that have historically been used to decrease abnormally profuse perspiration, known as hyperhydrosis. It is a well-known lactifuge, and the cold tea is taken to reduce production of breast milk when nursing mothers want to wean babies. Sage has also been employed to control hot flashes and night sweats occurring during menopause and in diseases like tuberculosis.

Sage preparations must be taken cold to diminish glandular secretions of fluids, including saliva, sweat, and breast milk. When using tincture, at least 20-30 drops taken 3 times a day are needed to reduce perspiration, and it should be added to cold water.

Studies on Sage tea and tincture dating back to 1896 demonstrate that constituents in the volatile oils suppress perspiration. Later experiments confirmed a 50% decrease in perspiration with maximum effects lasting about two hours after ingestion. Sage is recognized as standard treatment for profuse perspiration and menopausal hot flashes and night sweats in Germany, where a preparation of the oils called Salvysat is marketed as an antihydrotic (Tyler, 1993). Also helpful for men, a revealing study showed that Sage safely and effectively controlled hot flashes in 10 prostate cancer patients treated with androgen deprivation therapy. This is a standard treatment for prostate cancer that reduces testosterone levels, but causes debilitating hot flashes in men. The 10 patients consumed 150 mg of *S. officinalis* extract 3 times daily over a 3-week period without any side effects. Their hot flashes diminished significantly during the 3 weeks of herbal therapy, and continued to be controlled during medical treatment (Vandecasteele, 2012).

Women's Health: Beta-sitosterol and luteolin are phytoestrogens found in Sage leaves that have estrogen-like activity which helps balance hormone levels and regulate the female reproductive system (Rahte, 2013). The herb is recommended for amenorrhea (abnormal cessation of menses) and infertility. Sage exerts a tonic effect on the uterus by toning weak muscles.

For menstruating women, Sage is an emmenagogue with stimulating influence on the uterus that promotes menstruation and initiates delayed menstruation. The herb reduces menstrual cramping and excessive bleeding. All species of Sage are **contraindicated during pregnancy** due to the emmenagogue actions and thujone content.

Sage is a reliable ally for menopausal women due to its phytoestrogen content and antihydrotic properties that reduce the excessive perspiration of hot flashes. I combine equal parts *S. officinalis*, Blue Vervain (*Verbena hastata*), and Black Cohosh (*Cimicifuga racemosa*) for women having hot flashes and night sweats, and have heard countless success stories from many of these women.

An Italian study involving 30 menopausal women suffering from hot flashes, insomnia, dizziness, headaches, and heart palpitations documented that an extract of Sage and Alfalfa leaves (*Medicago sativa*) resulted in significant improvement of symptoms. Hot flashes completely disappeared in 20 of the women, while four women showed good improvement and the other six showed a reduction in symptoms (De Leo, 1998). Another trial assessed the efficacy of a fresh Sage preparation in treating hot flashes and other menopausal complaints in 71 menopausal women having at least five hot flashes a day. A daily tablet of fresh Sage leaves was given for 8 weeks and was very well tolerated. There was a significant decline in the intensity of hot flashes by 50% of the women within 4 weeks and by 64% within 8 weeks. The number of mild, moderate, severe, and very severe hot flashes decreased by 46%, 62%, 79%, and 100% respectively (Bommer, 2011).

Antibacterial and antifungal properties of Sage are helpful for vaginal infections and discharges, including Candida yeast. For these problems, the tea or tincture should be ingested and the tea also used as a douche. The leaves may be combined with other appropriate herbs to make vaginal suppositories. Astringent tannins in Sage are helpful for the treatment of bleeding fibroids.

External Applications for Wounds and Bleeding: The antiseptic and antifungal constituents in the leaves reduce infections and heal wounds, skin ulcers, and all types of sores. Volatile oils that ease inflammation and pain help relieve sore muscles, arthritic joint pain, and carpal tunnel pain in the wrists. The astringent tannins reduce external and internal bleeding and bruises. The herb is reputed to be a hair tonic that stimulates hair growth, eliminates dandruff, and helps keep hair from turning gray. Apply Sage as a wash, poultice, oil, salve, or liniment for external problems. Ingesting the tea or tincture is also helpful.

Teachings from the Sage Deva

"Greetings, dear one. I am the deva of the Sage. There are many different plants in my tribe, and I will speak to you of the one you use for medicine and call Garden Sage. This plant balances the elements of fire, air, and water in the human body. My energy is initially stimulating, moving, expansive, balancing, and finally restoring and calming; my influence works on the cells and tissues in that order. My plants are under Jupiter's domain, the planet of expansive movement, and are influenced by Sagittarius, the sign of the archer who takes aim with intention and direction.

"Held within this plant, my stimulating energies are balancing and restoring to the human body. My medicine integrates and restores all parts of the body into light-filled wholeness. The bluish-purple color of my flowers is a signature of my beneficial influence and affinity with the nerves and glands of the endocrine system. And so I balance and restore these great regulators of your body. To feel into my essence, you are invited to sit in a patch of my blooming plants, to rest in the cooling, relaxing bluish-green light within my leaves, and to experience your mind's freedom in the great expanse radiating from the brilliant sky-blue radiance of my flowers. Let yourself relax and be held within the gentle, caring arms of my plants.

"My healing power within the plants is strong and it can permeate through your tissues. The oils are the strength behind my movement through the body. My plants control and regulate the waterways, especially at the level of the skin, where the body interacts with air. For I regulate and normalize the amount of fluid that passes through the skin pores. When an excess of fluids comes out through the pores, my medicine tightens and shuts them down, like turning off a leaky faucet. When doing this, I also help maintain correct temperature for human bodies. If there is too much heat from within, a cold tea or other preparation of my leaves will cool the body. But if coolness pervades the tissues, my medicine should be taken hot and it will allow more blood to flow and warm the outer body.

"My balancing and restoring energies also keep the digestive channels and air passages open, adjusting for optimal movement of food, air, and gases. My balancing and restorative energies are especially beneficial to the nerves and endocrine glands, and instill a deep support of calm that influences the mind and emotional experience of humans. The power of my medicine protects and preserves the cells of the nerves and restores them to function to their capacity to serve your needs. Ingesting my flowers and leaves calms the mind and emotions while also sharpening mental acuity, thought processes, and recall or memories, as you would say. A mind that is clear and awake has no limit of vision or perception, and my flowers are especially helpful to open the mind beyond its normal boundaries and programmed perceptions of 'self' and reality.

"The offering of my flowers is for the visionary, one with calm, clear mind and heart, who rests in balance and equilibrium, no longer pulled by polarities of good or bad, big or small, beautiful or ugly, me or you. For within this space of equilibrium is the twilight between the worlds of form and formlessness, where the mind and its thoughts are unhindered and freely move without confinement to these polarized points of reference. In this space, great awakenings are born and visions arise. This is a sacred space – accessible to all – a part of all of us, deva and human alike. So claim your birthright and partake of the gifts of my plants to assist you on this journey. It is a journey into the fully illuminated light of your own being, which is the being of all. My plants offer health and blessings on your journey. Be in peace and brilliance, dear one!"

Saint John's Wort

Hypericum perforatum
Hypericaceae (St. John's Wort) Family

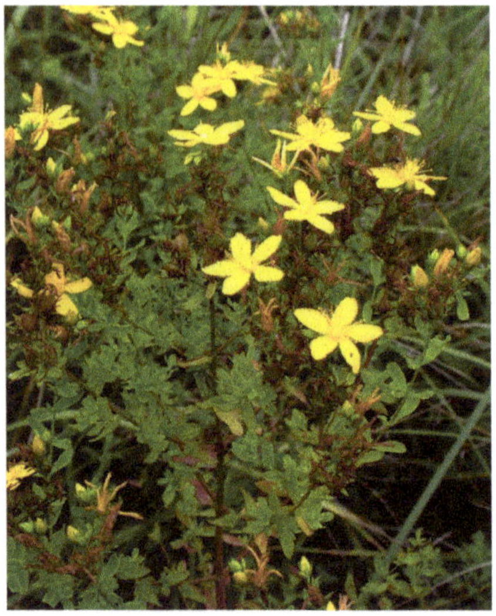

Common Names

Klamath weed, goat weed, amber, and Tipton weed are common names. Grace of God and Fuga Demonum (meaning devil's scourge) refer to the ancient belief that St. John's Wort is a sacred plant with the power to dispel evil.

Medicinal Part of the Plant

The flower heads and upper leaves contain the greatest concentration of medicinal constituents.

Range and Habitat

Hypericum is a large genus containing an estimated 370-400 species that grow worldwide. Many species contain identical phytochemicals and are utilized for similar medicinal purposes. *Hypericum perforatum* is the species commonly used in Western herbalism. Native to all parts of Europe, England, and temperate zones of Asia, it was introduced and has naturalized in North and South America, Africa, and Australia. The plant grows in sunny fields, grasslands, and along open edges of woodlands and roadsides.

Description of the Plant

H. perforatum is a beautiful wildflower and a hardy perennial herb growing 1-3′ tall. Several smooth, erect stems emerge from the fibrous roots. Many simple, entire, sessile leaves clasp the stalk opposite each other along the length of each stem. The small leaves grow up to 1″ long and are oblong to linear in shape, pinnately veined, and glabrous (smooth and hairless). A multitude of branching stalks in the upper portion of the plant end in a loose, rounded, or flat-topped compound cyme arrangement of several attractive bright-yellow, star-shaped flowers. The small flowers are about 1/2″ in diameter and consist of 5 petals, 5 sepals, the central pistil, and several long, yellow stamens. Yellow blossoms appear around the summer solstice during the third week of June and continue blooming through August and September. Each ovary develops into the fruit, which is an oval-shaped capsule containing a lot of very tiny, round, brown seeds.

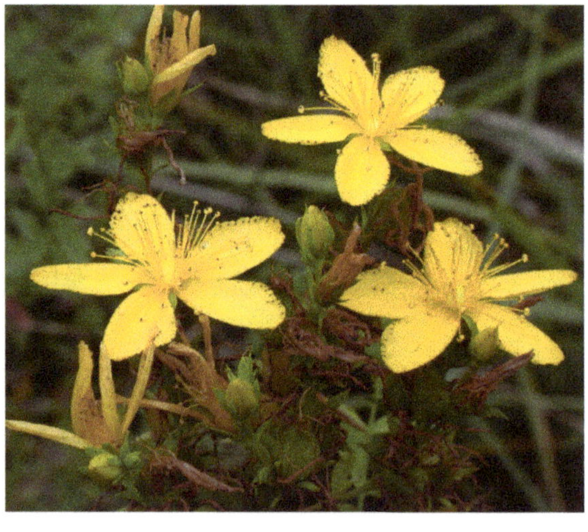

In several species of St. John's Wort, including *H. perforatum,* the leaves and edges of the flower petals are covered with oil glands appearing as tiny, reddish-brown pinholes that can be seen when held up to the sunlight. These are the perforations that inspired the species name *perforatum,* and they are a helpful clue to identifying the plant. These dark dots contain the medicinally active phytochemical hypericin, the red pigment that leaves a stain on the skin when the leaves and flowers are pinched and rubbed between the fingers. Hypericin is also responsible for the beautiful burgundy-red color of St. John's Wort tea, tincture, and oil.

Cultivation

The vibrant, golden-yellow flowers are a visual delight that brings cheer to the heart and makes St. John's Wort a favorite garden ornamental. It will grow in poor clay or sandy soil, but thrives best in mild to moderately alkaline sandy soil (6.8-7.2 pH) with at least average fertility, good drainage, and full sun. The herb naturally reproduces from seeds that fall to the ground in autumn and from spreading rhizomes. Germination rates can be rather poor but improved by washing the seeds with running water, cold conditioning (stratification), and/or brief exposure to high temperatures around 210°F. These are helpful methods to deactivate natural germination inhibitors in the seeds. Mimic nature and cold condition the seeds by planting them in autumn in an outdoor nursery bed and allowing them to winter over for better springtime germination. Or for spring planting, seeds can be cold conditioned by taking them in and out of refrigeration (33-38°F) for several weeks before planting. Use a sandy loam potting soil for best germination.

Seeds are light-dependent and require exposure to sunlight to germinate. They should be pressed into soil rather than covered. Germination is enhanced by high temperatures and can take between 3-4 weeks or several months. New seedlings are extremely tiny and delicate, so water them gently with a mist sprayer to avoid damage. When they are 4-6″ tall, the wispy seedlings can be transplanted into a permanent bed and spaced singly or in clusters of 3-5 seedlings planted 1′ apart. As each seedling matures, it grows many stems and branches to form an attractive, showy bush. First-year seedlings may produce some flowers but will be most prolific in the second year. Reduce watering during the flowering stage to increase production of the medicinal oils. Seeds can remain viable for many years.

Insect predators are not usually problematic for herbs, but the Klamath weed beetle (*Chrysolina quadrigemina*), a small, shiny, bluish-black beetle, loves to eat St. John's Wort. Native to South America, it was introduced into the western United States in a program to eradicate large, invasive populations of *H. perforatum* that can be toxic to grazing animals. Unfortunately, the beetle has spread throughout the country.

St. John's Wort is also susceptible to a type of fungus blight that turns the entire plant brown, beginning at the stem base, and eventually kills it. Blights can infest an entire area, so all diseased plants should be removed immediately to avoid contamination.

Harvest

The fresh flowering tops, consisting of upper leaves, flowers and unopened buds, contain the greatest concentrations of medicinal hypericin and flavonoids. The flowers and flower buds contain more hypericin than the leaves. Hypericin rapidly decreases after the flowers have bloomed, so harvest the upper leaves and flower heads when the plant is in full bloom for optimal medicinal properties when preparing tea and tincture. To make oil or salve for external use, let the plants get a bit older and harvest the flower heads after they start developing green seedpods because hyperforin, which has excellent wound healing properties, is at highest concentration during this stage. Harvest by pruning 6-8″ off the tops of the plant, leaving some flower heads so plants can complete their growing cycle and produce seeds.

> *For internal use, harvest leaves and flowers when in full bloom.*
>
> *For external use, harvest as the green seedpods are developing.*

Harvest seeds when seedpods are dry and brown. Cut stems below each seed head and put them upside down in a large paper bag. When thoroughly dry, shake and pound the bag to dislodge the seeds, hold the bag upside down, gather the open end into a funnel shape, and shake so the seeds fall out.

Warning: Hypericin is easily absorbed through the skin and is known to cause sunburns and blisters in some sensitive, fair-skinned people after they apply the tincture or oil to their skin or after spending several hours handling the plant in full sun. Wear gloves when handling large amounts of freshly harvested St. John's Wort to protect your skin.

Preparation of Plant Medicine and Dosages

St. John's Wort yields its properties to hot water, oil and alcohol, but alcohol is the best extractor of the medicinal constituents. Teas yield about 6-10% of the available hypericin, while tinctures made with 70-80% alcohol contain much more hypericin. Only freshly harvested flowers and leaves should be used to make top-quality tea, tincture and oil, but they can be dried for future tea preparations. When purchasing or creating St. John's Wort preparations, remember that well-made alcohol extracts and oils provide much greater potency than pills and capsules made with the dried herb, which deteriorates over time, especially when exposed to light and heat. The concentration and potency of hypericin and other biologically active constituents drop significantly when the plant is dried and stored for more than 6 weeks (Upton, 1997).

If you do want to dry some of the flower heads, tie them in small bundles and hang them in a well-ventilated, shady area or place them on screens. When dry, rub them between your hands or on a screen to separate the herb from stems.

Remember: Wear gloves to protect your skin when handling the plant for an extended time, and avoid long exposure to sunlight after taking a large dose of this herb or if you are using it for a period of time.

PREPARATIONS

Infusion: Steep 1-2 teaspoons of the fresh or dried upper leaves and flowers in 1 cup of boiling water. Dosage: 1-3 cups a day as needed. The German Commission E herbal regulatory agency recommended 2-4 grams of the whole herb per day. The tea has a mild, pleasant flavor. A strong tea can be applied externally as a wash or fomentation for wounds and injuries.

Tincture: Cover freshly harvested, finely chopped upper leaves and flowers with 75% 190-proof grain alcohol and 25% distilled water. It is a beautiful sight when the liquid menstruum is poured over the herb and it immediately turns red from the hypericin pigments. As the tincture processes, it becomes a deeper burgundy-red color indicative of the potency and quality of the preparation. Dosage: 20-60 drops or 2-4 mL 1-4 times a day as needed. As treatment for allergic reactions or poisoning, take 60-90 drops every 10 minutes in 8 ounces of water for up to 5 doses or until symptoms are relieved.

Oil: Put fresh, finely-chopped flower heads and upper leaves into a stainless steel bowl, cover with olive oil, and stir. Bake in an oven at 200°F for 2-3 hours. Remove from the oven and allow the herb and oil mixture to sit in full sun for several hours to increase yields of medicinal flavonoids, including rutin and quercetin (Upton, 1997). Strain the cooled oil from the herb, bottle, and store in a cool, dark place. The hypericin pigment imparts a beautiful red color to the oil. Oil will last for at least 2 years, and longer if kept cool. Apply to skin as needed. Dosage for internal use: 1 teaspoon twice daily.

Salve: St. John's Wort is a marvelous ingredient for salve. Prepare the oil and add beeswax to thicken.

Standardized Preparations: Most commercial preparations of St. John's Wort pills, capsules, and liquid extracts are standardized to contain 0.125-0.3% hypericin and/or 2-5% hyperforin. The typical dosage for depression and other problems is 300 mg taken 3 times daily (900 mg a day).

Chemical Constituents

The most biologically active compounds in St. John's Wort are the naphthodianthrones consisting of hypericin (3% in flowers and 1-1.8% in leaves), hyperforin, pseudohypericin, isohypericin, and emodin-anthrone; flavonoids (11.71% in flowers); and essential oils (0.059-0.35%) (Upton, 1997). Hypericin and pseudohypericin are responsible for the characteristic red pigment in the plant and for antidepressant, antiviral, anticarcinogenic, antileukemic, and antitumor effects. Hyperforin has analgesic, antibiotic, anti-inflammatory, anticarcinogenic, antidepressant, sedative, and wound healing capacity (Brondz, 1982).

Flavonoids are typically diuretic, calming, anti-inflammatory, antioxidant, and anticarcinogenic. They include rutin, quercetin (anti-allergy), isoquercetin (antibacterial, hypotensive), isorhamnetin, amentoflavone (anti-inflammatory), luteolin (good for the eyes, anti-atherosclerotic), kaempferol, and hyperin/hyperoside (analgesic, antibacterial, antidermatitis, antiflu, hepatoprotective, antiviral, hypotensive).

Volatile oils are generally antibacterial, anticarcinogenic, antioxidant, antispasmodic, and anti-inflammatory. They include caryophyllene (anti-sinusitis, anti-ulcer, vulnerary), humulene, myrcene (diuretic, analgesic, anticonvulsant, fungicide), limonene (antiflu, antilithic, antiviral, expectorant, antifungal, sedative), nonane, decanal, pinene (expectorant, fungicide), terpineol, and geraniol.

Tannins are astringent and reduce diarrhea and bleeding. Epicatechin is anti-anaphylactic, antibacterial, antihepatitis, anti-HIV, anti-inflammatory, antileukemic, antiviral, antioxidant, and cardiotonic. Other compounds include caffeic, chlorogenic, coumaric, ferulic and gentisic acids, carotenoids, xanthones, beta-sitosterol, choline, pectin, beta-carotene (plant source of vitamin A, and ascorbic acid (vitamin C). Several protein amino acids are present, including cysteine, glutamine, leucine, lysine (antiherpes), ornithine, proline, threonine, and GABA (0.7 mg/gm), which acts as a calming neurotransmitter (Upton, 1997).

Safety, Contraindications, and Drug Interactions

St. John's Wort is considered a safe herb that most people can use without problems. There is no evidence of acute or accumulated toxicity or decrease in effectiveness when taken over extended periods of time. Children and the elderly can safely use this herb for acute or chronic conditions. Side effects are uncommon, but include mild stomach upset, dizziness, dry mouth, anxiety, restlessness, insomnia, constipation, allergic reactions, fatigue, and photosensitivity (sensitivity to the sun).

The effectiveness and side effects of a 4-week treatment with hypericum extract LI 160 were investigated in 3,250 patients (ages 20 to 90 years) diagnosed with mild depression (49%), moderate depression (46%), or severe depression (3%). In about 30% of the patients, depression decreased and moods improved during the therapy. Side effects were reported in 79 (2.4%) patients, and 48 (1.5%) discontinued the herbal therapy. The most common side effects were gastrointestinal discomfort (0.6%), allergic reactions (0.5%), fatigue (0.4%), and restlessness (0.3%) (Woelk, 1994).

Photosensitivity: St. John's Wort has an interesting relationship with the sun. The oil is an effective topical treatment for all types of burns. Yet some sensitive, fair-skinned people get severe sunburns when they consume excessively large doses (1,800 mg/day) of St. John's Wort or apply the tincture or oil to exposed skin before spending several hours in the sun. There are rare accounts of people who harvest the plant for several hours on sunny days and develop burns wherever the oil resin gets on their skin. This photosensitivity is one of the most publicized and serious side effects, so caution is advised. Exposure to ultraviolet light therapy after using or handling St. John's Wort should be avoided.

Photosensitivity can also be problematic for livestock that eat the herb while grazing in full sunlight. The interaction of sun and oxygen with the hypericin pigment in the plant can cause welts, burns, and other symptoms of toxicity in cows, sheep, goats, horses, and other grazing animals.

Safety for Depression: The clinical efficacy of standardized St. John's Wort extracts in the treatment of mild to moderate depression has been evaluated in over 38 controlled clinical trials and at least two meta-analyses. Sixteen post-marketing surveillance studies involving 34,804 patients recorded a low incidence of side effects ranging from 0-6%, which were mild and transient in most of the cases. Of these studies, the four large-scale surveillance studies consisting of 14,245 patients documented very low occurrences of adverse effects ranging from 0.1-2.4% (Schultz, 2006). A clinical trial designed to evaluate effects of high doses of hypericin (up to 1.5 mg) and pseudohypericin (up to 3.16 mg) were studied in 13 healthy volunteers using oral ingestion of St. John's Wort extract over a two-week period. Treatment with Hypericum extract, even in high doses, was well tolerated (Kerb, 1996).

St. John's Wort and antidepressant selective serotonin reuptake inhibitors (SSRIs) both increase serotonin levels in the brain. Hypothetical allegations warn that combining these may cause excessive serotonin levels known as serotonin syndrome. However, many clinical herbalists, myself included, have observed good results when people take St. John's Wort while successfully weaning off their prescription antidepressants.

Monoamine oxidase (MAO) inhibitor: Researchers initially thought that St. John's Wort reduces depression by inhibiting monoamine oxidase (MAO), but subsequent studies proved this theory to be incorrect.

Bipolar and Mania: Antidepressant drugs are known to precipitate mania or cause rapid cycling between depressive and manic episodes in some people with bipolar syndrome. These drugs may elicit a negative, paradoxical impact and contribute to treatment-resistant bipolar depression. There are four reported cases in which the use of St. John's Wort has caused manic episodes (Bone, 2001). Therefore, people with bipolar disorder should use this herb with caution and awareness of these potential problems.

Pregnancy and Lactation: There are no known harmful effects when women who are pregnant or breast feeding ingest moderate doses of St. John's Wort, and studies have demonstrated it to be safe during pregnancy and lactation (Moretti, 2009; Lee, 2003). Herbalist midwives have traditionally recommended it to pregnant women if needs arise. The German Commission E and other herbal authorities do not place restrictions on using the herb during pregnancy or lactation. However, since it has mild emmenagogue effects, it is safer to use in moderate doses after the first trimester of pregnancy.

Herb-Drug Interactions: St. John's Wort interacts with an important enzyme system of the liver called cytochrome P-450, which is involved in the metabolism of pharmaceutical drugs. The herb is a potent inducer of cytochrome P-450 enzymes that metabolize and inactivate several drugs. Recent studies show that the degree of enzyme induction and diminished drug action correlates strongly with the amount of hyperforin found in St. John's Wort preparations (Madabushi, 2006; Pal, 2006). Over 50 papers have been published investigating potential interactions between St. John's Wort and prescription drugs.

It is generally agreed that St. John's Wort should not be taken concurrently with coumarin-type anticoagulants, immunosuppressants, or protease and reverse transcriptase inhibitors used in cancer, HIV, and AIDS therapy. Co-medication with the herb has resulted in decreased blood levels of amitriptyline, cyclosporine, digoxin, fexofenadine, amprenavir, indinavir, irinotecan, lopinavir, ritonavir, saquinavir, benzodiazepines, theophylline, irinotecan, midazolan, warfarin, phenprocoumon, alprazolam, dextrometorphane, and simvastatin (Jobst, 2000; Piscitelli, 2000). When regular use of St. John's Wort is combined with oral contraceptives, the herb increases estrogen clearance from the liver and may reduce contraceptive effects. It has been reported to cause breakthrough bleeding and increase the risk of unwanted pregnancy (Hall, 2003; Pfrunder, 2003).

Medicinal Uses

History of the Plant

St. John's Wort has a colorful history and has been employed in similar ways by different cultures since ancient times. Many of its current therapeutic uses originate from ancient Greek medicine and were documented by renowned herbal physicians of that era, including Hippocrates, Theophrastus, Pliny the Elder, Dioscorides, and Galen. They recommended the herb for a host of ailments such as depression, anxiety, wounds, burns, nerve pain and injuries, inflammation, ulcers, parasites, and venomous bites, stings, and other poisons. Dioscorides used St. John's Wort to treat painful battle wounds and stop bleeding when he was a physician for the Roman army, and he recognized its diuretic effects. He wrote, "The seed drunk for the space of forty days together, cureth the sciatica, and all aches that happen in the hips" (Dioscorides, 1959).

The famous English herbalist John Gerard (1545–1612) wrote that St. John's Wort tea increases the flow of urine and is helpful for treating kidney and bladder stones. He prepared a wine tincture and olive oil-based ointment of the leaves and flowers to treat deep wounds, burns, ulcers, poisonous bites and stings, and painful muscles. He claimed, "I know in the world there is not a better . . . natural balm" (Gerard, 1633). The English apothecary and physician Nicholas Culpeper (1616–1654) prescribed it for these traditional purposes and determined that this cheerful herb with yellow flowers is ruled by the Sun and is under the influence of the astrological sign Leo.

St. John's Wort was a popular herb among the common folk in Europe, and Catholic monks grew it in their monastery gardens for medicine and protection. During the Dark and Middle Ages, Europeans were possessed with the fear of witches, witchcraft, and the devil. Many people believed that certain plants held magical powers capable of warding off evil and protecting them from demonic possession. St. John's Wort was regarded as a holy herb and was one of the more popular protector plants. Its name refers to John the Baptist, and the red pigment in the leaves and flowers is associated with the blood of his beheading. The plant was traditionally harvested every year on June 24, which is celebrated as St. John's Day to commemorate the saint's beheading, and the leaves and flowers were hung in homes and churches to ward off evil spirits, witchcraft, and lightning strikes.

There are two explanations for the origin of the genus name *Hypericum*. One claims that the herb was named for Hyperion, god of the sun in Greek mythology, which is appropriate since the yellow flowers have such a strong relationship with the sun. The genus name is also believed to originate from two Greek words, *hyper* and *eikon*, meaning "over an apparition," referring to the belief that ingesting or wearing the herb repulses evil spirits and drives them away. "Wort" is an Anglo-Saxon term meaning "medicinal herb." St. John's Wort was used to cure insanity and bizarre behavior, especially if the patient was thought to be possessed by the devil or evil spirits. It is probable that many people diagnosed as being "possessed" were actually suffering from imbalances in brain chemistry, which the herb helped to normalize.

Early European settlers introduced *H. perforatum* and its medicinal uses in North America during the colonial period. During the early 1800s and 1900s in Europe and North America, it was a popular homeopathic preparation for treating anxiety, depression, nerve injuries, sharp pain, inflammation, and lockjaw (a symptom of tetanus). Eclectic physicians prescribed the tincture for similar problems and applied it externally for all types of injuries. Eclectic physician Finley Ellingwood (1852–1920) used it specifically for muscular bruises, swelling, burning pain, spinal injuries, concussions, painful lacerations, and deep puncture wounds. John King, M.D. (1813–1893) wrote in his *American Family Physician*, "The tops and flowers possess astringent, sedative, and diuretic properties, and have been used in infusion, in suppression of the urine, chronic urinary affections, diarrhea, dysentery, worms, jaundice, hysterics [an antiquated term for mood swings, depression, irritability, and anxiety associated with menstrual cycles and menopause], excessive menstruation, and nervous irritability" (King, 1864).

In 1984, Germany approved St. John's Wort for relief of mild to moderate depression, anxiety, dyspepsia (impaired digestion), soft tissue injuries, bruising, muscle pain, and first-degree burns. As continual studies documented its effectiveness, it became the leading antidepressant in Germany. Its popularity in the United States soared in 1997, when newspaper headlines and national television news reported it to be an effective antidepressant, and it became one of the top-selling medicinal herbs almost overnight. One of the most researched herbs in the world, tremendous amounts of data from laboratory and clinical studies investigating St. John's Wort phytochemicals and their biological effects have confirmed many of its traditional uses. It continues to be one of the most widely used herbs for depression in Europe and the United States.

Healing Qualities

Alterative, analgesic, antibacterial, anticarcinogenic, antidepressant, anti-inflammatory, antioxidant, antiseptic, antispasmodic, antitoxin, antiviral, astringent, diuretic, hepatic, nervine, sedative, and vulnerary.

Traditional Chinese Medicine (TCM) Perspective

According to TCM, St. John's Wort is cooling and drying. It strengthens Wei Qi (immunity) and benefits the liver and kidneys. It calms and restores the nervous system and helps maintain balanced brain chemistry. The herb promotes the harmonious movement of Qi throughout the body, and relieves constrained Qi manifesting as nervous tension, depression, spasms, muscle and spinal aches, and pain. It is helpful for Bladder Qi constraint causing scanty urination and bed-wetting, and for Kidney and Liver Qi Stagnation with metabolic toxicity that contributes to headaches, irritability, inflammation, and the development of cysts and tumors. Painful and irregular periods, cramps, and menopausal symptoms can result from Uterine Qi constraint, which the herb addresses. TCM often regards depression as mental stagnation manifesting from liver imbalance and congestion. Because St. John's Wort has a protective, detoxifying, and stimulating influence on the liver, which reduces congestion and promotes movement of Qi and blood throughout the body, this action on the liver contributes to the plant's antidepressant properties.

Primary Actions

St. John's Wort has a healing influence on the nervous system and affects several neurotransmitters that normalize brain chemistry, moods, and mental cognition. It is most popular for treating depression, yet this is only one aspect of its beneficial actions. It also detoxifies the liver and blood, eases nerve pain, and is a powerful antiviral that is remarkably effective against the herpes family of viruses, which attacks nerve cells.

When using St. John's Wort as an antidepressant, it is extremely important to realize that depression is a symptom of imbalance and a signal that underlying causes need to be resolved. If depression results from being in a miserable relationship or job, or because one's life purpose is not being realized, real healing is achieved by making different choices and changing the situation. Taking herbal or pharmaceutical antidepressants can be helpful coping tools while the basic causes of depression are being addressed, but they will never cure the underlying issues. Brain chemistry is greatly affected by our thoughts and emotions. Indulging in chronic anger, bitterness, grief, frustration, and other disturbing states can create imbalanced brain chemistry over time, manifesting as depression, anxiety, or poor cognitive function. Daily practice to develop calm thoughts and emotions is paramount to a happy and healthy life, so be sure to combine this with a nutritious diet and appropriate herbal therapy when treating depression and other mood disorders.

The ancient myths surrounding St. John's Wort focus on its protective qualities as a talisman against danger and negative forces (or low-frequency energies). I learned about this protection many years ago when someone broke into my home several times and stole different items. I decided to hang a bundle of freshly picked St. John's Wort flowers over the entry door of my log cabin home. As I prepared the bundle, I stated the intention that anyone entering my house with malicious intentions would get confused, leave, and not return. The intruder returned one more time, but did not take anything. That bundle of herbs hung over the door for several years, and no one ever broke in again.

Nervous System: St. John's Wort is a restorative nerve tonic. Its strong influence on nerve tissue is calming, protective, and restoring to the entire nervous system. By helping to normalize brain chemistry and moods, the herb gently energizes and stimulates the nervous system when it is depressed, or relaxes it in conditions of hyperstimulation and anxiety. St. John's Wort has long been used for treating psychiatric and neurological conditions, including depression, insomnia, poor cognitive function, migraine headaches, and trigeminal neuralgia. Although most attention has focused on the herb's antidepressant properties, it also benefits anxiety, obsessive-compulsive disorder (OCD), and post-traumatic stress disorder (PTSD). Research has shown that a St. John's Wort extract significantly reduced anxiety over a 6-week period with excellent tolerance in 151 out-patients suffering from pain and symptoms arising from psychiatric problems (Volz, 2002). The calming ability of St. John's Wort eases nerve and muscle tension, and procyanidin components in the herb have vasorelaxant actions that relax blood vessels and increase circulation (Nahrstedt, 1997).

St. John's Wort's Mechanisms of Action in the Brain and Nervous System: Many research studies and clinical trials have been conducted to identify and understand the various modes of action that St. John's Wort exhibits. It affects several neurotransmitters, which are specialized chemicals in the brain and nervous system that regulate cognitive function, mood, and behavior. Serotonin and GABA (gamma-amino-butyric acid) are neurotransmitters that promote relaxation, while dopamine, epinephrine (adrenaline), and norepinephrine excite the nervous system. Glutamate (also called glutamic acid) provides energy necessary for normal brain function and has an energizing influence. Neurotransmitter levels are reduced by enzymes that break them down during the process called reuptake, in which they are inactivated. St. John's Wort appears to influence this regulatory mechanism. Depression, anxiety, insomnia, and a host of other mood and neurological problems are usually caused by insufficient and/or excessive amounts of specific neurotransmitters. Several pharmaceutical drugs called selective serotonin reuptake inhibitors (SSRIs) have been developed to inhibit the reuptake of this neurotransmitter, resulting in greater concentrations of serotonin and nervous system relaxation.

Much European research has been conducted with the St. John's Wort extract called LI 160, which is standardized to contain 0.31% hypericin and pseudohypericin. *In vitro* and *in vivo* research using LI 160 demonstrates that hyperforin and hypericin have an affinity for many neurotransmitter receptors. This means that they attach to receptors on cells and influence their activity. Hyperforin and hypericin inhibit the enzymatic breakdown and reuptake of serotonin, GABA, dopamine, epinephrine and glutamate, which increases levels of these neurotransmitters and enhances mood and greater feelings of well-being (Butterweck, 2003; Chatterjee, 1998; Muller, 1997; Neary, 1999). One *in vitro* test showed that LI 160 reduces the destruction of tryptophan, the amino acid that converts into serotonin (Winkler, 2004). Serotonin increases relaxation, and a deficiency can result in depression, insomnia, anxiety, and sugar cravings. Researchers have also observed that phytochemicals in St. John's Wort (amentoflavone and other flavonoids) have strong affinity with GABA receptors (Baureithal, 1997). GABA is the calming neurotransmitter that specifically reduces obsessive thinking during the day and when trying to sleep at night. The herb binds to GABA receptor sites on cells, inhibits the reuptake of GABA, and increases its levels (Muller, 1996; Cott, 1997). Interestingly, studies show that whole herb extracts are much more effective than isolated hypericin in binding to GABA receptors. Small amounts of GABA also naturally occur in the plant.

St. John's Wort has been shown to inhibit the activity of interleukin-6, an inflammatory cytokine that may contribute to increased cortisol production often occurring during major depression (Thiele, 1994). Cortisol is an adrenal hormone that increases blood pressure and blood sugar levels, suppresses the immune system, and is secreted in greater amounts during stress. *In vivo* research shows that extracts of *H. perforatum* significantly reduced cortisol and corticosterone (another adrenal steroid hormone) in frontal cortex tissue of the brain. Since an increase in cortisol is frequently observed in depression and stress, the herb's ability to reduce cortisol levels and stabilize the adrenal glands is another mode of its antidepressant and anti-anxiety action (Franklin, 2004).

Monoamine oxidase (MAO) is a class of enzymes that breaks down serotonin, norepinephrine, epinephrine (adrenaline), and dopamine. MAO inhibitor drugs are a popular class of pharmaceutical antidepressants. It was once believed that the antidepressant activity of St. John's Wort resulted from its ability to increase norepinephrine by inhibiting monoamine oxidase (MAO), but new research has refuted this notion. In a study lasting 7 days, 16 healthy volunteers ingested either St. John's Wort (300 mg), imipramine (50 mg to increase norepinephrine levels), or a placebo 3 times a day. St. John's Wort did not increase blood concentrations of norepinephrine and had no effect on blood pressure or heart rate, which are typically increased under the influence of norepinephrine and imipramine. However, concentrations of dihydroxyphenylacetic acid (the main metabolite of dopamine) increased in every subject. This indicates that the herb's mode of action is partly due to its ability to increase levels of dopamine, the stimulating neurotransmitter that reduces depression and elevates mood and feelings of well-being (Schroeder, 2004).

St. John's Wort's sedative properties, helpful for insomnia, are also supported by small amounts of melatonin (4.39 mcg/gm) occurring in the fresh flowers (Murch, 1997). Melatonin is a hormone that promotes sleep and is produced in the brain by the pineal gland. Serotonin is an important calming neurotransmitter necessary for the production of melatonin. An increase in melatonin production was observed after administration of a St. John's Wort extract for 3 weeks (Demisch, 1991).

As a soothing and protective herb, St. John's Wort may be taken before bedtime to encourage restful sleep and eliminate nightmares. Blend it with Scullcap (*Scutellaria lateriflora*), Hops (*Humulus lupulus*), and Valerian (*Valeriana officinalis*) for an excellent sedative, analgesic, and restorative remedy to the nervous system.

Depression: In recent years, St. John's Wort has emerged as a leading herbal antidepressant. I have given the tincture to many people who have reported improvement in their depression and emotional well-being without any side effects when using 60 drops 2-3 times daily. For clients who want to discontinue their prescription antidepressants, I usually recommend that they start using the herb and gradually wean themselves off the prescription medicine over 3-6 weeks. This approach usually works quite well. The effectiveness of St. John's Wort increases over time and usually requires 3-6 weeks of use to obtain its full potential for relieving depression.

Extensive research over several decades confirms the efficacy and safety of St. John's Wort in treating mild to severe depression. Researchers have compared it to several pharmaceutical anti-depressants and found it to be an effective alternative with significantly fewer side effects. A meta-analysis of 23 controlled clinical studies involving 1,757 outpatients diagnosed with mild to moderate depression stated that St. John's Wort extract was significantly superior to placebo, and was comparably effective to prescription antidepressants with fewer adverse effects. Most studies lasted 4-8 weeks. Side effects were reported in 19.8% of the participants taking the herb and in 52.8% of those taking drugs. St. John's Wort preparations used in these studies were standardized to contain 0.3% hypericin in doses of 0.4-2.7 mg of hypericins per day (Linde, 1996). Another more recent meta-analysis of 30 research studies obtained similar results when the herb showed significantly better results than placebo and similar efficacy compared to prescription antidepressants. The herb caused fewer side effects than the drugs with a lower rate of drop-outs (Roder, 2004).

> *St. John's Wort effectively reduces all types of depression by normalizing neurotransmitters that regulate nerve function and brain chemistry.*
>
> *Most notably, the herb enhances levels of serotonin, GABA, and dopamine to reduce depression and stabilize moods and well-being.*

A 6-week clinical trial comparing a standardized St. John's Wort extract with amitriptyline (Elavil) revealed that 3 daily doses of 300 mg of the extract was as effective in treating mild to moderate depression in 165 participants with fewer side effects than 75 mg of Elavil (Wheatley, 1997). An 8-week study comparing the herb with imipramine (Tofranil) in 263 people diagnosed with moderate depression found that 350 mg of St. John's Wort taken 3 times a day was as effective in reducing symptoms as 100 mg of Tofranil taken daily. Those using the herb reported fewer side effects (Philipp, 1999). Several studies have compared the effects of St. John's Wort extract to fluoxetine (Prozac). One study involved 240 people with mild to moderate depression. Over a 6-week period, 128 people ingested a 250 mg tablet of the herb twice a day and 114 people took 20 mg of Prozac once a day. Improvements in mood were confirmed to be equal in both groups with significantly fewer side effects in the herbal group (28%) compared to 72% in the Prozac group (Schrader, 2000). A multi-center study involving 241 patients diagnosed with moderate depressive disorder demonstrated that daily doses of 612 mg of a St. John's Wort extract had the same beneficial effects as 50 mg of sertraline (Zoloft) after a 12- and 24-week trial period (Gastpar, 2005).

Although primarily used for mild to moderate depression, research confirms St. John's Wort's ability to reduce major depression. A clinical study involving 209 patients diagnosed with severe depression found that 3 daily doses of 600 mg of St. John's Wort (1,800 mg daily) or 50 mg of imipramine (Tofranil) (150 mg daily) exerted similar antidepressant effects over a 6-week period. These are large doses, and side effects were reported by 23% of the herb group compared to 41% of the Tofranil group (Vorbach, 1997). A multi-center trial involving 251 patients diagnosed with moderate to severe depression confirmed that the herb was as effective as paroxetine (Paxil) and better tolerated (Szegedi, 2005). In another trial with 135 patients diagnosed with major depression, half received the standardized LI-160 extract at 900 mg a day and the other half took 20 mg of Prozac daily. After 12 weeks, 38% of the herbal group experienced higher rates of remission than the Prozac group, which reported 30% improvement. St. John's Wort was significantly more effective while being safe and well tolerated (Fava, 2005). Assessing a meta-analysis of 29 trials (5,489 patients) comparing St. John's Wort extracts with prescription antidepressants, researchers concluded that the herb causes fewer side effects and is as effective as antidepressants for major depression (Linde, 2008).

Twenty patients with seasonal affective disorder (SAD), which is precipitated by cloudy winter months of sun deprivation, reported that 300 mg of St. John's Wort taken 3 times a day improved their depression during a 4-week trial. The improvement was as effective as bright light therapy with no reported adverse reactions (Martinez, 1994). For best results in treating SAD, combine St. John's Wort with Lemon Balm (*Melissa officinalis*).

Obsessive-Compulsive Disorder (OCD): This is an anxiety disorder characterized by uncontrollable repetitive behaviors and thoughts. Insomnia is frequently caused by an overactive mind that will not stop thinking, even though the body is physically tired. The ability of St. John's Wort to attach to GABA receptors quiets the mind and is helpful in reducing obsessive thoughts and behaviors throughout the day.

Recent studies have shown that selective serotonin reuptake inhibitor (SSRI) antidepressants are effective in treating OCD, and researchers conducted a small clinical study involving 13 people who had been diagnosed with OCD for at least one year to determine if St. John's Wort would be helpful. Participants received 450 mg of a standardized 0.3% hypericin preparation twice daily for 12 weeks. Reported side effects included diarrhea in three people, restless sleep in two, and one dropped out of the study due to a rash, leaving 12 participants. At the end of the trial, participants and researchers evaluated that OCD symptoms were "much" or "very much improved" in 42% (five people), "minimally improved" in 50% (six participants), and 8% (one person) did not experience any benefit (Taylor, 2000).

Nerve Injury, Inflammation, and Pain Relief: Called the "arnica of the nervous system," St. John's Wort provides soothing analgesic and restorative actions on nerve cells and the nervous system. The herb reduces nerve pain and inflammation, and has a long history of use as an effective remedy for all types of injuries and damage to the nerves and spinal cord.

Researchers have validated the presence of analgesic, antioxidant, and anti-inflammatory constituents in alcohol extracts of *H. perforatum* (Herold, 2003). The extracts decreased levels of several inflammatory compounds, including myeloperozidase (an enzyme promoting inflammation), and have demonstrated similar modes of action as prescription anti-inflammatories when tested on human white blood cells (Pabuccuoglu, 2003; Tedeschi, 2003). Hypericin's antioxidant actions decrease free radical damage to cells, which reduces inflammation and preserves cells (Lavie, 1995). St. John's Wort extracts have also inhibited the release of inflammatory arachidonic acid, leukotrienes, and interleukins (Panossian, 1996).

Taken as a tonic over time, the herb is beneficial for nerve injuries and degeneration, peripheral neuropathies, head and spinal injuries, concussions, falls on the coccyx, crushing injuries, backaches, sore muscles and ligaments, muscle spasms, myalgia (muscle pain), and Reynaud's disease. It eases many types of neuralgia (nerve pain), including headaches, migraines, sciatica, arthritis pain, surgical wounds, phantom limb pain, trigeminal neuralgia, fibromyalgia, and palsy (paralysis). Research data suggest that St. John's Wort may be helpful for degenerative nerve conditions like multiple sclerosis, Alzheimer's, and Parkinson's disease because it protects the nerves from trauma, oxidation, and other damage (Lu, 2004; Silva, 2004).

St. John's Wort is one of my favorite herbs for serious injuries and nerve problems. For these conditions, drink the fresh tea or tincture and apply St. John's Wort oil or tincture to the affected area. It works synergistically when taken with Scullcap (*Scutellaria lateriflora*) to reduce pain and heal nerve injuries.

Antiviral Activity against the Herpes Family and Other Viruses: I have repeatedly found that a potent tincture of the crude herb promotes significant and often amazing reductions in symptoms and recovery time for many people suffering from the herpes family of viral infections. These include facial cold sores (caused by herpes simplex type 1), genital lesions (caused by herpes simplex type 2), shingles (from herpes zoster), cytomegalovirus, and mononucleosis (caused by the Epstein-Barr virus, also implicated in chronic fatigue syndrome). Many clients and friends consistently report that applying a few drops of St. John's Wort tincture to skin lesions, in addition to ingesting a dose of 60 drops in water 3-4 times throughout the day, cleared their herpes outbreak faster and noticeably reduced discomfort. The herb's analgesic and anti-inflammatory properties ease pain. Taking 5-10 drops of tincture on a daily basis can prevent future herpes outbreaks from occurring. St. John's Wort is reliable in treating the herpes virus because it has a special influence and relationship with nerve cells, and herpes is a virus living in the nervous system, either in an active or dormant state.

> *A combination of St. John's Wort and Lemon Balm is specific for attacking the herpes virus.*

Several *in vitro* and *in vivo* studies demonstrate that hypericin and pseudohypericin attack several viruses. These include the herpes family, vesicular stomatitis (caused by a virus in the same family as the rabies virus, which St. John's Wort is known to treat), parainfluenza virus (causes croup, bronchitis, and pneumonia), influenza A and B (causes the flu), HIV, and hepatitis B and C (Lopez-Bazzocchi, 1991; Meruelo, 1988; Weber, 1994; Wood, 1990). Two separate clinical trials were designed to examine the effects of an orally administered St. John's Wort pill compared to placebo for treating people with recurrent facial and genital herpes. Over a 90-day period, participants ingested an herbal tablet 3 times a day when they were free of symptoms, and took a double dose (2 tablets 3 times daily) during herpes outbreaks. The herb significantly reduced outbreaks and offered symptomatic relief in both trials (Mannel, 2000).

Human Immunodeficiency Virus (HIV): Researchers have observed that hypericin and pseudo-hypericin in St. John's Wort exhibit strong antiviral activity against retroviruses by disrupting and inactivating their replication. Retroviruses mutate quickly and become resistant to antiviral vaccines and drugs. Since retroviruses are difficult to eradicate, they can result in chronic infections. Human immunodeficiency virus (HIV) is a retrovirus causing acquired immunodeficiency syndrome (AIDS). Other retroviruses include human T-cell lymphotropic virus type 1 and 2, causing specific leukemias and lymphomas. When researchers at Upstate Medical University in Syracuse, New York, designed an analytical, *in vitro* study to determine immune activity of 10 common herbs, St. John's Wort showed consistent immunostimulatory activity on lymphocytes (white blood cells) (Wilasrumee, 2002).

The hypericins exhibit impressive ability to inhibit and destroy HIV during *in vitro* studies. Researchers at New York University Medical Center and Weizmman Institute of Science in Israel reported that *in vitro* tests demonstrated hypericin's ability to prevent healthy T-lymphocytes (white blood cells that provide immunity and are attacked by HIV) from becoming infected by HIV (Meruelo, 1988; Lavie, 1989). Research in which HIV-infected animals were given hypericins (orally or by injection) showed that they reduced the spread of HIV without observed side effects. The scientists concluded that hypericins may interfere with the virus's reproduction. Another mode of action may involve a protein in St. John's Wort that suppressed expression of the HIV-1 genome during *in vitro* testing, resulting in decreased viral replication of HIV-1-infected cells (Darbinian-Sarkissian, 2006).

The possibility that hypericin may be beneficial in treating HIV has inspired several clinical trials to investigate the efficacy and tolerance of St. John's Wort preparations for treating HIV-infected people. Many of these studies have resulted in mixed outcomes, which have not been as successful as those in laboratory *in vitro* experiments. On the positive side, however, one of the primary researchers at New York University Medical Center, Dr. Daniel Meruelo, Ph.D., found that hypericin exerts significant activity against HIV, hepatitis, and herpes viruses in some human clinical trials. Typical dosages in these trials were 0.5 mg/kg or 35 mg/day, which are extremely high doses compared to those used to treat depression. The high doses resulted in more side effects and dropout rates in many of the trials. Interestingly, alcohol extracts of hypericin derived from St. John's Wort plants were more effective and caused fewer side effects than the synthetic hypericin (Mulry, 1999).

Clinical trials have demonstrated the ability of St. John's Wort to improve the psychological moods of HIV-infected patients while increasing their energy levels and general sense of well-being (James, 1989). In a study lasting 40 months, 18 patients diagnosed with AIDS were treated with hypericin by intravenous administration. Sixteen patients remained clinically stable with a majority experiencing improvements in viral markers. Only two of the 16 participants experienced opportunistic infections during the trial period (Steinbeck, 1993).

A small study designed to investigate the safety and antiviral activity of St. John's Wort used oral and injectable forms of synthetic hypericin. Not only did this fail to show antiviral activity, but about half of the 30 AIDS participants developed severe sunburn caused by phototoxicity (Gulick, 1999). Since the synthetic version does not reflect the true biological effects of the herb, it is likely that the failure of this test and high incidence of sunburn were caused, at least in part, by use of a synthetic form rather than an extract of the plant.

One major problem with attempting to use St. John's Wort for HIV/AIDS treatment involves its interactions with several drugs used in conventional HIV/AIDS medical therapy, including protease inhibitors (indinavir) and immunosuppressants (cyclosporin). The herb inactivates these drugs and lowers effective blood levels. **Do not use St. John's Wort in conjunction with these HIV/AIDS drugs.**

Cancer: Several *in vitro* and *in vivo* studies have demonstrated that isolated hypericin and hyperforin extracted from the herb, or their synthetic forms, exhibit significant anticancer and antitumor activity. Both phytochemicals have killed cancer cells in cultured human tissue. They reduced inflammation and inhibited both neovascularization (the formation of new microvascular networks of veins and capillaries) and angiogenesis (the new growth of capillaries from pre-existing blood vessels), which are necessary for the growth and nutrient supply of cancer cells and tumors. Hypericin and hyperforin also induced apoptosis (programmed cell death) in tumor cells and inhibited cancer metastasis in lab studies. When live mice were injected with hyperforin, inflammation diminished, neovascularization was inhibited, and the size of tumors decreased while the animals exhibited healthy and active behavior (Dona, 2004).

Researchers have designed *in vitro* tests that demonstrate hyperforin's strong ability to inhibit angiogenesis by interfering with several key events in the process of capillary development. Hyperforin also reduced the ability of cancer to invade endothelial cells lining the interior surface of blood and lymphatic vessels. The researchers concluded that hyperforin is a promising compound that should be investigated for its potential role in the treatment of cancer, to inhibit metastasis, and for angiogenesis-related pathologies (Martinez-Poveda, 2005).

Hypericin is especially effective against glioma tumors and leukemia. A glioma is a type of tumor composed of nerve tissue that originates in the brain or spine. Gliomas make up about 30% of all brain and spinal tumors and 80% of all malignant brain tumors. *In vitro* research showed that when glioma cells were treated with hypericin in tissue cultures for 48 hours, their growth was inhibited and hypericin induced apoptosis (programmed cell death) that killed the glioma cells (Couldwell, 1994).

Several *in vitro* studies found that an alcohol extract of the whole herb showed significant ability to inhibit and kill leukemia cancer cells during incubation when compared to isolated hypericin, which showed very weak effects (Roscetti, 2004; Kapsokalyvas, 2005).

The Digestive System: St. John's Wort's ability to increase levels of serotonin (the neurotransmitter necessary for healthy digestive function) calms and restores the nerves of the solar plexus to regulate digestion and optimize actions of the stomach, liver, gallbladder, pancreas, and intestines. The herb is helpful in treating stomachaches, gastritis, colic, stomach and intestinal ulcers, inflammatory bowel syndromes, diarrhea, dysentery, and hemorrhoids. Ingesting the tincture or tea decreases inflammation, pain, spasms, and bleeding throughout the digestive tract. The German herbalist Rudolf Weiss, M.D., recommended one teaspoon of St. John's Wort oil taken twice a day on an empty stomach to heal gastritis and gastric ulcers.

Liver and Detoxifying Actions: Since ancient times, St. John's Wort has been used as a powerful blood cleanser, an antidote for ingested poisons, a remedy for venomous bites and stings, and for rabies inflicted from bites of infected animals. St. John's Wort's protective and antioxidant effects on the liver are mechanisms for these abilities.

The herb detoxifies the liver. Its stimulating actions improve metabolic functions of the liver, increase bile production, and clear excess estrogen from the body. An *in vivo* study using rats that were fed a cholesterol-rich diet showed that a St. John's Wort extract significantly lowered their blood levels of total cholesterol, triglycerides, and low density lipoproteins. Levels of superoxide dismutase (SOD), a potent antioxidant produced by cells in the body, were increased in their blood and liver tissues (Zou, 2005).

St. John's Wort clears toxins from the liver and blood.

Combine it with Milk Thistle seeds and Dandelion, Yellow Dock and Burdock roots for an exceptional remedy.

Years ago, I successfully ingested large amounts of St. John's Wort tincture when I developed severe food poisoning that resulted in anaphylactic shock a few hours after eating a mango. I awoke in the middle of the night when swelling in my throat made breathing difficult. My body was beet red and I knew the choices were either a trip to the hospital emergency room or a good dose of herbal blood and liver cleansers. Of course, I opted for the herbs and started drinking 2 teaspoons of St. John's Wort tincture with 2 teaspoons of a root tincture of Dandelion, Yellow Dock, and Burdock in a cup of water every 10 minutes for almost an hour. My symptoms improved and I returned to bed, waking up three hours later feeling and looking normal. I was impressed! Since then, I have recommended the same herbs to different people suffering from severe food poisoning, Brown Recluse spider bites, and exposure to chemical solvents, resulting in impressive outcomes. Milk Thistle seeds (*Silybum marianum*) are also excellent to detoxify the liver and can be included in the blend.

Urinary Tract: St. John's Wort's calming and normalizing influence on the nerves regulating the urinary tract is excellent for bladder spasms and irritation, pain, bleeding, cystitis (bladder infection), and interstitial cystitis (chronic bladder inflammation with urinary urgency and frequency). The herb seems to improve nerve and muscle control of the bladder sphincter to normalize the voiding reflex. Diuretic properties increase urine output and excretion of waste products and toxins. One interesting *in vitro* study found that hypericins in an alcohol extract of the herb demonstrated significant cytotoxic activity against cancer cells in the bladder (Skalkos, 2005).

Another traditional use of St. John's Wort is to reduce bed-wetting in children. A cup of tea or 10-20 drops of tincture in water are taken before bedtime. Emotional trauma and deep-seated fear can be an underlying cause of bed-wetting, so be sure the emotional life of the child and other family members is healthy. Take a tincture of the herb over time as a tonic for chronic bladder weakness and other problems, or short-term for spasms and infections.

The Lungs and Respiratory System: St. John's Wort has historically been used as a remedy for lung and bronchial infections, congestion, bleeding, and inflammation. Using *in vivo* tests, researchers found that a crude extract of the herb reduced bronchial spasms and promoted relaxation during spontaneous and induced spasms, which is similar to the actions of opiate drugs prescribed for cough suppression (Gilani, 2005). The tea or tincture is ingested for these problems, while a gargle of the tea is helpful for sore throats. Combine St. John's Wort with other lung herbs such as Elecampane (*Inula helenium*), Horehound (*Marrubium vulgare*), and Pleurisy Root (*Asclepias tuberosa*).

Women's Health: St. John's Wort helps normalize irregular menses and decrease premenstrual syndrome (PMS) symptoms, pelvic pain, and menstrual cramping. I usually recommend the tincture to women who have uterine fibroids and ovarian cysts with good results, especially when combined with Yarrow (*Achillea millefolium*) and Chasteberry (*Vitex agnus-castus*).

As previously mentioned, **women using contraceptive drugs should not use St. John's Wort** because it can interfere with the metabolism of pharmaceutical hormones and stimulate clearance of excess estrogen from the liver, making birth control pills less effective. This has caused breakthrough bleeding and increases the risk of unwanted pregnancy (Hall, 2003; Pfrunder, 2003).

Clinical observations show that St. John's Wort is safe to use in small doses during pregnancy (Moretti, 2009), but is safest to ingest after the first trimester because it is a mild uterine stimulant. During childbirth the tincture or tea helps reduce labor pains and afterbirth pains caused by strong contractions of the uterus as it returns to normal size. St. John's Wort also helps reduce uterine hemorrhage. It may be applied externally as an oil, salve, fomentation, or the tea is used in a sitz bath to heal perineal tears and sore, inflamed tissues following delivery.

A clinical trial involving 144 women recovering from cesarean delivery documented that the topical application of *H. perforatum* ointment around the incision safely facilitated wound healing while minimizing scar formation. The women were divided into 3 groups: a treatment group that applied the herbal ointment 3 times a day for 16 days, a placebo group, and a control group that received no intervention. Women using the ointment also reported significantly less pain and pruritus (itching) (Samadi, 2010). Nursing mothers can also apply the oil or ointment to sore or caked breasts, as long as it is wiped off before nursing. A study involving 33 nursing mothers showed that the herb is safe for mothers and their infants while breast-feeding (Lee, 2003).

St. John's Wort is also helpful during menopausal changes that can trigger irritability and anxiety. One research trial designed to assess the effects of the herb on problematic symptoms involved 106 menopausal women who took a tablet of a standardized extract containing hypericin (300 mg) 3 times a day for 12 weeks. None of the women were on hormone therapy. At the start of the trial, 80-90% of participants complained of moderate to severe menopausal symptoms that included irritability, anxiety, depression, headaches, heart palpitations, and hot flashes. About 70% of the women experienced significant improvement in their symptoms at the conclusion of the trial, while 80% happily reported their sexuality was noticeably enhanced (Grube, 1999). Other clinical studies have validated the herb's efficacy for mood disorders related to menopause (Geller, 2005). In one study, 301 women experiencing menopausal hot flashes with depression and irritability were given alcohol extracts of St. John's Wort and Black Cohosh (*Cimicifuga racemosa*) or placebo for 4 months. Researchers concluded that the herbal combination significantly alleviated menopausal complaints and was superior to the placebo (Uebelhack, 2006).

Wounds, Skin Infections, and Dermatitis: St. John's Wort is a wonderful and sometimes miraculous external healer that I have included as a main ingredient in my herbal salve for over 35 years. Hyperforin occurring in the leaves, flowers, and immature seedpods has antibiotic, anti-inflammatory, and vulnerary properties excellent for treating deep and superficial wounds. Astringent properties reduce or eliminate bleeding and bruising, especially when applied immediately after injuries occur. Antibacterial properties of the herb have traditionally been employed as antiseptics for wound healing to prevent and treat infection. Laboratory studies show that St. John's Wort extracts have broad-spectrum antimicrobial activity against Gram-negative and Gram-positive bacteria, including *Staphylococcus aureus, Streptococcus mutans, Proteus vulgaris, Escherichia coli,* and *Pseudomonas aeruginosa* (Barbagallo, 1987; Sakar, 1990). Combining it with Yarrow for external healing works especially well.

This remarkable vulnerary is a first aid remedy that is also beneficial for chronic problems. Apply it as a liniment using the tincture, a fomentation (wash of the tea), poultice, oil, or salve to decrease pain, inflammation, and swelling. Using external applications of St. John's Wort while ingesting the tincture is a specific treatment for painful herpes skin lesions, including cold sores, genital lesions, and shingles. External applications of the herb are helpful for impetigo, a very contagious staphylococcal skin infection. It is healing and reduces pain for sore muscles (myalgia), sprains, carpal tunnel, deeply lacerated and punctured wounds, venomous bites and stings, boils, bruises, varicose veins, hemorrhoids, skin ulcers, urticaria (hives), and some types of tumors. St. John's Wort may be applied to gums around painful teeth and works well combined with Clove oil for toothaches. It is interesting that although oral and topical use of the herb can cause photosensitivity and sunburns, it is a well-known treatment for easing pain, promoting healing, and reducing scarring for many types of burns such as sunburns, radiation and chemical burns.

A German study revealed that the application of a St. John's Wort preparation (made by extracting 5 grams of the fresh flowers in 100 grams of olive oil for 10 days at 68°F) greatly increased the rate of healing in first-, second-, and third-degree burns, and significantly reduced scarring. First-degree burns healed within 48 hours, while second- and third-degree burns healed at least three times faster than burns treated by conventional therapies (Saljic, 1975).

The herb can also be healing and relieve pain and inflammation caused by different types of dermatitis like eczema and psoriasis, especially when applied as an oil or salve and combined with other appropriate herbs. A study involving 21 patients suffering from mild to moderate eczema revealed that a cream of *Hypericum* extract standardized to contain 1.5% hyperforin significantly reduced the eczema lesions and *Staphylococcus aureus* bacteria when patients received treatment twice daily over a 4-week period (Schempp, 2003).

Teachings from the St. John's Wort Deva

"Greetings. I am the deva of the St. John's Wort plants. I am a protector and mediator, helping people to interact within their environment and to live peacefully doing so. I am a regulator of the solar plexus, a primary energy center in the body. This is the center and consciousness of physical power that is each person's identity as an individual self. This physical power and sense of self enable people to be fully present and connected with the strength of their unique being to interact in the world and with others in balanced, life-promoting, empowered ways. My golden-yellow flowers point to this affinity with the solar plexus energy; for the powerful energies of my plants (ruled by Leo and the Sun) energize the solar plexus nerve center. There is a direct link of communication between the nerve 'bundle' in the solar plexus and the one in the head that you call the brain. The medicines of my plants harmonize and balance these two nerve centers and the communication network between them, assisting with their balanced flow of energies, allowing the body and mind to adapt to the constantly changing dramas and circumstances of daily life. For the solar plexus monitors the energetic frequencies of the 'outer world' and is constantly interpreting and assimilating the surrounding environment and people. Through the nervous system network, messages are relayed to the brain, which adjusts and creates the chemicals necessary for the body to maintain balance. I help the body make adjustments to assimilate and accommodate the outer world with the inner world of the individual. This is a primary aspect of my protective energies.

"I am under the domain of the Sun and Jupiter. My powerful medicine comes from the forces of the Sun and is carried through the tissues of your body by the expansive movement of Jupiter. The actions and personality of my plants are masculine in nature, and they are ruled by the elements of fire and air. These two elements together hold and carry the spark of light and life, as manifested in the nervous system of animal and human bodies. My medicines protect, energize, and restore the light essence of the human body. They assist the light essence as it is condensed into the solid structure of nerve tissues that carry the frequencies of life-giving light through the body. This 'translation' of essence into structure requires the fine-tuning of frequencies within the tissues, and a certain 'tension' between the polarities must be maintained for the system to work correctly; for it is a finely tuned instrument.

"My medicine promotes the smooth, harmonious movement of energies throughout the body – in nervous energy allowing smooth movement of muscles and peaceful thoughts and emotions; in the smooth flow of food through the digestive tract; in the smooth passage of water through the waterways and blood vessels; and in the gentle flow of air through the airways.

"The great power and force of the Sun are reflected within my plants, which can destroy and eliminate persistent viruses, poisons, and toxins. This purification is another outcome of the balanced energy between the solar plexus and brain. Of all the tissues in the body, I provide great purification and healing to the liver, which must always battle with toxins and unwanted substances from the external world.

"The medicine of my flowers is as powerful as my leaves, and the flowers are especially suited for those with a weak heart and feelings of helplessness and hopelessness. My protective and restorative qualities will heal from the inside out, from the essence to the form. And so I assist in the manifestation of energy and light essence into human form. I heal from the space of essence to normalize and harmonize the frequencies of the emotions and thoughts emitted from the body and mind.

"The teaching I offer reflects my healing and harmonious blending of nerve networks in the solar plexus and brain. Humans are now called upon to evolve as a global family and develop balance between the center of individual personal power grounded in the solar plexus with the higher centers of the compassionate heart and clear mind of awareness. For when the heart and mind evolve, the old perspective of a self-contained individual separate from others transforms into the experience of being connected and at one with all of life. With this perspective of existence, no one and no thing is truly separate from ourselves, and people treat each other, all creatures upon the earth, and the earth itself with greater kindness. The relationship with self and the outside world is peacefully resolved in unity. My medicines help to reconnect the broken fragments of 'self' back together, to mend and make whole. This is also one of my abilities in healing injuries of broken and crushed tissues.

"When the brute force and power contained within the solar plexus are calm and aligned rather than chaotic and destructive, harmony is restored and peace prevails. Just as the delightful, sunny-golden aura of my flowers elicits beauty, great joy arises. And so, dear one, breathe deeply of life. Feel the spark and movement of the sacred and mysterious force of life lighting up your body. Learn to be at peace in this vast space of awareness, where reference points of 'self' and 'other' melt and merge into oneness. Rest dear one, and know that you are the essence of radiance and calm."

Scullcap

Scutellaria lateriflora
Labiatae (*Lamiaceae*) (Mint) Family

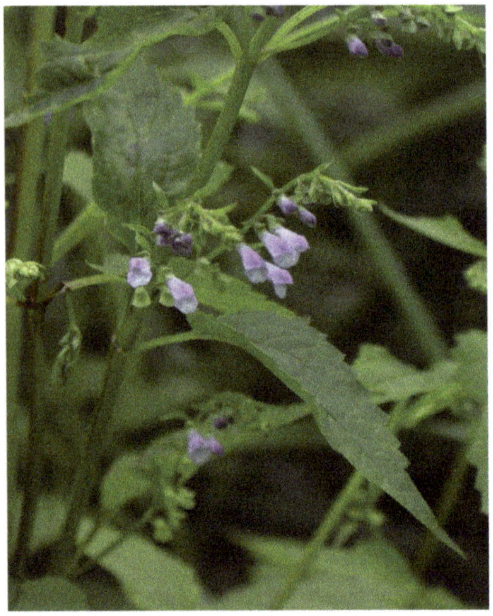

Common Names

Skullcap, helmet flower, hood wort, hooded willow herb, and blue pimpernel are descriptive of the shape and color of the flowers. Mad dog scullcap, mad dog weed, and mad weed originate from its use in treating rabies from the bites of infected animals.

Medicinal Part of the Plant

The leaves and flowers contain the active phytochemicals.

Range and Habitat

More than 300 species of *Scutellaria* grow throughout temperate and tropical regions worldwide, including about 100 species occurring in North America. Indigenous to central and eastern North America, *Scutellaria lateriflora* is the medicinal variety commonly used and marketed in the United States and Europe. It grows in moist, shady areas along banks of streams and lakes, but also does well in partial or full sun. Many *Scutellaria* species are medicinal and include *S. baicalensis* and *S. barbata* native to China, and *S. integrifolia* and *S. incana* indigenous to North America.

Description of the Plant

S. lateriflora is a beautiful perennial herb growing 2-3′ tall. The fibrous roots produce several square, erect, smooth stalks with many opposite branches. The green stalks are tinged with a reddish-maroon color that increases over the growing season.

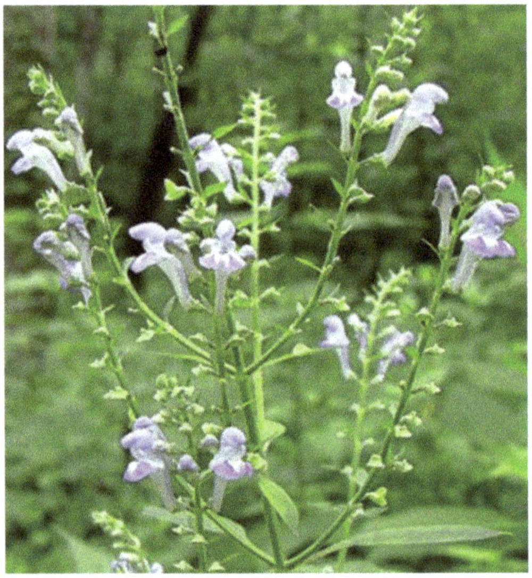

The 1-3″ long leaves climb the stalks in an opposite pattern and are attached by petioles. Leaves are simple with pinnate veins, lanceolate to ovate in shape with serrated margins and pointed tips.

Blooming from June through August, the pale bluish-purple flowers appear in several slender racemes 2-6″ long. The species name *lateriflora*, meaning "flowering on the side," refers to the way flowers grow along one side of the upper stalks. The small flowers are ¼″ long and consist of a tubular corolla ending in two lips (bi-labiate). The upper lip has a hood-shaped, helmet-like protuberance and the lower lip consists of two rounded lobes. The common name "Scullcap" emerged because these two-lobed flowers resemble a soldier's helmet or cap. All *Scutellaria* species have flowers with this characteristic bi-lobed shape. When the corolla dries and falls off, an accordion-shaped, bi-lobed pod is left containing tiny, dark seeds. The genus name comes from the Latin word *scutella*, meaning "little dish" or "platter," referring to the shape of the seedpod.

Cultivation

Scullcap prefers complete or partially shaded areas, but tolerates sun. It thrives in consistently moist, fertile soil. It is a delicate perennial, and in my experience the plant seldom lives more than 3-4 years. It will self-sow its seeds and the rapidly growing root system sends up many stems.

Cultivation by sowing seeds, which have a high germination rate, is fairly easy. They can be directly sown into the garden in early spring or started in greenhouse flats in March. Seeds are very tiny, so pat them into the soil rather than burying them. Transplant seedlings to a permanent bed when they are 2-3″ high, spacing them 6-10″ apart. Apply dried mulch around the seedlings and keep the roots moist. The beautiful Chinese species, *S. baicalensis* and *S. barbata,* are also easy to grow in my southern Indiana gardens.

Harvest

Prune the upper leaves and flowers when the plant is blooming. Do not over-prune, as this can severely damage and kill the plant. Since this is a relatively short-lived perennial, always harvest some seeds to replant the following spring.

Preparation of Plant Medicine and Dosages

Ensure a potent remedy by preparing tincture or tea from freshly harvested leaves and flowers, because the herb's medicinal constituents rapidly decline after drying. Dried tea, pills, and capsule preparations of *S. lateriflora* often have little therapeutic effect, but tinctures are quite potent and do not deteriorate.

PREPARATIONS

Tincture: Process the freshly harvested leaves and flowers in 75% 190-proof grain alcohol and 25% distilled water. Dosage: 10-60 drops up to 4 times a day as needed. Small doses consisting of 10-30 drops can be ingested during the day, while larger doses are taken at night for insomnia and greater sedation. For severe anxiety, pain or spasms, large doses of 90 drops may be taken up to 4 times a day.

Tea: Cover 1-2 teaspoons of the fresh herb with 1 cup of boiling water and steep for 10-15 minutes. Dosage: 1 cup up to 4 times a day as needed. The tea has a pleasant, mild flavor.

Chemical Constituents

The therapeutic effects of *S. lateriflora* are primarily due to its flavonoids that include scutellarin (sedative, antispasmodic, cardiovascular tonic), scutellarein, baicalin (antioxidant, anticarcinogenic), baicalein, lateriflorin, ikonnikoside, apigenin, hispidulin, luteolin, and wogonin. Baicalin was identified in a 50% alcohol extract (40 mg/gm) and baicalein was present in a 95% alcohol extract (33 mg/gm), as well as the amino acids GABA (gamma-aminobutyric acid) in water and alcohol extracts (approximately 1.6 mg/gm) and glutamine (31 mg/gm) in a water extract (Awad, 2003). Melatonin (the pineal hormone promoting sleep) and serotonin have been identified in the leaves (Cole, 2008). GABA and serotonin are the primary calming neurotransmitters, and glutamine supports muscles, the immune system, intestinal health and digestion.

Volatile oils include limonene, terpineol, cadinene, caryophyllene, and humulene. Hentriacontane is anti-inflammatory and diuretic. Lignins decrease cholesterol and have antibacterial, antioxidant, antitumor, antiviral, and laxative effects. Nutrients include calcium, potassium, magnesium, chromium, iron, manganese, selenium, zinc, ascorbic acid (vitamin C), beta-carotene (vitamin A), niacin (vitamin B3), and riboflavin (B2).

Safety, Contraindications, and Drug Interactions

Scullcap is a safe herb with no known toxicity. Due to its relaxing action on the nervous system, it can increase the effects of sedating and antidepressant drugs when taken together. There have been reports of liver damage and toxicity attributed to Scullcap, which were actually caused by Germander (*Teucrium* spp.) plants that were mistakenly harvested and marketed as Scullcap. Claims have been made that an overdose of Scullcap can cause giddiness, stupor, mental confusion and twitching, but I have never seen or heard of any actual cases, and these symptoms may be caused by adulteration with Germander. Unfortunately, Germander adulteration is common, but the herb industry is attempting to correct the problem. When possible, grow your own Scullcap to know that you have the correct medicinal species. If you purchase the tincture, be sure that it is harvested and produced by a reliable company.

Medicinal Uses

History of the Plant

Although several species of *Scutellaria* are indigenous to Britain and Europe, they do not appear in the old herbals of Dioscorides, Gerard, or Culpeper. When Europeans immigrated to North America, woodland tribes, including the Iroquois, Penobscot and Cherokee, were using indigenous Scullcap species for medicinal purposes. The Cherokee drank the tea as part of a combination to treat suppressed menses, breast pain, and diarrhea. Dr. Charles Millspaugh wrote that the Scullcaps "are valued by the aborigines of countries in which they grow as antihydrophobics [remedies for rabies]" (Millspaugh, 1887).

S. lateriflora was introduced into North American medicine in 1773 by Dr. Lawrence Van Derveer of New Jersey, who is credited with using it to successfully treat over 400 cases of rabies in people and 1,000 cases in cattle over a 40-year period with only two reported deaths. Although there is some controversy over the validity of the doctor's claim, Scullcap was widely used for treating rabies by physicians in colonial America.

During the 1800s, *S. lateriflora* was administered for its sedating properties by all North American schools of medicine and was especially extolled by the Eclectic physicians. Harvey Felter, M.D. (1865–1927) wrote that doctors primarily prescribed it as a tranquilizer and sedative for insomnia and all types of nervous conditions, including mental and physical exhaustion, anxiety, neuralgia (nerve pain), convulsions, muscle spasms, tremors, chorea (involuntary spasms in the face, legs, and arms), tetanus, epilepsy, and delirium tremens caused by advanced alcoholism. Scullcap was a remedy for intermittent fevers of malaria, infant irritability and pain caused by teething, and for anxiety due to hormonal changes in women (Felter, 1898). The herb was listed as a tranquilizer and nervine in the *U.S. Pharmacopoeia* from 1860–1900 and in the

National Formulary from 1916–1947.

A popular herb in North America and Europe, *S. lateriflora* is a primary ingredient in many sleep formulas. Only a few studies have investigated the biological effects of *S. lateriflora*, while most research has been on *S. baicalensis* (Chinese Scullcap). Both species have similar phytochemicals and biological effects of calming the nervous system.

Healing Qualities

Analgesic, anti-inflammatory, antioxidant, antispasmodic, mild diuretic, febrifuge, hypotensive, nervine, sedative, and tonic for the nervous system.

Traditional Chinese Medicine (TCM) Perspective

S. lateriflora is mildly bitter, cooling, and drying. Its relaxing, restoring, and stabilizing actions especially benefit the nervous system, brain, heart, and liver. The herb eases constrained Qi throughout the body to relieve general anxiety, pain, spasms, tremors, and to allow the release of heat and toxins. By reducing Qi constraint in the heart and blood vessels, Scullcap eases chest pains, palpitations, irritability and hypertension, and promotes circulation. It is therapeutic for Heart and Kidney Yin deficiency that can cause night sweats, palpitations, insomnia, panic attacks, and tinnitus. Its cooling and restoring nature clears empty heat caused by Yin deficiency. Scullcap addresses nervous tension, exhaustion, anxiety, and "burn-out" caused by Qi constraint in the kidneys and adrenal glands. It is specific for internal Wind and Liver Wind conditions responsible for spasms, tremors, tics, convulsions, facial paralysis, and restless leg syndrome.

More than 90 species of Scullcap grow in China. *S. baicalensis*, known as Baical Scullcap and Huang-qin, is native to China and northern Asia, and is the most widely used and researched species in TCM. The root (rather than leaves and flowers) is prescribed for damp heat conditions and is anti-inflammatory, antibiotic, cholagogue, antihypertensive, and sedating. Research shows it is effective against some cancers. Scutellarin, a flavonoid occurring in both species, is widely used in treating various cardiovascular diseases in TCM.

Primary Actions

The nervous system regulates all activities and functions in the body. Insufficient or excessive nerve stimulation has many ramifications. In this chaotic world, the nervous system is easily depleted and stressed into dysfunction, making Scullcap a wonderful ally for many of us! The herb's relaxing and tonifying actions on the nerves throughout the body makes it one of the finest nervine and antispasmodic herbs. It has been the primary ingredient in my "Nerve Tonic and Insomnia Relief" tincture formula for over 35 years. Based on personal experience and observation of friends and clients using the tincture, I have found *S. lateriflora* to be a gentle, consistently reliable herb, and am continually grateful for its healing gifts. It is my all-time favorite nervine and sedative to restore and calm the nerves, and it always has a place in my medicine cabinet at home and medicine bag when traveling.

I will always remember when, many years ago, I received news so shocking and horrifying that I experienced a type of hysteria in which I lost control and went into a terrified panic that felt very scary. I had enough wits to take about 90 drops of *S. lateriflora* tincture in water and was amazed at the quick energetic switch I felt as the muscles in my chest and abdomen relaxed, followed by deeper breathing and a hint of inner calmness. It had felt like I was uncontrollably exploding outward during the fit of hysteria, and then I felt the action of Scullcap pulling me back into my center, and I calmed down within 20 minutes.

Nervous System: Scullcap is one of the most effective and dependable sedative and nervine herbs. As a sedative it is relaxing, and as a nervine it nourishes, soothes, and revitalizes the central nervous system. A unique characteristic of this restorative tonic is its dualistic ability to either relax or stimulate the nerves. It is calming and relaxing for all types of anxiety and nervous tension, overstimulation and hyperactivity, muscle rigidity, spasms, and obsessive compulsive behavior. As a stimulating nervine, it can energize and restore a weak, depleted nervous system, and is helpful for depression and nervous exhaustion.

The tincture is wonderful for nerve and muscle pain, cramps, inflammation, stress headaches, fibromyalgia, trigeminal neuralgia (facial nerve pain), sciatica, tics, twitching, tremors, restless leg syndrome, and Parkinson's disease. It has historically been prescribed for the treatment of convulsions, epilepsy and seizures, palsy (paralysis), meningitis (inflammation of the membranes covering the brain and spinal cord), and delirium tremens (uncontrollable tremors and impaired brain function due to alcohol addiction and withdrawal). Scullcap normalizes and calms the nervous system during any kind of drug or alcohol withdrawal, including the cessation of caffeine and nicotine. Medium to large doses (60-90 drops) of tincture can be taken 4-6 times throughout the day for these more serious conditions. Scullcap reduces pain and should be combined with other analgesics such as Willow bark (*Salix* spp.), Meadowsweet (*Filipendula ulmaria*), and St. John's Wort (*Hypericum perforatum*) for optimal strength and pain relief. Research shows that inflammation is reduced by wogonin, a flavonoid in Scullcap that decreases inflammation by inhibiting the release of histamine and leukotrienes (both cause allergic reactions and inflammation). Wogonin also reduced blood levels of IgE, a component of the immune system that rises in response to allergic reactions (Lim, 2003).

Scullcap tincture provides deep, refreshing sleep without hangovers or possibility of addiction, and is helpful for many cases of insomnia, restless sleep, and nightmares. For these problems, take 30 drops before bedtime. The dosage may be increased to 60-90 drops, and Scullcap may be combined with other sedatives like Hops (*Humulus lupulus*), Catnip (*Nepeta cataria*), Chamomile (*Matricaria recutita*), and Valerian (*Valeriana officinalis*). Valerian is a warming herb and Scullcap is cooling, so they have a balancing effect.

Scullcap is a remedy for adrenal exhaustion and "burn-out" because it calms the sympathetic nervous system while supporting and normalizing the adrenal medulla. This inner core of the adrenal gland secretes epinephrine (adrenaline) and norepinephrine during the "fight or flight" response to stress. These both act as stimulating hormones and neurotransmitters that are involved in rapid increases in nerve and metabolic activity. Scullcap's strong calming influence reduces the excitatory actions of these adrenal hormones.

Researchers have identified several compounds in *S. lateriflora* leaves and their mechanisms of action contributing to their relaxing and restorative abilities. Baicalin, baicalein, and the amino acids GABA (gamma-aminobutyric acid) and glutamine are found in water and alcohol extracts of the herb (Awad, 2003).

Baicalin and baicalein bind to GABA receptors on cell membranes (the same sites used by benzodiazepine drugs), eliciting a relaxing effect on the nervous system. GABA is a primary inhibitory neurotransmitter that has powerful relaxing, anti-anxiety action on the nervous system. GABA is necessary for normal brain function and mood regulation, and it reduces obsessive thinking. Glutamine is a source of cellular energy, providing fuel for normal brain and muscle function. It protects the cells lining the digestive tract and supports gut immunity. Serotonin (another primary calming neurotransmitter) and melatonin (the pineal hormone promoting sleep) are also present in the leaves (Cole, 2008). Flavonoids (scutellarin, lateriflorin, and ikonnikoside) that were extracted from the leaves in boiling water and 70% alcohol extracts bound to serotonin receptors on cell surfaces and elicited a strong calming influence in studies (Gafner, 2003).

One small clinical study with 19 healthy subjects demonstrated the effectiveness of *S. lateriflora* in reducing anxiety. The participants took a single dose of 1 or 2 capsules of freeze-dried Scullcap extract (100 mg/capsule) or a placebo. Although participants were not suffering from anxiety, everyone who took the Scullcap reported a noticeable relaxing effect (Wolfson, 2003). Another clinical trial involved 43 people, of whom 81% experienced mild anxiety. The volunteers took freeze-dried Scullcap leaves (350 mg) or a placebo 3 times a day for 14 days. Those taking Scullcap experienced significant improvement in their anxiety without fatigue or loss of energy. Five people also reported improvement in chronic conditions (irritable bowel, painful menstruation, hay fever, and eczema) during Scullcap treatment (Brock, 2014).

University researchers in Canada designed a test to determine the ability of *S. lateriflora* to inhibit seizures in rats. After inducing epilepsy in male rats, they were divided into five groups. Three groups were given a weak extract of Scullcap with Gelsemium (*Gelsemium sempervirens*) and Jimson Weed (*Datura stramonium*) (both contain toxic alkaloids) in their water supply continuously for 30 days. The fourth group received minerals in water and the fifth control group received only water. The number of seizures in all the rats were recorded each day. Those that drank the herbal extract displayed no seizures during the treatment, while many seizures were recorded in the other two groups. However, when the herbal extract was discontinued, the rats displayed many spontaneous seizures comparable to the two control groups. Although Scullcap was used in combination with two toxic herbs, this test strongly suggests the calming and antispasmodic effects of *S. lateriflora* on the nervous system (Peredery, 2004).

Researchers have explored the ability of *S. lateriflora* to protect nerve cells from oxidative stress, a major contributor to nerve degeneration and neuropsychiatric conditions like anxiety, depression, Alzheimer's, and Parkinson's disease. Water and alcohol extracts of the herb exhibited significant antioxidant action by destroying free radicals that cause oxidation and by protecting nerve tissues from damage (Lohani, 2013).

The sedative and nervine properties of Scullcap are beneficial for neurasthenic conditions, which are nerve-related problems anywhere in the body caused by underlying anxiety and nervousness. The herb helps relieve nervous tension, spasms, and pain in the digestive, cardiovascular, and genitourinary systems.

Digestive System: Scullcap is helpful in treating nervous indigestion, "butterflies" in the stomach, spastic bowels, diarrhea, and hiccups, which are spasms of the diaphragm muscle. The amino acid glutamine, occurring in the leaves, supports healthy digestion by helping the body to rebuild and protect the mucosa (the thin lining) of the digestive tract. Glutamine soothes and heals inflamed, ulcerated tissues in the stomach and intestines, and it reduces the risk of irritable bowel and leaky gut problems in the intestines.

Cardiovascular System: Scullcap helps relax, normalize, and restore the muscular layers of blood vessels, making it an effective vasodilator that promotes increased circulation, reduces vascular spasms, and relieves stress-induced headaches and hypertension. Since the heart is primarily a muscular organ regulated by the nervous system, Scullcap can be beneficial for palpitations and arrhythmias. Baicalin and scutellarin extracted from Scullcap are widely used in TCM to treat and prevent cardiovascular diseases, including hypertension and arteriosclerosis. Baicalin is a strong antioxidant that protects cells from injury and reduces blood clot formation (Huang, 2005).

Scutellarin is widely used in treating various cardiovascular diseases in TCM. In clinical trials involving 634 people suffering from cerebral embolisms, thrombosis (blood clots), and paralysis following a stroke, a scutellarin extract of the herb improved blood flow in more than 88% of the participants when it was given orally or by muscular and intravenous administration (Peigen, 1987).

Genitourinary System: Scullcap relaxes nerves and muscles in the pelvis and genitourinary tract to help problems caused or worsened by nervous agitation and overstimulation. As a mild diuretic, it increases kidney activity and urine output. The herb relaxes a spastic bladder and helps urinary incontinence. Combine it with St. John's Wort and Mullein root (*Verbascum thapsus*) for this purpose. The tea or tincture relaxes the ureters, helping to decrease the excruciating spasms and pain during the passage of kidney stones.

Researchers have conducted in *vitro tests* exploring the ability of different herbs to reduce renal fibrosis, the scarring and excessive amounts of connective tissue that promote kidney disease. *S. lateriflora* demonstrated strong antioxidant effects in protecting kidney cells, and reduced the amounts of fibroblasts that produce excess connective tissue and cause scarring (Wojcikowski, 2009).

Women's Health and Young Children: Scullcap relaxes pelvic muscles and the tissues of reproductive organs, promoting healthy circulation and calming anxiety and nervous tension occurring with premenstrual syndrome (PMS) and menopause. The herb is a helpful remedy for suppressed menstruation caused by anxiety, and it relieves menstrual cramps.

Scullcap may be taken in small amounts during pregnancy and during childbirth for pain relief. When combined with Lobelia (*Lobelia inflata*) tincture, I have seen it assist laboring mothers by relaxing the cervical os, allowing for greater dilation. Scullcap is also beneficial for postpartum depression, especially when combined with appropriate herbs and glandular supplements providing endocrine gland support.

Young children can safely take pediatric doses of Scullcap for painful teething, irritability, restlessness, insomnia, and other problems caused by overstimulation (see page 148 for pediatric dosages).

Cancer Research: Researchers discovered that scutellarein extracted from *S. lateriflora* has anticancer potential for fibrosarcoma, an aggressive and highly metastatic cancer of the connective tissue. *In vitro* studies revealed that scutellarein suppressed the proliferation rate of human fibrosarcoma cells by inducing apoptosis (programmed cell death). *In vivo* experiments using mice showed that the volume and weight of the tumors were markedly reduced and metastasis was inhibited after scutellarein treatment (Shi, 2015).

Teachings from the Scullcap Deva

"Greetings, dear one. It is the deva of the beautiful Scullcap herb that speaks to you. I am a being of sweetness and gentle peace. I am feminine in nature and my embracing, mothering ways are alive in my healing plants. I calm the soul and bring sweetness to the bitterness and difficult times in life. My presence on this planet is to soothe people and the animals. The purple-blue color of my flowers calms the visual and nervous centers in the body. With this calming action comes relaxation followed by the expansive, flowing movement of the sacred life force.

"My plants are ruled by the feminine energies of Venus and the expansive, joyful frequencies of Jupiter that carry and enhance the healing powers offered by Venus. For Venus affects the emotional body of humans and animals, offering gifts of balance and harmony manifesting as strong, healthy tissues in well-functioning organs. Having a joyful, grateful attitude in one's life enlivens a radiant frequency of energy that brings the spark of life to the cells of your body. My plants assist in this process. And although the energies of my plants are expansive, they bring calm and balance to the body, heart and mind, and the experience of deep, inner peace and oneness to the soul.

"The indigenous people who once walked upon this land called my plants 'of the beauty way.' Beauty below me, beauty above me, beauty in front of me, beauty behind me. Beauty is me. Beauty. Please sow my seeds and grow my plants so you may sit with them as they bloom into their magnificent glory. For you can feel the healing essence of these sweet ones by simply being in their presence. By sitting with my plants and drinking the medicine of the leaves and flowers, they will assist you in healing a wounded heart. My calming energies restore and make whole the fragments of a broken heart to bring it back to the healing space of deep peace and reconnection with the heart of the Great Mother, to be comforted and made whole.

"I have great compassion for the ills of humans and wish to soothe and comfort you, and to teach you to be present in your heart. This means to quietly sit, feeling into and focusing upon your heart. Breathe. Relax. Move toward the feeling of calmness. Whatever thoughts or feelings arise that interfere with your sense of calm, gently breathe into them, allowing tension to dissipate. Keep your attention on your own heart and feelings rather than dwelling on the object of your thoughts and feelings. Make this a daily practice, and eventually the thoughts and feelings that interrupt your experience of calm can be resolved and dissolved by this powerful practice.

"I am a being in service to the heart. The medicines offered by my plants calm the nerves and tissues of the body so the heart may live and pulsate in joyful, expansive expression of compassion and love. For this is the essence of a happy, healthy heart. I offer my blessings to you, dear one. It is our wish that you be joyful and content in your heart."

Senna

Senna marilandica
Leguminosae (*Fabaceae*) (Legume or Pea) Family

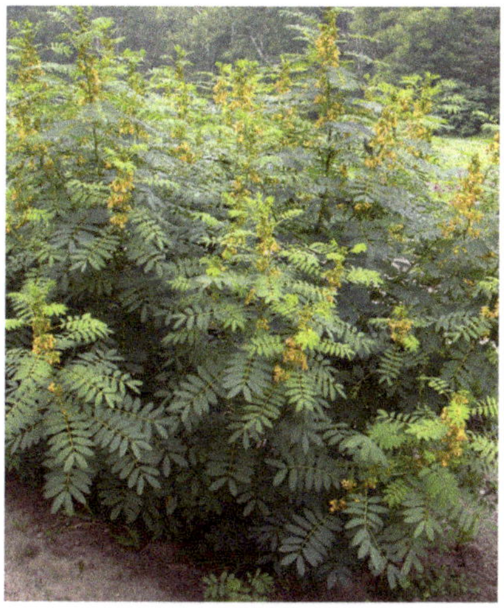

Senna marilandica

Common Names

American Senna, Maryland Senna, Wild Senna, and locust plant are common names for North American varieties of Senna.

Medicinal Part of the Plant

The leaves and seedpods are used medicinally.

Range and Habitat

Several varieties of Senna are native to India, Pakistan, China, southwest Asia, North Africa, and North and South America. *Senna angustifolia* grows in India, other parts of Asia, and the Middle East. Alexandrian Senna is known as *Senna alexandrina, Cassia senna,* and *Cassia acutifolia*. The North American species, *Senna marilandica* (Maryland or American Senna) and *Senna hebecarpa* (Wild Senna), are therapeutically similar to Alexandrian Senna. *Senna marilandica* is also called *Cassia marilandica* (an older name). Dwindling populations of North American species are found in central and eastern United States.

Senna is a hardy plant that tolerates a variety of growing conditions and soils (clay, sandy, and loamy). It grows in full or partial sun in thickets, meadows, prairies, and disturbed areas. The herb lives in dry or moist soil, and established plants can tolerate drought.

Description of the Plant

S. marilandica is a vibrantly colorful and attractive perennial shrub that reaches a height of 4-6′ in fertile soil. The stout stems are round and slightly hairy. Pinnately compound leaves are 6-10″ long and consist of 6-12 pairs of oblong, blunt leaflets. Each leaflet is entire, pinnately veined, and 1-2″ long. A conspicuous club-shaped gland sits near the base of each leaf petiole. The bright-yellow flowers bloom from June through September, appearing in attractive, loose raceme clusters that emerge from the leaf axils. The showy flowers are about ¾″ long and consist of 5 irregular petals that vary in shape and 10 stamens with distinct, brown anthers. Seedpods look like typical legumes and grow to a length of 2-4″. They are very flat and segmented by multiple joints that are twice as wide as they are long. *S. hebecarpa* has a similar appearance to *S. marilandica,* except the seedpods are divided into segments that are longer than they are wide, and the flowers have styles with long spreading hairs compared to the short hairs of *S. marilandica*.

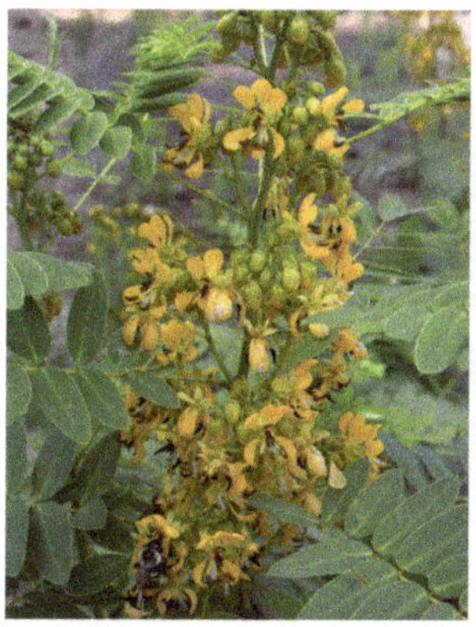

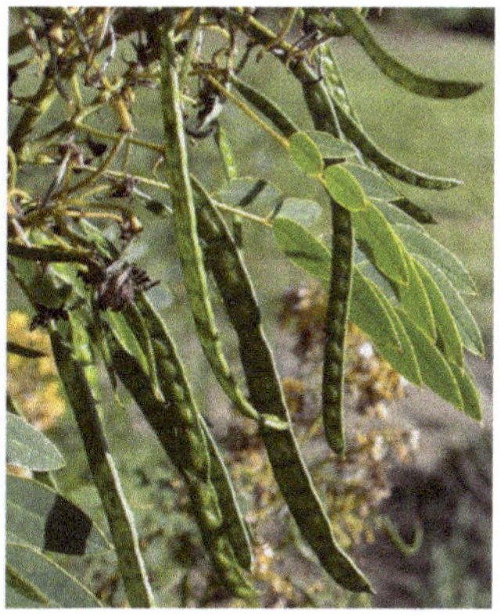

Flowers of *S. marilandica* and seedpods

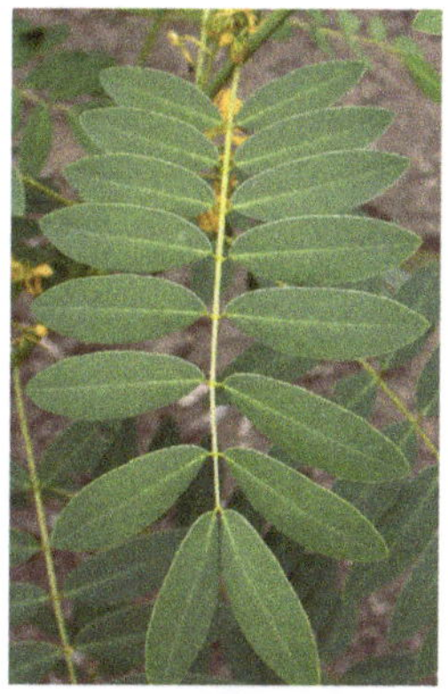

***S. marilandica* leaf with eight pairs of leaflets**

Cultivation

To produce the most vigorous shrubs, plant Senna seeds in early spring under full sun in moist, sandy-loam soil with good drainage. Senna is easy to grow from its large seeds that have a hard, thick covering. Germination is improved by scarification, the method of nicking or scratching seeds to enhance water absorption. Scarify the seeds by rubbing them between two pieces of sandpaper and soaking them in water for 3-5 hours. Then plant them in trays or directly into a fertile garden bed. Seeds germinate in 2-3 weeks. If planted in trays, transplant the seedlings into a garden when they are 2-3″ tall and space them 2′ apart. Adult plants readily self-sow, and the seeds germinate the following year.

Harvest

Gather leaves when the flowers are in bloom. Harvest seedpods when they are fully ripe and green, before they dry and turn brown.

Preparation of Plant Medicine and Dosages

Freshly harvested seedpods and leaves have the greatest potency, but may be dried for future use. Alcohol and hot water extract the phytochemicals, making tincture and tea beneficial preparations. Senna leaves contain about half the amount of active phytochemicals as the seedpods, but have much stronger cathartic properties due to resinous oils that cause intestinal pain and spasms. For this reason, **make preparations for internal use with the seedpods** which are slower and more gentle-acting, and **use leaves for external applications**.

Senna is a bitter-tasting herb and most people prefer taking a pill, capsule, or a few sips of tincture rather than drinking a cup of the bitter tea. Standard doses usually result in bowel movements within 5-10 hours. Many people prefer taking Senna at night before going to bed, which usually stimulates bowel movements the next morning. Due to its strong nature, use Senna on a short-term basis, no longer than 1-2 weeks at a time.

Commercial Senna preparations are available in powders, granules, tablets, tea, tincture, and syrups. Senna is sometimes sold in combination with psyllium fiber from the seeds of *Plantago ovata*, which adds bulk to bowel contents and must be taken with lots of water.

PREPARATIONS

Tincture: Chop freshly harvested seedpods, place in a glass jar, and cover with 50% 190-proof grain alcohol and 50% distilled water. Dosage: 20-30 drops 1-3 times a day as needed.

Tea: Steep 1-2 teaspoons of chopped seedpods in a cup of water for 15-20 minutes. Dosage: 1 cup of tea over the course of a day or ½ cup before bedtime. Do not drink more than 1 cup a day.

Pills and Capsules: These are prepared from seedpods or purchased. To make your own, dry and grind the seedpods into fine powder, which may be packed into gelatin capsules or processed into pills. Dosage: For adults (including the elderly) and children age 12 and over, the usual dose is 15-17 mg daily. Take no more than 34 mg daily. The recommended dose for children 6 to 12 years old is typically 9 mg a day. Correct fluid intake, dietary issues, and other underlying causes of constipation.

When emptying the bowels in preparation for a colonoscopy, the usual dose of Senna is 130 mg taken the day before the procedure. This large dose usually produces complete emptying of the bowels.

External Uses: The leaves are prepared as tea used as a wash and fomentation, or as a poultice or salve to apply to skin diseases, ringworm, and acne.

Chemical Constituents

The primary phytochemicals providing laxative effects are anthraquinone glycosides. These include sennosides A and B (rhein dianthrones), sennosides C and D (rhein aloe-emodin heterodianthrones), and numerous minor sennosides. These act on the colon to stimulate contractions. Emodin is antibacterial, anticarcinogenic, diuretic, immunosuppressive, and vasorelaxant (relaxes and dilates blood vessels). Senna leaves contain about 1.5-3% anthraquinones and the seedpods contain about 2-5%. The plant also contains flavonoids (including isorhamnetin and kaempferol), naphthalene glycosides, and polysaccharides including 7-10% mucilage (galactose, arabinose, rhamnose, and galacturonic acid) that has a soothing effect on tissues it contacts. Other carbohydrates include mannose, fructose, glucose, pinitol, and sucrose. Salicylic acid (anti-inflammatory, analgesic), saponins, tannins, resins, and traces of volatile oils are also present.

Safety, Contraindications, and Drug Interactions

Senna seedpods are gentler than the leaves, resulting in the American Herbal Products Association's warning against long-term use of Senna leaf, but not the seedpod. The anthraquinone glycosides in Senna stimulate uterine contractions and **should not be ingested during pregnancy and in cases of endometriosis, uterine fibroids, or excessive uterine bleeding**. The herb is **contraindicated during lactation** because anthraquinone glycosides can pass from mother's milk into the infant to cause diarrhea. Senna, especially the leaf, is contraindicated in cases of diarrhea, abdominal pain, fecal impaction, kidney inflammation and damage, and irritable and inflammatory bowel conditions such as Crohn's disease, ulcerative colitis, diverticulosis, appendicitis, intestinal obstructions, and hemorrhoids. Senna **should not be ingested by children younger than 6 years of age**, and should be cautiously used by all children and the elderly.

Do not take Senna for more than 10-14 days at a time. Excessive use can cause colic, cramping, abdominal pain, nausea, vomiting, diarrhea and copious liquid stools, and eventual loss of muscle tone and the ability to propel contents through the small and large intestines. Continual consumption of this laxative herb for chronic constipation should also be avoided because the intestines can become dependent on its stimulating action to function. Constant use of Senna has been reported to cause subacute cholestatic hepatitis (obstructed bile secretion into the small intestine), jaundice, and elevated levels of bilirubin and liver enzymes (Sonmez, 2005). Herbal and pharmaceutical laxatives stimulate the contents of the intestines to move quickly, which may reduce absorption of food nutrients and prescription drugs.

Medicinal Uses

History of the Plant

People have taken Senna as a laxative for many centuries and it continues to be one of the most widely used laxative herbs in modern medicine. The medicinal properties of the plant were first described in the writings of Arabian physicians during the ninth century, when it was introduced into European herbalism. It remains an important herb in North American and European medicine, and in the Chinese, Indian Ayurvedic, and Islamic Unani medical traditions. Senna's cleansing actions have been used in the treatment of constipation, atherosclerosis, anemia, jaundice, bronchitis, skin eruptions due to toxins, wounds, hemorrhoids, and ringworm and other fungal infections.

The American Eclectic physicians prescribed it as a laxative during the 1880s–1930s. Harvey Felter, M.D. (1865–1927) wrote, "Its influence is chiefly exerted on the small intestines, augmenting their mucous secretions, exciting increased peristaltic motion, and producing loose, yellowish-brown evacuations. A nursing infant may be purged by the milk of the mother who has taken senna, and so susceptible are some persons to its action, that its odor is said to induce a cathartic action" (Felter, 1898).

Sennosides from Alexandrian Senna (*S. alexandrina*) are used by the pharmaceutical and herbal supplement industries worldwide for their laxative effect. The phytochemicals in Senna and their laxative properties have been extensively researched.

Healing Qualities

The leaves and seedpods have anti-fungal, cathartic, stimulating laxative, and vermifuge properties.

Traditional Chinese Medicinal (TCM) Perspective

Senna is a very strong, Yang-acting herb that is bitter and cooling. By stimulating downward draining movement in the intestinal tract, it purges obstructions and clears Intestinal Qi stagnation that causes constipation. Senna's stimulation is irritating to intestinal membranes, which increases blood flow and muscular wave-like intestinal contractions, called peristalsis, that propel food and waste through the intestinal tract. The cooling nature of Senna helps relieve excess heat in the intestines, which has a drying, constipating effect. The herb's stimulating action can also increase uterine contractions and bleeding.

Primary Actions

Senna is known for its strong laxative action and is indicated for sluggish intestines. It is used to treat mild to severe constipation and to empty the intestines before surgeries and diagnostic tests such as colonoscopies.

This herb should only be taken on a temporary basis while underlying causes of constipation are explored and addressed. Typical causes of chronic constipation include 1) insufficient water intake; 2) a lack of high-fiber foods including fresh fruits, vegetables, whole grains and legumes; 3) food allergies and sensitivities to gluten, dairy, or other common foods; 4) a deficiency of digestive enzymes including stomach acids, pancreatic enzymes and bile, which are all necessary to break food into tiny particles for complete digestion and normal bowel movements, which should occur 1-2 times a day; 5) chronic stress which causes muscle rigidity and a sluggish gut; and 6) some medicines including analgesics and opiates. It is imperative that these factors are corrected rather than only depending on herbal laxatives.

Senna is less expensive than the other well-known laxative, Cascara Sagrada (*Rhamnus purshiana*), but has the tendency to cause more intestinal cramps and spasms. For this reason, Senna is often combined with soothing anti-inflammatory and antispasmodic herbs like Fennel (*Foeniculum vulgare*), Peppermint (*Mentha x piperita*), Cardamom (*Elettaria cardamomum*), Coriander (*Coriandrum sativum*), and Ginger (*Zingiber officinale*).

Senna is an FDA-approved nonprescription laxative. Commercial Senna preparations typically contain the dried seedpods or leaves of *Senna alexandrina*.

Intestinal Cleanser and Laxative: Senna is a powerful, reliable, and stimulating laxative for sluggish intestines and resulting constipation. It can also be used to soften stools and prevent constipation when people have anal fissures, hemorrhoids, and after rectal surgeries. Senna may be taken with other vermifuge herbs and food-grade diatomaceous earth to kill and expel intestinal parasites. The herb's laxative, cleansing actions are beneficial to use as part of a detox program.

In vivo research confirms Senna's ability to promote gastrointestinal motility (Wang, 2002). Sennosides in the leaves and seedpods promote colon activity by increasing nerve stimulation that promotes peristalsis, the series of wave-like contractions causing intestinal muscles to contract and move food through the digestive tract. When ingested, the sennosides in Senna remain largely inactive until they reach the large intestine, where beneficial bacterial enzymes convert them into bowel stimulating compounds called aglycones (rheinanthrones). These aglycones stimulate a nerve network, Auerbach's plexus, which causes peristalsis resulting in a bowel movement, typically within 6 to 12 hours. The sennosides help to temporarily prevent fluid from being absorbed from the large intestine, contributing to softer stools. They also increase the secretion of acidic stomach enzymes to promote digestion. Sennosides are not well-absorbed through the intestinal walls, and about 90% are excreted in the feces (Vanderperren, 2005).

Many clinical trials have validated Senna's efficacy in relieving constipation. Thirty geriatric patients ages 65-94 participated in a trial that examined Senna and a bulk laxative (Agiolax) in the treatment of chronic constipation. Lactulose (a popular laxative) was used as the reference medicine. The bulk laxative plus Senna (14.8 gm daily) produced about twice as many bowel movements than lactulose (20.1 gm daily). Both laxatives proved to be safe for use (Kinnunen, 1993). Another clinical study was conducted to determine treatment and cost efficiency for Senna compared to lactulose in 91 terminal cancer patients treated with opiate narcotics, which often result in difficult constipation. Participants were divided into two groups, one treated with Senna (starting with 0.4 mL daily) and the other treated with lactulose (starting with 15 mL daily) for a 27-day period. The final scores for general health status were similar in both groups. Given that the two treatments had similar efficacy and adverse effects, a recommendation was made for the use of Senna because it is less expensive than lactulose (Agra, 1998).

Research trials reveal that Senna effectively cleans the intestines prior to surgical interventions (Bailey, 1991; Ziegenhagen, 1992; Brouwers, 1980). In a multicenter study, the ability of Senna to clean the colon and rectum prior to surgery was compared with polyethylene glycol, a pharmaceutical laxative. The study involved 523 patients who were preparing for surgery to treat colon cancer, rectal cancer, or diverticular disease. On the evening before surgery, 262 patients received Senna (a package diluted in a glass of water) while 261 patients received polyethylene glycol (2 packages diluted in 2-3 liters of water). Data showed that Senna resulted in better colon cleanliness with less risk for fecal soiling during surgery compared to the pharmaceutical drug. Senna caused fewer side effects and was better tolerated, especially in people with intestinal blockages. Abdominal distention was a problem in 15 patients using polyethylene glycol compared to only 8 people taking Senna (Valverde, 1999). A study of 345 patients undergoing colonoscopies assessed the efficacy of magnesium citrate (a laxative) combined with Senna versus magnesium citrate alone. In patients receiving only magnesium citrate, 6.9% had to reschedule the colonoscopy due to inadequate bowel evacuation. Only 4.4% of the patients also receiving Senna required rescheduling. Adequate visualization during the colonoscopy occurred in 81.3% of patients receiving combination therapy compared with 67.5% receiving magnesium citrate alone (Vradelis, 2009).

Teachings from the Senna Deva

"Greetings, dear one. I am the deva of the Senna plants. I am a spit-fire of energy and my sassy plants are alive with forceful medicine. They are very masculine in nature with strong, fiery, Yang energies that call forth swift, stimulating movement in the solar plexus and lower abdomen of the human body. Although my golden-yellow flowers are beautiful and soothing to behold, my medicine is anything but gentle – it is a mover and pusher of all blockages and propels food through the bowels in a powerful, forceful way. For the power of my plants to act upon the body in this way comes from the same power deep within the earth that spews molten rock and gases through the surface like a volcano. The power of my plants is a miniature reflection of the vast power of the earth when huge land shifts occur and earthquakes shake with a mighty impact. Thus, the power making the earth move and shift in these ways is the same force of my plants that pushes food through the bowels of your body. And so, when using my plants for creating movement in the bowels to purge and make them clean, remember that my medicine must be taken in small amounts with respect for its power.

"The essence of my flowers helps those who are psychologically and emotionally stuck, lacking the ability and momentum to move forward. My flowers are for those who are caught in old patterns so deeply that they cannot see their dilemma and become somewhat paralyzed energetically. Those who are so lost to themselves that they are blinded to self-understanding can benefit from my offerings. I bring stimulus and clarity to provide momentum to these lost ones who lack their own inner drive to push forward. A few drops of the essence of my flowers is good medicine for those who are chronically 'constipated' in unhappy and unfulfilling circumstances, but seem unable to create change.

"Consider my yellow flowers to be like rays of sunlight flying freely through space lacking any restraints. For my plants are blessed with the powerful light and force of the Sun to pierce through all blockages and obstructions – those in the physical body, emotional body, and mental body. My energetic being and the plants emerging from my essence are under the domain of the Sun and astrological sign Leo, and also of Mars and Aries. Aries is of the fire element and ruled by Mars, the planet of powerful, bold, and aggressive warrior energy of fiery action that pushes forward without fear or hesitation.

"When the energies of the Sun and Mars join forces, it is a power to behold, as is the medicine of my plants with their masculine, brute force. This is why many plant people combine my plant medicine with gentle, feminine herbs to create balance. Use my plants wisely, dear one; for they are good teachers in learning how to implement power in your own life by developing the powerful forces of life within yourself."

Stinging Nettle

Urtica dioica

Urticaceae (Nettle) Family

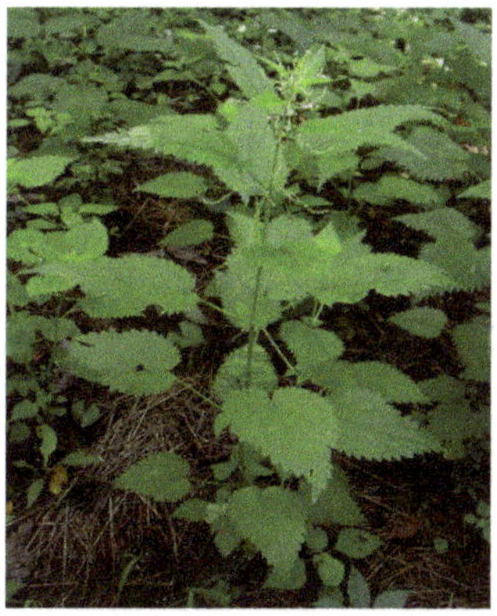

Common Names

Nettle, common Nettle, greater Nettle, wild spinach, and devil leaf (referring to the painful nettle sting) are common names for *Urtica dioica*.

Medicinal Part of the Plant

The leaves are used for food and medicine. The roots are specific for inflammation, prostate, and urinary tract problems. Old herbals recommend using the seeds as a poison antidote, to nourish the endocrine glands, and for treating goiters, tuberculosis, and malarial fevers.

Range and Habitat

The genus *Urtica* contains 40-50 species that grow throughout the world, and many are harvested for food and medicine. Several species have similar medicinal properties and are used interchangeably, but Stinging Nettle (*U. dioica*) is the most popular for healing purposes. It is native to temperate regions of Europe and Asia, and has naturalized in North America and globally. Nettle plants prefer damp, rich soil and full or partial shade, but will grow in sun if soil is moist. *U. dioica* grows in large patches in meadows, woodlands, lowlands, along streams, and other moist areas.

Description of the Plant

Stinging Nettle is a hardy perennial growing 2-4′ tall. The erect, square stems emerge from yellow fibrous roots that are hardy underground creepers branching out to form large patches. The deep-green leaves are opposite and grow 2-4″ long. Ovate leaves have pointed tips, heart-shaped bases, deeply serrated teeth, and are pinnately veined. Stinging Nettle is named for the tiny, silica-tipped hairs covering the leaves and stems. The sharp tips of the hollow hairs, called nettles, penetrate the skin like tiny hypodermic needles and break off to release stinging, irritating chemicals. The genus name *Urtica* is derived from the Latin verb *urere*, meaning "to burn," because of the pain inflicted by the stinging hairs. The English word "nettle" is derived from the Anglo-Saxon word *noedl*, which means "needle".

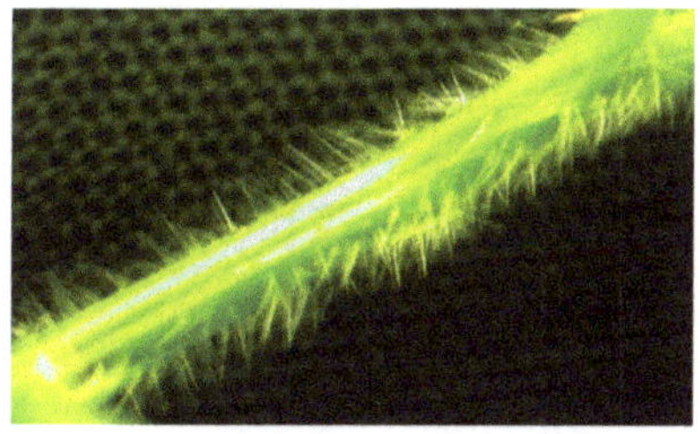

Nettle hairs on the stem

The tiny, inconspicuous, greenish-white flowers droop down from the upper leaf axils in slender, branching panicle clusters. They appear from June through September, depending on the climate. *U. dioica* is dioecious, meaning that individual plants have either male flowers or female flowers, but not both. These flowers lack petals and are unisexual, meaning that they do not have both stamens and pistils. Instead, male flowers have only stamens that release pollen and they appear in loose sprays or racemes. Female flowers have the seed-producing pistil and are more densely clustered together. This characteristic is reflected in the species name *dioica,* which means "two houses" and refers to male and female flowers being on separate plants.

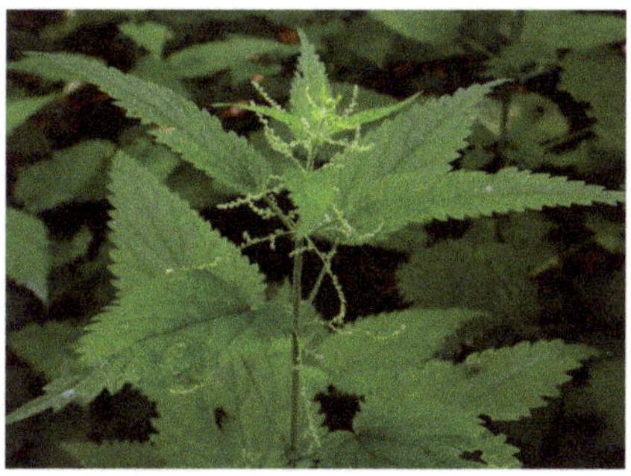

***Urtica dioica* flowers**

U. urens is an annual known as Dwarf Nettle and grows only 1′ tall. It is a monoecious herb, and male and female flowers occur on the same plant. This species, introduced to North America from its native habitat in Europe and Asia, has similar medicinal properties as *U. dioica* and they are used interchangeably in European herbalism.

In the United States, *U. dioica* is classified as a subspecies, *U. dioica* ssp. *dioica*, while European herbalists do not make such a distinction. The subspecies *U. dioica* ssp. *gracilis*, native to North America, is called American or California Nettle. **Do not to confuse *Urtica* plants with *Laportea canadensis* (Wood Nettle) because it irritates the kidneys.**

Cultivation

Stinging Nettle grows naturally in many areas and can be wildcrafted, so cultivation may not be necessary. If you do grow it, remember that the perennial roots are creeping and the herb can spread out rapidly. Plant Nettle where it can have free range without being invasive to other plants. The soil should be high in nitrogen and organic matter naturally occurring in undisturbed woodlands. It is best to plant the herb in full or partial shade. The roots need plenty of moisture, especially if grown under more sun.

The herb can be propagated from seed or root division. Plant seeds in autumn or early spring because they need cold, moist conditioning to germinate. For propagation by root division, it is best to wait until autumn when the leaves have died back to divide the roots. It is said that planting Stinging Nettle with aromatic herbs like Sage, Peppermint, Lavender, and Rosemary increases their production of fragrant oils.

Harvest

Always harvest Nettle leaves in early spring before the flowers bloom because older leaves may cause kidney and urinary tract irritation. Clip the stems 1-3" above the ground and put them upside down in a paper bag, making it easier to handle them. When harvesting and handling fresh Nettles, **protect yourself from the irritating sting and cover your skin** by wearing long pants, socks, a long-sleeved shirt, and gloves.

Harvest the roots in autumn from plants that are at least two years old. Collect seeds in summer when they are dry. The easiest way to harvest seeds is to cut off the top of the plant when the seed heads are mature and brown, and leave them in an open paper bag in a sunny location so that the seeds will fall to the bottom of the bag when they are thoroughly dried.

Preparation of Plant Medicine and Dosages

The freshly harvested leaves can be prepared as tea, tincture, or a poultice. To dry leaves, tie the stems into a bundle and hang them upside down to dry. The thin leaves dry quickly in a shady, well-ventilated area. The seeds and fresh or dried roots are prepared as tea and tincture. **The irritating sting of the nettles on freshly harvested plants is eliminated when they are dried, cooked, or prepared in alcohol as tincture.**

Stinging Nettle can safely and effectively be taken in relatively large doses. Use it as a tonic for an extended period of time for best results.

PREPARATIONS

Nettle Leaf:

Tea: Steep 1 heaping tablespoon of fresh or dried leaf in 1-2 cups of boiled water for 20-60 minutes, or put ¼ cup of leaves in a quart jar and fill it with boiling water. To prepare sun tea, put leaves in a glass jar full of warm water and place it in the sun to brew for 12-24 hours. The dark-green tea has a mild, pleasant flavor. Liven up the taste by combining it with other teas like Green tea, Ginger, Holy Basil (Tulsi), Raspberry, Lemon Balm, or Peppermint. Dosage: 1-3 cups daily.

Tincture: Put freshly harvested, finely chopped leaves in a glass jar, cover with 70% 190-proof grain alcohol and 30% distilled water. Dosage: 1-2 teaspoons 1-3 times a day.

Freeze-dried Capsules: Dosage: 120-600 mg a day.

Fomentation and Poultice: Prepare a strong tea in the usual manner for external application.

Nettle Root:

Decoction Tea: Gently simmer 1 tablespoon of chopped root in 2 cups of water for 10 minutes and steep for 30 minutes. Dosage: 2-3 cups a day.

Tincture: Prepare freshly harvested roots with 70% 190-proof grain alcohol and 30% distilled water. Dosage: 1-1½ teaspoons 1-3 times a day.

Solid Extract: 1-2 grams 1-3 times a day.

Nettle Seeds:

Tea: Crush about 20 seeds and steep in a cup of water for 30 minutes. Dosage: 1-2 cups a day.

Tincture: Crush seeds and cover with 85% 190-proof grain alcohol and 15% distilled water. Dosage: 20-30 drops 1-3 times a day.

Culinary Uses

Stinging Nettle is one of the most nutritious herbs and an excellent source of plant protein. It contains such an abundance of easily digested vitamins, minerals, and protein that it is an excellent food enjoyed by people of many cultures. Young leaves on early spring shoots taste best, but they must first be cooked or dried to eliminate their sting. The fresh, young leaves have a mildly pleasant flavor similar to that of spinach. They can be lightly steamed in a little water, sautéed in oil, or added to soups and casseroles. The dried leaves add a healthy boost when sprinkled over vegetables, salads, or soup.

Chemical Constituents

Nettle leaves are a rich source of minerals and vitamins, including calcium, magnesium, potassium, iron, selenium, chromium, phosphorus, zinc, copper, sulfur, boron (promotes calcium utilization, strong bones, and increased estrogen levels), silica (a building block of tissue in the body), beta-carotene (plant form of vitamin A), vitamins C, D, K, the vitamin B complex, and fiber. The leaves contain higher concentrations of protein (up to 24%) than other plants. The high chlorophyll content gives the tea a dark-green color while providing excellent nourishment and detoxification. The seeds are a rich source of essential fatty acids.

Chemical analysis shows that the stinging hairs contain formic acid, acetic acid, butyric acid, leukotrienes, histamine (causes inflammatory allergic responses), 5-hydroxytryptamine (precursor of serotonin), and acetylcholine (another neurotransmitter) (Collier, 1956). Histamine and acetylcholine are lost after the leaves have been air-dried (Maitai, 1980), but freezing preserves these substances and 5-hydroxytryptamine (Saxena, 1965). Rapid enzymatic breakdown of serotonin occurs in extracts of Stinging Nettle. Formic acid is released from the hairs when brushed against bare skin and causes the stinging sensation. However, formic acid quickly deteriorates and loses its stinging properties when the plant is dried or heated in water.

The leaves contain phenolic acids, such as chlorogenic and caffeic-malic acids, which are anti-inflammatory and have been shown to inhibit the production of inflammatory compounds known as prostaglandins and leukotrienes. Roots and leaves contain flavonoids (kaempferol, quercetin, isohamnetin, and rutin), minerals, coumarins including scopoletin (anti-inflammatory, antispasmodic, antibacterial), and stigmasterol, campesterol, and beta-sitosterol (helps inhibit cell division and growth in prostate cells).

Nettle roots are the source of different lignans including a lectin called *Urtica dioica* agglutinin, and oleanolic acid, phenolic acids, and polysaccharides (Hiermann, 1989). Research indicates that lignans decrease testosterone levels by blocking sex hormone binding globulin (SHBG), which reduces prostate inflammation (Schottner, 1997).

Safety, Contraindications, and Drug Interactions

Stinging Nettle is a safe herb for people of all ages with no known toxicity, contraindications, or drug interactions. Side effects from excessive consumption are rare but include mild gastrointestinal upset and urticaria (hives). Stop ingesting the herb if side effects occur, drink lots of water, and the problem will clear.

Nettle is notorious for its temporary but painfully irritating sting occurring when hairs on fresh plants brush against bare skin. The sting leads to temporary itching and development of red welts usually lasting for several minutes, or longer in sensitive individuals, and numbness is occasionally reported. The stinging sensation can be relieved by quickly rubbing the juice from torn or mashed leaves of Jewelweed (*Impatiens capensis, I. pallida*), Plantain (*Plantago* spp.), or Yellow Dock (*Rumex crispus*) on the affected area. Medicinal extracts of nettle do not cause the stinging reaction because the hairs are destroyed in processing.

Do not ingest preparations made from mature Nettle leaves harvested after the appearance of seeds. **Older leaves can promote the formation of tiny cystoliths** (calcium carbonate crystals) that irritate the kidneys and promote stone formation.

Keep in mind that the herb is a diuretic that can be drying to mucous membranes and skin if taken in sufficient amounts, especially by people who naturally have dry skin. Combine it with moisturizing herbs like Marshmallow (*Althaea officinalis*), Chickweed (*Stellaria* spp.), or Plantain to counteract this quality.

Medicinal Uses

History of the Plant

Stinging Nettle has a rich history and people throughout the world have used different species for fiber, food, and medicine for thousands of years. According to ancient legends, Milarepa, the great yogi of Tibet, survived on a diet of Nettles while meditating and living in Himalayan caves during the first century. In the Ayurvedic medical tradition of India, Asian varieties of Nettle are traditionally used for blood purification, abnormal bleeding such as uterine hemorrhage, and skin eruptions like eczema and hives.

Throughout European history, Nettles have been cultivated for food and medicine to treat arthritis, gout, kidney disease, coughs, tuberculosis, and problematic skin conditions. In ancient Greece, Hippocrates (*circa* 460 – *c.* 377 B.C.) and other physicians applied Nettle leaf juice to venomous bites and stings, and prescribed the tea as an antidote for animal and plant poisons. The Greek physician Pliny the Elder (A.D. 23–79) noticed the plant's ability to stop all types of bleeding. Dioscorides (*c.* A.D. 40 – *c.* 90) and Galen (*c.* 131 – *c.* 200) recommended it as a diuretic and treatment for nosebleeds and infected wounds. Early European herbalists used Nettle for coughs and tuberculosis, and smoked the leaves to relieve asthma. Nettle was one of the primary herbal remedies in the wise women healing tradition. The tea was ingested as a remedy for scurvy, a vitamin C deficiency, and Nettle juice was a popular hair growth stimulant. The 17th century English astrologer, herbalist, and apothecary Nicholas Culpeper (1616–1654) wrote that Mars has dominion over the herb. He applied fresh Nettle leaves to the skin to treat painful gout, arthritis, and sciatica. Culpeper recommended that the roots and leaves be boiled or juiced and taken for wheezing, shortness of breath, excess phlegm, and throat inflammation. A tea of the seeds was given for poisonous bites and stings. He used Nettle for urinary problems and wrote, "It provoketh urine, and expelleth the gravel and stone in the reins or bladder" (Culpeper, 1992). Culpeper and other healers from many cultures applied fresh Nettle leaves to painful, inflamed joints, and used the stems and leaves for a whipping therapy called "urtification" or "urtication." Whipping paralyzed limbs and arthritic joints with fresh Nettle is known to stimulate muscles and diminish pain.

Nettle stems have extremely strong fibers. Like Hemp (*Cannabis sativa*) and Flax (*Linum usitatissimum*), they can be spun and woven into durable thread and fabric, once known as nettle-cloth, which is much stronger than cotton. Nettles were once grown for their fiber content in Europe, Asia and Central America, and were used to make paper, clothes, burial shrouds, rope, fishing lines, and sails for boats.

In North America, many Native Americans employed Nettle for food and medicine. The Cherokee and Lakota Sioux used it for upset stomachs, and the Paiute prepared it for sore, swollen joints. Native women ate and drank it as a nutritious tonic during pregnancy and lactation.

During the 1880s–1930s, American Eclectic physicians prescribed the leaves and roots of *U. dioica* and *U. urens*. John King, M.D. (1813–1893) and Harvey Felter, M.D. (1865–1927) found the root decoction valuable for treating diarrhea and dysentery, hemorrhoids, various types of hemorrhage, feverish conditions, eruptive skin conditions like eczema and hives, chronic cystitis (bladder infection), kidney problems including stones, and childhood ailments. Seeds were prescribed for goiter, gas, and parasites (Felter, 1922). Finley Ellingwood, M.D. (1852–1920) also prescribed the herb for bleeding ulcers, post-partum hemorrhage, and for chronic diseases of the mucous membranes lining the organs and passageways of the respiratory, gastrointestinal, and urinary tracts.

U. dioica continues to be a popular medicinal herb and subject of modern research, much of which has focused on the ability of the root to treat benign prostatic hyperplasia (BPH) and related urinary problems.

Healing Qualities

Leaves are alterative (blood purifying), antacid, anti-catarrhal, antihistamine, anti-inflammatory, antioxidant, antiscorbutic, antiseptic, antispasmodic, anti-uric, astringent, depurative, diuretic, exanthematous, expectorant, galactagogue, hemostatic, nephritic, nutritive, pectoral, restorative, rubefacient, and tonic.

Roots are antacid, antihistamine, anti-inflammatory, anti-uric, astringent, depurative, diuretic, lithotropic (dissolves kidney and gallbladder stones), nephritic (used for kidney problems and diseases), and restorative.

Seeds are anthelmintic, anti-goiter, diuretic, and nephritic.

Traditional Chinese Medicine (TCM) Perspective

Stinging Nettle is mildly cooling and drying and removes excess dampness. The nutritiously fortifying leaves can be classified as a Yin tonic, even though they are drying rather than moisturizing. Nettle nourishes Liver Yin and is beneficial for blood deficiency (anemia), excessive Lung dampness manifesting as respiratory and sinus congestion, Lung Yin deficiency manifesting as asthma, dry cough and emphysema, and Intestinal dampness resulting in diarrhea. The roots and leaves are specific for Kidney Qi stagnation causing edema, kidney stones, metabolic toxicity, gout, skin eruptions, fatigue, and urinary tract infections.

Primary Actions

The nutrients in Stinging Nettle help tone, strengthen, and restore all tissues of the body, and sipping a quart of the tea throughout the day as a general tonic is highly recommended. The herb enriches the blood and benefits the endocrine glands, offering a vast array of applications. When taken continually as a tonic, it benefits many types of chronic, deficiency, and degenerative conditions like chronic fatigue, muscle weakness, and fibromyalgia. The abundant levels of alkalizing minerals in the leaves and roots support the kidney's ability to excrete excess acids (normal waste products of metabolism) from the blood and tissues. The herb is valuable for treating conditions related to excessive acidity that promote joint and tissue inflammation, gout, excessive mucous production in the lungs and nasal sinuses, and dermatitis. Modern research has confirmed the presence of anti-inflammatory substances and their ability to reduce production of many inflammatory chemicals known as prostaglandins (Obertreis, 1996). There is also significant research on the herb's superb action in reducing symptoms of hay fever and benign prostatic hyperplasia (BPH).

Regular use of the tea or tincture over an extended period of time is a great way to maintain optimal health while also improving many chronic ailments. The pleasant flavor of the tea provides an enjoyable drink that may be combined with other herbs. Remember that Nettle is slightly drying, so combining it with moisturizing herbs may be appropriate for people with dry skin and warmer, dry constitutions.

Respiratory System and Allergies: Various Stinging Nettle species have been used for centuries by many cultures for lung and sinus problems, including bronchitis, coughs, chest congestion, asthma, and allergic rhinitis (hay fever). The herb exerts an astringent effect that reduces profuse discharges from mucous membranes in the nasal sinuses and lungs, and its expectorant properties help expel excess mucous. Nettle's antihistamine actions reduce histamine release, which decreases mucous production, tissue inflammation, spasms and wheezing, while opening up congested bronchial and nasal passages.

The nutritive qualities of Nettle leaves benefit chronic lung conditions when they are consumed on a continual basis as tea or steamed greens. It is most effective when combined with other appropriate respiratory herbs such as Mullein (*Verbascum thapsus*), Horehound (*Marrubium vulgare*), Elecampane (*Inula helenium*), Pleurisy Root (*Asclepias tuberosa*), Wild Cherry bark (*Prunus serotina*), and Lobelia (*Lobelia inflata*) for chronic lung problems. Stinging Nettle is specific for asthma when taken daily for extended periods of time. To reduce asthma symptoms, it works best when combined with a dairy- and gluten-free diet, Mullein tea (2-3 cups a day), and Lobelia tincture (2-5 drops up to 5 times a day).

For hay fever, Nettle leaves are most effective when taken a few weeks before the allergy season starts. Substantial amounts of the tea (2-3 cups daily) or freeze-dried capsules (4-8 daily) should be ingested over a period of time for best results. In a study at the National College of Naturopathic Medicine in Portland, Oregon, involving 69 people suffering from hay fever, 57% of the participants found that 2 capsules (300 mg each) of freeze-dried Stinging Nettle leaves were moderately or highly effective in improving their allergy symptoms compared to a placebo (Mittman, 1990).

Blood, Lymphatic, Heart, Cholesterol, Diabetes, Anti-inflammatory, and Antioxidant Benefits: The rich supply of minerals, vitamins, and protein makes Stinging Nettle one of the best blood-building tonics to improve energy and vitality. An excellent treatment for anemia, the iron in Nettle is easily digested and increases hemoglobin levels in blood. By reducing acids, alkalizing minerals tend to decrease inflammation and the body's susceptibility to infections. The abundance of chlorophyll in the leaves increases magnesium and oxygen levels, which relaxes and nourishes muscles and is very detoxifying to the blood, lymphatic fluids, and skin. Nettle leaf tea is a beneficial tonic for nourishing and restoring a sluggish liver, which is also beneficial for maintaining healthy blood and skin.

Astringents occurring in the leaves and roots, along with vitamin K which promotes blood coagulation, help decrease bleeding and hemorrhage from injuries, excessive menstrual flow, nosebleeds, hemorrhoids, bleeding ulcers, bloody diarrhea, and bloody coughs. Applying a poultice of the leaves can relieve inflamed varicose veins.

Researchers have studied the ability of Stinging Nettle tincture to reduce cardiovascular risk factors in a clinical trial involving 50 overweight patients (men and women) diagnosed with diabetes type 2. Participants were divided into a control group receiving a placebo or a treatment group receiving 5-6.7 mL of the Nettle tincture (depending on their body weight). The patients took either the placebo or Nettle tincture 3 times daily following meals. After 8 weeks, levels of total cholesterol, low density lipoproteins (LDL), triglycerides, and systolic blood pressure showed a significant decrease, while beneficial high density lipoproteins (HLD) increased in those taking the Nettle tincture compared to the placebo group. The Nettle tincture reduced fasting blood sugar levels from an average of 129 mg/dL to 112 mg/dL after 8 weeks, while the average blood sugar for the placebo group did not change. Hemoglobin A1c, a measure of long-term glucose control, improved from an average of 7.3% to 6.1% in the Nettle group (Namazi, 2011-a). Several markers for inflammation were measured during this clinical trial. C-reactive protein (CRP) indicates degrees of systemic inflammation. Those taking Nettle tincture for 8 weeks had a significant reduction in CRP (from an average of 2.52 mg/dL to 1.37 mg/dL), indicating less inflammation throughout their bodies. Interleukin 6, another inflammatory marker, dropped from 3.52 to 1.19 pg/mL in the treatment group (Namazi, 2011-b). Lowering oxidative stress also greatly reduces the risk of cardiovascular disease. The Nettle group experienced improvement in markers measuring oxidative stress and inflammation after 8 weeks of treatment. Levels of superoxide dismutase (a potent antioxidant) in their red blood cells improved, rising from 1,200 to 1,500 U/mg Hb, but remained unchanged in the placebo group. The total antioxidant capacity of the patient's serum almost tripled in the Nettle group, while no improvement occurred in the placebo group (Namazi, 2012).

In another study, 30 patients with diabetes type 2 who took *Urtica dioica* extract (100 mg/kg) 3 times daily for 8 weeks benefited with significantly improved insulin concentration and decreased insulin resistance. The 30 diabetics who received a placebo did not experience these improvements (Khajeh-Mehrizi, 2014).

Digestion: Nettle leaf tea and cooked greens are healing to a weak, dysfunctional digestive system. They soothe and nourish mucous membranes lining the digestive tract and reduce inflammation. The herb helps to tone and normalize the stomach, liver, gallbladder, spleen, and intestines. It can be used in a formula to treat excess stomach acid, stomach and intestinal ulcers, and chronic intestinal problems. Ingesting the tea and soaking in it as a sitz bath helps shrink and heal hemorrhoids. Eclectic physicians prescribed it for diarrhea, dysentery, and excess stomach acids with belching and vomiting.

Adrenals and Thyroid: Stinging Nettle leaves nourish and restore the endocrine glands to benefit the entire system. Long-term use of the herb is specific for adrenal exhaustion. Eclectic physicians highly recommended the seeds as a remedy for goiter resulting from underactive thyroid function, and prescribed doses of 14-16 seeds taken 3 times daily or 1-10 drops of the tincture prepared with 100% alcohol. Nettles can be helpful for Hashimoto's disease, an autoimmune condition of hypothyroidism.

Kidneys and the Urinary Tract: Stinging Nettle is an excellent non-irritating kidney tonic, restorative, and alkalizing diuretic that strengthens and normalizes the kidneys to benefit the entire urinary tract. The herb reduces pain and inflammation in the kidneys, ureters, bladder, and urethra. Nettle root improves urine flow and reduces frequency of urination and nocturia (night-time urination). The leaves and roots are taken for all types of kidney and bladder pain and inflammation, acute and chronic urinary tract infections, urethritis, kidney stones, and painful urination with hematuria (bloody urine). The herb may also be helpful to people on dialysis. For urinary tract problems, add Stinging Nettle to a formula with other herbs specific for the problem-at-hand. Nettle seeds are very restorative to kidney function and help slow the progression of degenerative kidney disease, including glomerulonephritis and chronic nephritis (kidney inflammation).

The German Commission E herbal regulatory agency recommended drinking several cups of Nettle root tea on a daily basis to treat inflammatory diseases of the urinary tract and to prevent and treat kidney stones. Uric acid is a metabolic waste product that promotes the development of gout, arthritis, skin rashes, kidney stones, and other inflammatory problems. Nettle extract, juice, and tea draw uric acid out of the tissues into the bloodstream where it is excreted by the kidneys. In China, the herb is prescribed for kidney infections, inflammation, and cystitis (bladder infection). Early American Eclectic physicians recognized Nettle root as a diuretic and prescribed it for kidney, bladder, and urinary tract infections and inflammation, nephritis, and chronic cystitis with mucous discharges.

The high potassium content in Nettle leaves provides a safe diuretic that does not leach minerals from the body. The herb can be taken for edema and other conditions of fluid excess, including high blood pressure, cardiac edema, congestive heart failure, and premenstrual bloating. In a 14-day clinical study, a daily dose of Nettle leaf juice (15 mL) was given to 32 patients with myocardial or chronic venous insufficiency. This produced significant diuretic effects, including minor decreases in body weight and systolic blood pressure (Kirchhoff, 1983).

Prostate Health: Stinging Nettle root is effective in treating prostatitis (prostate inflammation) and benign prostatic hyperplasia (BPH). BPH is a non-cancerous swelling of the prostate and a common problem for many men over the age of 50. Testosterone is necessary for the development and growth of prostate cells. In the prostate, testosterone is broken down and converted into its metabolite, dihydrotestosterone (DHT), by the enzyme 5-alpha-reductase. High levels of DHT are associated with prostate enlargement, inflammation, and prostate cancer. The prostate gland normally wraps around the urethra below the bladder, but when the prostate enlarges, it constricts the urethra causing obstructed urine flow, incomplete emptying of the bladder, and increased frequency of urination. The German Commission E herbal regulatory agency recommended daily consumption of Nettle root as an effective treatment for BPH, related urinary problems, and early stages of prostate adenoma (a benign tumor). The typical dose for these problems is 4-6 grams of the root taken daily in divided doses or 1-1½ teaspoons of the tincture taken 3 times a day.

Numerous research studies have focused on the beneficial actions of Stinging Nettle root on the prostate. Water soluble polysaccharides, scopoletin, and the lectin known as *Urtica dioica* agglutinin (UDA) have anti-inflammatory activity that reduces symptoms of BPH (Wagner, 1994 & 1995). Beta-sitosterol and other sterols in the roots help to inhibit the conversion of testosterone to DHT, and large doses of isolated beta-sitosterol (20 mg taken 3 times daily) have reduced BPH symptoms (Berges, 1995). In a large study involving over 4,000 men in all stages of BPH, participants experienced improved urinary flow and significant decrease of residual urine and frequency of night-time urination after 8 weeks of treatment with Stinging Nettle root extract in daily doses of 1,200 mg (Stahl, 1984). During a longer study in which 558 men with BPH received a water extract of Nettle root (120 mg) or a placebo 3 times daily, 81% of the Nettle group reported improvement in urinary problems and moderate reduction in prostate size compared to only 16% of the placebo group (Safarinejad, 2005).

Stinging Nettle root is often combined with Saw Palmetto fruit (*Serenoa repens*) and Pygeum bark (*Pygeum africanum*) because their synergistic activity is greater than their individual benefits for BPH. Nettle root and Pygeum extracts partially block the actions of 5-alpha-reductase (the enzyme that converts testosterone to DHT) and aromatase (the enzyme that converts testosterone to estradiol, a form of estrogen that can promote BPH and reproductive cancers). Aromatase levels tend to increase as men age, leading to higher levels of estradiol and prostate enlargement. *In vitro* tests confirm that a combination of Nettle root and Pygeum extract was more effective in blocking DHT and 5-alpha-reductase to reduce BPH symptoms than either of the individual extracts (Hartmann, 1996). A substance known as 9-hydroxy-10-trans-12-cis-octadecadienic acid (HOA) occurring in Nettle root inhibits aromatase in prostate tissue (Kraus, 1991).

Several clinical studies validate the ability of Stinging Nettle root to relieve symptoms of BPH by reducing prostate size and inflammation, urinary frequency, and nocturia (night-time urination), and by improving the flow of urine and complete emptying of the bladder. In a study comparing the effects of different doses of *U. dioica* root and Pygeum, 72 men diagnosed with BPH took 2 capsules twice daily of an extract of Stinging Nettle root (300 mg) with Pygeum (25 mg). The second group of 72 men took half this amount. After 28 and 56 days, both dosages promoted significant improvements in symptoms, including better urine flow and reduced residual urine and nocturia. There were no problematic side effects (Krzeski, 1993). Another study was conducted by researchers at the Institute of Urology in Moscow and involved 257 men with urinary problems caused by BPH. Half of the participants took one capsule of Nettle root (120 mg) and Saw Palmetto (160 mg) twice a day, and the other half received a placebo. After 24 weeks, urinary symptoms and discomfort diminished in those receiving the herbal combination (Lopatkin, 2005).

A large study in Germany involving the practices of 419 urology specialists investigated 2,080 patients with BPH who were treated with a combination of Stinging Nettle and Saw Palmetto. A before-and-after comparison documented improvements in pathological findings, pain, ability to urinate, and general quality of life. The physicians assessed the efficacy and tolerability of the herbal preparations to be "good" or "very good," and only 15 patients developed mild side effects (Schneider, 1995).

Researchers have also compared the actions of these herbs to pharmaceutical drugs in treating BPH. Finasteride (Proscar) is a popular drug prescribed for BPH because it inhibits 5-alpha-reductase and reduces DHT levels. In a clinical trial lasting 48 weeks, 543 men with BPH were given daily doses of a Stinging Nettle root (240 mg) and Saw Palmetto (320 mg) combination or Proscar (5 mg). Both groups experienced improved increases in urinary flow rate. The herbal combination was as effective as the drug in treating BPH, however, the herbal therapy was better tolerated and participants reported significantly fewer adverse side effects, cases of erectile dysfunction, and headaches (Sokeland, 1997 & 2000). In a 60-week study involving 140 men, daily doses of Stinging Nettle (240 mg) and Saw Palmetto (320 mg) were compared to tamsulosin

(Flomax) (0.4 mg daily) for the relief of urinary symptoms associated with BPH. The researchers concluded that the herbal combination was slightly more effective with fewer side effects than Flomax (Engelman, 2006). Considering the wealth of documentation, it appears that men with prostate and urination problems would be wise to use these safe and effective herbs.

Skin Problems and Eczema: The leaves have historically been employed for the treatment of acute and chronic eruptive skin problems like eczema and various types of dermatitis, hives and other rashes, acne, measles, and chicken pox. A compress of the tea or diluted tincture applied to burns helps heal the skin and reduce inflammation and scarring. The herb can also be taken internally for relief from burn pain and to promote healing from the inside. Many factors contribute to its ability to improve skin conditions, such as its abundance of alkalizing minerals, blood-building properties, toning and detoxifying influence on the kidneys, liver and blood, and anti-inflammatory and antihistamine actions. Nettles were traditionally taken as a spring tonic to cleanse the liver and blood, and were ingested and used as a wash or poultice for chronic skin problems. Some people have found that their warts disappear when fresh Nettle juice is rubbed on them 3-4 times a day for a few weeks.

Stinging Nettle is an excellent remedy for childhood and adult eczema. The Eclectic physicians documented good results by applying olive oil to remove crusted skin and washing the affected area with Nettle tea. They also recommended internal use of the tea. Stinging Nettle combines well with Burdock root (*Arctium lappa*) and Chamomile (*Matricaria recutita*) for eczema.

Joint Inflammation, Arthritis, and Gout: The leaves of Stinging Nettle are traditionally ingested for joint problems, and freshly harvested leaves are applied as a poultice on affected areas. Just like physicians of the past, the German Commission E herbal regulatory agency recommended *U. dioica* and *U. urens* for arthritis and other inflammatory joint conditions. In a multicenter study, 152 patients suffering from degenerative joint disease ingested 1.54 grams of a dry Nettle leaf extract daily. After 3 weeks, 70% of the people reported improvement in their symptoms (Ramm, 1995).

Urtication is a unique treatment in which the fresh plant is directly applied to the arthritic joint by striking or flogging the area with the stem and leaves. Over the centuries, people have discovered that the stinging of Nettle decreases their gout and arthritic pain while improving joint movement. The formic acid released from Nettle hairs instantly irritates and inflames the skin on contact to produce hot, red, raised welts. This counter-irritation stimulates an increased blood supply in the area, which eases deeper arthritic pains. The formic acid in Nettle hairs is also found in the stinging venom of bees and ants, and bee venom therapy has also been shown to reduce pain and inflammation when bees are allowed to sting arthritic joints. Several research studies have demonstrated significant improvement in arthritic joint symptoms after urtication with fresh Nettle leaves (Randall, 1994, 1999, & 2000).

The abundance of minerals in the leaves fortify the blood with nutrients to reduce acidity and inflammation, making Stinging Nettle helpful for joint swelling and pain, including tendonitis and bursitis. Laboratory tests suggest other factors responsible for Nettle's ability to reduce pain and inflammation. The herb inhibits COX-1 and COX-2 because it blocks activity of cyclooxygenase and 5-lipoxygenase, which are substances promoting inflammation. In a study designed to investigate the herb's anti-inflammatory mechanisms in arthritic conditions, blood was obtained from six healthy men and incubated with lipopolysaccharide (LPS). LPS is a strong activator of tumor necrosis factor (TNF) and interleukin-1 (IL-1) secretion by white blood cells. These inflammatory cytokines are implicated in the development of osteoarthritis and rheumatoid arthritis. The men's blood was also incubated with different concentrations of a tincture extract of Nettle leaves. The study demonstrated that the 5 mg/mL concentration of Nettle extract significantly inhibited TNF secretion by 51% and IL-1 secretion by 100% after 24 hours (Obertreis, 1996).

Nettle's ability to eliminate uric acid through the kidneys can improve symptoms of gout arising from excessive uric acid that settles in the big toe joint to cause pain and inflammation. Dandelion (*Taraxacum officinale*) also increases elimination of uric acid and may be combined with Nettle when treating gout. People have reported that striking their painful, gouty toe with fresh Nettle provides temporary pain relief.

Hair Growth: The juice, tea, and tincture of Stinging Nettle root have a long history of use for stimulating hair growth and eliminating dandruff when applied to the scalp on a regular basis. Drinking tea made from the leaves or eating them steamed is encouraged to nourish the blood with protein and minerals necessary for healthy hair. Modern research provides interesting evidence linking male pattern baldness with elevated levels of the enzyme 5-alpha-reductase, which converts testosterone to dihydrotestosterone (DHT). Increased levels of DHT that promote prostate enlargement are also found in the scalps of men experiencing hair loss. The ability of Stinging Nettle to reduce DHT levels may be a mechanism for its effectiveness in promoting healthy scalps and hair growth (Dean, 2000).

Nervous System: The abundant concentration of minerals in the leaves nourish and calm the nervous system, and are helpful for anxiety and hyperactive conditions. Researchers have documented that the leaves exert depressant activity on the central nervous system and inhibit drug-induced convulsions in animal studies (Broncano, 1987). Relaxing, anti-inflammatory actions can be helpful for easing migraine headaches when the leaves are ingested daily. Calming, diuretic effects may also reduce hypertension. Researchers at the University of Pisa, Italy, found that water and alcohol extracts of Nettle root relax and dilate blood vessels during *in vitro* testing, and may be helpful to improve circulation and reverse high blood pressure (Testai, 2002).

Women's Health: Nettle leaves are an excellent and safe ally for women to enjoy during all stages of reproductive life. The herb is a uterine tonic that helps normalize the menstrual cycle and reduce excessive menstrual bleeding and cramps. As a nutritive tonic that encourages iron-rich blood, it can help promote fertility and treat amenorrhea (the abnormal cessation of menses). Its diuretic effects reduce water retention and bloating during menses and pregnancy.

A daily cup of tea during pregnancy nourishes the mother and infant. It increases energy levels and reduces anemia and fatigue during pregnancy and the post-partum period. Nettle's vitamin K content helps decrease hemorrhage during and after childbirth. It is an excellent galactagogue because the powerhouse of nutrients promotes production of rich breast milk. Native American women ate and drank Nettle leaves during pregnancy for nourishment, to ease childbirth, and to enrich milk production.

Stinging Nettle is helpful for menopausal hot flashes and night sweats. Significant amounts of calcium, magnesium, phosphorous, silica, and boron contribute to strong bones and prevention of osteoporosis. Boron helps bones absorb and retain calcium.

Teachings from the Stinging Nettle Deva

"Greetings, dear one. I am the deva of the Stinging Nettle. My essence embodies the fullness of the feminine qualities of abundance, compassion, and nurturing. Just as the Great Mother provides all that is required by her children to grow and prosper, my plants embody the earth element and contain the nutrients necessary for strong human bodies. My plants synthesize or blend together the other elemental forces of fire, water, and air to meet the needs of your physical body.

"My teaching and the offering of my medicine is 'protection through radiance and vitality of being.' This means that my plants protect the body by making it radiant and vital in life force. By the miraculous power of light and the spark of life, my plants transform sunlight into energy that nourishes them and provides the physical structure of their roots, stems, leaves, and flowers. The abundance of green chlorophyll in their leaves produces oxygen that contributes to life on this planet. Their roots also draw upon and absorb the minerals and nutrients within soil to transform them into the bodies of my plants. And so, rich and strong in the elements of the sun and earth, my plants provide the nutrients necessary for healthy blood and strong bones, tissues, and organs in the human body. When the blood and tissues are healthy, they exist and vibrate at their normal frequencies of light and energy, which radiate out from the body into the surrounding environment. This radiance is what people call the 'aura' or 'field of energy' that is the essence of every person. The aura is a direct reflection and radiance of the health of the physical, emotional, and mental bodies of each person. When the body is fatigued or in a state of 'dis-ease,' the frequency of the aura is reduced – like dark, gray clouds that hide the sun and reduce the brilliant rays of sunlight. When you have a strong, vibrant aura, it helps protect you against harmful people and circumstances, just as light naturally dispels darkness. A healthy physical body enhances clarity of mind and peaceful emotions. In this way, my nourishing medicine offers protection and good health on all levels.

"My healing gifts balance opposing energies to bring humans health and comfort, and my piercing needles are a signature of this quality. For although they inflict pain and irritation when brushed against the skin, when used as medicine, the substances injected from these tiny needles actually relieve painful inflammation and irritation in the tissues and joints of the body. This talent of balancing opposite energies is a power behind my healing abilities.

"My plants live within the domain of Mars and Venus. Mars is the forceful masculine planet that supports the physical body and activity, which my plants accomplish so beautifully. The powerful force of Mars is tempered and directed by the gentle, feminine, heartfelt nature of Venus, bringing balance and peace to those partaking of my medicines. The essence of the planet Mercury blends and equalizes the energies of these masculine and feminine powers.

"The aura radiating out into the world from of my plants is bright orange-red, golden-yellow, and the same deep-green color as my leaves. My medicine supports the lower three chakras of the body involved with developing a strong physical body, personality, and sense of 'individual self.' Each little plant is an example of how humans may live in this world – offering an abundance of healing nourishment, while being armored with protection and ready to meet challenges and difficulties as they arise. I am a calm and peaceful deva whose wish is to provide complete nourishment. My luscious green plants are common, my gifts are the nutrients and essence in simple leaves. Yet with this simplicity comes great peace and happiness; for when the body is fully nourished it is at peace."

Thyme

Thymus vulgaris
Labiatae (Lamiaceae) (Mint) Family

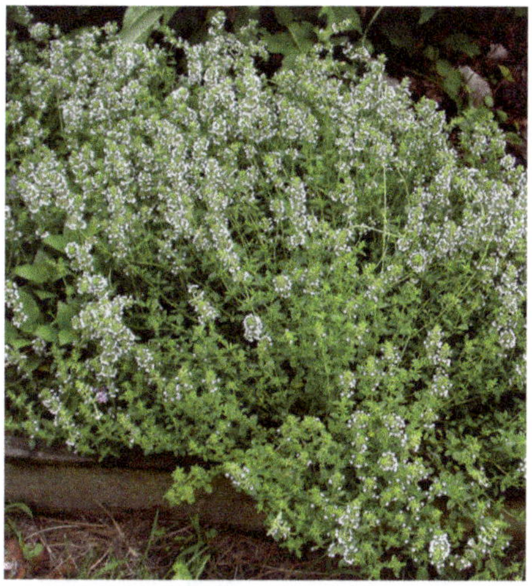

Common Names

Common Thyme, garden Thyme, and French, German, and English Thyme are common names for *Thymus vulgaris.*

Medicinal Part of the Plant

The upper leaves and flowering tops are used for culinary and medicinal purposes.

Range and Habitat

T. vulgaris is native to the Mediterranean region. It has been introduced and cultivated in the United States and many other temperate areas around the world.

Description of the Plant

The genus *Thymus* is a large family containing about 400 species, including many cultivars. The different species are small, perennial, strongly aromatic evergreens. Many species contain similar constituents and are used interchangeably for medicinal purposes. *T. serpyllum* (known as Wild Thyme, Creeping Thyme, and Mother of Thyme) is a low-growing, thick, creeping ground cover with medicinal properties similar to those of *T. vulgaris*.

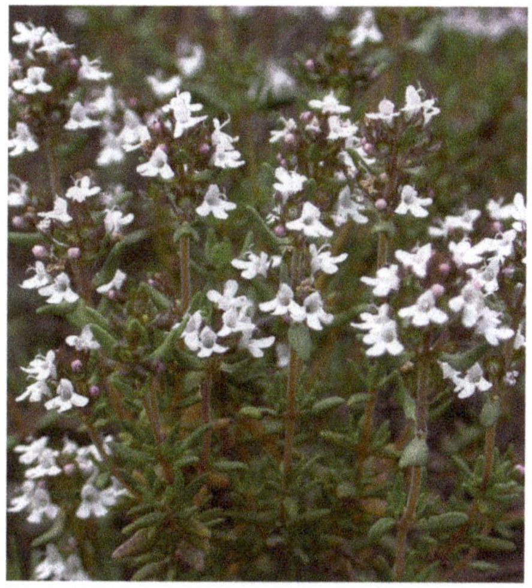

T. vulgaris is considered the most potent species for medicinal purposes and is the one most commonly used in North America. It is a dense, low-growing, creeping plant growing 8-16″ tall. Emerging from a fibrous root system, many small stems spread out into a large mass as the plant ages. Younger stems are square and pubescent (covered with barely visible soft, fine hairs) with many branches, while older stems get woody at their base.

The tiny leaves are 1/4-1/3″ long, entire (lacking teeth), smooth, and appear in a variety of shapes from oval to lanceolate or linear. Leaves emerge opposite each other along the stems and are covered with oil glands responsible for their fragrance. Along the upper portion of the stems, clusters of miniature flowers emerge in short spikes from the stem tips. Blooming from late spring through summer, flowers appear in colors from pinkish white to light purple. The flower corolla is tubular with 5 petals held within a cup-shaped calyx. A delicate-looking plant, Thyme is an attractive addition to rock gardens or cascading down a rock wall.

Cultivation

Thyme needs fertile soil because it is a heavy feeder that thrives with periodic fertilization. It likes loamy, sandy, well-drained soil, so avoid heavy, wet soils that promote fungal diseases and root rot. Grow Thyme under full sun for maximum production of the medicinal volatile oils. It is most easily propagated from seed, but stem cuttings and root division can also work.

The seeds are very tiny and should be started in planting trays or greenhouse flats in early spring for best results. They are light-dependent germinators, so spread seeds on the soil surface and gently tap them down rather than covering with dirt. A temperature of 65-70°F is necessary for germination, which takes 2-4 weeks in ideal conditions. When seedlings are 3-4″ tall, transplant them 6-12″ apart in a permanent bed. The patch will eventually fill in with Thyme due to its dense, spreading root system. Keep soil around the herb moist, weeded, and mulched.

Roots from older, well-established plants can be divided into halves or thirds in early spring and transplanted 12″ apart in a prepared bed. To develop plants from stem cuttings, snip 3″ pieces from stems with new growth and put them in a container filled with wet, sandy, potting mix. Be sure there are drainage holes in the container. Put it in a shady area and keep the mix very moist. When roots appear in a few weeks, plant the cuttings in moist soil, mulch around the cuttings, water, and keep the soil moist.

Thyme is a good companion plant to grow alongside Lavender, Sage and Hyssop, attracting bees that hum a droning chant as they collect pollen from the flowers. Mulch Thyme plants with grass clippings to protect the roots over winter in climates where temperatures dip below 10°F.

Harvest

Gather leaves and flowers just as blooming begins because thymol, the primary medicinal phytochemical, reaches its highest concentration and potency at this stage. Harvest by gently grabbing handfuls of the tops of the stems and pruning the upper 3-4″ of leaves and flowers. The second growth of flowers that develops may be harvested or allowed to go to seed. When seedpods are brown and dry, collect the seeds for planting by pruning the upper 3-4″ of the stems and putting them in a small paper bag or box, which will hold the tiny seeds as they fall out of their pods.

Preparation of Plant Medicine and Dosages

Thyme yields its medicinal phytochemicals to boiling water and alcohol, so tea and tincture prepared from freshly harvested leaves and flowers provides potent preparations. It is a wonderful ingredient to be included in cough syrups, oils, and salves for external application, or it may dried for future use.

PREPARATIONS

Tea: Steep 1-2 teaspoons of the leaves and flowers in 1 cup of boiled water for 15 minutes. Dosage: 1-2 cups per day. The tea has a pleasantly mild flavor.

Tincture: Chop leaves and flowers, pack in a glass jar, and cover with 70% 190-proof grain alcohol and 30% distilled water. Dosage: 10-60 drops 3 times a day as needed.

Oil: Put chopped leaves and flowers in a glass or stainless steel bowl, cover with olive oil, and bake at 250°F for 3 hours. Separate the herb from the oil, bottle the oil, and store in a cool, dark place.

Salve: Add melted beeswax to the oil to make a thick ointment.

Cough Syrup: Prepare a strong tea using 1 ounce of the herb per 1 pint of water. Add honey. Preserve the syrup by storing it in the refrigerator or freezer. Dosage: 1-2 teaspoons up to 5 times a day as needed for coughs, colds, and sore throats. For a stronger-acting syrup, Thyme may be combined with other herbs (refer to "The Index of Health Issues and Herbal Recommendation" for suggestions).

Essential oil: This is produced by steam distillation of fresh leaves and flowers. It must be used cautiously because the thymol content is toxic in large amounts. Only 1-2 drops of essential oil should be ingested in a day.

Bath Additive: Make a gallon of strong tea and add it to bath water for a relaxing, aromatic soak. The essential oil may be added to a bath, but do not exceed 5-6 drops – too much of the highly concentrated essential oil may cause skin irritation, burning, or other adverse reactions.

Culinary Uses

Thyme is enjoyed as a flavorful culinary herb that can be added to many food, including meats, fish, sauces, salads, vegetables, and soups. The leaves contain antioxidants that inhibit cellular death and decay, and were packed around meat and fish to preserve them prior to refrigeration.

Chemical Constituents

Thymol is a primary medicinal constituent in the volatile oils that impart the characteristic odor and pungent taste of the herb. Thymol is used as an analgesic, antiseptic, mouthwash, deodorant, and anthelmintic for hookworms and other parasites. It helps prevent blood clots and is an antioxidant that protects cells from inflammation and damage. The volatile oils also contain carvacrol, cineole, citral, thymene, borneol (analgesic, febrifuge, hepatoprotective, sedative), eugenol (anticonvulsant, diuretic, carminative, febrifuge, hepatoprotective, vasodilator), geraniol, linalool, bornyl, camphor (analgesic, carminative, decongestant), cymene, anethole (antitumor, carminative, estrogenic, expectorant, immunostimulant, protective to kidneys), terpineol (anti-asthmatic, diuretic, sedative, vulnerary), terpinene (diuretic), and pinene (antiflu, expectorant, sedative). Thymol, carvacrol, and other components of the volatile oils and flavonoids (including luteolin, apigenin, and thymonin) are antioxidant, anti-inflammatory, antimicrobial, antiparasitic, break up mucous congestion, reduce coughing and bronchial spasms, promote normal breathing, and relieve indigestion and gas.

Linolenic acid is an antihypertensive, anti-inflammatory, immunostimulant, vasodilator, and anti-aggregant that reduces blood clots. Apigenin reduces blood platelet aggregation and allergic symptoms, and is antibacterial, antihistamine, anti-inflammatory, antioxidant, antiviral, sedating, and a vasodilator. Caprylic acid is a fungicide and candidicide. Rosmarinic acid and related caffeic acid derivatives exert choleretic, analgesic, diuretic, antihistamine, antioxidant, antibacterial, and antiviral actions in addition to inhibiting the production of inflammatory leukotrienes and prostaglandins (Skenderi, 2003). Tryptophan (a precursor to the calming neurotransmitter serotonin) has been identified and has antidepressant and sedative effects. The leaves contain significant amounts of chromium, iron, silicon, calcium, manganese, magnesium, selenium, and boron (a mineral that is involved in the metabolism of calcium, necessary for calcium uptake in bones, and promotes strong bones).

Safety, Contraindications, and Drug Interactions

Long historic use and current research verify the safety of Thyme when it is used as a culinary herb or taken medicinally in recommended doses. The tea and tincture are safe for children and adults with no known contraindications, side effects, or drug interactions.

The essential oil of Thyme, which contains thymol, can be toxic in large doses and should be taken in small amounts diluted with water for internal uses and with vegetable oil for external applications. Ingesting more than a few drops of the oil or taking excessive amounts of the tea and tincture over time can eventually lead to symptoms of toxicity, overstimulation of the thyroid glands, vomiting, depression, fatigue, dizziness, and difficulty breathing. When using the distilled essential oils for a bath, only add 5-6 drops to the water because too much can cause skin irritation and burning. Before applying essential oil to the skin, be sure it is sufficiently diluted by putting some on a small area to test for any reactions

Although excessive amounts of Thyme stimulate the uterus, pregnant and lactating women can safely drink a cup of the mild tea a few times a week after the first trimester. The distilled essential oil should be avoided during pregnancy and lactation, and by young children.

Medicinal Uses

History of the Plant

Thyme is a traditional symbol of strength, courage, and grace. The genus name *Thymus* is thought to derive from the Greek word *thumus* or *thymon*, meaning "courage and strength." It may also stem from *thyo*, meaning "perfume," because it was burned as incense to purify the air in homes and during ceremonies due to its strong aromatic and antiseptic qualities. Egyptians used Thyme to make fragrant soaps and perfumes and as an embalming ingredient. The Greeks added it to their baths and massage oils, and Roman soldiers bathed in Thyme water to instill themselves with strength and bravery. During the Middle Ages, European women embroidered sprigs of Thyme into clothing as a symbol of their knights' bravery and courage. According to old legends, drinking Thyme tea allows people to see fairies and watch them dance in beds of Thyme.

Pliny (A.D. 23–79), Dioscorides (*circa* 40 – *c.* 90), and other early Greek physicians used *Thymus vulgaris* and *T. serpyllum* to treat asthma, coughs, colds, the flu, nervous conditions, depression, stomach problems, gas, colic, parasites, warts, rheumatism, to promote stalled menstruation, and to dissolve blood clots. It was grown in monastery gardens and eaten as a favorite kitchen herb by common people, who added it to food for flavoring and to preserve meat.

Hildegard of Bingen (1098–1179) was a German Benedictine nun and herbalist who employed Thyme to heal leprosy, paralysis, and kill body lice. Later European physicians, including John Gerard (1545–1612) and Nicholas Culpeper (1616–1654), prescribed the herb as a remedy for coughs, excess phlegm, and other lung problems; to treat nervous disorders, indigestion, parasites, bites, stings, and 4pelvic pain; and for women during childbirth to ensure safe and speedy delivery. Culpeper wrote, "It is a noble strengthener of the lungs. It purges the body of phlegm, and is an excellent remedy for shortness of breath. It kills worms in the belly, and being a notable herb of Venus, provokes the terms [stimulates menstruation], gives safe and speedy delivery to women in travail, and brings away the after-birth [placenta]. It is so harmless you need not fear the use of it. An ointment made of it takes away hot swellings and warts, helps the sciatica and dullness of sight; it is excellent for those that are troubled by gout; as also, to anoint the testicles that are swelled. The herb taken any way inwardly, comforts the stomach much, and expels wind [gas]" (Culpeper, 1992).

In 1719, German chemist Caspar Neumann discovered and isolated Thyme oil, which was eventually sold in apothecary stores as "oil of origanum." It became a popular antiseptic applied to wounds, bruises, sprains, and infections.

European immigrants brought *T. vulgaris* to North America where it naturalized and became a popular herbal remedy. The Eclectic physicians prescribed it in their clinical practice during the 1980s–1930s. *King's Dispensatory*, one of the popular Eclectic texts, notes, "Thyme is tonic, carminative, emmenagogue, and antispasmodic. The cold infusion is useful in dyspepsia, with weak and irritable stomach, and as a stimulating tonic in convalescence from exhausting diseases. The warm infusion is beneficial in hysteria [anxiety and mood swings associated with menstrual cycles], dysmenorrhoea [painful menstruation], flatulence, colic, headache, and to promote perspiration. Occasionally the leaves have been used externally, in fomentation. The oil is valuable as a local application to neuralgic and rheumatic pains" (Felter, 1898).

Oil of Thyme and thymol were listed as official medicines in the *U.S. Pharmacopoeia* from 1880–1947, and were widely used as antiseptics for battle wounds during World War I. Thyme remains a popular medicinal and culinary herb in North America and Europe.

Healing Qualities

Antibiotic, anti-catarrhal, antifungal, anti-inflammatory, antioxidant, antiseptic, antispasmodic, antiviral, antitussive, astringent, carminative, diaphoretic, diuretic, emmenagogue, expectorant, febrifuge, nervine, pectoral, rubefacient (essential oil only), mild sedative, stomachic, vasodilator, vermifuge, and vulnerary.

Traditional Chinese Medicine (TCM) Perspective

Thyme is a warming and drying herb that improves cold, damp conditions and breaks up Qi stagnation. It benefits the lungs, nerves, adrenals, digestive organs, intestines, and uterus. It restores and relaxes the nervous system, while also stimulating digestion and circulation of blood and Qi throughout the body.

The herb is recommended for Wind Cold conditions causing chills, muscle aches, wheezing, mucous excess, watery sinus drainage, coughs, and sore throats. In the lungs and sinuses, it resolves excess phlegm accompanying congestion, coughs, and bronchitis. Thyme's stimulating action relieves Lung Qi constraint causing chronic lung problems like asthma and emphysema.

In the digestive tract, its warming and Qi tonic properties stimulate normal digestion and reduce dampness causing nausea, indigestion, gas, and yeast overgrowth. Thyme also warms the uterus and restores the flow of Qi to promote normal cycles and menstrual periods that are free of cramps and spasms.

Primary Actions

T. vulgaris is a restorative, warming tonic for the whole system. The potent volatile oils have broad-spectrum benefits on the nervous system, organs, glands, and tissues throughout the body with a special affinity for the respiratory and digestive systems. It exerts a balancing action of relaxing an overly stressed nervous system or gently stimulating and tonifying a depleted, exhausted system. I add Thyme to respiratory formulas and combine it with other antiviral herbs when treating viral infections, including herpes.

Tea, tincture, pills, or capsules are potent remedies that are safe to use and easily prepared at home. Although the concentrated essential oils are the most potent preparations for healing, they must be used cautiously because they can be toxic even in moderate doses.

Antimicrobial Actions for Internal and External Infections: Thymol and other components in the volatile oils are broad-spectrum antimicrobials that can inhibit and destroy many types of bacteria (Hersch-Martinez, 2005), viruses, and fungi when ingested or applied externally. Laboratory research shows that the oil permeates cellular membranes to destroy infectious organisms. It exhibits specific activity against upper respiratory infections, septicemia (blood toxicity), meningitis, *Listeria monocytogenes* (a dangerous bacterial source of food poisoning), and *Staphylococcus aureus*, which is responsible for many types of skin and deep tissue infections, such as impetigo and septicemia (Nguefack, 2004).

Thyme helps reduce fevers and pain. When taken hot, it stimulates perspiration by bringing internal heat to the surface to be released. These febrifuge and analgesic properties have been demonstrated in mice after ingesting extracts of Thyme (Mohsin, 1989).

The herb is a strong antiseptic for infected wounds, promoting cell growth and repair. When applied to injured tissues, the essential oil acts as a rubefacient that dilates blood vessels to increase blood flow and delivery of healing blood components. Thyme is beneficial for inflammation, bruises, sprains, and arthritis. Continual application of the tincture or essential oil helps kill parasites on and under the skin, including crabs, lice, and scabies.

For external infections, the herb may be ingested and applied externally using the diluted essential oil, tincture, salve, poultice, or a fomentation made from a strong tea. The tea, diluted oil, or diluted tincture can be used as a mouthwash for thrush (a yeast infection in the mouth), gingivitis (inflamed, infected gums), and other gum problems caused by tooth decay or infection. Synthetically produced thymol is an ingredient in Listerine mouthwash and other dental and topical products.

As an antiviral, the herb is ingested and applied externally to treat painful herpes outbreaks, including shingles. Thyme is specific for treating herpes infections because it has an affinity with the nerves, and herpes is a virus living in the nervous system. *In vitro* studies demonstrate that water extracts (tea) of Thyme have strong antiviral activity against Herpes simplex 1 and 2 when applied to the lesions (Nolkemper, 2006). Combine Thyme with St. John's Wort (*Hypericum perforatum*) and Lemon Balm (*Melissa officinalis*) for best results when treating the herpes virus. Warts are viral infections that can be treated with applications of Thyme oil or tincture combined with other appropriate antiviral herbs, such as Bloodroot (*Sanguinaria canadensis*) and the white latex juice of many members of the Milkweed (*Asclepiadaceae*) family.

Several *in vitro* studies show that Thyme's volatile oils induce irreversible damage to fungal cells by damaging their outer membranes (Rasooli, 2005) and demonstrate strong ability to treat fungal infections including Candida yeast (Bonjar, 2004; Giorgani, 2004; Pina-Vaz, 2004). A clinical trial involving 64 women diagnosed with candida vaginitis revealed that a vaginal cream containing Thyme and Garlic was as effective as clotrimazole vaginal cream (an antifungal pharmaceutical) in eliminating their yeast infections (Bahadoran, 2010). Thyme is taken internally and the oil is applied externally to treat athlete's foot, ringworm, and other fungal infections. It is known to reduce phlegm and excess dampness in the body, which can encourage fungal growth. Researchers have verified the antifungal and antioxidant activity of the volatile oils and their capacity to reduce damaging free radicals and lipid peroxidation, which damages cells and makes them vulnerable to infection (Agbor, 2005; Bozin, 2006; Proestos, 2005).

Thyme baths are prepared by adding a gallon of tea or 5-6 drops of concentrated essential oil to bath water. This is a wonderfully soothing treatment for achy joints and muscles, fibromyalgia, bruises, sprains, muscle spasms, arthritic pain, and anxiety.

Respiratory System: Thyme has a special affinity with the lungs and is an excellent remedy for many bronchial problems. The volatile oils are helpful for coughs due to their stimulating expectorant action and antispasmodic effects on the bronchioles. The oil's antimicrobial, anti-inflammatory, anti-catarrhal, diaphoretic, and febrifuge properties are also valuable when treating sinus and bronchial infections involving fevers and excessive mucous production. Synthetically produced thymol is an ingredient in Vick's VapoRub, an ointment that is applied to the chest to break up mucous congestion and reduce coughs.

The herb is an excellent bronchodilator, antispasmodic, expectorant, and antitussive helpful for labored breathing, bronchial spasms, and acute and chronic coughs with thick phlegm. The tea or tincture is taken to treat sore throats, the common cold, influenza (the flu) mucous congestion, acute and chronic sinusitis, bronchitis, laryngitis, tonsillitis, and whooping cough (also known as pertussis, an acute, highly contagious bacterial infection). Emphysema and asthma can be eased by combining Thyme with 2-4 drops of Lobelia (*Lobelia inflata*) tincture. Gargle and drink Thyme tea for sore throats and laryngitis. Thyme works well combined with Echinacea, Boneset (*Eupatorium perfoliatum*), Elecampane (*Inula helenium*), Pleurisy Root (*Asclepias tuberosa*), and Fenugreek (*Trigonella foenum-graecum*) for respiratory problems. Remember that Thyme is drying, so combine it with moistening herbs like Marshmallow root (*Althaea officinalis*) or Chickweed (*Stellaria* spp.) when treating dry coughs.

The German Commission E herbal regulatory agency approved *T. vulgaris* for bronchitis, whooping cough, and mucous congestion in the upper respiratory tract. Several multicenter studies in Germany have investigated the benefits of Thyme for respiratory conditions. Researchers studied the effects of a *T. vulgaris* and Primula or Cowslip root (*Primula veris*) dried extract (marketed as Bronchipret ®) compared to synthetic drugs for the treatment of acute bronchitis in 7,783 patients. The study revealed that the herbal combination was more effective in treating bronchitis with fewer side effects than the synthetic drugs (Ernst, 1997). Another multicenter study assessed the efficacy and tolerability of a Thyme and English Ivy leaf (*Hedera helix*) syrup compared to a placebo in 361 outpatients suffering from acute bronchitis and productive coughs. During the 11-day treatment, the participants received 5.4 mL of the Thyme and English Ivy syrup (sold as Bronchipret Saft ®) or placebo syrup 3 times daily. Those taking the herbal combination experienced a 68.7% reduction in their coughing on the seventh and ninth days compared to a 47.6% reduction in the placebo group (Kemmerich, 2006). The same researcher conducted a later study consisting of 361 outpatients with acute bronchitis and productive coughs to assess the efficacy and tolerability of a dry extract of Thyme and Primula root (*Primula veris*) marketed as Bronchipret TP FCT ®. The outpatients were divided into a treatment group receiving 1 tablet of the herbal combination 3 times daily for 11 days or a group receiving 3 placebo tablets daily. Those receiving the herbal treatment experienced 67% reduction in coughing on days 7 to 9 compared to 51% reduction in the placebo group. In the Thyme-Primrose combination group, a 50% reduction in coughing fits from baseline was reached about 2 days earlier compared to the placebo group (Kemmerich, 2007).

Nervous System: Thyme is a calming nervine, mild sedative, and antispasmodic herb helpful for many problems caused by nervous overstimulation and hyperactivity. It helps restore adrenal function and treat adrenal exhaustion caused by chronic stress and anxiety. Researchers using *in vitro* studies found that thymol has an affinity with GABA (gamma-aminobutyric acid) receptor sites on human cells and binds to them, eliciting a calming response (Priestley, 2003). GABA is a neurotransmitter that reduces hyperstimulation and anxiety, and the ability of thymol to increase GABA activity is one mechanism of Thyme's relaxing action. The flavonoids and volatile oils relax smooth muscle (Boskabady, 2006) and reduce smooth muscle spasms (Van Den Broucke, 1983).

The herb has historically been ingested to relieve tension headaches, aching muscles and spasms, nervous indigestion, sciatica pain, and neurasthenia (a condition involving abnormal fatigue, lack of motivation, depression, mental fog, and insomnia). Pillows stuffed with Thyme and Lavender are enjoyed for easing restless sleep and nightmares. Thyme is also used to treat bed-wetting during childhood.

Digestive System: The volatile oils in Thyme provide a soothing digestive tonic. The nervine and sedative properties are helpful for digestive problems stemming from anxiety. As a carminative, Thyme relieves flatulence (gas) and stimulates sluggish digestion. It reduces inflammation and has a long history of use in treating indigestion, chronic gastritis (stomach inflammation), stomatitis (mouth and tongue inflammation), halitosis (bad breath), anorexia, abdominal infections, and diarrhea. Antispasmodic properties in the oils relax smooth muscle and make this herb beneficial for abdominal cramps and hiccups, which are spasms in the diaphragm muscle.

Several *in vitro* tests validate the potent antimicrobial activity of the volatile oils that keep the digestive tract free of infectious organisms, including Candida yeast. An infusion of *T. vulgaris* has been shown to be effective against *Helicobacter pylori* bacteria promoting stomach ulcers (Tabak, 1996). Thyme oils have demonstrated strong ability to inhibit chicken and pig strains of *Escherichia coli*, *Salmonella enteritidis*, *S. essen*, *S. choleraesuis*, and *S. typhimurium*, which all cause intestinal infections and diarrhea (Penalver, 2005; Rota, 2004). Thyme oil also destroys parasites in the gastrointestinal tract and is specific for hookworms and roundworms (including ascarids) in children and adults.

Cardiovascular System: Thyme has a calming and normalizing action on the heart and blood vessels. *In vitro* studies demonstrate that it relaxes the muscular layers of blood vessels, causing vasodilation and improved blood flow (Grande, 2004). This helps to increase warmth in the extremities, normalize blood pressure, and prevent vascular diseases such as atherosclerosis. The herb may be helpful for migraine headaches and circulatory problems like Raynaud's disease and intermittent claudication (muscle pain and cramping in the calf muscle). Thymol inhibits aggregation or clumping together of red blood cells, which reduces blood clot formation contributing to heart attacks and strokes. (Okazaki, 2002; Duke, 1997). An *in vitro* and *in vivo* study on mice revealed that the juice of Thyme leaves has significant ability to protect against thrombosis (formation of blood clots) by inhibiting aggregation of blood platelets (Yamamoto, 2005).

Women's Health: Thyme relaxes uterine muscles and is an excellent emmenagogue that relieves stalled menstruation, eases menstrual cramps, and controls excessive blood flow. Two clinical studies have shown that *T. vulgaris* reduces menstrual pain and cramps as effectively as ibuprofen in women diagnosed with dysmenorrhea (painful menstruation). The first study involved 120 university students (Direkvand-Moghadam, 2012), and 84 students participated in the second (Salmalian, 2014).

Old European herbalists recommended Thyme to pregnant women, and Nicholas Culpeper wrote that it "provokes the terms" and gives safe and speedy delivery for women in labor. It helps expel a retained placenta, heal uterine inflammation and infections, and eases mastitis (breast inflammation and infection).

A Poem about Thyme

Woman: *I'm very fond of wild Thyme.*
Man: *I've had a wild time, too!*
Woman: *Grow it in your garden, won't you make a note.*
Man: *Yes, I'll grow it in the spot where I sowed a wild oat.*

Gertrude Lawrence

Teachings from the Thyme Deva

"Greetings, dear one. It is the deva of the Thyme plants that speaks to you. My essence is sweet and light, like thousands of bright little stars all shining. My essence embraces the vast oneness and wholeness of all the little individual parts of creation. My plants reflect this in that they do not live alone as a solitary stem with leaves and flowers. Rather, they always exist as members of a large patch that spreads over the ground like a beautiful blanket of life. My essence is the consciousness and experience of the great unification and completion of life – the full 'coming into being' of all parts of the whole to the extent that each individual part loses the identification of separation and merges into the experience of being in the oneness of life and existence. The reference point of the individual self merges into oneness. It is a great expanse of freedom to live in this awareness!

"My plants are dominated by the air element that fills all space without a focal point or time of reference. Air emerges and exists everywhere. My plants are influenced by the energies and expression of the air sign Aquarius, symbolized by the water-bearer pouring out the abundant, limitless water of life for all to partake. My affinity with the air element provides good medicine to keep open the air passages in the human body. My medicines assist in keeping all energies in the body open and flowing without obstruction, especially in the nervous, digestive, and urinary systems.

"The essence of my flowers helps people who wish to be unbound and free of their self-limited views and identity of self. Those who are wound too tightly and restricted and want to be released from the confines of their self-imposed restrictions should use my medicines. My flowers bring the spacious breath and experience of oneness into your being.

"The sign of Aquarius is ruled by Neptune and Uranus, the outer planets of our solar system that influence the higher consciousness in understanding that all is One. All contain the common bond and thread of light and life. Humans are ultimately a family living upon one home – called Earth. And just as a single cell within your body is part of your whole being, planet Earth is one body in the vast, limitless universe. As more individuals on your planet come into this awareness, they will treat each other as 'family,' and greater peace, happiness, and health will emerge. The change that so many people wait for arises from a shift and expansion in consciousness. This is essentially so simple, yet so vast in its complexity. Please remember, always, that all objects and forms, including you and your body, arise from that which is formless. And this formlessness is what the plant devas refer to as Oneness. To live in a physical body with the awareness and experience of being one with all brings great peace and freedom. My essence and the medicine within my plants hold and rest in this space of Oneness. How magnificent!"

Valerian

Valeriana officinalis
Valerianaceae (Valerian) Family

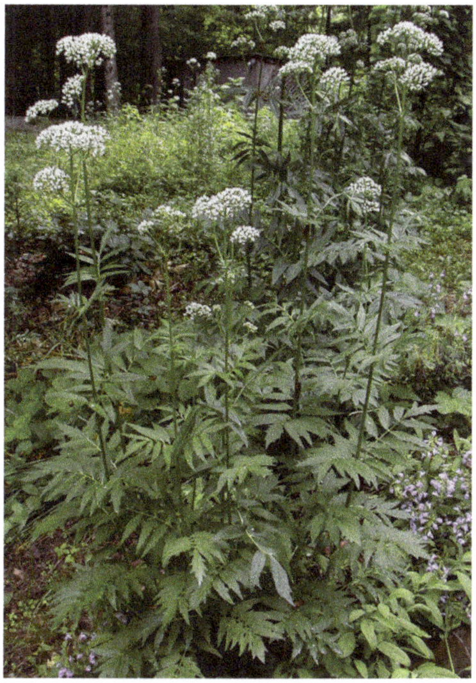

Common Names

English Valerian, German Valerian, fragrant Valerian, Amantilla, setwell, vandal root, all-heal, heal-all, garden heliotrope, Capon's tail, and phu or fu (referring to the stinky smell of the roots) are common names for *Valeriana officinalis*.

Medicinal Part of the Plant

The root is used medicinally.

Range and Habitat

V. officinalis is native to England, Europe, and temperate Asia. It is cultivated in many temperate areas worldwide and has escaped gardens to become naturalized. There are about 250 species of *Valeriana* and about 20 are indigenous to Europe. North America has about 16 native and naturalized species growing in Canada and northern United States. Its natural habitat includes woodlands, damp lowlands, marshes and stream banks, as well as dry pastures, grasslands, and mountainous areas.

Description of the Plant

V. officinalis is a tall, attractive plant and a hardy perennial. Mature plants reach heights of 3-5′ when flowering. The fibrous root is light tan on the outside and creamy-white inside. In spring, a rosette of fern-like leaves emerges from the root crown. The erect flower stalk is hollow, grooved, and predominately smooth with very short hairs around the leaf axils. Pinnately compound leaves grow opposite each other at wide intervals along the length of the stalk. Each leaf typically has 3-10 pairs of sessile leaflets that are 1–3″ long and grow opposite each other on both sides of the mid-stem. The leaflets at the base of the stalk are larger, broader, and more ovate in shape compared to leaflets on the upper portions, which are smaller and lance-shaped. A few large serrate teeth line the leaf margins. All leaflets have a very nettled, pinnate vein pattern. They are smooth with inconspicuous hairs on the underside of the leaf blade.

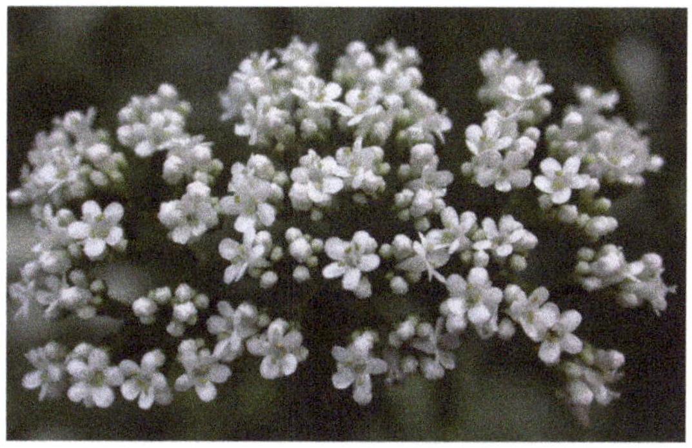

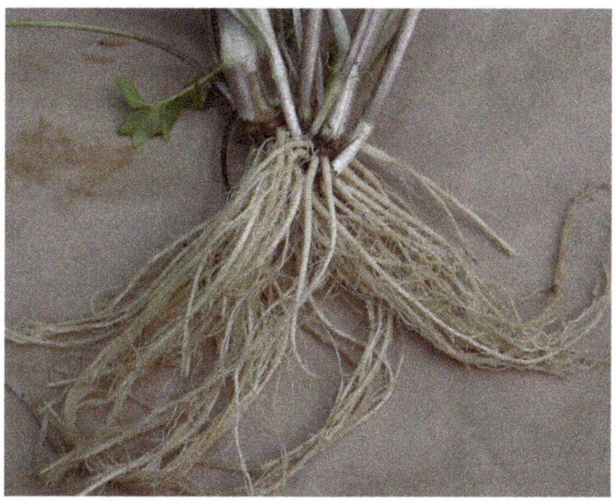

Flower heads grow from upper leaf axils and on top of the tall stalks. Tiny flowers form slightly rounded, compact umbrella-shaped clusters called panicled cymes. The buds are a delicate pink color and open into white flowers tinged with light pink. Each tubular flower has 5 lobed petals with 3 cream-colored stamens. Flower heads are 2-5″ wide and expand as the flowers open. Blossoms appear in May and June. Flowers mature into brown seeds with short hairy tufts that function like parachutes to carry them in the wind.

The roots have a characteristically distinctive odor that most people liken to dirty gym socks. Many authors write that this odor develops as the root dries, but all the roots I've dug up emit this aroma immediately, even very young plants. In contrast to the roots – and in all fairness to the plant – it should be mentioned that the flowers have a pleasantly sweet, musky fragrance.

Cultivation

Valerian thrives in fertile, loamy, moist soil under full sun, but will tolerate partial shade. Propagation is achieved by seed or root division. Once mature plants are established, they typically self-sow their seeds and many seedlings can appear around parent plants each spring. These can be transplanted or left alone. The seeds are generally viable for only one year and tend to germinate slowly with about a 30% success rate.

After the plants have flowered, harvest mature seeds and immediately sow them in planting trays or outdoor beds. They may also be planted early the following spring. Valerian seeds depend on light and constant moisture to germinate, so press them onto the soil surface rather than covering with dirt, and keep the soil continually moist. They will typically germinate in 10-20 days with warm conditions. Young seedlings sprout two rounded leaves (cotyledons) and do not develop their deep-toothed leaves until they are about a month old. Seedlings may be transplanted 12″ apart when 4-5″ tall.

Propagate Valerian by root division in early spring during dormancy or in early fall to allow sufficient root growth for winter survival. Dig up the roots of plants that are at least 3 years old. Break the large crowns into smaller starts and replant them. Keep young plants watered and mulched. Remember that the medicine is contained in the roots, which will grow larger if some flowering tops are cut off as they appear in spring.

I have been growing *V. officinalis* for many years, and this lovely plant always has a special place in my gardens. Once established, Valerian spreads out into large patches and develops into attractive and prominent plants that are a source of calming beauty.

Harvest

The medicinal essential oils in the roots reach their highest concentration and potency at the end of summer, and are ready to harvest in the autumn of their second year when leaves die back before the first frost. Roots may also be harvested in early spring after leaves appear. When harvesting older plants, be sure that the roots are succulent rather than woody, which makes them unfit for medicinal use. Chop off the stem and most of the root for medicinal preparations, leaving the root crown with some fibers attached to replant and propagate another plant.

Harvest the seeds when they are dry and have turned brown, and plant as soon as possible.

Preparation of Plant Medicine and Dosages

After harvesting the roots, break apart large clusters, remove dirt and debris with a strong water sprayer, and allow surface water on the roots to dry. Valerian imparts its properties to both water and alcohol, so teas and tinctures are reliable preparations. Always make tincture with freshly harvested roots to obtain the highest potency of chemical constituents and volatile oils, which begin to deteriorate after drying.

Although Valerian is a renowned sedative, its calming effects are not always consistent because it can elicit the opposite effect of stimulating rather than sedating the nervous system. Most people experience relaxation after ingesting Valerian, but a small percentage of the population responds with increased anxiety and insomnia. This stimulating effect primarily occurs in people who are hot natured with a red complexion, fast pulse, and require less clothing or bed covers than others. For this reason, it is best to start with small doses and gradually increase. If any undesirable effects are experienced, decrease the dosage or stop completely. Combining Valerian with other sedating herbs often reduces or eliminates this issue.

To obtain optimal sedating, antispasmodic and analgesic benefits, larger doses of Valerian are usually required, and can be repeated 2-3 times in 30-60 minute intervals as needed for severe conditions. It may be taken during the day for anxiety, spasms, and other related nerve problems, and taken at night 30-60 minutes before bedtime for insomnia. For chronic problems, some people may need to use the herb for 2-4 weeks to feel the full scope of its calming effects. Valerian is safe for children over 3 years of age when taken in smaller doses (refer to the chapter “How to Calculate Dosages” on page 148 for pediatric doses).

PREPARATIONS

Tea: Unlike most roots, Valerian should not be boiled or simmered because it reduces the potency of the medicinal essential oils. To make tea, pour a cup of boiling hot water over 1-2 teaspoons of chopped or powdered root, cover with a lid, and allow it to steep for 20-40 minutes. Dosage: 1 cup of tea up to 4 times a day as needed. The tea has a strong, bitter flavor.

Tincture: Prepare the root tincture in the standard way using 75% 190-proof grain alcohol and 25% distilled water. Dosage: 30-90 drops up to 4 times a day as needed in water or grape juice (to hide the taste). Start with a lower dose of 10-15 drops and increase the dosage until relaxing effects are adequate. Larger doses of 3 or more teaspoons may cause mild but temporary indigestion or light-headedness, although these side effects are rare.

Capsules or Tablets: These preparations are often the least effective due to deterioration after drying. Dosage: 300-500 mg 1-3 times a day.

Chemical Constituents

The sedative action of Valerian is attributed to the synergistic interaction of several chemical components, including the valepotriates (which are very unstable and break down in heat and moisture), kessyl esters, and the volatile oil containing sesquiterpenes that include valerenic acid (sedating, antispasmodic, anti-anxiety), valeronone, and kessane. The calming valepotriates regulate autonomic nervous function and are antispasmodic, anticonvulsant, vasodilating (relaxes and dilates blood vessels), and increase circulation to the heart. Baldrinals are only present in the dried roots and are produced as the valepotriates degrade when drying. The distinctive odor of the roots comes from valeric acid and terpinolene.

Other sedating constituents in the oil and roots are valerenal, beta-pinene (anti-inflammatory and antispasmodic), borneol (analgesic, anti-inflammatory, antispasmodic, choleretic), eugenol, limonene (anti-inflammatory, antispasmodic, muscle relaxant), and camphene (antioxidant, expectorant). Valeric acid has muscle relaxant, sedating, tranquilizing, and hypotensive actions. Bornyl acetate is an antispasmodic, expectorant, and muscle relaxant. Beta-caryophyllene is anti-inflammatory, antispasmodic, and diuretic.

Alkaloids include actinidine, chatinine, valerianine, and valerine (sedating). Amino acids include arginine, glutamine, alanine, tyrosine, and GABA (gamma-aminobutyric acid). Other constituents are formic acid, caffeic acid (analgesic, antidepressant, anti-inflammatory, sedative, diuretic), coumaric acid (antioxidant, antispasmodic), chlorogenic acid (analgesic, anti-inflammatory), linolenic acid (vasodilator, hypotensive), acetic acid (expectorant), beta-sitosterol (anticancer, diuretic, anti-inflammatory, antioxidant, antitumor), kaempferol (anti-inflammatory, antispasmodic, neuroprotective, vasodilator), the bioflavonoid quercetin, and minerals, including sodium, potassium, magnesium, and high concentrations of selenium and calcium.

Safety, Contraindications, and Drug Interactions

Valerian's historic use in well-established medical systems and current clinical research confirms its general safety. The German Commission E regulatory agency and other herbal authorities have reported no known contraindications, serious drug interactions, or side effects. **It is not recommended during pregnancy and lactation** due to lack of research and emmenagogue actions. The herb may increase the effects of alcohol and sedating drugs, and excessive doses may result in temporary side effects of lightheadedness, headache, agitation, stupor, indigestion, or nausea. As mentioned, people who are hot-natured may experience restlessness, anxiety, and insomnia. People have reported vivid dreams or nightmares after taking Valerian, but combining it with Passion Flower (*Passiflora incarnata*) helps prevent unpleasant dreams.

Normal dosages of Valerian do not impair the ability to drive or operate machinery, and do not produce a morning hangover. Several clinical trials show that it is an effective alternative to benzodiazepine tranquilizers such as Valium and Xanax, yet is not addictive and does not produce the drug-induced side effects of impaired coordination, confusion, lethargy, or rebound insomnia after withdrawal from the medication. One study involving 102 people confirmed that 600 mg of Valerian root taken nightly for 14 days did not cause these side effects and participants were alert the next morning (Kuhlmann, 1999). Despite the similar-sounding name, the prescription drug Valium is not related to or derived from Valerian.

The herb is safe for children and the elderly. The basic safety of Valerian was confirmed by a woman who took an overdose of 40-50 capsules of the powdered root (470 mg per capsule) in a suicide attempt. The usual dose for sleep is 2 capsules. After 30 minutes, she experienced fatigue, abdominal cramps, lightheadedness, chest tightness, tremors in her hands and feet, and dilated pupils. However, these side effects resolved within 24 hours, and her liver function and all other medical tests were normal (Willey, 1995).

Medicinal Uses

History of the Plant

Asian species of Valerian have been used as a popular medicinal for many centuries in Unani, Ayurvedic, and Chinese medicine. In European medicine, Hippocrates (*circa* 460 – *c.* 377 B.C.) was the first to document the use of *V. officinalis* root, and later the Greek physician and botanist Dioscorides (A.D. *c.* 40 – *c.* 90) recommended it for digestive problems, liver ailments, urinary tract illness, and as a diuretic and poison antidote. The early Greeks and Romans employed it for heart arrhythmias and palpitations, digestive disorders including gas and nausea, urinary tract problems, menstrual cramps, and epilepsy. Greek physician Galen (A.D. 131 – *c.* 200) affirmed its success in treating insomnia, cramps, convulsions and epilepsy in children and adults, headaches, poisoning, water retention, jaundice, chest congestion and coughs, mouth ulcers, and menstrual difficulties due to tension and anxiety. It was applied to cuts and wounds. Dioscorides and Galen called Valerian "Phu" due to the strong, stinky odor of the roots. Hildegard of Bingen (1098–1179) was a famous German Benedictine nun and herbal healer who recommended Valerian root as a sedative. During medieval times, the herb was such a popular remedy that it was known as "all-heal." English herbalist and astrologer Nicholas Culpeper (1616–1654) believed that it was ruled by the astrological influence of the planet Mercury. According to Swedish botanist Carl Linnaeus (1707–1778), the plant was named in honor of the Roman emperor Publius Valerianus, who ruled from A.D. 253–260. Valerian's common name is derived from the Latin words *valere* or *valeo*, meaning "to be healthy and strong," in reference to the plant's powerful healing ability and perhaps to the strong odor of the roots.

European immigrants brought *V. officinalis* to North America during the early 1600s, planting it in their herbal gardens where it escaped cultivation and naturalized. When the Europeans arrived, some American Indian groups were already using native species of Valerian to treat wounds. The Thompson Indians from British Columbia pulverized fresh roots and leaves to apply as a poultice directly on injuries, while the dried roots were used as an antiseptic powder.

Valerian's reputation as a primary herb for spasms and insomnia evolved during the 1600s and 1700s. The early American Eclectic physicians were aware of Valerian's action on the nervous system and employed it as a nervine for anxiety, headaches, spasms, and epilepsy. They recommended it for depression and poor blood circulation to the brain, and extolled it as one of best treatments for chorea, an old term for constantly rapid, jerky, involuntary movements. During World War I, the herb was prescribed to soldiers and civilians as a treatment for anxiety and "shell-shock" (currently known as post-traumatic stress disorder or PTSD). Until the advent of synthetic drugs during the 1940s, Valerian was listed as an official medicine in the *U.S. Pharmacopoeia* from 1820–1930 and in the *National Formulary* from 1888–1946.

The popularity of Valerian as a sedative herb has dramatically increased, and extensive research, most notably in Europe, has resulted in more than 200 published scientific studies validating many of its traditional uses. The herb is commercially grown, and the roots are a common ingredient in hundreds of over-the-counter preparations sold in the United States and Europe, especially in Germany. It is recognized by the World Health Organization as a mild hypotensive that lowers blood pressure.

Healing Qualities

Analgesic, antispasmodic, cardiotonic, carminative, emmenagogue, hypnotic, hypotensive, nervine, sedative, stimulating for stomach and intestinal motility, and tonic to the nervous system.

Traditional Chinese Medicine (TCM) Perspective

A warming and mildly drying root, Valerian disperses blocked, stagnant energy and calms the spirit. In TCM, it is a remedy for Qi deficiency conditions (caused by Qi restraint throughout the system) and for Yin deficiency conditions with empty heat, especially Heart and Kidney Yin deficiency. It is restoring and relaxing to the nervous system, and decongesting to "pent-up" nervous energy. The roots clear internal Wind that causes spasms and tremors, and their ability to disperse Qi in the nervous system reduces anxiety, restlessness, pain, and spasms. Valerian is specific for Heart Qi constraint causing palpitations, arrhythmias and hypertension, and for Lung Qi constraint responsible for labored breathing, coughs, wheezing, and asthma. Qi constraint in the genitourinary tract may cause irregular and painful menstruation, which Valerian also improves. The herb helps normalize Stomach, Liver, and Intestinal Qi Stagnation responsible for sluggish digestion, gas, spasms, and constipation.

Primary Actions

Valerian's restoring and calming influence on the nervous system benefits the whole body, helping reduce hyperstimulation, anxiety, insomnia, pain, spasms, and inflammation. The herb exhibits an affinity with GABA (gamma-aminobutyric acid) and serotonin, which are important inhibitory neurotransmitters that regulate and calm the central nervous system, promote relaxation and sleep, and stabilize moods. **Valerian is indicated for conditions of weakness and depletion rather than excess.** Its warming nature is specific for people with a pale complexion and cool skin, whose nervous system is frail and agitated due to emotional tension and possible nutritional deficiencies.

When using Valerian, always remember that it may have the **opposite effect of stimulating rather than sedating the nervous system** in some people who are hot-natured. For the best and most reliable results, I usually combine Valerian with other nervine and sedative herbs such as Scullcap (*Scutellaria lateriflora*), Hops (*Humulus lupulus*), Lemon Balm (*Melissa officinalis*), Passion Flower (*Passiflora incarnata*), Catnip (*Nepeta cataria*), Chamomile (*Matricaria recutita*), and St. John's Wort (*Hypericum perforatum*).

Nervous System: Valerian is one of the most popular herbs for calming and restoring the nervous system. It is specific for many physical and psychological problems resulting from acute or chronic nervous tension and overstimulation. By regulating the autonomic nervous system, which works automatically without our conscious control, Valerian inhibits hyperactivity and is beneficial for psychosomatic problems stemming from nervous system imbalance and agitation. By reducing overstimulation in the peripheral nerves, it is a muscle relaxant, mild analgesic, and antispasmodic. Research has confirmed that its antispasmodic properties specifically relax smooth muscles in the lungs, colon and uterus, and ease painful cramps and spasms throughout the body (Hazelhoff, 1982). A study involving 39 patients diagnosed with fibromyalgia revealed that soaking in Valerian whirlpool baths 10 times over a 3½ week period reduced the intensity of their general body pain and improved their quality of sleep and feelings of well-being (Ammer, 1999).

Valerian is indicated for acute or chronic stress, anxiety, restlessness, and depression. It improves cognitive function to promote clear thinking and is used for attention deficit disorder in both children and adults. Lignans and other constituents in the roots have antioxidant and vasorelaxant actions (relaxes muscles in blood vessels) (Piccinelli, 2004), and demonstrate ability to protect nerves against toxins and degenerative conditions (Malva, 2004). The herb's ability to dilate blood vessels, including cerebral vessels, make it specific for poor circulation, diminished blood flow to the brain, and hypertension due to nervous stress. The roots are an effective nerve tonic for long-term use and can be helpful for nerve deterioration and pain, such as arthritic pain, headaches, migraines, and trigeminal neuralgia. By relaxing hyperactive nerves and constricted muscles throughout the body, Valerian relieves a multitude of problems, including hyperactivity, nervous tics, trembling and tremors, alcohol and drug withdrawal (delirium tremens), convulsions, and epilepsy. Valerian is also a tranquilizing sedative that improves the quality of sleep and is excellent for insomnia. It reduces the amount of time it takes to get to sleep and promotes sound, restful sleep. It can also reduce or eliminate nightmares. I have found that taking Valerian helps people wean off of pharmaceutical sedatives and anti-anxiety drugs like Valium and Xanax, which tend to have side effects and can be addictive.

Many historic uses of Valerian are validated by numerous research studies that have identified chemical constituents and demonstrated the herb's influence on the nervous system. A primary mode of its sedating, anti-anxiety action involves the ability to bind to GABA (gamma-aminobutyric acid) receptors on cells in the nervous system. GABA is a primary inhibitory neurotransmitter that decreases overstimulation and promotes calm relaxation. Several studies show that valerenic acid (occurring in the roots) binds to GABA receptors to exert this calming effect (Benke, 2009; De Feo, 2003; Granger, 2005; Holzl, 1989; Mennini, 1993; Ortiz, 1999). Valerenic acid inhibits the enzyme that breaks down GABA, contributing to increased GABA levels in the body. Valerian also contains glutamine, an amino acid that provides fuel for the brain, helps the nervous system heal from the damage of drug and alcohol abuse, and support the digestive system (Santos, 1994).

Pharmaceutical sedatives like Valium and other benzodiazepines also work by binding to GABA receptors. GABA is the primary ingredient in several drugs prescribed for convulsions, epilepsy, and neuropathy due to nerve damage, such as Neurontin (gabapentin) and Lyrica (pregabalin).

Researchers know that Valerian also attaches to serotonin and melatonin cell receptors in the brain that promote relaxation (Abourashed, 2004; Dietz, 2005). Serotonin is another primary inhibitory neurotransmitter and its deficiency can cause depression, anxiety, insomnia, and poor digestive function. Melatonin, a hormone promoting deep sleep, is produced from serotonin and secreted by the pineal gland.

Many clinical trials have evaluated the efficacy and safety of Valerian combined with other nervine and sedative herbs. Several studies demonstrate that Valerian is a useful alternative to antidepressant and anti-anxiety drugs in the treatment of mild depression and anxiety, especially when combined with St. John's Wort (*Hypericum perforatum*). In a 2-week trial involving 100 patients diagnosed with anxiety, a combination of Valerian and St. John's Wort was more effective than diazepam (Valium) in treating anxiety (Panijel, 1985). In another research test lasting 6 weeks, 130 people diagnosed with depression took a combination of Valerian and St. John's Wort or amitriptyline (Elavil). During the study, 80% of the herb group and 88% of the drug group experienced a 50% reduction in their symptoms of depression. Although there were no significant side effects in the herb group, 5 patients receiving Elavil required a dosage reduction due to unpleasant side effects (Kneibel, 1988).

Formulas of Valerian and Lemon Balm (*Melissa officinalis*) are widely used as a treatment for insomnia and nervous tension. Researchers conducted a study of this combination with 98 healthy volunteers who took either 3 capsules of dry Valerian extract (480 mg per capsule) with Lemon Balm (240 mg per capsule) or a placebo 30 minutes before bedtime. Although the participants did not have insomnia, those taking the herbal mixture reported 33% improvement in their quality of sleep without problematic side effects (Cerny, 1999). A Valerian and Lemon Balm preparation was investigated in a multicenter study in Germany involving 918 children younger than 12 years old who were diagnosed with restlessness and nervous insomnia. Each child received 3-4 tablets daily of the herbal preparation containing 160 mg of Valerian root and 80 mg of Lemon Balm leaf. When their parents and the researchers evaluated the therapeutic efficacy and tolerability of the herbs after 30 days, they reported significant reduction in the severity of all symptoms. The core symptoms of insomnia and restlessness were reduced from "moderate/severe" to "mild" or "absent" in most of the children. A total of 80.9% who suffered from insomnia experienced improvement, and 70.4% of the children with restlessness demonstrated greater calmness. Parents and researchers reported the efficacy of the herbal therapy to be "very good" (60.5%) or "good" (67.7%) (Muller, 2006). The results of another multicenter study showed that daily intake of Valerian (640 mg) and Lemon Balm (320 mg) improved symptoms of attention deficit hyperactivity disorder (ADHD) in 136 children ages 6-11. After 7 weeks of treatment, 62% of the physicians reported "good" or "very good" improvement in hyperactivity, impulsiveness, social behavior, insomnia, and the ability to concentrate. The children's tolerance of the herbal treatment was rated as "very good" or "good" by 97% of the physicians (Gromball, 2014).

Clinical research shows that Valerian root improves overall sleep quality, shortens the length of time it takes to fall asleep, helps people sleep more soundly, and can be as effective as small doses of barbiturates and benzodiazepines without the side effects. A study of about 42 people suffering from insomnia showed that 800 mg of the root extract taken before bedtime significantly improved their ability to fall asleep and enhanced sleep quality (Leathwood, 1982). In a 4-week trial that included 121 participants with insomnia, those who took 600 mg of Valerian root extract an hour before bedtime reported significantly improved sleep quality, dream recall, and psychological well-being with less daytime fatigue and no side effects compared to those receiving placebo (Vorbach, 1996). Another study using electroencephalogram (EEG) testing to compare the effect of herbs with Valium concluded that 1,200 mg of Lavender and Valerian extract had similar effects as Valium on the brain waves of 23 women suffering from sleep disorders (Schulz, 1997).

In a 2-week clinical study, 78 elderly people suffering from sleep disturbances and nervous conditions experienced significant improvement in falling asleep and staying asleep without side effects when using Valerian before bedtime (Kamm-Kohl, 1984). A small but interesting study consisted of 5 boys (7-14 years old) who had severe insomnia, an IQ (intelligence quotient) of less than 70, and cognitive and neurological problems that included epilepsy, hyperactivity, and attention deficit disorder. A nightly dose of Valerian in tablet form (containing 500 mg of the root with 5.52 mg of valtrate and isovaltrate) significantly decreased sleep latency (the amount of time to fall asleep) and increased total sleep time without any adverse effects (Francis, 2002).

Several studies have focused on the therapeutic effects of Valerian combined with Hops (*Humulus lupulus*). In one test, researchers explored the ability of these two herbs to counteract the stimulating effects of caffeine (Schellenberg, 2004). Constituents in Valerian can bind to adenosine receptors in the central nervous system, which induces sleep. Caffeine also binds to these receptors, but has the opposite action of exciting the nervous system because it blocks adenosine from binding to these receptors. In this study involving healthy men, researchers found that when participants ingested 500 mg of Valerian combined with 120 mg of Hops, the stimulating effects of 200 mg of caffeine were reduced within one hour. A larger dose consisting of 1,500 mg of Valerian with 360 mg of Hops completely inhibited the caffeine reaction. Another clinical trial involving 30 people suffering from mild to moderate insomnia revealed that after 2 weeks of taking 500 mg of Valerian and 120 mg of Hops extracts before bedtime, insomnia was replaced by faster, restful, and refreshing sleep without adverse effects (Fussel, 2000).

In a multicenter study conducted in nine sleep disorder centers throughout the United States, the efficacy and safety of a Valerian and Hops combination was compared to diphenhydramine (Benadryl) for the treatment of mild insomnia in 184 adults. Participants were divided into three groups, and for 28 days they took either 374 mg of a standardized Valerian extract with 84 mg of Hops, Benadryl, or a placebo. The Benadryl group took 50 mg for 14 days followed by a placebo for 14 days. Study results revealed improvements of sleep parameters with the herbal combination and Benadryl, although Valerian and Hops promoted faster onset of sleep (Morin, 2005).

Valerian's activity has also been compared with the anti-anxiety drug oxazepam (Serax) in a multicenter study involving 202 adult outpatients diagnosed with insomnia. After 6 weeks of treatment, Valerian (600 mg taken daily) was shown to be as effective as oxazepam (10 mg daily) in significantly improving sleep quality. Mild to moderate side effects occurred in 29 patients (28.4%) receiving Valerian and 36 patients (36%) using oxazepam. In the Valerian group, 83% of the patients assessed their treatment as "very good" compared to 73% in the oxazepam group (Ziegler, 2002).

Valerian root was found to be helpful for obsessive-compulsive disorder (OCD) during a clinical trial involving 31 adult outpatients diagnosed with OCD. They were randomly assigned to receive either a capsule of the Valerian extract (765 mg) or a placebo every day for 8 weeks. The results showed a significant difference between the herbal extract and placebo at the end of treatment, revealing that Valerian reduced obsessive and compulsive behavior (Pakseresht, 2011).

For nervous overstimulation and anxiety problems, Valerian combines well with Lemon Balm, Scullcap, and Hops. For pain, combine it with St. John's Wort, Meadowsweet (*Filipendula ulmaria*), and Wood Betony (*Staychs officinalis*).

Cardiovascular System: Many heart and circulatory problems are directly related to stress and anxiety, which Valerian helps to correct. It relaxes nerves and muscles in the heart and blood vessels, and laboratory studies show that the root extract is a potent smooth muscle and blood vessel dilator. Researchers have found that the vasodilatory effect of Valerian is mediated by GABA (Fields, 2003). These attributes serve to increase circulation to the heart, brain, and tissues throughout the body.

Valerian tends to decrease and normalize rapid heart rate (tachycardia), while increasing the contracting force to efficiently pump blood. Current research has found anti-arrhythmic chemicals in the roots, validating its historic use in treating tachycardia. It is recommended for high blood pressure with constriction and resistance in blood vessels that is caused by anxiety. Valerian can be used as a tonic over time for heart and circulation problems related to anxiety, and should be combined with other cardiac tonics such as Hawthorn berries (*Crataegus* spp.) and Motherwort (*Leonurus cardiaca*).

In a large multicenter study involving 2,243 patients diagnosed with cardiovascular disorders and/or hypotension, researchers documented an 84% improvement rate when the patients used a combination of Valerian, Hawthorn, Camphor (*Cinnamomum camphora*), and Night-blooming Cereus (*Echinocereus grandiflorus*). Patients experienced a beneficially slight increase in blood pressure and decrease in heart rate (Busanny-Caspari, 1986).

When Chinese researchers gave a volatile oil preparation extracted from Valerian roots to 82 patients with coronary heart disease (CHD) and angina pectoris, it was 87.8% effective in reducing chest pressure and pain caused by oxygen deficiency in the heart muscles. The patients experienced fewer attacks of angina with shorter duration, and the herb helped restore blood supply to heart tissues. In addition, it was discovered that Valerian lowered blood plasma lipids as well. No toxic actions to the liver, kidneys, or other tissues were observed (Yang, 1994).

Gastrointestinal Tract: Valerian reduces nervous indigestion and related problems caused by chronic anxiety and muscle tension. Valerian relieves stomach and intestinal cramps and spasms, hiccups, and colic in infants. The bitter-tasting constituents stimulate enzyme secretion in the stomach and liver, and encourage intestinal peristalsis (movement) to help eliminate sluggish digestion, gas, bloating, and constipation. It has also been added to formulas for treating stomach and intestinal ulcers caused by anxiety. Valerian's choleretic properties promoting the production and secretion of bile from the liver and gallbladder are documented by research studies (Takeda, 1981).

Urinary Tract: Valerian decreases spasms in the kidneys, bladder, ureters, and urethra. This helps the expulsion of kidney stones by relaxing the ureters and allowing for easier, less painful passage.

Respiratory System: As an antispasmodic, Valerian may be added to cough formulas for its relaxing actions on nerves and muscles in the lungs. This eases spastic coughing and bronchial spasms, expectorates phlegm, and reduces shortness of breath.

Female Reproductive System: Valerian is an emmenagogue promoting menstruation. It reduces menstrual cramps and pain, and relaxes the pelvic muscles allowing greater blood flow. The herb relieves tension and anxiety during premenstrual syndrome (PMS) and menopause. Combine it with Ginger (*Zingiber officinale*), Black Cohosh (*Cimicifuga racemosa*), Cramp Bark (*Viburnum opulus*), and Motherwort (*Leonurus cardiaca*) for menstrual cramps.

Because Valerian is an emmenagogue, it is generally **not recommended during pregnancy or lactation**. Although it is documented that pregnant women have safely used small amounts of Valerian for anxiety, insomnia (Holst, 2008), and high blood pressure during pregnancy and childbirth, it is prudent to use other herbs for anxiety and insomnia which are known to be safe for mother and infant, specifically Skullcap (*Scutellaria lateriflora*), German Chamomile (*Matricaria recutita*), Lemon Balm (*Melissa officinalis*), and Passion Flower (*Passiflora incarnata*). Hawthorn berries (*Crataegus* spp.) are safe to take for hypertension.

Teachings from the Valerian Deva

"Greetings, dear one. It is the deva of the Valerian plants that speaks to you. My feathery leaves reflect the lightness of my nature; for my medicine removes the heavy, stagnant energies held within the human body – residues of emotional and mental turmoil. These energies manifest as disturbing thoughts and feelings of depression, hopelessness, helplessness, anxiety, anger, and all other causes of emotional and mental suffering. My medicine relaxes the nervous system, quiets the heart, and helps the tightly-wound ball of turmoil to slowly unwind. As the energies within the body open, expand and flow, peaceful harmony and ease of movement eventually allow the experience of gentle stillness.

"The white color of my flowers points to my activity of cleansing and purifying the emotional field of the human body, and also of the Earth. My plants help heal old wounds upon the land where brutal, heartless actions have occurred, leaving energetic scars. I heal this distorted, wounded energy for the Earth and for humans. I assist in healing the wounded warrior, drained and weakened from the long-embroiled battles of life. The pink tinge within the whiteness of my flowers points to my affinity with the heart and blood. My plants relax the tissues of the heart and blood vessels, allowing the easy and abundant flow of life-giving blood. My medicine allows the emotionally wounded, constricted heart to open and expand the rigid walls of self-protection, re-merging into the natural flow of life and love. I help transform and heal old scars so that the light and life force of the Earth and of humans can be fully radiant and flowing.

"My plants are a balanced blend of the merging of the four elements. My medicine merges all energies of existence to bring balance to the human body and to the Earth. Planting Valerian in open fields and along the edges of woodlands is healing and restoring to the Earth, so please do this!

"The musky, earthy odor emitted from my roots and the sweet fragrance of my flowers are reminders of my capacity to transform the foul aspects of life into beautiful sweetness. Use my flowers when preparing medicines from the roots; for the flowers will contribute to the healing essence, especially when cleansing and healing the wounded, exhausted emotional body.

"My essence is that of the visionary – one whose spirit is calm and at peace – who sees subtle energies and movements at the root of all actions; one who sees and feels the movement of these energies through time. There is wildness to my nature. For when humans live in this state of inner stillness, there is open expanse and freedom from limitations people place upon their way of perceiving and their very existence. With the purifying healing offered by my plants, people become prepared to sit comfortably in the presence of this vast stillness where peace reigns. The wisdom of the ancient, timeless sage and the fresh vitality of the newborn are both contained within my healing plants.

"And so, you are invited to partake of the calming influence and wisdom offered by my plants. As you use my medicine, which serves so well, please make an offering of gratitude to the Earth, your ultimate Mother, for giving you life and a body to live in. Enjoy your life. Be grateful for the blessings of Nature around you!"

Wood Betony

Stachys officinalis
(*Stachys betonica* and *Betonica officinalis* are older names)
Labiatae (*Lamiaceae*) (Mint) Family

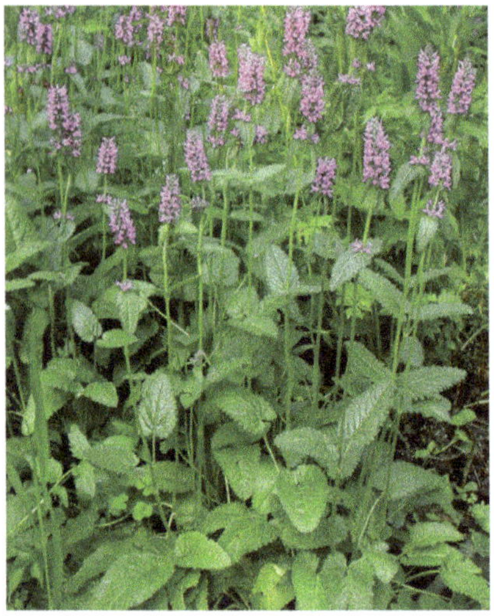

Common Names

Betony, purple betony, common betony, and bishopswort are common names.

Medicinal Part of the Plant

The leaves and flowers are medicinal.

Range and Habitat

Stachys officinalis is indigenous to Europe, western Asia and northern Africa, growing wild in woodlands, meadows, and sunny slopes. It is cultivated and has naturalized in some areas of the United States.

Description of the Plant

Wood Betony is a colorful, ornamental plant that offers both healing medicine and great beauty, making it a favorite plant of many gardeners. A multitude of single leaves grow directly out of the fibrous root system on long, square stems forming an attractive mound of deeply rich-green foliage. The leaves are simple and oblong at the base of the plant, becoming ovate higher on the stems. Leaves have a rounded, heart-shaped (cordate) base and a wrinkled texture. The leaf margins are crenate with many rounded teeth. Stems and leaves are sparsely covered with white hairs. Each mound of leaves produces several long flower stalks 1½-2′ tall. Each stalk has a few opposite, petiole leaves spaced at wide intervals and a beautiful whorled spike of flowers at the tip.

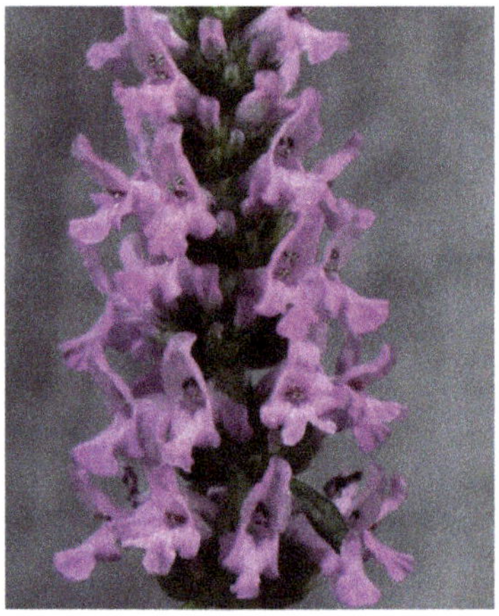

The vibrantly pinkish-purple flowers are ½-¾″ long and tubular. A curly bi-lobed upper lip and tri-lobed lower lip are held within 5 sepals forming a cup-like calyx. Flowers bloom from June through August, attracting butterflies, hummingbirds, and plant lovers! After the flower petals fall, 4 seed-like nutlets develop in the bottom of the calyx. Wood Betony is a hardy perennial herb that returns each spring to grace the landscape.

Cultivation

Wood Betony is easy to grow in sun or shade, although plants grown in full sun thrive best. The herb requires moderately fertile soil and good drainage. It propagates by seed and root division. Seeds are planted in flats in early spring and transplanted into a prepared bed when the seedlings are 3-4″ tall. Divide well-established roots in spring or early autumn and transplant.

Harvest

Harvest the leaves and flowers when the plant is in bloom for greatest concentrations of phytochemicals.

Preparation of Plant Medicine and Dosages

The freshly harvested leaves are made into tea, tincture and salve, or dried for future use. Tincturing is the best way to preserve potency and shelf life. I like to add freshly harvested flowers with the leaves when making herbal preparations.

PREPARATIONS

Tea: Steep 1-2 teaspoons of the leaves and flowers in 1 cup of boiling water. Dosage: 1-2 cups a day. The tea has a mild, pleasant flavor.

Tincture: Cover the fresh leaves and flowers with 75% 190-proof grain alcohol and 25% distilled water. Dosage: 10-30 drops 1-4 times a day as needed.

Salve: Chop the herb, cover with olive oil, and bake. Other herbs may be added (refer to "Skin Problems" on page 591 in the "Index of Health Issues and Herbal Recommendations" for suggestions).

Chemical Constituents

Wood Betony leaves contain alkaloids, including trigonelline (lowers blood sugar levels), turicin, and betonicine and stachydrine, which are both cholagogues and anti-inflammatory. Stachydrine is a cardiotonic, systolic depressant, and decreases arthritic pain. The flavonoid glycosides are hypotensive and sedating. Bitter principles include betolide and iridoids that have shown mild choleretic, hepatoprotective, anti-inflammatory, laxative, antibacterial, antifungal, and immunomodulant effects.

Rosmarinic acid and other caffeic acid derivatives inhibit inflammatory leukotrienes and prostaglandins, and are antioxidant, analgesic, choleretic, antibacterial, antiviral, immunostimulating, sedative, neuroprotective, and vulnerary. Tannins reduce bleeding and diarrhea. Other phytochemicals in the leaves include coumarins, choline, and betaine (cardioprotective, diuretic, emmenagogue, expectorant, hepatoprotective, lipotropic). The main constituents in the volatile oil are germacrene D, caryophyllene, alpha-pinene, and humulene.

Safety, Contraindications, and Drug Interactions

There are no known side effects or drug interactions. Since Wood Betony is a mild uterine stimulant, it **should not be used during the first or second trimester of pregnancy**.

Medicinal Uses

History of the Plant

Wood Betony was a popular, highly-esteemed herb during early Greek and Roman history and into the Renaissance era. Because of its great beauty and medicinal and protective qualities, it was widely cultivated by common folk and in monastery and apothecary gardens. A preparation of the leaves and flowers was reputed to be a panacea against all physical ills and to protect the soul. It was believed that drinking the tea would guard against dreaming of ghosts, monstrous night visitors, and nightmares. During the Middle Ages, when fear of the supernatural and devil was rampant, people thought Wood Betony had the power to exorcise demons. People wore the leaves and flowers as an amulet or talisman, and planted Wood Betony around their homes and churchyards for protection from malevolent spirits, witchcraft, and plagues.

The Greek physician and botanist Dioscorides (*circa* A.D. 40 – *c.* 90) recommended the herb to treat liver, spleen, kidney and bladder problems, convulsions and epilepsy, ingested poisons and bites of venomous snakes, pain, and as an emmenagogue to stimulate menstruation. John Gerard (1545–1612) used the herb in his medical practice for headaches, sciatic pain, and kidney and bladder pain and stones. He wrote, "It cleans the lungs and chest, it taketh away obstructions or stoppings of the liver and gallbladder, it is good against the yellow jaundice. It makes man have a good stomach and appetite . . . . It is also good for ruptures, cramps and convulsions, it is a remedy against the bitings of mad dogs and venomous serpents, being drunk and applied to the hurt" (Gerard, 1975).

English herbalist and apothecary Nicholas Culpeper (1616–1654) included Wood Betony in his pharmacy and mixed the powdered leaves with honey to treat coughs, colds, fevers, wheezing, and shortness of breath. He stated that the herb is astrologically ruled by Jupiter and Aries, and wrote in his herbal, "The decoction thereof made in wine and taken, killeth the worms in the belly, openeth obstructions both of the spleen and liver . . . helpeth bring down women's courses. It helpeth also to break and expel the stone, either in the bladder or kidneys." Culpeper mentioned Antonius Musa, a Roman physician serving Emperor Augustus Caesar, who regarded Wood Betony to be a cure for 47 diseases, including bites from snakes and rabid dogs, stomach and digestive problems, and plagues. Musa wrote a book about the virtues of Wood Betony, saying "that it preserveth the liver and bodies of men from the danger of epidemical diseases, and from witchcraft also. It helpeth the jaundice, falling sickness, the palsy, convulsions, or shrinking of the sinews, the gout, and those that are inclined to dropsy, those that have continual pains in the heads" (Culpeper, 1992).

With the advent of modern medicine, the beneficial properties of Wood Betony were virtually forgotten. Even today, this herb is not well known, although it continues to be used by many herbalists. Clinical studies on Wood Betony are lacking, but researchers have identified several phytochemicals that are responsible for many of the plant's healing actions.

Healing Qualities

Alterative, analgesic, anti-inflammatory, antiparasitic, antirheumatic, antiscorbutic, antiseptic, mild antispasmodic, astringent, carminative, diuretic, expectorant, mild laxative, nervine, sedative, tonic, and vulnerary.

Traditional Chinese Medicine (TCM)

Wood Betony leaves are cooling, drying, and slightly bitter. Their relaxing action is beneficial for all types of Qi constraint and the resulting tension and pain throughout the body. The herb circulates constrained Qi, which has a restoring and normalizing influence on the nervous system.

It specifically eases and releases constrained Qi in the digestive system. The leaves invigorate the stomach, resolve Liver and Kidney Qi Stagnation to prevent and treat sluggish indigestion, gas, constipation, and metabolic toxicity with gout, jaundice, skin rashes, arthritis, aches, and pains.

Wood Betony circulates Lung Qi to relieve labored breathing, asthma, bronchitis, and dispel white or yellow phlegm. It is used for Heart Qi constraint that can cause palpitations, anxiety, dizziness, headaches, visual disturbances, and hypertension. The herb is also specific for Uterine Qi constraint and congestion, and eases menstrual difficulties.

Primary Actions

I recommend Wood Betony for its restorative and normalizing benefits on the nervous system, and for nervous debility associated with anxiety and tension. It is a specific remedy for neck and head pain, including headaches and migraines, poor circulation, sinus congestion, and allergies. When taken over time as a tonic, Wood Betony normalizes and promotes the free flow of vital energy throughout the body, and it is indicated for people plagued by obsessive thinking and mental energy trapped in the head.

The herb also works through the solar plexus, the dynamic nerve center located in the abdomen that coordinates nerve messages throughout the body and brain. The solar plexus has been called the "brain of the stomach" because it specifically influences the digestive system. Many people hold excessive nervous tension in their solar plexus, which can feel like a tight knot and adversely affects the whole body, especially the digestive system, by restricting normal movement and function. Wood Betony strengthens the solar plexus by relaxing and easing nervous tension, allowing movement that unblocks rigid tissues and muscles in the digestive system and throughout the body. Strong solar plexus energy helps people establish emotional and psychological security by feeling connected and grounded within ourselves, our friends and family, and within the earth. This herb is specific for debilitated conditions and for frail, spacey people who have difficulty focusing and who feel cut off from other people and the world. By strengthening and normalizing the solar plexus and restoring calm cognitive function with the aid of Wood Betony, we become more centered, grounded, and radiant. In doing this, we protect ourselves against all types of negative influences. Perhaps this is related to the ancient beliefs that the herb protects against harmful forces.

This is a mild herb that is safe for the elderly and excellent for children suffering from "failure to thrive." I typically use Wood Betony in combination with other herbs.

Nervous System, Headaches, and Pain: Wood Betony is a relaxing and restorative nervine tonic that calms and strengthens the nervous system, and eases an overactive, obsessive mind. When taken daily for several weeks, it helps rebuild nerves after the damaging effects of fever, poisoning, drug abuse, and strokes. It is also a mild sedative that relaxes the system and promotes sleep. Wood Betony is beneficial for all types of nervous tension and anxiety, listlessness, inability to concentrate and other cognitive impairments, and has been used for childhood and adult epilepsy and convulsions.

The herb dilates cerebral arteries and improves general circulation, especially to the neck and head, which reduces ischemia (blood and oxygen deprivation) and pain. Wood Betony promotes normal brain and nerve function, and can be helpful for hypertension, dizziness, memory loss, cognitive decline, toothaches, and facial neuralgia (nerve pain and loss of muscle control) like Bell's palsy and trigeminal neuralgia. It is helpful for arthritis and can relieve lower back pain and sciatica, especially when combined with St. John's Wort (*Hypericum perforatum*). By relaxing nerves, muscle tone throughout the body is improved. *In vivo* research has demonstrated that the anti-inflammatory activities of Wood Betony leaf and flower water extracts (tea) are due, in part, to their iridoid content (ajugoside, aucubin, acetylharpagide, harpagide and harpagoside) (Háznagy-Radnai, 2012).

Wood Betony is specific for head and neck pain, including headaches and migraines. It is one of the best remedies for headaches due to its ability to dilate cerebral arteries and exert relaxing effects on the solar plexus. Many of my clients suffering from migraines report that equal parts of Wood Betony and Feverfew (*Tanacetum parthenium*) tincture with a small amount of Lavender (*Lavandula* spp.) reduce the frequency and pain of their headaches. Combining Wood Betony with Black Cohosh (*Cimicifuga racemosa*) and Jamaican Dogwood (*Piscidia piscipula*) also provides an excellent formula for headaches and migraines.

For a sedating effect, Wood Betony works well combined with Hops (*Humulus lupulus*), Scullcap (*Scutellaria lateriflora*), and Valerian (*Valeriana officinalis*). For nervous debility, combine Wood Betony with Scullcap, Motherwort (*Leonurus cardiaca*), Black Cohosh, and Valerian.

Cardiovascular System: Wood Betony exerts mild relaxation on the heart and blood vessels, allowing the vessels to dilate for improved circulation, especially to the head. This is excellent for ischemic (lack of blood flow) conditions affecting the head. When taken as a tonic over time, it may be helpful in preventing and treating strokes and pain in the face and head. In the past, during recuperation following a stroke, herbalists made a poultice from the leaves and applied it to damaged eyes for 8-10 hours to restore nerve function and muscle tone. Due to the constricting action of the tannins, regular ingestion and poultices of Wood Betony may reduce varicose veins.

One research study has demonstrated that glycosides in the herb have observable hypotensive actions (Zinchenko, 1962). Researchers have also found that alcohol extracts of the leaves exhibit substantial antioxidant properties with the ability to inhibit oxidation of fats and scavenge harmful free radicals responsible for cellular damage (Matkowski, 2006).

Digestive System: As a tonic to the digestive system, Wood Betony's restoring and strengthening actions on the solar plexus helps normalize all digestive functions, including production and secretion of enzymes, nutrient absorption, and adequate movement of food through the gastrointestinal tract. It is excellent for the stomach as it specifically eases nervous indigestion, stomach cramps, colic, and heartburn. Betony is indicated for gastrointestinal irritability and is antispasmodic to relieve cramping. Astringent tannins in the leaves help reduce internal bleeding and diarrhea. The tea or diluted tincture may be used as a mouthwash or gargle for sore, inflamed mouths and throats.

A tea or tincture of the leaves gently stimulates the liver and gallbladder to increase bile flow, which promotes digestion of fats and bowel elimination. Wood Betony improves debilitated digestion especially due to nervous tension. Appetite improves and indigestion, gas, and bloating are relieved. It is used for jaundice and constipation.

Urinary Tract: The herb has diuretic actions, and a strong infusion or tincture stimulates urination and can be taken for water retention and edema.

Allergies, Colds, and Coughs: Wood Betony is a mild astringent and demulcent that reduces sinus secretions and soothes irritated and inflamed mucous membranes. It strengthens weak lungs and is an expectorant for coughs. The herb works well for sinus congestion, allergic rhinitis and hay fever, sinusitis, colds, coughs, wheezing, asthma, bronchitis, and shortness of breath.

Women's Health: Wood Betony supports the female reproductive system by improving circulation to the uterus and ovaries and relaxing muscle tone. It eases the nervous tension and anxiety of premenstrual syndrome (PMS) and menopause, and has been used to treat amenorrhea (abnormal cessation of menses), menstrual cramps and pain, uterine prolapse, and excessive bleeding. It is a mild uterine stimulant that has been used during childbirth for difficult labor due to atonic muscles and insufficient nerve stimulus. The volatile oil in the herb has mild anti-yeast activity against *Candida albicans* (Lazarevi, 2013).

External Applications: Apply Wood Betony leaves as a salve or poultice to reduce pain and help heal wounds, sprains, swellings, achy muscles, painful joints, external ulcers, and old sores. Tannins in the leaves constrict tissues to stop bleeding and reduce bruising. For skin diseases and animal bites, ingest the tea or tincture for its blood cleansing properties while applying the leaves externally.

Teachings from the Wood Betony Deva

"Greetings. I am the deva of the Wood Betony plants and my essence is of the feminine nature. The color of my flowers points to my affinity with the heart and mental centers; for I relax and balance these areas in the human body. The pink color points to the heart and blood vessels, which my medicine relaxes while promoting constant powerful movements of the heart muscle and of the blood flowing through the body. The purple color of my flowers reflects my relationship with the head, brain, and nerves to calm and enhance their normal functioning.

"The nature of my medicine is gentle and soothing to remove stagnation and blockages in the flow of blood through the heart and vessels and in the flow of electrical energy along the nerves. For the blockage of blood or nerve energy ultimately results in pain and dysfunction.

"The medicine of my leaves and flowers enhances and empowers the capacity of the human heart to be relaxed, expansive, and capable of expressing love. At the 'heart' of my healing rests the power of loving unconditionally – love that automatically and spontaneously radiates outward to all beings without thought to oneself. Unconditional love is the most basic, primordial expression of self which, unfortunately, seems to be hidden from the awareness of so many people in this day and age. And so my most precious gift is in assisting to open the heart of human beings who are moving in this direction home to the center of their being – in true expression of their essence, you might say. A most beautiful gift, but one so seldom sought these days. Nonetheless, we are here for you and for the beauty of the planet and to benefit our animal friends in whatever ways we can. For my plants are radiant and joyous, and delight in bringing this offering of beauty and peace to the world.

"Jupiter is the ruling planet of my plants. Jupiter is the planet of expansive, forward movement guided and directed by optimistic perspective and intentional purpose to serve the highest good of all beings. And my plants are a balanced blend of all four elements: fire, earth, air, and water. My lovely flowers manifest this perfection in a state of completion and rest. When learning and experiencing the full spectrum of love without limitations, people are able to enjoy the peaceful, restful state of joyful completion and contentment that this brings forth. All is well."

Yarrow

Achillea millefolium

Compositae (Asteraceae) (Aster or Sunflower) Family

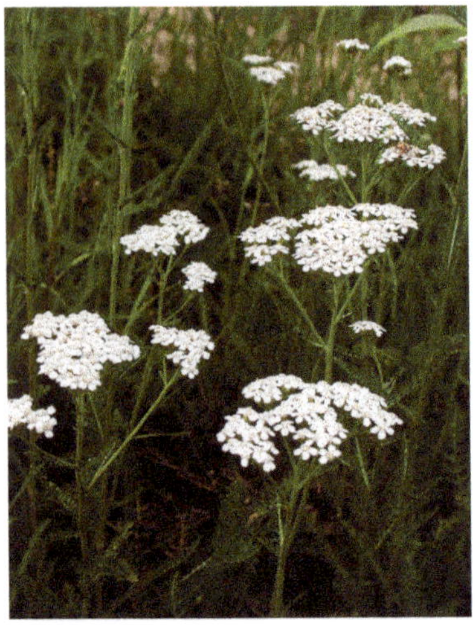

Common Names

Yarrow is called "milfoil" and "thousand leaf" in reference to its many tiny leaflets. Nosebleed, bloodwort, staunch wound, carpenter's weed, herbe militaris (military herb), and soldier's woundwort are common names derived from the herb's ability to stop bleeding and heal wounds.

Medicinal Part of the Plant

The leaves and flower heads contain the medicinal constituents.

Range and Habitat

The genus *Achillea* consists of about 85 species and many subspecies. *Achillea millefolium* is native to North America, Europe and Asia, including India and China. Growing in temperate regions all over the world, it is a sun-loving plant found in open fields and woods, prairies, grasslands, and along pathways and roadsides.

Description of the Plant

Yarrow is a hardy perennial. Delicate-looking leaves emerge from the fibrous root as a small rosette in early spring, and the leaf and flower stalks eventually reach a height of 1-2′. The tough, fibrous stem is erect, round, hollow, and covered with soft, white, fuzzy down. Leaves grow along the entire length of each stalk in an alternate arrangement. The finely divided compound bipinnate leaves are deep green, narrow, and grow 2-8″ long. The leaves consist of many tiny, thread-like leaflets, hence the species name *millefolium* (*milli*, meaning "many" and *folium*, meaning "leaf or foliage"). Yarrow leaves look like feathers, and this unique shape makes identification easy.

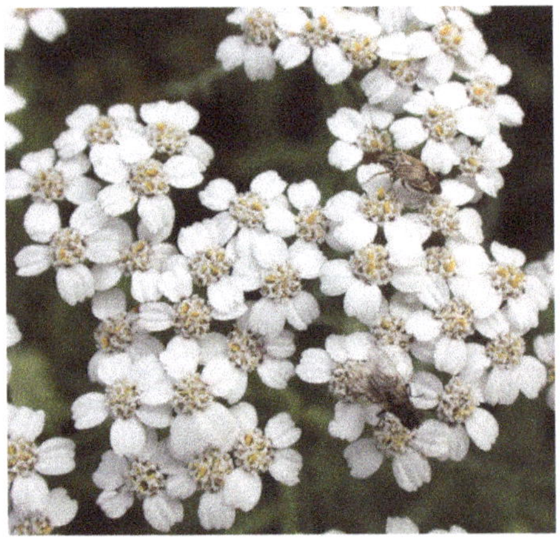

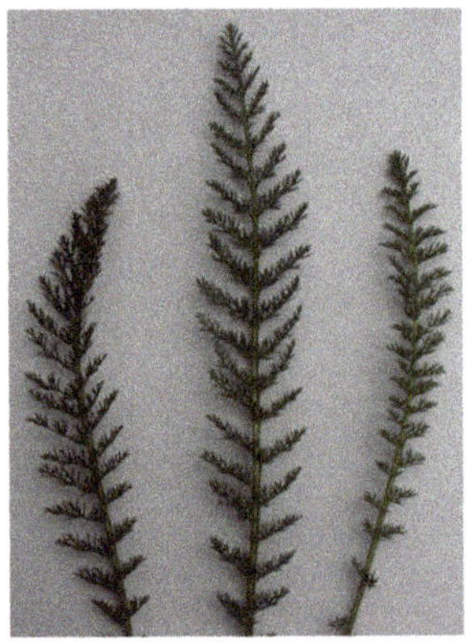

Mature plants have flat clusters of compound umbel flower heads on the end of the stalks. Flower heads are composed of tiny flowers, each one about 1/8″ in diameter. The flowers are white, and occasionally pale-pink varieties are found growing in the wild. Flowers consist of ray petals surrounding the central disc, and the tip of each ray petal has three distinct lobes. Yarrow blooms from late May through September. Hybrid varieties of Yarrow with yellow and pink flowers are used as garden ornamentals, but are not suitable for medicinal purposes.

Cultivation

A hardy, drought-resistant plant, Yarrow is easy to grow and requires little care. Requiring full sun to thrive, it will grow in almost any type of soil. Plants contain more medicinal phytochemicals when they are not fertilized. In many parts of the country, Yarrow can be found growing abundantly in the wild, making cultivation unnecessary. However, it may be cultivated by seed or root division. For root division, dig up and divide roots during wet weather in spring or fall. Mature plants have a cluster of basal leaf rosettes and each of these can be pulled apart and replanted.

It is easy to propagate this herb by planting seeds in early spring or in autumn. Press the seeds onto the surface of a prepared bed or seed flat. Do not cover the seeds with soil because they need light to germinate, which usually takes 2-3 weeks. When seedlings are about 4″ tall, transplant them to a permanent bed 12″ apart. Cultivated Yarrow tends to become bushier and can look different than the more spindly, single-stemmed plants growing in the wild. Yarrow roots secrete substances into the surrounding soil that can inhibit the growth of other plants, and the herb is a natural insecticide against many insects.

Harvest

Gather upper leaves and flowers as they start blooming, when the essential oil content is at its peak. The flowers are medicinally stronger than the leaves. Harvest the seeds for planting when flower heads are brown and dry.

Preparation of Plant Medicine and Dosages

Yarrow leaves and flowers are used fresh to make tea, tincture and salve, or dried for future use. The tea has a bitter taste.

PREPARATIONS

Tea: Steep 1-2 teaspoons of chopped leaves and flowers in 1 cup of boiled water for 10-15 minutes. Dosage: 1-3 cups a day. *For external use:* Simmer 3-4 tablespoons of the herb in 1 pint of water for 5 minutes, cool, and apply the tea to the skin as a wash or fomentation, or use it in a sitz bath.

Tincture: Cover freshly harvested leaves and flowers with 60% 190-proof alcohol and 40% distilled water and process in the usual way. Dosage: 10-40 drops 1-4 times a day as needed.

Salves and Poultices: Yarrow is an excellent primary ingredient for external healing.

Chemical Constituents

The volatile oils in Yarrow leaves and flowers have strong antiseptic, antimicrobial, anti-inflammatory, antispasmodic, and antioxidant actions. The oil contains chamazulene (analgesic, febrifuge, vulnerary), pinene (anti-acne, anticarcinogenic, expectorant, sedative), caryophyllene (anti-asthmatic, antitumor, sedative), eugenol, linalool, menthol, borneol (analgesic, choleretic, febrifuge, hepatoprotective, sedative), cineol (anthelmintic, anti-catarrh, expectorant, carminative, choleretic, hypotensive, sedative), camphor (analgesic, anti-acne, antiseptic, antispasmodic, carminative, decongestant, expectorant), and thujone (abortifacient, emmenagogue, neurotoxic, cerebro-depressant).

Flavonoids include quercetin (anti-inflammatory, anti-allergenic), rutin (anti-atherosclerotic, antihistamine, anti-inflammatory, vasodilator, strengthens capillaries, reduces bruising), kaempferol, luteolin (antibacterial, anticarcinogenic, antihistamine, anti-inflammatory, antioxidant, antispasmodic, choleretic, diuretic, estrogenic, vasodilator), and apigenin (reduces blood clotting, anti-arrhythmic, antibacterial, antihistamine, antiviral, anti-HIV, anti-inflammatory, antitumor, antioxidant, choleretic, diuretic, estrogenic, hypotensive, sedative, vasodilator). The flavonoid casticin has demonstrated anticancer activity (Haidara, 2006).

Tannins are astringents that reduce bleeding and diarrhea. Sabinene is antibacterial and eliminates *Helicobacter pylori*, which contributes to the development of stomach ulcers. Myrcene is analgesic, antibacterial, antioxidant, antispasmodic, diuretic, fungicidal, and a muscle relaxant. Bitter alkaloids include betaine, stachydrine (cardiotonic, emmenagogue, lactagogue), and achilleine (a strong hemostatic agent that coagulates blood and stops bleeding).

Phenolic acids include salicylic acid (analgesic, anti-inflammatory, febrifuge), caffeic acid (antiviral, antitumor, choleretic, diuretic, hepatoprotective), and rosmarinic acid (antioxidant, anti-inflammatory). Coumarins are blood thinners. Sesquiterpene lactones exhibit antimicrobial, anticancer, and anti-inflammatory activities. These include achillicin, achillin (herbicide and pesticide), and leucodin. Phytosterols reduce cholesterol levels and provide precursors for hormonal production, and include beta-sitosterol (anticarcinogenic, diuretic, antioxidant, hepatoprotective), campesterol, and stigmasterol (anti-inflammatory, antiviral, hepatoprotective).

Fatty acids include linoleic, myristic (antioxidant, anticarcinogenic), palmitic, oleic (anti-inflammatory, anticarcinogenic, choleretic), and stearic acid. Nutrients include potassium, calcium, magnesium, iron, phosphorus, selenium, chromium, choline, inositol, folic acid, ascorbic acid, and beta-carotene.

Safety, Contraindications, and Drug Interactions

Yarrow is a safe herb when taken in normal doses. Ingestion is **contraindicated during pregnancy**, especially in the first three months due to its stimulating emmenagogue effects, but can be taken in small amounts during lactation. There are no known interactions with drugs. Direct contact with the plant may produce temporary dermatitis and allergic sinus reactions in some people.

Medicinal Uses

History of the Plant

The genus name *Achillea* is derived from the name of the famous Greek hero and warrior, Achilles. During the Trojan War, Achilles followed the instructions of Chiron, the wise healer and centaur, and staunched the wounds of his soldiers with Yarrow to stop bleeding and infection. According to legend, when Achilles was born, his mother held him by the heel as she dipped him in a bath of Yarrow water for protection against all harm. Yarrow did protect him until he died from an arrow wound in his heel, the only part of his body not exposed to the herbal bath.

Yarrow has a long history of use in the healing traditions of many cultures around the world wherever it grows. It is universally employed to stop bleeding, heal deep wounds and burns, and treat inflammation in the digestive, urinary, and female reproductive systems. English herbalist and surgeon John Gerard (1545–1612) wrote about Yarrow in *The Herball or Generall Historie of Plantes*, saying that "the leaves of Yarrow do close up wounds, and keep them from inflammation, or fiery swellings: it staunchеth blood in any part of the body, and it is likewise put into baths for women to sit in." He wrote that the green leaves were chewed as a remedy for toothache (Gerard, 1975). Nicholas Culpeper (1616–1654) stated that the plant is under the domain of Venus, and used the tea boiled in white wine to stop bleeding, treat hemorrhoids and vaginitis, and ease pain. He applied a Yarrow ointment on ulcers, fistulas, and other wounds. During the Middle Ages in Europe, it was a popular herb used by the Wise Woman healers for many ailments and in ceremonies.

When Europeans arrived in North America, they discovered that the indigenous people's use of Yarrow was extensive. Many tribes employed it to stop bleeding and heal wounds, sprains, bruises, burns, skin rashes and itching, arthritic pain, toothaches, and sore gums. It was applied as poultice, tea fomentation, or powder of dried leaves and flowers for these problems. The Utes in southwestern North America, considered to be fierce warriors, relied on Yarrow to heal battle wounds and called it "wound medicine." The tea was ingested to increase sweating to reduce fevers and treat colds, coughs, bronchitis, throat irritations, internal bleeding, delayed menstruation, and diarrhea. The roots were taken to reduce pain and the tea was put in the ears for infection and earaches. The powdered leaves were inhaled as a nasal snuff to relieve headaches.

As well as relieving physical problems, people of many cultures believe that Yarrow has protective powers against harmful influences. In ancient Europe, it was used for divination, protection against evil forces, and was brought to weddings to ensure at least seven years of happiness in the marriage. Native American Indians used Yarrow in sweat lodges and other ceremonies for its aroma and purifying energies. For thousands of years, the Chinese have used Yarrow stalks for divination when consulting the Oracle of the ancient *I Ching* (*The Book of Changes*). Yarrow flower essence is taken homeopathically for psychic and physical protection.

During the American Civil War, many battles occurred in open meadows where Yarrow grew. After the fighting, physicians harvested Yarrow and applied the flowers and leaves to the soldiers' wounds to arrest bleeding and prevent infection. Later, during the 1880s–1930s, the Eclectic physicians prescribed it for fevers, coughs, chronic urinary infections, spasms, all types of internal and external bleeding, diabetes, hemorrhoids, female reproductive problems, diarrhea, and dysentery. Yarrow was listed in the *U.S. Pharmacopoeia* from 1863–1882 as an official tonic, stimulant, and emmenagogue drug.

Many *in vitro* and *in vivo* research studies have identified active medicinal constituents in the herb, but human clinical trials are lacking. Research has validated many of the historic and current medicinal uses of Yarrow in traditional health care systems.

Healing Qualities

Alterative, analgesic, antibiotic, antifungal, anti-inflammatory, antioxidant, antiseptic, antispasmodic, astringent, bitter tonic, carminative, cholagogue, diaphoretic, diuretic, emmenagogue, febrifuge, hemostatic, hypotensive, nephritic, nervine, sedative, stomachic, sudorific, vasodilator, and vulnerary.

Traditional Chinese Medicine (TCM) Perspective

Yarrow is cooling, drying, and bitter. It is a stimulating Yang herb that moves Qi and blood throughout the system to remove congestion, stagnation, and restore normal function. This is helpful for conditions of excess heat and congestion, and is specifically indicated when the pulse is rapid and full. Yarrow is beneficial for many female reproductive problems caused by Uterine Qi and Blood stagnation, including abnormal bleeding, irregular cycles, prolonged menstruation, uterine fibroids, cysts, and hormonal imbalances.

The leaves and flowers of Yarrow also help resolve Qi constraint in the heart and blood vessels, urinary tract, and digestive system, especially in the liver and intestines. It helps heal liver and spleen disharmony, and dispels Liver Yang heat rising to the head.

Primary Actions

One of the best wound healers, Yarrow is remarkable in its ability to stop bleeding and bruising, and is a primary ingredient in my herbal salve. The powerful and versatile healing properties of Yarrow tincture make it a personal favorite for treating infections, the common cold, flu, and fevers. I have found that its effectiveness is synergistically enhanced when combined with Boneset (*Eupatorium perfoliatum*) and Echinacea (*Echinacea purpurea*) for these acute problems. Yarrow tincture is extremely reliable and specific for pelvic issues and infections, and is a primary herb I recommend for many female gynecological problems.

Yarrow tincture may be used as a tonic taken over a period of time to alter imbalances and optimize health. Its normalizing effect on blood vessels and mucous membranes reduces excessive mucous secretions and bleeding. It promotes a balanced flow of nerve impulses and exerts a calming influence on the nervous system especially beneficial to the cardiovascular, digestive, urinary, and female reproductive systems.

Infections, Fevers, and Inflammation: Yarrow exerts strong antibiotic activity against many Gram-positive and Gram-negative bacteria. Several *in vitro* studies demonstrate its broad spectrum activity against *Staphylococcus aureus, Streptococcus pneumoniae, Clostridium perfringens, Escherichia coli, Klebsiella pneumoniae, Pseudomonas aeruginosa, Mycobacterium smegmatis, Salmonella enteritidis,* and two fungi including *Aspergillus niger* and *Candida albicans* (Molochko, 1990; Candan, 2003; Stojanovic, 2005). The tea and tincture are excellent in reducing symptoms and speeding up recovery from the common cold, influenza (flu), hay fever, sinusitis, and other infections specific to the respiratory, digestive, and genitourinary systems. Especially beneficial when taken in the early stages of acute illness, Yarrow helps reduce excessive mucous secretions and coughs.

The herb is also a cooling febrifuge and powerful diaphoretic that promotes perspiration to reduce fevers. When taken as a hot tea or tincture, volatile oils in Yarrow decrease body heat by stimulating and equalizing circulation, opening the sudoriferous sweat pores on the skin and producing perspiration that cools fevers and expels toxins. Yarrow also contains salicylic acid (the active ingredient in aspirin) that reduces fevers, pain, and inflammation. The blend of Yarrow, Peppermint (*Mentha x piperita*), and Elderberry flowers (*Sambucus* spp.) was once a popular remedy for the common cold, flu, and fevers. Sage (*Salvia officinalis*), Boneset, and Echinacea also combine well with Yarrow for these problems. Prior to modern medicine, Yarrow was used in treating eruptive diseases such as measles, chicken pox, smallpox, and typhoid fever.

Yarrow is traditionally employed to reduce inflammation, and this ability is substantiated by modern *in vivo* research demonstrating its effectiveness against several inflammatory agents, including histamine and prostaglandins (Goldberg, 1969; Shipochliev, 1984). In addition to the actions of salicylic acid, researchers found that volatile oils in *A. millefolium* reduce the inflammatory response by their strong antioxidant abilities of down-regulating damaging, inflammatory nitric oxide, cyclooxygenase-2 (COX-2), tumor necrosis factor, and interleukin-6 (Chou, 2013).

These cooling, anti-inflammatory, and analgesic qualities make Yarrow helpful for arthritis, especially when combined with other appropriate herbs. It may be ingested and applied externally for joint problems.

Nervous System: As a nervine and mild sedative, Yarrow exerts a relaxing influence throughout the body. It reduces pain and is a smooth muscle relaxant that resolves muscle tension and spasms, especially in the digestive, genitourinary, and cardiovascular systems. The tea or tincture can ease nervous headaches. Researchers have documented that volatile oils in the herb elicit relaxation in mice and rats, while inhibiting convulsions and inducing restful sleep (Kudrzycka-Bieloszabska, 1966).

Cardiovascular System and Blood: Yarrow's calming influence on the nervous system is beneficial for normal function of the heart and blood vessels. Flavonoids, volatile oils, and other constituents relax and dilate peripheral blood vessels, which promotes equalized circulation of blood that is especially helpful for people with chronically cold feet or hands. While the herb stops abnormal bleeding and hemorrhage, it also has blood thinning actions that break up congealed blood obstructing blood flow and causing thrombosis (formation of blood clots). These dual actions support optimal circulation and are specific for congestion and blockage in the cardiovascular system.

Yarrow is helpful for many vascular problems such as varicose veins, hemorrhoids, and phlebitis (vein inflammation). Anti-inflammatory, antispasmodic, and antioxidant properties promote healthy blood vessels with normal muscle tone. For these reasons, Yarrow helps decrease vascular rigidity and hypertension and is recommended for thrombosis and angina. The herb also exerts a protective mechanism on the blood. Research has demonstrated that 15 species of *Achillea* are effective in protecting human erythrocytes (red blood cells) and leucocytes (white blood cells) from oxidative damage and cell death (Konyalioglu, 2005).

Bleeding and Wounds: A classic hemostatic herb that stops bleeding, Yarrow is an exceptional vulnerary for all types of wounds and injuries. Achilletin and achilleine found in the leaves and flowers reduce bleeding, and achilleine decreased blood clotting time in rabbits by 32% without causing any toxicity when administered intravenously (Miller, 1954). Tannins in the herb are astringent and tighten tissues, which is helpful for boggy, overly relaxed tissues that lack tone and leak out blood and fluids.

The tea or tincture may be ingested to stop hemorrhage in the lungs, digestive and urinary tracts, and for excessive menstrual flow. Yarrow reduces bleeding from stomach ulcers, ulcerative colitis, and urinary tract infections causing bloody urine. Nosebleeds can be treated by stuffing the chopped leaves directly into the nostrils or using the tea as a nasal spray. Yarrow can be applied externally as a poultice or salve to stop bleeding wounds and will prevent the formation of bruises if applied immediately after injury occurs. In his *Book of Herbal Wisdom*, herbalist Matthew Wood writes, "Yarrow seems to help the arteries actually suck up blood that has flowed out through a torn vessel into the tissues. The importance of this should be considered in acute brain aneurisms and similar emergencies" (Wood, 1997). The cooling, antibacterial actions of Yarrow are also helpful to treat excess heat in the blood caused by blood congestion, fever, or toxins. According to Traditional Chinese Medicine, hemorrhage can result from excess heat in the blood, and bitter, cooling herbs such as Yarrow are used to counteract this imbalance.

Yarrow excels in treating internal and external wounds, and is specific for deep cuts and traumatic injuries. Its antiseptic, analgesic, and anti-inflammatory properties contribute to healing wounds, ulcers, boils, acne, hemorrhoids, and varicose veins. For these problems, it can be applied directly to the skin as a wash or fomentation made from tea, as a poultice, or an ointment. Yarrow and Chamomile (*Matricaria recutita*) tea can help clear up eczema when ingested and used as a wash on the affected area. Yarrow can be used to heal all types of burns, and is excellent for radiation burns and other deeply penetrating burns.

I have heard many accounts and personally experienced the amazingly swift action of Yarrow to stop bleeding and bruising. I once fell down a flight of stairs and scraped off a couple layers of skin from my shin. Luckily, a jar of my healing salve containing substantial amounts of Yarrow was on a table at the bottom of the stairs, and within seconds I quickly applied a liberal dose of salve to my injured leg. I bruise very easily, but much to my amazement, no bruising occurred and the pain and bleeding stopped almost immediately!

A similar experience happened several years later when I lost balance on a large granite boulder and tore about 8″ of skin off my shin. I always keep my salve in my bag, so I quickly applied it liberally. Once again, the wound immediately stopped bleeding and the pain subsided within a few minutes. My leg healed without bruising or scarring.

Digestive System: An excellent herb for the digestive system, Yarrow seems to have a balancing influence depending on what the various organs need. As a stimulating bitter tonic, it helps normalize a sluggish, atonic system by increasing production and release of digestive enzymes (saliva, stomach acids, pancreatic enzymes, and bile). This promotes movement throughout the digestive tract to clear stagnation responsible for indigestion, gas, bloating, and constipation. Yarrow reduces inflammation and contains chamazulene (a chemical also occurring in Chamomile) that helps relax smooth muscle and ease spasms. Several studies validate Yarrow's antispasmodic activity throughout the gut (Lemmens-Gruber, 2006; Benedek, 2007; Borrelli, 2012). As a carminative, it reduces flatulence by soothing and toning the stomach and intestines to relieve abdominal distention and pain. The astringent tannins tone the mucous membranes of the stomach and intestines, normalize excessive secretions throughout the entire digestive system, and are especially helpful for bleeding ulcers in the stomach and intestines, dysentery, diarrhea, and bloody stools. The herb's antibiotic activity addresses bacterial infections. Research studies show that water extracts of *A. millefolium* are effective in protecting the stomach lining of lab rats against acute lesions induced by alcohol and indomethacin (a drug used to treat arthritis), and in healing chronic stomach ulcers caused by acetic acid without any signs of toxicity, even during long exposure (Cavalcanti, 2006). Yarrow is an effective treatment for colic, *Helicobacter pylori* (implicated in stomach ulcers), ulcerative colitis, Crohn's disease, irritable bowel syndrome, diverticulitis, and inflammation in the stomach (gastritis), small intestines (enteritis), and large intestines (colitis).

Yarrow helps regulate and normalize liver function because it encourages optimal blood flow and its cholagogue property stimulates bile flow to break down fats, promote peristaltic movement propelling food through the intestines, and decrease stagnation resulting in constipation. Animal studies confirm the ability of Yarrow alcohol and water extracts to stimulate bile flow (Benedek, 2006). The herb also protects the liver from toxins and chemical damage, and can be used in treating hepatitis. Researchers found that a crude extract of *A. millefolium* showed antioxidant and hepatoprotective effects against hepatitis in mice. Yarrow protected the mice against toxins, prevented elevation of liver enzymes, and reduced abdominal spasms (Candan, 2003; Yaeesh, 2006).

Although it does not alter insulin secretion or uptake, Yarrow has been used for adult onset diabetes because it improves blood circulation to the abdominal cavity and removes stagnation and inflammation in the pancreas. Russian researchers have documented that Yarrow shows significant hypoglycemic and glycogen sparing properties in diabetic mice and rats (Molokovshii, 1989).

Yarrow stimulates the flow of digestive enzymes to improve digestion when taken 5-10 minutes before meals, and is taken after meals to relieve gas, bloating, and constipation. Combine it with tasty herbs that promote digestion such as Licorice (*Glycyrrhiza glabra*), Fennel (*Foeniculum vulgare*), Peppermint, Chamomile (*Matricaria recutita*), and Lemon Balm (*Melissa officinalis*). Yarrow works well with Goldenseal (*Hydrastis canadensis*) to eliminate infections in the digestive organs, and can be combined with Marshmallow (*Althaea officinalis*) root to decrease inflammation and heal ulcerated tissues.

Bladder and Kidneys: Yarrow has specific affinity with the urinary tract, toning and strengthening the kidneys, ureters, bladder, and urethra. In my clinical practice, I use the tincture for urinary tract problems with excellent results, recommending 30-60 drops 1-2 times daily for chronic problems and higher doses of 60-90 drops 3-4 times daily for acute infections. Yarrow exerts mild diuretic action helpful in correcting fluid imbalance and edema when the tea or tincture is taken cold. The antispasmodic, anti-inflammatory, antibacterial, antifungal, and analgesic properties are useful in treating all types of urinary tract spasms, inflammation, pain, urethral irritation, and infections such as cystitis (bladder infection) and Candida yeast. The herb blends well with the soothing properties of Marshmallow root for these problems. Astringent tannins in Yarrow stop bleeding by tightening and toning weak tissues, making it helpful for kidney and bladder hemorrhage with bloody urine, stress incontinence, bed-wetting, and bladder prolapse.

Yarrow can be used for mild kidney problems and more serious diseases like nephritis (kidney inflammation caused by infection, toxins, or autoimmune disease) and the progression of kidney failure. Early American herbalists used Yarrow for Bright's kidney disease (an older term for nephritis), and the Eclectic physicians prescribed it for chronic urinary tract diseases and propensity towards infections and incontinence.

Yarrow helps the kidneys clear creatinine, urea nitrogen, nitric oxide, and other harmful substances that build up in the blood due to kidney failure. A small study involving 31 patients with chronic kidney disease explored the ability of *A. millifolium* flower heads to reduce elevated blood levels of nitric oxide, a possible cause of bleeding in those suffering from chronic kidney disease. During a 2-month period, 16 patients received 1.5 grams of the powered flowers 3 days each week, while 15 patients received placebo. After 2 months, nitrite and nitrate blood levels showed a slight decrease in the group taking Yarrow, while these levels slightly increased in the placebo group (Vahid, 2012).

Women's Health: Yarrow, a remarkable tonic for many challenges during the menstrual and menopausal years, is one of my favorite and most dependable gynecological remedies. This women's ally tones the mucous membranes of the reproductive organs and normalizes the menstrual cycle by stimulating and improving circulation throughout the pelvic area. This removes blood congestion and stagnation, making the herb helpful for premenstrual symptoms (PMS), pelvic pressure, leg aches and muscle cramps, and stalled or suppressed menstrual periods, including amenorrhea (abnormal cessation of menses). Anti-inflammatory and antispasmodic properties ease pelvic and menstrual pain and cramps (dysmenorrhea).

The astringent tannins reduce excessive menstrual bleeding, abnormal bleeding between periods, and bleeding caused by uterine fibroids, endometriosis, and ruptured ovarian cysts. This plant has been used by midwives to stop hemorrhage during miscarriage and following childbirth. The astringent action tones a sluggish, atonic uterus to prevent or treat uterine prolapse.

Yarrow contains phytosterols with estrogen and progesterone-like activity (Innocenti, 2007) that help regulate normal hormonal levels and menstrual cycles. I have seen Yarrow help many women and consider it to be an herb-of-choice for treating endometriosis, uterine fibroids, ovarian cysts, and other conditions caused by blood congestion and estrogen-progesterone imbalance with estrogen dominance.

Yarrow is my favorite herb for treating vaginal infections, pelvic inflammatory disease (PID), and abnormal discharges, including Candida yeast. Drink the tincture and douche with a strong tea. To stop excessive bleeding after childbirth, combine Yarrow with other astringents such as Cranesbill (*Geranium maculatum*) or Shepherd's Purse (*Capsella bursa-pastoris*). Yarrow can be combined with Comfrey (*Symphytum officinale*) and used as a sitz bath after childbirth to heal perineal tears, prevent infection, relieve pain, and reduce varicose veins. The tea, poultice, or salve can be applied to sore and cracked nipples to relieve pain and promote fast healing when breast-feeding, but washed off before nursing.

Teachings from the Yarrow Deva

"Greetings. The deva of the Yarrow tribe speaks with you now. My healing plants were beloved by those once living upon this land – the Indians, as they are now called. My leaves and flowers were used to heal many ailments, and we were happy to be of service to those people who loved us and all upon the earth as brothers and sisters.

"Creator has been gracious in allowing my medicine plants to grow throughout a vast area of land to serve the needs of humankind. My plants hold the energy and action of the male warrior who protects others from harm. The strength of my medicine especially protects the female organs. The white color of my flowers reflects the purity I bring to the human body after my protection and cleansing actions have healed wounds, infections, and other imbalances in the tissues. The essence of my flowers brings the ability to stand strong and firm in the midst of difficulty and to move forward into action if necessary. My medicine helps maintain an inner core of strength and balance to guide all activity by compassionate wisdom. I direct the flow of energy and actions towards fruitful, fulfilling maturation.

"I maintain balance in the human body due to the equal influences of Venus, the planet of nurturing, beauty and the feminine, and Mars, the masculine planet and ruler of physical activity. My plants use the masculine power of Mars to enable the gentle, sublime feminine qualities to emerge in women and manifest in full force.

"The aura of my plants is a deep shade of blue like the lapis lazuli stone. As well as protecting and supporting the physical body, my medicine is also for the visionary – one whose sight pierces through time and space to perceive the deep mysteries of life while remaining rooted in calm stillness. My white flowers especially support the brain, providing clear, accurate vision and understanding. The essence of my flowers helps people see into the hidden and obscured, to clearly 'read' the energies for deeper, fuller meaning. This is, in part, the Scorpio aspect of my ruling planet, Mars. Scorpio can see into the hidden realms and also regulates the reproductive organs of creativity.

"My strong, rigid stems embrace the strength and power of my masculine nature. My delicate, feathery leaves reflect the lightness, flexibility, and fluidity of my feminine nature. And the cluster of white flowers reflects the purification and balance made possible by my medicine; for my plants live on this planet to assist humans in their health and ability to prosper. My lessons are to be of strong will and backbone to support yourself through the ups and downs of life, and to be fluid and flexible in your understanding and actions. Namaste, dear one. Be in health and peace. Enjoy and protect the great beauty of this planet that you are blessed to live upon for a short time."

Yellow Dock

Rumex crispus
Polygonaceae (Buckwheat) Family

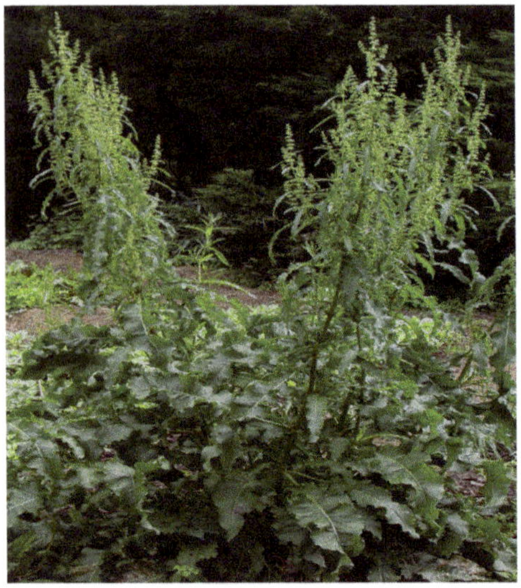

Rumex crispus

Common Names

Rumex crispus is known as curled or curly dock, narrow dock, sour dock, garden patience, and rumex.

Medicinal Part of the Plant

The roots contain the greatest concentrations of phytochemicals and are traditionally used for medicinal purposes, although the leaves can be applied topically for external healing.

Range and Habitat

Yellow Dock is native to Europe and northern Asia, and naturalized in North America after being introduced during the colonial period. It is a common herb growing abundantly in many fields and meadows, waste places, and along roadsides and pathways throughout the world. Many people, especially farmers, consider it to be an obnoxious weed due to its prolific nature.

Description of the Plant

R. crispus grows 3-4′ tall. The large, fleshy taproot grows 1-1½′ in length. The outer root is brown and the interior is a distinct yellow color, hence its common name of Yellow Dock. In early spring, the leaves appear in a basal rosette, and several erect stalks grow from the root crown as the season progresses. The round, fibrous stalk is smooth with many distinct vertical furrows along its entire length. The simple, lance-shaped, petiolate leaves (with stems) have one central vein with smaller pinnate veins. The leaf is glabrous (smooth and hairless). Leaf margins lack teeth and are distinguished by their curly, wave-like margins, giving the whole leaf a wrinkled appearance. Lower leaves are larger than the upper leaves, ranging from 6″-1½′ in length.

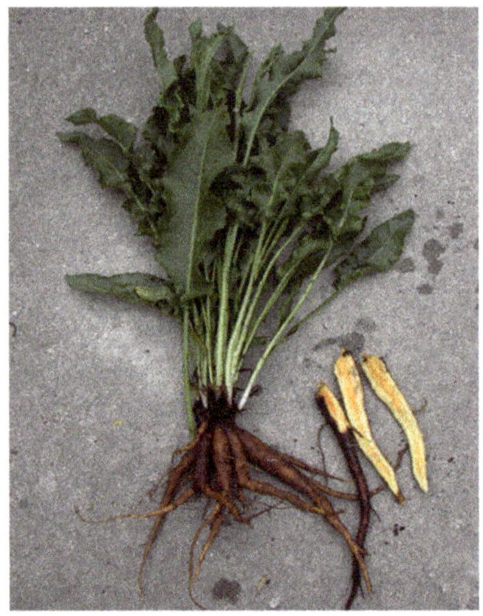

***Rumex crispus* root**

Yellow Dock blooms from May through July. The tiny, pale-green flowers are about 1/6″ long and grow on many long, slender raceme spikes forming large panicle clusters. Lacking petals, each flower consists of a 6-sepal green, white, or pinkish-red calyx with stamens and pistils. The green flower matures into a rusty reddish-brown seed that looks like a tear-shaped berry. The seed is a 3-winged, heart-shaped nut or capsule. As the seed pods mature, they dry into a dense, dark-brown mass.

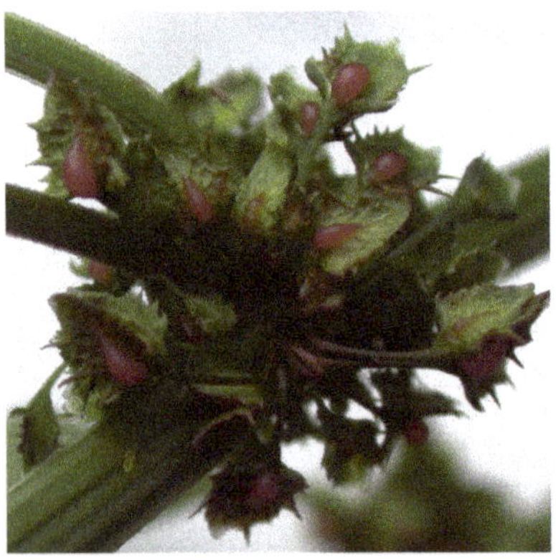

***Rumex crispus* seed**

There are many species of Dock but only a few are considered medicinal, including *Rumex hydrolapthum*, *R. britannica*, *R. acutus*, *R. aquaticus*, *R. patientia*, and *R. obtusifolius*, which are all perennials. *R. hydrolapthum* reaches a height of 5-6′ and is the tallest of all the Docks. This was a popular species used by Dioscorides, Pliny, and other ancient Greek physicians. *R. aquaticus* grows 3-5′ tall and is found in moist fields, meadows, and ditches. The leaves have crisped, wavy edges that are similar in appearance to *R. crispus*, but much broader.

R. obtusifolius, also introduced from Europe, is a large plant growing 2-4′ tall. Its long, broad, deep-green leaves are obtuse (rounded and blunt) at their tip and base, hence the species name *obtusifolius*. A distinguishing feature of this species is the reddish tinge in the veins at the leaf base. The leaves of *R. crispus* are more pointed, like a lance, without as much of the red tinge.

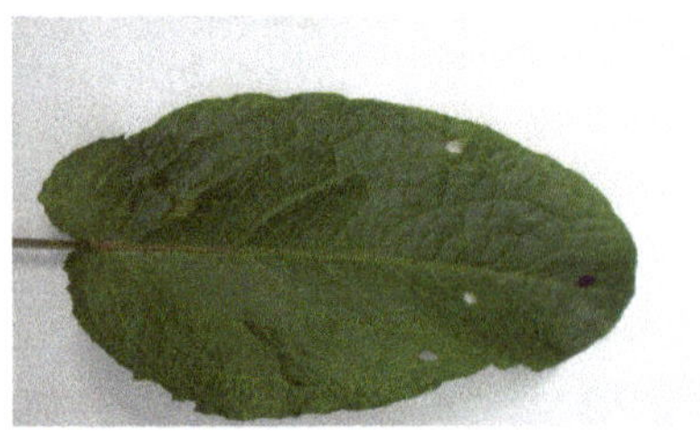

***Rumex obtusifolius* leaf**

All of these Dock species may be used interchangeably for medicinal purposes because they contain tannins and anthraquinone glycosides that have similar healing actions. Yellow Dock (*R. crispus*) remains the most popular species that is used by American herbalists and sold in the commercial market.

Cultivation

Cultivating Yellow Dock is usually unnecessary because it is such a prolific and commonly found medicinal weed that can be wildcrafted from many areas. If you do want to introduce a specific species into your garden or fields, broadcast the seeds in disturbed soil. They usually germinate quite readily after a few weeks of warm weather. Docks produce copious amounts of seeds and can quickly take over gardens.

Harvest

Roots can be harvested in spring, summer or fall, but usually contain the greatest amount of medicinal phytochemicals in late summer and early autumn, after storing nutrients over summer to survive the dormant months of winter. Darker shades of yellow in the inner root indicate greater concentrations of phytochemicals and stronger biological actions. Dig a fairly deep hole to harvest the entire taproot, which can extend 1-1½′ into the soil. Leaves may be collected anytime for external purposes.

Preparation of Plant Medicine and Dosages

Phytochemicals in the root are extracted by boiling water and alcohol. Fresh roots produce the most potent medicines and can be prepared as tincture, decoction tea, salve, or a poultice. Roots may also be dried, ground into powder, and stuffed into capsules or prepared as pills, suppositories, poultices, and tea. Most people prefer taking the herb in tincture, pill, or capsule preparations rather than drinking the bitter tea. The leaves are used for external healing as a salve or poultice, or made into tea for application as a compress, fomentation, or wash.

PREPARATIONS

Decoction Tea: Gently simmer 1 teaspoon of the finely chopped fresh root or ½ teaspoon of ground dried root in 1-2 cups of water for 10 minutes. Dosage: 1 cup taken 1-2 times a day as needed.

Tincture: Prepare roots in the usual way using 60% 190-proof grain alcohol and 40% distilled water. Dosage: 20-60 drops taken 1-2 times daily in water.

Capsules and Pills: Dosage: 1-2 capsules or pills 1-2 times a day as needed.

Salve, Poultice, Fomentation: The roots and leaves may be used alone or combined with other herbs (refer to "Skin Problems" on page 591 in the "Index of Health Issues and Herbal Recommendations").

Culinary Uses

Since ancient times, Dock leaves have been part of the cuisine of people all over the world, including Asians, Europeans, Native American tribes, and early American settlers. However, the leaves contain oxalic acid that can contribute to kidney stone formation and cause other health problems, so caution is advised.

To reduce the bitterness and oxalic acid content, collect young leaves in early spring when they are not so bitter. Chop the leaves, put them in a pan, cover with water, and bring it to a boil. This water is then discarded and the process is repeated to eliminate more of the oxalic acid. The leaves can be eaten like spinach and garnished with butter, salt, soy sauce, a little vinegar, or lemon juice. Native Americans cooked the seeds as a gruel.

Chemical Constituents

The roots and leaves contain easily digestible iron, calcium, magnesium, manganese, phosphorus, potassium, selenium, chromium, zinc, thiamine (vitamin B1), riboflavin (vitamin B2), niacin (vitamin B3), ascorbic acid (vitamin C), and beta-carotene (the plant form of vitamin A).

The root contains anthraquinone glycosides that are laxative and antimicrobial. Anthraquinones include chrysophanic acid (antispasmodic, fungicide, pesticide), emodin (antibacterial, anti-inflammatory, antileukemic, antilymphomic, antimutagenic, antineoplastic, antiplaque, antiseptic, antitumor, anti-ulcer, antiviral, cathartic, purgative, vasodilator), nepodin (fungicide), and physcion (antiseptic, purgative). Roots also contain astringent tannins, erucic acid (antitumor), and rumicin (given for scrofula, a type of tuberculosis involving the lymph nodes in the neck). More than 60 chemical components have been identified in the complex volatile oil. The leaves and root contain oxalic acid, which forms insoluble calcium salts that can disrupt calcium and potassium levels, kidney function, and blood coagulation. Prolonged ingestion of oxalic acid may cause metabolic acidosis, a dangerous blood disorder caused by excessive acids.

Safety, Contraindications, and Drug Interactions

Yellow Dock is generally safe to use in normal doses. It **should not be taken during pregnancy and lactation**, or in cases of bowel and gallbladder blockages. Overuse can cause stomach irritation, nausea, abdominal cramps, diarrhea, and excessive urination. People with kidney stones should avoid this herb due to its oxalic acid content. Sheep and other livestock have developed oxalic acid toxicity after eating large amounts of Dock leaves (Panciera, 1990). One fatal human poisoning was reported when a 53-year-old man experienced gastrointestinal distress, severe calcium deficiency, metabolic acidosis, and acute liver failure, and died 72 hours after ingesting Yellow Dock (Reig, 1990).

Medicinal Uses

History of the Plant

People throughout the world have used *R. crispus* and other Dock species for medicinal purposes. The genus name of the Dock tribe is *Rumex*, which is Latin for "lance," in reference to the long, pointed shape of their leaves. All Docks were formerly classified under the genus *Lapathum*, derived from the Latin term *lapazein*, meaning "to cleanse," alluding to their cleansing action on the liver, intestines, blood, and lymphatic fluids. Yellow Dock's species name *crispus* refers to the crisped or wavy edges of the leaves.

Greek botanist and physician Dioscorides (*circa* A.D. 40 – *c.* 90) employed *R. patientia* and *R. aquaticus* for dysentery, nausea, kidney stones, scorpion bites, and ear and tooth pain (Dioscorides, 1959). John Gerard (1545–1612), the English apothecary and surgeon, wrote about several species of Docks that he used for healing. The European astrologer-herbalists assigned Jupiter as the ruling planet of the Docks.

European colonists introduced Yellow Dock to the Native Americans, who incorporated the plant into their herbal pharmacies. Many native people pulverized the leaves and roots, using them as a poultice to relieve itching, skin problems, animal or insect bites and stings, and to draw toxins and pus from wounds and boils. The leaves and roots were bruised or crushed and directly applied to the affected area, or they were chopped and cooked in water or animal fat to create an ointment for external application. The plant was valued by many tribes, including the Cherokee, Cheyenne, Chippewa, Delaware, Navajo, Paiute and Zuni, and used for diarrhea, dysentery, constipation, sore throats, bleeding, urinary problems, jaundice and other liver ailments, blood purification, ulcers, and swellings (Erichsen-Brown, 1979; Moerman, 1998). The root was a favorite ingredient in herbal formulas of immigrant doctors, early settlers, and traveling "medicine men." Many people traditionally combined Yellow Dock with Dandelion (*Taraxacum officinale*) and Burdock (*Arctium* spp.) roots to drink as a cleansing spring tonic.

The American Eclectic physicians followed the traditions of the old European herbalists in prescribing the decoction tea, tincture, and dried powder made from the roots of *R. crispus* and *R. obtusifolius* as a remedy for dyspepsia (impaired stomach function), anemia, rheumatism, inflammation of the respiratory tract, sexually transmitted diseases, jaundice, and other liver and gallbladder problems. The Docks were given for conditions caused by blood toxicity, such as cancers, ulcers, enlarged lymph glands, lymph node inflammation and tumors, and for skin diseases and eruptive conditions such as eczema, psoriasis, boils, abscesses, acne, and leprosy. *R. obtusifolius* was listed in the *U.S. Pharmacopoeia* as an official laxative and astringent drug from 1820–1905, and *R. crispus* was listed from 1863–1905.

Reports of clinical research on Yellow Dock are lacking. Scientific studies have identified the presence of ascorbic acid (vitamin C), tannins and anthraquinone glycosides, validating the herb's historic use for the prevention and treatment of scurvy (a vitamin C deficiency disease) and its traditional role as a laxative and beneficial herb for the liver.

Healing Qualities

Alterative, mild antibiotic, antiscorbutic, mild astringent, bitter tonic, cholagogue, depurative, detergent, hepatic, laxative, nutritive tonic, and tonic for the liver, kidneys, and blood.

Traditional Chinese Medical (TCM) Perspective

Yellow Dock is bitter, cooling, and drying. The nourishing Yin qualities are provided by many vitamins and minerals in the roots, making this plant an excellent nutritive tonic. The stimulating Yang action of the herb clears congestion, stagnation, and damp toxic heat from the blood, lymphatic fluids and lymph nodes, liver, gallbladder, kidneys, uterus, and intestines. It is specific for Liver, Uterine, and Intestinal Qi Stagnation and damp heat. It is indicated for people with a red tongue covered with excess white or yellow fur coating, which shows excess heat and dampness in the body.

Primary Actions

Yellow Dock root is an excellent alterative that gradually helps restore normal function throughout the body. It is primarily used for decongesting and normalizing the liver, cleansing the blood, lymph and kidneys, for treating chronic and eruptive skin problems, and as a treatment for constipation or diarrhea. It promotes the elimination of toxins through the liver, kidneys, colon, and skin. The alkalizing minerals provide nutrients.

Yellow Dock is especially effective when combined with Dandelion and Burdock roots because they have similar qualities and act synergistically to provide an excellent liver, kidney, and detoxification remedy. I call these herbs the "Three Sisters" and have combined them (in tincture form) with St. John's Wort (*Hypericum perforatum*) in repeated doses every 10 minutes with remarkable success for severe anaphylactic shock I once experienced that was caused by food poisoning. A few hours after eating a mango for the first time, I woke in the middle of the night in distress when my skin had turned bright red and my inflamed windpipe made breathing difficult. My options were to go to the emergency room or use my herbs. I took five large doses of the tinctures, repeated every 10 minutes, each in one cup of water. I felt better as my breathing normalized and my skin started returning to its normal color. I went to sleep and felt fine the next day. This same formula helped a client who had been bitten by a brown recluse spider three days before seeing me, and was suffering from nausea, dizziness, fever, altered mental state, and severe pain at the site of injury. I suggested using 1½ teaspoons of the tincture combination every 2-3 hours and gave her a jar of my salve containing Yellow Dock, recommending continual application on the spider bite, which had become a large, raised welt 2″ in diameter and full of white pus. She reported feeling much better the next day and said that the welt fell off after three days of applying the salve, leaving healthy pink tissue underneath. I saw her a year later and she showed me a very faint scar left from the bite.

Liver and Digestive System: Yellow Dock is a bitter digestive stimulant that improves digestion and normalizes functions of the stomach, pancreas, liver, gallbladder, and intestines. Its cholagogue properties increase the production and flow of bile from the liver into the gallbladder and small intestines. This promotes the normal breakdown of fats and regular bowel movements, and protects against liver and gallbladder congestion that contributes to gallstones and elevated cholesterol levels. Anthraquinones in the roots have a gentle laxative effect that stimulates normal bowel elimination. This stimulating activity normalizes digestion and is helpful for conditions caused by a sluggish liver, stomach and pancreas, including chronic constipation, gas and bloating, difficulty digesting fats, a metallic taste in the mouth, liver and gallbladder problems including inflammation and jaundice, and tendencies towards food allergies. The roots have traditionally been used to treat malabsorption, excess stomach acids, and steatorrhea (a condition of excess fat in the feces caused by a deficiency of bile and pancreatic enzymes). Containing astringent tannins that are excellent in reducing diarrhea, Yellow Dock has been a traditional treatment for dysentery and enteritis (intestinal inflammation). The blood cleansing, astringent, and mild antibiotic properties of the roots can be helpful for stomach and intestinal ulcers, Crohn's disease and colitis, especially when combined with Marshmallow (*Althaea officinalis*) and Licorice (*Glycyrrhiza glabra*) roots.

Kidneys and Urinary Tract: The roots remove toxins, excess acids, and waste products from the blood by stimulating kidney function and promoting urination. European doctors and the American Eclectic physicians of the 1880s–1930s found Yellow Dock to be valuable in dissolving kidney stones and treating edema, cystitis (bladder infection), metabolic acidosis, and gout.

Blood and Lymphatic System: Yellow Dock is a renowned blood purifier because it improves the general quality of blood and lymphatic fluids by stimulating the entire body to eliminate waste products, excess acids, and toxins through the liver, kidneys, and intestines. It has a wonderful cleansing and normalizing action on the blood, lymphatic fluids, and lymph nodes. In describing the actions of Yellow Dock, Eclectic physician Finley Ellingwood, M.D., wrote, "The alterative properties of this agent are underestimated. It is a renal depurant [stimulates kidney action to filter the blood] and general alterative of much value when ulceration of mucous surfaces or disease of the skin results from impure blood. It acts directly in its restorative influence, purifying the blood, removing morbific material, and quickly cures the disease conditions" (Ellingwood, 1919).

Yellow Dock roots are a nutritive tonic supplying significant quantities of minerals that alkalize and enrich the blood and neutralize excess acids. Most notable are the high concentrations of easily digestible iron, an excellent remedy for anemia, especially when combined with other herbs containing substantial amounts of iron like Stinging Nettle (*Urtica dioica*) and Dandelion. The cooling nature of Yellow Dock reduces toxic heat in the blood, which can be a causal factor in the formation of tumors, cancers, inflammation, and skin diseases and eruptions. The astringent tannins in the roots and leaves constrict tissues and are used to stop internal and external bleeding.

The herb is excellent for the entire lymphatic system, including lymph fluid, nodes, and spleen (an immune system organ composed of lymphatic tissue). As a lymphatic decongestant, Yellow Dock cleanses and stimulates movement of the lymphatic fluid, and has historically been used for swollen, painful lymph nodes, glandular tumors, and tuberculosis of the lymph nodes in the neck called scrofula.

Yellow Dock and other alkalizing herbs like Dandelion root, Oregon Grape Root (*Mahonia aquifolium*), and Burdock can be beneficial for a wide range of conditions caused by excess acids in the bloodstream and inflammation, including canker sores, excess stomach acid and acid reflex, arthritis, gout, and eruptive skin diseases. Excess acids may also be a factor in vascular headaches caused by inflammation of blood vessels in the head. A blend of these alkalizing herbs combined with Scullcap (*Scutellaria lateriflora*) and Feverfew (*Tanacetum parthenium*) can be helpful in resolving vascular headaches.

Gout and Arthritis: Yellow Dock's cooling, anti-inflammatory, and cleansing actions can be helpful for joint problems. Alkalizing minerals in the roots reduce excessive acids in the blood, which is an underlying cause of joint inflammation and pain. The herb's beneficial action on the kidneys is helpful for gout. According to Traditional Chinese Medicine, the liver regulates joints and ligaments, and herbs supporting the liver generally tend to improve joint problems. In Tibet and China, different species of Dock leaves are sometimes used in moxibustion to treat arthritis. The dried leaves are rolled into small balls that are burned over painful arthritic joints to promote warmth and increase the flow of blood and energy (Qi). The leaves are also applied as a poultice over the affected area and a decoction tea of the roots is ingested.

Skin Problems: Many skin problems and chronic skin conditions originate from blood and lymphatic fluids that are laden with waste products and toxic metabolites from incomplete digestion, poor liver function, and environmental toxins. Yellow Dock's stimulating and cleansing action on the liver, kidneys, blood, and lymph help many types of problematic skin conditions. The astringent tannins constrict tissue to stop abnormal bleeding and can be applied to wounds, bruises, and hemorrhoids. Anthraquinones in the roots show mild antibacterial activity against Gram-positive bacteria (*Staphylococcus aureus* and *Mycobacterium smegmatis*) and Gram-negative bacteria, including *Escherichia coli* and *Shigella* spp. (Miyazawa, 1983).

When treating skin problems, ingest the root as tea, tincture or pills, and apply the leaves or root as a salve, poultice, wash, or fomentation. Yellow Dock provides a cooling poultice that draws out heat and toxins. The roots and leaves have been used for many chronic and acute skin problems such as bites, stings, itching, inflammation, skin blemishes like pimples and acne, hives, eruptive skin conditions such as rashes, boils, fistulas, abscesses, ulcers, eczema, impetigo (a streptococcal infection), and fungal infections that include ringworm, athlete's foot, and Candida yeast. Topical application relieves itching and irritation caused by physical contact with poison ivy, poison oak, and Stinging Nettle. Tea made from the roots can be used as a mouthwash and gargle for treating canker sores and other mouth sores, gingivitis, and sore, infected throats. The leaf may also be chewed into a pulpy mass and applied directly on the mouth sore.

Herbalist Stephen Buhner reports extensive use of Yellow Dock root to treat psoriasis, combining it with equal parts of the roots of Figwort (*Scrophularia nodosa*), Sarsaparilla (*Smilax ornata*), Dandelion, Burdock, and Oregon Grape Root (*Mahonia aquifolium*) (Buhner, 2006). Ingesting Yellow Dock and Sarsaparilla roots is specific for blood cleansing and treating glandular swellings and eruptive skin conditions.

Women's Health: Yellow Dock's stimulating and decongesting actions on the uterus help move and cleanse stagnated, toxic, hot blood in the pelvis and normalize reproductive function. Congested blood flow in the uterus can cause copious menstrual bleeding with blood clots, excessive menstrual pain and cramping, and abdominal pressure and bloating. The herb's astringent properties decrease excessive menstrual flow, while easily digested iron helps anemic conditions and replaces iron lost during menstruation. It is an excellent ingredient in formulas for premenstrual syndrome (PMS) and hormonal imbalances, and can be cooling for hot flashes.

Nursing mothers experiencing painful, inflamed, and engorged breasts can obtain relief by applying a leaf or root poultice. For vaginal issues, the root tea may be taken internally and prepared as a douche, and vaginal suppositories can be made with the dried, powdered root. These are used for the treatment of vaginal infections and discharges, Candida yeast infections, uterine fibroids, and ovarian cysts. The herb can help strengthen and tone weak muscles when treating uterine prolapse. Prior to the age of antibiotics, Yellow Dock was an esteemed remedy for syphilis and gonorrhea.

Teachings from the Yellow Dock Deva

"Greetings, dear one. I am the deva of the Yellow Dock tribe whose large roots reach deep into the earth to draw upon her essence of 'physicality.' For my plants support the structure of the physical body and the deeper organs. My plants and the power of their essence are dominated by Mars, ruler of the physical body and activity, and are also influenced by Scorpio's energies pervading the deeper, more hidden side of life. The reproductive powers of Scorpio are seen in the multitude of my prolific seeds. And the medicine in my roots helps the liver to be vibrantly healthy and perform its job of nurturing and regulating the reproductive system in men and women, which is ruled by Scorpio.

"The reddish pigment in the stems and veins of my plants reflects my value in keeping blood enriched and potent with minerals, and helping the blood to flow freely and nourish the cells in the human body. I am a great cleanser of living tissues, and the ultimate results of my cleansing abilities are vibrant bodies, happy hearts, and wise minds.

"My plants contain the cooling earth element. Their medicine helps you to feel grounded upon the earth, within your body, and within the light essence of your being. It is a complete journey, a spiraling circle of life, growth, and consciousness. Whether noticed or not, the light cannot be changed or diminished in any way. And so, dear one, behold the light that you are – the inner light – as the force of life shared and lived by all. The devas urge you to refine your thoughts, your feelings and habits – refine all aspects of your life, allowing your inner light to shine forth in full and complete radiance. For this, dear one, is essential to fulfill your time and purpose on this earth plane, and to be prepared for coming events and life on this planet. The old is falling and crumbling apart to make way for the new. My plant's medicine will assist you in this process. Live in the power and compassion of the light, dear one, and be in peace. This is the devas' wish for you; for we love humankind, despite much neglect and abuse from so many. It is our nature to be forgiving and compassionate in understanding the short-sightedness and suffering within the human race. And so we offer our humble gifts to you to make your journey easier and your heart more open to embrace loving kindness and acceptance."

SECTION THREE

Index of Health Issues and Herbal Recommendations

Herbs for Pregnancy, Childbirth and Lactation

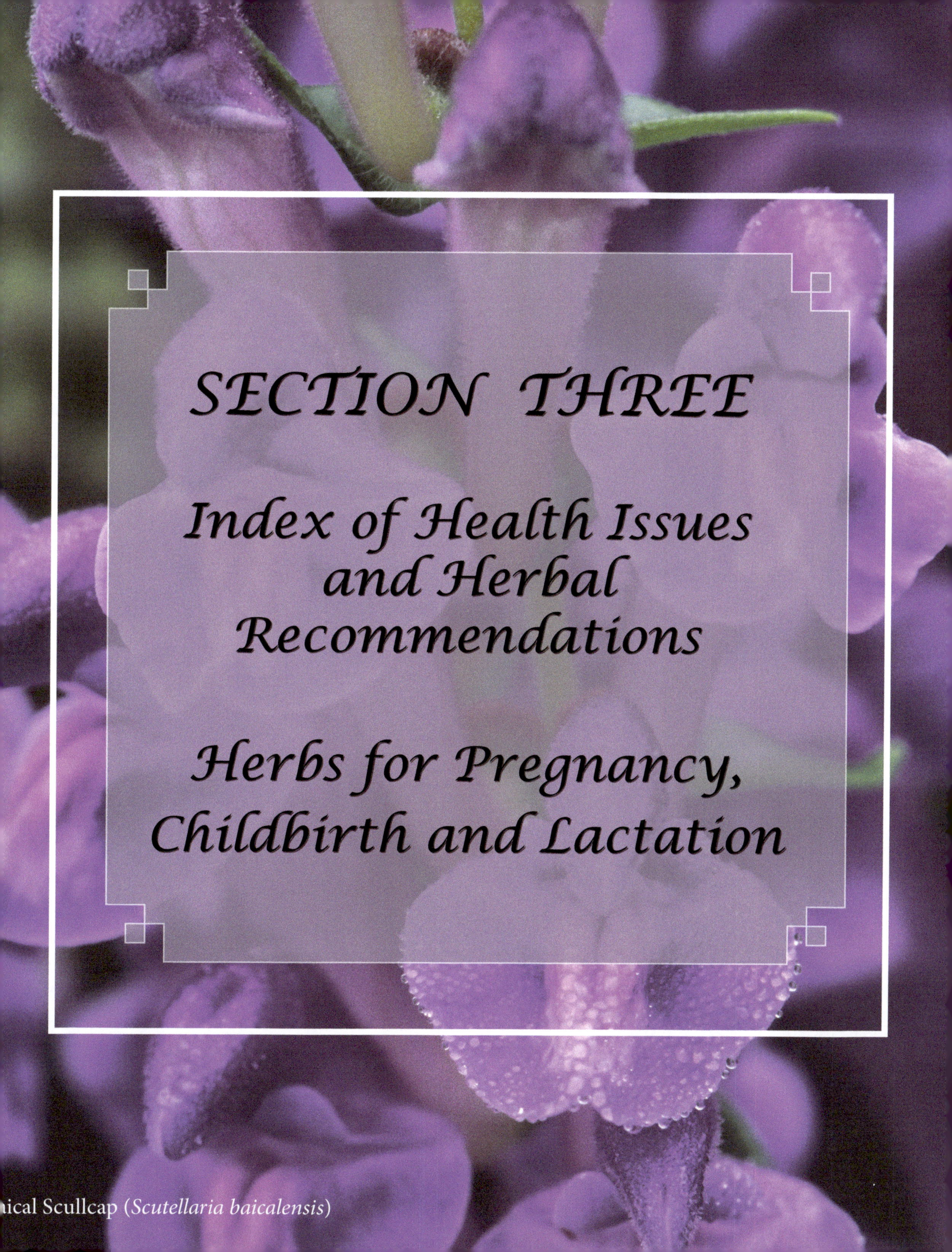

ical Scullcap (*Scutellaria baicalensis*)

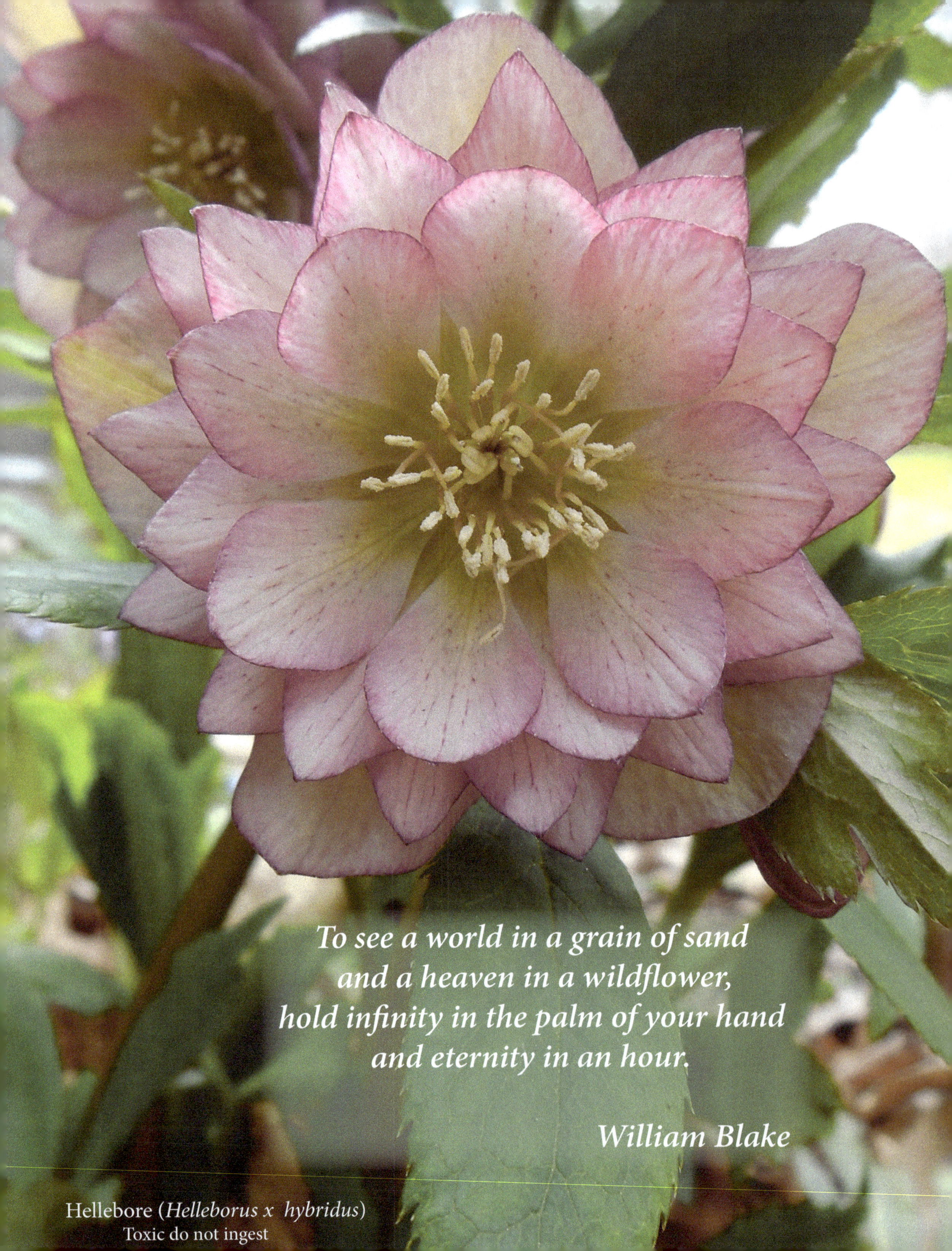
To see a world in a grain of sand
and a heaven in a wildflower,
hold infinity in the palm of your hand
and eternity in an hour.
William Blake

Hellebore (*Helleborus x hybridus*)
Toxic do not ingest

Index of Health Issues and Herbal Recommendations

This index is a helpful tool when deciding which herbs to use for specific health issues. The herbs listed under each health issue are found in the Materia Medica of this book, where greater detail and clarification are provided and thorough review is encouraged. Additional herbs not included in the Materia Medica are listed under *"Other Helpful Herbs"* and should also be further researched before being used. Another tool to assist in deciding appropriate herbs for specific health conditions is the last chapter in Section One titled "**Healing Qualities of Herbs**" (pages 180-189).

It is always important to research medicinal plants before using them to ensure safe and correct applications. In addition to your own research, it is wise to collaborate with a qualified health care practitioner when taking medicinal herbs, especially when working with more challenging health problems. See "**Media Resources for Herbal Research**" in the Appendix (pages 638-639) for a listing of websites, search engines, and literature most helpful for researching medicinal herbs.

Always remember that the most profound and lasting healing occurs when herbal therapy is combined with a holistic perspective; healthy lifestyle; an organic, non-GMO whole foods diet; a high-quality vitamin, mineral, and essential fatty acid supplement; and daily attention and awareness as to how our thoughts, emotions, and behaviors affect the health and disease of our body. Engaging in a daily practice of meditation or relaxation to gently and courageously explore our inner universe of thoughts, feelings, and "body consciousness" invites amazing opportunities for profound healing at causal levels. By understanding the holistic body/mind relationship, our healing potential is mobilized and empowered, making herbal therapies more effective. Refer to **"The Holistic Perspective ~ Living and Healing in Holism"** at the beginning of this book (pages xiii-xv) for a thorough explanation of holism and its application in health care and herbalism.

Abdominal Distention and Bloating: See Digestive System

Abortants (uterine stimulants to be avoided during pregnancy):

Black Cohosh ~ never use during pregnancy until the last 2-3 weeks before birth; large amounts can result in miscarriage, especially during the first trimester of pregnancy.

Blue Cohosh ~ never use during pregnancy until the last 2-3 weeks before the due date; large amounts can result in miscarriage, especially in the first trimester. Always use in combination with Black Cohosh.

Feverfew ~ a strong uterine stimulant that can stimulate a miscarriage.

Abscess: See Skin

Acid Reflux or Gastroesophageal Reflux Disease (GERD): See Stomach

Acidosis

Acidosis is a condition of excess acids and depletion of alkaline reserves in the blood and tissues causing imbalance and inflammation. Reduce intake of acid-forming foods (sugar, meat, dairy, fats, coffee, alcohol) and eat lots of vegetables (especially green), tree-ripened fruits, and a vitamin and mineral supplement to help to alkalize the body and reduce damaging inflammation.

American Centaury ~ a strong bitter that alkalizes blood and releases excess acids via the kidneys.

Astragalus ~ decreases excess stomach acids; helps reduce acid reflex, heartburn, and acidosis.

Blue Vervain ~ a bitter that stimulates kidney excretion of excess acids; helpful for gout and arthritis.

Boneset ~ a bitter that stimulates kidneys to excrete excess acids; relieves gout, arthritis, and muscle pain.

Burdock ~ a diuretic that reduces excessive acids in blood, including uric acid; helpful for gout and arthritis.

Chickweed ~ high in minerals that alkalize the system.

Dandelion ~ high in alkalizing minerals; stimulates kidneys to excrete excess acids; eases gout and arthritis.

Goldenseal ~ alkalizes the blood and neutralizes excess acids.

Horehound ~ alkalizes blood; promotes kidney excretion of excess acids; resolves general acidosis.

Stinging Nettle ~ high mineral content alkalizes blood and promotes kidney excretion of excess acids.

Other Helpful Herbs:

Chlorella (*Chlorella* spp.) and Spirulina (*Arthrospira platensis, A. maxima*) ~ highly nutritious freshwater algae that contain alkalizing minerals.

Acne: See Skin

Adhesions:

Chickweed ~ can prevent adhesions following surgery when taken as tea.

Adrenal Glands and Adaptogens:

Adaptogens are herbs that help the body adapt to and defend against acute and chronic environmental toxins and emotional, psychological, and physical stress. Taken as a daily tonic, adaptogens enhance and normalize functions of the adrenal, pituitary and hypothalamus glands, support immunity, increase vitality and endurance, and help normalize blood sugar levels during times of stress.

The adrenal medulla produces adrenaline (epinephrine) and noradrenaline (norepinephrine), which stimulate nervous system and metabolic activity. The adrenal cortex produces cortisol and hydrocortisone, which help regulate metabolism, immunity, and other processes. The cortex also produces aldosterone, which regulates urinary output.

Astragalus ~ an adaptogen; helps reduce adrenal exhaustion and "burn out," stress, and chronic fatigue.
Echinacea ~ stimulates adrenals to secrete hormones that improve immunity and ability to manage stress.
Holy Basil ~ an adaptogen; excellent for adrenal exhaustion, coping with stress, and high blood sugar levels.
Lobelia ~ small doses stimulate adrenal secretion of adrenaline.
Sage ~ strengthens the adrenals.
Saint John's Wort ~ reduces excessive cortisol produced by adrenals during stress; helps stabilize adrenals.
Scullcap ~ helps restore and normalize adrenal function; reduces adrenal "burn-out" from stress.
Stinging Nettle ~ minerals nourish adrenal glands; helps reduce adrenal exhaustion.
Thyme ~ helps restore adrenal function; beneficial for stress-related adrenal exhaustion.

Other Helpful Herbs:

Ashwagandha (*Withania somnifera*) ~ a tonic adaptogen; supports adrenal medulla; helps normalize cortisol levels; recommended for debility, nervous exhaustion, and convalescence.
Bacopa (*Bacopa monniera*) ~ an adaptogen that reduces stress and anxiety; antioxidant.
Bupleurum (*Bupleurum chinense*) ~ promotes optimal function; improves energy levels; supports weak adrenals and recovery after corticosteroid treatment; taken with Licorice and Ginseng in Chinese medicine.
Codonopsis root (*Codonopsis pilosula*) ~ an adaptogen; increases blood levels of corticosterone (the stress hormone) produced by the adrenals to restore deficient cortisol; replenishes vital energy.
Eleuthero/Siberian Ginseng (*Eleutherococcus senticosus*) ~ an adaptogen; normalizes adrenal activity and decreases stress response; supports adrenal medulla; helps normalize cortisol production and reduce high levels; improves DHEA levels promoting production of androgens and estrogens (male and female sex hormones); improves vitality and physical endurance .
Ginseng, Asian (*Panax ginseng*) and American (*Panax quinquefolius*) ~ adaptogens; restore adrenal function; support the medulla; help body adapt to stress; used for deficiency conditions, weakness, and exhaustion.
Gotu Kola (*Centella asiatica*) ~ an adaptogen that increases energy and endurance and reduces stress.
Licorice (*Glycyrrhiza glabra*) ~ an adaptogen specific for adrenal exhaustion and insufficiency; roots contain glycyrrhizin, which has similar structure and activity as cortisol; valued treatment for Addison's disease (a serious condition in which adrenals do not produce enough cortisol and aldosterone).
Maca (*Lepidium meyenii*) ~ supports the hypothalamus-pituitary-adrenal (HPA) axis that controls metabolism and other primary body processes; helps nourish and improve adrenal function and reduces adrenal fatigue.
Rhodiola (*Rhodiola rosea*) ~ a cooling, stimulating adaptogen that restores weak adrenals; reduces stress responses by regulating cortisol levels and reducing excessive amounts; used for adrenal "burnout," chronic fatigue, debility, and convalescence; improves mental and physical performance and endurance.
Schisandra (*Schisandra chinensis*) ~ a tonic adaptogen; helps restore adrenals, improve physical strength and endurance, and reduce chronic fatigue; antioxidant properties protect cells from damage.
Turmeric (*Curcuma longa*) ~ restores cortisol balance and adrenal function in animal studies; antioxidant.

AIDS (Acquired Immune Deficiency Syndrome) and HIV (Human Immunodeficiency Virus):

Astragalus ~ antiviral; strengthens immune system and reduces secondary bacterial infections.
Bloodroot ~ a powerful antiviral and broad antimicrobial (use cautiously due to toxicity).
Burdock ~ stimulates immunity.
Calendula ~ antiviral; stimulates immunity.
Echinacea ~ antiviral; stimulates immunity; blood and lymphatic cleanser.
Elderberry ~ antiviral; stimulates immunity; blood and lymphatic cleanser.
Hyssop ~ exerts activity against HIV virus in laboratory studies.
Isatis ~ antiviral; may be helpful for HIV.
Saint John's Wort ~ antiviral that has potential activity against HIV; do not use with pharmaceutical drugs.

Other Helpful Herbs:

Cat's Claw (*Uncaria tomentosa*) ~ one of the best antiviral herbs to boost the immune system and fight viral infections, including HIV; anti-inflammatory, antimutagenic, and antioxidant.
Licorice (*Glycyrrhiza glabra*) ~ immunostimulant; research shows that glycyrrhizin inhibits HIV cell division.

Alcohol Withdrawal: See Drug and Alcohol Withdrawal

Allergies: See Sinus Problems

Alzheimer's Disease: See Brain and Cognitive Function

Anemia:

Herbs containing significant amounts of iron to reduce anemia include Burdock root, Catnip, Chickweed, Chlorella, Dandelion, Elderberries, Spirulina, Stinging Nettle, Yellow Dock root, and Beet root.

Antioxidants: See Oxidative Stress

Anxiety: See Nervous System
Arteriosclerosis: See Vascular System
Arthritis (Rheumatoid and Osteoarthritis):

Reducing intake of acidic foods (sugars, gluten, coffee, alcohol, meat, and dairy) and the nightshade family helps reduce inflammation, a primary cause of arthritis. A diet rich in organic vegetables, especially greens, and tree-ripened fruit provides alkaline minerals that reduce inflammation.

American Centaury ~ stimulates circulation; decreases heat and inflammation; alkalizes blood.
Black Cohosh ~ reduces joint inflammation and pain.
Blue Vervain ~ anti-inflammatory and analgesic.
Boneset~ anti-inflammatory; supports liver and kidney function to alleviate causes of arthritis.
Burdock~ reduces pain, inflammation, and excess acids; lubricates joints.
Catnip ~ used externally for painful joints.
Cayenne ~ relieves pain with external application.
Chamomile ~ anti-inflammatory; reduces pain; cooling; alkalizing.
Chickweed ~ alkalizing; soothing to inflamed, hot joints.
Cinquefoil ~ reduces inflammation; can be helpful for muscle and joint pain.
Dandelion ~ cooling; anti-inflammatory; reduces acids; supports liver and kidney function.
Echinacea ~ cooling; anti-inflammatory; improves lubrication of joints.
Elderberry ~ contains alkalizing minerals; cooling and anti-inflammatory.
Feverfew ~ anti-inflammatory; analgesic.
Holy Basil ~ anti-inflammatory COX-2 (cyclooxygenase-2) inhibitor; analgesic; increases circulation.
Hyssop ~ anti-inflammatory.
Lavender ~ anti-inflammatory; analgesic.
Lobelia ~ liniment can help relieve stiff, painful, inflamed joints.
Mugwort ~ cooling; anti-inflammatory; used internally and externally.
Mullein ~ leaves are used externally; cooling and anti-inflammatory.
Peppermint ~ oil or tincture is applied externally to reduce pain and inflammation.
Sage ~ anti-inflammatory; applied externally to relieve joint pain.
Stinging Nettle ~ an alkalizing, cooling, COX-2 inhibitor that reduces inflammation.
Thyme ~ analgesic and anti-inflammatory.
Yarrow ~ cooling, anti-inflammatory, analgesic.
Yellow Dock ~ a cooling anti-inflammatory; reduces excess acids in blood; supports liver function.

Other Helpful Herbs:

Alfalfa (*Medicago sativa*) ~ high mineral content decreases excess acidity and joint inflammation.
Andrographis (*Andrographis paniculata*) ~ antioxidant; decreases joint inflammation and pain.
Ashwagandha (*Withania somnifera*) ~ antioxidant; anti-inflammatory; decreases inflammatory COX-2.
Boswellia (*Boswellia serrata*) ~ reduces pain by inhibiting 5-LOX (5-lipoxygenase), the key enzyme of leukotriene production that promotes inflammation; inhibits connective tissue damage; increases blood supply to joints; specific for arthritic conditions.
Celery seed (*Apium graveolens*) ~ antioxidant and anti-inflammatory specific for rheumatoid arthritis, gout.
Devil's Claw root (*Harpagophytum procumbens*) ~ has NSAID-like effects by decreasing production of inflammatory prostaglandins.
Ginger (*Zingiber officinale*) ~ antioxidant; warming; inhibits inflammatory COX-2, LOX-2 (lipoxygenase 2), prostaglandins, and leukotrienes to ease painful, swollen joints.
Licorice (*Glycyrrhiza glabra*) ~ glycyrrhizin has similar anti-inflammatory, analgesic actions as hydrocortisone.
Meadowsweet (*Filipendula ulmaria*) ~ contains salicylic acid which is anti-inflammatory and analgesic.
Mormon Tea (*Ephedra nevadensis*, spp.) ~ does not contain ephedrine, but can be helpful for arthritis.
Oregano (*Origanum vulgare*) ~ strong anti-inflammatory and antioxidant that reduces arthritic pain; diluted oil may be applied to sore joints.
Rosemary oil (*Rosmarinus officinalis*) ~ topical application reduces pain, inflammation; strong antioxidant.
Turmeric (*Curcuma longa*) ~ decreases inflammatory COX-2, 5-LOX, prostaglandins, and leukotrienes; antioxidant; a primary herb taken to reduce chronic inflammation and pain.
Wild Yam (*Dioscorea villosa*) ~ helpful in relieving joint inflammation and pain.
Wintergreen (*Gaultheria procumbens*) ~ salicylic acid, the main substance in the oil, is analgesic and anti-inflammatory; oil is applied to relieve joint pain and inflammation.
Yucca (*Yucca* spp.) ~ anti-inflammatory specific for rheumatoid arthritis; over time it may dissolve abnormal bony bumps or nodules on the hand.

Asthma: See Lung and Bronchial Problems
Atherosclerosis: See Vascular System
Athlete's Foot: See Fungal Infections
Backache: See Pain
Bacterial Infections:

American Centaury ~ has mild antibacterial activity.

Astragalus ~ strengthens immune system to fight bacterial and viral infections.
Black Walnut ~ antibacterial against wounds and gastrointestinal infections.
Blue Vervain ~ helpful for all types of bacterial infections, including sinusitis and upper respiratory infections.
Boneset ~ excellent immunostimulant for fever, body aches, and bacterial infections; excellent combined with Echinacea.
Calendula ~ taken for gastrointestinal infections; a topical wound disinfectant.
Catnip ~ kills some Gram-positive bacteria, including MRSA (methicillin-resistant *Staphylococcus aureus*).
Cayenne ~ for all types of bacterial infections, including sinus, upper respiratory, and gastrointestinal.
Echinacea ~ stimulates immune system; excellent for bacterial infections.
Elecampane ~ specific for bacterial infections of the lungs, skin, and urinary and digestive tracts.
Feverfew ~ useful for bacterial infections.
Goldenrod ~ specific for urinary, intestinal, bronchial, and sinus infections.
Goldenseal ~ effective against bacteria on skin and in the respiratory, digestive, and genitourinary systems.
Holy Basil ~ immunomodulator; helpful for bacterial infections, including *Staphylococcus*.
Hops ~ effective against bacteria in the throat, lungs, skin, and digestive and urinary systems.
Hyssop ~ specific for bacterial infections in the respiratory and digestive tracts.
Isatis ~ a strong antibacterial; specific for lung and skin infections; very cooling, reduces fevers.
Lavender ~ a soothing antiseptic and antibacterial herb.
Lemon Balm ~ a mild antibiotic helpful for internal and external infections.
Motherwort ~ especially helpful for respiratory and sinus infections.
Mugwort ~ primarily used for intestinal and urinary tract infections, pneumonia, *Pseudomonas,* and staph.
Sage ~ antiseptic and antibacterial for skin, intestines, respiratory system, and genitourinary tract.
Saint John's Wort ~ antiseptic and antibacterial against some bacteria.
Thyme ~ antiseptic and antibacterial for the skin and respiratory and digestive systems.
Yarrow ~ antiseptic and antibacterial for skin, intestines, respiratory system, and genitourinary tract.

Other Helpful Herbs:

Clove (*Syzyygium aromaticum*) ~ the oil is applied externally; antiseptic and antibacterial for skin and gums.
Eucalyptus (*Eucalyptus* spp.) ~ antimicrobial oil is applied to skin; internally used for respiratory infections.
Garlic (*Allium sativum*) ~ a strong antiseptic and antibacterial for infections throughout the body.
Myrrh (*Commiphora myrrha*) ~ antimicrobial primarily used for inflammation and infection in the respiratory and gastrointestinal tracts and externally for wound healing; stimulates white blood cell production.
Oregon Grape Root (*Mahonia aquifolium*) ~ strong antimicrobial; specific for all mucous membranes.
Pau D'arco (*Tabebuia impetiginosa*) ~ an immunomodulator; antibacterial.
Rosemary (*Rosmarinus officinalis*) ~ antibacterial to skin and gastrointestinal and respiratory tract; kills staph.
Tea Tree oil (*Melaleuca alternifolia*) ~ applied externally for bacterial skin infections.
Wild Indigo (*Baptisia tinctoria*) ~ a strong antibacterial used for all types of infections and septic conditions of blood and tissues; use under guidance of a qualified herbalist due to toxicity of large doses.

Bad Breath (Halitosis): See Digestion (Sage and Thyme)
Bed-Wetting: See Bladder and Incontinence
Bladder:

Astragalus ~ promotes kidney and bladder function; diuretic; beneficial for <u>cystitis</u> (bladder infection), <u>urinary tract infections</u> (UTIs), bloody urine, incontinence, and preventing bladder prolapse.
Blue Vervain ~ helpful for bladder infections and inflammation; a mild diuretic.
Boneset ~ a mild diuretic; antibiotic against *E. coli*; helpful for cystitis and most UTIs.
Burdock ~ diuretic; used for cystitis and bladder inflammation.
Calendula ~ antibiotic and anti-inflammatory for cystitis.
Chickweed ~ soothing and cooling for bladder inflammation; a mild diuretic.
Cinquefoil ~ for urinary incontinence, bladder inflammation, ulceration, prolapse, and bloody urine.
Comfrey ~ soothing to inflamed, irritated, and ulcerated bladder; helpful for cystitis and bloody urine.
Cranesbill ~ reduces pus, mucous, and bleeding in the bladder.
Dandelion ~ an excellent diuretic; helpful for bladder infections; cooling and anti-inflammatory.
Echinacea ~ antibacterial for bladder infections.
Elecampane ~ antibacterial, diuretic, and anti-inflammatory for bladder infections.
Goldenrod ~ a diuretic used for inflammation, spasms, cystitis, difficult and scanty urination, bloody urine.
Goldenseal ~ antibacterial; anti-inflammatory; cooling and soothing to tissues; helps bladder prolapse.
Hops ~ relieves irritation, inflammation, spasms, and eases bladder infections.
Marshmallow ~ anti-inflammatory; antispasmodic; soothing for infections and painful or bloody urination.
Mullein root ~ anti-inflammatory; antispasmodic; used for infections and painful, bloody urination; reduces incontinence in children and adults, including bed-wetting, stress, and menopausal incontinence.
Sage ~ antibacterial; anti-inflammatory; beneficial for cystitis, bladder spasms, and bloody urine.
Saint John's Wort ~ for cystitis, bloody urine, bed-wetting; exhibits cytotoxic activity against bladder cancer.
Scullcap ~ relaxes painful spasms; reduces incontinence and bed-wetting caused by neurological problems.
Stinging Nettle ~ cooling; anti-inflammatory; used for bloody urine and cystitis.
Yarrow ~ reduces bladder spasms, inflammation, pain, infections, and bloody urine; excellent for cystitis.

Other Helpful Herbs:
Buchu (*Agathosma betulina*) ~ diuretic; antimicrobial; anti-inflammatory; helpful for cystitis.
Celery seed (*Apium graveolens*) ~ diuretic; anti-inflammatory; antiseptic for cystitis and other UTIs.
Cleavers (*Galium aparine*) ~ diuretic; anti-inflammatory; excellent for treating cystitis.
Corn Silk (*Zea mays*) and Plantain (*Plantago* spp.) ~ soothing demulcents; anti-inflammatory; ease cystitis.
Couch Grass (*Elymus repens*) ~diuretic; soothing; used for UTIs and cystitis; usually taken with other herbs like Yarrow, Uva-ursi, and Buchu.
Cranberry (*Vaccinium macrocarpon*) ~ prevents *E. coli* bacteria, the most common cause of cystitis, from adhering to tissues lining the bladder; unsweetened juice is a preventative and treatment for cystitis.
Gravel Root (*Eupatorium purpureum*) ~ diuretic; reduces incontinence; helps cystitis and burning urination; helps dissolve and eliminate kidney stones.
Hydrangea (*Hydrangea arborescens*) ~ diuretic; helpful for cystitis; helps dissolve and eliminate stones.
Juniper berry (*Juniperus communis*) ~ a stimulating diuretic; antibacterial for cystitis; avoid overuse.
Oregon Grape Root (*Mahonia aquifolium*) ~ antimicrobial, anti-inflammatory; healing for cystitis.
Parsley (*Petroselinum crispum*) ~ decreases bladder spasms; diuretic; helps treat cystitis.
Pau D'arco (*Tabebuia impetiginosa*) ~ antibacterial; used for cystitis and urethritis.
Uva-ursi/Bearberry (*Arctostaphylos uva-ursi*) ~ kills bacteria in urine; excellent for acute and chronic inflammation; diuretic; restores bladder tone; used for cystitis, incontinence, ulceration of urinary tract membranes.

Blood (also see Vascular System):
American Centaury ~ detoxifies blood due to action on liver and kidneys.
Astragalus ~ helps prevent anemia and blood clotting.
Black Walnut ~ cleans toxic blood and reduces chronic constipation by stimulating sluggish digestion.
Bloodroot ~ stimulates circulation; detoxifies blood; antiviral (use small doses cautiously due to toxicity).
Blue Vervain ~ helps eliminate toxins, excess acids, and heat in blood; stimulates circulation.
Burdock ~ detoxifies, mineralizes, and reduces excess acids in blood; iron content in roots reduces anemia.
Calendula ~ normalizes circulation; reduces excess heat in blood; stops hemorrhage; detoxifies blood.
Cayenne ~ normalizes blood flow; reduces abnormal clotting; stops internal and external hemorrhage.
Chamomile ~ thins blood by reducing blood platelet aggregation; a vasodilator (dilates blood vessels) that increases circulation.
Chickweed ~ alkalizing; cooling and cleansing to blood; high iron content reduces anemia.
Cinquefoil ~ excellent for all types of hemorrhage; used for septicemia (blood poisoning and infection).
Cranesbill ~ strong astringent that reduces abnormal bleeding and hemorrhage.
Dandelion ~ high iron and potassium content helpful to reduce anemia; detoxifies and removes excess heat and acids from blood; decreases abnormal blood clotting; promotes circulation.
Echinacea ~ antibiotic for septicemia from toxins, venom, pathogens; stimulates white blood cell production.
Elderberry ~ the berries alkalize, cool, cleanse, and fortify blood with minerals; helpful for treating anemia.
Elecampane ~ blood cleanser for toxic conditions and skin problems caused by toxicity.
Feverfew ~ acts on blood platelets to thin the blood and reduce abnormal clotting.
Goldenseal ~ cleanses and mineralizes blood; reduces toxicity; promotes circulation.
Holy Basil ~ anticoagulant properties help to prevent blood clot disorders.
Hops ~ cleansing to blood; antiplatelet activity inhibits abnormal blood clotting in vessels.
Isatis ~ reduces heat and pathogens in blood; detoxifying; used for septicemia.
Saint John's Wort ~ excellent blood cleanser for venom, toxins, chemicals, and food poisoning.
Stinging Nettle ~ reduces bleeding and toxins; nourishes and alkalizes blood; high iron content helps anemia.
Thyme ~ reduces abnormal blood clot formation; antimicrobial for septicemia.
Yarrow ~ excellent to stop abnormal bleeding; breaks up blood clots and promotes circulation.
Yellow Dock ~ mineralizes, alkalizes, and detoxifies the blood; high iron content reduces anemia.
Other Helpful Herbs:
Codonopsis root (*Codonopsis pilosula*) ~ promotes red blood cell production; helpful for anemia.
Garlic (*Allium sativum*) ~ helps prevent abnormal blood clotting by inhibiting blood platelet aggregation.
Ginger (*Zingiber officinale*) ~ thins blood, prevents abnormal clots, and improves circulation by inhibiting blood platelet aggregation and elevated levels of fibrinogen involved in blood clot formation.
Gotu Kola (*Centella asiatica*) ~ ability to detoxify blood helps heal skin eruptions, ulcers, eczema, psoriasis.
Red Clover (*Trifolium pratense*) ~ blood purifier used for chronic skin conditions; anticoagulant that reduces abnormal clotting; studies show that it increases elasticity of arteries to promote circulation.
Sarsaparilla (*Smilax ornata*) ~ purifies blood by binding to endotoxins (toxins excreted from bacteria) in the gut and prohibiting their absorption into the blood.
Turmeric (*Curcuma longa*) ~ blood thinner; inhibits blood platelets from clumping together to form clots.
Wild Indigo (*Baptisia tinctoria*) ~ a powerful antimicrobial for infections and septic conditions of the blood and tissues; use under guidance of a qualified herbalist due to toxicity of large doses.

Blood Pressure: See Hypertension or Hypotension
Blood Vessels: See Vascular System
Boils: See Skin

Bones and Osteoporosis:

Maintain strong bones by ingesting calcium-rich foods, a calcium supplement (hydroxyapatite is the best form for bone absorption and mineralization), and herbs containing substantial amounts of calcium.

Black Cohosh ~ estrogenic effects help prevent bone loss.
Boneset ~ can be helpful for mending broken bones.
Chasteberry ~ helpful to heal fractures and prevent osteoporosis.
Chickweed ~ contains substantial calcium and other minerals; supports strong bones to prevent osteoporosis.
Comfrey ~ helps mend broken and bruised bones; stimulates formation of new bone cells.
Dandelion ~ high mineral content promotes strong bones; helps prevent osteoporosis.
Hops ~ estrogenic effects inhibit breakdown of bones and may help prevent osteoporosis.
Mullein ~ external application may help reset broken bones and a herniated disc.
Stinging Nettle ~ high in minerals including calcium, magnesium, phosphorus, boron, and silica.

Other Helpful Herbs:

Alfalfa (*Medicago sativa*) ~ high in calcium and other minerals to promote strong bones.
Horsetail (*Equisetum arvense*, spp.) ~ contains silica that helps repair collagen in tissues and bones.
Red Raspberry leaf (*Rubus idaeus*) ~ high in calcium, phosphorus, and potassium for optimal bone health.
Estrogenic herbs that promote bone density ~ Dong Quai (*Angelica sinensis*), Licorice (*Glycyrrhiza glabra*), and Red Clover (*Trifolium pratense*), which also contains substantial levels of calcium and other minerals.

Brain and Cognitive Function:

Optimal brain function depends on adequate nutrients, blood supply, protective antioxidants, and balanced neurotransmitter levels. Neurotransmitters that regulate the nervous system are either inhibiting and calming (serotonin and GABA/gamma-aminobutyric acid) or excitatory and stimulating (epinephrine/adrenaline, norepinephrine, dopamine, glutamate, and phenethylamine or PEA). The pineal and pituitary endocrine glands, located in the center of the brain, are master regulators of the body and brain function.

Holy Basil ~ supports optimal brain, neurotransmitter, and neurological function; used for attention deficit hyperactivity disorder (ADHD), nerve deterioration, cognitive and memory loss, dementia, and depression.
Lavender ~ a calming brain tonic used for altered brain chemistry, mental imbalance, and neurosis.
Lemon Balm ~ a brain tonic that improves memory and cognitive function.
Lobelia ~ increases dopamine levels; harmonizes stimulating and inhibiting chemicals of the nervous system.
Passion Flower ~ increases GABA and relaxation; has normalizing effect on pituitary and pineal glands.
Sage ~ a brain tonic that vitalizes and restores nerve and brain function; enhances pituitary function, memory, and cognitive abilities; may help prevent and treat dementia and Alzheimer's disease.
Saint John's Wort ~ balances neurotransmitters to stabilize emotions and support cognitive function.
Scullcap ~ contains calming neurotransmitters that help regulate and normalize brain and nervous system function.
Thyme ~ a calming nervine that promotes optimal brain function; attaches to GABA cell receptor sites.
Valerian ~ increases levels of melatonin, glutamine, and inhibitory neurotransmitters GABA and serotonin.

Other Helpful Herbs:

Ashwagandha (*Withania somnifera*) ~ an antioxidant that protects nerve cells; improves cognitive function, disorders, and memory; shown to increase and normalize levels of GABA, a calming neurotransmitter.
Bacopa (*Bacopa monniera*) ~ antioxidant; protects and nourishes nerve cells; increases cerebral blood flow; balances neurotransmitter levels; enhances cognitive clarity and memory.
Eleuthero/Siberian Ginseng (*Eleutherococcus senticosus*) ~ improves diminished mental, cognitive abilities.
Ginkgo (*Ginkgo biloba*) ~ an antioxidant that protects nerves, brain tissues, blood vessels; promotes blood flow and oxygenation to brain; improves cognitive functions and memory; protects against dementia.
Ginseng, Asian (*Panax ginseng*) and American (*Panax quinquefolius*) ~ antioxidants; stimulating effects improve concentration, alertness, cognition, memory; helpful for treating ADHD, especially in children.
Gotu Kola (*Centella asiatica*) ~ improves cognition and memory; calms nervous system due to GABA support.
Rhodiola (*Rhodiola rosea*) ~ an antioxidant that protects nerve cells from damage and inflammation; improves cognition, attention span, and memory; small to medium doses are stimulating, increase levels of norepinephrine, dopamine and serotonin, and are taken for depression; larger doses relax and sedate to reduce anxiety.
Rosemary (*Rosmarinus officinalis*) ~ a strong antioxidant; nervine stimulant; improves cognition, memory, and blood circulation to the brain; reduces anxiety and depression.
Schisandra (*Schisandra chinensis*) ~ a nervine; improves mental alertness, performance, and cognition; an antioxidant that reduces oxidative damage and inflammation; sedating actions diminish anxiety.
Turmeric (*Curcuma longa*) ~ protects nerve cells; decreases oxidative damage, inflammation, and beta amyloid formation implicated in Alzheimer's disease; improves blood circulation and vascular stability in the brain; increases levels of serotonin (calming) and dopamine (improves cognition).

Breast and Breast-Feeding (also see pages 610-611 in "Herbs for Pregnancy, Childbirth, and Lactation"):

Black Cohosh~ helpful for mastitis and menstrual breast soreness; protects against breast cancer.
Blue Vervain ~ a galactagogue that increases milk supply and stimulates lactation.
Burdock~ used to heal breast cysts, breast soreness and tenderness related to PMS, and cancer; taken

internally and applied as a poultice to reduce inflammation and infection caused by mastitis.
Calendula ~ used for breast cysts, tumors, cancer, and fluid retention due to poor lymphatic drainage and post-mastectomies; applied as a salve for sore, cracked nipples and mastitis in nursing mothers.
Catnip ~ taken internally to stimulate lactation; used as a poultice for sore breasts and cracked nipples.
Chasteberry ~ helpful to reduce fibrocystic breast disease and tenderness due to estrogen dominance; a galactagogue that stimulates lactation and increases milk supply.
Chickweed ~ used internally and externally for breast cysts, cancers, and mastitis.
Comfrey ~ used externally for sore nipples and fissures; softens engorged breasts; healing for mastitis.
Dandelion ~ cooling and anti-inflammatory; reduces PMS breast tenderness, cysts, and tumors; a nutrient-rich galactagogue; a cooling and anti-inflammatory treatment for mastitis.
Echinacea ~ has been used for mastitis and breast cancer.
Elderberry ~ a tea of the flowers is cooling and applied to the breasts as a compress to treat mastitis and pain.
Hops ~ stimulates lactation to increase milk supply in nursing mothers.
Marshmallow ~ increases flow of breast milk; a cooling and anti-inflammatory treatment for mastitis.
Sage ~ a lactifuge that decreases breast milk production and is taken by nursing mothers to wean babies.
Saint John's Wort ~ applied externally to reduce pain and heal cracked and caked breasts of nursing mothers.
Stinging Nettle ~ increases nutrient content and volume of breast milk.
Thyme ~ anti-inflammatory; antibacterial; helpful for mastitis.
Yarrow ~ applied to sore, cracked nipples to relieve pain and promote fast healing when breast-feeding.
Yellow Dock ~ an externally applied poultice reduces breast inflammation.
Astringent lactifuge herbs that reduce milk flow when weaning ~ Cinquefoil, Cranesbill, Sage, and Yarrow.

Bronchitis: See Lung and Bronchial Problems

Bruises: See Skin

Burns:

Blue Vervain ~ antibiotic, anti-inflammatory, analgesic, cooling; specific for healing burns.
Burdock ~ applied externally for burns; cooling and anti-inflammatory.
Calendula ~ antiseptic; applied externally to promote tissue regeneration and reduce scar formation.
Chamomile ~ applied externally; cooling, anti-inflammatory, antiseptic; promotes tissue regeneration.
Chickweed ~ soothing, cooling, moisturizing, anti-inflammatory.
Cinquefoil ~ excellent when applied to burns to reduce pain and stimulate healing.
Comfrey ~ excellent external application for burns; soothing, cooling, moisturizing; promotes tissue growth.
Echinacea ~ used externally to reduce pain, inflammation, and prevent and treat infection.
Elderberry ~ berries are applied externally to soothe and heal tissues.
Goldenrod ~ applied externally as an antiseptic; heals and relieves the pain of burns.
Hops ~ antiseptic, soothing, cooling, and analgesic when applied to burns.
Lavender ~ antiseptic and analgesic; reduces scaring.
Lemon Balm ~ antiseptic, analgesic, and healing when applied to burns.
Marshmallow ~ soothing, cooling, and moisturizing.
Mullein ~ applied externally; cooling, anti-inflammatory, moisturizing, and analgesic.
Saint John's Wort ~ specific for burns when applied externally; analgesic; antiseptic.
Stinging Nettle ~ external application is healing, cooling, and anti-inflammatory.
Yarrow ~ excellent for all types of mild and severe burns; cooling, analgesic, and antiseptic.

Bursitis (inflamed bursa, the pad-like sacs containing synovial fluid that lubricates joints): See Arthritis

Cancer and Tumors:

Cancer cells begin as normal cells that become damaged or mutated and cease to function correctly. Normally, human cells grow and divide to form new cells as the body needs them. When cells age or become damaged, they are genetically programmed to die by a process called apoptosis, and are replaced by new healthy cells. In cancerous cells, DNA and RNA damage causes genetic changes and rapid, unchecked division of damaged, malfunctioning cells. Many cancer cells form solid tumors and some, like blood and lymphatic cancers, do not. Malignant tumors invade other tissues, but benign tumors do not.

Do your best to prevent cancer by 1) eating a healthy diet of organic, non-GMO whole foods; 2) avoiding man-made chemicals in food, water, body care products, home cleaners, pesticides, and herbicides; and 3) letting go of upsetting, harmful thoughts and emotions by developing a calm mind and compassionate heart.

***Always** enlist the aid of oncologists when dealing with cancer. Many herbs are used in treatment programs, including radiation and chemotherapy, to reduce side effects, nausea and pain, support immunity, and improve quality of life. Herbal adaptogens, antioxidants, anti-inflammatories, immunomodulators, and immunostimulants can be beneficial adjuvants in healing cancer.*

Astragalus ~ antiviral; immunostimulant; used during chemotherapy and radiation to decrease nausea, vomiting, weight loss, fatigue, and secondary bacterial infections.
Black Cohosh ~ studies show it protects against some estrogen-dependent cancers and inhibits proliferation of breast cancer cells.
Black Walnut ~ detoxifies blood and lymph; an antiviral that inhibits some cancers.
Bloodroot ~ historically used for internal and external cancers and tumors (be cautious of toxicity).
Blue Vervain ~ research shows it induces death of some cancer cells and may be helpful in treating leukemia.

Boneset ~ stimulates immunity and contains anticarcinogenic and antitumor phytochemicals.
Burdock ~ an ingredient in many cancer formulas, including Essiac and Hoxsey; contains anticarcinogens.
Calendula ~ stimulates immunity; detoxifies blood and lymph; historically used as a cancer treatment.
Cayenne ~ antioxidants help protect against cellular damage; some constituents may inhibit cancer.
Chasteberry ~ used for prostate cancer and female reproductive cancers related to hormonal imbalance.
Chickweed ~ detoxifies blood and lymph; alkalizing.
Dandelion ~ historically used in treating specific cancers; immunostimulant against some cancers.
Echinacea ~ specific for treatment of cancer due to immune stimulating activity, blood and lymphatic cleansing, and antiviral properties; used during chemotherapy and radiation.
Elderberry ~ berries are a highly nutritious cancer preventative.
Elecampane ~ research shows it reduces some tumors by destroying their energy-producing mitochondria.
Feverfew ~ parthenolide stimulates immune response and induces apoptosis (programmed destruction of cancerous cells).
Goldenrod ~ *in vivo* research shows activity against melanoma, prostate, breast, and lung cancers.
Goldenseal ~ research shows it stimulates white blood cells to destroy some types of cancerous cells.
Holy Basil ~ stimulates immunity; shows anticancer activity; protects cells against radiation damage.
Hops ~ found to inhibit cancer cells in lab testing; may be helpful against some cancers.
Isatis ~ may be helpful for some cancers, specifically prostate.
Lavender ~ antiviral; preliminary investigations demonstrate anticarcinogenic activity.
Motherwort ~ research shows potential for treating leukemia and breast, uterine, lung, and colon cancers.
Mugwort ~ research shows cytotoxic activity against leukemia and breast cancers.
Saint John's Wort ~ studies show ability to destroy some types of cancer cells and prevent metastasis.
Scullcap ~ studies show it may reduce fibrosarcoma cancer of the connective tissue.

Other Helpful Herbs:

Ashwagandha (*Withania somnifera*) ~ an immunomodulator; inhibits tumor growth; promotes apoptosis; used for breast, lung, and colon cancers; increases white blood cell count during chemotherapy.
Bupleurum (*Bupleurum chinense*) ~ immunomodulator; antioxidant; inhibits development and metastasis of tumor and cancer cells by increasing macrophage activity and apoptosis.
Ginseng, Asian (*Panax ginseng*) and American (*Panax quinquefolius*) ~ antioxidant; immunostimulant; studies indicate benefit for some cancers and tumors, including lung, liver, pancreas, stomach, and ovarian; used in conjunction with cancer treatments; protects healthy cells from radiation damage.
Licorice (*Glycyrrhiza glabra*) ~ immunostimulant; research shows cytotoxic action on some tumor cells.
Maitake (*Grifola frondosa*), Reishi (*Ganoderma lucidum*), Shiitake (*Lentinula edodes*), and Turkey Tail (*Trametes versicolor*) mushrooms ~ immunomodulators and immunostimulants; used for many conditions, including cancer; strengthen a weak immune system; helpful for autoimmune conditions.
Pacific Yew (*Taxus brevifolia*) ~ prevents cancer cells from replicating; can help treat many types of cancer.
Pau D'arco (*Tabebuia impetiginosa*) ~ an immunomodulator; can stimulate apoptosis and reduce metastasis.
Red Clover (*Trifolium pratense*) ~ excellent blood purifier; research shows it inhibits several types of cancers, including reproductive cancers.
Turmeric (*Curcuma longa*) ~ inhibits most aspects of cancer development; supports immunity; protects cells from toxin and radiation damage by reducing inflammation, oxidation, and free radical scavenging; promotes apoptosis; inhibits cancer cell replication; used for prevention and treatment in conjunction with medical therapies.

Candida Yeast: See Fungal Infections (yeast is a fungus)

Canker Sores: See Mouth

Carpal Tunnel: (also see Inflammation and Pain)

Cayenne ~ externally applied for pain relief; internally taken to increase circulation to the wrist.
Sage ~ oil, salve, or liniment are externally applied to relieve wrist inflammation.
Saint John's Wort ~ taken internally and applied externally to relieve pain and inflammation.

Cataracts: See Eyes

Cervical Dysplasia: See Uterus

Chicken Pox (caused by the herpes virus *Varicella zoster*): See Herpes Virus

Childbirth: See pages 608-610 in "Herbs for Pregnancy, Childbirth, and Lactation"

Cholesterol: See Liver

Chronic Fatigue Syndrome (CFS):

CFS is a systemic condition involving chronic immuno-endocrine deficiency and dysfunction, including impaired adrenal, thyroid, and liver function. Chronic infection of Epstein-Barr, cytomegalovirus (both members of the herpes family of viruses), and Candida yeast are possible causes of CFS, as are environmental toxins and food allergies. Treatment consists of a healthy diet, avoiding harmful chemicals, and using herbs that are adaptogens, antioxidants, and support immunity, the endocrine glands (especially adrenals and thyroid), and detoxify the liver and lymphatic system.

Astragalus ~ strengthens immunity and supports the endocrine glands.
Cayenne ~ has warming, stimulating actions on circulation; improves glandular functions and secretions.
Elderberry ~ berries are highly nutritious and fortifying; promote vitality and strengthen muscles.

Elecampane ~ stimulates normal organ and glandular function; addresses underlying causes of fatigue, especially when lung weakness is involved.
Holy Basil ~ restores adrenal function; nourishing and normalizing to nervous and endocrine systems.
Lemon Balm ~ can be effective against the Epstein-Barr virus implicated in CFS.
Motherwort ~ effective against the Epstein-Barr virus.
Saint John's Wort ~ a powerful antiviral against the Epstein-Barr virus; helpful for reducing depression.
Stinging Nettle ~ highly nutritious leaves nourish the system and promote vitality.

Other Helpful Herbs:

Eleuthero/Siberian Ginseng (*Eleutherococcus senticosus*) ~ an adaptogen; supports immunity; reduces the stress response.
Ginseng, American (*Panax quinquefolius*) and Asian (*Panax ginseng*) - adaptogens that energize the adrenals and reduce chronic fatigue.

Cigarette Smoking: See Nicotine Withdrawal

Circulation: See Blood and Vascular System

Colds (Rhinitis) and Flu (Influenza):

The common cold and flu are viral infections, requiring antiviral herbs. However, bacterial infections like sinusitis may also be present and require antibacterial botanicals. Use herbs that support the immune system and avoid mucous-forming foods (sugar, dairy, gluten in grains), red meat, and alcohol while ill.

Astragalus ~ stimulates the immune system; antiviral and antibacterial.
Blue Vervain ~ antibacterial and antiviral; decreases fever, inflammation, and excessive mucous discharge.
Boneset ~ a superior remedy and immunostimulant for colds, flu, and sinus infections; reduces fever, muscle aches, and mucous drainage and congestion.
Calendula ~ a mild antiviral and antibacterial; safe for children.
Catnip ~ helpful for colds, flu, fevers, and coughs; specific for infants and young children.
Cayenne ~ antibacterial for sinusitis; superb for coughs and colds; decreases mucous drainage and congestion.
Chamomile ~ stimulates immunity; mild antibacterial and antiviral; reduces mucous, inflammation, fevers.
Echinacea ~ strong immunostimulant, antiviral, antibacterial; reduces inflammation and mucous discharge.
Elderberry ~ berries and flowers are specific for viral infections, sinus drainage, coughs, and fevers.
Elecampane ~ specific for excessive mucous discharge and congestion; antiviral and antibacterial.
Feverfew ~ reduces mucous discharge; antibacterial.
Goldenrod ~ reduces excess mucous production; has antihistamine action.
Goldenseal ~ normalizes mucous secretion; antimicrobial; reduces sinus inflammation; a superb nasal spray.
Holy Basil ~ strengthens immunity; antiviral, antibacterial; reduces fevers and excessive mucous production.
Hyssop ~ antiviral and antibacterial; specific for respiratory distress, mucous congestion, and coughs.
Isatis ~ strong antiviral and antibacterial; cooling to reduce high fevers.
Lavender ~ antiviral against colds and flu; reduces fevers; analgesic for pain.
Lemon Balm ~ antiviral; reduces fevers and excessive mucous production; analgesic.
Motherwort ~ reduces mucous congestion in lungs and nasal sinuses; lowers fevers.
Mullein ~ tea is excellent for upper respiratory infections and the flu.
Peppermint ~ antimicrobial; reduces fevers; thins mucous, breaks up lung congestion; helpful for coughs.
Pleurisy Root ~ specific for lungs; reduces mucous congestion; helpful for dry or productive coughs.
Sage ~ antiviral; specific for fever, coughs, sore throats, and body aches that accompany colds and flu.
Thyme ~ antiviral; specific for the respiratory system; reduces fevers, excess mucous, and congestion.
Wood Betony ~ helpful for colds and sinus congestion.
Yarrow ~ excellent for flu and high fevers; analgesic; decreases excess mucous and breaks up congestion.

Other Helpful Herbs:

Angelica (*Angelica archangelica*) ~ anti-inflammatory; expectorant for coughs, bronchitis, cold, and flu.
Bupleurum (*Bupleurum chinense*) ~ helpful for colds, flu, fever, coughs, bronchitis, pneumonia, and asthma.
Eucalyptus (*Eucalyptus* spp.) ~ antimicrobial, expectorant, and anti-inflammatory for colds and flu.
Fenugreek seeds (*Trigonella foenum-graecum*) ~ a soothing expectorant; beneficial for bronchitis, colds, flu.
Garlic (*Allium sativum*) ~ a strong antibacterial and antiviral commonly taken for colds and flu.
Ginger (*Zingiber officinale*) ~ antibacterial; breaks up mucous congestion; diaphoretic action lowers fevers.
Linden (*Tilia* spp.) ~ decreases mucous; helpful to relieve sore throats, colds, flu, and coughs; lowers fevers.
Oregano (*Origanum vulgare*) ~ strong anti-inflammatory and antioxidant; antimicrobial for infections; expectorant; beneficial for sore throat, coughs with thick mucous, bronchitis, laryngitis, and pharyngitis.
Oregon Grape Root (*Mahonia aquifolium*) ~ strong antibacterial and antiviral; reduces excess mucous.
Pau D'arco (*Tabebuia impetiginosa*) ~ an immunomodulator; antibacterial and antiviral for colds and flu.
Rosemary (*Rosmarinus officinalis*) ~ antibacterial and antiviral; anti-inflammatory; specific for colds and flu.
Wild Indigo (*Baptisia tinctoria*) ~ strong immunostimulant and antimicrobial to treat colds and flu.

Cold Sores: See Herpes Virus (causes cold sores)

Colic: See Digestion, Infants, and Stomach

Colon: See Intestines

Constipation: See Intestines

Convulsions: See Seizures

Coronary Artery Disease: See Vascular System
Cough: See Lung and Bronchial Problems
Cramps and Spasms: See Muscle or Menstruation
Crohn's Disease: See Intestines
Cyst:

The body protects itself from the dangers of abnormal cells by encapsulating them in a closed sack, or cyst, in the form of fluids, fats, and other semi-solid material. There are many types of cysts and although most are benign, some may develop into cancer. Using herbs that are antioxidants, strengthen the immune system, and detoxify the liver, blood, and lymphatic system are important to reduce cysts and ensure vibrant health.

Burdock ~ helpful for breast and ovarian cysts.
Calendula ~ helpful in reducing all types of cysts.
Chasteberry ~ reduces breast and ovarian cysts caused by estrogen dominance.
Chickweed ~ helps dissolve and reduce cysts.
Dandelion ~ reduces toxic heat; helps liver clear excess estrogen promoting hormone-related cyst formation.
Saint John's Wort ~ detoxifying action; clears excess estrogen from the liver that promotes cyst formation.

Dandruff: See Hair
Dehydration:

Catnip ~ used for dehydration caused by high fevers.
Chickweed ~ very moisturizing; drink tea throughout the day to restore moisture to tissues.
Marshmallow ~ very moisturizing; drink tea throughout the day to rehydrate tissues.

Delirium Tremens: See Drug and Alcohol Withdrawal
Depression (also see Brain and Cognitive Function):

Depression is often the normal response to dealing with difficult people and situations in our life, and the best action is to take charge and make necessary adjustments. But depression may also be caused by imbalance of the endocrine glands (especially pituitary, thyroid, adrenal, and reproductive glands) and neurotransmitters, including deficiencies of serotonin (a calming neurotransmitter), adrenaline (epinephrine), norepinephrine, dopamine, or phenylalanine (excitatory, stimulating neurotransmitters). Urine and saliva tests are helpful in determining adrenal and neurotransmitter levels.

Black Cohosh ~ for dark, brooding depression, premenstrual syndrome (PMS), and menopausal depression.
Blue Vervain ~ for depression and anxiety, chronic fatigue, and a debilitated nervous system.
Holy Basil ~ especially helpful for depression caused by stress, exhaustion, and adrenal "burn-out."
Lavender ~ has a stimulating and uplifting effect on a depleted, depressed nervous system.
Lemon Balm ~ helpful for depression and seasonal affective disorder (SAD).
Saint John's Wort ~ a classic herb for depression; balances brain neurotransmitters, especially serotonin.
Valerian ~ has a restorative effect on a depleted nervous system.

Other Helpful Herbs:

Damiana (*Turnera diffusa*) ~ for mild depression with loss of libido.
Rosemary (*Rosmarinus officinalis*) ~ improves brain function; a stimulating nervine helpful for depression.

Dermatitis: See Skin
Detoxification (also see Blood, Intestines, Liver, and Lymphatic System):

In addition to waste products that the body produces from daily metabolic processes, people are constantly exposed to toxic chemicals in food, water, and the environment. The blood, lymphatic system, liver, kidneys, and intestines are the primary focus of detoxification. Ingesting organic foods, purified water, and periodic use of detoxifying herbs promotes healthy tissues and helps prevents disease.

American Centaury ~ has stimulating and cleansing actions on the liver, kidneys, and blood to remove toxins throughout the body.
Black Walnut ~ antimicrobial; a laxative that opens channels of elimination to clean blood and lymph.
Bloodroot ~ powerful cleanser of blood and tissues; strong immunostimulant specifically used for detoxification in cases of cancer; use cautiously in small doses due to toxicity.
Blue Vervain ~ stimulates and detoxifies the liver, kidneys, and bloodstream; reduces excess acids.
Boneset ~ detoxifies the liver, kidneys, and blood; reduces acids and excess heat in the bloodstream.
Burdock ~ stimulates detoxification of the liver, kidneys, blood, and lymph.
Calendula ~ excellent for liver, blood, and lymphatic cleansing.
Cayenne ~ stimulating action on blood circulation, sweat glands, liver, kidneys, and intestines promotes detoxification.
Chickweed ~ detoxifies blood and lymphatic fluids; cooling and moisturizing for hot, toxic conditions.
Cinquefoil ~ specific for septicemia and toxemia (toxins in the blood).
Dandelion ~ stimulates elimination; removes toxic heat and acids; cleanses blood, lymph, liver, kidneys.
Echinacea ~ stimulates the immune system to neutralize toxins, poisons, venoms, bacteria, viruses, and fungi; an excellent blood and lymphatic detoxifier.
Elderberry ~ berries stimulate elimination; excellent blood and lymphatic cleanser; alkalizing to blood.
Elecampane ~ helps normalize liver and kidney function to detoxify poisons and clear them from the body; a stimulating blood cleanser.

Goldenrod ~ promotes detoxification by removing waste products via the kidneys.
Holy Basil ~ a blood purifier that eliminates toxins, poisons and venom, including animal bites and stings.
Horehound ~ alkalizing; reduces excess acids in the blood and tissues; supports liver and kidney function; used to treat venomous bites and stings and bites from rabid animals.
Hyssop ~ cleansing to the liver, kidneys, blood, and skin.
Lemon Balm ~ protects cells from radiation and chemical damage by increasing levels of the body's natural antioxidants (superoxide dismutase/SOD, glutathione, and catalase), protecting cell membranes from lipid peroxidation (the destruction of fats in cell membranes), and protecting cellular DNA.
Lobelia ~ causes vomiting and is used for food poisoning; externally applied to venomous bites and stings.
Saint John's Wort ~ a powerful blood and liver cleanser; excellent antidote to treat acute reactions to toxins, poisons, venom, and rabies.
Senna ~ laxative actions are beneficial for colon cleansing; used during detox programs.
Stinging Nettle ~ supports release of wastes through kidneys; cleansing to blood, lymph, liver, and skin.
Yellow Dock ~ removes toxins by cleansing actions on the liver, kidneys, blood, lymph, and skin.
Other Helpful Herbs:
Chlorella (*Chlorella* spp.) and Spirulina (*Arthrospira platensis, A. maxima*) ~ high nutrient freshwater algae; reduce heavy metals and chemical toxins from bloodstream and tissues.
Ginkgo (*Ginkgo biloba*) ~ reduces oxidative stress and free radical damage in tissues; decreases chromosomal damage in cells following exposure to radiation.
Milk Thistle (*Silybum marianum*) ~ a primary liver detoxification herb that eliminates toxins in the liver and their release into the bloodstream, lymphatic fluids, and tissues throughout the body.
Turmeric (*Curcuma longa*) ~ antioxidant; detoxifies liver; protects cellular and DNA damage from toxins.
Diabetes (Hyperglycemia): See Pancreas
Diarrhea: See Intestines
Digestive System (also see Stomach, Pancreas, Liver, Gallbladder, and Intestines):
A well-functioning digestive system is fundamental to health and optimizes the healing potential of herbal therapy. Digestive enzymes secreted from the stomach and pancreas and bile produced in the liver determine how well food is broken down to be metabolized into usable energy at the cellular level. Normal stomach, pancreas, and liver activity are necessary for the health and functions of the intestines. Serotonin supports the nervous system of the solar plexus to promote optimal, harmonious function of the digestive system.
American Centaury ~ stimulates sluggish digestion by increasing production of stomach and pancreatic enzymes and bile from the liver; decreases gas, bloating, indigestion, nausea, heartburn, and constipation.
Astragalus ~ strengthens weak digestive organs; helps indigestion, abdominal bloating, and poor appetite.
Blue Vervain ~ a bitter, stimulating tonic that strengthens digestive organs, increases enzyme and bile production, and promotes intestinal movement; relieves indigestion, abdominal spasms, gas, and pain.
Boneset ~ increases enzymes and bile; stimulates sluggish digestion; eases gas and bloating; a mild laxative.
Burdock ~ supports the liver and gallbladder; reduces inflammation, excess stomach acid, and constipation.
Calendula ~ taken for stomachaches, indigestion, gastrointestinal ulcers, and liver problems.
Catnip ~ for nervous stomach, nausea, indigestion, gas, heartburn, ulcers, and irritable bowel conditions.
Cayenne ~ stimulates secretion of digestive enzymes and peristaltic movements in the intestines; reduces gas, bloating, indigestion, ulcers, and constipation; antibacterial; kills parasites.
Chamomile ~ for digestive problems caused by nervous tension, including indigestion, gas, bloating, cramps, spasms, diarrhea, stomach and intestinal ulcers and inflammation, and irritable bowel conditions.
Chickweed ~ soothing and moisturizing to tissues and mucous membranes; anti-inflammatory; heals ulcers.
Comfrey ~ tea is soothing and healing to all tissues it contacts; helpful for inflammatory bowel diseases, ulcers, heartburn, upset stomach, and constipation.
Dandelion ~ a gentle bitter that stimulates secretion of stomach and pancreatic enzymes and bile; normalizes digestion; beneficial for poor fat metabolism and relieving gas and indigestion.
Elderberry ~ stimulates production of enzymes and movement through the digestive tract; healing to ulcers.
Elecampane ~ a stimulating bitter; strengthens and tones a sluggish and congested digestive system; promotes enzyme production; helpful for indigestion, gas, bloating, diarrhea, and constipation.
Feverfew ~ a bitter tonic that stimulates normal digestion, secretion of enzymes, and bile flow; helpful for a sluggish digestive system, gas, indigestion, cramps, colic, and constipation.
Goldenrod ~ stimulating for sluggish digestion; reduces gas, diarrhea, and yeast overgrowth.
Goldenseal ~ anti-inflammatory; antimicrobial for gastrointestinal infections; normalizes mucous membranes.
Holy Basil ~ stimulates enzyme production; decreases indigestion, gas, bloating, vomiting, ulcers, spasms.
Hops ~ a stimulating bitter for sluggish digestion, gas, and bloating; increases enzyme secretions and intestinal movements; antibacterial; helpful for digestive problems caused by nervous anxiety.
Horehound ~ a stimulating bitter that increases enzymes and bile; for indigestion, gas, bloating, constipation.
Hyssop ~ anti-inflammatory; anti-bacterial; used for indigestion, gas, colic, and constipation.
Lavender ~ for indigestion and problems due to anxiety, including cramps, spasms, nausea, irritable bowel.
Lemon Balm ~ used for digestive problems caused by tension and anxiety, including indigestion, gas, cramps, nausea, vomiting, and stomachaches; antimicrobial against infections and Candida yeast.
Lobelia ~ relaxing and normalizing to nerves; benefits digestive problems and spasms caused by tension.

Marshmallow ~ helps relieve heartburn, ulcers, inflammatory conditions, spasms, and irritable bowel.
Motherwort ~ bitter tonic that improves digestion and helps digestive problems caused by anxiety.
Mugwort ~ helpful for infections, nervous stomach, spasms, diarrhea, constipation, and parasites.
Mullein ~ contains soothing mucilage; reduces inflammation and spasms.
Peppermint ~ anti-inflammatory; helpful for spasms, nausea, gas, bloating, and indigestion; contraindicated in cases of acid reflux and gastroesophageal reflux disorder (GERD).
Sage ~ antibiotic; reduces spasms and inflammation; stimulates production of digestive enzymes; used for nausea, indigestion, gas, bloating, diarrhea, and bad breath.
Saint John's Wort ~ helps regulate and calm the solar plexus and digestive organs; anti-inflammatory.
Thyme ~ for indigestion due to anxiety; antimicrobial; decreases bad breath, inflammation, cramps, and gas.
Valerian ~ helpful for indigestion, gas, bloating, spasms, and ulcers caused by anxiety.
Wood Betony ~ specific for nervous indigestion; eases cramps, colic, heartburn, gas, and bloating.
Yarrow ~ stimulates secretions of digestive enzymes; anti-inflammatory; reduces spasms; good for all types of indigestion, gas, bloating, and constipation or diarrhea.
Yellow Dock ~ a stimulating bitter tonic for sluggish digestion and constipation; increases bile production.

Other Helpful Herbs:

Andrographis (*Andrographis paniculata*) ~ a bitter, stimulating liver tonic; promotes production of digestive enzymes; antioxidant; anti-inflammatory; antibacterial; antiviral; used for indigestion, gas, bloating, diarrhea, gastroenteritis, irritable bowel, ulcerative colitis, Crohn's disease, dysentery, and intestinal worms.
Angelica (*Angelica archangelica*) ~ anti-inflammatory; a carminative that reduces gas and colic.
Anise (*Pimpinella anisum*) ~ carminative; relaxes and normalizes the digestive system, especially the stomach.
Blessed Thistle (*Cnicus benedictus*) ~ a strong bitter; a digestive stimulant that increases stomach, liver, and small intestine activity; improves sluggish liver and poor fat metabolism; helpful for hiatal hernia.
Cabbage, White (*Brassica oleracea*) ~ contains significant amounts of glutamine, an anti-inflammatory amino acid that supports and heals membranes lining the stomach and intestines; contains indole-3-carbinol, which enhances DNA repair in cells; drinking a quart of raw, freshly juiced white cabbage throughout the day for several weeks is very healing for stomach and intestinal ulcers.
Caraway (*Carum carvi*) ~ helpful for indigestion, gas, bloating, cramps, and irritable bowel syndrome.
Cardamom (*Elettaria cardamomum*) ~ reduces indigestion, gas, and cramps.
Codonopsis root (*Codonopsis pilosula*) ~ adaptogen and immunomodulator; antibacterial and antifungal; used for chronic inflammation of the gastrointestinal tract in Traditional Chinese Medicine.
Fennel (*Foeniculum vulgare*) ~ excellent for chronic indigestion, gas, bloating, spasms, and irritable bowel.
Fenugreek seed (*Trigonella foenum-graecum*) ~ soothing anti-inflammatory; for gastritis and irritable bowel.
Garlic (*Allium sativum*) ~ strong antimicrobial for stomach and intestinal infections and spasms.
Licorice (*Glycyrrhiza glabra*) ~ excellent for healing inflammation, spasms, ulcers, heartburn, and gastritis.
Linden (*Tilia* spp.) ~ relieves indigestion, heartburn, low stomach acidity, and constipation.
Oregano (*Origanum vulgare*) ~ strong anti-inflammatory and antioxidant; reduces spasms, cramps, and gas; antibacterial and antifungal (kills Candida yeast).
Oregon Grape Root (*Mahonia aquifolium*) ~ antimicrobial; anti-inflammatory; improves sluggish digestion.
Parsley (*Petroselinum crispum*) ~ decreases gastrointestinal spasms, gas, and colic.
Pau D'arco (*Tabebuia impetiginosa*) ~ for bacterial, viral, and fungal infection; helps gastritis and diarrhea.
Rosemary (*Rosmarinus officinalis*) ~ has toning and calming effect on the digestive system; especially effective in cases of nervous tension; beneficial for inflammation, spasms, indigestion, gas, and infections.
Wild Yam (*Dioscorea villosa*) ~ an anti-inflammatory and antispasmodic specific for the digestive tract.

Dizziness (Vertigo): See Ears

Drug and Alcohol Withdrawal:

Provide good nutrition and support the nervous and endocrine systems when working with addiction and recovery. Neurotransmitter levels and endocrine glands are negatively affected and should be a primary focus. To calm and restore the nervous system, use a high-potency vitamin B complex, calcium, magnesium, essential fatty acids, and herbs that are calming, antioxidant, and support liver and general detoxing.

Black Cohosh ~ used for delirium tremens from drug and alcohol withdrawal; calms and restores nerves.
Blue Vervain ~ restores debilitated nerves; relaxing sedative; helps delirium tremens; healing to the liver.
Cayenne ~ helps with tremors, hallucinations, mental confusion, and restlessness during withdrawal.
Chasteberry ~ can help withdrawal from drugs due to its ability to attach to dopamine cell receptors.
Feverfew ~ reduces spasms and delirium tremens.
Hops ~ sedating to the nervous system; reduces spasms and delirium tremens.
Lavender ~ sedating; analgesic; reduces tension, muscle cramps, and spasms.
Lemon Balm ~ sedating; improves cognitive function; reduces tension, anxiety, muscle cramps, and spasms.
Lobelia ~ sedating and restoring to the nervous system; reduces agitation, anxiety, muscle cramps, and spasms; helpful for withdrawal from drugs, especially nicotine.
Motherwort ~ calming and restoring to the nerves; reduces spasms; helpful for delirium tremens.
Passion Flower ~ calming; anti-anxiety; antispasmodic; helpful for delirium tremens.
Scullcap ~ excellent to ease and restore a depleted nervous system; helpful in treating delirium tremens.
Valerian ~ excellent sedative and nervine tonic to restore a depleted nervous system; helps delirium tremens.

Dysentery: See Intestines

Ears (Tinnitus, Vertigo):

Black Cohosh ~ specific for <u>tinnitus</u> (ringing in the ears).
Blue Vervain ~ for tinnitus and <u>vertigo</u> (dizziness).
Calendula ~ putting a few drops of oil made from the flowers into the ears reduces infection and pain.
Cranesbill ~ reduces fluid accumulation in the ears, which can cause tinnitus and diminished hearing.
Dandelion ~ a diuretic that can reduce edema in the inner ear, a cause of tinnitus and diminished hearing.
Echinacea ~ an effective antibiotic for ear infections.
Goldenseal ~ used as ear drops for infection, inflammation, and earaches.
Holy Basil ~ traditionally used for earaches; analgesic; anti-inflammatory; antibacterial.
Hops ~ a diuretic used to remove fluid from the ears; analgesic; antibacterial.
Mullein ~ drops of flower oil are placed in the ears to treat infections and earaches.
Sage ~ specific for vertigo with underlying nerve weakness and deterioration.

Other Helpful Herbs:

Bupleurum (*Bupleurum chinense*) ~ can be beneficial for treating tinnitus and vertigo.
Eclipta (*Eclipta prostata*) ~ helpful for dizziness caused by liver or kidney deficiency.
Garlic (*Allium sativum*) ~ antimicrobial; use the oil as ear drops for infection and pain.
Ginkgo (*Ginkgo biloba*) ~ increases blood circulation to the head; helps regenerate damaged nerves; used for ear-related problems such as vertigo, tinnitus, Meniere's disease, and hearing loss.
Privet (*Ligustrum lucidum*) ~ helpful for dizziness and tinnitus caused by liver or kidney deficiency.
Wild Indigo (*Baptisia tinctoria*) ~ antimicrobial; small amounts are taken internally; tea or diluted tincture are applied as ear drops.

Eczema:

Eczema is an inflammatory skin condition causing an itchy, red rash and is related to stress, toxic overload, and sensitivity to food and/or environmental allergies. The use of immunosuppressant steroid drugs is the most common conventional treatment for eczema, but this only masks symptoms rather than healing the underlying causes, and side effects can be more problematic than the skin condition. Herbal therapy combined with healthy diet, lifestyle, and a calm emotional environment can safely help correct underlying imbalances and reduce symptoms. A chemical-free diet and home are important. The most problematic foods to be avoided include sugar, dairy, eggs, gluten grains, corn, tomato, coffee, and chemical food additives.

American Centaury ~ decreases heat and inflammation in the skin; cleansing to blood, liver, and kidneys.
Astragalus ~ fortifies the blood; releases heat, toxins, and inflammation from the skin.
Black Walnut ~ beneficial for eczema related to a congested digestive system, constipation, and toxic excess.
Blue Vervain ~ healing for hot, red, irritated and inflamed skin conditions.
Burdock ~ a specific remedy for eczema; take internally and apply externally.
Calendula ~ decreases inflammation; cleansing to the blood, lymph, and liver.
Chamomile ~ specific for eczema; cooling; anti-inflammatory; take internally and soak skin with tea.
Chickweed ~ soothing, cooling, and cleansing to inflamed, irritated tissues.
Dandelion ~ reduces heat and inflammation; cleansing actions improve toxic conditions.
Echinacea ~ cleansing to the blood and lymphatic systems; cooling; reduces inflammation and toxic load.
Elderberry ~ berries are antioxidant, cooling, and cleansing to blood and lymph; alkalizing; fortifies blood.
Elecampane ~ detoxifies blood; helps heal inflammatory skin conditions.
Goldenrod ~ cleansing to blood; anti-inflammatory.
Goldenseal ~ cleanses the blood and lymphatic system; soothing and cooling to inflamed tissues.
Hops ~ cleansing; cooling; anti-inflammatory.
Isatis ~ cleansing; anti-inflammatory; cooling to system.
Lobelia ~ helpful when used as a skin wash and taken internally for underlying nervous tension.
Marshmallow ~ soothing and cooling to dry, inflamed skin.
Saint John's Wort ~ applied externally and taken internally for underlying nervous tension and detoxification.
Stinging Nettle ~ cleansing to blood and lymph; anti-inflammatory; specific for eczema.
Yarrow ~ cooling; anti-inflammatory.
Yellow Dock ~ cleansing to the blood and lymphatic system; soothing and cooling to inflamed tissues.

Other Helpful Herbs:

Cleavers (*Galium aparine*) and Red Clover (*Trifolium pratense*) ~ reduce toxins in blood and lymph.
Evening Primrose oil (*Oenothera biennis*) ~ gamma-linolenic acid (GLA) benefits dry, scaly skin conditions.
Licorice (*Glycyrrhiza glabra*) ~ has anti-inflammatory actions similar to hydrocortisone; reduces toxic overload in liver and blood; ingesting the root and using topical applications are beneficial for eczema.
Oregon Grape Root (*Mahonia aquifolium*) ~ antimicrobial; anti-inflammatory; helps scaly skin conditions.
Sarsaparilla (*Smilax ornata*) ~ helpful for skin diseases by binding to endotoxins (toxins excreted from bacteria) in the gut, prohibiting absorption; specific for scaly skin conditions such as eczema and psoriasis.

Edema (water retention in the tissues): See Kidneys

Endocrine Glands (also see Hypothalamus for endocrine gland support):

The seven endocrine glands include the pineal, pituitary, thyroid, thymus, pancreas, ovaries or testes, and adrenals. They are master regulators of the body and their health is important for all functions. The following herbs are general tonics that support and strengthen the endocrine glands and should be taken for several weeks. Adaptogen and antioxidant herbs provide excellent support for the endocrine system. High-quality glandular supplements are also very helpful in supporting and strengthening endocrine glands.

Astragalus ~ nourishes and tones endocrine glands; an adaptogen herb helpful for coping with stress.
Cayenne ~ a stimulating restorative for sluggish, underactive endocrine glands.
Chasteberry ~ helps restore function of the pituitary and pineal glands.
Elderberry ~ the highly nutritious, alkalizing berries are a revitalizing tonic to the endocrine glands.
Holy Basil ~ an excellent adaptogen and tonic for the endocrine system, especially the adrenals and pituitary.
Lobelia ~ small doses stimulate secretion of hormones by the endocrine glands.
Sage ~ vitalizes and restores the adrenals, pituitary, and ovaries.
Stinging Nettle ~ nourishes and tones the endocrine glands.

Endometriosis: See Uterus

Epilepsy: See Seizures

Epstein-Barr Virus:

Epstein-Barr, a member of the herpes family of viruses, is implicated as a cause of mononucleosis, fibromyalgia, chronic fatigue syndrome, and some cancers, autoimmune diseases, and other chronic degenerative conditions. Treatment consists of using antiviral and immune-enhancing herbs.

Astragalus ~ an immunostimulant specific for the herpes family of viruses.
Boneset ~ one of the best immunostimulants; specific for herpes viruses.
Echinacea ~ an immunostimulant specific for the herpes family of viruses.
Elderberry ~ the berries are antiviral for treating herpes viruses.
Feverfew ~ parthenolide suppresses growth of the Epstein-Barr virus.
Hyssop ~ an antiviral specific against the herpes virus family.
Isatis ~ a strong, cooling antiviral.
Lemon Balm ~ a primary herb that is specific against the herpes virus family.
Mugwort ~ active against the herpes virus family.
Saint John's Wort ~ primary antiviral specific against the herpes virus family; protects and supports the liver.

Other Helpful Herbs:

Cat's Claw (*Uncaria tomentosa*) ~ an immunomodulator and stimulant; increases lymphocyte production and phagocytosis to destroy pathogens; anti-inflammatory; antiviral against Epstein-Barr.
Pau D'arco (*Tabebuia impetiginosa*) ~ an immunomodulator; antiviral; used for herpes family, mononucleosis.

Eyes:

Only use herbs for eye care when they are prepared as tea that has been thoroughly filtered to remove all sediment, poured into sterile glass containers, and refrigerated. The tea is used as eye drops or eye wash. Never put tincture or oils in the eye.

Calendula ~ applied to the eyes for conjunctivitis, inflammation, and irritation.
Catnip ~ drinking the tea provides antioxidants that are helpful for cataracts.
Chickweed ~ application soothes inflammation and itching; used for conjunctivitis, styes, pollen irritation.
Comfrey ~ eye drops or wash soothes and helps cellular repair in irritated and injured eyes.
Echinacea ~ applied as eye drops or wash for irritated and infected eyes.
Goldenseal ~ superior for serious eye infections, styes, allergies, inflammation, irritation, and itching.
Hyssop ~ apply to eye for bacterial infections and inflammation.
Isatis ~ eye drops or wash is used for irritation and infections.
Marshmallow ~ soothing and healing when applied to irritated, inflamed, dry eyes.

Other Helpful Herbs:

Bilberry (*Vaccinium myrtillus*) ~ promotes circulation to the head and eyes to enhance vision; helps prevent and treat eye disorders, including macular degeneration, cataracts, retina damage, and night blindness.
Eyebright (*Euphrasia rostkoviana*) ~ eyewash of tea reduces inflammation, styes, and conjunctivitis.
Ginkgo (*Ginkgo biloba*) ~ oral intake increases blood flow to the head and eyes; can help glaucoma.
Oregon Grape Root (*Mahonia aquifolium*) ~ antibacterial for conjunctivitis and blepharitis (inflamed eyelid).

Fatigue (also see Adrenal Glands and Adaptogens, Antioxidant Support, and Chronic Fatigue Syndrome):

Astragalus ~ strengthens and normalizes endocrine glands and primary organs to address causes of fatigue.
Blue Vervain ~ eases depression and listlessness; helps restore normal energy levels.
Cayenne ~ stimulating to promote normal function of body systems.
Holy Basil ~ helps restore endocrine glands, especially adrenal function, and normal energy levels.
Lemon Balm ~ helps normalize and invigorate a depleted nervous system.
Peppermint ~ has a stimulating and revitalizing effect helpful for mental fatigue and physical exhaustion.
Sage ~ stimulating properties revitalize nervous system; beneficial for mental and physical exhaustion.

Other Helpful Herbs:

Ginseng, Asian (*Panax ginseng*) and American (*Panax quinquefolius*) ~ tonic used by the elderly for general fatigue, exhaustion, debility; helps restore physical and mental vitality.

Female Reproductive System: See Menstruation, Menopause, Breast, Ovary, Uterus, Vaginal Infections,

Infertility, Pregnancy, Childbirth, Postpartum, or Breast-Feeding

Other Helpful Herbs:

Bupleurum (*Bupleurum chinense*) ~ improves uterine blood flow; helps PMS, painful menses, depression related to PMS and menopause, and prolapsed uterus; potent antioxidant and cytotoxic action involving apoptosis protects ovarian cells from becoming cancerous; energetic clearing effects on the uterus help release chronically suppressed emotions such as anger, rage, shame, and guilt.

Dong Quai (*Angelica sinensis*) ~ uterine tonic; regulates estrogen and progesterone; helps gynecological disorders, infertility, chronic miscarriage, PMS, painful menses, and menopausal symptoms.

Ginseng, American (*Panax quinquefolius*) ~ helps reduce menopausal hot flashes; has estrogenic effects.

Licorice (*Glycyrrhiza glabra*) ~ contains phytoestrogens (estriol); improves estrogen levels.

Maca (*Lepidium meyenii*) ~ promotes hormonal balance, especially estrogen; promotes fertility; beneficial for menopausal difficulties, including depression and anxiety.

Red Clover (*Trifolium pratense*) ~ contains estrogenic isoflavones that help balance hormones; marketed for PMS and problems of estrogen excess in menstruating women, including fibroids, cysts, endometriosis; used by menopausal women for estrogen support; research shows it inhibits several types of cancerous cells, including cancers in the reproductive organs.

Wild Yam (*Dioscorea villosa*) ~ contains diosgenin which is chemically converted into progesterone or estrogen in laboratory settings; Wild Yam is converted into usable progesterone and marketed in cream-based products to increase progesterone levels.

Fever:

American Centaury ~ diaphoretic that reduces fevers by drawing internal heat to the skin where it is released.
Blue Vervain ~ a cooling diaphoretic that draws heat to the surface and stimulates perspiration.
Boneset ~ excellent for all fevers caused by viral and bacterial infections; stimulates perspiration.
Burdock ~ cooling; increases perspiration to reduce fevers, inflammation, and other heat conditions.
Calendula ~ a mild herb that promotes perspiration and lowers fevers.
Catnip ~ safe and specific for childhood illness and fevers.
Chamomile ~ cooling; promotes perspiration to reduce fevers.
Chickweed ~ the tea is cooling and moisturizing for hot, feverish conditions.
Cinquefoil ~ lowers fever; especially helpful for intermittent fevers that come and go.
Echinacea ~ an immunostimulant that fights infections causing fevers; decreases toxic heat.
Elderberry ~ promotes perspiration; reduces toxic heat in the blood.
Feverfew ~ antibiotic; promotes perspiration; as the name implies, it specific for fevers.
Goldenrod ~ a cooling diaphoretic that lowers fevers by promoting perspiration.
Goldenseal ~ cooling; reduces fevers caused by infectious pathogens.
Holy Basil ~ strengthens immunity; antimicrobial; lowers fevers by promoting perspiration.
Hyssop ~ reduces fevers; antiviral and antibacterial.
Isatis ~ very cooling to reduce fevers; a strong antibacterial and antiviral.
Lemon Balm ~ cooling to lower fevers; antibacterial and antiviral.
Lobelia ~ promotes perspiration to reduce fevers; calms agitation.
Marshmallow ~ cooling for high fevers; mucilage properties hydrate the body.
Motherwort ~ a diaphoretic that reduces fevers.
Mugwort ~ a bitter, cooling diaphoretic.
Peppermint ~ a diaphoretic that promotes perspiration to reduce fevers.
Sage ~ an excellent diaphoretic to lower fevers; antibacterial.
Thyme ~ antibacterial and antiviral; reduces fevers by increasing perspiration.
Yarrow ~ promotes perspiration; excellent for fevers; antibacterial.

Other Helpful Herbs:

Linden (*Tilia* spp.) ~ a diaphoretic that lowers fevers.

Fibromyalgia (also see Antioxidants, Muscle, Pain, and Epstein-Barr Virus):

Fibromyalgia is a complex chronic pain disorder characterized by severe muscle pain and various symptoms that include fatigue, depression, anxiety, insomnia, headaches, cognitive difficulties, low-grade fever, swollen lymph nodes, and abdominal pain. Causes of the generalized muscle pain are uncertain, but may result from a deficiency of the calming neurotransmitters serotonin and GABA and oversensitivity to pain, causing the brain and nerves to misinterpret or overreact to normal pain signals. Serotonin, GABA, the vitamin B complex, and magnesium may be helpful in addition to herbal therapy, which should include antioxidants. The Epstein-Barr virus (member of the herpes family) and toxic overload may also be involved.

Astragalus ~ boosts immunity; strengthens weak muscles; reduces fatigue.
Blue Vervain ~ reduces nerve and muscle pain and spasms.
Boneset ~ eases nerve and deep-seated muscle pain and spasms; strong immunostimulant.
Cayenne ~ warming and stimulating to the system; improves circulation and glandular activity.
Elderberry ~ berries enrich the blood and strengthen muscles; supports immunity.
Holy Basil ~ supports the nervous and endocrine systems; helps normalize neurotransmitter levels; analgesic.
Hops ~ calming to the nervous system; an analgesic that reduces muscle and nerve pain.

Lavender ~ analgesic; reduces anxiety, muscle pain, and stiffness.
Lemon Balm ~ reduces anxiety; supports the nervous system; analgesic; strong antiviral against Epstein-Barr.
Lobelia ~ normalizes and calms the nervous system; reduces muscle rigidity, spasms, and discomfort.
Passion Flower ~ calms the nervous system; reduces muscle tension and discomfort.
Peppermint ~ the volatile oils are relaxing and analgesic.
Saint John's Wort ~ restorative to nerves; supports serotonin; analgesic; strong antiviral against Epstein-Barr.
Scullcap ~ anti-inflammatory; antioxidant; contains calming neurotransmitters that ease pain.
Stinging Nettle ~ high levels of chlorophyll, vitamins, and minerals nourish muscles.
Thyme ~ analgesic; reduces muscle tension; antiviral against the herpes family.
Valerian ~ analgesic; relaxes nervous and muscular tension and spasms.
Other Helpful Herbs:
Ashwagandha (*Withania somnifera*) ~ antioxidant; anti-inflammatory; can be helpful for fibromyalgia.
Flu (Influenza): See Colds and Flu
Fungal Infections (Athlete's Foot and Ringworm) and Candida Yeast Infections (yeast is a fungus):
Black Walnut ~ specific for Candida yeast and fungi; cleanses blood and lymph; internal and external use.
Bloodroot ~ has strong activity against yeast and fungal infections; use externally with caution.
Boneset ~ taken internally for fungal and yeast infections.
Burdock ~ taken internally for fungal infections.
Calendula ~ taken internally and applied externally or used as a vaginal douche.
Cayenne ~ kills Candida yeast.
Chamomile ~ used externally as a wash or vaginal douche and taken internally as tea or tincture.
Cinquefoil ~ used as a douche for vaginal yeast infections.
Cranesbill ~ antifungal; taken internally and used as a douche for vaginal yeast infections.
Echinacea ~ stimulates the immune system to eliminate fungal and yeast infections.
Elecampane ~ used internally and externally to kill fungi and reduce excess dampness.
Feverfew ~ antifungal; taken internally.
Goldenrod ~ ingesting the herb reduces heat and excess dampness to eliminate yeast and fungi.
Goldenseal ~ internal and external applications are used for fungal infections; clears blood and lymph.
Holy Basil ~ used internally and externally to kill yeast and fungal growth.
Hops ~ used internally and externally for fungal and yeast infections; cooling and drying.
Hyssop ~ used internally and externally for fungal infections.
Isatis ~ used internally for yeast and fungal infections; cooling; cleansing to blood.
Lavender ~ antifungal; used internally and externally.
Lemon Balm ~ antifungal.
Marshmallow ~ external application to affected area reduces inflammation and discomfort.
Motherwort ~ taken internally and applied externally and as a douche to treat yeast and fungal infections.
Mugwort ~ kills fungi and yeast; used internally and externally.
Peppermint ~ volatile oils are antifungal; used internally and externally.
Sage ~ kills yeast and fungi.
Thyme ~ antifungal for ringworm, athlete's foot, yeast, and thrush.
Yarrow ~ cooling and drying; used internally and externally for fungal and yeast infections.
Yellow Dock ~ helps eliminate fungi and yeast; cleans blood and lymph; used internally and externally.
Other Helpful Herbs:
Clove (*Syzygium aromaticum*) ~ the diluted oil is applied externally for all types of fungal infections.
Garlic (*Allium sativum*) ~ a strong, broad-spectrum antifungal for Candida yeast, ringworm, athlete's foot; used internally and externally.
Myrrh (*Commiphora myrrha*) ~ may be used internally or externally for fungal infections.
Oregano (*Origanum vulgare*) ~ a strong antifungal used for athlete's foot, ringworm, and Candida yeast.
Oregon Grape Root (*Mahonia aquifolium*) ~ used internally or externally for fungal and yeast infections.
Pau D'arco (*Tabebuia impetiginosa*) ~ a strong antifungal; helpful for Candida; used internally and externally.
Tea Tree oil (Melaleuca alternifolia) ~ applied externally for fungal and yeast infections.
Gallbladder:
The gallbladder receives, concentrates and stores bile, an alkaline fluid continuously made by the liver. During digestion the gallbladder contracts and squirts bile into the small intestine duodenum to break down and digest fats. Gallbladder problems, including inflammation and gallstones, are often related to poor diet and compromised liver health.
American Centaury ~ stimulates bile flow into the gallbladder and intestines; helps prevent gallstones.
Blue Vervain ~ a bitter that relaxes bile ducts and stimulates bile flow; for gallstones and inflammation.
Boneset ~ relaxes bile ducts and stimulates bile flow.
Burdock ~ stimulates bile flow; helpful for inflammation and gallstones.
Calendula ~ stimulates bile flow.
Cayenne ~ stimulates liver and gallbladder activity and bile flow; helps prevent stone formation.
Dandelion ~ reduces gallbladder congestion, inflammation, and stone formation; stimulates bile flow.
Goldenseal ~ stimulates bile flow; reduces gallbladder inflammation, toxins, and stone formation.

Hops ~ a bitter that stimulates bile flow; reduces spasms, inflammation, and the formation of gallstones.
Horehound ~ a bitter that stimulates bile flow; reduces gallbladder spasms.
Hyssop ~ stimulates bile flow.
Marshmallow ~ soothes gallbladder inflammation and spasms.
Mugwort ~ taken for gallstones and jaundice.
Peppermint ~ relaxes bile ducts; stimulates bile flow; helps prevent and treat inflammation and gallstones.
Sage ~ stimulates bile flow; reduces gallbladder spasms and inflammation.
Yarrow ~ a bitter that stimulates flow of bile; reduces gallbladder inflammation and spasms.
Yellow Dock ~ stimulates bile flow.

Other Helpful Herbs:

Barberry (*Berberis vulgaris*) ~ contains berberine; promotes liver function and bile flow; reduces gallbladder inflammation and jaundice.
Fringe Tree (*Chionanthus virginicus*) ~ valuable for many liver and gallbladder problems, including gallstones and inflammation.
Gentian root (*Gentiana lutea*) ~ a strong bitter; increases bile production in liver and bile flow to gallbladder.
Oregon Grape Root (*Mahonia aquifolium*) ~ antimicrobial; anti-inflammatory; normalizes bile flow.
Turmeric (*Curcuma longa*) ~ anti-inflammatory; normalizes cholesterol levels, liver function, and bile flow.
White Oak bark (*Quercus alba*) ~ reduces inflamed, enlarged gallbladder; helps dissolve gallstones.

Gas: See Digestive System and Intestines

Gingivitis (gum inflammation): See Mouth

Gout (also see Arthritis):

Gout is a type of arthritis caused by excess uric acid in the blood that crystallizes and is deposited in joints, most often in the big toe, causing pain and inflammation. Eating meat, fish, sugar, coffee, and alcohol increase uric acid levels, and reducing their consumption usually improves gout symptoms.

American Centaury ~ promotes excretion of acids; decreases heat and inflammation; relieves gout pain.
Blue Vervain ~ improves kidney function to decrease acids in blood; helpful for gout pain and inflammation.
Boneset ~ normalizes kidney function and helps eliminate excess acids in blood.
Burdock ~ reduces uric acid levels and joint inflammation.
Cayenne ~ external application relieves joint pain.
Chamomile ~ cooling; reduces joint inflammation and pain.
Chickweed ~ high mineral content reduces acids and heat in the blood; decreases joint inflammation.
Dandelion ~ stimulates excretion of uric acid via the kidneys; cooling; anti-inflammatory.
Elderberry ~ berries are highly nutritious and alkaline; cooling; anti-inflammatory; supports kidney function.
Elecampane ~ stimulates normal kidney function and reduces gout pain.
Hops ~ supports kidneys in filtering and eliminating uric acid; relieves joint pain and inflammation; cooling.
Mugwort ~ anti-inflammatory; diuretic; helpful for gout.
Mullein ~ tea and externally applied poultices can help reduce painful joint swellings.
Stinging Nettle ~ promotes kidney excretion of uric acid; anti-inflammatory.
Yellow Dock ~ high mineral content reduces acids and heat in the blood; decreases joint inflammation.

Other Helpful Herbs:

Gravel Root (*Eupatorium purpureum*) ~ diuretic kidney action reduces uric acid levels and gout symptoms.

Gum Disease: See Mouth

Hair:

Protein, vitamins, minerals, and essential fatty acids are essential for the growth of healthy hair. Use natural hair care products free of harsh chemicals.

Black Walnut ~ external application is used to treat dandruff, cradle cap, and alopecia (hair loss).
Burdock ~ can stimulate hair growth and reduce dandruff.
Cinquefoil ~ may be helpful for hair loss related to toxic conditions or inner stress and tension.
Sage ~ helps to stimulate hair growth and reduce dandruff.
Stinging Nettle ~ large concentrations of nutrients in the leaves are helpful for hair growth and reducing dandruff; taken internally and applied to the scalp.

Other Helpful Herbs:

Gotu Kola (*Centella asiatica*) ~ increases circulation to scalp; blood purifier; can stimulate hair growth.
Rosemary (*Rosmarinus officinalis*) ~ oil applied to scalp stimulates circulation and hair follicle activity.

Halitosis (bad breath due to poor mouth hygiene or poor digestion): See Digestion (Sage and Thyme)

Hay Fever: See Sinus Problems

Headaches and Migraines:

Headaches have many causes that should be explored, including stress, hypoglycemia, food sensitivities, neurotransmitter imbalance, and blood vessel instability and inflammation which compromises circulation.

American Centaury ~ helps headaches caused by kidney and liver stagnation, excess heat, and toxicity.
Black Cohosh ~ specific for headaches caused by low estrogen levels during menopause and menstruation.
Blue Vervain ~ anti-inflammatory and analgesic; relaxes nerves and muscles; eases tension headaches.
Boneset ~ can help chronic headaches.
Burdock ~ can help chronic vascular headaches that are caused by blood vessel instability and inflammation.

Catnip ~ specific for stress headaches and muscle tension.
Cayenne ~ for migraines and headaches; used externally for pain relief and internally to normalize circulation.
Chamomile ~ eases stress headaches; thins blood and dilates blood vessels to normalize circulation.
Chasteberry ~ for headaches caused by estrogen dominance occurring around menstruation or menopause.
Feverfew ~ specifically addresses vascular instability and underlying causes of migraines; anti-inflammatory.
Holy Basil ~ relaxing and normalizing to nervous system; vasodilator (dilates blood vessels); analgesic.
Hops ~ taken for headaches caused by anxiety, overstimulated nervous system, or acid stomach.
Lavender ~ excellent for tension headaches; reduces pain, spasms, and inflammation; improves circulation.
Lemon Balm ~ eases tension headaches; dilates blood vessels; relaxes spasms; analgesic; anti-inflammatory.
Motherwort ~ a relaxing sedative; reduces spasms; specific for stress headaches.
Passion Flower ~ specific for weak, frail, debilitated people with headaches caused by anxiety and stress.
Peppermint ~ helpful for stress headaches; anti-inflammatory; reduces pain; relaxes and dilates blood vessels.
Sage ~ reduces spasms and inflammation; beneficial for stress headaches.
Saint John's Wort ~ analgesic; anti-inflammatory for headaches.
Scullcap ~ excellent for stress headaches; vasodilator that reduces vascular spasms; anti-inflammatory.
Stinging Nettle ~ nourishing and calming to the nervous system; dilates blood vessels.
Thyme ~ anti-inflammatory; antispasmodic; analgesic; vasodilator; taken for tension headaches.
Valerian ~ a relaxing sedative for nervous headaches; dilates blood vessels; reduces pain and spasms.
Wood Betony ~ for headaches and migraines; sedating; analgesic; vasodilator increases blood flow to head.

Other Helpful Herbs:

Ginger (*Zingiber officinale*) ~ analgesic; anti-inflammatory; normalizes blood circulation.
Ginkgo (*Ginkgo biloba*) ~ helps reduce headaches; antioxidant and anti-inflammatory properties protect blood vessels; vasodilating action on blood vessels improves blood flow to the head and reduces spasms.
Jamaican Dogwood (*Piscidia erythrina*) ~ excellent pain reliever for headaches and migraines.
Rosemary (*Rosmarinus officinalis*) ~ helps normalize circulation; antioxidant; anti-inflammatory; analgesic.
Turmeric (*Curcuma longa*) ~ helps normalize blood vessels and circulation; antioxidant; anti-inflammatory.

Heart (also see Vascular System):

Astragalus ~ a heart tonic helpful for palpitations, arrhythmias (irregular heartbeat), shortness of breath, angina, and congestive heart failure; helps recovery from heart attacks; protects heart from viral infections.
Black Cohosh ~ strengthens contractions and normalizes the pulse; can help relieve angina pain.
Blue Vervain ~ a calming heart tonic; vasodilator (dilates blood vessels); reduces rapid heart rate.
Calendula ~ strengthens and normalizes heart function; has gentle vasodilation action.
Cayenne ~ excellent tonic for cardiovascular problems; normalizes circulation and heart function; helps prevent heart attacks, congestive heart failure, arteriosclerosis, hypertension, abnormal blood clotting.
Dandelion ~ a diuretic that helps reduce edema from congestive heart failure; normalizes circulation.
Elderberry ~ highly nutritious berries strengthen heart muscles; protects against heart attacks.
Goldenseal ~ strengthens a weak heart; promotes normal muscle tone and heartbeat.
Holy Basil ~ relaxing to the nervous system; anticoagulant properties promote normal circulation.
Hops ~ sedating to the nervous system; calms palpitations and rapid heartbeat; reduces chest pressure.
Horehound ~ small amounts are calming to the nerves and heart; helps normalize arrhythmias.
Lavender ~ calming to the heart; beneficial for palpitations, shortness of breath, and angina.
Lemon Balm ~ benefits the cardiovascular system; taken for heart problems caused by anxiety, including chest pressure, heart palpitations, and arrhythmias.
Lobelia ~ larger doses are calming and can be helpful for rapid heart rate, arrhythmias, palpitations, chest pressure, angina, heart congestion, and labored breathing.
Motherwort ~ one of the best cardiac tonics; calming for anxiety and cardiovascular problems caused by tension, including palpitations, arrhythmias, rapid heart rate, and high blood pressure.
Mugwort ~ calming; reduces palpitations.
Passion Flower ~ dilates blood vessels; used for arrhythmias and heart problems caused by anxiety.
Peppermint ~ a calming heart tonic; strengthens heart muscles; helpful for palpitations; a mild vasodilator.
Pleurisy Root ~ a heart tonic that improves function, normalizes heart rate, increases blood output, and reduces palpitations and arrhythmias.
Scullcap ~ calming to the nervous system; strengthens the heart; reduces palpitations; a mild vasodilator.
Thyme ~ calming; normalizes heart rate; vasodilator activity increases blood flow; reduces blood clots.
Valerian ~ calming nervine and sedative that normalizes excessive heart rate and dilates blood vessels.
Wood Betony ~ calming nervine; vasodilator that improves circulation; reduces high blood pressure.
Yarrow ~ calming; vasodilator; normalizes circulation; blood thinner reduces clot formation; eases angina.

Other Helpful Herbs:

Dan Chen (*Salvia miltiorrhiza*) ~ used to increase coronary blood flow, reduce angina, and improve mild to moderate congestive heart failure.
Garlic (*Allium sativum*) ~ benefits cardiovascular system; helps prevent heart attacks and blood clots; lowers total cholesterol, LDL, triglycerides, and high blood pressure; dilates blood vessels; antioxidant protection.
Hawthorn berries (*Crataegus* spp.) ~ a classic heart tonic to prevent and treat coronary disease; improves heart function and contractions; normalizes heart rate and arrhythmias; increases blood flow and oxygen;

eases angina; benefits mild to moderate congestive heart failure.
Khella (*Ammi visnaga*) ~ smooth muscle relaxant; vasodilator; increases blood supply to heart; eases angina.
Linden (*Tilia* spp.) ~ calming nervine; dilates blood vessels; helps reduce hypertension and rapid heartbeat.
Night-Blooming Cereus Cactus (*Selenicereus grandiflorus*) ~ excellent heart tonic, normalizes arrhythmias.
Olive leaf (*Olea europaea*) ~ antioxidant; improves circulation; helps lower high cholesterol and triglyceride levels; reduces arrhythmias; supports heart function and helps protect from cardiac disease.
Schisandra (*Schisandra chinensis*) ~ a heart tonic; antioxidant protects cells from damage; reduces palpitations.

Heartburn: See Stomach

Hemorrhage: See Blood and Vascular System

Hemorrhoids:

Hemorrhoids are painful inflamed, bulging veins caused by weak anal muscles and increased pressure due to constipation or pregnancy. Vitamin C and rutin (a bioflavonoid) strengthen veins.

Astragalus ~ for chronic cases occurring with muscle weakness, loose stools, uterine or bladder prolapse.
Black Walnut ~ for hemorrhoids caused by sluggish digestion, chronic constipation, and toxic build-up.
Blue Vervain ~ reduces swelling to shrink hemorrhoids and lessens pain.
Calendula ~ used externally to heal hemorrhoids.
Catnip ~ used externally to shrink hemorrhoids and reduce pain and inflammation.
Cayenne ~ tones and normalizes blood vessels and circulation; decreases constipation.
Chamomile ~ reduces hemorrhoid pain and inflammation.
Chickweed ~ rutin in the leaves strengthens blood vessels to reduce hemorrhoid inflammation and swelling.
Cinquefoil ~ an astringent herb applied externally to shrink hemorrhoids.
Comfrey ~ used externally to shrink hemorrhoids and soothe painful, inflamed tissues.
Cranesbill ~ an astringent externally applied to shrink hemorrhoids.
Marshmallow ~ soothing and healing; reduces hemorrhoid inflammation and irritation.
Mullein ~ reduces pain and inflammation.
Saint John's Wort ~ reduces pain and inflammation; a mild astringent that can help shrink hemorrhoids.
Senna ~ reduces constipation and anal pressure that can promote hemorrhoids.
Stinging Nettle ~ external application reduces hemorrhoid swelling and inflammation.
Yarrow ~ an astringent that shrinks hemorrhoids and strengthens blood vessels.

Other Helpful Herbs:

Horse Chestnut (*Aesculus hippocastanum*) ~ excellent for hemorrhoids and phlebitis (inflamed veins); only use dried preparations because raw preparations are toxic.
Witch Hazel (*Hamamelis virginiana*) ~ external application constricts and shrinks hemorrhoids.

Hepatitis: See Liver

Herpes Virus:

The herpes family of viruses includes Herpes simplex type 1 (causes cold sores) and 2 (causes genital lesions), Varicella zoster (causes chicken pox and shingles), Epstein-Barr, and Cytomegalovirus.

Astragalus ~ an antiviral and immunostimulant.
Black Walnut ~ externally applied to lesions; antiviral.
Boneset ~ antiviral; a powerful immunostimulant.
Cayenne ~ used externally on lesions for pain relief.
Echinacea ~ strong antiviral specific for herpes viruses; immunostimulant; relieves painful lesions.
Elderberry ~ antiviral; stimulates immunity; soothes and cools herpes skin lesions.
Goldenseal ~ used for external application to heal lesions; anti-inflammatory to lesions.
Hyssop ~ antiviral specific for herpes.
Isatis ~ strong antiviral specific for the herpes family; reduces heat, inflammation, and skin lesions.
Lemon Balm ~ a primary herb specific against the herpes virus.
Motherwort ~ the Chinese bathe in Motherwort baths to ease the pain of shingles.
Mugwort ~ active against the herpes virus.
Peppermint ~ antiviral against the herpes virus.
Saint John's Wort ~ a classic antiviral herb specific for members of the herpes family; analgesic.
Thyme ~ antiviral for herpes viruses; analgesic.

Other Helpful Herbs:

Cat's Claw (*Uncaria tomentosa*) ~ an immunomodulator and stimulant; increases lymphocyte production and phagocytosis to destroy pathogens; anti-inflammatory; antiviral against the herpes family.
Licorice (*Glycyrrhiza glabra*) ~ research shows that glycyrrhizin permanently inactivates the herpes virus.
Pau D'arco (*Tabebuia impetiginosa*) ~ an immunomodulator; strong antiviral used against herpes viruses.

Hiccups (caused by muscle spasms of the diaphragm):

Boneset ~ reduces spasms in the diaphragm muscle.
Catnip ~ reduces muscle spasms; specific for the digestive system.
Chamomile ~ specific for relaxing nerves in solar plexus area and reducing spasms and hiccups.
Holy Basil ~ reduces spasms in the diaphragm to stop hiccups.
Hops ~ relaxes the nervous system; reduces muscle spasms.
Hyssop ~ calms nerves and eases muscle spasms.

Lemon Balm ~ sedating; reduces internal tension and muscle spasms.
Lobelia ~ calms the nerves and relieves muscle spasms.
Passion Flower ~ reduces muscle spasms; for hiccups caused by anxiety; works best for frail people.
Peppermint ~ calming to the nerves; reduces muscle spasms; avoid in cases of acid reflux and GERD.
Scullcap ~ calms anxiety; reduces muscular tension and spasms.
Thyme ~ antispasmodic actions are specific to the digestive tract.
Valerian ~ calms the nervous system and spastic muscles.

High Blood Pressure: See Hypertension

Hirsutism (excessive hair growth in women on the face and chest): See Menopause

HIV (Human Immunodeficiency Virus): See AIDS

Hives: See Skin

Hyperactivity: See Nervous System

Hypertension (High Blood Pressure):

Hypertension develops over time from several causes, which can include poor diet and unhealthy lifestyle; unresolved stress; nervous system overstimulation resulting in muscular tension and constricted, damaged blood vessels with reduced circulation; water retention; and dysfunction in the organs that regulate blood pressure (the heart, kidneys, liver, thyroid, and adrenal glands).

Astragalus ~ normalizes heart contractions; diuretic; a vasodilator (relaxes and dilates blood vessels).
Black Cohosh ~ calms the nervous system; relaxes and dilates blood vessels.
Blue Vervain ~ relaxes the nerves; vasodilator; diuretic that reduces water retention.
Burdock ~ a diuretic for hypertension related to water retention.
Cayenne ~ dilates blood vessels; helps normalize circulation, heart rate, and kidney function.
Dandelion ~ diuretic that helps normalize kidney function and reduce hypertension caused by fluid overload.
Holy Basil ~ calms the nerves and eases stress responses; vasodilator; diuretic; lowers elevated cholesterol.
Hops ~ decreases anxiety and stress; relaxes and dilates blood vessels to improve blood flow.
Horehound ~ a vasodilator that promotes circulation; mildly diuretic.
Hyssop ~ calming to the nervous system; improves circulation.
Lavender ~ calming to the nerves; relaxes muscles in blood vessels to dilate and increase circulation.
Lemon Balm ~ calming to the nerves and cardiovascular system; a vasodilator that improves circulation.
Lobelia ~ calming to the nerves; a vasodilator that improves circulation by restoring normal vascular tone.
Motherwort ~ calming; helps normalize heart function; vasodilator; diuretic.
Passion Flower ~ eases tension; vasodilator; normalizes heart rate.
Pleurisy Root ~ strengthens the heart muscle; vasodilator; reduces tension in the cardiovascular system.
Scullcap ~ relaxes the nervous system to ease stress; a vasodilator that increases blood flow.
Stinging Nettle ~ mildly diuretic; vasodilator.
Thyme ~ reduces nervous tension; vasodilator.
Valerian ~ calming; improves health and function of the heart and blood vessels; vasodilator.
Wood Betony ~ a calming sedative; vasodilator; diuretic.
Yarrow ~ a calming vasodilator; normalizes blood flow; improves circulation in kidneys and liver.

Other Helpful Herbs:

Garlic (*Allium sativum*) ~ improves circulation by reducing high levels of cholesterol and triglycerides, elevating protective HDL, dilating blood vessels, and reducing blood coagulation and abnormal clotting.
Hawthorn (*Crataegus* spp.) ~ a relaxing heart tonic; vasodilator; antioxidant; reduces hypertension.
Linden (*Tilia* spp.) ~ dilates blood vessels; a relaxing nervine; antioxidant; anti-inflammatory.
Olive leaf (*Olea europaea*) ~ antioxidant; vasodilator that improves circulation; helps reduce high cholesterol and triglyceride levels; supports heart function; used for mild hypertension.
Turmeric (*Curcuma longa*) ~ vasodilator; anticoagulant to reduce clots; reduces atherosclerosis blockage.

Hypoglycemia (Low Blood Sugar): See Pancreas

Hypotension (Low Blood Pressure):

Lobelia ~ small doses temporarily stimulate; helps revive after shock and sudden drop in blood pressure.

Other Helpful Herbs:

Ginseng, Asian (*Panax ginseng*) and American (*Panax quinquefolius*) ~ stimulating effects help raise and normalize abnormally low blood pressure.

Hypothalamus:

The hypothalamus is a structure in the brain responsible for regulating activities of the autonomic nervous system, pituitary gland, and homeostasis of the body. It is responsible for the production of essential hormones that control physiologic functions, including reproduction, growth and development, temperature regulation, immunity, and circadian rhythms. It enables communication between the nervous and endocrine systems via the hypothalamus-pituitary-adrenal (HPA) axis. This axis controls metabolism, which is the rate at which the body converts food and oxygen into energy and how energy is stored and expended. Slow metabolism causes general sluggishness with symptoms like weight gain, fatigue, and constipation. Fast metabolism over-stimulates and causes problems like anxiety, insomnia, and heart palpitations.

The HPA axis regulates digestion, stress reactions, mood and behavior, thirst, appetite, weight regulation, sleep, and sex drive. Dysfunctions of the HPA axis can lead to psychological and nervous disorders, chronic fatigue syndrome, digestive and irritable bowel conditions, and hot flashes. Use antioxidant and adaptogen herbs to strengthen and optimize hypothalamus function.

Cayenne ~ influences the cooling center in the hypothalamus to lower body temperature.

Chasteberry ~ acts directly on the hypothalamus and pituitary to promote their optimal function; increases luteinizing hormone and reduces high prolactin levels in women, which helps balance the ratio of progesterone to estrogen, slightly raising the levels of progesterone.

Lobelia ~ supports hypothalamus by regulating and harmonizing functions of the autonomic nervous system.

Other Helpful Herbs:

Eleuthero/Siberian Ginseng (*Eleutherococcus senticosus*) ~ adaptogen; supports and normalizes HPA axis.

Ginseng, Asian (*Panax ginseng*) and American (*Panax quinquefolius*) ~ adaptogens that nourish and support the hypothalamus and all glands in the endocrine system.

Maca (*Lepidium meyenii*) ~ sterols in the root nourish and stimulate the hypothalamus and pituitary to promote their optimal function, which improves the functioning of all the endocrine glands, including the adrenals, pineal, thyroid, pancreas, ovaries, and testicles.

Myrrh (*Commiphora myrrha*) ~ antioxidant; stimulates the hypothalamus; increases oxygen by receptor sites near the hypothalamus, pineal, and pituitary; has a calming effect on the emotional center in hypothalamus.

Schisandra (*Schisandra chinensis*) ~ stimulates the hypothalamus by directly increasing dopamine levels.

Other herbs that support or activate the hypothalamus and HPA axis ~ Ashwagandha (*Withania somnifera*), Bupleurum (*Bupleurum chinense*), Corydalis (*Corydalis bulbosa*), Licorice (*Glycyrrhiza glabra*), Reishi mushroom (*Ganoderma lucidum*), Rehmannia (*Rehmannia chinensis*), and Rhodiola (*Rhodiola rosea*).

Immune System (also see Lymphatic System):

The immune system is the body's complex defense system that protects against cancers and microbial pathogens, including bacteria, viruses, fungi, yeast, and parasites. The immune system consists of lymphatic fluid, vessels, nodes and glands, the thymus gland, spleen, tonsils, adenoids, bone marrow, leukocytes (white blood cells), and other cellular components.

Three primary classes of herbs are used to strengthen and support immunity. Adaptogens strengthen and normalize the immune system, increasing the body's resistance to illness and ability to cope with physical and emotional stress. Immunomodulators regulate and normalize the immune system, stimulating immunity when appropriate and inhibiting it when there is overstimulation. Immunomodulators can be especially beneficial for chronic degenerative and malignant diseases. In conditions of immune dysfunction or autoimmune disorders, they calm an overactive immune system and bring it back into a healthy balance. Immunostimulants increase production and activation of white blood cells and specific immune compounds targeted at destroying infectious organisms. They are generally used during times of active infections, cancers, and immunodeficiency diseases. Immunostimulants are contraindicated for autoimmune diseases, organ transplants, and hypersensitivity reactions.

Astragalus ~ an immunomodulator; fights infections, cancer, and HIV/AIDS; may help autoimmune disorders.

Boneset ~ one of the most effective immunostimulants that neutralizes viral and bacterial pathogens.

Burdock ~ a blood and lymphatic cleanser; anticarcinogenic; supports immunity; may help autoimmunity.

Calendula ~ stimulates white blood cell activity; antiviral and antibacterial.

Chamomile ~ stimulates phagocytosis to destroy pathogens.

Echinacea ~ one of the best herbs to stimulate and enhance the immune system.

Elderberry ~ an immunostimulant; antiviral; berries are cancer preventatives.

Elecampane ~ stimulates immunity; antibacterial; antifungal; blood cleanser.

Goldenseal ~ increases the number of white blood cells to fight infections and toxins.

Holy Basil ~ an immunomodulator; antimicrobial.

Isatis ~ strengthens and stimulates immunity.

Other Helpful Herbs:

Ashwagandha (*Withania somnifera*) ~ an immunomodulator; may help with autoimmune conditions; used in treating cancer and tumors; helps restore white blood cell count during chemotherapy.

Bupleurum (*Bupleurum chinense*) ~ an immunomodulator; increases number and activation of macrophages; antiviral; antitumor; used for lupus and other autoimmune diseases in Chinese medicine.

Cat's Claw (*Uncaria tomentosa*) ~ an immunomodulator and stimulant; increases lymphocyte production and phagocytosis to destroy pathogens; anti-inflammatory; antiviral.

Chlorella (*Chlorella* spp.) ~ high nutrient freshwater algae; immunostimulant; increases macrophage activity and interferon production; supports endocrine glands; reduces levels of heavy metals and chemical toxins.

Codonopsis (*Codonopsis pilosula*) ~ root is adaptogen and immunomodulator; increases phagocytosis to destroy pathogens; antibacterial and antifungal.

Eleuthero/Siberian Ginseng (*Eleutherococcus senticosus*) ~ an immunomodulator and immunostimulant; increases T-lymphocyte count and natural killer cells; used for recovery after radiation and chemotherapy.

Ginseng, Asian (*Panax ginseng*) and American (*Panax quinquefolius*) ~ immunomodulators; immunostimulants; increase T-lymphocytes, macrophages, natural killer cells, interferon; used in cancer therapy.

Licorice (*Glycyrrhiza glabra*) ~ immunostimulant; immunomodulator; increases T-lymphocytes, interferon, macrophages; strong antiviral specific for herpes, HIV, and hepatitis.

Maitake (*Grifola frondosa*), Reishi (*Ganoderma lucidum*), Shiitake (*Lentinula edodes*), and Turkey Tail (*Trametes versicolor*) mushrooms ~ immunomodulators; immunostimulants; increase counts of B- and T-lymphocytes, macrophages, natural killer cells, tumor necrosis factor, interleukin, interferon, and production of granulocytes and blood platelets in bone marrow; strengthen a weak immune system but are also helpful for autoimmune conditions.
Pau D'arco (*Tabebuia impetiginosa*) ~ an immunomodulator; antibacterial; antifungal; inhibits some tumors.
Privet/Ligustrum (*Ligustrum lucidum*) ~ an immunostimulant.
Schisandra berry (*Schisandra chinensis*) ~ immunomodulator; increases lymphocytes.
Turmeric (*Curcuma longa*) ~ immunostimulant; anti-inflammatory; antioxidant.
Wild Indigo (*Baptisia tinctoria*) ~ a powerful immunomodulator and immunostimulant; increases white blood cells, interleukin-1, and macrophages; strong antimicrobial for all types of infections and septic conditions of blood and tissues; use under guidance of a qualified herbalist due to toxicity of large doses.

Impetigo (a skin infection caused by *Staphylococcus aureus* or *Streptococcus* bacteria):
Black Walnut ~ an antibacterial for external application.
Calendula ~ taken internally and applied externally.
Echinacea ~ an internal and topical antibacterial for staph and strep infections.
Elecampane ~ specific for staph infections.
Goldenseal ~ external application is specific for staph and strep infections.
Isatis ~ a strong, cooling antibiotic taken internally and applied externally for staph infections.
Lavender ~ an antibiotic for internal and external use; the oil may be applied to the skin for staph infection.
Peppermint ~ the oil is applied externally.
Saint John's Wort ~ analgesic; antibacterial against strep and staph infection; used internally and externally.
Thyme ~ antibacterial against staph infections; analgesic.
Yarrow ~ antiseptic and antibacterial for staph and strep infections; analgesic.
Yellow Dock ~ an antibacterial against staph infection; for external application.

Incontinence (Urinary) and Bed-Wetting (also see Bladder and Kidneys):
Astragalus ~ helps to eliminate problems causing incontinence.
Cinquefoil ~ helps reduce incontinence and emotional tension and stress often accompanying this problem.
Mullein root~ reduces incontinence in adults and children.
Saint John's Wort ~ helps incontinence and bed-wetting caused by anxiety and neurological problems.
Scullcap ~ may help incontinence and bed-wetting caused by anxiety and neurological problems.
Thyme ~ reduces anxiety and may be helpful for bed-wetting.
Yarrow ~ a calming, mild diuretic that can help these problems.

Other Helpful Herbs:
Gravel Root (*Eupatorium purpureum*) ~ diuretic; improves kidney function; can be helpful for incontinence.
Horsetail (*Equisetum arvense*) ~ diuretic and astringent actions help reduce incontinence and bed-wetting.
Uva-ursi/Bearberry (*Arctostaphylos uva-ursi*) ~ diuretic and astringent; can reduce bed-wetting.

Infants and Young Children:
Determine pediatric doses according to the child's weight (use Clark's Rule for Dosages on page 148).
Calendula ~ a very mild, safe herb for infant infections and skin and digestive problems.
Catnip ~ excellent for colic, gas, colds, flu, fevers, teething, restlessness, insomnia, and persistent crying.
Chamomile ~ helps colic, gas, diarrhea, colds, flu, fevers, earaches, teething, restlessness, and insomnia.
Echinacea ~ safe to give to infants for all types of infections, including the common cold and flu.
Lemon Balm ~ safe to give for colic, nausea, childhood infections, flu, fevers, teething, and restlessness.
Lobelia ~ a few drops of the tincture have been used to resuscitate newborns and for childhood convulsions.
Marshmallow ~ safely given for fevers, coughs, colic, nausea, vomiting, dehydration, and constipation.
Passion Flower ~ for anxiety, insomnia, muscle spasms, colic, painful teething, and childhood convulsions.
Peppermint ~ taken for anxiety, colds, flu, fevers, colic, and painful teething.
Scullcap ~ calming to the nervous system; reduces overstimulation; eases pain during teething.

Other Helpful Herbs:
Clove oil (*Syzygium aromaticum*) ~ excellent to reduce pain and gum inflammation when teething.

The following herbs contain substantial vitamins and minerals and can be enjoyed as tasty teas:
Fennel seeds (*Foeniculum vulgare*) ~ soothing to gastrointestinal tract; reduces inflammation, gas, and colic.
Ginger (*Zingiber officinale*) ~ helps colds, flu, coughs, sore throats, and stomach aches and nausea.
Raspberry leaf (*Rubus idaeus*) ~ decreases diarrhea.
Red Clover (*Trifolium pratense*) ~ an excellent blood purifier historically used for chronic skin problems in children and adults, such as eczema, psoriasis, chronic hives, and other eruptive conditions.
Rose hips (*Rosa* spp.) ~ contain vitamin C to prevent and treat the common cold and flu; helps reduce constipation.

Infertility, Female (also see pages 603-4 in "Herbs for Pregnancy, Childbirth, and Lactation"):
Astragalus ~ nourishes and tones the endocrine glands to promote fertility.
Black Cohosh ~ tones and restores the reproductive system, endocrine glands, and female hormones.
Burdock ~ helpful in restoring ovarian function.
Chasteberry ~ one of the most dependable herbs to normalize the hormonal reproductive system by

balancing and supporting the hypothalamus and pituitary glands; increases luteinizing hormone and reduces high prolactin levels, which helps balance the ratio of progesterone to estrogen, increasing progesterone levels when too low; promotes fertility and prevents miscarriage.
Holy Basil ~ used in India to increase fertility in men and women.
Motherwort ~ a uterine tonic; improves blood flow to the pelvis; helps normalize the menstrual cycle.
Sage ~ has normalizing and stimulating actions on the reproductive system that can help reverse infertility.
Stinging Nettle ~ tones and restores the endocrine glands and nourishes the whole system.

Inflammation:

Chronic inflammation is the root of many health problems and is caused by stress, toxic chemicals, sugar, alcohol, gluten grains, red meat, food sensitivities, allergies, and oxidative damage to tissues.

American Centaury ~ reduces heat; used for internal inflammation and external wounds, rashes, dermatitis.
Astragalus ~ releases heat and toxins from the interior and the skin.
Blue Vervain ~ taken to relieve inflamed muscles, organs, and wounds.
Boneset ~ reduces inflammation and heat throughout the body.
Burdock ~ cooling properties reduce inflammation.
Calendula ~ applied to heal inflammation and wounds.
Cayenne ~ antioxidants reduce inflammation throughout the body.
Chamomile ~ cooling; an excellent anti-inflammatory.
Comfrey ~ contains cooling, soothing mucilage that decreases inflammation.
Dandelion ~ a cooling anti-inflammatory specific for the liver, gallbladder, pancreas, spleen, and kidneys.
Echinacea ~ cooling and anti-inflammatory; used internally and externally.
Elecampane ~ taken to reduce inflammation, especially in the lungs and gastrointestinal tract.
Feverfew ~ strong anti-inflammatory specific to blood vessels and uterus; COX-2 inhibitor; cooling; analgesic.
Goldenseal ~ cooling and anti-inflammatory to all tissues it directly contacts, especially mucous membranes.
Holy Basil ~ anti-inflammatory; a COX-2 inhibitor; analgesic.
Hops ~ cooling and anti-inflammatory.
Hyssop ~ cooling and anti-inflammatory.
Lobelia ~ used internally and externally to relieve inflammation and nerve and muscle spasms.
Marshmallow ~ used internally and externally for its cooling, soothing, and anti-inflammatory mucilage.
Mullein ~ analgesic; contains mucilage that is cooling, soothing, and anti-inflammatory.
Peppermint ~ analgesic; anti-inflammatory.
Sage ~ analgesic; anti-inflammatory; reduces spasms.
Saint John's Wort ~ analgesic and anti-inflammatory.
Stinging Nettle ~ cooling; a COX-2 inhibitor; anti-inflammatory.
Thyme ~ analgesic; anti-inflammatory specific to the digestive, respiratory, and nervous systems.
Yarrow ~ analgesic; anti-inflammatory; eases spasms.

Other Helpful Herbs:

Ashwagandha (*Withania somnifera*) ~ antioxidant; decreases inflammatory COX-2 and chronic inflammation.
Bupleurum (*Bupleurum chinense*) ~ strong anti-inflammatory and antioxidant for organs and blood vessels.
Codonopsis (*Codonopsis pilosula*) ~ used for chronic inflammation of the gastrointestinal (gastritis and ulcers), genitourinary (chronic nephritis), and upper respiratory tracts (bronchitis and asthma).
Devil's Claw (*Harpogophytum procumbens*) ~ has NSAID-like effects; decreases inflammatory prostaglandins.
Garlic (*Allium sativum*) ~ inhibits activity of inflammatory prostaglandins and thromboxanes.
Ginger (*Zingiber officinale*) ~ antioxidant; anti-inflammatory; inhibits production of COX-2 and 5-LOX (lipoxygenase) involved in the production of inflammatory prostaglandins, cytokines, and leukotrienes; inhibits inducible nitric oxide (iNOS) that can promote inflammation.
Licorice (*Glycyrrhiza glabra*) ~ excellent anti-inflammatory; glycyrrhizin's action is similar to corticosteroids and supports the body's release of cortisol; inhibits inflammatory prostaglandins and leukotrienes.
Meadowsweet (*Filipendula ulmaria*), Willow bark (*Salix* spp.), and Wintergreen (*Gaultheria procumbens*) contain salicylic acid which is anti-inflammatory and analgesic.
Oregano (*Origanum vulgare*) ~ strong anti-inflammatory and antioxidant; inhibits production of inflammatory prostaglandins and leukotrienes; specific for gastrointestinal and respiratory systems and arthritis.
Oregon Grape Root (*Mahonia aquifolium*) ~ anti-inflammatory, especially for mucous membranes.
Pau D'arco (*Tabebuia impetiginosa*) ~ decreases inflammatory COX-2; helps reduce pain and arthritis.
Turmeric (*Curcuma longa*) ~ a primary antioxidant and anti-inflammatory; inhibits production of COX-2 and lipoxygenase (5-LOX) involved in the production of inflammatory prostaglandins, cytokines, and leukotrienes; inhibits inducible nitric oxide (iNOS) that can promote inflammation.

Insect Bites, Stings, and Venom:

American Centaury ~ stimulates the liver and kidneys to detoxify blood.
Calendula ~ externally applied and internally taken to detox the liver, blood, and lymphatic system.
Catnip ~ applied externally to pull toxins from tissues.
Chickweed ~ soothes itching and irritation.
Echinacea ~ an immunostimulant; excellent for neutralizing venomous bites and stings.
Elecampane ~ a wound healer; stimulates immunity; detoxifies blood against venom and poisons.

Goldenrod ~ taken internally to eliminate toxins by urination; applied externally for healing.
Holy Basil ~ taken internally and applied externally for relief of bites and stings.
Horehound ~ historically used for venomous bites, stings, and rabies.
Lemon Balm ~ a wound healer; antimicrobial; analgesic; historically taken for venomous bites and stings.
Lobelia ~ applied externally to draw toxins out of the tissues.
Saint John's Wort ~ blood and liver cleanser; antidote for ingested poisons, venom, and rabies; analgesic.
Yellow Dock ~ used internally to neutralize toxins; applied externally to draw toxins out of tissues.

Insect Repellents:

Everything applied to the skin is absorbed into the tissues and can get into the bloodstream, so beware of toxic, chemical-based insect repellents. Several herbs offer safe protection from mosquito and other insect bites when applied every 2-3 hours.

Herbal insect repellents include Eucalyptus, Holy Basil, Hyssop, Lavender, Lemon Balm, and Citronella oil (*Cymbopogon nardus*), which is one of the most popular and effective mosquito and insect repellents.

Insomnia (also see Nervous System):

Blue Vervain ~ a mild sedative that relieves tension and anxiety.
Catnip ~ a mild sedative; decreases insomnia, restless sleep, nightmares; specific for young children.
Chamomile ~ a mild sedative; helpful for restless sleep and nightmares.
Holy Basil ~ especially helpful for insomnia due to stress and adrenal exhaustion.
Hops ~ a hypnotic and sedative excellent for calming an agitated nervous system and treating insomnia.
Hyssop ~ sedating.
Lavender ~ calming and sedating; helpful for nightmares.
Lemon Balm ~ sedating and calming to the nerves; reduces tension causing insomnia and nightmares.
Mugwort ~ used in Chinese medicine to cure sleepwalking.
Passion Flower ~ calms the nerves; helpful for insomnia from mental turmoil and obsessive thinking.
Scullcap ~ one of the best sedative herbs to induce relaxing sleep; helpful for restlessness and nightmares.
Valerian ~ specific for insomnia by increasing levels of GABA and melatonin, which promotes sleep.
Wood Betony ~ sedative; nervine; reduces anxiety.

Other Helpful Herbs:

Jamaican Dogwood (*Piscidia piscipula*) ~ sedating; analgesic; for insomnia due to nervous tension and pain.
Linden (*Tilia* spp.) ~ a relaxing nervine helpful for insomnia.

Intermittent Claudication (leg cramps caused by insufficient circulation): See Vascular System

Intestines, Small and Large:

Probiotics and normal function of the stomach, pancreas, liver, and gallbladder promote intestinal health.

American Centaury ~ stimulates bile flow and intestinal motility; reduces gas, bloating, and constipation.
Astragalus ~ helpful for chronic loose stools and diarrhea.
Black Walnut ~ antimicrobial specific for killing yeast and parasites; taken for constipation and diarrhea.
Blue Vervain ~ a bitter that stimulates bile flow; used for gas, bloating, constipation, cramps, spasms, pain, and inflammation; helps colitis and other inflammatory irritable bowel problems.
Boneset ~ helpful for constipation, spasms, and bacterial and viral intestinal infections.
Burdock ~ reduces inflammation, constipation, infections, and irritable bowel and ulcerative conditions.
Calendula ~ helps heal ulcerated and inflamed tissues; used for diarrhea.
Catnip ~ helpful for all irritable bowel conditions; reduces ulcers, spasms, and diarrhea.
Cayenne ~ stimulates peristaltic movement to reduce constipation; antibiotic; kills parasites.
Chamomile ~ used for diarrhea, intestinal spasms, ulcerative colitis, and other inflammatory conditions.
Chickweed ~ soothing for inflammation and ulcers; adds moisture to bowels to reduce constipation.
Cinquefoil ~ tones tissues to ease diarrhea, dysentery, bleeding, and inflammatory and ulcerative conditions.
Comfrey ~ soothing for inflammatory bowel diseases and ulceration; moisturizing to reduce constipation.
Cranesbill ~ used for diarrhea, ulcers, inflammatory bowel conditions, bloody stools, and hemorrhoids.
Dandelion ~ stimulates bile flow; mild laxative; anti-inflammatory; can help colitis and colon cancers.
Echinacea ~ antibiotic for intestinal infections; cooling and anti-inflammatory to ulcerated tissue.
Elecampane ~ promotes regular bowel movements; maintains beneficial intestinal flora; used for indigestion, gas, bloating, and intestinal ulcers, infections, and parasites.
Feverfew ~ laxative; kills parasites; anti-inflammatory; reduces intestinal cramps and spasms.
Goldenrod ~ helpful for diarrhea, Crohn's disease, spasms, inflammation, infections, and yeast overgrowth.
Goldenseal ~ antibiotic for infections; kills yeast and parasites; beneficial for inflammation, irritable bowel conditions, ulcers, constipation due to a sluggish system, and diarrhea caused by bacteria and parasites.
Holy Basil ~ stimulates enzyme production; reduces spasms, gas, ulcers, diarrhea, constipation, parasites.
Hops ~ antibiotic; decreases parasites, dysentery, spasms, inflammation, and constipation.
Horehound ~ helpful for sluggish intestines, gas, bloating, and constipation; kills some intestinal parasites.
Hyssop ~ a mild laxative; kills parasites; reduces inflammation, spasms, gas, and bloating.
Lobelia ~ reduces inflammation, spasms, irritable bowel, and chronic constipation due to sluggish digestion.
Marshmallow ~ eases spasms, inflammation, constipation or diarrhea, hemorrhoids, and ulcerative colitis.
Mugwort ~ used for diarrhea or constipation; kills intestinal bacteria and parasites.
Mullein ~ cooling, soothing, anti-inflammatory; reduces bloody diarrhea; kills roundworms and tapeworms.

Peppermint ~ taken for inflammatory bowel problems, indigestion, gas, bloating, and diarrhea or constipation.
Sage ~ antibacterial; reduces gas, bloating, inflammation, spasms, bleeding, diarrhea, and colitis.
Senna ~ a strong laxative that stimulates peristalsis; used to treat constipation and intestinal parasites.
Stinging Nettle ~ anti-inflammatory; taken to treat ulcers and watery and/or bloody diarrhea.
Thyme ~ kills food-born infections and parasites; decreases diarrhea, spasms, and gas.
Valerian ~ reduces cramps, spasms, gas, and intestinal ulcers, especially for conditions involving anxiety.
Yarrow ~ helpful for gas, bloating, spasms, diarrhea or constipation, bleeding, infections, and inflammatory conditions like ulcerative colitis.
Yellow Dock ~ stimulates bile flow; may be helpful for Crohn's, ulcerative colitis, and diarrhea or constipation.

Other Helpful Herbs:

Carob bean (*Ceratonia siliqua*) ~ reduces diarrhea; the powdered bean tastes like chocolate and can be mixed in non-dairy milk, cookies, cakes, and other baked products; effective for young children and adults.
Fenugreek seeds (*Trigonella foenum-graecum*) ~ soothing mucilage reduces intestinal inflammation.
Ginger (*Zingiber officinale*) ~ anti-inflammatory; helps diarrhea, sluggish bowels, irritable bowel syndrome.
Khella (*Ammi visnaga*) ~ smooth muscle relaxant for gastrointestinal spasms and irritable bowel problems.
Licorice (*Glycyrrhiza glabra*) ~ excels in reducing inflammation and spasms and healing ulcerated tissue.
Oregon Grape Root (*Mahonia aquifolium*) ~ anti-inflammatory; antimicrobial; mild laxative.
Wild Yam (*Dioscorea villosa*) ~ intestinal anti-inflammatory and antispasmodic specific for irritable, inflamed bowels, ulcerative colitis, Crohn's disease, and diverticulitis.
Herbs that heal and restore integrity to the intestinal lining ~ Sarsaparilla (*Smilax aristolochiifolia*) and Turmeric (*Curcuma longa*) combination, Chamomile, Marshmallow, and Yarrow.
Other laxatives for constipation ~ Buckthorn bark (*Rhamnus cathartica*), Butternut bark (*Juglans cinerea*), Cascara Sagrada (*Rhamnus purshiana*), Culver's Root (*Veronicastrum virginicum*), Fennel (*Foeniculum vulgare*), Psyllium seed (*Plantago ovata*), and Turkey Rhubarb root (*Rheum palmatum*).

Irritable Bowel Syndrome: See Intestines

Kidneys and Edema:

The kidneys, major organs of the body's detoxification system, filter waste products out of the blood and eliminate them in urine. The kidneys also regulate fluid volume in the blood vessels and tissues.

American Centaury ~ stimulates blood flow in the kidneys; helps propel kidney stones through the ureters.
Astragalus ~ promotes normal function; diuretic; for infection, bloody urine, incontinence, and inflammation.
Black Cohosh ~ diuretic; eases painful kidney and ureter spasms during passage of kidney stones.
Blue Vervain ~ normalizes kidney function; mild diuretic; reduces inflammation, infections, and stones.
Boneset ~ normalizes kidney function; a mild diuretic to reduce fluid retention.
Burdock ~ excellent for kidney function; diuretic; used for kidney inflammation, infections, and stones.
Cayenne ~ antibiotic; stimulates increased blood flow to the kidneys and promotes normal function.
Chamomile ~ reduces BUN (blood urea nitrogen) levels.
Chickweed ~ soothing and cooling for infections and inflammation; a mild diuretic.
Comfrey ~ soothing and healing to painful, inflamed, ulcerated tissues; eases passage of kidney stones.
Dandelion ~ a favorite diuretic; excellent for urinary tract inflammation; helps prevent kidney stones.
Echinacea ~ excellent for all urinary tract infections, including kidney infections, cystitis, and urethritis.
Elderberry ~ an alkalizing diuretic that reduces edema.
Elecampane ~ diuretic, antibiotic, anti-inflammatory, and antispasmodic for urinary infections and stones.
Goldenrod ~ increases blood flow to kidneys and production of urine; for infections, inflammation, stones.
Goldenseal ~ anti-inflammatory; antibacterial for kidney infections; mildly diuretic.
Hops ~ diuretic; anti-inflammatory; antibiotic; reduces stone formation.
Horehound ~ a mild diuretic; improves blood flow through the kidneys.
Hyssop ~ a diuretic.
Lobelia ~ mild diuretic; reduces spasms, inflammation, and relaxes ureters during passage of kidney stones.
Marshmallow ~ mild diuretic; taken for inflammation, spasms, infections, and easier passage of stones.
Motherwort ~ stimulates sluggish kidneys; diuretic; reduces kidney inflammation and bloody urine.
Mullein Root ~ a diuretic that decreases edema and increases urine output while reducing frequency of urination; soothing, cooling, analgesic, anti-inflammatory; used for stones and incontinence.
Sage ~ reduces kidney inflammation and spasms; antibacterial.
Stinging Nettle ~ excellent diuretic and tonic for infections, inflammation, and reducing kidney stones.
Yarrow ~ excellent for all urinary tract infections; increases blood flow; reduces pain and inflammation.
Yellow Dock ~ supports the kidneys; promotes urination; helps eliminate excess acids.

Other Helpful Herbs:

Andrographis (*Andrographis paniculata*) ~ antioxidant; for nephritis (kidney disease and inflammation).
Barberry (*Berberis vulgaris*) ~ an antibacterial used for urinary tract infections (UTIs).
Buchu (*Agathosma betulina*) ~ diuretic; antibacterial; helps prevent UTIs; may reduce incontinence.
Bupleurum (*Bupleurum chinense*) ~ used for chronic nephritis; antioxidant actions protect kidneys from damage; promotes optimal blood flow through kidneys; strong anti-inflammatory.
Celery seed (*Apium graveolens*) ~ diuretic; anti-inflammatory; antibiotic for urinary tract.
Chicory (*Cichorium intybus*) ~ supports kidney function; diuretic; antioxidant; detoxifies kidneys and blood.

Cleavers (*Galium aparine*) ~ a primary diuretic that stimulates kidneys to remove waste products; improves blood filtration and urine production; clears heat, inflammation, and urinary tract infections (UTIs); helps nephritis (kidney disease and inflammation) following sepsis; safe to use as a tonic taken over time.
Couch Grass (*Elymus repens*) ~ diuretic; soothing; used for UTIs and kidney stones; usually taken with other herbs like Yarrow, Uva-ursi/Bearberry, and Buchu.
Dan Shen (*Salvia miltiorrhiza*) ~ a primary kidney herb in Traditional Chinese Medicine; antimicrobial; promotes blood flow; enhances urea (BUN) and creatinine clearance to reduce excessive levels.
Eclipta (*Eclipta prostata*) ~ a cooling kidney tonic; supports optimal function; anti-inflammatory; antibacterial; helpful treatment for bloody urine.
Goldthread (*Coptis chinensis*) ~ an antibacterial used for UTIs.
Gravel Root (*Eupatorium purpureum*) ~ diuretic; tones urinary membranes; very effective to loosen, dissolve, and eliminate sediment and stones in the urinary tract; used for decreasing excess albumin (protein) in urine, chronic nephritis, and later stages of kidney disease and kidney failure with edema and ascites (fluid retention in the abdominal cavity).
Hydrangea (*Hydrangea arborescens*) ~ diuretic; dissolves stones; helpful for UTIs and kidney inflammation.
Milk Thistle (*Silybum marianum*) ~ increases catalase and glutathione antioxidants that protect kidney cells from damage and toxins; protects from cancer; promotes apoptosis (programmed death of cancerous cells).
Oregon Grape Root (*Mahonia aquifolium*) ~ an antibacterial used for UTIs.
Parsley (*Petroselinum crispum*) ~ decreases spasms; diuretic; helps prevent formation of kidney stones.
Privet (*Ligustrum lucidum*) ~ a kidney tonic; antibacterial; anti-inflammatory; supports optimal function.
Schisandra (*Schisandra chinensis*) ~ a kidney tonic; helps correct diminished body fluids and excessive thirst; used for problems related to kidney weakness including incontinence, bed-wetting, night sweats, and chronic diarrhea.
Uva-ursi/Bearberry (*Arctostaphylos uva-ursi*) ~ antimicrobial; astringent; excellent for acute and chronic inflammation; used to treat nephritis, UTIs, ulceration of urinary tract membranes, and remove stones.
White Oak bark (*Quercus alba*) ~ astringent; antiseptic; helps to dissolve kidney stones.
Other diuretics ~ Corn Silk (*Zea mays*), Juniper (*Juniperus communis*), and Horsetail (*Equisetum arvense*).
Other helpful herbs for kidney stones ~ Barberry (*Berberis vulgaris*), Stone Root (*Collinsonia canadensis*), and Pellitory-of-the-Wall (*Parietaria officinalis*).

Lactation: See Breast-Feeding and pages 610-611 in "Herbs for Pregnancy, Childbirth, and Lactation"
Large Intestine: See Intestines
Laryngitis: See Throat
Liver: (also see Digestive System)

The liver is involved in a wide range of metabolic functions. It produces bile which digests fats and is stored in the gallbladder; processes nutrients absorbed by the intestines during digestion and converts them into forms that can be used by the body; metabolizes many toxins including alcohol, pharmaceutical and recreational drugs, and chemical toxins; stores vitamin A, iron, and glycogen (sugar); regulates the composition of blood, including the amounts of glucose, protein, and fat that enter the bloodstream; removes bilirubin, ammonia, toxins, and excessive estrogen from the blood; and produces cholesterol, triglycerides, albumin, hormones, many enzymes, and clotting factors necessary for blood to clot.

Toxic overload from alcohol, pesticides, chemical additives in water, food and other environmental sources, and the hepatitis virus are the primary causes of liver inflammation, jaundice, cirrhosis (scarring), and cancer. Hepatoprotective herbs protect the liver from many toxins and cellular damage.

American Centaury ~ stimulates bile production; helps indigestion, nausea, jaundice, and high cholesterol.
Astragalus ~ hepatoprotective; lowers high cholesterol levels; normalizes liver enzymes; helpful for hepatitis and other liver diseases; promotes liver cell regeneration.
Blue Vervain ~ increases bile flow; reduces gallstones, inflammation, jaundice, high cholesterol, and toxicity.
Boneset ~ stimulates sluggish liver and bile flow; normalizes liver function; helps jaundice and hepatitis.
Burdock ~ liver tonic and cleanser; promotes normal function and bile flow; lowers high cholesterol levels.
Calendula ~ promotes bile flow; healing and cleansing for jaundice, hepatitis, and liver toxicity.
Cayenne ~ stimulates blood and bile flow through the liver; normalizes liver function; reduces cholesterol.
Chickweed ~ soothing and moisturizing for liver inflammation and excess heat.
Dandelion ~ a superb liver tonic helpful for most liver problems, including high cholesterol levels, diminished bile flow, toxic overload, inflammation, hepatitis, and jaundice.
Elecampane ~ promotes bile production; helps conditions of congestion, including high cholesterol.
Goldenseal ~ stimulates bile flow; anti-inflammatory; used for normalizing liver function, cirrhosis, jaundice.
Holy Basil ~ reduces high cholesterol and triglycerides; used to treat hepatitis and jaundice.
Hops ~ a bitter stimulant; increases bile production; anti-inflammatory; helpful for hepatitis and jaundice.
Horehound ~ a bitter stimulant that increases bile flow; used for hepatitis and jaundice.
Hyssop ~ promotes bile flow; taken for jaundice and liver inflammation.
Isatis ~ antiviral; cooling; used for treating inflammation, jaundice, and hepatitis.
Lavender ~ helps normalize cholesterol levels, decrease LDL, and increase HDL cholesterol levels.
Mugwort ~ stimulates bile flow; inhibits hepatitis B and C; beneficial for sluggish liver and jaundice.
Peppermint ~ stimulates bile flow.

Sage ~ increases bile flow; stimulates a sluggish liver; lowers high cholesterol; protects liver against toxins.
Saint John's Wort ~ excellent liver herb that increases bile flow, stimulates a sluggish liver, and eliminates and protects against toxins.
Yarrow ~ protects liver from toxins and chemical damage; stimulates normal liver function; can be helpful for treating hepatitis.
Yellow Dock ~ a liver tonic and cleanser; promotes normal function and bile flow; lowers high cholesterol.

Other Helpful Herbs:

Andrographis (*Andrographis paniculata*) ~ bitter tonic; antioxidant; anti-inflammatory; hepatoprotective; eliminates toxins (used for venomous snake bites); improves bile function; used for liver damage, infections, hepatitis, jaundice, and cirrhosis.
Artichoke leaf (*Cynara scolymus*) ~ a bitter tonic that stimulates liver function; used for indigestion, nausea, gas, and bloating due to insufficient bile production; helps reduce elevated cholesterol and triglyceride levels; antioxidant; protects liver cells from alcohol, toxins, and other free radical damage; beneficial for treating hepatitis and cirrhosis; promotes regeneration of liver cells.
Ashwagandha (*Withania somnifera*) ~ used for chronic liver diseases; reduces total cholesterol and LDL.
Barberry (*Berberis vulgaris*) ~ contains berberine; improves liver function and bile flow; reduces jaundice.
Bupleurum (*Bupleurum chinense*) ~ primary hepatoprotective; anti-inflammatory; improves blood flow within liver; detoxifies liver and blood; lowers high cholesterol levels; antiviral; used for acute and chronic hepatitis, cirrhosis, hepatomegaly (enlarged liver); promotes repair of damaged cells; inhibits development of cancerous cells and tumors; energetically clears the liver and helps release chronically suppressed emotions such as rage, shame, and guilt.
Chicory (*Cichorium intybus*) ~ a mild bitter; supports liver function; helps normalize bile, cholesterol levels.
Eclipta (*Eclipta prostata*) ~ a cooling liver tonic; anti-inflammatory; reduces jaundice; used for liver diseases.
Fenugreek seeds (*Trigonella foenum-graecum*) ~ lowers elevated total cholesterol, LDL, and triglycerides.
Fringe Tree (*Chionanthus virginicus*) ~ valuable for jaundice and other liver problems including inflammation, enlargement, and pain; helpful for acute congestion and gallbladder problems.
Garlic (*Allium sativum*) ~ antioxidants help protect cells from damage; reduces elevated total cholesterol, LDL, and triglyceride levels; increases levels of protective HDL; promotes production and flow of bile.
Gentian root (*Gentiana lutea*) ~ stimulates liver function, bile flow; protects from toxins and viral infections.
Ginger (*Zingiber officinale*) ~ promotes bile flow; reduces high cholesterol levels.
Ginseng, Asian (*Panax ginseng*) and American (*Panax quinquefolius*) ~ antioxidant; protect liver from toxins and radiation exposure; reduce elevated total cholesterol and triglycerides; increase beneficial HDL.
Licorice (*Glycyrrhiza glabra*) ~ antioxidant; protects liver against toxic and viral damage; anti-inflammatory; promotes optimal function; helpful for hepatitis and cirrhosis; normalizes elevated liver enzymes.
Maitake (*Grifola frondosa*), Reishi (*Ganoderma lucidum*), and Shiitake (*Lentinula edodes*) mushrooms ~ used for alcohol damage, hepatitis, and cirrhosis; excellent immunomodulators that benefit the liver.
Milk Thistle (*Silybum marianum*) ~ classic liver herb; antioxidant that increases glutathione and superoxide dismutase (SOD) levels; protects liver, blood, and tissues from toxins; helps regenerate damaged liver cells; used in treatment of hepatitis, cirrhosis, and other liver problems.
Olive leaf (*Olea europaea*) ~ antioxidant; anti-inflammatory; hepatoprotective; helps reduce elevated cholesterol and triglyceride levels; used for alcohol damage, hepatitis, and cirrhosis.
Oregon Grape Root (*Mahonia aquifolium*) ~ antimicrobial; anti-inflammatory; helps normalize and stimulate liver function through mild irritation and should be used cautiously in chronic or acute liver disease.
Privet (*Ligustrum lucidum*) ~ hepatoprotective and tonic; anti-inflammatory; considered to be an excellent treatment for hepatitis in Traditional Chinese Medicine, and is often combined with Astragalus.
Schisandra (*Schisandra chinensis*) ~ promotes bile production and flow; anti-inflammatory; antioxidant; antiviral; beneficial for hepatitis and cirrhosis; lowers elevated liver enzymes indicative of liver damage; protects liver cells from effects of toxins and hepatitis; promotes regeneration of damaged liver cells.
Turmeric (*Curcuma longa*) ~ excellent liver herb; lowers elevated total cholesterol, LDL, and triglycerides; increases beneficial HDL; protects liver from alcohol and environmental toxin damage; helpful for treating most liver problems, including inflammation, jaundice, hepatitis, and cirrhosis.
Wild Yam (*Dioscorea villosa*) ~ supports liver function; promotes bile production; lowers elevated cholesterol, LDL, triglycerides, and raises beneficial HDL; anti-inflammatory.

Lung and Bronchial Problems:

Astragalus ~ antiviral and antibacterial for upper respiratory infections and the flu; strengthens lungs and immunity; beneficial for shortness of breath, allergies, chronic lung weakness, asthma, and emphysema.
Bloodroot ~ strong antibiotic, antiviral; expectorant for serious coughs and infections (be cautious of toxicity).
Blue Vervain ~ beneficial for viral and bacterial infections, coughs, asthma, lung spasms, and inflammation.
Boneset ~ strong immunostimulant and antimicrobial; used for bronchitis, pneumonia, asthma, emphysema.
Burdock ~ moisturizes lungs; for infections, dry coughs, bronchitis, pneumonia, asthma, and emphysema.
Catnip ~ specific for children; helpful for coughs, bronchitis and other respiratory infections, and asthma.
Cayenne ~ antibacterial; reduces excess mucous; excellent for coughs, spasms, shortness of breath, acute infections, and chronic lung problems including asthma and emphysema.
Chamomile ~ helps decrease congestion and coughs.

Chickweed ~ soothing and moisturizing for dry lung conditions, coughs, bronchitis, asthma, and emphysema.
Cinquefoil ~ an astringent that constricts tissues and reduces lung secretions and hemorrhage.
Comfrey ~ moisturizing, healing, and soothing for lung irritation and inflammation; cough expectorant.
Cranesbill ~ an astringent that constricts tissues and reduces lung secretions and hemorrhage.
Echinacea ~ an immunostimulant for upper respiratory tract infections, including bronchitis and pneumonia.
Elderberry ~ antiviral; specific for respiratory tract infections, coughs, flu, and fever.
Elecampane ~ specific for all lung problems, especially those related to excess phlegm; excellent for coughs, sinusitis, bronchitis, pneumonia; used for shortness of breath, emphysema, asthma, and tuberculosis.
Goldenrod ~ antihistamine actions help reduce excess mucous; used for infections, bronchitis, and the flu.
Goldenseal ~ specific for excessive mucous production and wet, productive coughs; anti-inflammatory; antibacterial for most upper respiratory infections, including tonsillitis, laryngitis, bronchitis, pneumonia.
Holy Basil ~ specific for excess mucous, colds, dry or wet coughs, bronchitis, asthma, and hay fever allergies.
Hops ~ antibiotic; anti-inflammatory; taken for coughs, pneumonia, and tuberculosis.
Horehound ~ specific for coughs, infections, cold and flu, excessive mucous discharge, congestion, asthma.
Hyssop ~ helpful for bacterial and viral respiratory infections, coughs, excess mucous, emphysema, asthma.
Isatis ~ specific for viral and bacterial respiratory infections; cooling properties lower fevers.
Lavender ~ antibacterial; calming actions reduce spasms and coughs and ease asthma.
Lemon Balm ~ antibiotic and antiviral; taken for coughs, excess mucous, and some types of asthma.
Lobelia ~ promotes easier breathing; herb of choice for many lung problems, including coughs, spasms, asthma, emphysema, bronchitis, pneumonia; helps to overcome nicotine addiction and stop smoking.
Marshmallow ~ moisturizes lungs; benefits dry coughs, bronchitis, pneumonia, emphysema, and asthma.
Motherwort ~ reduces spasms and mucous congestion; beneficial for bronchitis, coughs, and asthma.
Mullein ~ moisturizing; excellent for lung problems, including coughs, infections, asthma, and emphysema.
Peppermint ~ reduces congestion and thins mucous to reduce coughs.
Pleurisy Root ~ excellent for all respiratory problems, including coughs, infections, and excess phlegm.
Sage ~ antibacterial and antiviral; reduces phlegm and mucous; taken for coughs, spasms, and inflammation.
Stinging Nettle ~ antihistamine properties help coughs, congestion, bronchitis, asthma, and hay fever.
Thyme ~ taken for infections, coughs, excess mucous, bronchial spasms, bronchitis, emphysema, asthma.
Valerian ~ reduces coughing, bronchial spasms, and shortness of breath.
Wood Betony ~ soothes inflammation; expectorant; used for coughs, wheezing, bronchitis, and asthma.
Yarrow ~ antibacterial; reduces mucous, spasms, inflammation, and coughs.

Other Helpful Herbs:

Andrographis (*Andrographis paniculata*) ~ antibacterial; antiviral; reduces inflammation and fever; used for acute and chronic infections, including colds, flu, sore throat, coughs, bronchitis, and pneumonia.
Angelica (*Angelica archangelica*) ~ expectorant for coughs and colds with mucous congestion.
Anise (*Pimpinella anisum*) ~ a relaxing expectorant; reduces mucous, inflammation, and spasms; helpful for coughs, asthma, and emphysema.
Ephedra (*Ephedra sinica*) ~ stimulates norepinephrine release, which dilates bronchial air passages, improves breathing, and reduces spasms and mucous production; beneficial for bronchitis, hay fever, asthma, and emphysema.
Eucalyptus (*Eucalyptus* spp.) ~ anti-inflammatory, antimicrobial, and expectorant for respiratory infections.
Fennel (*Foeniculum vulgare*) ~ a soothing expectorant for coughs and bronchitis; reduces inflammation.
Fenugreek seed (*Trigonella foenum-graecum*) ~ soothing expectorant for sore throats, bronchitis, and coughs.
Garlic (*Allium sativum*) ~ antimicrobial for respiratory infections, including bronchitis, pneumonia, and whooping cough; reduces mucous production and eases coughs.
Ginger (*Zingiber officinale*) ~ decreases mucous congestion; expectorant; helps coughs, bronchitis, asthma.
Ginkgo (*Ginkgo biloba*) ~ anti-inflammatory; helpful for lung and breathing problems, especially asthma.
Ground Ivy (*Glechoma hederacea*) ~ commonly used in Europe as an expectorant, antiviral, antibacterial, and for treating hay fever, respiratory infections, and asthma.
Khella (*Ammi visnaga*) ~ a smooth muscle relaxant; bronchodilator for spastic lung conditions and asthma.
Licorice (*Glycyrrhiza glabra*) ~ anti-inflammatory and relaxing expectorant for coughs, bronchitis, asthma, and emphysema.
Linden (*Tilia* spp.) ~ reduces mucous production; used for treatment of coughs, sore throat, and bronchitis.
Oregano (*Origanum vulgare*) ~ anti-inflammatory, antioxidant, antibacterial, antiviral, and expectorant; beneficial for coughs with thick mucous, bronchitis, laryngitis, pharyngitis, and asthma.
Oregon Grape Root (*Mahonia aquifolium*) ~ antimicrobial; anti-inflammatory; reduces mucous production.
Pau D'arco (*Tabebuia impetiginosa*) ~ antibacterial, antiviral, and antifungal for respiratory infections.
Red Clover (*Trifolium pratense*) ~ expectorant; taken for colds, cough, bronchitis, whooping cough, asthma.
Schisandra (*Schisandra chinensis*) ~ a lung tonic; expectorant; antihistamine action; anti-inflammatory; antioxidant; antibacterial and antiviral for respiratory tract infections; beneficial for chronic coughs, shortness of breath, labored breathing, and asthma.
Wild Cherry bark (*Prunus serotina*) ~ calming bronchial tonic; expectorant; reduces spasms, sore throat, and mucous production; helps acute and chronic coughs, bronchitis, pneumonia, whooping cough, and asthma.

Lymphatic System (Lymphatic Fluid or Lymph, Lymphatic Vessels, Nodes, and Glands):

The lymphatic system is part of the circulatory system and a vital component of the immune system. Lymphatic fluid consists of about 95% water and 5% plasma, which contains proteins and lymphocytes (white blood cells involved in immunity). This clear fluid bathes the tissues and moves between cells to supply nutrients, remove toxins and metabolic waste products, and eliminate pathogens. Lymph is collected and transported through the lymphatic vessels, and is eventually dumped into subclavian blood veins. Lymph nodes are small, fibrous capsules of lymphocytes scattered along lymphatic vessels (most numerous in the armpit, neck, and groin) and in lymph tissues. Lymph nodes produce antibodies to fight infection and filter lymph fluids to remove pathogens like bacteria, toxins, and cancer cells. Lymph nodes and glands become swollen when infected. When lymph nodes become cancerous, they are known as lymphomas and include Hodgkin's disease. Lymphagogue herbs strengthen, detoxify, and stimulate lymph glands and the activity of the entire lymphatic system. They are helpful for many problems, including swollen glands, lymphatic congestion and cancers, and resolving chronic skin conditions.

Black Walnut ~ antibiotic and antiviral; stimulates movement and cleansing of lymph fluid and nodes.
Burdock ~ cleansing; stimulates lymph flow; promotes immunity; used for lymphatic infections and cancers.
Calendula ~ cleanses and promotes flow of lymph; helps infections, swollen nodes, and lymphatic cancers.
Chickweed ~ cleansing and detoxifying; promotes lymph circulation; reduces swollen lymph nodes.
Dandelion ~ cleansing; reduces lymph congestion and promotes circulation.
Echinacea ~ stimulates immunity; excellent for lymphatic cleansing, swollen nodes; for lymphatic cancers.
Goldenseal ~ detoxifies lymph; stimulates immunity; helps normalize spleen; taken for swollen nodes.
Isatis ~ antibacterial and antiviral; cooling and anti-inflammatory; used for swollen lymph glands and nodes.
Mullein ~ soothing and anti-inflammatory; detoxifies lymph; taken for swollen lymph nodes.
Pleurisy Root ~ promotes lymphatic circulation and drainage.
Stinging Nettle ~ cooling; anti-inflammatory; cleansing to lymph fluid and nodes.
Yellow Dock ~ cleanses and stimulates flow of lymph; used for lymphatic infections, swollen nodes, cancers.

Other Helpful Herbs:

Cleavers (*Galium aparine*) ~ one of the best tonics to detox and promote lymphatic circulation and drainage; effective for reducing swollen lymph nodes and glands, tonsillitis, and lymphedema after mastectomies.
Pau D'arco (*Tabebuia impetiginosa*) ~ supports entire lymphatic system; used for lymphatic congestion and detoxification; improves lymphatic circulation; antimicrobial against lymphatic infections.
Plantain (*Plantago* spp.) ~ antibacterial; promotes detoxification; reduces lymphatic congestion and inflamed, swollen lymph glands and nodes.
Poke root (*Phytolacca americana*) ~ one of the strongest, most reliable herbs for viral, fungal, and bacterial infections and acute or chronic hard, swollen lymph nodes and glands; stimulates flow of lymph fluids to remove toxins and metabolic waste products; use carefully as large doses cause vomiting and diarrhea.
Prickly Ash (*Zanthoxylum americanum*) ~ antimicrobial; has stimulating effect on lymphatic system.
Red Clover (*Trifolium pratense*) ~ excellent blood and lymph purifier; reduces swollen lymph glands, nodes.
Violet (*Viola papilionacea*, spp.) ~ lymphatic herb used for chronic swollen glands and nodes.
Wild Indigo (*Baptisia tinctoria*) ~ strong antimicrobial for lymphatic infection, congestion, and inflammation; reduces toxic overload; clears toxic heat; used for acute or chronic swollen glands and lymph nodes, tonsillitis, and septic infections; use under guidance of a qualified herbalist due to toxicity of large doses.
Woundwort (*Prunella vulgaris*) ~ has affinity for the lymphatic system; lymphatic decongestant; taken for swollen lymph nodes and glands and lingering infections.

Male Reproductive System (Prostate Gland and Testicles):

Black Cohosh and Blue Cohosh ~ exert estrogen-like activity that inhibits conversion of testosterone into dihydrotestosterone (DHT), the form contributing to benign prostatic hypertrophy (BPH), which is prostate inflammation and enlargement.
Burdock ~ reduces prostate swelling and inflammation.
Chasteberry ~ reduces excessive testosterone levels responsible for BPH.
Chickweed ~ helps decrease prostate inflammation; helpful for swollen, inflamed testicles and testicular and prostate cancers.
Echinacea ~ antibiotic, anti-inflammatory, and cooling for treatment of prostatitis (prostate inflammation).
Goldenrod ~ reduces prostate inflammation; promotes prostate health.
Goldenseal ~ reduces prostate inflammation.
Holy Basil ~ improves male fertility by increasing sperm count and motility.
Hops ~ reduces excessive libido, wet dreams, and premature ejaculation; estrogenic chemicals reduce testosterone levels as a treatment for BPH.
Sage ~ reduces hot flashes often caused by hormonal drug treatment when decreasing testosterone levels in men with BPH and prostate cancer.
Stinging Nettle ~ the roots are specific for prostate inflammation and BPH.

Other Helpful Herbs:

Buchu (*Agathosma betulina*) ~ diuretic; used for genitourinary infections and prostatitis.
Couch Grass (*Elymus repens*) ~ tea taken as a daily tonic helps reduce prostate swelling and inflammation.

Ginkgo (*Ginkgo biloba*) ~ improves circulation and can be helpful for erectile dysfunction.
Ginseng, Asian (*Panax ginseng*) and American (*Panax quinquefolius*) ~ can benefit impotence, erectile dysfunction, and increase sperm count and sexual stamina in older men.
Horny Goat Weed (*Epimedium sagittatum*) ~ studies show it can restore low testosterone levels; increases sexual energy and virility; used for infertility.
Horsetail (*Equisetum arvense*) ~ specific for prostate inflammation and BPH.
Hydrangea (*Hydrangea arborescens*) ~ diuretic; specific for prostate inflammation and enlargement.
Licorice (*Glycyrrhiza glabra*) ~ reduces BPH by inhibiting conversion of testosterone into dihydrotestosterone.
Maca (*Lepidium meyenii*) ~ improves libido, erectile dysfunction, sperm production, fertility; reduces BPH.
Muira Puama (*Ptychopetalum olacoides*) ~ improves libido and erectile dysfunction.
Pau D'arco (*Tabebuia impetiginosa*) ~ anti-inflammatory; helpful for prostatitis.
Pygeum (*Pygeum africanum*) ~ contains anti-inflammatory beta-sitosterols; improves symptoms of BPH.
Red Clover (*Trifolium pratense*) ~ studies show that estrogenic isoflavones inhibit development of BPH.
Saw Palmetto (*Serenoa repens*) ~ prevents and treats inflammation and BPH; inhibits conversion of testosterone to damaging dihydrotestosterone (DHT).

Mastitis: See Breast

Measles (also see Viral Infections):

Also called rubeola, measles is a highly contagious viral (Morbillivirus) infection of the respiratory tract that causes fever, flu-like symptoms, and an irritating skin rash that covers the body.

Burdock ~ reduces skin irritation and inflammation.
Catnip ~ specific for childhood illness; diminishes fever and skin irritation.
Chickweed ~ tea can soothe and cool hot, inflamed, irritated tissues; lowers fevers.
Echinacea ~ antiviral; immunostimulant; cooling and anti-inflammatory for skin eruptions.
Hyssop ~ antiviral; cooling; reduces fever.
Isatis ~ strong antiviral; cooling for fevers; soothing to skin eruptions.
Lemon Balm ~ antiviral; lowers fevers; analgesic.
Marshmallow ~ tea can soothe and cool hot, inflamed, irritated tissues and reduce fevers.
Stinging Nettle ~ used internally and externally to cool and soothe inflamed skin eruptions.
Yarrow ~ soothes and heals hot, inflamed tissues; analgesic; lowers fevers.

Other Helpful Herbs:

Olive Leaf (*Olea europaea*) ~ destructive to *Morbillivirus* causing measles; antioxidant.

Memory: See Brain and Cognitive Function

Meningitis (also see Viral Infections):

Meningitis is a life-threatening acute inflammation of the meninges, the protective membranes covering the brain and spinal cord, caused by viruses or bacteria. The most common symptoms are fever, headache, and neck stiffness. Pharmaceuticals are the necessary treatment, but herbs can be helpful additions.

Black Cohosh ~ reduces spinal stiffness, inflammation, and spasms.
Boneset ~ a strong immunostimulant to treat infections.
Cayenne ~ an antibiotic prescribed by the Eclectic physicians to treat meningitis.
Echinacea ~ immunostimulant; antibacterial and antiviral.
Goldenseal ~ effective against bacteria causing meningitis; stimulates immunity.
Isatis ~ a strong antibacterial; cooling for inflammation and high fevers.
Lobelia ~ reduces inflammation and spasms of meningitis; used by Eclectic physicians for meningitis.
Thyme ~ specific against bacteria causing meningitis; anti-inflammatory, antispasmodic, and analgesic.

Menopause:

Astragalus ~ can help reduce hot flashes.
Black Cohosh ~ excellent herb-of-choice for hot flashes, mood swings, irritability, depression, vaginal thinning and dryness, hirsutism (excessive hair growth on the face, neck, and chest in women), and other menopausal discomforts; an alternative for hormone replacement therapy (HRT).
Blue Vervain ~ decreases anxiety, nervous tension, and hot flashes; promotes hormonal balance.
Chasteberry ~ increases progesterone levels by supporting the hypothalamus and pituitary gland; increases luteinizing hormone and reduces high prolactin levels, which helps balance the ratio of progesterone to estrogen and increases progesterone levels when too low; excellent for infertility, estrogen dominance, polycystic ovarian syndrome (PCOS), and menopausal symptoms.
Dandelion ~ beneficial effects on the liver help reduce hot flashes, mood swings, and estrogen dominance.
Hops ~ exerts estrogenic activity; calming to nerves; may be beneficial to prevent or improve osteoporosis.
Motherwort ~ reduces menopausal anxiety, depression, heart palpitations, insomnia, and hot flashes.
Sage ~ reduces hot flashes, nervous tension, exhaustion, and other menopausal symptoms.
Saint John's Wort ~ helps ease menopausal symptoms and normalize moods.
Scullcap ~ excellent nervine and sedative to relieve anxiety, heart palpitations, and insomnia.
Stinging Nettle ~ cooling properties can ease hot flashes; minerals calm nerves and build bone.
Valerian ~ eases anxiety, tension, heart palpitations, and insomnia that may accompany menopause.
Yellow Dock ~ cooling properties and beneficial action on the liver can help relieve hot flashes.

Other Helpful Herbs:
Maca (*Lepidium meyenii*) ~ supports and normalizes the hypothalamus-pituitary-adrenal (HPA) axis; improves ovarian function; helps maintain estrogen and progesterone balance; can be helpful for PMS, menopause, hot flashes, increasing energy, and maintaining strong bones.

Menstruation:
American Centaury ~ stimulates menstruation; normalizes cycles; eases premenstrual syndrome (PMS).
Black Cohosh ~ normalizes the hormonal system; regulates menses; helpful for PMS, cramps, fluid retention.
Blue Cohosh ~ normalizes uterus and ovaries; regulates cycles; relieves PMS, cramps, and breast tenderness.
Blue Vervain ~ excellent for menstrual problems, including scanty or profuse bleeding, PMS, and cramps.
Burdock ~ a diuretic that helps reduce PMS bloating and breast tenderness; helps regulate menstrual cycles.
Calendula ~ promotes normal menstruation; relieves pelvic congestion, PMS discomforts, and cramps.
Catnip ~ relieves pelvic congestion; promotes menstruation; helps ease PMS and cramps.
Cayenne ~ increases circulation to the pelvic area; normalizes a sluggish reproductive system; reduces profuse menstrual bleeding and cramps.
Chamomile ~ taken for delayed and painful menstruation; eases uterine cramps and PMS tension.
Chasteberry ~ regulates and normalizes hormonal levels; helps most menstrual irregularities and problems.
Cinquefoil ~ an excellent astringent used to decrease excessive menstrual bleeding.
Cranesbill ~ an excellent astringent that decreases profuse menstrual bleeding.
Dandelion ~ beneficial effects on the liver help normalize menstruation and reduce mood swings, PMS, and cramps; a diuretic that relieves menstrual breast tenderness and fluid retention.
Elecampane ~ helpful for delayed, scanty menses, cramps, swollen breasts, and other PMS discomforts.
Feverfew ~ stimulates menstruation; reduces PMS and cramps; normalizes blood flow in pelvic organs.
Goldenrod ~ normalizes menstrual cycles; beneficial for painful and delayed menses; reduces cramps.
Holy Basil ~ eases menstrual cramps, PMS symptoms, and reduces tension in the pelvic area.
Hops ~ estrogenic; helps regulate menstrual cycles, reduce spasms and cramps, and ease irritability of PMS.
Horehound ~ stimulates menstruation; increases sluggish menstrual flow; relieves cramps.
Lemon Balm ~ relaxes pelvic muscles; relieves painful cramps; eases PMS mood swings.
Lobelia ~ relaxes pelvis muscles to reduce menstrual pain and cramps.
Motherwort ~ stimulates delayed menses; used for scanty flow, spasms, PMS, edema, emotional flare-ups.
Mugwort ~ normalizes cycles; stimulates menses; reduces PMS symptoms and excessive or spotty bleeding.
Peppermint ~ helpful for delayed and painful menstruation due to nervous tension and anxiety.
Pleurisy Root ~ beneficial for menstrual problems; increases circulation to pelvic organs.
Sage ~ stimulates delayed menses; reduces cramps and excessive bleeding; helps balance hormone levels.
Saint John's Wort ~ helpful for irregular, painful periods, depression, and moodiness.
Scullcap ~ eases menstrual anxiety and cramps.
Stinging Nettle ~ contains iron and nourishes the blood; can reduce excessive menstrual bleeding and cramps; helpful for infertility and amenorrhea (abnormal cessation of periods).
Thyme ~ a mild emmenagogue that stimulates suppressed and late menstruation; reduces uterine cramps.
Valerian ~ an emmenagogue; relaxes the pelvic muscles; eases cramps.
Wood Betony ~ helpful for PMS, menstrual cramps, and excessive bleeding.
Yarrow ~ normalizes periods and bleeding; helpful for cramps, bloating, and other PMS symptoms.
Yellow Dock ~ helpful for menstrual problems, including excessive bleeding, clots, bloating, and pain.
Other Helpful Herbs:
Evening Primrose oil (*Oenothera biennis*) ~ helpful for reducing PMS symptoms and breast pain and fullness; taken internally or applied externally.

Migraine: **See Headaches**

Miscarriage: **See pages 604-605 in "Herbs for Pregnancy, Childbirth, and Lactation"**

Moles:
Bloodroot~ a strong antiviral and caustic that can dissolve moles when externally applied (use with caution under guidance of an herbalist).

Mononucleosis: **See Epstein-Barr Virus (a cause of mononucleosis)**

Morning Sickness: **See page 605 in "Herbs for Pregnancy, Childbirth, and Lactation"**

Mouth, Tongue, and Gums:
The following herbs may be prepared as tea or diluted tincture and used as a mouthwash or gargle.
Bloodroot ~ helps prevent plaque formation, cavities, gum disease, and gingivitis (gum inflammation).
Burdock ~ reduces inflammation, painful canker sores in the mouth, and glossitis (tongue inflammation).
Calendula ~ soothes and heals mouth sores, gum disease, and inflammation.
Chamomile ~ used for gingivitis and toothaches.
Cinquefoil ~ helps inflamed, infected, and ulcerated mouth, tongue, gums, and throat.
Comfrey ~ a soothing gargle or mouthwash for canker sores, ulcers, tissue irritation, and inflammation.
Cranesbill ~ used as a gargle or wash for mouth ulcers, canker sores, thrush (Candida yeast), and sore throats.
Dandelion ~ alkalizing minerals reduce excess acids that cause painful canker sores.
Goldenseal ~ soothes and heals inflammation, canker sores, and infection of the tongue, gums, and mouth.
Sage ~ an antiseptic mouthwash for sore, ulcerated, and inflamed tongue, gums, and mouth.

Saint John's Wort ~ oil or tincture is applied for inflammation and pain in gums; eases toothaches.
Thyme ~ antiseptic, analgesic mouthwash for mouth sores and inflammation.
Yellow Dock ~ used for mouth and gum sores, canker sores, and inflammation.
Other Helpful Herbs:
Clove (*Syzygium aromaticum*) ~ the oil is a strong antiseptic and antibacterial for tooth and gum infections.
Garlic (*Allium sativum*) ~ antimicrobial for mouth and gum infections.
Myrrh (*Commiphora myrrha*) ~ antimicrobial for mouth inflammation and infections, including gingivitis.

Mucous Membranes:

These specialized mucous-secreting tissues line the inner surface of the respiratory, digestive and genito-urinary tracts, and are continuous with the skin at body openings such as the eyelids, ears, nose, mouth, urethra, vagina, and anus. Mucous membranes are a primary barrier between the external world and the interior of the body. Mucous is vital to hydrate, lubricate, and protect tissues.

Blue Vervain ~ normalizes sinus and bronchial mucous secretions; decreases mucous congestion.
Boneset ~ normalizes sinus and bronchial mucous secretions; drying; reduces drainage and congestion.
Burdock ~ normalizes mucous membrane secretion.
Chickweed ~ cooling, soothing, and moisturizing to mucous membranes; hydrates tissues.
Cinquefoil ~ astringent properties constrict membranes to reduce excessive secretion, bleeding, and diarrhea.
Comfrey ~ an exceptional healer; moistens and soothes mucous membrane irritation and inflammation.
Cranesbill ~ astringent properties constrict membranes to reduce excessive secretions, bleeding, diarrhea.
Elecampane ~ tones and normalizes mucous secretions; reduces phlegm; anti-inflammatory; antibacterial.
Feverfew ~ tones mucous membranes; reduces excessive mucous secretions.
Goldenrod ~ tones membranes to normalize secretions; antihistamine action reduces excessive mucous.
Goldenseal ~ normalizes mucous membranes; reduces excessive secretions; antimicrobial; anti-inflammatory.
Horehound ~ tones and normalizes mucous membranes in the respiratory, digestive, and urinary tracts.
Hyssop ~ normalizes mucous membranes, especially in the respiratory, digestive, and urinary tracts.
Lemon Balm ~ reduces excessive and chronic mucous production, drainage, and congestion.
Lobelia ~ helps normalize mucous membrane secretion and diminish mucous congestion.
Marshmallow ~ cools and moisturizes dry, inflamed mucous membranes; hydrates tissues; for dry conditions.
Motherwort ~ reduces excessive mucous secretions and congestion in the lungs and nasal sinuses.
Mullein ~ a mucilage that cools, soothes, and moisturizes mucous membranes and normalizes secretions.
Sage ~ tones mucous membranes and reduces excessive secretions.
Stinging Nettle ~ normalizes mucous membranes; reduces inflammation and excessive mucous secretions.
Yarrow ~ tones mucous membrane tissues to reduce excessive mucous secretions.
Other Helpful Herbs:
Oregon Grape Root (*Mahonia aquifolium*) ~ antimicrobial; anti-inflammatory; normalizes mucous membrane secretion and reduces mucous congestion.

Mumps (also see Viral Infections):

Mumps is typically a mild, short-term viral infection (rubulavirus) of the salivary glands occurring during childhood. Symptoms include painful inflammation and swelling of the salivary glands, headache, and fever.

Burdock ~ soothing and cooling to inflamed tissues.
Chickweed ~ the tea soothes and cools hot, inflamed, irritated tissues; lowers fevers.
Echinacea ~ antiviral; immunostimulant; cooling and anti-inflammatory.
Hyssop ~ antiviral, reduces fevers.
Isatis ~ a strong antiviral; cooling to reduce inflammation and fevers.
Marshmallow ~ cooling and anti-inflammatory.
Mullein ~ beneficial for swollen glands accompanying the mumps.
Stinging Nettle ~ cooling and anti-inflammatory.

Muscle:

Muscle cells contain protein fibers that slide past each another to produce contracting and relaxing movements that change the length and shape of the muscle. The three types of muscle are skeletal, cardiac, and smooth. Skeletal or voluntary muscle is attached to bones by tendons composed of collagen. It enables skeletal movement of the spine and extremities and maintains posture. Smooth or involuntary muscle is found within the walls of organs and structures such as the esophagus, stomach, intestines, diaphragm, bronchi, uterus, urethra, bladder, and blood vessels. Smooth muscle holds internal organs in place and is responsible for movement of internal organs, such as uterine contractions, inhalation and exhalation, and the movement of food through the digestive system. Cardiac muscle (myocardium) is found only in the heart.

Healthy muscle function depends on adequate nutrition (especially protein), blood and oxygen supply, and muscle tone, which is a state of balanced muscle contraction and relaxation while muscles are at rest. Muscle tone is influenced by the nervous system, and nervous hyperstimulation leads to muscle tension, cramps, spasms, and general discomfort. Lack of nerve stimulation results in muscle weakness and organ prolapse. Analgesic, antioxidant, and anti-inflammatory herbs support muscle health.

Astragalus ~ strengthens and tones muscles; beneficial for chronically weak muscles lacking tone, prolapsed organs (such as the bladder and uterus), and hemorrhoids.
Black Cohosh ~ relaxes tense muscles to reduce pain, inflammation, cramps, spasms and tremors;

strengthens weak muscles lacking normal tone and is helpful for uterine and bladder prolapse.
Blue Vervain ~ reduces muscle tension, spasms, sprains, pain; especially helpful for neck and back spasms.
Boneset ~ relaxing and analgesic for muscle tension, spasms, aches, and pain.
Catnip ~ analgesic; externally applied to reduce muscle sprains, spasms, and inflammation.
Cayenne ~ applied for muscle pain, sprains, and spasms; helps fibromyalgia and weak muscles lacking tone.
Chamomile ~ reduces muscular spasms and inflammation, especially in the digestive tract.
Cinquefoil ~ tones and strengthens weak, atonic muscles, prolapsed organs, hernias, and hemorrhoids.
Comfrey ~ excellent applied to sprains, bruises, torn ligaments; eases muscle pain, inflammation, backaches.
Cranesbill ~ tones and strengthens weak muscles; beneficial for prolapsed organs.
Elderberry ~ the berries fortify and enrich the blood to strengthen muscles.
Elecampane ~ beneficial for weak, atonic muscles.
Feverfew ~ anti-inflammatory; reduces spasms in smooth muscles of the blood vessels and organs.
Holy Basil ~ anti-inflammatory and analgesic; reduces spasms; helps ease pain of fibromyalgia.
Hops ~ reduces muscular tension, inflammation, and pain; helpful for muscle sprains and fibromyalgia.
Lavender ~ calming; eases muscle tension, spasms, sprains, cramps, and pain.
Lemon Balm ~ reduces pain, spasms, and inflammation; helpful for sprains and fibromyalgia.
Lobelia ~ a muscle relaxant for spasms, tics, inflammation, pain, and sprains.
Mugwort ~ calms nerves; used for spasms, uncontrollable shaking, tremors, seizures, and epilepsy.
Passion Flower ~ specific for frail, exhausted people with tight muscles due to nervous tension; reduces uncontrolled muscular movements like hiccups, tics, tremors, Parkinson's disease, and epilepsy.
Peppermint ~ the volatile oils reduce muscular inflammation, spasms, and pain.
Scullcap ~ a nervine and sedative that reduces muscle tension, spasms, nervous tics, and tremors.
Saint John's Wort ~ analgesic and anti-inflammatory.
Stinging Nettle ~ proteins, vitamins, and minerals in the leaves strengthen muscles; anti-inflammatory.
Thyme ~ eases muscular tension, pain, spasms, and inflammation; helpful for sprains and fibromyalgia.
Valerian ~ analgesic; reduces muscle tension, cramps, and spasms.
Wood Betony ~ relaxes the nervous system and muscles; reduces spasms and inflammation.

Other Helpful Herbs:

Kava Kava (*Piper methysticum*) ~ calms nervous system; analgesic muscle relaxant for spasms, fibromyalgia.
Rosemary (*Rosmarinus officinalis*) ~ increases blood flow to muscles; calming nervine; topical and internal applications relax smooth and skeletal muscle; decreases muscular pain, spasms, and inflammation.

Nausea: See Stomach

Nervous System (Anxiety, Stress, and Hyperactivity; also see Depression):

The nervous system is regulated by neurotransmitters, the hypothalamus, and the pineal, pituitary, thyroid, and adrenal endocrine glands, all interacting in a dynamic equilibrium. The hypothalamus connects and transfers communication between the endocrine and nervous systems. Neurotransmitters are either inhibiting and calming (serotonin and GABA/gamma-aminobutyric acid) or excitatory and stimulating (epinephrine/adrenaline, norepinephrine, dopamine, glutamate, and phenethylamine or PEA).

All psychological and physiological processes are intimately anchored in the nervous system. Our thoughts and emotions directly influence the nervous system, creating a multitude of effects ranging from calm relaxation to depression, anxiety or hyperstimulation, which manifest as healthy nerve function or lead to imbalances that cause disease. Engaging in daily relaxation and meditation practice is an empowering and effective way to manage stress and heal disturbing thoughts and emotions, which calms and normalizes the nervous system.

Nervine and sedative herbs specifically act on the nervous system. Nervine herbs strengthen, nourish, and restore the nerves. Some nervines are energizing and revitalizing, while others are calming relaxants. Sedative herbs calm the nervous system, reducing stress and tension throughout the body and promoting restful sleep. Many herbs have both nervine and sedative actions. Adaptogen, analgesic, anti-inflammatory, and antispasmodic herbs are also protective and beneficial to the nervous system, as well as calcium, magnesium, and the vitamin B complex.

Black Cohosh ~ a nervine; promotes mental calm and muscle relaxation; used to reduce anxiety, hyperactivity, pain, spasms, tremors, seizures, and epilepsy.
Blue Vervain ~ a nervine and mild sedative taken for depression, anxiety disorders, muscle spasms, pain, numbness, tics, tremors, and seizures.
Boneset ~ a calming and restoring nervine used for nervous exhaustion, anxiety, pain, and muscle spasms.
Catnip ~ mild sedative and nervine for anxiety, hyperactivity, spasms, and insomnia; specific for children.
Cayenne ~ helps relieve pain when applied externally; reduces spasms; calms and heals nervous system during withdrawal from drugs and alcohol.
Chamomile ~ nervine; mild sedative for anxiety, hyperactivity, nervous digestive system, and ADHD.
Holy Basil ~ helps restore nervous and endocrine systems; helpful for problems due to chronic anxiety.
Hops ~ a sedative for anxiety, panic attacks, insomnia, and spasms; analgesic for painful nerves.
Hyssop ~ a sedative and nervine that reduces nervous tension, hyperactivity, and insomnia.
Lavender ~ sedating and restoring to the nerves; analgesic; taken for nervous tics, spasms, convulsions, panic attacks, and problems caused by underlying emotional trauma and anxiety.

Lemon Balm ~ sedating and restoring; analgesic; used for spasms, anxiety, hyperactivity, and hyperthyroidism.
Lobelia ~ larger doses have a relaxing action on the entire nervous system and are helpful for spasms and conditions caused by underlying nervous tension.
Motherwort ~ calming to nerves and heart; for hyperactivity, spasms, and problems due to nervous tension.
Mugwort ~ small doses reduce nervous tension, mild depression, and conditions associated with stress.
Passion Flower ~ sedative and nervine; analgesic; taken for nervous tics and spasms, panic attacks, convulsions, Parkinson's disease, and problems caused by underlying trauma and anxiety.
Peppermint ~ calming and restoring to the nerves; helpful for anxiety and mental exhaustion.
Sage ~ excellent nervine to improve nerve deterioration and reduce exhaustion, depression, and anxiety.
Saint John's Wort ~ normalizes the nervous system by balancing neurotransmitters; calming; analgesic.
Scullcap ~ one of the best sedatives and nervines to normalize and revitalize the nervous system; analgesic; addresses a wide variety of problems caused by anxiety, stress, and trauma.
Thyme ~ a nervine and mild sedative that reduces nervous overstimulation; also energizes the nervous system when it is depleted by chronic stress and anxiety.
Valerian ~ a sedative and nervine that normalizes the nervous system; beneficial to relieve insomnia, anxiety, pain, spasms, and other uncontrollable movements.
Wood Betony ~ a sedative and nervine; may improve cognitive impairment; specific for head and neck pain.
Yarrow ~ a mild nervine and sedative; analgesic; anti-inflammatory.
Other Helpful Herbs:
Ashwagandha (*Withania somnifera*) ~ neuroprotective; sedative and nervine; shown to increase and normalize levels of the calming neurotransmitter GABA; beneficial for anxiety, insomnia, and Parkinson's; in Ayurvedic medicine it is taken for nervous exhaustion and to increase vitality and longevity.
Bacopa (*Bacopa monniera*) ~ an antioxidant and nervine that protects and nourishes nerve cells; helps normalize neurotransmitter levels.
Ginkgo (*Ginkgo biloba*) ~ studies show it helps regenerate damaged nerves and can be useful for peripheral neuropathy; an antioxidant that protects cellular membranes, specifically nerve and brain tissue.
Horsetail (*Equisetum arvense*) ~ supplies silica to strengthen and repair nerve cells.
Jamaican Dogwood (*Piscidia piscipula*) ~ sedating; relieves anxiety and panic; analgesic; reduces severe nerve pain throughout the body; eases insomnia caused by nervous tension and pain.
Kava Kava (*Piper methysticum*) ~ relaxes central nervous system while maintaining alert cognition; reduces physical and psychological anxiety; helpful for minor depression occurring with anxiety.
Linden (*Tilia* spp.) ~ a relaxing nervine taken for anxiety and insomnia.
Oat, fresh milky (*Avena sativa*) ~ one of the best nervine tonics to provide nutrients to nerve cells and support their structure; healing for nerve injuries; specific for nervous disability and exhaustion.
Rosemary (*Rosmarinus officinalis*) ~ a stimulating nervine; helps build and repair nerves; topical and internal applications reduce pain, spasms, inflammation; used for sciatica, anxiety, and depression.
Schisandra (*Schisandra chinensis*) ~ a nervine, sedative, and antioxidant; reduces anxiety and oxidative damage and inflammation of nerves.
Turmeric (*Curcuma longa*) ~ protects nerve cells; decreases oxidative damage and inflammation; increases neurotransmitters serotonin (calming) and dopamine (improves cognition).
For mild cases of Obsessive Compulsive Disorder (OCD) ~ combine Blue Vervain, Passion Flower, St. John's Wort, Scullcap, Blue Vervain, and Hawthorn berries.
For mild cases of ADD/ADHD ~ combine Eleuthero, German Chamomile, Hawthorn berries, Lemon Balm, Holy Basil, Linden, Milky Oats, and St. John's Wort.

Nicotine Withdrawal (also see Drug Withdrawal):
Lemon Balm ~ calming and restoring to the nervous system.
Lobelia ~ specific for nicotine withdrawal and reducing nicotine craving.
Mullein ~ the dried leaves may be smoked with dried Sage as a safe substitute for tobacco cigarettes.
Passion Flower ~ relaxes the nervous system during withdrawal.
Scullcap ~ relaxes and restores the nervous system; helps "burn-out" of nerve and adrenal exhaustion.

Nightmares and Sleepwalking: See Insomnia

Nose (also see Sinus Problems):
Bloodroot~ topical applications have been used to reduce nasal polyps; use caution due to tissue irritation.
Herbs that reduce nosebleeds ~ Calendula, Cayenne, Cinquefoil, Cranesbill, Stinging Nettle, and Yarrow.

Osteoarthritis: See Arthritis

Osteoporosis: See Bones

Ovaries:
Black Cohosh ~ helps restore normal ovarian function; may help polycystic ovarian syndrome (PCOS).
Blue Cohosh ~ used with Black Cohosh to normalize ovarian function.
Burdock ~ acts specifically on the ovaries to strengthen and normalize; helpful for ovarian tumors and cysts.
Calendula ~ taken to reduce ovarian cancers and cysts.
Chasteberry ~ restores normal ovarian function; helpful in treating PCOS, cysts, and problems caused by progesterone deficiency and estrogen dominance.
Other Helpful Herbs:

Maca (*Lepidium meyenii*) ~ helps balance and normalize hormones; can improve PCOS symptoms.

Oxidative Stress and Antioxidants

Oxidation is the constantly occurring chemical reaction in which oxygen combines with another molecule and causes electron loss. In the environment, oxidation happens when oxygen combines with iron to form iron oxide, or rust. In people, oxidation occurs throughout the body and at cellular levels, causing cellular damage and the aging process. Although oxidation is a controlled metabolic process of life, it also produces free radicals, which are unstable atoms and molecules that lack an electron and rob electrons from surrounding atoms and molecules to achieve stability. In their wake, free radicals generate even more unstable by-products known as reactive oxygen species (ROS) that cause further damage to healthy cells. Responding to oxidative damage throughout the body, our cells produce antioxidants (glutathione, superoxide dismutase/SOD, and catalase) that neutralize free radicals by donating electrons to them.

Oxidative stress occurs when the body's supply of antioxidants cannot keep up with the constant production of free radicals during normal metabolism and from environmental sources of oxidative damage, including toxic pollution in air, soil, water and food, tobacco, radiation, pharmaceutical and recreational drugs, and excessive exercise and exposure to sunlight. Oxidative stress damages and mutates cells, contributing to inflammation, the aging process, and development of many chronic degenerative diseases like Alzheimer's, Parkinson's, diabetes, rheumatoid arthritis, fibromyalgia, cancer, and neurological, autoimmune, and cardiovascular diseases.

As well as being produced by the body, antioxidants occur in herbs, vegetables, fruits, berries, nuts, seeds, dark chocolate, vitamins A (beta-carotene), C and E, and should be taken on a daily basis to promote optimum wellness and treat chronic illness.

Herbs containing significant amounts of antioxidants ~ Andrographis, Ashwagandha, Astragalus, Bacopa, Basil, Bilberry, Calendula, Catnip, Cat's Claw, Cayenne, Cinnamon, Cumin, Elder berries, Garlic, Ginger, Ginkgo, American and Asian Ginseng, Green Tea, Hawthorn berries, Holy Basil (Tulsi), Lemon Balm, Linden, Marjoram, Milk Thistle, Oregano, Parsley, Peppermint, Rose hips, Rosemary, Sage, St. John's Wort, Schisandra, Tarragon, Thyme, Turmeric, and Yarrow.

Pain (Neuralgia):

Pain is the normal response when tissues are damaged and inflamed. In addition to taking analgesic herbs, always address the causes of pain, which may involve improving lifestyle and dietary habits. Receiving physical therapy, massage, chiropractic adjustments, craniosacral therapy, and acupuncture are often very beneficial. Daily relaxation and meditation techniques are extremely valuable to relax the body and mind and reduce pain.

Black Cohosh ~ a nervine; eases the discomfort of sciatica, arthritis, fibromyalgia, and other nerve pain.
Blue Vervain ~ a nervine and analgesic used for pain, inflammation, spasms, arthritis, and fibromyalgia.
Boneset ~ a nervine for pain, spasms, inflammation, arthritis, and fibromyalgia.
Catnip ~ a mild analgesic; calming; reduces spasms; safe for children.
Cayenne ~ applied externally for nerve and muscle pain, including shingles, arthritis, sprains, gout, carpal tunnel, toothaches, headaches, and post-amputation pain.
Chamomile ~ helps relieve mild pain; reduces spasms and inflammation.
Elecampane ~ reduces pain, spasms, and inflammation; helpful for nerve injuries and sciatic pain.
Feverfew ~ analgesic; reduces inflammation throughout the body, including headache pain.
Holy Basil ~ anti-inflammatory; mild analgesic; reduces spasms; helpful for fibromyalgia.
Hops ~ anti-inflammatory; analgesic for nerve pain, sciatica, and fibromyalgia.
Lavender ~ analgesic for nerve and muscle pain; anti-inflammatory.
Lemon Balm ~ analgesic; anti-inflammatory; helpful for headaches and fibromyalgia.
Lobelia ~ calming and restoring to the nervous system; reduces pain, inflammation, and spasms.
Mugwort ~ eases pain; may reduce sciatic pain.
Mullein ~ a tincture of the roots and flowers is helpful for different types of facial nerve pain.
Passion Flower ~ eases pain, spasms, and nervous tics.
Peppermint ~ external application and ingestion of oil or tincture has analgesic effects and reduces spasms.
Sage ~ analgesic; decreases painful inflammation and spasms.
Saint John's Wort ~ strong analgesic that has an affinity with the nerves; anti-inflammatory.
Scullcap ~ analgesic; a sedating nervine that is restorative to the nerves.
Thyme ~ analgesic; anti-inflammatory; nervine; eases achy muscles, headaches, and sciatica.
Valerian ~ analgesic; relaxes overstimulated nerves and reduces spasms.
Wood Betony ~ specific for reducing pain in the head and neck; also used for sciatica and back pain.
Yarrow ~ analgesic; anti-inflammatory; especially helpful for external wound pain.

Other Analgesic Herbs:

Arnica (*Arnica montana*) ~ externally applied to inflamed and painful injuries, bruises, sprains, and arthritic joints. Do not apply to open cuts and wounds.
Jamaican Dogwood (*Piscidia piscipula*) ~ reduces severe nerve pain throughout the body, including painful menstruation, facial pain (Bell's palsy, trigeminal neuralgia, temporomandibular joint pain/TMJ), back pain, and spasms.
Kava Kava (*Piper methysticum*) ~ calms central nervous system; analgesic; muscle relaxant; reduces spasms.

Marijuana/ Hemp (*Cannabis sativa*) ~ cannabinoids are analgesic and reduce spasms; used internally and externally; Cannabidiol (CBD) oil helps relieve acute and chronic pain without inducing the "high" feeling.
Meadowsweet (*Filipendula ulmaria*) ~ contains salicylic acid which is analgesic and anti-inflammatory.
Rosemary (*Rosmarinus officinalis*) ~ helps repair and regenerate nerves; topical and internal applications reduce pain, spasms, and inflammation; used for many types of muscle and nerve pain, including sciatica.
Willow bark (*Salix* spp.) ~ contains salicylic acid which is analgesic and anti-inflammatory.
Wintergreen (*Gaultheria procumbens*) ~ salicylic acid, the main substance in the oil, is analgesic and anti-inflammatory; oil is applied for muscle, joint, and nerve pain and inflammation.

Pancreas, Diabetes and Hypoglycemia: (also see Digestive System)

The pancreas produces insulin, which regulates blood glucose levels, and digestive enzymes that break down and digest food. Protease enzymes digest proteins, lipase digests fats, and amylase digests carbohydrates. These enzymes are secreted into the upper small intestine duodenum when food is eaten.

American Centaury ~ tones and strengthens the pancreas; stimulates secretion of enzymes and insulin; helps maintain normal digestion and blood sugar levels.
Astragalus ~ helps normalize pancreatic function; helpful for hypoglycemia (low blood sugar) and diabetes (hyperglycemia or high blood sugar) by regulating blood sugar levels.
Blue Vervain ~ a bitter that stimulates increased production and secretion of pancreatic digestive enzymes.
Boneset ~ stimulates and restores normal pancreatic activity; increases secretion of digestive enzymes.
Burdock ~ supports the pancreas; reduces inflammation; helps normalize secretions of digestive enzymes and insulin.
Cayenne ~ stimulates secretion of digestive enzymes; externally applied to relieve diabetic neuropathy (nerve pain and deterioration caused by chronically elevated blood glucose levels).
Dandelion ~ supports the pancreas and promotes normal function; stimulates secretion of digestive enzymes; helps regulate blood sugar levels in people with diabetes and hypoglycemia.
Elecampane ~ tones and normalizes pancreatic function and secretion of enzymes; helpful for diabetes.
Goldenseal ~ tones and normalizes pancreatic function; stimulates secretion of enzymes; small amounts may improve blood sugar levels and lower insulin requirements.
Holy Basil ~ helps maintain normal blood sugar levels; stimulates production of digestive enzymes.
Hops ~ stimulates secretion of pancreatic enzymes.
Horehound ~ stimulates secretion of digestive enzymes; helps control blood sugar levels in diabetes type 2.
Hyssop ~ stimulates secretion of digestive enzymes.
Marshmallow ~ pectin in the roots helps normalize blood sugar levels.
Peppermint ~ promotes production and secretion of digestive enzymes.
Sage ~ supports pancreatic functions; increases secretion of digestive enzymes; helps reduce high blood sugar levels.
Yarrow ~ improves blood circulation to the pancreas; reduces stagnation and inflammation; helps normalize pancreatic functions of enzyme and insulin secretion; lowers high blood sugar levels.

Other Helpful Herbs:

Andrographis (*Andrographis paniculata*) ~ helps normalize blood sugar levels; beneficial for diabetes.
Artichoke leaf (*Cynara scolymus*) ~ stimulates secretion of pancreatic enzymes; an antioxidant that protects pancreatic cells from damage.
Ashwagandha (*Withania somnifera*) ~ improves cellular sensitivity to insulin and glucose uptake.
Bilberry (*Vaccinium myrtillus*) ~ reduces blood glucose levels; helps protect the blood vessels of diabetics.
Bitter Melon (*Momordica charantia*) ~ contains anti-diabetic substances, including charantin (lowers blood glucose), vicine, and polypeptide-p (an insulin-like compound); beneficial for diabetes type 1 and 2.
Blueberry fruit and leaf (*Vaccinium corymbosum*, spp.) ~ reduces blood sugar levels by improving insulin transport of glucose into cells.
Cinnamon (*Cinnamomum verum*) ~ improves blood glucose levels; increases insulin sensitivity.
Codonopsis root (*Codonopsis pilosula*) ~ tones and strengthens pancreas, especially the islets of Langerhans cells that produce insulin; used for diabetes type 2.
Fenugreek seeds (*Trigonella foenum-graecum*) ~ reduce symptoms of diabetes type 1 and 2 by improving glucose tolerance and lowering blood glucose levels.
Gentian root (*Gentiana lutea*) ~ a bitter that improves digestion; stimulates secretion of pancreatic enzymes.
Ginseng, Asian (*Panax ginseng*) and American (*Panax quinquefolius*) ~ reduce glucose levels in diabetes type 2; promote insulin release and increase cellular sensitivity to insulin and glucose uptake.
Gymnema (*Gymnema sylvestre*) ~ improves insulin production in diabetes type 2; improves insulin sensitivity and glucose uptake in type 1 and 2; reduces sugar craving.
Horsetail (*Equisetum arvense*) ~ silica content heals damaged tissues caused by inflammation from pancreatitis; animal studies indicate anti-diabetic properties.
Jerusalem Artichoke (*Helianthus tuberosus*) ~ helps pancreas metabolize glucose; helps prevent diabetes type 2.
Olive leaf (*Olea europaea*) ~ contains oleuropein which reduces inflammation of pancreatitis; studies show that it inhibits cellular damage and cancer cell proliferation in the pancreas.

Parasites:

Herbs that can eradicate intestinal parasites ~ American Centaury, Black Walnut (a primary herb to eliminate parasites and scabies), Blue Vervain, Cayenne, Elecampane, Feverfew, Goldenseal, Holy Basil, Hops, Horehound, Hyssop, Isatis, Lavender, Mugwort (also used for malaria, a mosquito-transmitted parasitic infection), Mullein (strong concentrations can kill roundworms and tapeworms), Sage, Senna, and Thyme.

Other Helpful Herbs:

Garlic (*Allium sativum*) ~ effective against parasites, specifically pinworms.

Oregon Grape Root (*Mahonia aquifolium*) ~ berberine in roots kills parasites, including giardia and amoeba.

Pau D'arco (*Tabebuia impetiginosa*) ~ kills some parasites.

Sweet Annie (*Artemisia annua*) ~ inhibits the life cycle of the malaria parasite; most popular herb for malaria.

Wormwood (*Artemisia absinthium*) ~ kills many parasites, including protozoa, roundworms, and pinworms.

Parkinson's Disease: See Nervous System

Peptic Ulcers: See Stomach

Perspiration (excessive perspiration is called hyperhydrosis and lack of perspiration is hypohydrosis):

Astragalus ~ helps reduce spontaneous sweating, menopausal hot flashes, and night sweats.

Black Walnut ~ used for excessive sweating on the palms of the hands and soles of the feet.

Burdock ~ normalizes perspiration and is used for excessive or deficient sweating, including night sweats.

Cayenne ~ stimulates sweat gland secretions that promote perspiration.

Cranesbill ~ an astringent that decreases excessive sweating.

Lobelia ~ small doses help reduce excessive perspiration, while larger doses stimulate normal perspiration.

Motherwort ~ used for excessive perspiration caused by hyperactivity, nervous tension, and hyperthyroidism.

Pleurisy Root ~ normalizes sweat glands to reduce excessive perspiration or increase scanty perspiration.

Sage ~ drying properties are helpful for excessive sweating.

Pineal Gland: See Brain and Cognitive Function, Endocrine Glands, and Hypothalamus

Pituitary Gland: See Brain and Cognitive Function, Endocrine Glands, and Hypothalamus

Pneumonia: See Lung and Bronchial Problems

Poison Antidotes: See Detoxification

Poison Ivy and Poison Oak: See Skin

Postpartum (the period of time following childbirth): See pages 610-611 in "Herbs for Pregnancy, Childbirth, and Lactation"

Pregnancy: See pages 599-610 in "Herbs for Pregnancy, Childbirth, and Lactation"

Premenstrual Syndrome (PMS): See Menstruation

Prolapsed Organs: See Muscle and Uterus

Prostate Gland and Benign Prostatic Hypertrophy (BPH): See Male Reproductive System

Psoriasis:

Psoriasis is a chronic inflammatory skin condition and metabolic disorder that causes skin cells to multiply too rapidly and accumulate, causing red patches of dry, scaly skin. It is an autoimmune disorder in which an overactive immune system produces excessive amounts of T cells (a type of lymphocyte that has a central role in cell-mediated immunity) in the blood and skin. Other frequent causes needing to be addressed include high blood and tissue levels of environmental toxins and endotoxins (toxins excreted from bacteria in the body); impaired liver function; incomplete protein digestion that causes proteins to break down into toxins that inhibit the formation of cAMP and increases skin cell proliferation; faulty glucose and/or fat digestion; poor diet and excessive consumption of animal fats, refined sugars, chemical additives, alcohol, and other food allergies or sensitivities; and chronic stress, trauma, and emotional, psychological, and spiritual factors. Some people with psoriasis develop psoriatic arthritis, also an inflammatory autoimmune condition.

The use of immunosuppressant steroid drugs is the most common conventional treatment for psoriasis, but this only masks symptoms and the side effects can be more problematic than the skin condition. Herbal therapy combined with healthy diet, lifestyle, and introspective exploration of one's inner life can safely help correct underlying causes of imbalances and reduce psoriasis outbreaks.

Burdock ~ cools and detoxifies blood and liver; an old treatment for psoriasis and other skin conditions.

Cayenne ~ is externally applied to relieve pain and itching.

Chickweed ~ helpful for hot, inflamed, irritated skin; cleansing to blood and lymphatic fluid.

Dandelion ~ cleansing to the liver and bloodstream; helpful for skin eruptions.

Holy Basil ~ helps clear skin diseases.

Yellow Dock ~ cleansing to liver, blood, lymphatic system; used for inflamed, irritated skin and skin eruptions.

Other Helpful Herbs:

Aloe (*Aloe vera*) ~ topical applications help clear psoriasis lesions in some people due to its ability to reduce heat, redness, and inflammation of the skin.

Bitter Melon (*Momordica charantia*) ~ antioxidant; anti-inflammatory; clears toxins from blood and tissues; decreases cGMP and rapid cell growth; helps reduce symptoms of autoimmune disorders including rheumatoid arthritis; drinking Bitter Melon juice and applying a paste of the dried, powdered seeds helps treat itching and skin conditions like psoriasis.

Cat's Claw ((*Uncaria tomentosa*) ~ used for psoriasis and psoriatic arthritis; inhibits the body's production of

inflammatory prostaglandins and tumor necrosis factor (TNF), an inflammatory metabolite produced by T cells in excessive amounts in autoimmune disorders like psoriasis and psoriatic arthritis.
Cleavers (*Galium aparine*) and Red Clover (*Trifolium pratense*) ~ reduce toxins in blood and lymph.
Dong Quai (*Angelica sinensis*) ~ contains psoralens which, when ingested, decrease skin cell production in the presence of sunlight and help clear psoriasis lesions.
Gingko (*Ginkgo biloba*) ~ helps treat psoriasis by increasing cAMP to reduce overgrowth of skin cells.
Licorice (*Glycyrrhiza glabra*) ~ reduces toxic overload in liver and blood; glycyrrhizin has anti-inflammatory actions similar to hydrocortisone; ingesting the root and using topical applications are beneficial to skin.
Milk Thistle (*Silybum marianum*) ~ one of the best herbs to detoxify and rejuvenate the liver; improves endotoxin removal by liver; inhibits abnormally high levels of cAMP phosphodiesterase and leukotrienes that occur in people with psoriasis; helps reduce the psoriasis rash by anti-inflammatory properties and ability to progressively reduce excessive proliferation of skin cells; inhibits T-cell activation occurring from an overactive immune system.
Oregon Grape Root (*Mahonia aquifolium*) ~ anti-inflammatory; antioxidant; roots contain berberine, berbamine and oxycathine, which inhibit rapid skin proliferation; berberine binds to endotoxins in the intestines to prevent toxins from circulating to the skin; has a long history of use for mild to moderate psoriasis and other scaly skin conditions; reduces redness in psoriasis lesions when used topically.
Pau D'arco (*Tabebuia impetiginosa*) ~ an immunomodulator and lymphogogue; anti-inflammatory.
Sarsaparilla (*Smilax ornata*) ~ helpful for skin diseases by binding to endotoxins in the gut and prohibiting their absorption; specific for scaly skin conditions such as eczema and psoriasis.
Turmeric (*Curcuma longa*) ~ a powerful anti-inflammatory and antioxidant; reduces TNF to improve symptoms; some people find it helpful in minimizing psoriasis and psoriatic arthritis flares.

Rashes: See Skin

Raynaud's Disease: See Vascular System

Respiratory Infections: See Lung and Bronchial Problems

Ringworm: See Fungal Infections

Sciatica: See Pain

Seizures, Convulsions, and Epilepsy:

These problems are conditions of excessive nervous system hyperstimulation. Treatment protocol includes the use of sedating and nervine herbs and supporting the calming neurotransmitters GABA (gamma-aminobutyric acid) and serotonin.

Black Cohosh ~ relaxing to the central nervous system; antispasmodic.
Blue Vervain ~ a nervine and sedative; reduces spasms.
Boneset ~ a relaxing nervine that reduces spasms; once used for epilepsy.
Catnip ~ calming to the nervous system; reduces spasms; once used for childhood convulsions.
Hyssop ~ a sedative and nervine; used for seizures and convulsions.
Lavender ~ calming and sedating to the nervous system; used for spasms and seizures.
Lobelia ~ calming and restoring to the nervous system; taken for spasms, seizures, convulsions, and epilepsy.
Motherwort ~ calming and restoring to nerves; relaxing to rigid and tense muscles; once used for epilepsy.
Mugwort ~ calms nerves; used for all types of uncontrollable shaking, seizures, epilepsy, and tremors.
Passion Flower ~ calming to the nervous system; used for spasms, epileptic seizures, and Parkinson's disease.
Scullcap ~ a calming sedative and nervine; helps restore the nervous system; used for spasms and epilepsy.
Valerian ~ a relaxing antispasmodic; historically used to treat seizures and epilepsy.
Wood Betony ~ a restorative nervine and sedative.

Shingles (*Herpes zoster*): See Herpes Virus

Shock (sudden drop in blood pressure):

Cayenne ~ very stimulating and reviving.
Lobelia ~ small doses revive the system.

Sinus Problems, Sinusitis, Allergies:

Sinusitis is usually a viral infection that causes inflammation in the mucous membranes lining the nose and sinuses with sinus pressure, runny, stuffy nose with thick yellow or green mucous, fever, cough, and fatigue. For all sinus problems, it is beneficial to eat a light diet of fruit, vegetables and vegetarian protein, while avoiding mucous-producing foods like dairy products, sugar, and gluten flours. Quercetin, a bioflavonoid, stabilizes mast cells (specialized immune cells that produce histamine and other inflammatory compounds in response to allergens) to reduce inflammation and allergic symptoms. Antimicrobial, anti-inflammatory, and immune enhancing herbs (immunomodulators) are helpful when treating sinus conditions.

Astragalus ~ an immunomodulator that strengthens immunity; reduces symptoms of allergic reactions.
Blue Vervain ~ antimicrobial; decreases mucous secretions and congestion.
Boneset ~ normalizes mucous secretions; relieves drainage and congestion; antimicrobial for infections.
Cayenne ~ drying; has antihistamine actions; reduces mucous drainage and congestion.
Chamomile ~ reduces histamine release and mucous production; stimulates immunity.
Dandelion ~ reduces excessive mucous and chronic sinus infections.
Echinacea ~ an antibiotic and antiviral for sinus infections, inflammation, and excessive mucous discharge; an immunomodulator that stimulates immunity; helps reduce environmental allergies including hay fever.

Elderberry ~ antiviral; decreases mucous production; beneficial for treating sinusitis.
Elecampane ~ stimulates immunity; antibiotic; decreases excessive mucous discharge.
Feverfew ~ reduces histamine release; tones mucous membranes and decreases excessive mucous discharge.
Goldenrod ~ antihistamine actions; reduces excess mucous secretions; helpful for sinusitis and allergies.
Goldenseal ~ excellent to reduce excess mucous drainage and congestion; anti-inflammatory; antimicrobial.
Holy Basil ~ reduces excess mucous; anti-inflammatory; stimulates immunity; antibacterial and antifungal.
Horehound ~ tones mucous membranes to reduce mucous congestion; antibacterial.
Hyssop ~ tones mucous membranes; reduces mucous congestion; antibacterial and antiviral.
Lemon Balm ~ antihistamine properties help reduce excess mucous discharge; antibacterial and antifungal.
Motherwort ~ reduces excessive mucous secretions in nasal sinuses and relieves congestion.
Mullein ~ smoking the leaves dries up draining sinuses and a runny nose (combines well with Sage leaves).
Peppermint ~ the volatile oils reduce mucous secretions and open airways.
Sage ~ specific for reducing excess mucous production, sinusitis, and hay fever allergies; smoking the leaves dries up draining sinuses and a runny nose (combine with Mullein leaves).
Stinging Nettle ~ antihistamine and anti-inflammatory actions are specific for relieving hay fever symptoms.
Thyme ~ reduces excessive mucous production and drainage; antimicrobial for infections.
Wood Betony ~ specific for sinusitis, allergies, and colds.

Other Helpful Herbs:

Butterbur (*Petasites hybridus*) ~ reduces inflammation by blocking histamine and leukotrienes; can be effective for relieving itchy eyes and sinus congestion.
Ephedra (*Ephedra sinica*) ~ stimulates norepinephrine release which relaxes and dilates the bronchi and bronchioles, allowing easier breathing and reduction of spasms and mucous production; beneficial for excessive mucous production, sinusitis, and hay fever.
Eucalyptus (*Eucalyptus* spp.) ~ antimicrobial, expectorant, and anti-inflammatory for sinusitis and allergies.
Eyebright (*Euphrasia rostkoviana*) ~ reduces inflammation and mucous production; helps hay fever, sinusitis.
Garlic (*Allium sativum*) ~ boosts immunity; antibacterial and antiviral; decongestant; anti-inflammatory; contains quercetin, a natural antihistamine; helps alleviate sinus infections and hay fever symptoms.
Ginger (*Zingiber officinale*) ~ a natural antihistamine; loosens phlegm to reduce chest and nasal congestion; strengthens the immune system; helpful for sinus infection and hay fever.
Licorice (*Glycyrrhiza glabra*) ~ supports adrenals to improve sinus and allergy problems; immunostimulant; reduces inflammation and congestion.
Oregon Grape Root (*Mahonia aquifolium*) ~ strong antimicrobial; normalizes mucous membrane secretions.
Turmeric (*Curcuma longa*) ~ prevents histamine release from mast cells; has similar activity to non-steroidal anti-inflammatory drugs (NSAIDs); alleviates allergic symptoms and reduces sinus congestion and drainage.
Wild Indigo (*Baptisia tinctoria*) ~ a strong antimicrobial for sinusitis and respiratory infections.

Skin Problems (also see Burns, Eczema, and Psoriasis):

American Centaury ~ for inflamed eruptions, hives, eczema, acne, ulcers, bites, stings, wounds, poison ivy.
Astragalus ~ promotes tissue regeneration; anti-inflammatory; helpful for chronic sores and wounds, ulcers, eczema, hives, and other eruptive dermatitis; helps release heat and toxins through the skin.
Black Walnut ~ reduces inflammation; antiseptic; used for rashes, dermatitis, eruptive skin diseases, wounds, ulcers, boils, abscesses, acne, and tumors caused by toxic conditions; kills yeast and fungal infections, including ringworm and athlete's foot; antiviral against warts.
Bloodroot ~ externally applied to eliminate warts, moles, fungal infections, cancers (use with caution).
Blue Vervain ~ antibiotic; anti-inflammatory; healing to old and new wounds, bruises, abscesses, burns, ulcers, and rashes.
Burdock ~ promotes healthy skin; healing for wounds, burns, bruises, rashes, hives, boils, acne, athlete's foot, ringworm, tumors, cysts, and dry, irritated, scaly skin conditions like eczema and psoriasis.
Calendula ~ reduces scar tissue; excellent for wounds, skin eruptions, rashes, acne, hives, eczema, fungal infections, burns, sprains, bruises, abscesses, chronic skin ulcers, and insect stings and bites.
Catnip ~ antiseptic; for painful swellings, sprains, bruises, acne, hives, poison ivy, and insect stings and bites.
Cayenne ~ antibiotic; applied to bruises, sprains, painful skin lesions such as herpes, shingles, and psoriasis.
Chamomile ~antiseptic; used for wounds, inflammation, burns, skin ulcers, rashes like hives and eczema.
Chickweed ~ soothing anti-inflammatory helpful for most skin problems, including acne, boils, burns, insect bites, abscesses, ulcers, hives and rashes, poison ivy, eczema, psoriasis, chicken pox, measles, and mumps.
Cinquefoil ~ stops bleeding; healing to acne, wounds, ulcers, burns, bruising, toxic rashes, and skin eruptions.
Comfrey ~ encourages cell growth and repair of damaged and injured tissues; for acute or slow-healing wounds, gangrene, bruises, burns, inflamed rashes, abscesses, insect bites, diaper rash, and skin ulcers.
Cranesbill ~ stops bleeding; anti-inflammatory; healing to ulcers, fungal infections, and bruises.
Dandelion ~ helpful for skin diseases, inflammation, boils, abscesses, acne, fungal infections, warts, and eruptive conditions like hives and eczema caused by toxins and excess heat and acids in the blood.
Echinacea ~ antiseptic; anti-inflammatory; promotes tissue healing to deep and superficial wounds; helpful for ulcers, acne, abscesses, boils, folliculitis, cellulitis, rashes, dermatitis, eczema, and psoriasis.
Elderberry ~ externally applied to wounds, skin infections, rashes, dermatitis, eczema, acne, boils, rosacea, burns, bruises, poison ivy, and eruptive skin conditions like mumps and chicken pox.

Elecampane ~ antiseptic; analgesic; anti-inflammatory; blood detoxifier; used for chronic skin diseases, fungal infections, wounds, rashes, eczema, skin ulcers and eruptions, scabies, and toxic bites and stings.
Feverfew ~ antiseptic; anti-inflammatory; analgesic for wounds, ulcers, and insect bites and stings.
Goldenrod ~ antiseptic; heals wounds, ulcers, sprains, and bruises; decreases inflammation.
Goldenseal ~ antiseptic; antifungal; cooling anti-inflammatory; excellent for wounds, infections, abscesses, rashes, itching, impetigo, ulcers, acne, eczema, ringworm, athlete's foot, and diaper rash.
Holy Basil ~ used for skin infections and diseases, fungal infections, abscesses, boils, bites, and stings.
Hops ~ antiseptic against staph; anti-inflammatory; eases pain; healing to wounds, bruises, boils, abscesses, burns, old ulcers, tumors, itching, bites and stings, acne, eczema, and yeast and fungal infections.
Horehound ~ antibacterial; anti-inflammatory; healing to wounds, skin eruptions, ulcers, bites, and stings.
Hyssop ~ antiseptic; anti-inflammatory; healing to wounds, burns, insect bites, strains, and sprains.
Isatis ~ antiseptic; a cooling anti-inflammatory that is helpful for wounds, staph infections, abscesses, boils, rashes, scabies, and eruptive skin conditions like eczema.
Lavender ~ a wound healer; antiseptic; analgesic; for skin ulcers, inflammation, bruises, acne, bites, burns.
Lemon Balm ~ antiseptic; antifungal; analgesic; anti-inflammatory; helps wounds heal.
Lobelia ~ topical application draws pus and infection from boils, insect bites, and abscesses; used for eruptive skin conditions like herpes, eczema, and ringworm.
Marshmallow ~ cooling and soothing for dry, inflamed skin conditions, wounds, burns, dermatitis, and boils.
Mugwort ~ used for bacterial and fungal skin infections, boils, abscesses, eczema, and itchy skin.
Mullein ~ leaves and flowers reduce pain and swelling, burns, varicose veins, and promote wound healing.
Sage ~ antiseptic; analgesic; anti-inflammatory; reduces bleeding and bruising; healing to ulcers and wounds.
Saint John's Wort ~ antiseptic; analgesic; reduces bleeding; used for wounds, burns, injuries, and dermatitis.
Stinging Nettle ~ specific for eczema, burns, dermatitis, acne, hives, and other rashes.
Thyme ~ antiseptic; kills lice; healing to bruises and wounds.
Yarrow ~ excellent for all wounds and deep cuts; stops bleeding and bruising; antiseptic; analgesic.
Yellow Dock ~ draws venom and toxins from the skin; beneficial for inflammation, wounds, bites and stings, ulcers, acne, eczema, psoriasis, boils, hives, and fungal infections.

Other Helpful Herbs:

Cleavers (*Galium aparine*) ~ excellent lymphatic detoxifier; used for acute and chronic skin conditions.
Gotu Kola (*Centella asiatica*) ~ antiseptic; strong anti-inflammatory; excellent topical wound healer; increases collagen production in tissues without creating scar tissue; used for reducing scar tissue and treating burns ulcers, scleroderma, eczema, and psoriasis.
Horsetail (*Equisetum arvense*) ~ silica content heals wounds, strengthens connective tissue, nourishes skin.
Khella (*Ammi visnaga*) ~ used as treatment for skin diseases, specifically vitiligo and psoriasis.
Oregon Grape Root (*Mahonia aquifolium*) ~ antimicrobial; anti-inflammatory; helps scaly skin conditions.
Plantain (*Plantago* spp.) ~ excellent wound healer; antiseptic; anti-inflammatory; contains soothing and healing mucilage; beneficial for healing boils, bites, poison ivy, and different types of dermatitis.
Red Clover (*Trifolium pratense*) ~ an excellent blood purifier historically used for chronic skin problems in children and adults, including eczema, psoriasis, chronic hives, and other eruptive skin conditions.
Sarsaparilla (*Smilax ornata*) ~ beneficial for skin diseases by binding to endotoxins (toxins excreted from bacteria) in the gut and prohibiting their absorption into the bloodstream; specific for scaly skin conditions such as eczema and psoriasis.
Tansy (*Tanacetum vulgare*) ~ used externally as a wash to kill lice and scabies.
Tea Tree oil (*Melaleuca alternifolia*) ~ antiseptic and antimicrobial; the oil is applied to bacterial and fungal skin infections.
Woundwort (*Prunella vulgaris*) ~ antibacterial; a classic wound healer; stops bleeding and inflammation.

Small Intestine: See Intestines

Spasms: See Muscle

Spleen:

The spleen is an important organ of the lymphatic and immune systems. It is the largest lymphatic organ and its structure is similar to a large lymph node. It manufactures B- and T-lymphocytes (white blood cells) that produce antibodies to kill foreign microorganisms and fight infections. Acting as a blood filter, the spleen removes bacteria, cellular debris, and damaged red blood cells and platelets from the bloodstream. It also recycles old red blood cells and iron, and stores blood platelets and white blood cells.

Astragalus ~ stimulates immune activity of the spleen; promotes regeneration of spleen cells.
Blue Vervain ~ antibiotic; anti-inflammatory; restores and stimulates the spleen.
Boneset ~ stimulates and normalizes normal function and blood flow through the spleen.
Burdock ~ has a cleansing and normalizing effect on the spleen.
Dandelion ~ stimulates and normalizes function and blood flow through the spleen.
Echinacea ~ stimulates the spleen to produce lymphocytes, antibodies, and other immune components to fight infection; enhances the spleen's ability to filter and clean blood.
Goldenseal ~ stimulates immunity and blood filtration of the spleen; cleansing and normalizing to spleen.
Isatis ~ stimulates and supports immune function.

Sprains: See Muscle

Stomach: (also see Digestive System)

The stomach produces an acidic mixture of hydrochloric acid, the enzymes pepsinogen and gastric lipase, and mucus that protects the stomach lining. Hydrochloric acid dissolves and breaks down minerals. When pepsinogen mixes with powerful acids in hydrochloric acid, it is converted into pepsin, which reduces proteins into amino acids. Gastric lipase breaks down fats.

Symptoms of deficient or excess stomach acid can be similar. Many people taking antacids actually lack stomach acids, which normally decrease as people age. Generally, excess stomach acid irritates the stomach lining and causes pain when the stomach is empty. Eating food reduces the pain by absorbing acids and reducing irritation. When stomach acids are deficient, food does not digest well, causing bloating, belching, and general discomfort. Excessive acid production is often due to anxiety and nervous overstimulation, which are reduced with the use of nervine and sedative herbs. Soothing herbs for the stomach lining are also beneficial. A deficiency of stomach acids can be improved by taking herbal bitters. Antibacterial herbs reduce overgrowth of Helicobacter pylori, which contributes to the development of ulcers.

American Centaury ~ a bitter; stimulates production of stomach acids; for indigestion, gas, bloating, nausea.
Astragalus ~ decreases excess stomach acids; taken for indigestion, heartburn, acid reflux, stomach ulcers.
Blue Vervain ~ relaxes stomach tension; stimulates production of stomach acids; helpful for indigestion.
Boneset ~ relaxes a nervous stomach; stimulates enzyme production; for indigestion, gas, bloating, hiccups.
Burdock ~ helpful for indigestion, inflammation, ulceration, pain, heartburn, and acid reflux.
Calendula ~ beneficial for infections, indigestion, cramps, ulcers, and nausea.
Catnip ~ helps reduce indigestion, heartburn, nausea, gas, colic, and stomach ulcers; safe for infants.
Cayenne ~ stimulates production of enzymes and hydrochloric acid; beneficial for indigestion, gas, bloating, nausea, vomiting, and ulcers; antibiotic for infections and excessive growth of *H. pylori.*
Chamomile ~ reduces inflammation, spasms, ulcers, gas, and indigestion; promotes enzyme production.
Chickweed ~ soothing for heartburn, acid reflux, stomach inflammation, and ulcers.
Cinquefoil ~ reduces bleeding ulcers and stomach cramps.
Comfrey ~ soothing and healing for stomach inflammation, heartburn, acid reflux, and ulcers.
Cranesbill ~ healing for ulcers and inflammation; decreases excess stomach acids; stops abnormal bleeding.
Dandelion ~ stimulates secretion of stomach acids to improve digestion.
Elderberry ~ healing to ulcers; helps indigestion, colic, sluggish digestion, and gas.
Elecampane ~ strengthens and tones stomach to improve digestion; helps indigestion and stomach ulcers.
Feverfew ~ taken for indigestion; anti-inflammatory; decreases cramps and spasms.
Goldenrod ~ beneficial for indigestion and stomach ulcers.
Goldenseal ~ antibacterial against *H. pylori*; anti-inflammatory; normalizes stomach enzyme secretion; helps indigestion, ulcers, heartburn, nausea, and gas.
Holy Basil ~ anti-inflammatory; helpful for nervous indigestion, gas, bloating, ulcers, and heartburn.
Hops ~ calms a nervous stomach; beneficial for indigestion, inflammation, spasms, and excess acids.
Horehound ~ a bitter that stimulates production of digestive enzymes; benefits indigestion, gas, and bloating.
Hyssop ~ a bitter that stimulates enzyme production; helpful for indigestion, gas, spasms, and colic.
Lavender ~ specific for problems due to underlying tension, including nausea, gas, colic, and cramps.
Lemon Balm ~ excellent for problems caused by stress, including stomachaches, gas, spasms, and nausea.
Marshmallow ~ a healing and soothing mucilage that reduces stomach inflammation, ulcers, and heartburn.
Mugwort ~ small doses ease a nervous stomach and reduce spasms.
Peppermint ~ specific for nausea, vomiting, stomachaches, indigestion, gas, and colic; do not use in cases of acid reflux because it can worsen the problem.
Sage ~ relieves nausea, indigestion, gas, bloating, and inflammation; kills *H. pylori* in the stomach.
Stinging Nettle ~ helps reduce excess stomach acid; healing to ulcers; anti-inflammatory.
Thyme ~ eases indigestion due to anxiety; used for gas, stomach inflammation, ulcers, and anorexia.
Wood Betony ~ calms tension in solar plexus; helps ease a nervous stomach, indigestion, and heartburn.
Yarrow ~ antibiotic; protects the stomach lining; stops bleeding from ulcers; stimulates enzyme secretion.

Other Helpful Herbs:

Angelica root (*Angelica archangelica*) ~ a warming bitter used for deficient hydrochloric acid, nausea, colic.
Fennel (*Foeniculum vulgare*) ~ soothing anti-inflammatory; stimulates and improves digestion; reduces gas.
Fenugreek seeds (*Trigonella foenum-graecum*) ~ a soothing mucilage that reduces stomach inflammation.
Gentian root (*Gentiana lutea*) ~ a bitter that improves digestion by stimulating secretion of hydrochloric acid.
Ginger (*Zingiber officinale*) ~ helps most stomach problems; for gas, heartburn, nausea, vomiting, and colic.
Licorice (*Glycyrrhiza glabra*) ~ excels in reducing and healing stomach inflammation and spasms; antibacterial against *H. pylori*; helpful in treating ulcers, heartburn, and gastritis.
Linden (*Tilia* spp.) ~ relieves indigestion and heartburn; improves low stomach acidity.
Meadowsweet (*Filipendula ulmaria*) ~ contains salicylic acid which is analgesic and anti-inflammatory; helps reduce excess hydrochloric acid; strengthens stomach.
Oregon Grape Root (*Mahonia aquifolium*) ~ antimicrobial against *H. pylori*; anti-inflammatory; helps normalize stomach enzyme secretion; taken for indigestion, heartburn, nausea, gas, and ulcers.
Plantain (*Plantago* spp.) ~ antibacterial; anti-inflammatory; soothing to mucosal membranes lining the

stomach; helps reduce excess hydrochloric acid and protects stomach lining from irritation and damage.
Herbs that kill H. pylori ~ Garlic (*Allium sativum*), Goldenseal (*Hydrastis canadensis*), Oregon Grape Root (*Mahonia aquifolium*), Rosemary (*Rosmarinus officinalis*), and Turmeric (*Curcuma longa*).
Herbs that reduce excess hydrochloric acid ~ Slippery Elm (*Ulmus* spp.) and Aloe Vera.

Stress: See Nervous System

Stroke: See Brain and Cognitive Function

Sweating: See Perspiration

Teeth:

Bloodroot ~ helps prevent plaque formation, cavities, and gum disease; use cautiously due to toxicity.
Catnip ~ the leaves may be chewed to help relieve toothaches.
Cayenne ~ external application is helpful for painful toothaches and gum infection.
Chamomile ~ external application eases the pain of toothaches and gum inflammation.
Passion Flower ~ can be helpful during infant teething to reduce pain and irritability.
Peppermint ~ oil or tincture is applied on the gums to reduce pain.
Saint John's Wort ~ oil or tincture is applied on the gums to reduce painful toothaches.

Other Helpful Herbs:

Clove oil (*Syzygium aromaticum*) ~ apply oil on the gums; excellent to reduce infection, inflammation, and nerve pain in teeth and gums.

Testicles: See Male Reproductive System

Throat:

American Centaury ~ reduces throat congestion and tightness and the inhibition of voice and self-expression.
Boneset ~ the tea is used as a gargle and ingested to heal a sore, infected throat.
Burdock ~ beneficial to soothe a sore and infected throat.
Calendula ~ the tea is taken as a gargle for sore throats, tonsillitis, and laryngitis.
Cayenne ~ an antibiotic taken for sore throats.
Chickweed ~ the tea is used as a gargle for sore throats, ulcerations, and hoarseness.
Cinquefoil ~ used as a gargle for sore, inflamed, ulcerated throats, laryngitis, and tonsillitis.
Comfrey ~ makes a soothing, moisturizing gargle for sore, inflamed throats and hoarseness.
Cranesbill ~ used as a gargle for sore, inflamed, ulcerated throats.
Echinacea ~ antibiotic and antiviral actions help heal sore throats, strep infections, tonsillitis, and laryngitis.
Elderberry ~ the flowers are antiviral; the tea is used as a gargle.
Goldenrod ~ the tea and tincture are used as a gargle for sore, infected throats and tonsillitis.
Goldenseal ~ antibiotic and anti-inflammatory for sore throats, strep infections, tonsillitis, and laryngitis.
Hops ~ antibiotic for sore throats and strep infections.
Horehound ~ specific for treating sore throats and infections.
Hyssop ~ beneficial for sore throats and tonsillitis.
Isatis ~ cooling and anti-inflammatory; helpful for sore, swollen, infected throats and laryngitis.
Marshmallow ~ excellent to soothe and moisturize dry, inflamed sore throats; eases hoarseness and laryngitis.
Mullein ~ a cooling anti-inflammatory for sore, swollen, infected throats, laryngitis, and swollen glands.
Peppermint ~ helpful for sore throats and laryngitis.
Sage ~ an excellent gargle for sore, infected, ulcerated and inflamed throats, laryngitis, and tonsillitis.
Thyme ~ an antiseptic gargle for sore throats, laryngitis, and tonsillitis.

Other Helpful Herbs:

Ginger (*Zingiber officinale*) ~ the tea is used as a gargle and ingested to soothe sore, infected throats.
Licorice (*Glycyrrhiza glabra*) ~ the tea is used as a gargle and drunk for sore throats and infections.
Wild Indigo (*Baptisia tinctoria*) ~ a strong antimicrobial for throat, nose, and sinus infections; reduces excess mucous; use under guidance of a qualified herbalist due to toxicity of large doses.

Thrush: See Fungal Infections

Thrush is a yeast overgrowth in the mouth. Yeast is a fungus treated with antifungal herbs.

Thymus:

The thymus is an endocrine gland located in the chest beneath the sternum (breastbone). Composed of lymphatic tissue, it regulates the immune system by stimulating the production and activity of T-lymphocytes (white blood cells). Immature T-lymphocytes are made in bone marrow and migrate to the thymus gland, where they are programmed into mature T-lymphocytes that orchestrate the immune response to seek and destroy invading pathogens and cancer cells.

The thymus is most active during youth and begins to atrophy (shrink) and produce less lymphocytes after age 20. A poorly functioning thymus gland weakens the immune response, resulting in more illness. Thymus function can be improved with a healthy diet and antioxidant and lymphatic herbs. Even in older people, well-made thymus glandular supplements greatly enhance thymus function and strong immune response.

Astragalus ~ promotes DNA and RNA synthesis for regeneration of thymus cells; strengthens immunity.
Echinacea ~ stimulates production of lymphocytes and antibodies to fight infection; strengthens immunity.

Thyroid:

The thyroid gland regulates the body's metabolism and expenditure of energy. The main thyroid hormones are thyroxine (T4), which must be converted to usable triiodothyronine (T3). When released into the bloodstream, T4 and T3 reversibly bind to plasma proteins, yet only the free (unbound) hormones are able to be used by cells. Hypothyroidism (underactive thyroid) is a deficiency of thyroid hormones, and is the most common type of thyroid disorder. It causes physical and mental sluggishness resulting in weight gain, low body temperature, dry skin and hair, thin brittle nails, lethargy, depression, and digestive problems such as constipation. Hashimoto's disease is an autoimmune disorder in which the immune system creates antibodies that attack and damage the thyroid, impairing production of T4 and T3 and causing hypothyroidism. Goiters (enlarged thyroid gland) and nodules may also form, with or without hormone deficiency. Goiters usually cause hypothyroidism and are related to iodine deficiency.

Hyperthyroidism is an overactive metabolic state in which the body's processes accelerate due to excessive T3 and T4 levels. Graves' disease, the most common cause of hyperthyroidism, is an autoimmune disease in which antibodies attack and stimulate thyroid tissue to secrete excess hormones, often resulting in an enlarged thyroid. Symptoms of hyperthyroidism include increased heat intolerance and perspiration, weight loss, insomnia, hand tremors, heart palpitations, nervousness, agitation, hyperactivity, bulging eyeballs, increased appetite, and digestive problems, including rapid transit and poor absorption of food and diarrhea.

Black Walnut ~ increases thyroxine (T4) levels in hypothyroidism, but should not be taken on a regular basis.
Lemon Balm ~ helpful in treating hyperthyroidism and Graves' disease.
Motherwort ~ for hyperthyroidism, Graves' disease, and hyperactivity; inhibits conversion of T4 into T3.
Stinging Nettle ~ eating the seeds is an old treatment for goiters resulting from an underactive thyroid.

Other Helpful Herbs:

Ashwagandha (*Withania somnifera*) ~ an adaptogen; used for hypothyroidism; supports the thyroid in making hormones; increases T4 in mice studies; enhances conversion of T4 into T3.
Bugleweed (*Lycopus americanus*) ~ classic herb for hyperthyroidism and Graves' disease; inhibits thyroid stimulating hormone (TSH) and conversion of T4 into T3; helps block action of antibodies attacking the thyroid; has a calming action on the nervous system and heart; discontinue slowly.
Eleuthero/Siberian Ginseng (*Eleutherococcus senticosus*) ~ adaptogen; immunomodulator; helpful for hypothyroidism.
Gromwell (*Lithospermum officinale*) ~ helpful for treating hyperthyroidism; lab and animal studies show it binds to TSH and inhibits the conversion of T4 to usable T3.
Guggul (*Commiphora mukul*) ~ used for hypothyroidism; enhances the conversion of T4 into usable T3.
Maca (*Lepidium meyenii*) ~ nourishes and stimulates the hypothalamus and pituitary, which improves thyroid function and may be helpful to normalize an underactive thyroid.
For cases of Hashimoto's Disease ~ use herbs listed under Epstein-Barr Virus (a cause of Hashimoto's).

Tics and Tremors: See Nervous System
Tinnitus (ringing in the ears): See Ears
Tongue: See Mouth
Tonsillitis: See Throat
Tumors: See Cancer
Ulcerative Colitis: See Intestines
Ulcers: See Skin, Mouth, Stomach, and Intestines (depending on location of ulcer)

Urethritis (inflammation and/or infection of the urethra):

Chickweed ~ the tea soothes painful, inflamed tissues of the urethra.
Comfrey ~ soothing and healing to inflamed tissues.
Dandelion ~ reduces tissue inflammation.
Echinacea ~ antibiotic and anti-inflammatory.
Goldenrod ~ reduces inflammation and spasms; antibacterial.
Goldenseal ~ antibacterial; anti-inflammatory.
Marshmallow ~ mucilage is cooling and soothing to inflamed, irritated tissues.
Mullein ~ mucilage is cooling and soothing.
Stinging Nettle ~ anti-inflammatory; beneficial for all urinary tract infections and bloody urine.
Yarrow ~ one of the best antibiotic herbs for the urinary tract system; anti-inflammatory; analgesic.

Other Helpful Herbs:

Buchu (*Agathosma betulina*) ~ diuretic; used for genitourinary infections and urethritis.
Couch Grass (*Elymus repens*) ~ diuretic; soothing; used for urinary tract infections and urethritis.
Gravel Root (*Eupatorium purpureum*) ~ diuretic; helpful for urinary tract infections and urethritis.
Hydrangea (*Hydrangea arborescens*) ~ diuretic; used for genitourinary infections and urethritis.
Pau D'arco (*Tabebuia impetiginosa*) ~ a strong antimicrobial for urinary tract infections; anti-inflammatory.

Urinary Tract Infection (UTI): See Bladder and Kidneys

Uterus:

American Centaury ~ promotes menstruation; reduces uterine fibroids and endometriosis caused by estrogen excess.
Astragalus ~ helpful for uterine prolapse and excessive or abnormal bleeding.
Black Cohosh ~ helps normalize the uterus, tones and relaxes uterine muscle; helpful during childbirth; beneficial for reducing cramps, abnormal bleeding, fibroids, endometriosis, and uterine prolapse.

Black Walnut ~ antiviral and antimicrobial; a douche may be helpful for cervical ulcers and lesions.
Blue Cohosh ~ tones uterine muscles; used for cramps, spasms, inflammation, pain, and prolapsed uterus; helpful during childbirth when combined with Black Cohosh to promote uterine contractions.
Burdock ~ may be helpful for uterine prolapse and cysts.
Calendula ~ normalizes the menstrual cycle; beneficial for treating uterine fibroids, cysts, and cancer.
Catnip ~ improves uterine blood circulation; reduces cramps and spasms; promotes normal menstruation.
Cayenne ~ antibiotic; increases circulation to the uterus, yet decreases excessive bleeding; used to reduce pain, spasms, and bleeding uterine fibroids.
Chamomile ~ reduces menstrual pain and cramps; stimulates delayed menstruation.
Chasteberry ~ normalizes the menstrual cycle; helps reduce fibroids, endometriosis, cervical dysplasia, and other conditions caused by estrogen excess and progesterone deficiency.
Chickweed ~ a blood cleanser; anti-inflammatory; may help reduce uterine cysts.
Cinquefoil ~ reduces excessive menstrual bleeding and abnormal bleeding due to fibroids and endometriosis; decreases uterine prolapse by toning weak muscles.
Cranesbill ~ decreases abnormal bleeding; strengthens uterine muscles and prevents or reduces prolapse.
Dandelion ~ helps clear excess estrogen; helpful for uterine fibroids, endometriosis, and difficult menses.
Elderberry ~ stimulates blood flow to the uterus; anti-inflammatory.
Elecampane ~ clears excessive mucous discharge and uterine infections.
Feverfew ~ normalizes uterine blood flow and delayed menstruation; anti-inflammatory; reduces cramps.
Goldenrod ~ anti-inflammatory; used to normalize uterine blood flow, regulate cycles, and reduce spasms.
Goldenseal ~ anti-inflammatory; reduces excessive menstrual bleeding and blood loss from fibroids and endometriosis; used for reducing and healing cervical erosion and dysplasia.
Hops ~ anti-inflammatory; soothing to the nerves; reduces uterine spasms; exerts estrogenic activity.
Motherwort ~ a uterine tonic; used to increase blood flow to the uterus, reduce spasms, promote menstruation, and stimulate contractions during childbirth.
Sage ~ promotes normal blood flow to the uterus and reduces excessive menstrual bleeding; helpful for easing uterine pain, cramps, and spasms.
Saint John's Wort ~ decreases pelvic pain; normalizes regular menstruation; beneficial for uterine fibroids.
Thyme ~ reduces uterine cramps and spasms; normalizes blood flow; antimicrobial.
Valerian ~ increases uterine blood flow; reduces pain, cramps, and spasms.
Yarrow ~ excellent for fibroids, uterine and menstrual problems, excessive bleeding, cramps, and spasms.
Yellow Dock ~ decreases heavy menstrual flow, blood clots, menstrual pain, cramps, and fibroids.

Vaginal Health and Infections (also see Fungal Infections):

Black Cohosh ~ reduces vaginal thinning and dryness occurring with menopause.
Black Walnut ~ a douche of the tea is helpful for bacterial, viral, yeast, parasitic, and amoebic infections.
Calendula ~ a douche of the tea is used to treat vaginal infections and Candida yeast.
Cayenne ~ an antibiotic helpful for vaginal infections and discharge.
Cinquefoil ~ used as douche for infections and discharge.
Comfrey ~ tea is used as a douche to soothe pain and irritation from Candida and other vaginal infections.
Cranesbill ~ tea is used as douche for vaginal discharge from bacterial infections and Candida yeast.
Echinacea ~ antibacterial; antiviral; anti-yeast; used for vaginitis and all pelvic inflammatory diseases.
Elecampane ~ antibacterial and antifungal for yeast infections, vaginitis, and vaginal discharges.
Goldenrod ~ antibacterial; antifungal; used for Candida yeast and other vaginal infections; dries discharges.
Goldenseal ~ used as a douche or suppository for yeast infections, vaginitis, discharges, cervical dysplasia.
Hops ~ helps eradicate *Trichomonas vaginalis* (a parasite causing vaginal and urethral infection).
Horehound ~ helpful for vaginal infections and discharges.
Isatis ~ a strong antibacterial and anti-yeast.
Lavender ~ antibacterial for treating vaginal infections, yeast, and *Trichomonas vaginalis.*
Motherwort ~ a douche of the tea is beneficial for treating vaginal infections and Candida yeast.
Mugwort ~ a douche of the tea is used to eliminate vaginal infections and Candida yeast.
Sage ~ antibacterial and antifungal against bacterial and yeast infections.
Yarrow ~ a strong antibiotic; kills Candida yeast; a cooling anti-inflammatory.
Yellow Dock ~ a douche of the tea is used to treat vaginal infections and Candida yeast.

Other Helpful Herbs:

Garlic (*Allium sativum*) ~ strong antibacterial and antifungal for infections and yeast; ingest and douche.
Oregon Grape Root (*Mahonia aquifolium*) ~ strong antibacterial and antifungal for infections and yeast.
Uva-ursi/Bearberry (*Arctostaphylos uva-ursi*) ~ antimicrobial; astringent; used for vaginal infections.

Varicose Veins: See Vascular System

Vascular or Circulatory System (also see Blood and Hypertension):

The vascular or circulatory system includes all veins, arteries, and capillaries that carry blood throughout the body to supply organs and tissues with oxygen, nutrients, enzymes, hormones, and a variety of other substances. Blood vessels also carry waste products that are eliminated through the kidneys.

Vascular diseases are typically caused by inflamed vessels, blood clots, and atherosclerosis, which is a buildup of plaque, deposits of fatty substances, cholesterol, cellular waste products, calcium, and fibrin in the inner lining of an artery. Plaque narrows blood vessels and decreases or completely blocks blood flow.

Eating a healthy diet of fresh fruits and vegetables and taking supplements of calcium, magnesium, the B vitamin complex, vitamin C and bioflavonoids, and EPA-DHA fatty acids supports healthy blood vessels. Herbs that are antioxidant, anti-inflammatory, and relax the nervous system benefit the vascular system.

American Centaury ~ helps reduce varicose veins.

Astragalus ~ a vasodilator (relaxes and dilates blood vessels) that improves circulation; reduces abnormal clotting, varicose veins, and hypertension.

Black Cohosh ~ a vasodilator; improves circulation; reduces hypertension.

Blue Vervain ~ relaxes the nerves and dilates blood vessels to improve circulation; reduces hypertension.

Boneset ~ a vasodilator that improves circulation.

Calendula ~ vasodilator; benefits circulation, varicose veins, spider veins, phlebitis (inflammation of a vein, usually in the leg), and intermittent claudication (leg pain due to narrowing of the arteries and insufficient oxygen supply to the leg muscles).

Catnip ~ a mild vasodilator beneficial to circulation.

Cayenne ~ improves circulation; tones and strengthens blood vessels; decreases abnormal hemorrhage and clotting; improves vascular problems including phlebitis, arteriosclerosis, varicose veins, hemorrhoids, peripheral vascular disease, and Raynaud's disease (cold extremities due to poor circulation).

Chamomile ~ a vasodilator and blood thinner; helps diminish varicose veins and hemorrhoids.

Cinquefoil ~ stops abnormal bleeding; helps reduce varicose veins and hemorrhoids.

Comfrey ~ helps restore normal muscle tone to blood vessels; used for varicose veins, hemorrhoids, phlebitis.

Cranesbill ~ stops abnormal bleeding; used for varicose veins and hemorrhoids.

Echinacea ~ a vasodilator and blood cleanser; may help shrink varicose veins.

Feverfew ~ promotes blood vessel stability; normalizes blood flow, especially in the head and uterus; specific for vascular headaches; inhibits blood clots from forming.

Goldenseal ~ normalizes muscle tone in blood vessels; equalizes circulation; helps varicose veins, phlebitis.

Holy Basil ~ dilates blood vessels and improves blood flow; an anticoagulant that helps prevent blood clots.

Horehound ~ a vasodilator.

Hyssop ~ improves circulation and venous insufficiency.

Lavender ~ improves circulation by its calming influence that relaxes and dilates blood vessels.

Lemon Balm ~ relaxes nervous tension in blood vessels, allowing vasodilation and improved circulation.

Lobelia ~ a vasodilator that promotes greater circulation.

Motherwort ~ relaxes and dilates blood vessels; helpful for vascular problems caused by nervous tension or vascular congestion and blockage.

Passion Flower ~ relaxes nerves and muscles to dilate blood vessels and reduce hypertension.

Peppermint ~ relaxes and dilates blood vessels.

Pleurisy Root ~ a vasodilator; normalizes and equalizes circulation; helps lower hypertension.

Sage ~ relaxes blood vessels to increase circulation and general body warmth.

Scullcap ~ relaxes blood vessels; a vasodilator; reduces stress-induced hypertension.

Stinging Nettle ~ relaxes blood vessels; astringent; reduces hemorrhage and varicose veins.

Thyme ~ vasodilator; helpful for hypertension, Raynaud's, intermittent claudication, other vascular problems.

Valerian ~ relaxes and dilates blood vessels; stimulates circulation; reduces hypertension.

Wood Betony ~ relaxes and dilates blood vessels; used for hypertension.

Yarrow ~ vasodilator; stimulates and normalizes circulation; reduces blood clots; stops abnormal bleeding.

Other Helpful Herbs:

Bilberry (*Vaccinium myrtillus*) ~ strong antioxidant; helpful for circulatory disorders; strengthens vessels; used in preventing and treating blood clots, varicose veins, atherosclerosis, and peripheral vascular insufficiency; stabilizes leaky and permeable capillaries to reduce edema.

Bupleurum (*Bupleurum chinense*) ~ optimizes blood flow throughout the body; warms extremities; a strong antioxidant that reduces inflammation and protects the heart and blood vessels; inhibits blood coagulation to reduce abnormal clotting.

Butcher's Broom (*Ruscus aculeatus*) ~ tones and strengthens blood vessels; improves elasticity; reduces inflammation, varicose veins, phlebitis, hemorrhoids; constricts blood vessels to stop hemorrhage.

Garlic (*Allium sativum*) ~ antioxidant; vasodilator; reduces cholesterol and triglyceride levels; helps prevent and treat thrombosis (blood clots that form in and block blood vessels), atherosclerosis, Raynaud's disease, and intermittent claudication.

Ginger (*Zingiber officinale*) ~ stimulates circulation; reduces clots, thrombophlebitis, and atherosclerosis.

Ginkgo (*Ginkgo biloba*) ~ antioxidant; anti-inflammatory; regulates tone and elasticity of blood vessels; has vasodilating action on endothelium of blood vessels; helps restore circulation in cases of vascular spasms; helps prevent abnormal blood clotting by decreasing blood platelet aggregation; widely used for peripheral arterial disorders, including intermittent claudication, Raynaud's disease, and atherosclerosis.

Ginseng, American (*Panax quinquefolius*) and Asian (*Panax ginseng*) ~ promote circulation by dilating peripheral blood vessels and inhibiting abnormal blood clotting; provide antioxidant protection.

Gotu Kola (*Centella asiatica*) ~ promotes optimal circulation; reduces vascular inflammation; used for chronic venous insufficiency, varicose veins, and hypertension due to constricted blood vessels.

Hawthorn (*Crataegus* spp.) ~ vasodilator; antioxidant; improves circulation; excellent for most circulatory problems, including atherosclerosis, varicose veins, intermittent claudication, Raynaud's disease, and hypertension.

Horse Chestnut (*Aesculus hippocastanum*) ~ vasotonic (tones blood vessels and promotes normal elasticity); classic remedy for chronic venous insufficiency, varicose veins, hemorrhoids, phlebitis; only dried preparations are used.

Linden (*Tilia* spp.) ~ vasodilator; reduces hypertension; supports cardiovascular system.

Olive leaf (*Olea europaea*) ~ a peripheral vasodilator; antioxidant; anti-inflammatory; reduces high cholesterol and triglyceride levels; promotes optimal circulation; protects against atherosclerosis and hypertension.

Prickly Ash bark (*Zanthoxylum clava-herculis*) ~ stimulates peripheral and capillary circulation; helps most circulatory problems, including varicose veins, intermittent claudication, and Raynaud's disease.

Rosemary (*Rosmarinus officinalis*) ~ has tonic effect on circulatory system; strengthens capillaries; increases peripheral circulation; beneficial for chronic circulatory insufficiency.

Turmeric (*Curcuma longa*) ~ improves circulation and prevents atherosclerosis by 1) reducing fibrinogen and abnormal clotting; 2) increasing endothelial nitric oxide (eNOS) which dilates blood vessels; 3) anti-inflammatory properties; and 4) antioxidant actions.

Vertigo (Dizziness): See Ears

Viral Infections:

Viruses must enter a living cell and "hijack" it in order to reproduce, and some do this by inserting their own DNA or RNA into that of the host cell. Many herbs contain antiviral chemicals that are very effective against human viruses.

Astragalus ~ supports and strengthens the immune system; can be effective against viral infections and flu.
Bloodroot ~ a powerful antiviral (be cautious of toxicity).
Blue Vervain ~ helpful in treating viral infections, including colds and flu (influenza).
Boneset ~ a powerful immunostimulant excellent for viral infections, fevers, and body aches.
Calendula ~ a mild antiviral.
Echinacea ~ effective against viral infections due to immunostimulant actions.
Elderberry ~ antiviral; promotes immunity.
Goldenseal ~ contains antiviral berberine and hydrastine.
Holy Basil ~ antiviral against hepatitis.
Hyssop ~ an antiviral used for the flu and herpes virus.
Isatis ~ an antiviral taken for the flu and other viral infections.
Lemon Balm ~ antiviral against the flu and herpes virus.
Motherwort ~ effective against the Epstein-Barr virus, flu, and common cold.
Sage ~ effective against the flu.
Saint John's Wort ~ an antiviral specifically effective in eradicating herpes lesions and suppressing the virus.
Thyme ~ an antiviral.

Other Helpful Herbs:

Cat's Claw (*Uncaria tomentosa*) ~ one of the best antiviral herbs to boost the immune system and fight viral infections, including the herpes virus, Epstein-Barr virus, HIV (human immunodeficiency virus), HPV (human papilloma virus), and warts (which are viral); anti-inflammatory, antimutagenic, and antioxidant.

Garlic (*Allium sativum*) ~ strengthens the immune system; a potent antiviral, antibacterial, and antifungal.

Ginger (*Zingiber officinale*) ~ supports the immune system; antiviral for the common cold and flu.

Licorice (*Glycyrrhiza glabra*) ~ enhances immunity by increasing interferon, which attacks and destroys many types of viruses.

Olive leaf (*Olea europaea*) ~ antiviral against colds, flu, Epstein-Barr, and herpes viruses.

Oregano (*Origanum vulgare*) ~ antiviral used for colds, flu, herpes, and other viral infections.

Oregon Grape Root (*Mahonia aquifolium*) ~ contains antiviral berberine and hydrastine.

Pau D'arco (*Tabebuia impetiginosa*) ~ a strong antiviral taken for the flu, common cold, and herpes viruses.

Wild Indigo (*Baptisia tinctoria*) ~ strong antiviral; use under guidance of a qualified herbalist due to toxicity of large doses.

Warts (caused by one of the many types of human papillomavirus or HPV):

Antiviral herbs specific to killing HPV when applied to warts for an extended time include Black Walnut, Bloodroot (be careful of caustic actions), Calendula, Dandelion, Stinging Nettle, Thyme, and the latex juice of the Common Milkweed (*Asclepias syriaca*).

Worms: See Parasites

Wounds, External: See Skin

Yeast Infection: See Fungal Infections

Herbs for Pregnancy, Childbirth and Lactation

Several medicinal plants that are historically validated and renowned for their benefits during pregnancy, birth, and lactation are discussed in this chapter. These herbs provide excellent nutritional support, tone and prepare the uterus for birth, ease discomforts of pregnancy, support labor, birth and lactation, and reduce the potential for complications that may arise during this special time in a woman's life. Many midwives and pregnant women from different cultures around the world rely on ancient and modern traditions of herbalism. Midwives from most herbal traditions typically use their specific pharmacy of local herbs that have been passed on from mother to daughter and teacher to student, and validated for their safety and effectiveness over many generations. We are fortunate to have access to this wisdom with reasonable assurance of the long-term safety of these herbs, which have passed the empirical test of time.

A good rule when using medicinal herbs during pregnancy is to ingest small amounts and never be excessive. The safest herbs are **tonic** and **nutritive teas**, which are generally mild-tasting with gentle biological activities. Avoid herbs with strong, bitter flavors indicating the presence of alkaloids and other chemicals too strong for pregnant women and developing infants. Examples of traditionally used tonic and nutritive herbs include the leaves of Alfalfa, Stinging Nettle, Dandelion, Red Raspberry and Peppermint, German Chamomile flowers, and Oat Straw. Pregnant women can safely enjoy a cup of these teas on a regular basis.

Emmenagogue herbs promote menstruation and are generally avoided during pregnancy, although some are very mild and can safely be taken in moderate amounts. **Abortifacients** stimulate expulsion of the fetus from the uterus, causing miscarriage, and are contraindicated during pregnancy. Some plants in this category (specifically Black Cohosh and Blue Cohosh) are traditionally taken only during the last two weeks of pregnancy to prepare the uterus for childbirth, strengthen contractions, and promote easier and faster delivery.

Teas are one of the best ways to ingest herbs during pregnancy and lactation. Pills or capsules also work well. When using **tinctures** (which contain alcohol), always evaporate the alcohol by putting the tincture in a small amount (1/2 cup) of boiling water and allowing it to sit for 10 minutes while stirring occasionally. Most of the alcohol will evaporate, making tinctures safe for pregnancy.

To make an **infusion tea** using leaves or flowers, put 1-2 teaspoons of dried herb or 2-3 teaspoons of finely chopped fresh herb in 1 cup of boiling water. Cover with a lid. Allow the herbs to steep for 5-15 minutes (the longer it steeps, the stronger the flavor and effects), and then strain out the herbs. To make a **decoction tea** using roots or bark, use 1 teaspoon of powdered or chopped bark or root per 1 cup of water. Gently simmer the herb for 8-10 minutes in a covered pan, cool, and strain. (For more details on making tea, refer to pages 124-126).

Enjoy the calm, nurturing ritual of preparing and ingesting medicinal plants during pregnancy. In addition to using herbs, remember that organic, high-nutrient foods, prenatal vitamin and mineral supplements from a reliable company, moderate exercise, and a joyful heart and peaceful mind are all necessary to grow healthy babies and enjoy the miraculous experience of pregnancy and childbirth. Avoid "junk" foods, chemical additives, and uncomfortable, unhealthy environments. Cultivating radiant emotional and mental health is much easier when surrounded with cheerful, supportive people. Enlist the aid of family, friends, midwives, and an obstetric physician. Be connected with your body, mind, emotions, and the infant within your womb. Nurturing your child and developing a relationship begins during pregnancy.

Herbs for Safe Use During Pregnancy

Pregnancy is a time of heightened sensitivity in a woman's body, and utmost care must be taken to ensure the safety of mother and developing infant. Some of the most widely used and historically validated herbs that are safe to take during pregnancy are listed below. I have experienced or witnessed the actions of many of these herbs during my years as a midwife-in-training, when pregnant with my two sons, and in my clinical practice as a registered nurse and herbalist, and can attest to their beneficial qualities.

The following herbs have been used for centuries and withstood the tests and trials of time by thousands of pregnant women. Modern researchers have identified many chemical constituents in plants, often confirming their historical uses. However, confusion can occur when some herbs that have safely been consumed by pregnant women over many centuries, such as Peppermint, German Chamomile and Red Raspberry, are sometimes contraindicated during the first trimester or the entire pregnancy due to their mild emmenagogue effects. These cautions are often speculative and not based on clinical evidence or other reports of harm to mother or infant. When pregnant, it is especially important to be confident in choosing what to eat and drink, so thoroughly investigate the herbs you use. Refer to "The Safety of Medicinal Herbs" in Section One for more considerations in understanding herbal safety. Try to find a knowledgeable herbalist for assistance, and let your physician, midwife, and other health professionals know which herbs you are using.

There are so many medicinal plants that are questionable or not safe to use during pregnancy that I recommend taking only the following herbs, which have a long historic "track record" of safety.

Materia Medica of Herbs for Pregnancy

Alfalfa leaves (*Medicago sativa*) are a rich source of vitamins and minerals, and have traditionally been enjoyed as a tonic and nutritive tea. Midwives often recommend it for nutritional deficiencies, anemia, and fatigue. *Dosage:* A cup of tea daily as needed. *Contraindications:* Alfalfa contains isoflavones and coumestans having estrogenic activity. Although this activity is slight and there is no clinical data of adverse effects when taken as tea in normal amounts during pregnancy, it is currently contraindicated by some references based on speculation. However, tea made from the leaves has a very long historic record of safety.

Black Haw bark (*Viburnum prunifolium*) is a well-known uterine tonic and restorative that may safely be taken throughout pregnancy and was once highly revered and prescribed by American Eclectic physicians. The bark contains scopoletin, which regulates the calming neurotransmitter serotonin that reduces anxiety and depression. Black Haw calms the nervous system, is a powerful uterine relaxant, decreases high blood pressure, and eases cramps and spasms in the pelvis and legs. It is helpful for morning sickness. Astringent constituents help stop spot-bleeding and blood loss after birth. The herb is especially effective in preventing habitual or threatened miscarriage. It reduces premature contractions and false labor pains, and eases uterine spasms after childbirth. Uses for Black Haw are similar to those for Cramp Bark (*Viburnum opulus*). *Dosage:* For general use during pregnancy, drink 1-2 cups of tea, 20-40 drops of tincture, or 2-3 capsules daily. *Contraindications:* None. Black Haw has a long history of safe and beneficial use throughout pregnancy.

Blackberry leaves (*Rubus fructicosus*) are traditionally enjoyed in Europe as a pregnancy tonic and have similar benefits as Red Raspberry leaf tea, although not as strong. Blackberry leaves are nutritious, and astringent properties reduce diarrhea, varicose veins, and hemorrhoids. *Dosage:* A cup of tea daily as needed. The tea may be soaked in a cloth and applied to varicose veins and hemorrhoids. *Contraindications:* None.

Burdock root (*Arctium lappa*) contains nourishing vitamins and minerals, and is eaten as a cooked vegetable in Asia. It is an excellent ovarian, liver and kidney tonic, and is helpful for anemia, edema, and blood cleansing. The roots are cooling and helpful for fevers, skin eruptions, toxic overload, and other heat conditions. *Dosage*: 1-2 cups of tea daily as needed. *Contraindications*: Animal research shows it exerts weak uterine stimulation, and some references speculate it is best to take it in small amounts after the first trimester. However, Burdock root is non-toxic and there are no reports of problems in the literature. (For more information about Burdock, refer to pages 266-274.)

Cayenne fruit (*Capsicum annuum*) can safely be taken in small amounts for bacterial and sinus infections, coughs, and the common cold. Cayenne breaks up mucous congestion and is also used to reduce hypertension, arthritis, muscle spasms in the upper torso, neuralgia (nerve pain), shingles, and abnormal bleeding. It stimulates digestion and is anti-inflammatory. *Dosage*: Pinches of the powder may be sprinkled on food sparingly. Since it is warming to any tissue it contacts, be sure to take it with food to prevent stomach upset. *Contraindications*: Due to its very warming nature, avoid use in cases of heartburn or fever, and do not take Cayenne on an empty stomach or apply it to a break in the skin, the eyes, or sensitive tissue. There are no currently known restrictions during pregnancy and lactation when used in very small amounts. (For more information about Cayenne, refer to pages 287-295.)

German Chamomile flowers (*Matricaria recutita*) are a source of easily digested calcium and other minerals. They are calming to the nervous system and helpful for anxiety, digestive problems (especially related to stress), morning sickness, gas, stomach and intestinal ulcers, insomnia, headaches, spasms, and inflammation. *Dosage*: Steep 1-2 teaspoons of the flowers in a cup of water and drink a cup daily as needed. The tea may be used as a wash for skin irritations, infections, and eczema. *Contraindications*: Large amounts stimulate the uterus, but drinking a daily cup of the flowers is safe and no problems have been reported. **Roman Chamomile (*Chamaemelum nobile*)** is an abortifacient and should never be used during pregnancy. (For more information about German Chamomile, refer to pages 296-302.)

Chasteberry (*Vitex agnus-castus*) is an excellent tonic for normalizing reproductive hormones and organs, and is specific for promoting fertility and preventing miscarriage. It normalizes hormones by increasing progesterone in relationship to estrogen. It benefits the pituitary and hypothalamus glands, and stimulates release of luteinizing hormone (LH), which triggers ovulation. Chasteberry also eases morning sickness. *Dosage:* 40 drops of tincture 1-2 times a day or 1-2 cups of tea. *Contraindications:* None. (For more information about Chasteberry, refer to pages 303-309.)

Chlorella (*Chlorella regularis*) is a freshwater algae that is packed with easily digested nutrients and draws many types of toxins, including heavy metals, out of the body. It contains 50-70% protein and an abundance of vitamins, minerals, and nucleic acids RNA and DNA. It supports the endocrine glands, enhances immunity, and benefits all organs. *Dosage:* 1-2 teaspoons of powder in a daily smoothie drink or mixed in food, or 2-4 pills or capsules with each meal. *Contraindications:* Chlorella is extremely safe with no toxicity. It may cause slight nausea if taken on an empty stomach, so always take it with food and start with small amounts.

Cramp Bark (*Viburnum opulus*) is a uterine tonic and restorative, and like its relative Black Haw (*Viburnum prunifolium*), it is excellent to prevent habitual or threatened miscarriage. Astringent actions improve poor muscle tone in the pelvic organs (including uterine prolapse and cervical weakness), help prevent spot bleeding, and reduce excessive bleeding after birth. Cramp Bark eases morning sickness and is a strong muscle relaxant that decreases leg cramps, uterine spasms, and premature contractions. It has been used to treat seizures during pregnancy. *Dosage:* Make tea by simmering 2 teaspoons of the bark in a cup of water and drink 1-4 cups daily as needed. Or use 20-60 drops of tincture 1-4 times daily. *Contraindications:* Cramp bark has a long history of safe use when taken in small amounts throughout pregnancy to support gestation, labor, and delivery. It should not be taken with blood thinning drugs because it contains coumarin constituents. It may lower blood pressure in people who are hypotensive. Do not ingest the toxic berries.

Dandelion leaves and roots (*Taraxacum officinale*) are an excellent liver tonic that gently stimulates liver activity and is helpful for most liver and gallbladder problems. Dandelion is a mild diuretic and laxative, and is beneficial for reducing skin rashes and outbreaks, edema, anemia, arthritis, gout, hypertension, and high cholesterol. It helps prevent pre-eclampsia (edema, hypertension, and protein in urine). The leaves and roots are a potent source of vitamins and minerals, especially vitamin A, iron, potassium, and calcium. *Dosage:* Gently simmer 2 teaspoons of the chopped or powdered root in a pint of water for 8 minutes and sip 1-2 cups daily as needed. The young leaves may be steeped in a tea or eaten like vegetables when steamed or sautéed. *Contraindications:* Do not use Dandelion in cases of bile duct obstruction or excess stomach acidity (heartburn). There are no currently known restrictions during pregnancy and lactation when taken in moderate doses. (For more information about Dandelion, refer to pages 332-340.)

Echinacea leaves, flowers, and roots (*Echinacea purpurea, E. angustifolia*) enhance immune function and are excellent for bacterial and viral infections, common colds, flu, fever, upper respiratory tract infections, and Candida yeast. Use at the first signs of illness. *Dosage:* The tincture form is far superior to tea and pills, so put it in boiling water to evaporate the alcohol. Use 60 drops of tincture in water 3-5 times daily as needed for infections. *Contraindications:* Echinacea may exacerbate autoimmune diseases such as AIDS, HIV, lupus, and multiple sclerosis. There are no currently known restrictions during pregnancy and lactation, and both empirical evidence and modern research demonstrate its safety during pregnancy and lactation (Gallo, 2000 & 2001). (For more information about Echinacea, refer to pages 341-352.)

Elderberry flowers and berries (*Sambucus canadensis, S. nigra*) have a long history of use for treating coughs, the common cold, flu, and fevers. Diuretic properties reduce water retention. *Dosage:* The dried flowers are used in teas, tinctures, tablets, and cough syrup. For pregnancy, 1-2 cups of tea daily or cough syrup (follow directions on bottle) are recommended. *Contraindications:* There are no currently known restrictions during pregnancy or lactation. (For more information about Elderberry, refer to pages 353-359.)

Fennel seed (*Foeniculum vulgare*) is anti-inflammatory, soothing to the stomach and digestive tract, a gentle laxative, and relieves gas and colic in infants and adults. It reduces excess mucous in the respiratory tract. *Dosage:* 1-2 cups of tea, 30-60 drops of tincture, or 5-7 grams in pills or capsules may be taken daily when necessary. *Contraindications:* None. Moderate amounts are safe during pregnancy and lactation.

Flaxseed (*Linum usitatissimum*) is excellent for the cardiovascular system, helps lower elevated cholesterol levels, and is a gentle laxative. Its mucilage soothes inflamed, irritated tissues and helps irritable bowels, stomach inflammation, and rheumatoid arthritis. The seeds contain lignans (plant estrogens) and substantial amounts of essential fatty acids, especially Omega-3. *Dosage:* Grinding whole flax seeds into a fine powder using an electric coffee bean grinder is the best method of preparation. Refrigerate the powder to preserve freshness. Use one tablespoon daily sprinkled over food or add to drinks. Or take 1-2 capsules daily. *Contraindications:* None. Flaxseed is safe to use as a food during pregnancy and lactation.

Garlic (*Allium sativum*) benefits the cardiovascular system and helps regulate cholesterol levels, blood pressure, and blood glucose levels. It kills bacteria, viruses, parasites, Candida yeast and other fungi, and is used for the common cold, coughs and mucous congestion, the flu, and other infections. *Dosage:* Use small amounts of freshly chopped Garlic and add to foods. *Contraindications:* Garlic is very warming and should not be taken with fevers, heartburn, gastric acidity, inflammation, and other conditions of excess heat. There are no currently known restrictions, but it should only be ingested in small amounts with food during pregnancy. It is not recommended during lactation because the strong odor can affect breast milk.

Ginger root (*Zingiber officinale*) is warming and stimulates circulation of blood and energy throughout the body. It has an extensive global history as one of the most popular herbs taken for the nausea of morning sickness and motion sickness. It benefits the entire digestive system, relieving cramps, spasms, indigestion, and gas. In the respiratory tract, it clears mucous congestion and is helpful for colds, flu, sore throats, and coughs. Ginger clears congestion in the reproductive system by increasing blood flow to the pelvis, and relaxes muscles to ease spasms and cramps. *Dosage:* 1-2 cups of tea daily. Ginger is a delicious tea and can be enjoyed with a little honey and lemon juice, which also clears phlegm. Limit intake of capsules or pills to 250 mg 1-2 times a day. *Contraindications:* Ginger is traditionally used to stimulate menstruation, so there have been questions about its ability to cause miscarriages. Two Japanese studies in the 1980s indicated that 6-gingerol, one of the compounds isolated from Ginger roots, had mutagenic activity *in vitro* at high doses (Namakura, 1982; Nagabhushan, 1987). However, other compounds in the roots exhibit anti-mutagenic actions that counteract these. Since these two studies were published, recommendations against using Ginger during pregnancy have appeared, although there is no clinical research or medical evidence that normal amounts of Ginger cause any harm to the fetus or mother. On the contrary, many published studies validate its ability to effectively and safely relieve nausea during pregnancy without any side effects.

Hawthorn berries (*Crataegus* spp.) contain proanthocyanidins having antioxidant activity that protects cells from damage. The berries dilate blood vessels, and extensive research confirms beneficial effects for the heart, circulation, and hypertension. The late master herbalist and naturopathic doctor John Christopher successfully combined Garlic and Hawthorn berries to treat high blood pressure. Hawthorn can relieve hot flashes during pregnancy and help the placenta disengage following labor. *Dosage:* A cup of tea daily as needed during the second and third trimesters. *Contraindications:* There are no currently known restrictions during pregnancy and lactation when used in small amounts after the first trimester.

Lemon Balm leaves (*Melissa officinalis*) calm the nervous system and reduce insomnia, headaches, anxiety, and depression. The herb helps ease morning sickness, gas and dizziness, especially when combined with Ginger tea. Lemon Balm primes the uterus for labor and helps expel a retained placenta. *Dosage:* 1 cup of tea daily as needed. *Contraindications:* Lemon Balm is a mild emmenagogue (due to its relaxing effects on the uterus), but moderate amounts of tea have been used safely throughout pregnancy for centuries. (For more information about Lemon Balm, refer to pages 426-433.)

Marshmallow root (*Althaea officinalis*) contains soothing and anti-inflammatory mucilage that heals irritated and injured tissues in the mouth, throat, gastrointestinal tract, lungs, kidneys, and bladder. It is helpful for morning sickness and vomiting, and neutralizes excess acids to ease heartburn. The roots are nourishing, and usually an upset stomach will accept this tea when all else fails. It is helpful for coughs, fevers, and bladder infections. *Dosage:* Drink the powdered or chopped root as a tea. Sip on 1-3 cups daily as needed. *Contraindications:* This is a very safe herb with no restrictions during pregnancy and lactation. (For more information about Marshmallow, refer to pages 444-449.)

Milk Thistle seeds (*Silybum marianum*) excel in detoxifying the liver, neutralizing and eliminating poisonous and allergy-inducing substances, and rejuvenating liver cells. The seeds are used for toxic liver damage, chronic inflammatory liver disease, viral liver infections, and cirrhosis. *Dosage:* 200-400 mg daily as needed. *Contraindications:* There are no currently known restrictions during pregnancy and lactation.

Mullein leaves (*Verbascum thapsus*) are excellent for coughs and lung problems. Oil made from the **flowers** is combined with Garlic oil and works well for ear infections and pain. *Dosage*: Prepare tea with the leaf and drink 1-2 cups daily as needed. *Contraindications:* None. (For more information about Mullein and directions for preparing oil for ear drops, refer to pages 462-467.)

Oat Straw and fresh milky Oats (*Avena sativa*) contain silica, calcium, magnesium, and other minerals that support bone growth and the nervous system, calm anxiety, and strengthen blood vessels. They are helpful for varicose veins and hemorrhoids, and the tea may be used as a bath for inflamed, itchy, and seborrheic skin diseases (over-secretion of sebaceous glands). *Dosage:* The dried leaf, stem, and unripe grain are made into tea. Drink 1-2 cups daily as needed. *Contraindications:* There are no currently known restrictions during pregnancy and lactation.

Partridge Berry (Squaw Vine) leaf and root (*Mitchella repens*) has a long history of use as a valuable uterine tonic and restorative, and is often combined with Red Raspberry leaf or Black Haw to tone the uterus for childbirth and facilitate easier, more effective labor. Partridge Berry may be taken throughout pregnancy. It is calming and vitalizes the blood, removes uterine congestion, and diuretic properties help reduce edema. Known to normalize female hormones, it is recommended for prevention of miscarriage in women with prior history, and should be taken in early pregnancy for this problem. Towards the end of pregnancy, it tones the uterus, is helpful during labor, and promotes lactation. Native American Indian women drank a cup of the decoction tea 2-3 weeks before the due date to promote safe and less painful births. It was considered a specific and superior herb to prepare the uterus for labor by the American Eclectic medical physicians during the 1800s and early 1900s. It is a cooling herb that combines well with Ginger, which is warming. *Dosage*: To tone the uterus or prevent habitual miscarriage, use 1 cup of tea or 15-30 drops of tincture 1-3 times daily. For threatening miscarriage, take 50 drops of tincture every 20-30 minutes until contractions stop. *Contraindications*: None.

Passion Flower leaves and flowers (*Passiflora incarnata*) are a calming nervine and mild sedative helpful for hormonal adjustments occurring during pregnancy. The herb eases anxiety, nervous exhaustion, cramps and spasms, and may reduce hypertension related to stress. It diminishes after-pains of childbirth. *Dosage:* A cup of tea or 10-40 drops of tincture (evaporate the alcohol) are safe daily doses. *Contraindications:* Although recent speculative warnings have been cited after isolated harman and harmaline constituents caused uterine stimulation in animal studies, pregnant and lactating women have been drinking Passion Flower tea for centuries without known problems. The German Commission E herbal regulatory agency determined it to be safe during pregnancy and lactation. (For more information about Passion Flower, refer to pages 468-473.)

Peppermint leaves (*Mentha x piperita*) calm and ease painful spastic conditions in the gastrointestinal tract, gallbladder, and bile ducts. The herb helps reduce morning sickness and nausea, indigestion, gas, spasms, irritable bowel problems, anxiety, headaches, colds, flu, fevers, and coughs. *Dosage:* A cup of tea daily as needed. *Contraindications:* Although it is a very mild emmenagogue, pregnant women worldwide have safely used Peppermint tea to relieve morning sickness and other discomforts of pregnancy. Peppermint oil is too strong to ingest. Avoid Peppermint in cases of acid reflux or heartburn because it relaxes the muscle sphincter between the stomach and esophagus, allowing stomach contents to empty into the esophagus and cause burning. (For more information about Peppermint, refer to pages 474-480.)

Red Raspberry leaf (*Rubus idaeus*) has a specific affinity for the uterus and is one of the most popular herbal teas enjoyed by pregnant women. It is a uterine tonic, and regular use during pregnancy tones and strengthens uterine and pelvic muscles, improves blood circulation in the uterus, helps prevent miscarriage, and prepares the uterus for labor. Red Raspberry leaves reduce morning sickness, ease labor pains, promote a safe, speedy, and easy delivery, and mild astringent properties help prevent postpartum hemorrhage. The herb soothes the nervous system, reduces stress, promotes sleep, tones mucous membranes throughout the body, and reduces diarrhea. It is extremely nourishing, containing calcium, magnesium, iron, and other minerals and vitamins. Drinking the tea after delivery improves milk production. *Dosage:* 1-2 cups of the pleasant-tasting tea may be taken daily throughout pregnancy and lactation. *Contraindications:* Raspberry leaf tea has a long history of safe use during pregnancy and lactation and is commonly recommended by midwives and herbalists. Some sources have recently recommended not using it during pregnancy, but this is a hypothetical speculation unsubstantiated by real-life evidence. Confirming the safety of Red Raspberry, two studies involving 243 pregnant women who took Red Raspberry during their pregnancies found a decreased likelihood of premature and overdue labor, a slightly shorter duration of the second stage of labor, and fewer forceps deliveries (Parsons, 1999; Simpson, 2001).

Scullcap leaves and flowers (*Scutellaria lateriflora*) are excellent to calm the nervous system and help reduce anxiety, mood swings, headaches, nerve pain, insomnia, and hypertension. *Dosage:* 1-2 cups of tea or 10-40 drops of tincture (evaporate alcohol with boiling water) 1-2 times daily as needed. *Contraindications*: None. (For more information about Scullcap, refer to pages 506-510.)

Slippery Elm bark (*Ulmus rubra*) contains mucilage that soothes all tissue it contacts. It neutralizes stomach acids and is excellent for nausea, vomiting, heartburn, and coughs. It has similar properties as Marshmallow root, and may be used interchangeably since many Slippery Elm trees have died from Dutch Elm disease. *Dosage:* Drink as a tea because the mucilage qualities are extracted best by hot water. Steep 1-2 tablespoons of chopped or powdered root in a quart of hot water for 30-60 minutes and drink up to a quart daily as needed. *Contraindications*: None. This is a very safe and mild herb for mothers and infants.

Spearmint leaves (*Mentha spicata*) reduce morning sickness, gas, spasms, hemorrhoids, and anxiety. *Dosage:* A cup of tea daily as needed. *Contraindications*: None.

Stinging Nettle leaves (*Urtica dioica*) are an extremely nutritious source of many vitamins, calcium, iron, and other minerals, and help prevent anemia. A favorite herb of many midwives, it relaxes leg cramps and other muscle spasms; improves elasticity of varicose veins; relieves hemorrhoids, kidney and bladder infections, inflammation, and rheumatoid arthritis; and helps balance blood sugar levels. It contains anti

histamines to reduce allergy symptoms, and gentle diuretic effects are helpful for water retention. Native American women ate and drank Stinging Nettle as a pregnancy tonic, to prevent hemorrhage during and after birth, and to enrich and increase the flow of breast milk. *Dosage*: A cup of tea daily as needed. *Contraindications:* Recent scientific studies show that Stinging Nettle has very mild emmenagogue properties. However, it has a long historic record of safe use during pregnancy and no adverse effects are reported in the literature. (For more information about Stinging Nettle, refer to pages 515-522.)

Wild Yam root (*Dioscorea villosa*) contains diosgenin, a phytosterol having progesterone effects. It is beneficial for morning sickness and halting threatened miscarriage and premature labor associated with low progesterone levels. Wild Yam reduces spasms, helps relieve general pain during pregnancy, and is relaxing to the nerves. *Dosage*: 20-30 drops of tincture (evaporate alcohol with boiling water) 1-4 times daily, or sip 1-2 cups of tea throughout the day. Wild Yam root is also prepared as a topical cream that may be purchased and applied on the skin twice daily. *Contraindications:* None. Since Wild Yam improves hormone levels, it should be used in cases of low progesterone.

Herbs that Promote Fertility

When women have difficulty becoming pregnant, it is best to seek the counsel of a healthcare provider who can help identify the underlying causes. Simple blood tests can determine if hypothyroidism or imbalanced hormone levels are problems. Progesterone deficiency is a common cause of infertility, especially in older women, and can safely be corrected with the use of specific herbs.

To promote optimal fertility, it is vital to eat nutritious food; avoid chemicals and toxins in your food, body care products, household cleaners, and lawn care products; check for possible food allergies and sensitivities; and, very importantly, cultivate a calm mind and happy, peaceful emotions.

The following herbs help normalize estrogen and progesterone levels to enhance fertility. When pregnancy occurs stop taking Dong Quai, Licorice, Motherwort, and Sarsaparilla. Chasteberry and Wild Yam root may be continued during pregnancy in cases of low progesterone levels.

Chasteberry (*Vitex agnus-castus*) is an excellent tonic specific for promoting fertility by enhancing progesterone levels. *Dosage:* 40 drops of tincture 1-2 times daily or 1-2 cups of tea until pregnancy occurs. *Contraindications:* Chasteberry may be taken during pregnancy, especially when progesterone levels tend to be low. (For more information about Chasteberry, refer to pages 303-309.)

Dong Quai root (*Angelica sinensis*) is an excellent hormonal tonic to normalize the reproductive system and tone the uterus. Studies show that it exerts estrogenic effects (Circosta, 2006). In China, it is traditionally used in combination with other herbs. *Dosage:* A cup of tea or 30-40 drops of tincture twice daily. *Contraindications:* Discontinue when pregnant.

Licorice root (*Glycyrrhiza glabra*) contains phytoestrogens that exert mild estrogen-like activity. Licorice is best taken during the pre-ovulatory phase of the menstrual cycle (which begins on the first day of menstrual bleeding and ends about 14 days later with ovulation) when estrogen levels are low. *Dosage:* Drink a daily cup of Licorice tea beginning on the day menstruation ends until day 14 of your cycle and then stop. This may be repeated each month. *Contraindications:* Take the deglycyrrhized form of Licorice to avoid any side effect of hypertension, water retention, or cardiovascular problems. Discontinue when pregnant.

Motherwort (*Leonurus cardiaca*) has been used to promote fertility when taken over a period of several weeks or months. It is most effective when combined with other fertility herbs. *Dosage:* 40 drops of tincture 2-3 times daily. *Contraindications:* Do not use in cases of heavy menstrual bleeding because it may worsen the problem. Most importantly, Motherwort is contraindicated during pregnancy, so stop using it before actively trying to become pregnant. (For more information about Motherwort, refer to pages 454-455.)

Sarsaparilla root (*Smilax aristolochiifolia,* spp.) contains phytosterols having progesterone activity and is used to improve fertility when progesterone levels are low. *Dosage:* Drink 1-2 cups of tea daily starting on day 14 of your cycle until day 28, or until your period starts, then stop. If your period does not start, you may be pregnant. In that case, you may continue drinking 1/2 cup of tea each day to promote the pregnancy for 2-3 more weeks. If your period does resume, simply begin drinking the tea again, and be patient. *Contraindications:* Discontinue when pregnant.

Wild Yam root (*Dioscorea villosa*) provides precursors to progesterone and safely increases low levels to support pregnancy. *Dosage:* 1-2 cups of tea daily or 30-40 drops of tincture twice daily. The topical cream may be applied to the skin twice daily. *Contraindications:* Small amounts may be continued during pregnancy to reduce morning sickness and protect against miscarriage, especially when progesterone levels are low.

Uterine and Pregnancy Tonics

The following herbs have safely been used over the centuries and are recommended to provide important nutrients that help tone the uterus, grow healthy babies, and prepare the uterus for childbirth. These herbs may be taken alone or blended together and taken as tea, tincture, pills, or capsules. Most of these combine well into a tasty tea. When preparing tea, blend a few herbs together to make a quart of tea and enjoy this throughout the day. Tincture preparations are excellent to use, but remember to evaporate the alcohol by adding it to boiled water or tea. More information on each herb can be found above in the "Materia Medica of Herbs for Pregnancy."

Alfalfa leaves are a rich source of nutrients.
Black Haw is a uterine tonic.
Blackberry leaves are nutritional.
Chlorella contains many nutrients and safely removes some heavy metals from the body.
Cramp Bark is a uterine tonic.
Flaxseed contains essential fatty acids necessary for fetal development, specifically Omega-3 fatty acids.
Partridge Berry is a valuable uterine tonic that blends well with Red Raspberry leaf.
Red Raspberry leaf is the most widely used and safest uterine tonic.
Stinging Nettle leaf contains high amounts of chlorophyll and other nutrients.

Herbs to Prevent Miscarriage and Premature Labor

Progesterone deficiency is one of the major causes of infertility and miscarriages, and I have found this to be true with several pregnant women who came to my office concerned about repeating their history of past miscarriages. I recommended Chasteberry and a topical cream containing Wild Yam (both herbs increase progesterone levels), and they all gave birth to healthy, full-term babies.

Premature labor is often caused by weak muscle tone in the uterus and cervix and by premature contractions. Spot bleeding is an indication of possible problems. Black Haw and Cramp Bark are especially helpful in reversing these problems. False Unicorn is mentioned because it was widely used for its effectiveness, but it is now an endangered species and difficult to find.

The herbs listed below may be combined for greater efficacy, and should be used with the supervision of a qualified health care practitioner and herbalist.

Black Haw bark (*Viburnum prunifolium*) is especially effective in preventing habitual or threatened miscarriage, and during the 1800s it was listed in most pharmacy books and widely used for this purpose. *Dosage:* To prevent habitual miscarriage, simmer 2 teaspoons of the dried bark in a cup of water for 10 minutes and drink 1-3 cups daily. Or take 5-10 ml (1 ml equals 15 drops) of tincture 3 times daily. If using capsules, the daily dose is 2.5-5 grams. For threatened miscarriage, drink a cup of tea every hour. If using tincture, take 1 teaspoon every hour or 15 drops every 15 minutes until contractions stop. *Contraindications:* Black Haw has a long history of safe and beneficial use throughout pregnancy.

Chasteberry (*Vitex agnus-castus*) increases progesterone levels due to pituitary stimulation and the balancing of FSH (follicle stimulating hormone) and LH (luteinizing hormone). The berries work amazingly well to provide necessary progesterone needed to maintain pregnancy. *Dosage*: 1-2 cups of tea or 20-30 drops of tincture in water daily at the beginning or throughout pregnancy. *Contraindications:* The berries are safe when used in recommended doses. (For more information, refer to pages 307-308.)

Cramp Bark (*Viburnum opulus*) is excellent in preventing habitual or threatened miscarriage, and has stronger actions than the related species Black Haw (*Viburnum prunifolium*). Cramp Bark improves poor muscle tone in the uterus, strengthens a weak cervix, and stops spot bleeding, uterine spasms, and premature contractions. It is a relaxing nervine that eases cramps and spasms. *Dosage:* To prevent habitual miscarriage, put 2 teaspoons of the dried bark in a cup of water and simmer for 10 minutes. Drink 1 cup of the tea 3 times a day. Or take 20-75 drops of tincture 1-4 times daily. If using capsules the dose is 2-4 grams daily. For threatened miscarriage, take 1 teaspoon of tincture every hour as needed, or 15 drops every 15 minutes until contractions stop. *Contraindications:* Use cautiously with blood thinning drugs because it contains coumarins. It may lower blood pressure in people who are hypotensive. Do not ingest the toxic berries.

False Unicorn Root (*Chamaelirium luteum*) is an ovarian and uterine tonic. It tightens and strengthens pelvic and uterine muscles, and is especially helpful for women with habitual miscarriages due to incompetent cervix from weak muscle tone. *Dosage:* To prepare tea, use 1-2 teaspoons of root per cup of water and gently simmer 10-15 minutes. Drink 1-3 cups daily. Or take 30-60 drops of tincture diluted in water 3 times daily. If using the dried root, take 1/4-1/2 teaspoon (1-2 grams) 3 times daily. *Contraindications:* The long history of use is evidence of safety, however there is no research confirming this. As mentioned, this is an endangered plant that is difficult to find and rarely used today.

The late herbalist and naturopathic doctor John Christopher prescribed a combination of False Unicorn Root (3 parts) and ***Lobelia inflata*** (1 part) to halt threatened miscarriages. He prescribed 1 teaspoon of this combination in a cup of water, giving a half a cup every 30 minutes until bleeding stopped. Patients drank half a cup every hour for the rest of the day, then 3 times daily for the next 3 days.

Partridge Berry (*Mitchella repens*) has been widely used to prevent miscarriages in women with prior history, and should be taken in early pregnancy for this problem. *Dosage:* To tone the uterus or prevent habitual miscarriage, use 1 cup of tea or 15-30 drops of tincture 1-3 times daily. For threatened miscarriage, take 50 drops of tincture every 20-30 minutes until contractions stop. *Contraindications:* None.

Red Raspberry leaf (*Rubus idaeus*) helps prevent miscarriage and premature labor when taken daily as tea. *Dosage:* 1-2 cups of tea daily throughout pregnancy. *Contraindications:* None.

Wild Yam root (*Dioscorea villosa*) helps stop threatened miscarriage and premature labor associated with low progesterone levels. It is relaxing and eases spasms and morning sickness. *Dosage:* For threatened miscarriage, use 1/2-1 teaspoon of tincture every half hour or 4 ounces of tea every half hour until contractions subside. *Contraindications:* None.

Herbs for Common Problems During Pregnancy

Eating nutritious foods, living a healthy lifestyle, and engaging in kind and loving relationships naturally promotes a safe and enjoyable pregnancy, and safeguards against many problems that may be encountered during this time. For issues that do arise, many herbs can safely and effectively be taken either throughout pregnancy or during specific stages of pregnancy. More information on the use, dosage, and contraindications of each herb listed below can be found above in the "Materia Medica of Herbs for Pregnancy."

Morning Sickness and Indigestion

Morning sickness (nausea occurring during the first trimester of pregnancy) is a common problem many women experience. Morning sickness may be caused by hormonal imbalances (especially low progesterone levels), low blood pressure, thyroid weakness, low blood sugar or food sensitivities, so these possibilities need to be explored. Eat several small but nutritious meals throughout the day to maintain balanced blood sugar levels. Have some protein with each meal, including plant proteins such as raw nuts and seeds, soy, amaranth, and quinoa. Avoid spicy and greasy foods, chemical additives, and excessive meat, sugar, and grains containing gluten. The B vitamin complex is necessary for digestion, adequate energy levels, and growing a strong baby. Get daily fresh air and exercise, and sip on some of the herbal teas listed below to prevent and relieve morning sickness.

The following herbs have been used for centuries to safely reduce morning sickness and indigestion:

Black Haw
Chasteberry
Cramp Bark
Dandelion
Fennel
Flaxseed
German Chamomile
Ginger
Lemon Balm
Marshmallow
Peppermint
Red Raspberry leaf
Slippery Elm
Spearmint
Wild Yam

Heartburn

Pregnant women may experience heartburn, usually occurring in the later months of pregnancy, due to hormonal changes and the growing uterus pushing against the stomach and other abdominal organs. It is helpful to eat small, frequent meals and avoid spicy and acidic foods, cane and corn syrup sugars, heavy fats, refined and processed foods, and grains containing gluten. Papaya fruit, juice, or tablets can be very soothing. Milk (dairy or non-dairy), yogurt, and kefir neutralize stomach acids to reduce heartburn. Avoid Peppermint because it may worsen esophageal reflux.

Fennel, Marshmallow, and **Slippery Elm** teas are excellent to ease heartburn.

Anemia (Iron Deficiency)

Eat plenty of foods containing iron, including dark-green vegetables and leafy greens, beets, molasses, prunes, raisins, cherries, blackberries, apricots, figs, eggs, meat, and raw nuts and seeds. Take a natural, high-quality vitamin and mineral supplement purchased from a health food store or health professional. The best form of iron for easy digestion is ferrous bis-glycinate. It does not cause the side effects of ferrous sulfate, an inorganic form of iron notorious for causing stomach distress and constipation in some people. Vitamin C enhances iron absorption.

Herbs containing substantial amounts of easily digested iron include:

Alfalfa
Burdock
Chlorella
Dandelion
Elder Berries
Hawthorn berries
Red Raspberry leaf
Stinging Nettle

Constipation

Avoid constipation by drinking plenty of water and herbal teas. Eat a diet of whole grains (gluten-free), fresh fruits, and vegetables for fiber. Grape, cherry, and prune juice are safe laxatives, as are prunes, raisins, and figs. Avoid meat and refined flour products when constipated. Be sure your prenatal vitamin and mineral formula does not contain the ferrous sulfate form of iron because it can cause constipation, as does calcium carbonate. Calcium citrate and hydroxyapatite (the best for bone health) are better calcium sources.

Moderate daily exercise promotes good bowel activity. Gentle abdominal massage in a clockwise direction will promote peristaltic activity in the intestines. Do not use strong laxative herbs like Senna or Cascara Sagrada during pregnancy due to uterine irritation they may promote.

Non-irritating, gentle laxatives that are safe to take during pregnancy and lactation include:

Burdock
Dandelion root
Fennel
Flaxseed
Marshmallow
Slippery Elm

Diarrhea

Eating orange foods (cooked carrots, sweet potatoes, and squash) and **carob** powder baked in cookies, brownies, and cakes are a pleasant way to reduce diarrhea.

Blackberry leaves and **Strawberry leaves** are gentle astringents that can be taken as tea to reduce diarrhea.

Edema (Water Retention)

The following herbs support the kidneys to reduce water retention throughout the body:

Burdock
Dandelion
Elderberry flower
Partridge Berry
Stinging Nettle

Colds, Flu, Coughs, and Infections

Avoid dairy, sugar, and gluten foods when sick because they promote mucous production, which contributes to sinus and lung congestion and provides a nourishing environment for viruses, bacteria, and fungi. Sugar depresses the immune system. Red meat should also be avoided during illness.

Herbs are most effective when taken at the initial phase of any sickness. Use the recommended dosages in regular intervals throughout the day. Sipping on appropriate teas is helpful and comforting. The following herbs are safe to use for illness during pregnancy and lactation with the exception of Garlic, which should not be eaten during lactation because its strong flavor can negatively affect breast milk:

Burdock root
Cayenne
Echinacea
Elderberry flower
Garlic
German Chamomile
Ginger
Milk Thistle
Mullein
Peppermint

Goldenseal (*Hydrastis canadensis*) should not be ingested during pregnancy, but making tea with the root and using it as a nasal spray is safe and one of the most effective remedies for sinus infections and allergies. The filtered tea is also excellent to apply as eye drops for eye infections, including conjunctivitis or pink eye. (For more information about the preparation of Goldenseal nasal spray and eye drops, refer to pages 384 and 387.)

Varicose Veins and Hemorrhoids

Both of these conditions are caused by muscle weakness in the blood vessels causing them to enlarge. Vitamin E, the vitamin B complex, vitamin C, and bioflavonoids strengthen blood vessels. Rutin is the most effective bioflavonoid taken for this purpose, but should only be taken after the first trimester.

Astringent herbs constrict tissues to improve muscle tone and reduce varicosities and hemorrhoids. They may be taken internally and some are best applied externally.

Blackberry leaves
Oatstraw
Plantain leaves (*Plantago major, P. lanceolata*) are astringent and anti-inflammatory and can be applied topically to varicosities and hemorrhoids.
Spearmint
Stinging Nettle
Witch Hazel (*Hamamelis virginiana*) is a strong astringent that tightens tissues to reduce swelling and pain. It may be purchased at a drug store. Soak gauze in Witch Hazel and apply it directly to varicose veins and hemorrhoids. Witch Hazel can be combined with a strong tea of **White Oak bark (*Quercus alba*)** and applied topically or used as a sitz bath to treat hemorrhoids.

Other herbs that should not be ingested during pregnancy but are safe for topical application include **Calendula (*Calendula officinalis*), Comfrey (*Symphytum officinale*), St. John's Wort (*Hypericum perforatum*), Shepherd's Purse (*Capsella bursa-pastoris*),** and **Yarrow (*Achillea millefolium*)**. Use seperately or combine several of these herbs and apply them as a salve or make a strong tea to use as a compress, wash, or sitz bath. Tinctures of these herbs may be added to the teas to use for external applications.

Nervous Tension, Anxiety, Headaches, and Insomnia

The following herbs are calming, support the nervous system, and are beneficial for many types of nervous conditions and overstimulation:

Black Haw
German Chamomile
Lemon Balm
Oat Straw and fresh milky Oats
Passion Flower
Peppermint
Red Raspberry leaf
Scullcap
Spearmint

Hypertension

Some women have high blood pressure before becoming pregnant, and some may experience gestational hypertension characterized by a steady rise in blood pressure after the 28th week of pregnancy, which requires medical supervision and close monitoring of blood pressure.

Lifestyle and dietary modifications are helpful in addition to herbal support. Reduce emotional and physical stress as much as possible. Practice deep relaxation and meditation techniques to increase inner calm. Moderate daily exercise along with adequate rest is important. Avoid all stimulants in foods and drinks, including caffeine and nicotine, and increase consumption of plant protein and fresh fruits and vegetables.

The following herbs can be helpful in safely reducing hypertension:

Black Haw
Cayenne
Dandelion
Garlic
German Chamomile
Hawthorn
Lemon Balm
Passion Flower
Red Raspberry leaf
Scullcap

Muscle Cramps

Muscle cramps often occur due to nutritional deficiencies. Take calcium citrate or hydroxyapatite (1500 mg) and magnesium (500-800 mg) daily. One of the most effective forms of magnesium for quick absorption and cramp relief is magnesium bis-glycinate.

Herbs that contain calcium, magnesium, and potassium to relax the nervous system to ease cramps include:

Alfalfa
Black Haw
Burdock
Cramp Bark
Dandelion
German Chamomile
Ginger
Red Raspberry leaf
Scullcap
Stinging Nettle

Herbs to Prepare for Childbirth

The following herbs have traditionally been taken in small amounts 1-2 weeks before the due date to prepare the uterus for effective and forceful contractions and ease the discomforts of labor. Blue Cohosh and Black Cohosh are contraindicated earlier in pregnancy due to their stimulating effect on the uterus, but are beneficial shortly before birth.

Black Cohosh root (*Cimicifuga racemosa*) and **Blue Cohosh root (*Caulophyllum thalictroides*)** are taken in combination to tone and prepare the uterus for safe and effective labor. *Dosage:* 10 drops Blue Cohosh with 30 drops Black Cohosh in a tincture preparation 1-2 times daily in water for 1-2 weeks prior to the due date. Blue Cohosh is taken in small amounts (10 drops) and is always combined with Black Cohosh rather than taken alone. *Contraindications:* Do not use Blue Cohosh in cases of hypotension or hypertension. (For more information about Black Cohosh refer to pages 220-231, and for Blue Cohosh refer to pages 246-252.)

Evening Primrose oil (*Oenothera biennis*) is warmed and applied directly around the vaginal opening to tone and promote elasticity of the tissues. This helps prevent tearing during the pushing and crowning phase of labor. *Dosage:* Oil is applied once or twice daily a few weeks before delivery date. *Contraindications:* None. The oil contains healthy essential fatty oils and is safe for mother and infant.

Mugwort (*Artemisia vulgaris*) ~ in Traditional Chinese Medicine acupuncturists use Mugwort leaves with moxabustion to correct breech presentations. (For more information, refer to pages 460-461.)

Helpful Herbs During Childbirth

Several types of herbs contribute to easier and faster childbirth. **Parturient** herbs safely stimulate productive uterine contractions for easier, faster, and less painful birth. They are wonderful allies during the birthing process, but are avoided during pregnancy due to their stimulating effects on the uterus. Parturient herbs are beneficial for delayed onset of labor, stalled labor, and ineffective contractions. Other herbs are used to relax and nourish the mother, reduce discomfort and hemorrhage, and promote a safe birth. Many years ago when attending home births (twenty-two in total, including the births of my two sons), I had the opportunity to witness how effectively these herbs worked each time they were used with successful outcomes of healthy newborns and happy mothers.

Birthroot or Trillium root (*Trillium* spp.) stimulates production and release of the hormone oxytocin, which promotes strong, effective contractions. Trillium helps initiate stalled labor, deliver a retained placenta, and prevent postpartum hemorrhage. It strengthens and normalizes weak pelvic tissues that have lost their muscle tone, causing uterine prolapse and abnormal bleeding. Roots contain the steroidal saponins diosgenin and trillarin, which have these hormonal effects. *Dosage:* 1/4-1/2 teaspoon of tincture with water every 30-60 minutes during labor as needed. *Contraindications:* Do not use during pregnancy until labor begins.

Black Cohosh root (*Cimicifuga racemosa*) tincture is specific for difficult, prolonged, and painful labor with irregular contractions. It promotes cervical softening and dilation, strengthens and normalizes contractions, eases pain, and helps prevent hemorrhage during and after birth. It relaxes the smooth muscle of blood vessels to increase blood flow to the uterus. The combination of Black and Blue Cohosh was used by many Native American women to facilitate labor, and modern-day herbal midwives continue using this combination 1-2 weeks prior to and during birth. *Dosage:* Usual dose during labor is 10-30 drops of tincture in water every 30-60 minutes as needed. Start with small doses and gradually increase as necessary. *Contraindications:* Large amounts, especially during the first trimester, can induce labor and thus it is contraindicated until the last 1-2 weeks before the due date. (For more information, refer to page 229.)

Blue Cohosh root (*Caulophyllum thalictroides*) tincture stimulates oxytocin release and is used to initiate labor, increase blood flow to the pelvis, and stimulate and strengthen the force of contractions. It tones and strengthens weak uterine muscles and relaxes spastic uterine muscles. Blue Cohosh is specific for difficult, painful labor with failure to progress and for retained placenta. It eases labor pain and the "after pains" of childbirth. It is always used in combination with Black Cohosh and never taken by itself. The tincture is more dependable than tea or pills because the active ingredients of both Cohoshes are alcohol soluble, not water soluble, and tinctures have an indefinite shelf life. *Dosage:* To support childbirth and induce labor or treat stalled labor, take 10 drops of tincture every hour (with 10-30 drops Black Cohosh) until labor resumes. *Contraindications:* Blue Cohosh is never taken alone, but in combination with Black Cohosh. It is a strong uterine stimulant that is never taken until 1-2 weeks before the due date. Ingesting Blue Cohosh earlier in pregnancy has been implicated in infant cardiovascular problems. As Blue Cohosh starts to work, there may be a noticeable increase in fetal heartbeats, in which case it should be discontinued. (For more information, refer to page 251.)

Evening Primrose oil (*Oenothera biennis*) is applied directly to a rigid os to soften and promote elasticity of the tissues, allowing dilation and easier passage of the infant's head. The oil contains healthy essential fatty oils, including GLA (gamma-linoleic-acid), which benefits the female reproductive system and hormonal balance. *Dosage*: The oil is squeezed out of several capsules (3 capsules daily help ripen the cervix) and rubbed around the os. *Contraindications*: None. The oil is safe to apply or ingest.

Flaxseed oil (*Linum usitatissimum*) may be applied to the cervix to help soften and dilate it. *Dosage:* 1 teaspoon of the oil is applied to the cervical os as needed. *Contraindications:* None.

Ginger (*Zingiber officinale*) tea energizes laboring mothers during long, exhausting labor by increasing energy and aiding mental focus. It supports the laboring uterus with its warming quality and ability to increase the circulation of blood and Qi (energy) to the pelvis. *Dosage*: Sip 1-2 cups of tea during labor or take 5-10 drops of tincture every 30 minutes as needed. *Contraindications:* Ginger increases circulation to the uterus and may increase chances of postpartum hemorrhage if used within an hour of delivery.

Ginseng (*Panax* spp.) is energizing and helps sustain the mother during a long, exhausting labor. *Dosage:* 1 capsule every hour with a maximum 6 capsules or 1 liquid vial every 60-90 minutes. *Contraindications:* Avoid in cases of hypertension and anxiety.

Lavender *(Lavandula* spp.) leaves bring healing energy into the birthing room. Midwives traditionally hang a fresh sprig of Lavender leaves and flowers on the birthing bed to promote calm, harmonizing energies conducive to childbirth. Taken internally, Lavender promotes productive contractions, relaxes the mother, and eases birthing pain.

Lobelia (*Lobelia inflata*) is specific for difficult and painful labor, failure to progress, and rigidity of the cervical os and perineum. Lobelia is very dependable in relaxing smooth muscle, dilating the cervix, and facilitating effective uterine contractions. It works well when taken with Blue and Black Cohosh. *Dosage:* 3-10 drops of tincture every 15-30 minutes as needed. Start with small doses and increase as needed. *Contraindications:* Larger doses can cause nausea and vomiting, so it is best to use in small repeated doses. Do not use during pregnancy. (For more information, refer to page 442.)

Motherwort (*Leonurus cardiaca*) stimulates oxytocin release that promotes strong, productive contractions to facilitate the birthing process. Motherwort relaxes the mother and eases labor pains, especially when combined with St. John's Wort (*Hypericum perforatum*). *Dosage:* 10-20 drops of each tincture every 20-30 minutes as needed during labor and postpartum. *Contraindications:* Motherwort and St. John's Wort are not used during pregnancy, but are safe to ingest during labor and postpartum. (For more information, refer to page 455.)

Red Raspberry (*Rubus idaeus*) tea facilitates labor, provides nutrients, reduces pain and uterine swelling, and decreases bleeding after childbirth. *Dosage:* The tea may be drunk freely throughout the birthing process. *Contraindications:* None.

St. John's Wort (*Hypericum perforatum*) tincture reduces pain during labor and also afterbirth pain. The oil is soothing and analgesic when applied to the perineum during labor and after delivery to heal perineal bruising, inflammation, tearing, and episiotomy repair. *Dosage:* 20-30 drops of tincture every 30 minutes as needed. *Contraindications:* None. It is safe to use internally and externally during labor. (For more information, refer to pages 503-504.)

Scullcap (*Scutellaria lateriflora*) is excellent for helping to relax tense muscles, dilate the cervical os, and relieve pain during childbirth. It combines well with Motherwort and St. John's Wort for pain. *Dosage:* 10-20 drops of Scullcap tincture every 20-30 minutes as needed. *Contraindications:* None. Scullcap is very safe, just remember it is sedating. (For more information, refer to page 510.)

Tasty Herbal Teas Providing Nutrients and Energy for the Laboring Mother

Alfalfa, Catnip (also helps to expel the placenta), Ginger, Holy Basil (*Ocimum sanctum*), Lemon Balm, Peppermint, Red Raspberry, Spearmint, and Stinging Nettle teas may be sipped throughout labor.

Herbs Helping to Prevent Hemorrhage

Drinking Alfalfa, Stinging Nettle, and Red Raspberry leaf tea on a regular basis throughout pregnancy helps increase vitamin K and hemoglobin (transports iron) levels in the blood. Several cups of tea during labor also decrease the chance of hemorrhage.

Herbs to Stop Hemorrhage After Delivery

Lemon Balm (*Melissa officinalis*), Mugwort (*Artemisia vulgaris*), and Thyme (*Thymus vulgaris*) help the uterus expel a retained placenta. The following astringent herbs may be ingested separately or combined for stronger blood clotting activity:

Shepherd's Purse (*Capsella bursa-pastoris*) is well known for its blood coagulant and vasoconstrictor actions that promote uterine contractions and decrease bleeding. It is the traditional favorite herbal midwives use to stop postpartum hemorrhage. *Dosage:* Tinctures made from the fresh leaves and flowers are most potent, and 20-40 drops are ingested every 5 minutes as needed until bleeding normalizes. Most commercial tinctures are made from dried herbs requiring larger doses of 1 teaspoon (about 150 drops). *Contraindications:* None. This is a safe herb used after delivery.

Cinquefoil (*Potentilla* spp.) is a strong astringent excellent for all types of hemorrhage. *Dosage:* 10-30 drops of tincture every 10-20 minutes until bleeding is normalized. *Contraindications:* None. (For more information, refer to pages 318-319.)

Cranesbill (*Geranium maculatum*) is a reliable astringent excellent for all types of excessive bleeding, including postpartum hemorrhage. *Dosage:* 10-30 drops of tincture every 10-20 minutes until bleeding normalizes. *Contraindications:* None. (For more information, refer to page 331.)

Motherwort (*Leonurus cardiaca*) contracts uterine muscles following delivery, which decreases bleeding and helps expel the placenta. *Dosage:* 10-15 drops of tincture every 10-30 minutes immediately after birth. *Contraindications:* None. Motherwort is safe to use during and after childbirth, but not during pregnancy. (For more information, refer to page 455.)

Yarrow (*Achillea millefolium*) is a remarkable women's ally, including its ability to reduce postpartum hemorrhage. *Dosage:* 10-30 drops of tincture every 10-20 minutes as needed. *Contraindications:* Although not recommended to ingest during pregnancy, it is very safe to use following delivery. (For more information, refer to page 545.)

Herbs for Postpartum Support

Wound-Healing Herbs for Perineal Tears, Episiotomy, and C-section

Apply ice immediately after perineal repair is complete to decrease swelling and inflammation. Expose the wound to air and sunlight to promote healing. Take sitz baths or apply a compress using strong, filtered teas of Calendula (*Calendula officinalis*), Comfrey (*Symphytum officinale*), Goldenseal (*Hydrastis canadensis*), Echinacea spp., Saint John's Wort (*Hypericum perforatum*), and Yarrow (*Achillea millefolium*). (Refer to page 130 for sitz bath instructions.)

Postpartum Discomfort, Depression, and Restoration

Postpartum depression may be caused by nutritional deficiencies, an imbalance of reproductive hormones, and/or imbalances in neurotransmitters (chemicals regulating brain chemistry and moods). Be sure to eat nutritious food to nourish the body and produce rich breast milk. The following herbs help to safely ease afterbirth discomfort, pain and depression, and to restore hormonal balance. Continue to evaporate alcohol from tinctures during postpartum and lactation.

Astragalus (*Astragalus membranaceus*) is excellent for postpartum weakness and depression. It supports the endocrine system, tones and strengthens pelvic muscles to prevent uterine and bladder prolapse and hemorrhoids, and fortifies blood to prevent anemia. *Dosage:* 1-2 cups of tea or 60 drops of tincture daily. *Contraindications:* None.

Black Cohosh (*Cimicifuga racemosa*) helps balance and restore female reproductive hormones and organs. The roots tone pelvic muscles to prevent prolapse of the uterus and bladder. *Dosage*: 5-10 drops of tincture in water 2-3 times throughout the day. *Contraindications*: None.

Blue Vervain (*Verbena hastata*) balances the reproductive hormones, eases depression, anxiety and nervous conditions, and is a muscle relaxant for cramps and spasms. *Dosage*: 20-30 drops of tincture 2-3 times daily is preferred over the bitter-tasting tea. *Contraindications*: None.

Hops (*Humulus lupulus*) reduces uterine spasms and after-pains following childbirth. *Dosage:* 20-30 drops of tincture 2-3 times a day. *Contraindications*: None.

Lemon Balm (*Melissa officinalis*) is a gentle calming herb for depression, anxiety, insomnia, stress headaches, and spasms. It is also soothing to the digestive system. *Dosage*: 1-2 cups of tea daily. *Contraindications*: None. Women with hypothyroidism (low thyroid function) should use this herb sparingly since it could possibly worsen the condition.

Motherwort (*Leonurus cardiaca*) reduces pain following labor and helps restore hormonal balance. Its calming actions ease depression, anxiety, irritability, and mood swings. *Dosage*: 10-20 drops of tincture 2-3 times daily. The tea is very bitter. *Contraindications*: None.

Passion Flower (*Passiflora incarnata*) is a calming nervine that helps relieve after-birth pain, anxiety, and depression. *Dosage*: 1-2 cups of tea or 30 drops of tincture 1-2 times a day. *Contraindications*: None.

St. John's Wort (*Hypericum perforatum*) increases serotonin levels and is well known for its anti-depressant effects. It is excellent for treating nerve pain, the herpes virus, and other viral infections. *Dosage*: The tincture form is more potent than tea or pills. Take 10-25 drops of tincture 2-3 times daily. This works well when taken with Lemon Balm tea. *Contraindications*: St. John's Wort makes some people feel sleepy, but this is usually not a problem.

Herbs that Support Lactation

The following herbs, known as **galactogogues**, safely increase production and flow of breast milk and have a long history of use. Most have a pleasant flavor and work best when prepared as tea that is sipped throughout the day. Drink these teas, separately or combined, and plenty of water rather than soda pop and caffeinated drinks lacking nutrients. Fresh vegetable juices (carrot, celery, cucumber, kale, and chard) are delicious and make nutrient-rich breast milk. Organic fruits and vegetables (especially leafy greens) and whole grains (gluten-free grains are not inflammatory and reduce chances of allergic responses) also promote milk production. (For more information and suggestions for herbs that are helpful during lactation, refer to "Breast-Feeding" on pages 558-559 in the "Index of Health Issues and Herbal Recommendation.")

Alfalfa leaf (*Medicago sativa*) stimulates lactation and improves nutritional quality of breast milk.
Anise seeds (*Pimpinella anisum*) are crushed to make a tasty licorice-flavored tea.
Blessed Thistle (*Cnicus benedictus*) stimulates blood flow to the mammary glands and is one of the best herbs to increase and enrich milk production.
Blue Vervain (*Verbena hastata*) is a bitter herb that stimulates lactation and increases milk supply.
Calendula (*Calendula officinalis*) ~ applying the salve or ointment to the breast heals irritated and cracked nipples and reduces pain and soreness from nursing.
Catnip leaf (*Nepeta cataria*) increases flow of breast milk and stimulates the "let-down" response.
Chasteberry (*Vitex agnus-castus*) promotes prolactin levels necessary for milk production in nursing mothers, and helps correct underlying problems in women having insufficient milk production. *Dosage:* 1-2 cups of tea daily or 40 drops of tincture 1-2 times daily. *Contraindications*: None. (For more information on Chasteberry and breast milk production, refer to pages 304 and 308.)
Dandelion root and leaf (*Taraxacum officinale*) stimulates milk production. The nutrient-rich herb enriches breast milk and reduces jaundice in infants.
Fennel seed (*Foeniculum vulgare*) is crushed and steeped as tea to increase milk production.
Fenugreek seed (*Trigonella foenum-graecum*) is steeped for 4-5 minutes as a tea (longer steeping creates a bitter taste). The seed contains phytoestrogens and diosgenin, which increase milk flow.
Goat's Rue leaf and flower (*Galega officinalis*) have strong galactagogue actions shown to increase production and flow of breast milk by as much as 50% in some women. It may also stimulate development of mammary glands. *Dosage:* For tea, steep 2 teaspoons of the dried herb in 2 cups water for 10-15 minutes and drink throughout the day. For tincture, take 15-30 drops 3 times daily. For capsules, take 70-500 mg daily. *Contraindications:* None. Goat's Rue may reduce elevated blood sugar levels and increase the action of hypoglycemic drugs.
Hops strobules (*Humulus lupulus*) increase and enrich milk production.
Marshmallow root (*Althaea officinalis*) increases flow of milk.
Oat straw and fresh milky oats (*Avena sativa*) increase milk flow and provide nutrients that enrich milk.
Red Raspberry leaf (*Rubus idaeus*) has an extremely high vitamin and mineral content for rich milk. However, the astringent qualities may diminish the amount of milk in some women.
Stinging Nettle leaf (*Urtica dioica*) contains an array of nutrients that enrich milk.

Herbs for Weaning

Lactifuge herbs decrease milk production and typically have strong astringent properties that dry up milk secretions. Lactifuge herbs are dependable during the weaning process to naturally decrease milk production, and may be used alone or combined for increased effectiveness. Small amounts of tea (1/2 cup) or tincture (20 drops) should be taken every 2-3 hours for a continual effect.

Sage (*Salvia officinalis*), Parsley (*Petroselinum* spp.), and **Yarrow (*Achillea millefolium*)** are the most popular and commonly used lactifuge herbs.

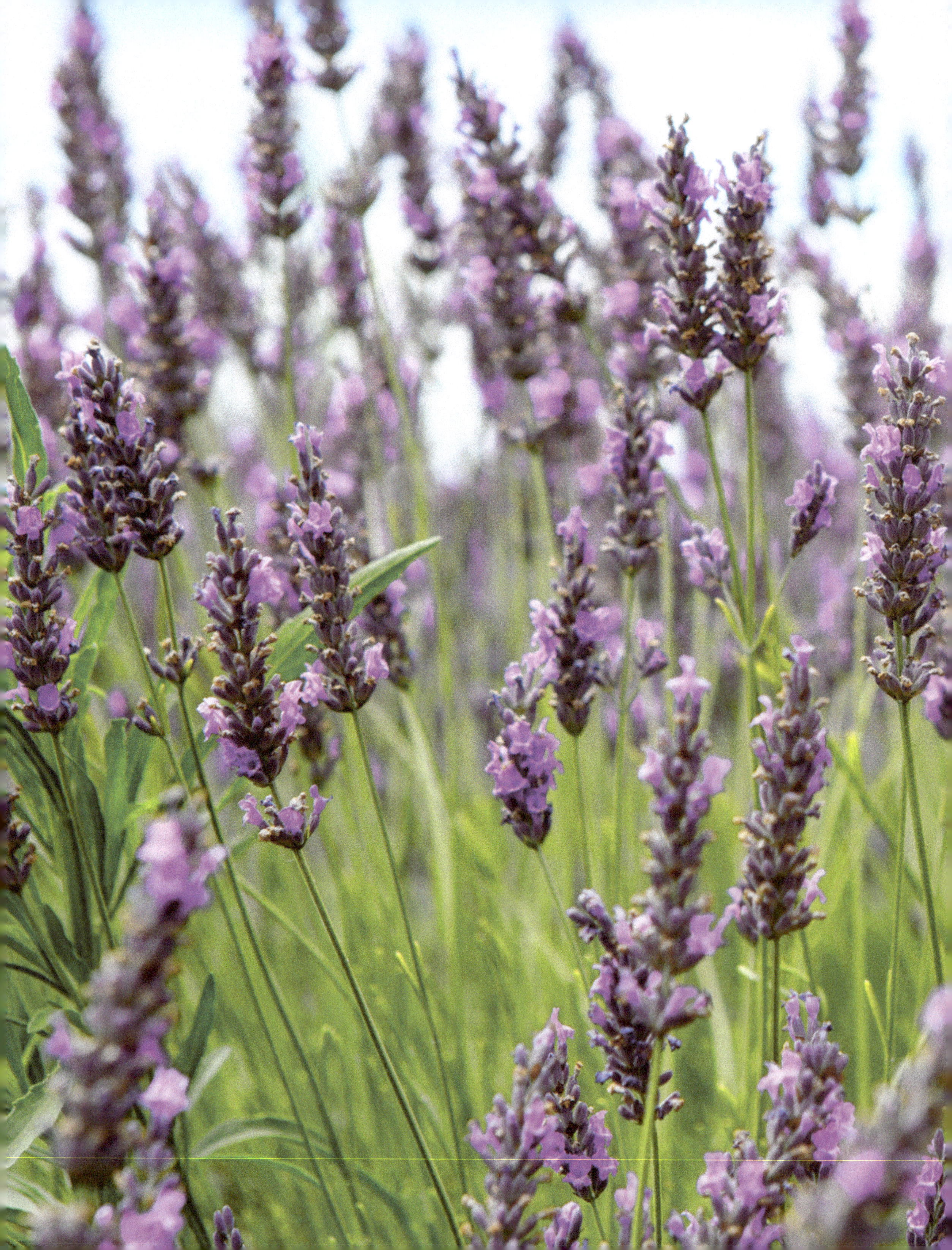

APPENDICES

Glossary

Cross-Reference of Common and Botanical Plant Names

Media Sources for Herbal Research

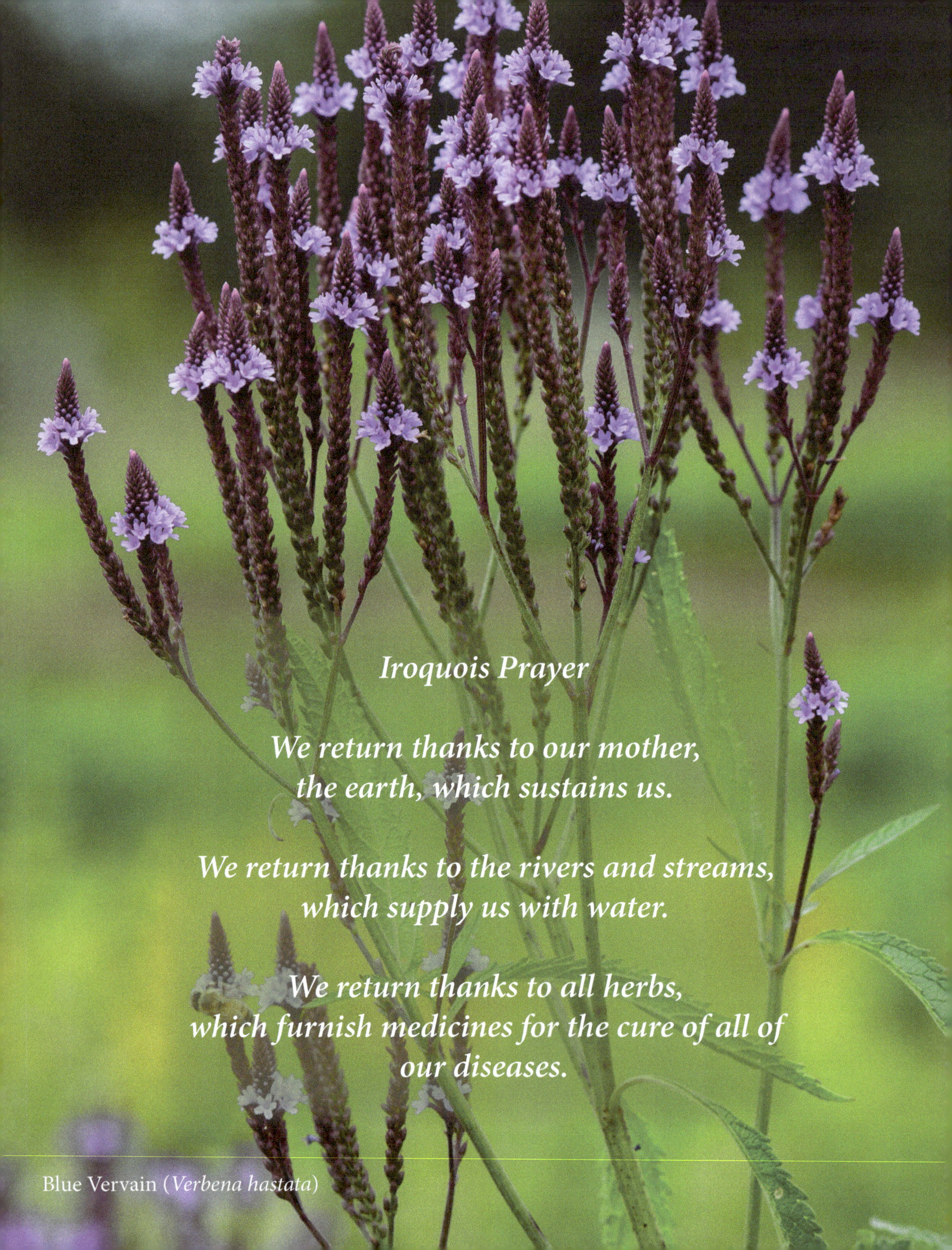

Iroquois Prayer

We return thanks to our mother,
the earth, which sustains us.

We return thanks to the rivers and streams,
which supply us with water.

We return thanks to all herbs,
which furnish medicines for the cure of all of
our diseases.

Blue Vervain (*Verbena hastata*)

APPENDIX ONE

Glossary

abortifacient: a plant or drug that induces abortion.
abscess: a collection of pus and dead tissue localized in a cavity that separates it from the rest of the body.
acetylcholine: a neurotransmitter that activates muscle movement at neuromuscular junctions throughout the body, relaxes cardiac muscle, and enhances brain function by improving sensory perception, attention, learning, and memory. It is used to treat the severe muscle weakness of myasthenia gravis.
acetlycholinesterase: an enzyme present in nervous tissue, muscle, and red blood cells that breaks down acetylcholine to choline and acetic acid. Acetylcholine is released when a nerve impulse reaches a myoneural junction, causing the muscle fibers to contract. Acetylcholinesterase stops stimulation and activation of muscle fibers.
acid: a compound that produces hydrogen ions in water. On the pH scale of 1-14, acidic substances have a pH between 1-6, with a pH of 1.0 being the most acidic. Hydrochloric acid produced in the stomach and vinegar are examples of strong acids.
acid reflux: refers to stomach acids escaping into the esophagus, causing burning sensations and inflammation.
acidosis: an excessive amount of acids and hydrogen ions in the blood and tissues caused by acid accumulation or depletion of alkaline reserves. Metabolic acidosis, respiratory acidosis, and diabetic acidosis are the most common forms of acidosis.
acute illness: any illness with rapid onset and short duration, such as the common cold and the flu. In contrast, chronic illnesses persist over a period of time.
adaptogen: an herb that stabilizes physiological processes by helping the body (especially the adrenals, pituitary, and hypothalamus) adapt to stress and "burn-out." Adaptogens support immunity.
adenocarcinoma: a malignant tumor of glandular origin found in epithelial tissues lining internal and external surfaces of the body.
adenoma: a benign tumor of epithelial tissue with glandular origin and/or glandular characteristics. Adenomas can grow from the adrenal glands, pituitary gland, thyroid, prostate, and other glands.
adjuvant: an herb added to formulas that enhances their beneficial activity by increasing circulation and assisting in transporting other herbs to their target tissues and organs. Cayenne and Ginger are examples of adjuvants often used in formulas.
adrenaline: a hormone and neurotransmitter secreted by the adrenal medulla that produces quick energy and the "fight-or-flight" response; also called epinephrine.
agonist: a chemical that binds to a cell receptor and activates the receptor to produce a biological response. An agonist promotes an action compared to an antagonist, which blocks actions.
ague: an old term for intermittent fevers and chills occurring with malaria and occasionally the flu.
alanine aminotransferace (ALT), also known as serum glutamic-pyruvic transaminase (SGPT): a liver enzyme that leaks into the bloodstream when liver cells are damaged. Elevated levels indicate liver damage.
aldosterone: the main mineralocorticoid steroid hormone secreted by the adrenal cortex. It regulates electrolyte and water balance by promoting the retention of sodium and excretion of potassium.
alkaline: any base compound with a pH between 7-14. It forms salts with acids and can neutralize acids.
alkaloid: a large group of nitrogen-containing substances in plants that are alkaline, bitter-tasting, and often exert powerful physiologic activity. Examples are cocaine, nicotine, morphine, and caffeine.
allergen: a substance that causes allergic and hypersensitive reactions in the blood and tissues.
allopathic or allopathy: the current system of Western medical practice that primarily treats disease and illness with pharmaceutically produced chemical substances, modern technology, and surgery.
alterative: herbal tonics that gradually normalize body functions and restore health and vitality.
alternate: refers to the arrangement of buds, flowers, or leaves that grow in an alternating pattern on stems, as compared to an opposite pattern.
amenorrhea: the abnormal absence or cessation of menstruation.
anaerobic: organisms that live and grow in the absence of free oxygen.
analeptic: herbs that restore normal cellular and tissue function and are nutritionally fortifying.
analgesic: an herb or drug that relieves the sensation of pain; also called anodyne.
androgen or androgenic: refers to steroid hormones that are produced in the testes, ovaries, and adrenal glands. The principal androgens, testosterone and androstenedione, are present in much higher levels in men than women, and play an important role in the development of male characteristics and reproduction. Other androgens include dihydrotestosterone (DHT) and dehydroepiandrosterone (DHEA). In women, one of the main purposes of androgens is to be converted into estrogens.
angiogenesis: the formation and development of new blood vessels from pre-existing blood vessels.
anhydrotic: an herb or other agent that stops excessive sweating; also called antihydrotic.
annual: plants that produce seeds and complete their life cycle in one year and then die.

anodyne: an herb or drug that relieves pain; also called analgesic.
antacid: a substance that neutralizes excess acid in the stomach and small intestines.
anthelmintic: an agent that destroys and expels parasites; also called vermicide, vermifuge, antiparasitic, and parasiticide.
anthrax: a serious and sometimes life-threatening bacterial infection caused by *Bacillus anthracis*.
anti-aggregate: an herb or drug that decreases aggregation or clumping together of blood platelets and inhibits blood clotting.
anti-arrhythmic: an agent that normalizes abnormal, irregular heartbeats.
anti-atherosclerotic: an agent that reduces narrowing of arteries caused by deposits of plaque, cholesterol, fats, and other substances on the blood vessel walls.
antibacterial: an agent that destroys and inhibits bacterial growth.
anticarcinogenic: an herb or drug that inhibits the development and/or growth of cancerous cells.
anti-catarrhal: an agent that reduces the formation and secretion of mucous. Catarrh is an old term for phlegm and mucous secreted from irritated membranes, particularly in the respiratory tract.
anticholinesterase: an enzyme that inhibits destruction of the neurotransmitter acetylcholine.
anticoagulant: an herb or drug that prevents the coagulation or clotting of blood.
anti-edemic: an agent that reduces fluid retention (edema) in the tissues by stimulating kidney activity.
anti-emetic: an herb or drug that decreases nausea and vomiting.
antigen: any foreign substance that stimulates the immune system to activate lymphocytes (white blood cells) and produce antibodies for defense against allergens and pathogens.
antihemolytic: an agent that prevents hemolysis, which is the destruction of red blood cells.
antihistamine: an agent that reduces the tissue release of histamine (a protein causing allergic reactions).
antihydrotic: a plant or drug that reduces excessive perspiration; also called anhydrotic.
antihypertensive: an herb or drug that reduces high blood pressure.
anti-inflammatory: a substance that soothes and reduces inflammation, heat, and irritation in tissues.
antilithic: an herb that prevents, dissolves, and eliminates kidney, bladder and gallbladder stones, and dissolves mineral deposits in joints. It is similar in meaning and action as lithotryptic.
antilymphomic: an herb or drug used for the prevention and treatment of lymphatic infections and cancers.
antimicrobial: an agent with broad spectrum activity against bacteria, viruses, fungi, yeast, and parasites.
antimitotic: an herb or drug that reduces or interferes with cell division (mitosis).
antimutagenic: a substance that reduces cellular dysfunction and mutation leading to cancerous growths.
antineoplastic: an agent that stops abnormal and uncontrolled growth of benign and malignant cells.
antineuralgia: an herb or drug that reduces nerve pain (neuralgia).
antioxidant: a substance that reduces cellular damage caused by the oxidative process and free radical damage. Antioxidants (glutathione, superoxide dismutase/SOD, and catalase) are produced in the body and occur in vegetables, fruits, berries, nuts, seeds, vitamins A, C and E, and many herbs.
antiparasitic: an agent that kills parasites; also called vermicide, vermifuge, anthelmintic, and parasiticide.
antiperiodic: an herb or drug that relieves alternating fevers and chills typically seen in malaria.
antipyretic: a cooling herb or drug that dispels excess heat and fever; also called febrifuge or refrigerant.
antirheumatic: an herb or drug that reduces the causes and/or symptoms of arthritic joint pain.
antiscorbutic: herbs and foods containing vitamin C, which prevents the deficiency disease known as scurvy.
antiseptic: a substance that is applied to the skin to kill bacterial growth and infection.
antispasmodic: an herb or drug that relaxes muscles and prevents or relieves muscle spasms.
antitussive: an herb or drug that suppresses coughs.
anti-uric: an agent that promotes the excretion of excess uric acid through the urine; protects against gout.
anti-uricaemic: same meaning as anti-uric.
aperient: a mild bowel stimulant that acts as a gentle laxative.
aperitive: an herb or drug that stimulates the appetite.
aphrodisiac: an herb or drug that stimulates and improves sexual desire and vitality.
apoptosis: the biological "time clock" and physiologically regulated process of cellular suicide necessary for the maintenance of healthy tissues. Genetically programmed into every cell, apoptosis is the process of programmed cell death that protects the body by destroying and eliminating damaged or dysfunctional cells. Apoptosis protects against uncontrolled cell division and proliferation, which is characteristic of all cancer cells. The process of apoptosis reduces cancerous and other dysfunctional cells into fragments that phagocytes engulf and destroy.
aromatic: descriptive of herbs containing volatile oils that emit a strong, pleasant fragrance.
arrhythmia: abnormal heart beat.
aspartate aminotransferase (AST), also called serum glutamic-oxaloacetic transaminase (SGOT): an enzyme found in cells of the liver, heart, kidneys, muscle, and brain. When these cells are damaged, AST leaks out into the bloodstream.
astringent: an herb that constricts and tones tissues and blood vessels; used to treat diarrhea, bleeding, hemorrhoids, and sore throats. Astringents are also called hemostatics and styptics.
athlete's foot: a fungal skin infection of the toes and feet.
atony or atonic: refers to weak muscles and tissues that lack normal tone. Atonic muscles in blood vessels

expand into hemorrhoids and varicose veins. Atonic muscles in the pelvis are unable to hold organs (such as the bladder or uterus) in their normal position, causing them to sag or prolapse.

B-cells or B-lymphocytes: a type of white blood cell that is formed in bone marrow and provides humoral immunity against infections. B-cells attach to antigens (foreign substances) and produce antibodies to destroy them. Antibodies circulate through the bloodstream providing future immunity.

bacteriocide or bacteriostatic: an herb or drug that stops the development and growth of bacteria.

balsam: a resinous semisolid or viscous mass exuded from plants; also refers to a soothing and healing herb.

beta-carotene: a non-toxic, fat-soluble antioxidant occurring in fruits and vegetables that converts into vitamin A in the liver.

biennial: plants that complete their life cycle in two years. Typically the roots and leaves develop during the first year, and flowers and seeds mature during the second year.

binomial: the system of naming plants and animals in which each species is classified by two names. The first identifies the genus and the second is the species. Binomials are typically written in *italics*.

bitter tonic or bitters: bitter-tasting herbs that promote digestion by acting on mucous membranes lining the mouth and stomach to stimulate the normal flow of saliva, acids, bile, and pancreatic enzymes.

boil: the contagious bacterial infection of a hair follicle usually caused by *Staphylococcus aureus* or *Streptococcus pyogenes*. A cluster of boils is called a carbuncle.

botanical: a medicine made from plants.

bronchodilator: a drug or herb that relaxes and opens bronchial passages to allow for greater breathing.

broncho-relaxant: a drug or herb that relaxes smooth muscle in bronchial passages to enhance breathing.

candidicide: an herb or other medicine that kills yeast infections, including Candida yeast.

capillary permeability or vascular permeability: the ability of fluids to move through capillary walls. Increased permeability causes edema (fluid retention) in the tissues.

carbuncle: a cluster of boils that become infected around hair follicles and drain pus onto the skin. Boils and carbuncles are usually caused by *Staphylococcus aureus* or *Streptococcus pyogenes*, which are contagious bacterial infections that can become serious.

carcinogenic: any substance capable of causing cellular dysfunction and damage leading to cancer.

cardiac: a substance that tones and helps restore normal heart rhythm and function.

cardiotonic: a tonic herb that normalizes and improves heart function.

cardiovascular: the circulatory system consisting of the heart and blood vessels.

carminative: an herb containing volatile oils that promote normal digestion, relieve stomach and intestinal gas, spasms and inflammation, and stimulate peristalsis or movement through the digestive system. It is similar in activity to a stomachic herb.

catalase: a primary antioxidant produced by all cells in the body; protects the life and integrity of cells.

catarrh: excessive thick mucous or phlegm secreted by mucous membranes.

cathartic: a strong laxative that stimulates rapid bowel evacuation. Laxatives are gentle compared to stronger-acting cathartics and purgatives.

caustic: a corrosive plant or other substance that is able to burn or dissolve tissue; similar in meaning to escharotic, epispastic, and vesicant. Poison Ivy and Bloodroot (*Sanguinaria canadensis*) are examples.

cell-mediated immunity: the immune response that fights infections, allergens, and other foreign substances by activating macrophages, phagocytes, natural killer cells, T-lymphocytes, and different cytokines. Cell-mediated immunity does not involve antibodies (see humoral immunity).

cellulitis: a serious infection, inflammation, and edema of the skin and underlying tissues caused by *Streptococci, Staphylococci*, and other bacteria.

cephalic: pertaining to the region of the head.

cervical os: the mouth of the uterus that must dilate to allow the passage of infants during childbirth.

chakra: one of seven energy centers located along the spine and in the brain that receive vital life energy. The seven chakras manifest in physical form as the seven endocrine glands, which are master regulators of all body functions.

chlorophyll: the green pigment in plants that allows plants to absorb energy from sunlight and is essential for photosynthesis.

cholagogue: an herb that promotes bile production in the liver and stimulates gallbladder contraction for release of bile into the small intestines. Cholagogues improve digestion of fats and promote normal bowel movements.

cholera: an acute intestinal infection caused by *Vibrio cholerae*, a bacteria carried in urine, feces or vomit, and transmitted to others in contaminated food and water. It causes severe vomiting, diarrhea, and dehydration that may be fatal if untreated. It has virtually been eliminated in North America and Europe, but remains a danger in many parts of the world, especially the tropics and India.

choleretic: same meaning as cholagogue.

clinical trial: a systematic investigation formulated according to the scientific method that is used to determine the efficacy and safety of herbs and drugs within a specific human population.

colic: pain caused by gas and spastic contractions in the digestive and urinary tracts; common in infants.

colitis: inflammation of the large intestines causing pain, spasms, and diarrhea.
constituents: chemicals in herbs that are necessary for the life processes of the plant. Many botanical constituents exert biological activity in animals and people.
contraindication: any condition that renders a particular treatment to be unsafe or undesirable.
controlled trial: a clinical study in which one group of participants receives the experimental herb or drug while another group gets a placebo or an approved drug therapy.
corticosteroids: hormones produced by the cortex of the adrenal gland.
COX-2 (Cyclooxygenase-2): an enzyme that promotes inflammation, which is the body's normal response to heal injury. However, when inflammation gets out of control (such as with arthritis and other chronic inflammatory disorders) chronic pain occurs. COX-2 produces thromboxane and prostaglandins responsible for inflammation and pain. COX-2 inhibitors reduce inflammation.
cystitis: inflammation and infection of the bladder.
cytokines: a group of small proteins that act as chemical messengers between cells. Cytokines include chemokines, lymphokines, interleukins, interferon, and tumor necrosis factor. These are critical to the development and function of the immune system, and become activated in response to inflammation, infections, sepsis, and immunological diseases like cancer. Cytokines can be anti-inflammatory or pro-inflammatory. They are produced by a broad range of cells, including immune cells like macrophages, T- and B-lymphocytes, and mast cells. Cytokines moderate the balance between humoral and cell-mediated immune responses, and are important in health and disease.
cytotoxicity: refers to the quality of being toxic to cells. Chemotherapy uses cytotoxic chemicals to kill cancer cells.

decoction: a tea made with plant roots or bark that is gently simmered or boiled in water.
decongestant: an herb or drug that decreases mucous production and congestion in nasal sinuses and lungs.
delirium tremens: severe muscular twitching, trembling, restlessness, hallucinations, psychological delusions, and incoherence caused by neurological and chemical imbalances from chronic alcohol or drug addiction. Delirium tremens often occur during alcohol and drug withdrawal.
demulcent: an herb containing moisturizing and protective mucilage which soothes irritated and inflamed tissues; similar in meaning to emollient and mucilage.
deobstruent: an herb that removes obstructions in the body by opening natural passages of elimination.
depressant: an herb or drug that decreases nervous stimulation and physical activity; similar to a sedative.
depurative: an herb that cleans and purifies the blood and organs by promoting elimination.
dermatitis: skin inflammation, irritation, or eruptions causing itching and pain.
detergent: an herb or drug that is cleansing to the skin and conditions such as boils, ulcers, and wounds.
deva: the etheric intelligence, spiritual forces, and light beings in nature and plants.
diaphoretic: herbs that promote perspiration and elimination of waste products through the skin; also called sudorific.
diatomaceous earth (food-grade): consists of fossilized remains of diatoms, a hard-shelled algae that contains silica crystals and is ingested to kill intestinal parasites. The silica crystals pierce the bodies of parasites to destroy them without hurting the digestive tract of people or animals.
dilate: to expand and broaden; often refers to blood vessels being expanded.
diphtheria: an acute, highly contagious throat infection caused by *Corynebacterium diphtheriae* bacteria. It was once one of the most fatal childhood diseases but has practically been eliminated in countries where immunization is practiced.
discutient: an herb or drug that dissolves and removes tumors; similar in meaning to resolvent.
dispensatory: a book describing officially recognized medicines and their preparation, dosages, and uses.
diuretic: an herb or drug that increases the production and flow of urine by promoting kidney activity; used to reduce water retention (edema) and high blood pressure.
Doctrine of Signatures: an ancient doctrine widely cited in literature about medicinal plants. According to the doctrine, a plant's structure, appearance, color, smell, and other characteristics are signs that reveal its healing attributes and therapeutic value. Pliny the Elder, Dioscorides, and other early classical scholars held this belief, and it was further developed and popularized by Paracelsus during the Middle Ages, and later by Nicholas Culpeper.
dopamine: a primary neurotransmitter necessary for normal muscle movement. A deficiency can cause tremors and motor impairments, as seen in Parkinson's disease which involves dopamine deficiency. Dopamine has a stimulating action on the nervous system and promotes a sense of well-being.
double-blind study: a method used during research trials to prevent against bias by ensuring that neither the researchers nor participants know when the experimental agent or placebo are being used.
dysentery: intestinal inflammation, pain, and diarrhea often mixed with blood and mucous. Dysentery is caused by chemical toxins and bacterial, viral, or parasitic infections.
dysmenorrhea: painful and difficult menstruation; has same meaning as menorrhalgia.
dyspepsia: indigestion with abdominal pain, gas, bloating, and sometimes nausea and vomiting.
dysplasia: abnormal and pathological cellular growth typically associated with cancerous tissues.

Eclectic physicians: a group of American medical doctors who embraced holistic perspectives and prescribed herbal preparations in their clinical practice. They were an important sector of the medical system during the 1880s to 1930s, but became obsolete due to political and economic pressure.
eczema: an inflammatory skin condition causing redness, itching, irritation, weeping sores, and scaling.
edema: excessive accumulation and retention of water in the tissues. Dropsy is an old name for edema.
eicosanoids: derived from arachidonic acid and polyunsaturated fatty acids such as omega-3 and omega-6. Eicosanoids act in diverse ways to regulate body functions, and can increase or decrease inflammation, allergic symptoms, fevers, and other immune responses. Subfamilies of eicosanoids include prostaglandins, thromboxanes, and leukotrienes.
emetic: an agent that induces vomiting and is taken when a poison has been ingested; similar to nauseant.
emmenagogue: an herb or drug that promotes and regulates menstruation; contraindicated during pregnancy.
emollient: an herb or other substance externally applied to soften and protect skin and soothe inflammation; has similar meaning and qualities as mucilage and demulcent.
emphysema: a chronic lung condition of excess mucous congestion and diminished tissue elasticity causing difficult breathing, especially exhalation.
endogenous: substances naturally produced within the body as opposed to exogenous or "from outside the body."
endometriosis: an abnormal condition in which uterine tissue grows outside the uterus throughout the pelvic cavity and causes pain, pressure, and abnormal bleeding and menstrual cycles.
enteritis: inflammation of the intestines caused by bacteria, viruses, toxicity, chemicals, and other factors.
Enterobacteria: a large family of Gram-negative bacteria that includes many of the more common pathogens such as *Salmonella, Escherichia coli, Yersinia pestis, Klebsiella, Shigella, Proteus, Enterobacter, Serratia*, and *Citrobacter*.
epispastic: a corrosive herb or other substance that burns or dissolves tissue and can cause blisters; similar meaning as caustic, escharotic, and vesicant.
escharotic: a caustic or corrosive herb that burns and destroys tissue that it contacts.
essential oil: volatile oil in plants responsible for their odor and many of their medicinal properties.
estriol: one of the three estrogens produced by the body, primarily as a metabolite or product of estradiol. Estriol is the main estrogen secreted by the placenta during pregnancy and is the form of estrogen typically excreted in the urine of pregnant women.
estrogenic: an herb, food, or other substance that elicits estrogen responses in human and animal tissues.
ethnobotany: the botanical traditions of different ethnic cultures.
exanthematous: an herb that is healing to skin diseases and eruptions; similar in meaning to herpatic.
expectorant: an agent that makes coughing easier and enhances the expulsion of mucus and phlegm.

febrifuge: an herb or drug that reduces fever; similar in action to antipyretic and refrigerant herbs.
fibroids: non-malignant tumors and fibrous tissues occurring in the uterus and breast.
fibromyalgia: a stress-related, neuromuscular condition characterized by several specific areas of muscular pain and inflammation, chronic fatigue, and poor immunity.
flower essence: a homeopathic-like remedy specifically prepared by infusing the vibrational essence of flowers into pure water, which is then ingested to heal at emotional and spiritual levels.
folliculitis: a contagious bacterial infection and inflammation of hair follicles that is usually caused by *Staphylococcus aureus* or *Streptococcus pyogenes*.
fomentation: an external application of warm herbal tea soaked in a cloth that is laid on the affected area.
free radical: a highly reactive oxygen-containing molecule with unpaired electrons that roams the body in search of healthy cells to "steal" their electrons. Free radicals cause oxidative stress that promotes cellular damage and aging, inflammation, scar tissue formation, and chronic degenerative conditions. Antioxidants occurring in many herbs and foods protect cells from oxidative and free radical damage.
fungicide or fungistatic: an herb or drug that kills fungus.

galactagogue: an herb that increases breast milk in nursing mothers; also called lactagogue.
garble: the process of separating leaves and flowers from the stems of plants, and removing dirty and damaged plant parts before making herbal preparations.
gastritis: an acute or chronic inflammation of the stomach lining due to food poisoning, toxins, drugs, bacteria, viruses, or alcohol.
genus: a specific classification of plants ranked according to similarities in characteristics. There are usually several species of plants within each genus. The plural form of genus is genera.
German Commission E: a regulatory agency that consisted of a committee of physicians, pharmacologists, toxicologists, and lay people appointed by the German government in 1978 for the purpose of assessing the safety and efficacy of herbal medicine. The Commission evaluated over 380 medicinal herbs and provided guidelines for the European Union in establishing regulations governing the sale and dispensing of over-the-counter and prescription herbal medications. The Commission's work and recommendations have been translated into English by the American Botanical Council and

published as *The German Commission E Monographs*, a book that has become a standard herbal reference for many herbal practitioners. The German Commission E no longer exists.
glabrous: leaves that have a smooth surface without hairs.
glacous: leaves that have a thin, waxy, or whitish powdery coating on their surface.
glutathione: one of the body's primary antioxidants that protects cells from oxidative damage.

hemolysis: the rupture and destruction of red blood cells caused by several conditions, including bacterial infections, parasites, autoimmune and genetic disorders, and toxic chemicals.
hemostatic: substances that stop hemorrhaging and usually have astringent properties; similar to styptic.
hepatic: agents that protect and support normal liver function; used to treat liver weakness and disease.
hepatoprotective: herbs that protect the liver from damage and support its normal function.
herb or herbaceous plants: fleshy seed-bearing plants with non-woody stems that typically grow close to the ground and up to 6-7′ tall. To herbalists, an herb refers to any plant with medicinal properties.
herpatic: a remedy for skin eruptions, rashes, and dermatitis; similar in meaning to exanthematous.
hiatal hernia: a bulging protrusion of the stomach that pushes upward through weak diaphragm muscles.
histamine: a nitrogen compound in most body tissues that increases capillary dilation and permeability, lowers blood pressure, and accelerates heart rate and constriction of most smooth muscles. Histamine is released in response to contact with allergens and causes allergic reactions, including edema, inflammation, itching, hay fever, and hives. Antihistamines are used to counteract these effects.
Hodgkin's disease: cancer of lymph nodes, spleen, and lymphoid tissue that spreads throughout the body.
homeopathy or homeopathic: a therapeutic system founded by Samuel Hahnemann (1755-1843) that is based on the theory that "like cures like." Diseases are treated with substances that in healthy people are able to produce symptoms similar to those of the disease being treated. Homeopathic medicines are taken in extremely minute, diluted dosages.
humoral immunity: the type of immunity that fights bacteria and viruses with proteins called immunoglobulins (known as antibodies) that are produced by B-lymphocytes.
hypertensive: an herb or drug that increases blood pressure.
hypnotic: a strong sedative herb or drug that induces sleep; similar in meaning to soporific.
hypoglycemic: substances that decrease elevated blood sugar levels and are used to treat diabetes.
hypotensive: remedies that lower abnormally high blood pressure.
hypothalamus: a gland in the midbrain involved with autonomic nervous system regulation of involuntary body functions, including body temperature, water balance, sleep, thirst, hunger, emotions, metabolism of protein, fats and carbohydrates, development of secondary sex characteristics, and sexual activity. It regulates the endocrine system and secretion of endocrine hormones.

immunomodulator or immunoregulator: an herb or drug that regulates, normalizes, and strengthens the immune system; it is not necessarily stimulating. In conditions of immune dysfunction or autoimmune disorders, they calm an overactive immune system and bring it back into a healthy balance, while also promoting overall health and wellness.
immunostimulant: an herb or drug that stimulates the immune system by activating or increasing white blood cells and other components of immunity.
impetigo: a contagious Staphylococcus skin infection typically occurring around the nose and mouth.
in vitro: is Latin for "in glass," referring to an artificial environment designed for laboratory research that is constructed outside a living plant or animal. *In vitro* testing typically involves the use of test tubes and petri dishes.
in vivo: is Latin for "in life" and refers to laboratory research done within the living body of animals or humans. *In vivo* studies are carried out in human clinical trials and animal studies.
influenza: an acute viral infection of the respiratory tract that is also called the flu and grippe.
innervate: to affect or stimulate cells, tissues, and organs with nerve impulses.
interferons: proteins produced by cells of the immune system that interfere with the ability of bacteria, viruses, parasites, and cancerous cells to multiply. Interferons belong to the large class of immune substances known as cytokines.
interleukins: a type of cytokine essential for communication between all cells and components of the immune system and for normal immune function. Several different interleukins are involved in various immune responses, and interleukin deficiencies or dysfunctions result in autoimmune diseases or immune weakness.
interleukin-2 (IL-2): a beneficial interleukin that regulates white blood cells (leukocytes) responsible for immunity. IL-2 is part of the body's natural response to microbial infections, and is used in pharmaceutical drug therapy to treat viral infections, cancers, and HIV/AIDS.
interleukin-6 (IL-6): one of the most problematic inflammatory cytokines that damages cells and causes inflammatory conditions throughout the body. Levels increase during inflammatory episodes.
interleukin-10 (IL-10) an anti-inflammatory cytokine.
intermittent claudication: pain in calf muscles caused by vascular problems and insufficient circulation.
irritant: an herb, drug, or other agent that causes itching, inflammation, or abnormal sensitivity in tissues.

ischemia: restricted blood supply to tissues causing reduced oxygen and glucose uptake and tissue damage and dysfunction. Ischemia usually occurs due to problems within blood vessels.

lactagogue: an herb or other substance that promotes breast milk production; similar action as galactagogue.
lactifuge: an herb or drug that decreases or stops the production of breast milk.
laxative: an herb or drug that promotes evacuation of the bowels; a gentle purgative used for constipation.
leukocyte or leucocyte: white blood cells that protect the body against infections and foreign substances by secreting chemicals (antibodies, histamine) and the process of phagocytosis, in which pathogens are surrounded and destroyed. Leukocytes occur in all tissues, blood, and the lymphatic system.
leukotrienes: belong to the family of eicosanoid inflammatory mediators, and are produced in white blood cells from the oxidation of arachidonic acid. Leukotrienes regulate immune and inflammatory responses, and their production is usually accompanied by the production of histamine and prostaglandins, which also act as inflammatory mediators.
lipid: a fatty substance such as fatty acids, phospholipids, waxes, prostaglandins, and steroids.
lipid peroxidation: the oxidative degradation of lipids (fats). It is the process in which free radicals "steal" electrons from the lipids in cell membranes, resulting in cell damage. It most often affects polyunsaturated fatty acids
lipotropic: compounds involved in the metabolic break down and removal of fats from the liver.
lipoxygenase (5-LOX): a group of enzymes involved in the production of inflammatory prostaglandins and leukotrienes. 5-LOX inhibitors reduce painful inflammation.
lithotropic or lithotryptic: agents that dissolve and eliminate kidney, bladder, and gallbladder stones; similar to antilithic.
lupus: an autoimmune connective tissue disease affecting the skin and other connective tissues in the body.
lymphadenopathy: a disease of the lymph nodes in which they are inflamed, swollen, firm, and tender. Common causes of lymphadenopathy include infections, autoimmune diseases, and cancers.
lymphagogue: an herb or drug that strengthens, detoxifies, and stimulates lymph glands and activity of the entire lymphatic system; beneficial for treating swollen glands and lymphatic illness.
lymphatic system: consists of lymph tissue, nodes, fluid and lymphatic vessels, and the appendix, tonsils, and spleen. Lymphatic tissue produces beneficial while blood cells and other immune components.
lymphoma: cancer of lymphatic tissue; includes Hodgkin's disease.

macrophage: a type of phagocyte and specialized cell of the immune system that searches for pathogens and foreign substances to surround, digest, and destroy in the process known as phagocytosis.
mastitis: breast inflammation, pain, and tenderness caused by fibrocystic breast disease, bacterial infection, or engorged milk ducts during lactation.
materia medica: a Latin term meaning "medical material" that describes a text of collected knowledge about the therapeutic properties of herbs and drugs used in medical remedies.
melatonin: a hormone that promotes sleep. It is synthesized from serotonin and secreted by the pineal gland.
Meniere's disease: a disorder of the inner ear causing tinnitus (ringing), hearing loss, and vertigo (dizziness).
meningitis: a serious, acute inflammation of the meninges (the protective membranes covering the brain and spinal cord) usually caused by bacterial or viral infection.
menorrhalgia: difficult and painful menstruation; same meaning as dysmenorrhea.
menses: another name for menstruation.
meridian: according to Traditional Chinese Medicine, a meridian is a pathway of energy movement in the body. Acupuncture points are specific areas along the meridians.
metabolite: a small molecule resulting from chemical reactions during the degrading or breakdown of different substances; metabolites are formed during normal metabolic reactions in the body.
monograph (herbal): a scholarly book or treatise on a single herb.
mucilage or mucilaginous: a gummy or gelatinous substance in some plants that is soothing and cooling to inflamed and irritated tissues; similar in meaning to demulcent and emollient.
mucolytic: an agent that denatures and reduces the viscosity (thickness, stickiness) of mucous secretions.
mucosa or mucous membranes: specialized mucous-secreting tissues lining all hollow organs and cavities that open on to the skin, including the nasal passages, throat, and mouth. Mucous is vital to lubricate and protect tissues throughout the body.
myalgia: muscle pain.

narcotic: an agent that depresses the central nervous system and is used to relieve pain and induce sleep.
National Formulary: a book of official standards for regulating pharmaceuticals and medicines.
natural killer (NK) cell: a type of white blood cell involved in the first line of defensive immune response that quickly recognizes, attacks, and destroys viruses and cancerous cells. NK cells trigger apoptosis (programmed cell death) in cells invaded by viruses and cancer.
naturopathy: a branch of holistic medicine that improves health by addressing lifestyle, diet, mind/body connection, and by using remedies other than pharmaceutical drugs and surgery. These include herbal therapy, acupuncture, body work, and other alternative/complementary therapies.

nephritic: the class of herbs or drugs used for kidney weakness and disease.
nephritis: a damaging kidney disease involving inflammation and reduced blood filtration, which allows blood and proteins (albumin) into urine; also called Bright's disease.
nervine: herbs that have a calming, soothing effect on the nerves. They have similar actions to sedative herbs, but nervines also tone, nourish, heal, and restore the nerves.
neuralgia: nerve pain and inflammation.
neurasthenia: abnormal fatigue, lack of energy and motivation, depression, mental fog, and insomnia.
neuritis: inflammation of the nerves causing pain, pins-and-needles, numbness, and/or weakness.
neuropathy: functional disturbances and/or pathological changes in the peripheral nervous system.
neurotransmitters: are powerful chemical messengers. They either excite (glutamate, epinephrine/adrenaline, norepinephrine, dopamine, phenethylamine/PEA) or inhibit (serotonin, gamma-aminobutyric acid/GABA) nerve impulses. Neurotransmitters regulate the nervous system and mental processes and affect moods, cognition, coping skills, energy levels, sleep, and many other body functions.
nitric oxide synthase (NOS): takes two forms in the body, endothelial (eNOS) and inducible (iNOS). The endothelium (inner lining) of blood vessels uses nitric oxide to signal smooth muscle relaxation, resulting in vasodilation and increased blood flow. eNOS also protects blood vessels by inhibiting platelet aggregation leading to abnormal blood clotting. People with atherosclerosis, diabetes, and hypertension often show impaired eNOS pathways. iNOS is involved in the immune response and phagocytic destruction of bacteria, viruses, cancerous cells, and parasites. However, iNOS can promote excessive inflammation.
nomenclature: the scientific system of assigning names to describe, define, and classify plants and animals.
Nrf2 (Nuclear factor-like 2): a protein found in all cells of the body that activates the production of antioxidants (glutathione, superoxide dismutase/SOD, catalase) to protect against oxidative damage.
nutritive: an herb that nourishes the body to sustain life and assists in food digestion and assimilation.

opthalmicum: an herb or drug used to treat eye inflammation, infections, and diseases.
oxidative stress: occurs when the body's supply of antioxidants cannot keep up with the constant production of free radicals during normal metabolism in addition to environmental sources of oxidative damage that include pollution, tobacco, radiation, pharmaceutical and recreational drugs, and excessive exercise and exposure to sunlight. Oxidative stress damages and mutates cells, contributing to inflammation, the aging process, and development of many chronic degenerative diseases.
oxytocic: an agent that stimulates the release of oxytocin hormone from the pituitary gland, which produces uterine contractions to facilitate labor and childbirth and stimulates breast milk production.

parasiticide: a remedy that kills parasites; similar in action to vermicide, vermifuge, and anthelmintic.
parasympathomimetic: an herb or drug that activates the parasympathetic nervous system and has a generalized relaxing effect throughout the body.
parturient: a substance that induces strong uterine contractions during childbirth; similar to oxytocic.
pathogen: viruses, bacteria, fungi, parasites, and other agents causing infection and disease.
pectoral: a remedy for lung and cardiopulmonary problems.
perennial: plants that live for many years and have roots that are dormant during winter.
peripheral vascular disease: are diseases of the blood vessels and include arteriosclerosis, atherosclerosis, Raynaud's disease, thrombophlebitis, and intermittent claudication.
peristalsis: wave-like contractions in the muscles of the gastrointestinal tract and in tubular organs that move their contents. In the stomach and intestines, peristalic movement propels food downward.
peritonitis: life-threatening inflammation of the serous membranes (called the peritoneum) lining the surfaces of organs in the abdominal cavity and the inner surface of the abdominal cavity itself, often caused by infection.
petiole: the small stem of a leaf that attaches to a larger stalk. Petiolate leaves attach to stalks by small stems.
pH: a measure of the acidity or alkalinity of substances based on a scale of 1 (extreme acid) to 14 (extreme alkaline or base). The pH of pure water is 7.0, which is neutral. All life forms exist within specific ranges of pH.
phagocytes: a group of specialized white blood cells that protect the body by surrounding, ingesting, and destroying harmful foreign particles, bacteria, viruses, cancerous cells, and dead or dying cells. Phagocytes are essential for fighting infections and for subsequent immunity
phagocytosis: a primary immune response in which phagocytes seek out, identify, engulf, digest, and destroy bacteria, viruses, toxins, and cancerous cells.
pharmaceutical: a manufactured drug or medication that is sold by a pharmacy.
pharmacopoeia: an official treatise and publication listing drugs, their preparation, and dosages.
phlebitis: inflammation of a vein most often occurring in the legs.
phlegm: another word for mucous or sputum.
phyto: means "coming from a plant" or "plant-based," and refers to herbal medicines.
phytochemical: chemicals plants produce that are necessary for their survival and protection against pathogens and predators. Responsible for characteristic colors, flavors, and odors of plants, many

phytochemicals provide antibiotic, antiviral, and other beneficial medicines for human health.

phytoestrogens: substances occurring in many plants that have a similar chemical structure to estrogen and elicit estrogen-like activity or effect estrogen metabolism in humans. Although phytoestrogens are less potent than estradiol and other endogenous estrogens (human forms of estrogen), they act via similar mechanisms and compete with estradiol for estrogen receptor sites in breast, uterine and ovarian cells, producing similar but weaker effects. When endogenous estrogens are low during menopause, phytoestrogens bind to estrogen receptor sites in cells to increase estrogen activity. For conditions of excess estrogen (such as fibroids, endometriosis, and reproductive cysts and cancers), phytoestrogens bind to receptor cites and block more potent estrogens. Phytoestrogens are safe, healthy alternatives to potentially dangerous synthetic estrogens.

The major phytoestrogen groups are isoflavones (genistein, daidzein, glycitein, formononetin in soy and legumes); flavones (luteolin); coumestans (coumestrol in soy and legumes); stilbenes (resveratrol); lignans (secoisolariciresinol, matairesinol, pinoresinol, lariciresinol); and sterols or phytosterols (beta-sitosterol, diosgenin).

phytomedicine or phytotherapy: plant-based medicine.

phytosterols: the most potent type of phytoestrogen, these are naturally occurring plant steroids with chemical structures similar to cholesterol that reduce intestinal cholesterol absorption. Phytosterols include beta-sitosterol, campesterol, stigmasterol, and diosgenin. Phytosterols provide raw materials for the production of hormones, and are chemically manipulated in labs to create estrone, progesterone, and testosterone.

phytotherapy: the European and Western term for the practice of herbal medicine.

placebo: a substance with no inherent pharmacological activity that is used in research studies.

pleurisy: inflammation of the pleura lining the lungs caused by infection, trauma, cancer, or lung diseases like pneumonia, influenza (the flu) and tuberculosis. Pleurisy causes coughing and painful breathing.

polyp: a benign growth on mucous membranes typically occurring in the nasal passages and intestines.

postpartum: the transitional period of time following childbirth.

poultice: a preparation of crushed or powdered plant material that is applied to the skin for the treatment of external wounds, rashes, joint and muscle pain, and other ailments.

prolactin: a hormone in all mammals necessary for milk production in females. It is secreted from the pituitary gland in response to ovulation, estrogen treatment, mating, and nursing. Prolactin plays an essential role in metabolism, regulation of the immune system, and pancreatic development.

prolapse: the downward fall and displacement of organs due to weak muscles that are unable to hold the organs in their normal anatomical positions.

prostaglandins: a large group of lipid compounds found in most tissues of the body that exert a wide range of influence in many physiological functions. Some dilate blood vessels and others constrict, and many are involved in immune responses that inhibit or promote inflammation.

prostatitis: inflammation of the prostate gland.

psoriasis: a chronic, autoimmune skin condition characterized by rapid cell growth of the skin with red, irritated, dry, scaly patches.

pubescent: the downy texture of fine, short, soft hairs on the surface of some leaves.

purgative: a strong laxative producing vigorous emptying of bowels that usually causes watery evacuation.

pustule: a small pimple filled with pus (indicative of infection) that can form on the skin and is most commonly associated with acne.

pyorrhea: periodontal mouth disease involving infection and discharge of pus from the gums.

Qi: In Traditional Chinese Medicine, Qi generally refers to the energy or life force that manifests on physical or material planes and on the nonphysical or etheric levels. Qi within the body provides warmth, movement, conscious awareness, and the ability to continually generate new cells.

randomized clinical trial: a type of trial that randomly divides participants into at least two groups to study specific conditions that they all share by comparing different treatments and their outcomes.

Raynaud's disease: a vascular disorder of insufficient circulation in the extremities causing fingers and toes to be cold and turn blue.

refrigerant: herbs or drugs having a cooling effect that reduces fevers; same action as febrifuge and antipyretic.

resolvent: an herb or drug that dissolves and removes tumors; similar in action to discutient.

restorative: herbs that restore normal function and vitality; similar in action to analeptic.

retrovirus: a more resistant type of virus whose genetic material contains RNA instead of the usual DNA.

rheumatism: inflammation and degeneration of the joints causing pain, stiffness and immobility; includes rheumatoid arthritis (an autoimmune condition), osteoarthritis, bursitis, and gout.

rhinitis: inflammation of the mucous membranes lining the nose and sinus cavities caused by bacterial, viral, or allergic reactions. The common cold and hay fever are types of rhinitis.

ringworm: a contagious skin infection caused by different types of fungi. It is also called tinea.

rosacea: a skin disease marked by chronic redness (erythema) and flushing on the face that can include the presence of hard pimples (papules) or pus-filled pimples (pustules), and small spider-like veins.

rubefacient: an agent that is applied externally to stimulate capillary dilation, which promotes increased blood flow and local redness on the skin. It is used to cleanse, heal, and ease pain and swelling.

salve (herbal): a preparation for external use prepared by baking herbs in oil and adding bees wax to harden the oil into a thick ointment.

scabies: a contagious infestation of the skin by the human itch mite (*Sarcoptes scabiei* var. *hominis*). The microscopic scabies mite burrows into the upper layer of the skin where it lives and lays eggs. The most common symptoms are intense itching and a pimple-like skin rash. The scabies mite usually is spread by direct, prolonged, skin-to-skin contact with a person who has scabies.

scarification: the process of scratching, cutting, and softening a thick seed coat to enhance germination.

scarlet fever: an acute contagious childhood disease caused by *Streptococci* bacteria.

sciatica: nerve pain along the sciatic nerve affecting the lower back and legs.

sebaceous glands: develop with hair follicles in the skin and secrete sebum to lubricate, moisturize, and protect the hair and skin.

seborrhea: a type of dermatitis involving excessive secretion by sebaceous glands that causes greasy scales or cheesy plugs on the skin, and is usually accompanied with irritation, itching, or burning.

sedative: an herb or drug that calms and sedates the central nervous system; used for insomnia and anxiety.

septic: a generalized toxic condition caused by infectious bacteria and their toxins.

septicemia: blood poisoning caused by infectious pathogens or their toxins.

serous membranes: specialized cells lining the abdominal and pelvic cavities that secrete fluids to moisten and lubricate tissues.

serum glutamic-oxaloacetic transaminase (SGOT): see aspartate aminotransferase (AST).

serum glutamic-pyruvic transaminase (SGPT): see alanine aminotransferace (ALT)

sessile: the type of leaf that attaches directly to stems and lacks a connecting stalk.

shelf-life: the period of time in which herbs retain their potency and effectiveness after being harvested.

shingles: extremely painful skin eruptions and lesions caused by the *Herpes zoster* virus.

sialogogue: a remedy that stimulates secretion of saliva in the mouth and aids carbohydrate digestion.

sinusitis: infection and inflammation of the nasal sinus cavities.

smooth muscle: the type of muscle found in blood vessels, organs, and glands. Smooth muscle is involuntary and controlled by the autonomic nervous system.

soporific: sedative herbs or drugs that induce deep sleep; similar to hypnotic and somnifacient.

sp. and spp.: abbreviations that mean "species plural" and "all species in a genus," and are used to specify one or several species of a genus, respectively.

standardized: an herbal preparation guaranteed to contain a specified amount of active phytochemicals.

stomachic: a digestive aid that strengthens, heals, and improves stomach function; similar to carminative.

stye (also spelled sty, plural is styes or sties): the inflammation of a sebaceous gland on an eyelid.

styptic: an astringent, hemostatic agent that stops bleeding by contracting tissues and blood vessels.

sudoriferous glands: sweat glands on the skin.

sudorific: agents that promote profuse sweating when taken hot, and act as a tonic when taken cold. They are used for fevers and detoxification; similar in action to diaphoretic.

superoxide dismutase (SOD): a primary antioxidant enzyme produced by all cells in the body to protect against oxidative and free radical damage and destruction to cells.

synergestic: the harmonious interaction between substances that enhances their overall effect and counter-balances possible side effects. Synergestic herbs have greater activity when used together than separately.

systemic: affecting the entire body.

T-cell or T-lymphocyte: a type of white blood cell that is produced in bone marrow and matures in the thymus gland. T-cells attack foreign antigens by the process of cell-mediated immunity in which the antigen is slowly destroyed by the T-cell or by a toxin released from the T-cell.

tetanus: a potentially fatal disease caused by *Clostridium tetani* bacteria that causes severe muscle spasms and convulsions.

tetany: the continuous and painful spasm and contraction of a muscle.

Thomsonian: a system of early American herbal medicine developed by Samuel Thomson (1769-1843).

thrombophlebitis: phlebitis or vein inflammation caused by blood clots.

thrombosis: the formation of blood clots in blood vessels.

thromboxane: a substance formed from prostaglandins that promotes blood clotting by constricting blood vessels and increasing blood platelet aggregation.

thrush: a Candida yeast infection in the mouth and throat.

tincture: a liquid herbal preparation typically made by alcohol extraction of plant material.

tincturing: the process of soaking the marc (plant material) in a menstruum solution (usually alcohol) to create an herbal tincture.

tinnitus: ringing in the ears.

tonic: an herb taken over time to restore normal function and strengthen specific organs or the entire body.

toxemia: the accumulation of toxins and waste products in the blood.
trigeminal neuralgia: facial pain caused by irritation and inflammation of the fifth cranial (trigeminal) nerve.
tumor necrosis factor (TNF): a multifunctional cytokine that affects lipid metabolism, blood coagulation, insulin resistance, the function of endothelial cells lining blood vessels, and immune responses during cellular damage and infections. TNF can induce necrosis (death) of tumor cells. Drugs that block the action of TNF reduce inflammation in many inflammatory diseases such as Crohn's disease and rheumatoid arthritis.
typhoid fever: a bacterial infection caused by *Salmonella typhi* that is transmitted by water, food, and shellfish. The bacteria multiply in the bloodstream and eventually localize in the intestinal tract and gallbladder to cause fever and diarrhea.
typhus: an acute infectious disease caused by *Rickettsia* parasites transmitted from infected rats and other rodents to people by lice, fleas, ticks, and mites.

United States Pharmacopoeia (UPS): a legally recognized compendium of standards for drugs and botanical products, including assays and tests to determine their strength, quality, and purity. It was established in 1820 and is recognized as the official U.S. organization empowered to establish standards for pharmaceuticals, health care technologies, and dietary supplements, including herbs.
urethritis: inflammation of the urethra (the tubular passage carrying urine from the bladder out of the body) usually due to infection or obstructions.
uterotonic: an herb that strengths and tones the uterine muscles and promotes normal uterine function.

vaginitis: inflammation of the vagina caused by infection or irritants, resulting in pain and discharge.
vascular: pertaining to the blood vessels.
vascular impermeability: see capillary impermeability.
vascular tonic: nourishes and supports normal function of blood vessels.
vasoconstrictor: an herb or drug that tightens and constricts blood vessels; used for hemorrhaging.
vasodilator: an agent that relaxes and dilates blood vessels to improve circulation and reduce hypertension.
vasoprotective: remedies that protect and strengthen blood vessels.
vegan: a type of diet that excludes all animal products, including dairy, eggs, meat, and fish.
vermicide: an herb or drug that destroys worms and parasites in the gastrointestinal tract and on skin; also called anthelmintic, parasiticide, and vermifuge.
vermifuge: destroys and expels worms and parasites.
vesicant: a substance that produces blisters upon local contact; also called caustic, escharotic, and epispastic.
vulnerary: herbs that promote wound healing by stimulating cell growth and repair and protecting against infection.

wildcraft: to harvest herbs naturally occurring in the wilds, as opposed to those that are cultivated.

yang: a term used in Traditional Chinese Medicine referring to the qualities and polarity of the masculine; light, energy, fire, heat, activity, and function.
yellow fever: an acute infectious viral disease transmitted by certain species of female mosquitoes in tropical areas. Symptoms include fever, jaundice due to liver destruction, and albuminuria (excess protein in the urine).
yin: a term used in Traditional Chinese Medicine referring to the qualities and polarity of the feminine; darkness, rest, cold, water, and nourishment.

APPENDIX TWO

Cross-Reference of Common and Botanical Plant Names

The first section of this cross-reference lists the common name or names of a plant followed by the Latin botanical, which includes the genus and species written in italics. In the second section beginning on page 632, the Latin names appear first and are followed by the common names.

If several species in a genus are used medicinally, the abbreviation "spp." is written, such as *Trillium erectum*, spp. or *Trillium* spp. Synonyms of Latin names appear in brackets to indicate alternate or obsolete scientific names. An example is the Latin name of Almond trees *Prunus dulcis [P. amygdalus]*.

COMMON NAME	BOTANICAL NAME
Abscess Root	***Polemonium reptans***
Aconite, Monkshood	*Aconitum napellus*
Agar-agar (red algae)	*Gelidium amansii*, spp.
Agave, Century Plant	*Agave americana*
Agrimony	*Agrimonia eupatoria, A. gryposepala*, spp.
Alfalfa	*Medicago sativa*
Allspice Tree	*Pimenta dioica*
Almond Tree	*Prunus dulcis [P. amygdalus]*
Aloe Vera	*Aloe vera*
Alumroot	*Heuchera americana*, spp.
Amaranth	*Amaranthus* spp.
American Centaury	*Sabatia angularis*
Andrographis	*Andrographis paniculata*
Angelica,	*Angelica archangelica*
American Angelica	*A. atropurpurea*
Wild Angelica	*A. sylvestris*
Anise, Aniseed	*Pimpinella anisum*
Anise Hyssop	*Agastache foeniculum*
Anise Root	*Osmorhiza longistylis*
Apple Tree	*Malus pumila [M. domestica]*
Apricot Tree	*Prunus armeniaca*, spp.
Arnica	*Arnica montana*, spp.
Artichoke	*Cynara scolymus*
Arugula	*Eruca sativa, E. vesicaria*
Ashwagandha	*Withania somnifera*
Asparagus	*Asparagus officinalis*
Astragalus	*Astragalus membranaceus*
Atractylodes	*Atractylodes macrocephala*
Avens, Wood Avens	*Geum urbanum*
Bacopa	***Bacopa monnieri***
Balloonflower	*Platycodon grandiflorus*
Balm of Gilead	*Commiphora gileadensis*
Balmony, Turtlehead	*Chelone glabra*
Balsam of Tolu, Tolu Balsam	*Myroxylon balsamum*
Baneberry, Bugbane	*Actaea pachypoda [A. alba]*
Barberry	*Berberis vulgaris, B. canadensis*
Barley	*Hordeum vulgare*
Basil	*Ocimum basilicum*
Basswood, Linden	*Tilia americana, T. cordata*

COMMON NAME	BOTANICAL NAME
Bay Laurel	*Laurus nobilis*
Bayberry	*Myrica cerifera*
Bearberry, Uva-ursi	*Arctostaphylos uva-ursi*
Bedstraw, Cleavers	*Galium aparine*
Beebalm (Lavender), Wild Bergamot	*Monarda fistulosa*
Beebalm (Scarlet), Oswego Tea, Red Bergamot	*Monarda didyma*
Belladonna, Deadly Nightshade	*Atropa belladonna*
Benzoin Tree	*Styrax benzoin*
Bergamot (Red), Scarlet Beebalm, Oswego Tea	*Monarda didyma*
Bergamot (Wild), Lavender Beebalm	*Monarda fistulosa*
Betony, Lousewort	*Pedicularis canadensis*
Bilberry	*Vaccinium myrtillus*
Birthroot, Bethroot	*Trillium erectum*, spp.
Bistort	*Polygonum bistorta*
Bitter Melon	*Momordica charantia*
Bittersweet (American)	*Celastrus scandens*
Black Cohosh	*Cimicifuga racemosa [Actaea racemosa]*
Black Current	*Ribes nigrum*
Black Haw	*Viburnum prunifolium*
Black Pepper	*Piper nigrum*
Black Root, Culver's Root	*Veronicastrum virginicum [Leptandra virginica]*
Black Tea, Green Tea	*Camellia sinensis*
Black Walnut (American)	*Juglans nigra*
Black Walnut (English)	*Juglans regia*
Blackberry	*Rubus villosus, R. fruticosus*
Blackberry Lily, Leopard Flower	*Belamcanda chinensis [Iris domestica]*
Black-eyed Susan	*Rudbeckia hirta*
Bladderwrack	*Fucus vesiculosus*
Blessed Thistle	*Cnicus benedictus*
Bloodroot	*Sanguinaria canadensis*
Blue Cohosh	*Caulophyllum thalictroides*
Blue Flag	*Iris versicolor*

Common Name	Botanical Name
Blue Vervain	*Verbena hastata*
European Vervain	*Verbena officinalis*
Blueberry	*Vaccinium corymbosum,* spp.
Bogbean	*Menyanthes trifoliata*
Boldo	*Peumus boldus*
Boneset	*Eupatorium perfoliatum*
Borage	*Borago officinalis*
Boswellia	*Boswellia serrata*
Bouncing Bet, Soapwort	*Saponaria officinalis*
Broad-leafed Dock	*Rumex obtusifolius*
Bryony (White)	*Bryonia alba*
Buchu	*Agathosma betulina [Barosma betulina]*
Buckbean	*Menyanthes trifoliata*
Buckthorn	*Rhamnus cathartica*
Buckwheat	*Fagopyrum esculentum*
Bugbane, Baneberry	*Actaea pachypoda [A. alba]*
Bugle	*Ajuga reptans*
Bugleweed, Gypsywort	*Lycopus americanus, L. virginicus, L. europaeus*
Bupleurum, Thorowax	*Bupleurum chinense*
Burdock	*Arctium lappa, A. minus*
Burnet (Great)	*Sanguisorba officinalis*
Butcher's Broom	*Ruscus aculeatus*
Butterbur	*Petasites hybridus*
Butterfly Weed, Pleurisy Root	*Asclepias tuberosa*
Butternut	*Juglans cinerea*
Cajeput Tree	***Melaleuca cajeputi, M. leucadendra***
Calamint	*Calamintha sylvatica,* spp.
Calamus, Sweet Flag	*Acorus calamus [A. americanus]*
Calendula	*Calendula officinalis*
California Bay Laurel	*Umbellularia californica*
California Poppy	*Eschscholzia californica*
Camphor	*Cinnamomum camphora*
Caraway	*Carum carvi*
Cardamom	*Elettaria cardamomum*
Cardinal Flower	*Lobelia cardinalis*
Carob	*Ceratonia siliqua*
Carrot (Wild)	*Daucus carota*
Cascara Sagrada	*Rhamnus purshiana*
Castor Oil Plant	*Ricinus communis*
Catnip	*Nepeta cataria*
Cat's Claw	*Uncaria tomentosa*
Cayenne	*Capsicum annuum*
Celandine (Greater)	*Chelidonium majus*
Celery	*Apium graveolens*
Centaury (American)	*Sabatia angularis*
Centaury (European)	*Centaurium erythraea [Erythraea centaurium]*
Century Plant, Agave	*Agave americana*
Chamomile (German)	*Matricaria recutita [M. chamomilla, Chamomilla recutita]*
Chamomile (Roman, English)	*Anthemis nobilis [Chamaemelum nobile]*
Chaparral	*Larrea tridentata*
Chasteberry, Vitex	*Vitex agnus-castus*
Cherry (Wild)	*Prunus serotina*
Chervil	*Anthriscus cerefolium*
Chickweed	*Stellaria media,* spp.
Chicory	*Cichorium intybus*
Chinese Knotweed, Fo-ti	*Polygonum multiflorum*
Chinese Scullcap	*Scutellaria baicalensis*
Chinese Yam	*Dioscorea batata*
Chives	*Allium schoenoprasum*
Chlorella	*Chlorella regularis,* spp.
Cicely (European)	*Myrrhis odorata*
Cicely (Sweet)	*Osmorhiza claytonii*
Cinnabar Sage, Red Sage, Dan-Shen	*Salvia miltiorrhiza*
Cinnamon	*Cinnamomum verum,* spp.
Cinquefoil (Common)	*Potentilla recta, P. tormentilla*
Cinquefoil (Creeping)	*Potentilla reptans*
Clary Sage	*Salvia sclarea*
Cleavers, Bedstraw	*Galium aparine*
Clove	*Syzygium aromaticum*
Clover (Red)	*Trifolium pratense*
Clover (Sweet), Yellow Melilot	*Melilotus officinalis,* spp.
Clover (Sweet White)	*Melilotus alba*
Clover (White)	*Trifolium repens*
Clubmoss	*Lycopodium clavatum*
Coca (cocaine source)	*Erythroxylum coca*
Cocoa (chocolate)	*Theobroma cacao*
Codonopsis, Dang Shen	*Codonopsis pilosula*
Coffee	*Coffea arabica,* spp.
Colic Root, True Unicorn Root	*Aletris farinosa*
Coltsfoot	*Tussilago farfara*
Comfrey	*Symphytum officinale*
Russian Comfrey	*Symphytum x uplandicum*
Coneflower	*Echinacea purpurea,* spp.
Coptis, Chinese Goldthread,	*Coptis chinensis*
American Goldthread, Canker Root	*Coptis trifolia*
Cordyceps, Chinese Caterpillar Fungus	*Cordyceps sinensis*
Coreopsis	*Coreopsis tinctoria*
Coriander	*Coriandrum sativum*
Corn, Corn Silk	*Zea mays*
Corydalis	*Corydalis bulbosa,* spp.
Costmary	*Tanacetum balsamita [Chrysanthemum balsamita]*
Couch Grass	*Elymus repens [Elytrigia repens, Agropyron repens]*
Cowslip, Primula	*Primula veris [P. officinalis]*
Cramp Bark	*Viburnum opulus*
Cranberry	*Vaccinium macrocarpon, V. oxycoccos,* spp.
Cranesbill	*Geranium maculatum*
Culver's Root, Black Root	*Veronicastrum virginicum [Leptandra virginica]*
Cumin	*Cuminum cyminum*
Damiana	***Turnera diffusa***
Dan Shen, Cinnabar Sage	*Salvia miltiorrhiza*
Dandelion	*Taraxacum officinale*

Common Name	Botanical Name
Dang Shen	*Codonopsis pilosula*
Datura, Jimson Weed	*Datura stramonium*
Deadly Nightshade	*Atropa belladonna*
Devil's Claw	*Harpagophytum procumbens*
Devil's Club	*Oplopanax horridus [Echinopanax horridus]*
Dill	*Anethum graveolens*
Dodder	*Cuscuta epithymum*, spp.
Dong Quai	*Angelica sinensis*
Dragonroot	*Arisaema dracontium*
Dragon's Blood	*Daemonorops draco*
Dyer's Woad, Isatis	*Isatis tinctoria*
Echinacea, Coneflower	***Echinacea purpurea, E. angustifolia, E. pallida*, spp.**
Eclipta	*Eclipta alba [E. prostata]*
Elderberry (American)	*Sambucus canadensis*
Elderberry (Black)	*Sambucus nigra*
Elderberry (Dwarf)	*Sambucus ebulus*
Elderberry (Red)	*Sambucus racemosa*
Elecampane	*Inula helenium*
Eleuthero, Siberian Ginseng	*Eleutherococcus senticosus*
Ephedra, Ma Huang	*Ephedra sinica*
Eucalyptus	*Eucalyptus globulus*, spp.
Evening Primrose	*Oenothera biennis*
Eyebright	*Euphrasia rostkoviana, E. stricta [E. officinalis]*, spp.
False Solomon's Seal	***Smilacina racemosa [Maianthemum racemosum]***
False Unicorn Root, Helonias Root	*Chamaelirium luteum [Veratrum luteum]*
Fennel	*Foeniculum vulgare*
Fenugreek	*Trigonella foenum-graecum*
Feverfew	*Tanacetum parthenium [Chrysanthemum parthenium]*
Field Mint, Wild Mint	*Mentha arvensis*
Fig	*Ficus carica*, spp.
Figwort	*Scrophularia nodosa*, spp.
Flax, Flaxseed	*Linum usitatissimum*
Fo-ti, Chinese Knotweed	*Polygonum multiflorum*
Foxglove	*Digitalis purpurea*
Frankincense	*Boswellia serrata*
Fringe Tree	*Chionanthus virginicus*
Fumitory	*Fumaria officinalis*
Garcinia	***Garcinia cambogia***
Gardenia	*Gardenia jasminoides*, spp.
Garlic	*Allium sativum*
Gentian	*Gentiana lutea*, spp.
Geranium (Wild), Cranesbill	*Geranium maculatum*
Germander	*Teucrium canadense*, spp.
Ginger	*Zingiber officinale*
Ginger (Wild)	*Asarum canadense*
Ginkgo	*Ginkgo biloba*
Ginseng (American)	*Panax quinquefolius*
Ginseng (Asian)	*Panax ginseng*
Ginseng (Siberian)	*Eleutherococcus senticosus*
Goat's Beard	*Aruncus dioicus*
Goat's Rue	*Galega officinalis*
Goldenrod	*Solidago odora*, spp.
Goldenseal	*Hydrastis canadensis*
Goldthread (Chinese)	*Coptis chinensis*
Goldthread, Canker Root (North America)	*Coptis trifolia*
Gotu kola	*Centella asiatica [Hydrocotyle asiatica]*
Gravel Root, Joe Pye Weed, Queen of the Meadow	*Eupatorium purpureum*
Great Blue Lobelia	*Lobelia siphilitica*
Greek Valerian	*Polemonium reptans*
Green Dragon	*Arisaema dracontium*
Green Tea, Black Tea	*Camellia sinensis*
Grindelia, Gumweed	*Grindelia squarrosa*, spp.
Gromwell	*Lithospermum officinale*
Ground Ivy, Gill-over-the-Ground	*Glechoma hederacea*
Guar bean, Guar gum	*Cyamopsis tetragonoloba*
Guarana	*Paullinia cupana*
Guggul	*Commiphora mukul*
Gum Arabic Tree	*Acacia senegal*
Gumweed, Grindelia	*Grindelia squarrosa*, spp.
Gymnema	*Gymnema sylvestre*
Gypsywort	*Lycopus europaeus*
Hawthorn	***Crataegus monogyna, C. oxyacantha [C. laevigata]***
Heal-all, Selfheal, Woundwort	*Prunella vulgaris*
Hellebore (False)	*Veratrum viride*
Hellebore (White)	*Veratrum album*
Helonias Root, False Unicorn Root	*Chamaelirium luteum [Veratrum luteum]*
Hemlock (Poison)	*Conium maculatum*
Henbane (Black)	*Hyoscyamus niger*
Henbane (White)	*Hyoscyamus alba*
Hepatica, Liverwort	*Hepatica acutiloba*, spp.
Herb Robert	*Geranium robertianum*
Hibiscus	*Hibiscus* spp.
Hollyhock	*Alcea rosea [Althaea rosea]*
Holy Basil, Tulsi	*Ocimum sanctum [O. tenuiflorum]*
Holy Thistle	*Cnicus benedictus*
Hops	*Humulus lupulus*
Horehound (Black)	*Marrubium nigra [Ballota nigra]*
Horehound (White)	*Marrubium vulgare*
Horny Goat Weed	*Epimedium sagittatum*
Horse Chestnut	*Aesculus hippocastanum*
Horsemint	*Monarda punctata*
Horseradish	*Armoracia rusticana [A. lapathifolia, Cochlearia armoracia]*
Horseradish (Japanese)	*Wasabia japonica [Eutrema japonicum]*
Horsetail	*Equisetum arvense*
Hydrangea (Wild)	*Hydrangea arborescens*
Hyssop	*Hyssopus officinalis*
Iceland Moss	***Cetraria islandica***

Common Name	Botanical Name
Indian Snake Root	*Rauwolfia serpentina*
Indigo (True)	*Indigofera tinctoria*
Indigo (Wild)	*Baptisia tinctoria*
Ipecac	*Cephaelis ipecacuanha*
Irish Moss	*Chondrus crispus*
Isatis, Dyer's Woad	*Isatis tinctoria*
Ivy (English, Common)	*Hedera helix*
Jacob's Ladder	***Polemonium reptans***
Jamaican Dogwood	*Piscidia piscipula [P. erythrina]*
Jasmine	*Jasminum officinale*, spp.
Jerusalem Artichoke	*Helianthus tuberosus*
Jewelweed (Orange)	*Impatiens capensis [I. biflora]*
Jewelweed (Yellow)	*Impatiens pallida*
Jimsonweed	*Datura stramonium*
Joe Pye Weed, Gravel Root, Queen of the Meadow	*Eupatorium purpureum*
Juniper Berry	*Juniperus communis*
Kava Kava	***Piper methysticum***
Kelp	*Laminaria* spp.
Khella	*Ammi visnaga*
Kola Nut	*Cola nitida, C acuminata*
Kudzu	*Pueraria montana, P. edulis, P. tuberosa, P. phaseoloides*
Lady's Bedstraw	***Galium verum***
Lady's Mantle	*Alchemilla vulgaris*
Lady's Slipper (Pink)	*Cypripedium acaule*
Lady's Slipper (Yellow)	*Cypripedium pubescens*
Lamb's Quarters	*Chenopodium berlandieri*
Lapacho, Pau D'arco	*Tabebuia impetiginosa [T. avellanedae]*
Lavender	*Lavandula angustifolia [L. officinalis, L. vera]*, spp.
Leek	*Allium ampeloprasum*
Lemon Balm	*Melissa officinalis*
Lemon Verbena	*Aloysia citriodora [A. triphylla, Lippia citriodora, Verbena citriodora]*
Lemongrass	*Cymbopogon citratus*
Leopard Flower, Blackberry Lily	*Belamcanda chinensis [Iris domestica]*
Lettuce (Wild)	*Lactuca virosa, L. canadensis*
Licorice	*Glycyrrhiza glabra*
Ligustrum, Chinese Privet	*Ligustrum lucidum*
Lily-of-the-Valley	*Convallaria majalis*
Lime	*Citrus aurantifolia*
Linden, Basswood	*Tilia americana*
European Linden	*T. cordata, T. platyphyllos*
Liverwort, Hepatica	*Hepatica acutiloba*, spp.
Lobelia, Indian Tobacco	*Lobelia inflata*
Great Blue Lobelia	*L. siphilitica*
Cardinal Flower	*L. cardinalis*
Lomatium	*Lomatium dissectum*
Loosestrife (Purple)	*Lythrum salicaria*
Lotus (Sacred)	*Nelumbo nucifera*
Lousewort, Betony	*Pedicularis canadensis*
Lovage	*Levisticum officinale*

Common Name	Botanical Name
Lungwort	*Pulmonaria officinalis*
Ma Huang	***Ephedra sinica***
Maca	*Lepidium meyenii [L. peruvianum]*
Maidenhair Fern	*Adiantum capillus-veneris, A. pedatum*
Maitake Mushroom	*Grifola frondosa*
Male Fern	*Dryopteris filix-mas*
Mandrake (European)	*Mandragora officinarum*
Manzanita	*Arctostaphylos manzanita*
Marijuana	*Cannabis sativa, C. indica*
Marjoram	*Origanum majorana*
Marsh Trefoil	*Menyanthes trifoliata*
Marshmallow	*Althaea officinalis*
Mayapple	*Podophyllum peltatum*
Meadowsweet	*Filipendula ulmaria*
Melilot (White), Honey Clover, White Sweet Clover	*Melilotus albus*
Melilot (Yellow), Yellow Sweet Clover	*Melilotus officinalis*
Milk Thistle	*Silybum marianum*
Milkweed (Common)	*Asclepias syriaca*
Milkweed (Swamp)	*Asclepias incarnata*
Mint (American Wild)	*Mentha canadensis*
Mint (Wild or Field)	*Mentha arvensis*
Mistletoe (American)	*Phoradendron leucarpum*
Mistletoe (European)	*Viscum album*
Monarda	*Monarda didyma* (red), *M. fistulosa* (lavender)
Monkshood, Aconite	*Aconitum napellus*
Mormon Tea	*Ephedra nevadensis*, spp.
Motherwort	*Leonurus cardiaca*
Mugwort	*Artemisia vulgaris*
Mugwort (Chinese)	*Artemisia argyi*
Muira Puama	*Ptychopetalum olacoides*
Mullein	*Verbascum thapsus*
Mustard (Black)	*Brassica nigra [Sinapis niger]*
Mustard (White)	*Brassica alba [Sinapis alba]*
Myrrh	*Commiphora myrrha, C. molmol*, spp.
Narrow-leaf Coneflower	***Echinacea angustifolia***
Neem	*Azadirachta indica*
Nettle (Stinging)	*Urtica dioica*
New Jersey Tea, Red Root	*Ceanothus americanus*
Night-Blooming Cereus	*Cactus grandiflorus [Selenicereus grandiflorus], Echinocereus grandiflorus*
Nightshade (Black), European Nightshade	*Solanum americanum, S. nigrum*
Nightshade (Deadly), Belladonna	*Atropa belladonna*
Noni	*Morinda officinalis*
Nutmeg	*Myristica fragrans*
Oak Trees	***Quercus* spp.**
White Oak	*Quercus alba*
Oat, Oatstraw	*Avena sativa*
Old Man's Beard	*Usnea barbata, U. florida*

Common Name	Botanical Name
Olive leaf	*Olea europaea*
Onion	*Allium cepa*
Oregano	*Origanum vulgare*
Oregon Grape Root	*Mahonia aquifolium [Berberis aquifolium]*
Orris root	*Iris florentina, I. germanica, I. pallida*
Osha	*Ligusticum porteri*
Oswego Tea, Red Bergamot, Scarlet Beebalm	*Monarda didyma*
Pale Coneflower	***Echinacea pallida***
Papaya	*Carica papaya*
Parsley	*Petroselinum crispum*
Partridge Berry, Squaw Vine	*Mitchella repens*
Pasque Flower, Pulsatilla	*Pulsatilla vulgaris*
Passion Flower	*Passiflora incarnata*
Pau D'arco, Lapacho	*Tabebuia impetiginosa [T. avellanedae]*
Pawpaw	*Asimina triloba*
Pellitory	*Anacyclus pyrethrum*
Pellitory-of-the-Wall	*Parietaria officinalis*
Pennyroyal (American)	*Hedeoma pulegioides*
Pennyroyal (European)	*Mentha pulegium*
Pepper (Black)	*Piper nigrum*
Peppermint	*Mentha x piperita*
Peruvian Bark, Cinchona	*Cinchona officinalis*
Peyote	*Lophophora williamsii*
Pine Trees	*Pinus* spp.
White Pine	*Pinus strobus*
Pineapple Weed	*Matricaria discoidea [M. matricarioides, Chamomilla suaveolens]*
Pipsissewa	*Chimaphila umbellata*
Plantain (broad leaf)	*Plantago major*
Plantain (narrow leaf)	*Plantago lanceolata*
Platycodon, Balloon Flower	*Platycodon grandiflorus*
Pleurisy Root, Butterfly Weed	*Asclepias tuberosa*
Poison Ivy	*Toxicodendron radicans*
Poison Oak	*Toxicodendron diversilobum*
Poke Root	*Phytolacca americana [P. decandra]*
Pond Lily (White)	*Nymphaea alba*
Pond Lily (Yellow)	*Nymphaea lutea*
Poppy (California)	*Eschscholzia californica*
Poppy (Opium)	*Papaver somniferum*
Prickly Ash (Northern)	*Zanthoxylum americanum*
Prickly Ash (Southern)	*Zanthoxylum clava-herculis*
Prickly Pear Cactus	*Opuntia humifusa,* spp.
Primrose	*Primula vulgaris*
Primula, Cowslip	*Primula veris [P. officinalis]*
Privet (Chinese), Ligustrum	*Ligustrum lucidum*
Psyllium	*Plantago psyllium, P. ovata*
Pulsatilla, Pasque Flower	*Pulsatilla vulgaris*
Purple Coneflower	*Echinacea purpurea*
Purple Loosestrife	*Lythrum salicaria*
Purslane	*Portulaca oleracea*
Pygeum	*Pygeum africanum*
Queen Anne's Lace, Wild Carrot	***Daucus carota***
Queen of the Meadow Gravel Root, Joe Pye Weed	*Eupatorium purpureum*
Queen's Root	*Stillingia sylvatica*
Quinine, Peruvian Bark	*Cinchona officinalis*
Ragweed	***Ambrosia artemisiifolia***
Ragwort	*Senecio aureus [Packera aureus]*
Ramp, Wild Leek	*Allium tricoccum*
Raspberry (Red)	*Rubus idaeus*
Rauwolfia	*Rauvolfia serpentina*
Red Clover	*Trifolium pratense*
Red Root, New Jersey Tea	*Ceanothus americanus*
Rehmannia	*Rehmannia glutinosa, R. chinensis*
Reishi Mushroom	*Ganoderma lucidum*
Rhodiola	*Rhodiola rosea*
Rhubarb	*Rheum rhabarbarum*
Rooibos	*Aspalathus linearis*
Rose, Rose hips	*Rosa rugosa, R. canina, R. majalis, spp.*
Rosemary	*Rosmarinus officinalis*
Rue	*Ruta graveolens*
Sage (Cinnabar), Dan Shen	***Salvia miltiorrhiza***
Sage (Garden)	*Salvia officinalis*
Sage (Spanish)	*Salvia lavandulifolia*
Sage (White)	*Salvia apiana*
Sagebrush	*Artemisia tridentata*
Saint John's Wort	*Hypericum perforatum*
Sanicle (American)	*Sanicula marilandica, S. canadensis*
Sanicle (European)	*Sanicula europaea*
Sarsaparilla	*Smilax aristolochiifolia, S. ornata, S. officinalis,*spp.
Sarsaparilla (Wild)	*Aralia nudicaulis*
Sassafras	*Sassafras albidum*
Savory (Summer)	*Satureja hortensis*
Savory (Winter)	*Satureja montana*
Saw Palmetto	*Serenoa repens [S. serrulata, Sabal serrulata]*
Schisandra, Schizandra	*Schisandra chinensis*
Scotch broom	*Cytisus scoparius*
Scouring Rush	*Equisetum hyemale*
Scullcap, Skullcap	*Scutellaria lateriflora*
Scullcap (Chinese)	*Scutellaria baicalensis, S. barbata*
Selfheal, Heal-all, Woundwort	*Prunella vulgaris*
Seneca Snakeroot	*Polygala senega*
Senna	*Senna alexandrina [S. marilandica, Cassia marilandica, C. senna, C. angustifolia]*

Common Name	Botanical Name
Sheep's Sorrel	*Rumex acetosella*
Shepherd's Purse	*Capsella bursa-pastoris*
Shiitake Mushroom	*Lentinula edodes*
Siberian Ginseng, Eleuthero	*Eleutherococcus senticosus*
Siberian Motherwort	*Leonurus sibericus*
Silverweed	*Potentilla anserina [Argentina anserina]*
Skullcap, Scullcap	*Scutellaria lateriflora*
Skunk Cabbage	*Symplocarpus foetidus*
Slippery Elm	*Ulmus rubra [U. fulva]*
Soapwort, Bouncing Bet	*Saponaria officinalis*
Solomon's Seal	*Polygonatum biflorum*
Solomon's Seal (False)	*Smilacina racemosa [Maianthemum racemosum]*
Sorrel (Common)	*Rumex acetosa*
Southernwood	*Artemisia abrotanum*
Soybean	*Glycine max*
Spearmint	*Mentha spicata [M. viridis]*
Speedwell	*Veronica officinalis*
Spicebush	*Lindera benzoin*
Spikenard (American)	*Aralia racemosa*
Spirulina	*Arthrospira platensis, A. maxima*
Squaw vine, Partridge Berry	*Mitchella repens*
Squill	*Urginea maritima [Drimia maritima, Scilla maritima]*
St. John's Wort	*Hypericum perforatum*
Stevia	*Stevia rebaudiana*
Stillingia	*Stillingia sylvatica*
Stinging Nettle	*Urtica dioica*
Stone Root	*Collinsonia canadensis*
Sumac (red berry)	*Rhus glabra*
Sundew	*Drosera rotundifolia*, spp.
Sunflower	*Helianthus annuus*
Sweet Annie	*Artemisia annua*
Sweet Cicely	*Osmorhiza claytonii*
European Cicely	*Myrrhis odorata*
Sweet Flag, Calamus	*Acorus calamus, A. americanus*
Sweet Woodruff	*Galium odoratum*
Sweetgrass	*Heirachloe odorata*
Tansy	***Tanacetum vulgare***
Tarragon	*Artemisia dracunculus*
Tea Tree oil	*Melaleuca alternifolia*
Teasel	*Dipsacus sylvestris*
Tennessee Coneflower	*Echinacea Tennesseensis*
Thorowax	*Bupleurum chinense*
Thyme (Garden)	*Thymus vulgaris*
Toadflax, Butter-and-Eggs	*Linaria vulgaris*
Tobacco	*Nicotiana tabacum*, spp.
Tolu Balsam, Balsam of Tolu	*Myroxylon balsamum*
Tormentil, Cinquefoil	*Tormentilla erecta [Potentilla erecta, P. tormentilla]*
Trillium, Birthroot	*Trillium* spp.
True Unicorn Root	*Aletris farinosa*
Tulsi, Holy Basil	*Ocimum sanctum [O. tenuiflorum]*
Turkey Rhubarb	*Rheum palmatum*
Turkey Tail mushroom	*Trametes versicolor*
Turmeric	*Curcuma longa*
Turtlehead, Balmony	*Chelone glabra*
Twinleaf	*Jeffersonia diphylla*
Una de Gato, Cat's Claw	***Uncaria tomentosa***
Usnea, Old Man's Beard	*Usnea barbata, U. florida*, spp.
Uva-ursi, Bearberry	*Arctostaphylos uva-ursi*
Valerian	***Valeriana officinalis***
Venus Fly Trap	*Dionaea muscipula*
Vervain (Blue)	*Verbena hastata*
Vervain (European)	*Verbena officinalis*
Violet	*Viola papilionacea, V. odorata*, spp.
Virginia Snakeroot	*Aristolochia serpentaria*
Vitex, Chasteberry	*Vitex agnus-castus*
Walnut Tree (American),	***Juglans nigra***
(English)	***J. regia***
Water Lily (White)	*Nymphaea alba, N. odorata*
Water Lily (Yellow)	*Nymphaea lutea*
Water Mint	*Mentha aquatica*
Wild Angelica	*Angelica sylvestris*
Wild Carrot, Queen Anne's Lace	*Daucus carota*
Wild Indigo	*Baptisia tinctoria*
Wild Leek, Ramp	*Allium tricoccum*
Wild Mint, Field Mint	*Mentha arvensis*
Wild Yam	*Dioscorea villosa*, spp.
Willow Tree (Black)	*Salix nigra*
Willow Tree (White)	*Salix alba*
Wintergreen	*Gaultheria procumbens*
Witch Hazel	*Hamamelis virginiana*
Woad, Isatis	*Isatis tinctoria*
Wolfbane	*Aconitum vulparia*
Wood Avens	*Geum urbanum*
Wood Betony	*Stachys officinalis [S. betonica, Betonica officinalis]*
Wood Sorrel	*Oxalis corniculata*
Woodruff (Sweet)	*Galium odoratum*
Wormwood	*Artemisia absinthium*
Woundwort, Heal-all, Selfheal	*Prunella vulgaris*
Yam (Chinese)	***Dioscorea batata***
Yam (Wild American)	*Dioscorea villosa, D. quaternata*, spp.
Yarrow	*Achillea millefolium*
Yellow Dock Broad-leaf Dock	*Rumex crispus, R. obtusifolius*
Yellow Jasmine	*Gelsemium sempervirens*
Yerba Mansa	*Anemopsis californica*
Yerba Mate'	*Ilex paraguariensis*
Yerba Santa	*Eriodictyon californicum*
Yew (Pacific)	*Taxus brevifolia, T. baccata*
Yohimbe	*Pausinystalia yohimbe*
Yucca, Soapweed	*Yucca glauca, Y. filamentosa*, spp.

Cross-Reference of Botanical and Common Plant Names

BOTANICAL NAME	COMMON NAME
Acacia senegal	**Gum Arabic Tree**
Achillea millefolium	Yarrow
Aconitum napellus	Monkshood, Aconite
Aconitum vulparia	Wolfbane
Acorus calamus [A. americanus]	Calamus, Sweet Flag
Actaea pachypoda [A. alba]	Baneberry, Bugbane (white)
Actaea racemosa	Black Cohosh
Adiantum capillus-veneris, A. pedatum	Maidenhair Fern
Aesculus hippocastanum	Horse Chestnut
Agastache foeniculum	Anise Hyssop
Agathosma betulina	Buchu
Agave americana	Century Plant, Agave
Agrimonia eupatoria, A. gryposepala, spp.	Agrimony
Agropyron repens	Couch Grass
Ajuga reptans	Bugle
Alcea rosea	Hollyhock
Alchemilla vulgaris	Lady's Mantle
Aletris farinosa	True Unicorn Root, Colic Root
Allium ampeloprasum	Leek
Allium cepa	Onion
Allium sativum	Garlic
Allium schoenoprasum	Chives
Allium tricoccum	Ramp, Wild Leek
Aloe vera	Aloe Vera
Aloysia citriodora [A. triphylla]	Lemon Verbena
Althaea officinalis	Marshmallow
Althaea rosea	Hollyhock
Amaranthus spp.	Amaranth
Ambrosia artemisiifolia	Common Ragweed
Ammi visnaga	Khella
Anacyclus pyrethrum	Pellitory
Andrographis paniculata	Andrographis
Anemopsis californica	Yerba Mansa
Anethum graveolens	Dill
Angelica archangelica	Angelica
Angelica atropurpurea	American Angelica
Angelica sinensis	Dong Quai
Angelica sylvestris	Wild Angelica
Anthemis nobilis	Roman/English Chamomile
Anthriscus cerefolium	Chervil
Apium graveolens	Celery
Aralia nudicaulis	Wild/False Sarsaparilla
Aralia racemosa	American Spikenard
Arctium lappa	Greater Burdock
Arctium minus	Lesser Burdock
Arctostaphylos manzanita	Manzanita
Arctostaphylos uva-ursi	Bearberry, Uva-ursi
Argentina anserina	Silverweed
Arisaema dracontium	Dragonroot, Green Dragon
Aristolochia serpentaria	Virginia Snakeroot
Armoracia rusticana [A. lapathifolia]	Horseradish
Arnica montana	Arnica
Artemisia abrotanum	Southernwood
Artemisia absinthium	Wormwood
Artemisia annua	Sweet Annie
Artemisia argyi	Chinese Mugwort
Artemisia dracunculus	Tarragon
Artemisia tridentata	Sagebrush
Artemisia vulgaris	Mugwort
Arthrospira platensis, A. maxima	Spirulina
Aruncus dioicus	Goat's Beard
Asarum canadense	Wild Ginger
Asclepias incarnata	Swamp Milkweed
Asclepias syriaca	Common Milkweed
Asclepias tuberosa	Pleurisy Root, Butterfly Weed
Asimina triloba	Pawpaw
Aspalathus linearis	Rooibos
Asparagus officinalis	Asparagus
Astragalus membranaceus	Astragalus
Atractylodes macrocephala	Atractylodes
Atropa belladonna	Belladonna, Deadly Nightshade
Avena sativa	Oat, Oatstraw
Azadirachta indica	Neem
Bacopa monnieri	**Bacopa**
Ballota nigra	Black Horehound
Baptisia tinctoria	Wild Indigo
Barosma betulina	Buchu
Belamcanda chinensis	Leopard Flower, Blackberry Lily
Berberis aquifolium	Oregon Grape Root
Berberis vulgaris, B. canadensis	Barberry
Betonica officinalis	Wood Betony
Borago officinalis	Borage
Boswellia serrata	Boswellia, Frankincense Tree

Botanical Name	Common Name
Brassica alba	White Mustard
Brassica nigra	Black Mustard
Bryonia alba	White Bryony
Bupleurum chinense	Bupleurum, Thorowax
Cactus grandiflorus	**Night-Blooming Cereus**
Calamintha sylvatica	Calamint
Calendula officinalis	Calendula
Camellia sinensis	Black Tea/Green Tea
Cannabis sativa, C. indica	Cannabis, Marijuana, Hemp
Capsella bursa-pastoris	Shepherd's Purse
Capsicum annuum	Cayenne
Carica papaya	Papaya
Carum carvi	Caraway
Cassia marilandica [C. senna, C. angustifolia]	Senna
Caulophyllum thalictroides	Blue Cohosh
Ceanothus americanus	New Jersey Tea, Red Root
Centaurium erythraea	European Centaury
Centella asiatica	Gotu Kola
Cephaelis ipecacuanha	Ipecac
Ceratonia siliqua	Carob
Cetraria islandica	Iceland Moss
Chamaelirium luteum	False Unicorn Root, Helonias Root
Chamaemelum nobile	Roman/English Chamomile
Chamomilla recutita	German Chamomile
Chamomilla suaveolens	Pineapple Weed
Chelidonium majus	Greater Celandine
Chelone glabra	Balmony, Turtlehead
Chenopodium berlandieri	Lamb's Quarters
Chimaphila umbellata	Pipsissewa
Chionanthus virginicus	Fringe Tree
Chlorella regularis, spp.	Chlorella
Chondrus crispus	Irish Moss
Chrysanthemum balsamita	Costmary
Chrysanthemum parthenium	Feverfew
Cichorium intybus	Chicory
Cimicifuga racemosa	Black Cohosh
Cinchona officinalis, spp.	Peruvian Cinchona Tree (source of quinine)
Cinnamomum spp.	Cinnamon
Cinnamomum camphora	Camphor
Cnicus benedictus	Blessed Thistle, Holy Thistle
Cochlearia armoracia	Horseradish
Codenopsis pilosula	Dang Shen, Codonopsis
Coffea arabica, spp.	Coffee
Cola nitida, C. acuminata	Kola Nut
Collinsonia canadensis	Stone Root
Commiphora gileadensis	Balm of Gilead (Middle East)
Commiphora mukul	Guggul
Commiphora myrrha, C. molmol, spp.	Myrrh
Conium maculatum	Poison Hemlock
Convallaria majalis	Lily-of-the-Valley
Coptis chinensis	Chinese Coptis, Chinese Goldthread
Coptis trifolia	American Goldthread, Canker Root
Cordyceps sinensis	Cordyceps, Chinese Caterpillar Fungus
Coreopsis tinctoria	Coreopsis
Coriandrum sativum	Coriander
Corydalis bulbosa, spp.	Corydalis
Crataegus monogyna, C. oxyacantha [C. laevigata]	Hawthorn
Cuminum cyminum	Cumin
Curcuma longa	Turmeric
Cuscuta epithymum	Dodder
Cyamopsis tetragonoloba	Guar bean, Guar gum
Cymbopogon citratus	Lemongrass
Cynara scolymus	Artichoke
Cypripedium acuale	Lady's Slipper (pink flowers)
C. pubescens	(yellow flowers)
Cytisus scoparius	Scotch broom
Daemonorops draco	**Dragon's Blood**
Datura stramonium	Jimsonweed, Datura
Daucus carota	Queen Anne's Lace, Wild Carrot
Digitalis purpurea	Foxglove
Dionaea muscipula	Venus Fly Trap
Dioscorea batata	Chinese Yam
Dioscorea villosa	American Wild Yam
Dipsacus sylvestris	Teasel
Drimia maritima	Squill
Drosera rotundifolia	Sundew
Dryopteris filix-mas	Male Fern
Echinacea angustifolia	**Echinacea, Narrow Leaf Coneflower**
Echinacea pallida	Pale Coneflower
Echinacea purpurea	Purple Coneflower
Echinacea tennesseensis	Tennessee Coneflower
Echinocereus grandiflorus	Night-Blooming Cereus
Echinopanax horridus	Devil's Club
Eclipta alba [E. prostata]	Eclipta
Elettaria cardamomum	Cardamom
Eleutherococcus senticosus	Eleuthero, Siberian Ginseng
Elymus repens [Elytrigia repens]	Couch Grass
Ephedra nevadensis	Mormon Tea

Ephedra sinica	Ma Huang, Ephedra
Epimedium sagitttatum	Horny Goat Weed
Equisetum arvense	Horsetail
Equisetum hyemale	Scouring Rush
Eriodictyon californicum	Yerba Santa
Eruca sativa, E. vesicaria	Arugula
Erythraea centaurium	European Centuary
Erythroxylum coca	Coca (source of cocaine)
Eschscholzia californica	California Poppy
Eucalyptus globulus, spp.	Eucalyptus
Eupatorium perfoliatum	Boneset
Eupatorium purpureum	Gravel Root, Joe Pye Weed, Queen of the Meadow
Euphrasia rostkoviana, E. stricta [E. officinalis], spp.	Eyebright
Fagopyrum esculentum	**Buckwheat**
Ficus carica	Fig
Filipendula ulmaria	Meadowsweet
Foeniculum vulgare	Fennel
Fucus vesiculosus	Bladderwrack
Fumaria officinalis	Fumitory
Galega officinalis	**Goat's Rue**
Galium aparine	Cleavers, Bedstraw
Galium odoratum	Sweet Woodruff
Galium verum	Lady's Bedstraw
Ganoderma lucidum	Reishi mushroom
Garcinia cambogia	Garcinia
Gardenia jasminoides	Gardenia
Gaultheria procumbens	Wintergreen
Gelidium amansii, spp.	Agar-agar (from red algae)
Gentiana lutea	Gentian
Geranium maculatum	Cranesbill, Wild Geranium
Geranium robertianum	Herb Robert
Geum urbanum	Wood Avens, Avens
Ginkgo biloba	Ginkgo
Glechoma hederacea	Ground Ivy, Gill-over-the-Ground
Glycine max	Soybean
Glycyrrhiza glabra	Licorice
Grifola frondosa	Maitake Mushroom
Grindelia squarrosa	Grindelia, Gumweed
Gymnema sylvestre	Gymnema
Hamamelis virginiana	**Witch Hazel**
Harpagophytum procumbens	Devil's Claw
Hedeoma pulegioides	American Pennyroyal
Hedera helix	English Ivy, Common Ivy
Heirachloe odorata	Sweetgrass
Helianthus annuus	Sunflower
Helianthus tuberosus	Jerusalem Artichoke
Hepatica acutiloba, spp.	Hepatica, Liverwort
Heuchera americana	Alumroot
Hibiscus spp.	Hibiscus
Hordeum vulgare	Barley
Humulus lupulus	Hops
Hydrangea arborescens	Wild Hydrangea
Hydrastis canadensis	Goldenseal
Hydrocotyle asiatica	Gotu Kola
Hyoscyamus alba	White Henbane
Hyoscyamus niger	Black Henbane
Hypericum perforatum	Saint John's Wort
Hyssopus officinalis	Hyssop
Ilex paraguariensis	**Yerba Mate'**
Impatiens capensis [I. biflora]	Orange Jewelweed
Impatiens pallida	Yellow Jewelweed
Indigofera tinctoria	True Indigo
Inula helenium	Elecampane
Iris domestica	Blackberry Lily, Leopard Flower
Iris germanica, I. florentina, I. pallida	Orris Root
Iris versicolor	Blue Flag
Isatis tinctoria	Isatis, Woad
Jasminum officinale	**Jasmine**
Jeffersonia diphylla	Twinleaf
Juglans cinerea	Butternut Tree
Juglans nigra	American Black Walnut
Juglans regia	English Black Walnut
Juniperus communis	Juniper Berry
Lactuca virosa, L. canadensis	**Wild Lettuce**
Laminaria spp.	Kelp
Larrea tridentata	Chaparral
Laurus nobilis	Bay Laurel
Lavandula angustifolia [L. officinalis, L. vera, L. spica], spp.	Lavender
Lentinula edodes	Shiitake mushroom
Leonurus cardiaca	Motherwort
Leonurus sibericus	Siberian Motherwort
Lepidium meyenii [L. peruvianum]	Maca
Leptandra virginica	Culver's Root, Black Root
Levisticum officinale	Lovage
Ligusticum porteri	Osha
Ligustrum lucidum	Ligustrum, Chinese Privet
Linaria vulgaris	Toadflax, Butter-and-Eggs
Lindera benzoin	Spicebush
Linum usitatissimum	Flax
Lippia citriodora	Lemon Verbena
Lithospermum officinale	Gromwell
Lobelia cardinalis	Cardinal Flower
Lobelia inflata	Lobelia, Indian Tobacco
Lobelia siphilitica	Great Blue Lobelia

Lomatium dissectum	Lomatium
Lophophora williamsii	Peyote
Lycopodium clavatum	Clubmoss
Lycopus americanus, L. virginicus	Bugleweed
Lycopus europaeus	Gypsywort, European Bugleweed
Lythrum salicaria	Purple Loosestrife
Mahonia aquifolium	**Oregon Grape Root**
Maianthemum racemosum	False Solomon's Seal
Malus domestica [M. pumila]	Apple Tree
Mandragora officinarum	European Mandrake
Marrubium nigra	Black Horehound
Marrubium vulgare	White Horehound
Matricaria discoidea [M. matricarioides]	Pineapple Weed
Matricaria recutita [M. chamomilla]	German Chamomile
Medicago sativa	Alfalfa
Melaleuca alternifolia	Tea Tree (source of Melaleuca Oil)
Melaleuca cajeputi, M. leucadendra	Cajeput Tree
Melilotus albus	White Melilot, White Sweet Clover, Honey Clover
Melilotus officinalis	Yellow Melilot, Yellow Sweet Clover
Melissa officinalis	Lemon Balm
Mentha aquatica	Water Mint
Mentha arvensis	Field Mint, Wild Mint
Mentha canadensis	American Wild Mint
Mentha x piperita	Peppermint
Mentha pulegium	European Pennyroyal
Mentha spicata [M. viridis]	Spearmint
Menyanthes trifoliata	Bogbean, Buckbean, Marsh Trefoil
Mitchella repens	Partridge Berry, Squaw Vine
Momordica charantia	Bitter Melon
Monarda didyma	Red Bergamot, Oswego Tea, Scarlet Beebalm
Monarda fistulosa	Lavender Beebalm, Wild Bergamot
Monarda punctata	Horsemint
Myrica cerifera	Bayberry
Myristica fragrans	Nutmeg
Myroxylon balsamum	Tolu Balsam, Balsam of Tolu
Myrrhis odorata	Sweet Cicely (European)
Nelumbo nucifera	**Sacred Lotus**
Nepeta cataria	Catnip
Nereocystis luetkeana	Kelp
Nicotiana tabacum	Tobacco
Nymphaea alba, N. odorata	White Water Lily, White Pond Lily
Nymphaea lutea	Yellow Water Lily, Yellow Pond Lily
Ocimum basilicum	**Basil**
Ocimum sanctum [O. tenuiflorum]	Holy Basil, Tulsi
Oenothera biennis	Evening Primrose
Olea europaea	Olive leaf
Oplopanax horridus	Devil's Club
Opuntia humifusa	Prickly Pear Cactus
Origanum majorana	Marjorum
Origanum vulgare	Oregano
Osmorhiza claytonii	Sweet Cicely
Osmorhiza longistylis	Anise Root
Oxalis corniculata	Wood Sorrel
Packera aureus	**Ragwort**
Panax ginseng	Asian Ginseng
Panax quinquefolius	American Ginseng
Papaver somniferum	Opium Poppy
Parietaria officinalis	Pellitory-of-the-Wall
Passiflora incarnata	Passion Flower
Paullinia cupana	Guarana
Pausinystalia yohimbe	Yohimbe
Pedicularis canadensis	Betony, Lousewort
Petasites hybridus	Butterbur
Petroselinum crispum	Parsley
Peumus boldus	Boldo
Phoradendron leucarpum	American Mistletoe
Phytolacca decandra [P. americana]	Poke
Pimenta dioica	Allspice
Pimpinella anisum	Anise, Aniseed
Pinus spp.	Pine Trees
Pinus strobus	White Pine
Piper methysticum	Kava Kava
Piper nigrum	Black Pepper
Piscidia piscipula [P. erythrina]	Jamaican Dogwood
Plantago lanceolata	Narrow-leaf Plantain
Plantago major	Broad-leaf Plantain
Plantago psyllium, P. ovata	Psyllium seed
Platycodon grandiflorus	Balloonflower
Podophyllum peltatum	Mayapple
Polemonium reptans	Greek Valerian, Abscess Root, Jacob's Ladder
Polygala senega	Seneca Snakeroot
Polygonatum biflorum	Solomon's Seal
Polygonum bistorta	Bistort
Polygonum multiflorum	Fo-ti, Chinese Knotweed
Portulaca oleracea	Purslane
Potentilla spp.	Cinquefoil
Potentilla anserina	Silverweed
Potentilla recta, P. tormentilla	Common Cinquefoil, Tormentil
Potentilla reptans	Creeping Cinquefoil
Primula veris	Cowslip, Primula
Prunella vulgaris	Selfheal, Heal-all, Woundwort
Prunus armeniaca	Apricot Tree
Prunus dulcis [P. amygdalus]	Almond Tree
Prunus serotina	Wild Cherry Tree

Ptychopetalum olacoides	Muira Puama
Pueraria montana, P. edulis, P. tuberosa, P. phaseoloides	Kudzu
Pulmonaria officinalis	Lungwort
Pulsatilla vulgaris	Pulsatilla, Pasque Flower
Pygeum africanum	Pygeum
***Quercus* spp.**	**Oak Trees**
Quercus alba	White Oak Tree
Rauvolfia serpentina	**Rauwolfia, Indian Snake Root**
Rehmannia glutinosa [R. chinensis]	Rehmannia
Rhamnus cathartica	Buckthorn
Rhamnus purshiana	Cascara Sagrada
Rheum palmatum	Turkey Rhubarb
Rheum rhabarbarum	Rhubarb
Rhodiola rosea	Rhodiola
Rhus glabra	Red Sumac, Smooth Sumac
Ribes nigrum	Black Currant
Ricinus communis	Castor Oil Plant
Rosa rugosa, R. canina, R. majalis, spp.	Rose, Rose hips
Rosmarinus officinalis	Rosemary
Rubus idaeus	Red Raspberry
Rubus villosus, R. fruticosus	Blackberry
Rudbeckia hirta	Black-eyed Susan
Rumex acetosa	Common Sorrel
Rumex acetosella	Sheep's Sorrel
Rumex crispus	Yellow Dock
Rumex obtusifolius	Broad-leafed Yellow Dock
Ruscus aculeatus	Butcher's Broom
Ruta graveolens	Rue
Sabal serrulata	**Saw Palmetto**
Sabatia angularis	American Centaury
Salix alba	White Willow
Salix nigra	Black Willow
Salvia apiana	White Sage
Salvia lavandulifolia	Spanish Sage
Salvia miltiorrhiza	Cinnabar Sage, Dan Shen
Salvia officinalis	Garden Sage, Common Sage
Salvia sclarea	Clary Sage
Sambucus canadensis	American Elderberry
Sambucus ebulus	Dwarf European Elderberry
Sambucus nigra	Black Elderberry
Sambucus racemosa	Red Elderberry
Sanguinaria canadensis	Bloodroot
Sanguisorba officinalis	Great Burnet
Sanicula europaea	European Sanicle
Sanicula marilandica, S. canadensis	American Sanicle
Saponaria officinalis	Soapwort, Bouncing Bet
Sassafras albidum	Sassafras
Satureja hortensis	Summer Savory
Satureja montana	Winter Savory

Schisandra chinensis	Schisandra, Schizandra
Scilla maritima	Squill
Scrophularia nodosa	Figwort
Scutellaria baicalensis	Chinese Scullcap, Baical
Scutellaria barbata	Chinese Scullcap
Scutellaria lateriflora	Scullcap, Skullcap
Selenicereus grandiflorus	Night-Blooming Cereus
Senecio aureus	Ragwort
Senna alexandrina [S. marilandica]	Senna
Serenoa repens [S. serrulata]	Saw Palmetto
Silybum marianum	Milk Thistle
Sinapis alba	White Mustard
Sinapis niger	Black Mustard
Smilacina racemosa	False Solomon's Seal
Smilax ornata, S. aristolochiifolia, S. officinalis	Sarsaparilla
Solanum nigrum, S. americanum	Black Nightshade
Solidago odora, spp.	Goldenrod
Stachys officinalis [S. betonica]	Wood Betony
Stellaria media, spp.	Chickweed
Stevia rebaudiana	Stevia
Stillingia sylvatica	Stillingia, Queen's Root
Styrax benzoin	Benzoin Tree
Symphytum officinale	Comfrey
Symphytum x uplandicum	Russian Comfrey
Symplocarpus foetidus	Skunk Cabbage
Syzygium aromaticum	Clove
Tabebuia impetiginosa [T. avellanedae]	**Pau D'arco, Lapacho**
Tanacetum balsamita	Costmary
Tanacetum parthenium	Feverfew
Tanacetum vulgare	Tansy
Taraxacum officinale	Dandelion
Taxus brevifolia	Pacific Yew
Teucrium canadense	Germander
Theobroma cacao	Cocoa (source of chocolate)
Thymus vulgaris	Common Thyme, Garden Thyme
Tilia cordata, T. platyphyllos	Linden, (European)
T. americana	American Linden, Basswood
Tormentilla erecta	Common Tormentil, Cinquefoil
Toxicodendron diversilobum	Poison Oak
Toxicodendron radicans	Poison Ivy
Trametes versicolor	Turkey Tail mushroom
Trifolium pratense	Red Clover
Trifolium repens	White Clover
Trigonella foenum-graecum	Fenugreek

Trillium erectum, T. sessile, spp.	Birthroot, Bethroot, Trillium
Turnera diffusa	Damiana
Tussilago farfara	Coltsfoot
Ulmus rubra [U. fulva]	**Slippery Elm**
Umbellularia californica	California Bay Laurel
Uncaria tomentosa	Cat's Claw, Una de Gato
Urginea maritima	Squill
Urtica dioica	Stinging Nettle
Usnea barabta, U. florida, spp.	Old Man's Beard, Usnea
***Vaccinium corymbosum,* spp.**	**Blueberry**
Vaccinium macrocarpon, V. oxycoccos, spp.	Cranberry
Vaccinium myrtillus	Bilberry
Valeriana officinalis	Valerian
Veratrum album	White Hellebore
Veratrum viride	False Hellebore
Verbascum thapsus	Mullein
Verbena citriodora	Lemon Verbena
Verbena hastata	Blue Vervain
Verbena officinalis	European Vervain
Veronica officinalis	Speedwell
Veronicastrum virginicum	Culver's Root, Black Root
Viburnum opulus	Cramp Bark
Viburnum prunifolium	Black Haw
Viola papilionacea, V. odorata, spp.	Violet
Viscum album	Mistletoe
Vitex agnus-castus	Chasteberry, Vitex
Wasabia japonica	**Japanese Horseradish**
Withania somnifera	Ashwagandha
***Yucca glauca, Y. filamentosa,* spp.**	**Yucca**
Zanthoxylum americanum	**Prickly Ash (Northern)**
Zanthoxylum clava-herculis	Prickly Ash (Southern)
Zea mays	Corn, Corn Silk
Zingiber officinale	Ginger

APPENDIX THREE

Media Sources for Herbal Research

The following is a list of websites, databases, and online search engines that provide information for further research of medicinal herbs and holistic healing.

PubMed.com or ncbi.nlm.nih.gov/pubmed/: a free search engine of the US National Library of Medicine (NLM) at the US National Institutes of Health (NIH). It includes over 16 million citations from MEDLINE and other scientific journals.

nccih.nih.gov/: provides information and resources on medicinal herbs and health from the National Center for Complementary and Integrative Health at the US National Institutes of Health (NIH).

medlineplus.gov: the Medline Plus site from the US National Institute of Health (NIH) that provides information on health conditions and wellness issues.

abc.herbalgram.org: website of the American Botanical Council (ABC), a leading international, nonprofit educational organization that researches many aspects of medicinal plants. The American Botanical Council publishes the authoritative medicinal herb journal *HerbalGram*. Also see the American Botanical Council's Educational Link at cms.herbalgram.org/edlinks/index.

unitedplantsavers.org: website of United Plant Savers, a grassroots nonprofit organization whose mission is to protect native medicinal plants in the United States and Canada and their native habitat, to ensure abundant renewable supplies of medicinal plants for generations to come, and to advance herbal research and education.

ars-grin.gov/duke/ and phytochem.nal.usda.gov: a phytochemical and ethnobotanical database compiled by the late James Duke, PhD, a leading international authority of medicinal herbs. The website provides an extensive database of medicinal herbs and their chemical constituents, bioactivity, and ethnobotany using scientific and common names.

herbs.org: website of the Herb Research Foundation that is dedicated to herbal research and education.

americanherbalistsguild.com: website of the American Herbalists Guild, which is a nonprofit, educational organization representing the goals and voices of herbalists.

henriettes-herb.com: Henriette's herbal is one of the oldest and largest herbal medicine websites. It's been online since 1995 and is run by Henriette Kress, a herbalist in Helsinki, Finland.

herbnet.com: a very comprehensive website about medicinal herbs.

napralert.org: NAPRALERT (Natural Products Alert) is a database containing scientifically validated data on natural products, including medicinal plants. It was founded by the late Professor Norman R. Farnsworth, renowned pharmacognosist, internationally respected medicinal plant researcher, and head of the Department of Pharmacognosy and Pharmacology in the College of Pharmacy at the University of Illinois at Chicago.

medherb.com: an excellent website of the North American Institute of Medical Herbalism, founded by

Paul Bergner, medical herbalist and clinical nutritionist. The website provides links to herbal resources and education.

swsbm.com: website of the Southwest School of Botanical Medicine founded by the late herbalist, Michael Moore. It is an excellent site that includes links to the works of the American Eclectic physicians, who prescribed herbs in their medical practice and recorded their clinical experience.

healthy.net: an extensive source of information about integrative medicine and medicinal herbs.

naturalmedicinalherbs.net: this search engine has information on hundreds of medicinal herbs.

herbmed.org: an interactive herbal database providing hyperlinked access to scientific data underlying the use of herbs. It is an evidence-based information resource provided by the Alternative Medicine Foundation.

rmhiherbal.org: The Rocky Mountain Herbal Institute offers this directory of mostly online information on herbal sciences, health topics, research and educational resources, distributors of herbal textbooks, and more.

dogpile.com: Dogpile search engine is powered by Metasearch technology and provides the best results from leading search engines on a wide variety of subjects, including medicinal herbs.

Bibliography

INTRODUCTION

Eckhart Tolle quote is from the book *Stillness Speaks*. Copyright ©2003 by Eckhart Tolle. Reprinted with permission of New World Library, Novato, CA. www.newworldlibrary.com.

Section One: Fundamentals of Medicinal Herbalism

THE HISTORY OF HERBALISM AND EARLY MEDICINE

Achterberg, J. *Imagery in Healing: Shamanism and Modern Medicine*. Boston, MA: New Science Library, 1985.
Akerele, O. Summary of WHO Guidelines for the Assessment of Herbal Medicines. *HerbalGram*. 1993;28:13-20.
Arber, A. *Herbals: Their Origin and Evolution*. Darien, CT: Hafner Publishing Company, 1938.
Bensky, D., Gamble, A. *Chinese Herbal Medicine (Materia Medica)*. Seattle, WA: Eastland Press, 1986.
Berman, A., Flannery, M. *America's Botanico-Medical Movements*. New York, NY: Pharmaceutical Products Press, 2001.
Bettmann, O. *A Pictorial History of Medicine*. Springfield, IL: Charles C. Thomas Publisher, 1962.
Blumenthal, M. ESCOP, European Harmony in Phytotherapy. *HerbalGram*. 1992;24:41-2.
____________. Congress Passes Dietary Supplement Health & Education Act (DSHEA) of 1994. *HerbalGram*. 1994;32:18-20.
____________. FDA Proposes New Rules on Dietary Supplement Structure-Function Claims. *HerbalGram*. 1998;43:26-8.
____________. Congress Increasingly Active on Herbs and Dietary Supplements. *HerbalGram*. 2004;61:56-9.
____________. Market Report: Herbal Supplement Sales Rise in All Channels in 2009. *HerbalGram*. 2010;86:62-5.
____________. Herb Sales Continue Growth-Up 3.3% in 2010. *HerbalGram*. 2011;90:64-7.
Boyle, W. *Herb Doctors: Pioneers in 19th Century American Botanical Medicine*. East Palestine, OH: Buckeye Naturopathic Press, 1988.
Brown, E. *Arabian Medicine*. London, England: Cambridge University Press, 1921.
Buhner, S. *Sacred Plant Medicine: The Wisdom of Native American Herbalism*. Rochester, VT: Bear & Company, 2006.
Campbell, D., Kegan, P. *Arabian Medicine*. England: Trench, Trubner & Company, 1926.
Castleman, M. *The Healing Herbs*. Emmaus, PA: Rodale Press, 1991.
Cavaliere, C. Herbal Supplement Sales Experience Slight Increase in 2008. *HerbalGram*. 2009;82:58-61.
Coulter, H. *Divided Legacy: A History of the Schism in Medical Thought* (Vol. 3). Washington, DC: McGrath Publishing Company, 1973.
Cranz, H. Medicinal Plants and Phytomedicines Within the European Community. *HerbalGram*. 1993;30:50-3.
Dash, R., Sharma, V. *Caraka Samhita*. Chowkhamba Varanasi, India: Sanskrit Series Office, 1976.
Desai, P. *Health and Medicine in the Hindu Tradition*. New York, NY: Park Ridge Center, 1989.
Dioscorides, P. *The Greek Herbal of Dioscorides* (edited and published by Robert Gunther in 1933). Latest edition reprinted in New York, NY: Hafner Publishing Company, 1959.
___________. *De Materia Medica*. Translated by Lily Y. Beck. New York, NY: Olms-Weidmann, 2005.
Duke, J. *Handbook of Northeastern Indian Medicinal Plants*. Lincoln, MA: Quarterman Publications, 1986.
Ehrenreich, B., English, D. *Witches, Midwives and Nurses: A History of Women Healers*. New York, NY: Feminist Press, 1973.
Eisenberg, D. et al. Trends in Alternative Medicine Use in the United States, 1990-1997. *JAMA*. Nov. 11, 1998;(280):1569-1575.
Erichsen-Brown, C. *Use of Plants for the Past 500 Years*. Aurora, Canada: Breezy Creek Press, 1979.
Flannery, M. Archives of Phytomedicine: The Collection of the Lloyd Library and Museum in Cincinnati. *Herbalgram*. 1996;36:42-48.
_________. *John Uri Lloyd: The Great American Eclectic*. Carbondale, IL: Southern Illinois University Press, 1998.
Graves, J. *The Language of Plants: A Guide to the Doctrine of Signatures*. Great Barrington, MA: Lindisfarne Books, 2012.
Griggs, B. *Green Pharmacy: History of Western Herbal Medicine*. Rochester, VT: Healing Arts Press, 1991.
Gulick, R. et al. Phase I studies of hypericin, the active compound in St. John's Wort, as an antiretroviral agent in HIV-infected adults. *Annals of Internal Medicine*. 1999 Mar 16;130(6):510-4.
Hall, M. *Paracelsus: His Mystical and Medical Philosophy*. Los Angeles, CA: Philosophical Research Society, 1964.
Haller, J. *Kindly Medicine: Physio-Medicalism in America*. Kent, OH: Kent State University Press, 1997.
_______. *A Profile in Alternative Medicine: The Eclectic Medical College*. Kent, OH: Kent State University Press, 1999.
_______. *The People's Doctors: Samuel Thomson and the American Botanical Movement, 1790-1860*. Carbondale, IL: Southern Illinois University Press, 2000.
Hamdard, J. *Al-Qanun Fi'al-Tibb*. New Delhi, India: 1989.
Hamilton, B. *The Medieval Inquisition*. New York, NY: Holmes & Meier, 1981.
Hartman, F. *The Life of Paracelsus and the Substance of his Teachings*. London: 1887. Reprinted edition: San Diego, CA: Wizard's Bookshelf, 1985.
Hippocrates, Heracleitus. (Ed. W. Jones). *The Nature of Man*. Cambridge, MA: Harvard University Press (Loeb Classical Library, No. 150), 1931.
Israelsen, L., Blumenthal, M. FDA Issues Final Rules for Structure/Function Claims for Dietary Supplements Under DSHEA, *HerbalGram*. 2000;48: 32-8.
Jee, Bhagwat Sinh. *A Short History of Aryan Medical Science*. Nai Sarak, Delhi, India: New Asian Publishers, 1978.
Jouanna, J. *Hippocrates*. London, England: John Hopkins University Press, 1992.
Kane, Kenny. Personal interviews during 1998-2003 with Kenny Kane, a full-blood Lakota Sioux and descendent of Crazy Horse.
Kapoor, L. *CRC Handbook of Ayurvedic Medicinal Plants*. Boca Raton, FL: CRC Press, 1990.
King, J. *The American Family Physician*. Indianapolis, IN: A.D. Streught, 1864.
Kirchfeld, F., Boyle, W. *Nature Doctors*. Portland, OR: Medicina Biologica, 1994.
Lame Deer, J., Erodes, R. *Lame Deer Seeker of Visions*. New York, NY: Simon & Schuster, Inc., 1972;144. Reprinted with publisher's permission.
Liu, Salmon, J. Herbal medicine regulation in China, Germany, and the United States. *Integrative Medicine*. 2010;9(6):42-49.
Loudon, I. (Ed.) *Western Medicine: An Illustrated History*. New York, NY: Oxford University Press, 1997.
Mann, W. *Hippocratic Writings*. London, England: Penguin Books, 1950.
Martin, M. *The Genius of Arab Civilization* (2nd ed.). London, England: Eurabia Publishing, 1983.
McCalb, M. FDA Publishes Proposed Regulations for Good Manufacturing Practices for Dietary Supplements. *HerbalGram*. 1997;40:24-6.
_________. President's Commission on Dietary Supplement Labels Issues Final Report. *HerbalGram*. 1997;41:24-6.
Mills, S. *The Dictionary of Modern Herbalism*. Wellingbourgh, NY: Thorsons Publishing, 1985.
Moerman, D. *Native American Ethnobotany*. Portland, OR: Timber Press, 1998.
Molyneaux, M. Consumer Attitudes Predict Upward Trends for the Herbal Marketplace. *HerbalGram*. 2002;54:64-5.
Nunn, J. *Ancient Egyptian Medicine*. Norman, OK: University of Oklahoma Press, 1996.
O'Brien, J. *The Inquisition*. New York, NY: Macmillan Company, 1973.
Ondrizek, R. et al. An Alternative Medicine Study of Herbal Effects on the Penetration of Zona-free Hampster Oocytes and the Integrity of Sperm DNA. *Fertility and Sterility*. 1999;71(3):517-22.
Parke, Davis and Company. *Great Moments in Medicine*. The stories and paintings in the series *A History of Medicine in Pictures*. Text by George A. Bender and paintings by Robert A. Thom. Detroit, MI: Northwood Institute Press, 1966.
____________________. *Great Moments in Pharmacy*. The stories and paintings in the series *A History of Pharmacy in Pictures*. Text by George A. Bender and paintings by Robert A. Thom. Detroit, MI: Northwood Institute Press, 1966.
Payne, J. *English Medicine in the Anglo-Saxon Times*. Oxford, England: Clarendon Press, 1904.
Pliny the Elder. *Natural History*. London, England: Penguin Books, 1991.
Priest, A., Priest, L. *Herbal Medication: A Clinical and Dispensary Handbook*. London, England: Fowler & Co. Ltd, 1982.

Priyadaranjan, R., Gupta, H., Roy, M. *Susruta Samhita*. New Delhi, India: Indian National Science Academy, 1980.
Sarton, G. *Galen of Pergamon*. Lawrence, KS: University of Kansas Press, 1954.
Schauss, A. A Review of the European Food Supplements and Traditional Herbal Medicines Directive. *HerbalGram*. 2004;63:64-9.
Sigerist, H. *A History of Medicine* (Vol. 1). New York, NY: Oxford University Press, 1951.
Soller, W., Bayne, H., Shaheen, C. The Regulated Supplement Industry: Myths of an Unregulated Industry Dispelled. *HerbalGram*. 2012;93:42-57.
Solomon, P. et al. Ginkgo for memory enhancement: a randomized controlled trial. *JAMA*. 2002;287:1807-14.
Steele, E., Blumenthal, M. DSHEA at Five Years: A Review of Structure-Function Claims. *HerbalGram*. 1999;47:38-9.
Storm, H. *Seven Arrows*. New York, NY: Ballantine Books, 1972.
Stuart, M. *Encyclopedia of Herbs and Herbalism*. New York, NY: Crescent Books, 1979.
Sumner, J. *The Natural History of Medicinal Plants*. Portland, OR: Timber Press, 2000.
Swerdlow, J. *Nature's Medicine: Plants That Heal*. Washington, DC: National Geographic Society, 2000.
Thakkur, C. *Ayurveda: the Indian Art and Science of Medicine*. New York, NY: A.S.I. Publishers, 1974.
Thom, Dark Rain. *Kohkumthena's Grandchildren: The Shawnee*. Zionsville, IN: Guild Press of Indiana, 1994.
_____________. Personal interviews with Dark Rain Thom of the Shawnee Nation in November 2002 and August 2005.
Tyler, V. Natural Products and Medicine: An Overview. *Herbalgram*. 1993;28:40-45.
______. Phytomedicines in Western Europe. *HerbalGram*. 1994;30:24-7.
Upton, R. International Symposium of ESCOP. *HerbalGram*. 1999;46:58-60.
Wheelwright, E. *Medicinal Plants and Their History*. New York, NY: Dover Publications, 1974.
Wicke, R. *A World History of Herbology and Herbalism: Oppressed Arts*. RMH-Publications Trust, 1995.
Wilder, A. *History of Medicine*. New Sharon, ME: New England Eclectic Publishing Company, 1899.
Wong, K., Wu, L. *The History of Chinese Medicine*. Shanghai, China, 1936. Reprinted New York, NY: AMS Press, 1973.
Woodward, M. *Gerard's Herball*. London, England: R. & R. Clark, LTD. Edinburgh for Gerald Howe, 1927. Edited from the original edition of Thomas Johnson, 1636.
Vogel, V. *American Indian Medicine*. Norman, OK: University of Oklahoma Press, 1970.
Yarnell, E., Abascal, K. Dilemmas of Traditional Botanical Research. *HerbalGram*. 2002;55:46-5.

Books on Traditional Chinese Medicine

Beinfield, H., Korngold, E. *Between Heaven and Earth: A Guide to Chinese Medicine*. New York, NY: Ballantine Books, 1992.
Bensky, D., Gamble, A., Clavy, S., Stoger, E. *Chinese Herbal Medicine* (3rd ed.) Seattle, WA: Eastmand Press, 2004.
Kaptchuck, T. *The Web That Has No Weaver*. Chicago, IL: Contemporary Books, 2000.
Maciocia, G. *Foundations of Chinese Medicine*. New York, NY: Churchill Livingstone, 1989.
Molony, D. *The American Association of Oriental Medicine's Complete Guide to Chinese Herbal Medicine*. New York, NY: Berkeley Books, 1998.
Reid, D. *Complete Book of Chinese Health and Healing*. Boston, MA: Shambala, 1994.
Tierra, M. *The Way of Chinese Herbs*. New York, NY: Pocket Books, 1998.

References to Pictures in History Chapter

p. 1 Image by Robert Thom, "Before the Dawn of History" from Parke, Davis and Company's *Great Moments in Pharmacy*, 1966. Used with permission from Pfizer Inc. All rights reserved.
p. 2 Clay statue of a fertility goddess found in excavations of Catal Huyuk in central Turkey. Lyons, A., Petrucelli, J. *Medicine–An Illustrated History*. New York, NY: Harry N. Abrams, Inc. 1987;19.
p. 3 Image by Robert Thom, "Pharmacy in Ancient Babylonia" from Parke, Davis and Company's *Great Moments in Pharmacy*, 1966. Used with permission from Pfizer Inc. All rights reserved.
p. 4 Image by Robert Thom, "Days of the Papyrus Ebers" from Parke, Davis and Company's *Great Moments in Pharmacy*, 1966. Used with permission from Pfizer Inc. All rights reserved.
Statue of Imhotep. Osler, W. *The Evolution of Modern Medicine*. New Haven, CT: Yale University Press, 1921;10.
Statue of Serqet from 18th dynasty around 1550 B.C. Cairo Museum. Nunn, J. *Ancient Egyptian Medicine*. Norman, OK: University of Oklahoma Press, 1996;100.
p. 5 Painting of Chiron the Centaur from a mid-ninth century manuscript. U.S. National Library of Medicine, Bethesda, MD.
Image by Robert Thom, "The Temple and Cult of Asclepius" from Parke, Davis and Company's *Great Moments in Medicine*, 1966. Used with permission from Pfizer Inc. All rights reserved.
The Healing Cult of Asclepius–Incubation. A marble relief of Asclepius with a sleeping patient from the early fourth century. Loudon, I. (Ed.). *Western Medicine: An Illustrated History*. New York, NY: Oxford University Press, 1997;28.
p. 6 Asclepius standing with his staff; a detail from a ceremonial ivory diptych carved in the late Roman style. Loudon, I. (Ed.). *Western Medicine: An Illustrated History*. New York, NY: Oxford University Press, 1997;27.
p. 7 Hippocrates: a composite portrait designed from a study of ancient coins and medals by Swiss artist Albert Anker. U.S. National Library of Medicine, Bethesda, MD.
Schematic arrangement illustrating the properties and relationship of the four humors and four elements in Greek science. From *The Nature of Man* by Hippocrates & Heracleitus (Ed. W. Jones). Cambridge, MA: Harvard University Press (Loeb Classical Library, No. 150), 1931.
p. 8 Aristotle. U.S. National Library of Medicine, Bethesda, MD.
Theophrastus: a marble bust from the Torlonia Collection in Rome.
p. 9 Image by Robert Thom, "Dioscorides - a Scientist Looks at Drugs" from Parke, Davis and Company's *Great Moments in Pharmacy*, 1966. Used with permission from Pfizer Inc. All rights reserved.
A page from *De Materia Medica* by Dioscorides Pedanius of Anazarbos. Translated by Lily Y. Beck. New York, NY: Olms-Weidmann, 2005.
Galen by artist Vignernon. U.S. National Library of Medicine in Bethesda, MD.
p. 10 A 16th-century woodcut from H. Brunschwig in Strassburg, 1537. U.S. National Library of Medicine in Bethesda, MD.
p. 11 Image by Robert Thom, "Monastic Pharmacy" from Parke, Davis and Company's *Great Moments in Pharmacy*, 1966. Used with permission from Pfizer Inc. All rights reserved.
Fresco of St. Benedict healing a monk by Spinella Aretino. Lyons, A., Petrucelli, J. *Medicine–An Illustrated History*. New York, NY: Harry N. Abrams, Inc. 1987;278.
p. 12 Image by Robert Thom, "The First Apothecary Shops" from Parke, Davis and Company's *Great Moments in Pharmacy*, 1966. Used with permission from Pfizer Inc. All rights reserved.
p. 13 Wise Women in herbal gardens. Bettmann, O. *A Pictorial History of Medicine*. Springfield, IL: Charles C. Thomas, 1962;50.
p. 14 A manuscript illustration showing Hippocrates, Galen, and Avicenna from an edition of Galen's works published in Lyons, France in 1528. U.S. National Library of Medicine in Bethesda, MD.
Astrologer making calculations from an almanac known as *Prognosticons* and published by European universities during the 1500s. Osler, W. *The Evolution of Modern Medicine*. New Haven, CT: Yale University Press, 1921;120.
p. 15 Picture of Paracelsus from the first edition of the *Philosphia Magna* by Colon A. Birckmann and published in 1567. U.S. National Library of Medicine in Bethesda, MD.
European apothecary by artist Amman Jost (1539–1591). U.S. National Library of Medicine in Bethesda, MD.
Physicians discuss treatment at the bedside of a dying man. U.S. National Library of Medicine in Bethesda, MD.
p. 16 Title page of Gerard's *Herball: The Essence Thereof Distilled by Marcus Woodward* by John Gerard and Marcus Woodward (from the edition of Thomas Johnson). Originally published in London, England: R & R Clark LTD., 1637.
p. 17 Title page of one of Culpeper's books. Osler, W. *The Evolution of Modern Medicine*. New Haven, CT: Yale University Press, 1921;123.
Carolus Linnaeus by artist J. Chapman. U.S. National Library of Medicine in Bethesda, MD.
p. 18 Images by Robert Thom: upper left is "The Development of Chemotherapy" and lower right is "Pharmaceutical Manufacturing Comes of Age" from Parke, Davis and Company's *Great Moments in Pharmacy*, 1966. Used with permission from Pfizer Inc. All rights reserved.
p. 19 Page from an Islamic herbal book. Bettmann, O. *A Pictorial History of Medicine*. Springfield, IL: Charles C. Thomas, 1962;112.
p. 20 Page of a 15th-century Italian manuscript of *The Canon of Medicine* by Avicenna (written in Hebrew). U.S. National Library of Medicine, Bethesda, MD.

Picture of Rhazes on the title page of a 1529 Venetian printing of his book *Comprehensive Book of Medicine.* U.S. National Library of Medicine in Bethesda, MD.
p. 21 Image by Robert Thom, "Avicenna – the Persian Galen" from Parke, Davis and Company's *Great Moments in Pharmacy*, 1966. Used with permission from Pfizer Inc. All rights reserved.
p. 21 Avicenna. From a 1522 Venetian edition of *The Cannon of Medicine.*
p. 22 Painting of Medicine Man, Performing His Mysteries over a Dying Man by George Catlin. Courtesy of Smithsonian American Art Museum, Gift of Mrs. Joseph Harrison, Jr.
p. 23-28 Photographs of Dark Rain Thom by author Susan Clearwater and Dale Edson taken during her interview, September 2005.
p. 28 Image by Robert Thom: "Louis Herbert: Apothecary to New France" from Parke, Davis and Company's *Great Moments in Medicine*, 1966. Used with permission from Pfizer Inc. All rights reserved.
p.29 Images by Robert Thom: "The Governor Who Healed the Sick" and lower right is "First Hospital Pharmacy in Colonial America" from Parke, Davis and Company's *Great Moments in Pharmacy*, 1966. Used with permission from Pfizer Inc. All rights reserved.
p. 32 Picture of John King, M.D. from his book *The American Family Physician.* Indianapolis, IN: A.D. Streight, 1864.
Title page of John King's book *The American Family Physician.* Indianapolis, IN: A.D. Streight, 1864.
p. 33 Photograph of herbal preparations manufactured by the Lloyd Brothers Pharmaceutical Company taken by author Susan Clearwater at the Lloyd Library in Cincinnati, Ohio.
Photograph of the Lloyd Library and Museum in Cincinnati, Ohio. Taken by author Susan Clearwater.
p. 40 Image by Robert Thom: "Pharmacy in Ancient China" from Parke, Davis and Company's *Great Moments in Pharmacy*, 1966. Used with permission from Pfizer Inc. All rights reserved.
Portrait of Shen Nong. Courtesy of Wellcome Trustees, London.
p. 41 Portrait of Huang Ti. Courtesy of Wellcome Trustees, London.
p. 42 Photographs of Chinese pharmacists measuring herbs and herbs in the market taken by author Susan Clearwater in Hangzhou, China.
p. 44 Image by Robert Thom: "Sushruta-Surgeon of Old India" from Parke, Davis and Company's *Great Moments in Medicine*, 1966. Used with permission from Pfizer Inc. All rights reserved.

NOMENCLATURE AND CLASSIFICATION OF PLANTS

Cronquist, A. *The Evolution and Classification of Flowering Plants* (2nd ed.). Bronx, NY: The New York Botanical Garden, 1988.
Elpel, T. *Botany In a Day: Herbal Field Guide to Plant Families*. Pony, MT: HOPS Press, 1996.
Fuller, H., Tippe, O. *College Botany*. New York, NY: Henry Holt and Company, 1954.
Glimn-Lacy, J., Kaufman, P. *Botany Illustrated: Introduction to Plants, Major Groups, Flowering Plant Families*. New York, NY: Van Nostrand Reinhold,1984.
Hufford, T. *Botany, Basic Concepts in Plant Biology*. New York, NY: Harper & Row Publishers, 1978.
Langenheim, J., Thimann, K. *Botany, Plant Biology and Its Relation To Human Affairs*. New York, NY: John Wiley & Sons, 1982.
Raven, P., Ray, E., Eichhorn, S. *Biology of Plants* (6th ed.). New York, NY: W. H. Freeman & Company/ Worth Publishers, Inc., 1999.
Stafford, L. The Plant List: The First Comprehensive Inventory of Most Known Plant Species. *HerbalGram*. 2011:89;17-18.
Sumner, J. *The Natural History of Medicinal Plants*. Portland, OR: Timber Press, 2000.
Trehane, P. et al. *International Code of Nomenclature for Cultivated Plants*. Wimborne, UK: Quarterjack Publishing, 1995.
Weier, T., Stocking, C., Barbour, M., Rost, T. *Botany: An Introduction To Plant Biology* (6th ed.). New York, NY: John Wiley & Sons, 1982.
Image of Carolus Linnaeus on page 48 is from the painting by Lizars. U.S. National Library of Medicine.
Photographs on page 54 by author Susan Clearwater.

BOTANY FOR HERBALISTS

Capon, B. *Botany For Gardeners*. Portland, OR: Timber Press, 1990.
Corntenay, B., Zimmerman, J. *Wildflowers and Weeds*. London, England: Prentice Hall, 1978.
Fahn, A. *Plant Anatomy* (4th ed.). Elmsford, NY: Pergamon Press, 1990.
Fuller, H., Tippe, O. *College Botany*. New York, NY: Henry Holt & Company, 1954.
Gibbons, B. *The Secret Life of Flowers, A Guide To Plant Biology*. London, England: Blandford Press, 1984.
Hufford, T. *Botany, Basic Concepts in Plant Biology*. New York, NY: Harper & Row Publishers, 1978.
Kindersley, D. *The Visual Dictionary of Plants*. New York, NY: Dorling Kindersley, Inc., 1992.
Kolek, J., Konzinka, V. (Eds.). *Physiology of the Plant Root System.* Boston, MA: Kluwer Academic Publishers, 1992.
Langenheim, J., Thimann, K. *Botany, Plant Biology and Its Relation To Human Affairs*. New York, NY: John Wiley & Sons, 1982.
Mabberley, D. *The Plant Book: A Portable Dictionary of the Vascular Plants* (2nd ed.). New York, NY: Cambridge University Press, 1997.
Marinelli, J. (Ed.). *The Brooklyn Botanic Garden: Gardener's Desk Reference*. New York, NY: Henry Holt & Company, 1998.
Metcalfe, C., Chalk, L. *Anatomy of the Dicotyledons* (Vol. 1, 2nd ed.). Oxford, England: Clarendon Press, 1979.
Newcomb, L. *Newcomb's Wildflower Guide*. Boston, MA: Little, Brown and Company, 1977.
Niering, W. *The Audubon Society Field Guide to North American Wildflowers*. New York, NY: Chanticleer Press, 1979.
Peterson, L. *A Field Guide To Edible Wild Plants of Eastern/Central North America*. Boston, MA: Houghton Mifflin Company, 1977.
Raven, P., Evert, R., Eichhorn, S. *Biology of Plants* (6th ed.). New York, NY: W. H. Freeman & Company, Worth Publishers, 1999.
Weier, T., Stocking, C., Barbour, M., Rost, T. *Botany: An Introduction to Plant Biology* (6th ed.). New York, NY: John Wiley & Sons, 1982.
All line drawings and the photographs on pages 72 and 75 by author Susan Clearwater.

ENDANGERED MEDICINAL HERBS ~ BOTANICAL SANCTUARIES TO THE RESCUE

Cech, R. Balancing Conservation With Utilization: Restoring Populations of Commercially Valuable Medicinal Herbs in Forests and Agroforests. *HerbalGram*. 1999;45:18.
_______. Why "At-Risk"? *United Plant Savers Newsletter*, Fall 2000.
Gladstar, R., Hirsch, P. (Eds.). *Planting the Future: Saving Our Medicinal Herbs.* Rochester, VT: Healing Arts Press, 2000.
Johnston, B. Major Diversity Loss: One in Eight Plants in Global Study Threatened. *HerbalGram*. 1998;43;54.
Robbins, C. Medicinal Plant Conservation-A Priority at TRAFFIC. *HerbalGram.* 1998;44:52-4.
United Plant Savers (UpS) www.UnitedPlantSavers.org.

CULTIVATING MEDICINAL HERBS

Balter, G. *Gardening With Soul*. Fayetteville, AR: Learning Tree Books, 2003.
Blakley, T., Sturdivant, L. *Medicinal Herbs in the Garden, Field & Marketplace*. Friday Harbor, WA: San Juan Naturals, 1999.
Foster, C. *Plants-a-Plenty: How to Multiply Outdoor and Indoor Plants.* Emmaus, PA: Rodale Press, 1977.
Foster, S. *Herbal Bounty*. Salt Lake City, UT: Peregrine Books, 1984.
Miller, E. *Organic Gardening: A Comprehensive Guide to Chemical-Free Growing.* New York, NY: IDG Books Worldwide, Inc., 2000.
Phillips, H. *Growing and Propagating Wild Flowers*. Chapel Hill, NC: University of North Carolina Press, 1985
Powell, E. *From Seed To Bloom: How to Grow Over 500 Annuals, Perennials and Herbs*. Pownal, VT: Storey Books, 1995.
Raven, P., Evert, R., Eichhorn, S. *Biology of Plants* (6th ed.). New York, NY: W. H. Freeman & Company/ Worth Publishers, 1992.
Rodale, J. et al. (Eds.). *The Encyclopedia of Organic Gardening*. Emmaus, PA: Rodale Press, 1978.
Smillie, J., Gershuny, G. *The Soul of Soil: A Soil-Building Guide for Master Gardeners and Farmers*. White River Junction, VT: Chelsea Green Publishing Company, 1999.
Tyler, H. *Organic Gardening Without Poisons*. New York, NY: Van Nostrand Reinhold Company, 1970.
Wallace, D. et al. *Getting the Most from Your Garden: Advanced Intensive Gardening Techniques.* Emmaus, PA: Rodale Press, 1980.
Wolf, R. *Organic Farming*. Emmaus, PA: Rodale Press, 1977.
Wright, M. *Perelandra Garden Workbook: Complete Guide to Gardening with Nature Intelligences.* Warrenton, VA: Perelandra, 1987.
Yepsen, R. *Organic Plant Protection*. Emmaus, PA: Rodale Press, 1976.
All photographs and garden log by author Susan Clearwater.

SUSTAINABLE HARVESTING OF MEDICINAL HERBS

Two images on page 115 are from *The Herbalist Almanac,* Indiana Botanic Gardens. Hammond, IN. 1939; cover page and page 21.

All photographs by author Susan Clearwater.
BOOKS FOR IDENTIFYING HERBS:
Bremness, L. *Herbs*. New York,NY: Dorling Kindersley, 1994.
Foster, S., Duke, J. *Medicinal Plants and Herbs*. New York, NY: Houghton Mifflin Company, 2000.
Newcomb, L. *Newcomb's Wildflower Guide*. Boston, MA: Little, Brown and Company, 1977.
Niering, W. *The Audubon Society Field Guide to North American Wildflowers*. New York, NY: Chanticleer Press, 1979.
Peterson, L., Peterson, R. *A Field Guide to Edible Wild Plants*. Boston, MA: Houghton Mifflin Company, 1977.
Peterson, R., McKenny, M. *Peterson Field Guides: Wildflowers*. Boston, MA: Houghton Mifflin Company, 1968.
Wharton, M., Barbour, R. *A Guide to the Wildflowers & Ferns of Kentucky*. Lexington, KY: University Press of Kentucky, 1971.
Yatskievych, K. *Field Guide to Indiana Wildflowers*. Bloomington, IN: Indiana University Press, 2000.

DRYING AND STORING MEDICINAL HERBS

All photographs by author Susan Clearwater.

CREATING HERBAL PREPARATIONS

Blumenthal, M., Hall, T. What is Herb Standardization? *HerbalGram*. 2001;52:25.
Bone, K. Standardized Extracts. *HerbalGram*. 2001;53:50-9.
Patterson, E. Standardized Extracts: Herbal Medicine of the Future? *Herb Market Review*. Oct 23:10,1997.
Tilgner, S. Standardized Herbs: A Hot Topic. *Herbal Transitions*. 2001;4(1):13-17.
All photographs by author Susan Clearwater.

WEIGHTS AND MEASUREMENTS FOR THE HERBALIST

Blumenthal, M. (Ed.). *The Complete German Commission E Monographs*. Austin, TX: American Botanical Council, 1998.
Curren, A., Munday, L. *Math for Meds*. San Diego, CA: Wallcur, Inc., 1986.
Miller, B., Keane, C. *Encyclopedia and Dictionary of Medicine, Nursing, and Allied Health*. Philadelphia, PA: W. B. Saunders Company, 1983.

THE SAFETY OF MEDICINAL HERBS

Ames, B. et al. Ranking Possible Carcinogenic Hazards. *Science*. April 1987;236:271-280.
Bates, D. et al. The costs of adverse drug events in hospitalized patients. *JAMA*. 1997;277:307-311.
Blumenthal, M. et al. *The Complete German Commission E Monographs: Therapeutic Guides to Herbal Medicines*. Austin, TX: American Botanical Council, 1998.
Booker, S. Report on International Workshop to Evaluate Research Needs on the Use and Safety of Medicinal Herbs. *HerbalGram*. 1999;46:61-4.
Bradley, P. (Ed.). *British Herbal Compendium* (Vol. 1). Dorset, England: British Herbal Medicine Association, 1992.
Brinker, F. *Herb Contraindications & Drug Interactions* (3rd ed.). Sandy, OR: Eclectic Medical Publications, 2001.
Buhner, S. *The Lost Language of Plants: The Ecological Importance of Plant Medicines to Life on Earth*. White River Junction, VT: Chelsea Green Publishing, 2002;83-113.
Castleman, M. *The Healing Herbs*. Emmaus, PA: Rodale Press, 1991.
Classen, D. et al. Adverse drug events in hospitalized patients: excess length of stay, extra costs, and attributable mortality. *JAMA*. 1997;277:301-306.
DeSmet, P. et al. (Eds.). *Adverse Effects of Herbal Drugs* (Vols. 1 and 2). New York, NY: Springer-Verlag, 1992-93.
Duke, J. *The Green Pharmacy Herbal Handbook*. New York, NY: St. Martin's Paperbacks, 2000;19.
Edison, R., Muenke, M. Statin drugs induce malformations. *New England Journal of Medicine*. April 8, 2004;1579-1582.
Farnsworth, N. The Relative Safety of Herbal Medicine. *HerbalGram*. 1993;29:36.
__________. *Utilization of Medicinal Plants*. Philadelphia, PA: World Health Organization, 1993.
Fetrow, C., Avila, J. *Complementary and Alternative Medicines*. Springhouse, PA: Springhouse Corporation, 1999.
Foster, S., Duke, J. *Peterson Field Guide to Medicinal Plants and Herbs* (2nd ed.). New York, NY: Houghton Mifflin Company, 2000;10.
GAO/PEMB-90-15. *FDA Drug Review: Post approval Risks* 1976-1985;3. Published April 26, 1990.
Hoffmann, D. *Medical Herbalism: The Science and Practice of Herbal Medicine*. Rochester, VT: Healing Arts Press, 2003.
Kingsbury, J. *Poisonous Plants of the United States and Canada*. Englewood Cliffs, NJ: Prentice-Hall, 1964.
Larson, A. et al. Acetaminophen-induced acute liver failure: Results of a U. S. multicenter, prospective study. *Hepatology*. 2005;42(6):1364-1372.
Lazarou, J., Pomeranz, B., Corey, P. Incidence of adverse drug reactions in hospitalized patients. *JAMA*. 1998;279(15):1200-1205.
Leung, A., Foster, S. *Encyclopedia of Common Natural Ingredients Used in Food, Drugs and Cosmetics*. New York, NY: John Wiley & Sons, 1996.
Lindstrom, A. National Poison Control Center Database Annual Report Reflects Safety of Dietary Supplements. *HerbalGram*. 2011;91,18.
Litovitz, L., Klein-Schwartz, W., Felberg, L., White, S. 1995 Annual Report of the American Association of Poison Control Centers Toxic Exposure Surveillance System. *American Journal of Emergency Medicine*. 1996;14(5):487-537.
Litovitz, L., Klein-Schwartz, W., Dyer, S., et al. 1997 Annual Report of the American Association of Poison Control Centers Toxic Exposure Surveillance System. *American Journal of Emergency Medicine*. 1998;16(5): 443-497.
McCaleb, R., Leigh, E., Morien, K. *The Encyclopedia of Popular Herbs*. Rosefield, CA: Prima Health, 2000;31,33.
McGuffin, M., Hobbs, C., Upton, R., Goldberg, A. *Botanical Safety Handbook*. New York, NY: CRC Press, 1997.
Muenscher, W. *Poisonous Plants of the United States*. New York, NY: Macmillan Company, 1951.
Stargrove, M., Treasure, J., McKee, D. *Herb, Nutrient, and Drug Interactions*. St. Louis, MO: Mosby, 2005.
Stephans, H. *Poisonous Plants of the Central United States*. Lawrence, KS: University Press of Kansas, 1980.
Tess Annual Report of 1998. *American Journal of Emergency Medicine*. 1999;17(5):435-87.
Topol, E. Failing the public health—rofecoxib, Merck, and the FDA. *New England Journal of Medicine*. Oct. 21, 2004;351(17):1707-9.
Upton, R. Safety and Toxicity Issues Related to Botanical Drugs. *Medicines from the Earth*. 2004;112,123.
U.S. News and World Report. May 16, 1988;79.
WHO. *Guidelines for the Assessment of Herbal Medicines*. World Health Organization, 1992 &1998.
Wolfe, M. et al. Gastrointestinal Toxicity of Nonsteroidal Anti-inflammatory Drugs. *New England Journal of Medicine*. 1999;340(24).

CHEMICAL CONSTITUENTS IN PLANTS

Bergner, P. Inulin. *Medical Herbalism*. 1997;9(2):20-21.
Dewick, P. *Medicinal Natural Products: A Biosynthetic Approach*. West Sussex, England: John Wiley & Sons, Ltd., 2002.
Duke, J. web site: www.ars-grin.gov/duke/.
Elpel, T. *Botany in a Day*. Pony, MT: HOPS Press, 1996.
Evans, W. *Trease and Evans' Pharmacognosy* (13th ed.). London, England: Baillere Tindall, 1989.
Gilleland, M. *Introduction to General, Organic, and Biological Chemistry*. St. Paul, MN: West Publishing Company, 1982.
Harborne, J., Baxter, H. *Phytochemical Dictionary: Handbook of Bioactive Compounds from Plants*. Washington, DC: Taylor & Francis, 1993.
Heldt, H. *Plant Biochemistry and Molecular Biology*. New York, NY: Oxford University Press, 1997.
Herrmann, K., Weaver, L. The Shikimate Pathway. *Annual Review of Plant Physiology and Plant Molecular Biology*. 1999;50:473-503.
Hoffman, D. *The Holistic Herbal*. Scotland: Findhorn Press, 1983.
__________. *Medical Herbalism: The Science and Practice of Herbal Medicine*. Rochester, VT; Healing Arts Press, 2003.
Holmes, P. *The Energetics of Western Herbs* (Vols. 1 and 2). Boulder, CO: Snow Lion Press, 1989.
Ikan, R. *Natural Products: A Laboratory Guide*. New York, NY: Academic Press, 1991.
Raven, P., Evert, R., Eichhorn, S. *Biology of Plants*. New York, NY: W. H. Freeman and Company, 1999.
Rodman, M., Karch, A., Boyd, E., Smith. *Pharmacology & Drug Therapy in Nursing*. New York, NY: Lippincott Company, 1985.
Sumner, J. *The Natural History of Medicinal Plants*. Portland, OR: Timber Press, 2000.
Swerdlow, Joel. *Nature's Medicine: Plants that Heal*. Washington, DC: National Geographic Society, 2000;330-1. Reprinted by arrangement with National Geographic Partners, LLC.
Thompson, R. *The Chemistry of Natural Products*. New York, NY: Blackie Academic & Professional, 1993.
Tyler, V. *Pharmacognosy*. Philadelphia, PA: Lea & Febiger, 1981.
Willard. T. *Textbook of Advanced Herbology*. Alberta, Canada; Wild Rose College of Natural Healing, 1992.
Wood, M. *The Book of Herbal Wisdom: Using Plants as Medicine*. Berkeley, CA: North Atlantic Books, 1997.

Section Two: The Materia Medica

References for many of the cited research studies can be found online at PubMed.com and abc.herbalgram.org (web site of the American Botanical Council). **GENERAL REFERENCES** are listed numerically under each herb in the Materia Medica.

GENERAL REFERENCES

1) Blumenthal, M. et al. (Eds.). *The Complete German Commission E Monographs*. Austin, TX: American Botanical Council, 1998.
2) Blumenthal, M., Goldberg, A., Brinckmann, J. *Herbal Medicine: Expanded Commission E Monographs*. Newton, MA: Integrative Medicine Communications, 2000.
3) Brinker, F. *Herb Contraindications and Drug Interactions*. Sandy, OR: Eclectic Medical Publications, 2001.
4) Brown, D. *Herbal Prescriptions for Better Health*. Rocklin, CA: Prima Publishing, 1996.
5) Castleman, M. *The Healing Herbs*. Emmaus, PA: Rodale Press, 1991.
6) Cech, R. *Making Plant Medicine*. Williams, OR: Horizon Herbs Publication, 2000.
7) ______. *Growing At-Risk Medicinal Herbs*. Williams, OR: Horizon Herbs Publication, 2002.
8) Christopher, J. *School of Natural Healing*. Springville, UT: Christopher Publications, 1976.
9) Cook, W. *The Physiomedical Dispensatory: Therapeutics, Materia Medica, and Pharmacy*. Cincinnati, OH: Wm Cook, 1869.
10) Crellin, J., Philpott, J. *Herbal Medicine Past and Present: Reference Guide to Medicinal Plants*. London, England: Duke University Press, 1989.
11) Culpeper, N. *Culpeper's Complete Herbal and English Physician*. England: Magna Books, 1992. Originally published in 1826.
12) Dioscorides, P. *The Greek Herbal of Dioscorides*. Edited and published by Robert Gunther in 1933. Latest edition reprinted in New York, NY: Hafner Publishing Company, 1959.
13) Duke, J. *Handbook of Medicinal Herbs*. Boca Raton, FL: CRC Press, 1985.
14) ______. *The Green Pharmacy*. Emmaus, PA: Rodale Press, 1997.
15) ______. *Dr. Duke's Essential Herbs*. Emmaus, PA: Rodale Press, 1999.
16) ______. *The Green Pharmacy Herbal Handbook*. Emmaus, PA: Rodale Press, 2000.
17) ______. *Dr. Dukes Phytochemical and Ethnobotanical Database*, USDA-ARS-NGRL, Beltsville Agricultural Research Center, Beltsville, MD. Available at: www.ars-grin.gov/duke/
18) Ellingwood, F. *American Materia Medica, Therapeutics, and Pharmacognosy* (11th ed.). Portland, OR: Eclectic Medical Publications, 1983 (reprinted from the 1919 original).
19) Erichsen-Brown, C. *Medicinal and Other Uses of North American Plants*. New York, NY: Dover Publications, 1979.
20) Felter, H., Lloyd, J. *King's American Dispensatory* (18th ed.). Portland, OR: Eclectic Medical Publications, 1986 (reprinted from the 1898 original).
21) Felter, H. *The Eclectic Materia Medica, Pharmacology and Therapeutics*. Cincinnati, OH: J. K. Scudder, 1922.
22) Fetrow, C., Avula, J. *Professional's Handbook of Complementary and Alternative Medicines*. Springhouse, PA: Springhouse Corp., 1999.
23) Foster, S. *Herbal Renaissance*. Salt Lake City, UT: Gibbs-Smith Publisher, 1993.
24) ______. *101 Medicinal Plants*. Loveland, CO: Interweave Press, Inc., 1998.
25) Foster, S., Johnson, R. *Desk Reference to Nature's Medicine*. Washington, D.C.: National Geographic Society, 2006.
26) Foster, S., Chongxi, Y. *Herbal Emissaries: Bringing Chinese Herbs to the West*. Rochester, VT: Healing Arts Press, 1992.
27) Foster, S., Duke, J. *Peterson Field Guide to Eastern/Central Medicinal Plants and Herbs* (2nd ed.). Boston, MA: Houghton Mifflin, 2000.
28) Frawley, D., Lad, V. *The Yoga of Herbs*. Twin Lakes, WN: Lotus Press, 1986.
29) Gerard, J. *The Herball or Generall Historie of Plantes*. Edited by Thomas Johnson and reprinted in New York, NY: Dover Publications, 1975. Originally published in London, England in 1633.
30) Gladstar, R. *Herbal Healing for Women*. New York, NY: Simon & Schuster, 1993.
31) ________. *Family Herbal: A Guide to Living Life with Energy, Health and Vitality*. North Adams, MA: Storey Books, 2001.
32) Gladstar, R., Hirsh, P. (Eds.). *Planting the Future: Saving our Medicinal Herbs*. Rochester, VT: Healing Arts Press, 2000.
33) Grieve, M. *A Modern Herbal* (Vols. 1 and 2). New York, NY: Dover Publications, 1971.
34) Hobbs, C., Keville, K. *Women's Herbs, Women's Health*. Loveland, CO: Interweave Press, 1998.
35) Hoffman, D. *The Holistic Herbal*. Forres, Scotland: Findhorn Press, 1983.
36) _________. *Medical Herbalism, the Science and Practice of Herbal Medicine*. Rochester, VT: Healing Arts Press, 2003.
37) Holmes, P. *The Energetics of Western Plants: Treatment Strategies Integrating Western and Oriental Herbal Medicine* (Vols. 1 and 2). Boulder, CO: Snow Lotus Press, 1989.
38) Hutchens, A. *Indian Herbology of North America*. Ontario, Canada: Merco, 1973.
39) Hylton, W. (Ed.). *The Rodale Herb Book*. Emmaus, PA: Rodale Press, 1984.
40) Kindscher, K. *Medicinal Wild Plants of the Prairie*. Lawrence, KS: University Press of Kansas, 1992.
41) King, J. *The American Family Physician*. Indianapolis, IN: A.D. Streight Publishers, 1864.
42) Kloss, J. *Back to Eden*. New York, NY: Beneficial Books, 1971.
43) Lininger, S., Gaby, A., et al. *The Natural Pharmacy: Complete Home Reference to Natural Medicine*. Rocklin, CA: Healthnotes, Inc., 1999.
44) Lust, J. *The Herb Book*. New York, NY: Bantam Books, 1974.
45) McCaleb, R., Leigh, E., Morien, K. *The Encyclopedia of Popular Herbs*. Roseville, CA: Prima Health, 2000.
46) McGuffin, M., Hobbs, C., Upton, R., Goldberg, A. (Eds.). *Botanical Safety Handbook*. New York, NY: CRC Press, 1997.
47) Meyer, J. *The Herbalist*. Hammond, IN: The Hammond Book Company, 1918.
48) Mitchell, W. *Plant Medicine in Practice: Using the Teachings of John Bastyr*. Seattle, WA: Churchill Livingstone, 2003.
49) Moerman, D. *Native American Ethnobotany*. Portland, OR: Timber Press, 1998.
50) Molony, D., Molony, M., Burke, N. *The American Association of Oriental Medicine's Complete Guide to Chinese Herbal Medicine: How to Treat Illness and Maintain Wellness with Chinese Herbs*. New York, NY: Berkeley Books, 1998.
51) Mowrey, D. *The Scientific Validation of Herbal Medicines*. New Canaan, CT: Keats Publishing, 1986.
52) ________. *Herbal Tonic Therapies*. New Canaan, CT: Keats Publishing, 1993.
53) Murray, M. *The Healing Power of Herbs*. Rocklin, CA: Prima Publishing, 1992.
54) Murray, M., Pizzorno, J. *Encyclopedia of Natural Medicine*. Rocklin, CA: Prima Publishing, 1991.
55) Newall, C., Anderson, L., Phillipson, J. *Herbal Medicines: a Guide for Health-Care Professionals*. London, England: Pharmaceutical Press, 1996.
56) Newcomb, L. *Newcomb's Wildflower Guide*. Boston, MA: Little, Brown and Company, 1977.
57) Pedersen, M. *Nutritional Herbology*. Bountiful, UT: Pederson Publishing, 1991.
58) Phillips, R., Foy, N. *Herbs*. New York, NY: Random House, 1990.
59) Potterton, D. (Ed.). *Culpeper's Color Herbal*. New York, NY: Sterling Publishing, 1983.
60) Rafinesque, C. *Medical Flora or Manual of Medical Botany in the United States*. Philadelphia, PA: Atkinson and Alexander, 1828.
61) Scudder, J. *Specific Medication and Specific Medicines*. Cincinnati, OH: Wilstach, Baldwin & Company, 1870.
62) Skenderi, G. *Herbal Vade Mecum*. Rutherford, NJ: Herbacy Press, 2003.
63) Tierra, M. *The Way of Herbs*. New York, NY: Pocket Books, 1980.
64) _______. *Planetary Herbology*. Twin Lakes, WI: Lotus Press, 1988.
65) _______. *The Way of Chinese Herbs*. New York, NY: Pocket Books, 1998.
66) Tilgner, S. *Herbal Medicine from the Heart of the Earth*. Creswell, OR: Wise Acres Press, 1999.
67) Treben, M. *Health from God's Garden*. Rochester, VT: Healing Arts Press, 1988.
68) Tyler, V. *The Honest Herbal*. New York, NY: Pharmaceutical Products Press, 1993.
69) ______. *Herbs of Choice: The Therapeutic Use of Phytochemicals*. New York, NY: Pharmaceutical Products Press, 1994.
70) Vogel, V. *American Indian Medicine*. Norman, OK: University of Oklahoma Press, 1970.

71) Weed, S. *Wise Woman Herbal for the Childbearing Year.* Woodstock, NY: Ash Tree Publishing, 1985.
72) _______. *Wise Woman Herbal: Healing Wise.* Woodstock, NY: Ash Tree Publishing, 1989.
73) _______. *Menopausal Years: The Wise Woman Way*. Woodstock, NY: Ash Tree Publishing, 1992.
74) Weiner, M. *Earth Medicine, Earth Food: Plant Remedies, Drugs & Natural Foods of the North American Indians*. New York, NY: Collier Books,1972.
75) Weiss, R. *Herbal Medicine*. Beaconsfield, England: Beaconsfield Publishers, 1988.
76) Werbach, M., Murray, M. *Botanical Influences on Illness: A Sourcebook of Clinical Research.* Tarzana, CA: Third Line Press, 1994.
77) Willard, T. *Textbook of Advanced Herbology*. Calgary, Alberta Canada: Wild Rose College of Natural Healing, 1992.
78) ________. *Textbook of Modern Herbology*. Calgary, Alberta Canada: Wild Rose College of Natural Healing, 1997.
79) Williamson, E. *Potter's Herbal Cyclopaedia.* Essex, England: C. W. Daniel Company, 2003 (originally published in 1907).
80) Wood, M. *The Book of Herbal Wisdom*. Berkeley, CA: North Atlantic Books, 1997.
81) Yarnell, E., Abascal, K., Hooper, C. *Clinical Botanical Medicine*. Larchmont, NY: Mary Ann Liebert, Inc. 2003.
82) Yemm, J. (Ed.). *The Medical Herbalist.* Great Britain: National Association of Medical Herbalists of Great Britain, 1935.

HOW TO USE THE MATERIA MEDICA

Duke, J. *Dr. Dukes Phytochemical and Ethnobotanical Database*, USDA-ARS-NGRL, Beltsville Agricultural Research Center, Beltsville, MD. Available at www.ars-grin.gov/duke/
Hoffman, D. *Medical Herbalism: The Science and Practice of Herbal Medicine*. Rochester, VT; Healing Arts Press, 2003.
Illustration on page 202 created by artist Kevin Morgan. Used with permission by United Plant Savers, who are the owners of the illustration.
BOOKS ABOUT PLANT DEVAS:
Buhner, S. *The Secret Teachings of Plants: The Intelligence of the Heart in the Direct Perception of Nature*. Rochester, VT: Bear & Company, 2004.
Cowan, E. *Plant Spirit Medicine*. Newberg, OR; Swan/Raven & Company, 1995.
Montgomery, P. *Plant Spirit Healing: A Guide to Working with Plant Consciousness*. Rochester, VT: Bear & Company, 2008.
Summer Deer, T. *Wisdom of the Plant Devas. Herbal Medicine for a New Earth*. Rochester, VT: Bear & Company, 2011.
Wright, M. *Perelandra Garden Workbook: A Complete Guide to Gardening with Nature Intelligences.* Jeffersonton, VA: Perelandra Publishing, 1987.

AMERICAN CENTAURY

GENERAL REFERENCES: 1) p. 106; 8) pp. 448-50; 9) p. 673; 11) p. 230; 20) p. 1689; 33) p. 182; 36) p. 537; 37) p. 402; 44) p. 95; 47) p. 7; 58) p. 141; 59) p. 41; 61); 62) p. 89; 64) p. 208; 75) p. 247; 79) p. 108; 82) pp. 7, 17, 53, 97, 116.
Berkan, T. et al. Antiinflammatory, analgesic, and antipyretic effects of an aqueous extract of *Erythraea centaurium. Planta Med*. 1991 Feb;57(1):34-7.
Bianchini, F., Corbetta, F. *Health Plants*. New York, NY: Crescent Books, 1975;18.
Haloui, M. et al. Experimental diuretic effects of *Rosmarinus officinalis* and *Centaurium erythraea. J Ethnopharmacol*. 2000 Aug;71(3):465-72.
Kumarasamy, Y. et al. Bioactivity of secoiridoid glycosides from *Centaurium erythraea. Phytomedicine*. 2003 May;10(4):344-7.
Lacroix, R. et al. Algerian pharmacopeia: 2 plants with antipyretic properties: *Ptychotis ammoides & Erythraea centaurium*. *Tunis Med.* 1973;51(5):327.
Mabey, R. *The New Age Herbalist*. New York, NY: Macmillan Publishing, 1988;59-60.
Mroueh, M., Saab, Y., Rizkallah, R. Hepatoprotective activity of *Centaurium erythraea* on acetaminophen-induced hepatotoxicity in rats. *Phytother Res*. 2004 May;18(5):431-3.
Tuluce,Y. et al. Gastroprotective effect of small centaury (*Centaurium erythraea* L) on aspirin-induced gastric damage in rats. *Toxicol Ind Health*. 2011 Sep;27(8):760-8.
Valentao, P. et al. Hydroxyl radical and hypochlorous acid scavenging activity of small centaury (*Centaurium erythraea*) infusion. A comparative study with green tea (*Camellia sinensis*). *Phytomedicine*. 2003;10(6-7):517-22.

ASTRAGALUS

GENERAL REFERENCES: 3) pp. 34, 246; 6) p. 106; 14) pp. 147-8, 327, 544; 16) p. 40; 17); 24) p. 24; 25) p. 28; 26) p. 27; 36) p. 532; 43); 46) p. 17; 50) p. 88; 62) p. 24; 64) p. 294; 65) p. 174; 66) p. 35; 77) pp. 82-3, 91; 79) p. 34; 81) pp. 44, 61, 194.
Anetai, M. et al. Chemical evaluation of Astragalus radix. *Natural Medicine*. 1994;48(4):244-52.
Bensky, D., Gamble, A., Kaptchuk, T. *Chinese Herbal Medicine Materia Medica*. Seattle, WA: Eastland Press, 1993;318.
Buhner, S. *Healing Lyme: Natural Healing and Prevention of Lyme Borreliosis and Its Coinfections.* Silver City, NM: Raven Press, 2005.
Chang, H., But, P. *Pharmacology and Applications of Chinese Materia Medica* (Vol. 2). Hong Kong: World Scientific, 1987;1320.
Chen, H., Weng, L. Comparison on efficacy in treating liver fibrosis of chronic hepatitis B between *Astragalus Polygonum* anti-fibrosis decoction and jinshuibao capsule. *Zhongguo Zhong Xi Yi Jie He Za Zhi*. 2000;20(4):255-7.
Chen, K. et al. Reducing fatigue of athletes following oral administration of huangqi jianzhong tang. *Acta Pharmacology Sin*. 2002;23(8):757-61.
Chen, L., Liao, J., Guo, W. Effects of *Astragalus membranaceus* on left ventricular function and oxygen free radicals in acute myocardial infarction patients and mechanism of its cardiotonic action. *Hung Kuo Chung Hsi I Chieh Ho Tsa Chih*. 1995;15(3):141-3.
Cheng, Y. et al. Astragalus polysaccharides lowers plasma cholesterol through mechanisms distinct from statins. *PLoS One*. 2011;6(11):e27437.
Chevallier, A. *The Encyclopedia of Medicinal Plants*. New York, NY: DK Publishing, 1996.
Chu, D. et al. Immunotherapy with Chinese medicinal herbs. I. Immune restoration of local xenogeneic graft-versus-host reaction in cancer patients by fractionated *Astragalus membranaceus in vitro*. *J Clin Lab Immunology*. 1998;25:119-23.
Cui, R., Wang, B., et al. Suppressive effect of *Astragalus membranaceus* bunge on chemical hepatocarcinogenesis in rats. *Cancer Chemotherapy Pharmacology*. 2003;51(1):75-80.
Du, X. et al. Astragalus polysaccharides enhance humoral and cellular immune responses of hepatitis B surface antigen vaccination through inhibiting expression of transforming growth factor B and frequency of regulatory T cells. *FEMS Immunol Med Microbiol*. 2011;63(2):228-35.
Duan, P., Wang, Z. Clinical study on effect of Astragalus in efficacy enhancing and toxicity reducing of chemotherapy in patients of malignant tumor. *Zhongguo Zhong Xi Yi Jie He Za Zhi*. 2002;22(7):515-7.
Enqin, Z. (Ed.). *Chinese Materia Medica*. Shanghai, China: Publishing House of Shanghai College of TCM, 1988;376.
Fan, T., Fu, X., Zhang, G. The inhibitory effect of some herbs on hepatitis B virus replication *in vitro* and its mechanism. *Chinese Journal Exper Clin Virology*. 1996;10(1):27-30.
Foster, S., Leung, A. *Encyclopedia of Common Natural Ingredients Used in Food, Drugs and Cosmetics*. New York, NY: John Wiley & Sons, 1996.
Hikino, H. et al. Validity of Oriental Medicine. 2. Hypotensive principle of Astragalus and Hedysarum roots. *Planta Medica*. 1976;30:297.
Hou, Y., Zhang, Z. et al. Interferon induction and lymphocyte transformation stimulated by *Astragalus membranaceus* in mouse spleen cell cultures. *Zhonghua Weisheng Wuxue Hemian Yixue Zazhi*. 1981;1(2):137-9.
Huang, K. *The Pharmacology of Chinese Herbs* (2nd ed.). New York, NY: CRC Press, 1999.
Huang, L. et al. *Astragalus membranaceus* lectin induces caspase-dependent apoptosis in human leukemia cells. *Cell Prolif*. 2012 Feb;45(1):15-21.
Jiang, Xiao. *Handbook of Planta Medica*. Beijing, China: People's Health Publishers, 1986;127.
Jin, X. Clinical investigation on 30 cases of senile benign renal arteriolosclerosis treated by huang qi gu jing yin. *Journal of TCM*. 2001;21(3):177.
Li, S., Yuan, R., Gao, H. Clinical observation on the treatment of ischemic heart disease with *Astragalus membranaceus*. *Chung Kuo Chung Hsi I Chieh Ho Tsa Chih*. 1995;15(2):77-80.
Lin, Y., Wang, B., Luo, X. Clinical study of astragalus's preventing the recurrence of asthma in children. *Zhongguo Zhong Xi Yi Jie He Za Zhi*. 2011 Aug;31(8):1090-2.
Matkovic, Z. et al. Efficacy and safety of *Astragalus* in the treatment of patients with seasonal allergic rhinitis. *Phytotherapy Res*. 2010;24(2):175-81.
Mavligit, G. et al. Local xeno-genetic graft-vs-host reaction: a practical assessment of T-cell function among cancer patients. *Journal of Immunology.* 1979;123(5):2185-8.
McCaleb, R. Astragalus and Viral Heart Disease. *HerbalGram*. 1991;24:20.
McKenna, D., Hughes, K., Jones, K. Astragalus. *International Journal of Integrative Medicine*. October 2002;4(5):40-6.
Nalbantsoy, A. et al. Evaluation of the immunomodulatory properties in mice and *in vitro* anti-inflammatory activity of cycloartane type saponins from Astragalus species. *J Ethnopharmacol*. 2012 Jan 31;139(2):574-81.
Rou, M., Renfu, X. The effect of radix Astragali on mouse marrow hemopoiesis. *Journal of Traditional Chinese Medicine*. 1983;3(3):199-204.
Tang, L. et al. Clinical and experimental effectiveness of Astragali compound in the treatment of chronic viral hepatitis B. *J Internat Med Research*. 2009;37:662-667.
Tang, W., Eisenbrand, G. *Chinese Drugs of Plant Origin: Chemistry, Pharmacology, and Use in Traditional and Modern Medicine*. Berlin: Springer-

Verlag, 1992;1056.
Upton, R. *Astragalus Root Monograph*. Santa Cruz, CA: American Herbal Pharmacopoeia, August 1999.
Verotta, L. et al. Cycloartane saponins from *Astragalus peregrinus* as modulators of lymphocyte proliferation. *Fitoterapia*. 2001;72(8):894-905.
Wang, D. et al. Studies on protective effect of total flavonoids of Astragalus on liver damage. *Zhongguo Zhong Yao Za Zhi*. 2001;26(7):483-6.
Wassef, F. Astragalus: Spanning Eastern and Western Medicine. *American Journal of Natural Medicine*. June 1998;5(1):26-9.
Wei, H. et al. TCM Astragalus reverses predominance of TH2 cytokines and their upstream transcript factors in lung cancer patients. *Oncology Rep*. 2003;10(5):1507-12.
Yang, Y. et al. *Chinese Medical Journal*. 1987;197(7):595.
Ye, M. et al. Effects of Astragalus polysaccharide on proliferation and Akt phosphorylation of the basal-like breast cancer cell line. *Zhong Xi Yi Jie He Xue Bao*. 2011 Dec;9(12):1339-46.
Yuan, W. et al. Effect of *Astragalus membranaceus* on electrical activities of cultured rat beating heart cells infected with Coxsackie B-2 virus. *Chinese Medical Journal*. 1990;103(3):177-82.
Zhang, Y. et al. Effects of Astragalus on experimental liver injury. *Yaoxue Yuebao*. 1992;27(6):401-6.
Zhao, L. et al. Characterization of polysaccharide from Astragalus radix as the macrophage stimulator. *Cell Immunol*. 2011;271(2):329-34.
Zhao, X. Effects of *Astragalus membranaceus* and *Tripterygium hypoglaucum* on natural killer cell activity of peripheral blood mononuclear in systemic lupus erythematosus. *Zhongguo Zhongxi Yixue*. 1992;12(11):645,669-71.
Zuo, L. et al. The curative effects of *Astragalus membranaceus* bunge in combination with acyclovir on mice infected with HIV. *Virol. Sin*. 1995.

BLACK COHOSH

1) p. 90; 2) p. 22; 3) pp. 40, 92, 271; 5) p. 75; 6) p. 108; 7) p. 11; 8); 9) p. 341; 13); 14) p. 393; 16) p. 51; 17); 20) p. 528; 21) p. 466; 23) p. 47; 25) p. 54; 27) p. 64; 30) pp. 178, 231-2; 36) p. 539; 37) p. 578; 38); 41) p. 633; 42) p. 206; 43); 45) p. 76; 46) pp. 29-30, 183, 188; 48) p. 307; 49); 50) pp. 99, 183; 51); 54); 55); 62) p. 51; 63) p. 107; 64); 65) pp. 144, 166; 66) p. 37; 75) pp. 316, 318; 79) p. 129; 80) p. 219; 82) pp. 7 ,8, 16, 18, 53, 187.
American Botanical Council Staff. ABC-AHP-NCNPR Botanical Adulterants Program Publishes Black Cohosh Lab Guidance Document. *HerbalGram*. 2016;109:22-3.
Beer, A., Neff, A. Differentiated Evaluation of Extract-Specific Evidence on *Cimicifuga racemosa's* Efficacy and Safety for Climacteric Complaints. *Evidence Based Complementary Alternative Medicine*. 2013;2013:860602.
Benoit, P., Fong, H., Farnsworth, N. Biological and Phytochemical Evaluation of Plants, Anti-inflammatory Evaluation of 163 Species. *Lloydia*. 1976;19(2-3):160-171.
Bensky, D., Gamble, A., Kaptchuk, T. *Chinese Herbal Medicine Materia Medica*. Seattle, WA: Eastland Press, 1993;50.
Beuscher, N. *Cimicifuga racemosa* –Black Cohosh. *Zeitschrift fur Phytotherapie*. 1995;16:301-10.
Blumenthal, M. Australian TGA Publishes Liver Warning Policy for Black Cohosh. *HerbalGram*. 2006;71:60-1.
___________. European Health Agencies Recommend Liver Warnings on Black Cohosh Products. *HerbalGram*. 2006;72:56-8.
Bodinet, C., Freudenstein, J. Influence of *Cimifuga racemosa* on the proliferation of estrogen receptor-positive human breast cancer cells. *Breast Cancer Research Treatment*. 2002;76(1):1-10.
Briese, V., Stammwitz, U., Friede, M., Henneicke-von Zepelin, H. Black cohosh with or without St. John's wort for symptom-specific climacteric treatment-Results of a large-scale, controlled, observational study. *Maturitas*. 2007;57(4):405-414.
Burdette, J., Farnsworth, N. et al. Black cohosh acts as a mixed competitive ligand and partial agonist of the serotonin receptor. *J Agric Food Chem*. 2003 Sep 10;51(19):5661-70.
Burke, B., Olson, R., Cusack, B. Randomized, controlled trial of phytoestrogen in the prophylactic treatment of menstrual migraines. *Biomedical Pharmacotherapy*. 2002;56(6):283-8.
Chung, D. et al. Black cohosh and St. John's wort for climacteric symptoms. *Yonsei Medical Journal*. 2007;48(2):289-294.
Compton, J. et al. Phylogeny of *Actaea* including *Cimicifuga* (*Ranunculaceae*) inferred from nrDNA ITS sequence variation. *Biochemical Systematics and Ecology*. 1998;26:185-197.
Crawford, A. *The Herbal Menopause Book*. Berkeley, CA: Crossing Press, 1997.
Duker, E., Kopanski, L., Jarry, H., Wuttke, W. Effects of Extracts from *Cimicifuga racemosa* on Gonadotropin Release in Menopausal Women and Ovariectomized Rats. *Planta Medica*. 1991;57:420-4.
Einbond, L., Wen-Cai, Y. et al. Growth inhibitory activity of extracts and compounds from *Cimicifuga* species on human breast cancer cells. *Phytomedicine*. 2008 June;15(6-7):504-11.
Foldes, J. The Actions of an Extract of *Cimicifuga racemosa*. *Arzneimittel Forschung*. 1959;13(12):623-4.
Foster, S. *Black Cohosh: Cimicifuga racemosa*. P.O. Box 201660, Austin, TX 78720-1660: American Botanical Council, Series #314, 1998.
_______. Black Cohosh: *Cimicifuga racemosa*, A Literature Review. *HerbalGram*. 1999;45:35-50.
_______. Exploring the Peripatetic Maze of Black Cohosh Adulteration. *HerbalGram*. 2013;98:32-51.
Fritz, H. et al. Black cohosh and breast cancer: a systematic review. *Integrative Cancer Ther*. 2014 Jan;13(1):12-29.
Frontier Organic Research Herb Farm. *Black Cohosh: Grower's Crop Monograph*. 3027 78th St., Norway, IA, 52318.
Fugh-Berman, A., Awang, D. Black Cohosh. *Alternative Therapies in Women's Health*. 2001;3(11):81-88.
Genazzani, E., Sorrentino, L. Vascular Action of Acteina: Active Constituent of *Actaea Racemose*. *Nature*. 1962;194(4828):544-5.
Gladstar, R., Hirsh, P. (Eds.). *Planting the Future: Saving our Medicinal Herbs*. Healing Arts Press, Rochester, VT: 2000; 64-71.
Henneicke-von Zepelin, H. et al. Isopropanolic black cohosh extract and recurrence-free survival after breast cancer. *Int J Pharmacol Ther*. 2007 Mar;45(3):143-54.
Hernandez Munoz, G., Pluchino, S. *C. racemosa* for treatment of hot flashes in women surviving breast cancer. *Maruritas*. 2003;44(1): S59-65.
Jarry, H., Wuttke, W. et al. *Cimicifuga racemosa* extract BNO 1055 inhibits proliferation of the human prostate cancer cell line LNCaP. *Phytomed*. 2005;12:178-182.
Jiang, B. et al. The value of plant collections in ethnopharmacology: a case study of an 85-year-old black cohosh (*Actaea racemosa L.*) sample. *Journal of Ethnopharmacology*. 2005;96:521-528.
Kamel, H. Role of phyto-oestrogens in ovulation induction in women with PCOS. *Eur J Obstet Gynecol Reprod Biol*. 2013 May;168(1):60-3.
Li, J. et al. *In vitro* metabolic interactions between black cohosh (*Cimicifuga racemosa*) and tamoxifen via inhibition of cytochromes P450 2D6 and 3A4. *Xenobiotica*. 2011 Aug 9.
Liske, E. Therapeutic Efficacy and Safety of *Cimicifuga racemosa* for Gynecological Disorders. *Advances in Natural Therapy*. 1998;15(1):45-53.
Liu, Z. et al. Estrogenic effects of *Cimicifuga racemosa* (Black Cohosh) in mice and on estrogen receptors in MCF-7 cells. *Journal of Medicinal Food*. 2001;4(3):171-8.
McKenna, D. Black Cohosh: Efficacy, Safety, and Use in Clinical and Preclinical Applications. *Alternative Therapies*. May 2001;7(3):93.
Murphy, R. *Homeopathic Medical Repertory: Modern Alphabetical Repertory*. Pagosa Springs, CO: Hahnemann Academy of North America, 1993.
Murray, M. Remifemin: Answers to Some Common Questions. *American Journal of Natural Medicine*. 1997;4(3):3-5.
Nadaoka, I. et al. Oral administration of *Cimicifuga racemosa* extract attenuates psychological and physiological stress responses. *Biomed Res*. June 2012;33(3):145-152.
Osmers, R. et al. Efficacy and safety of isopropanolic black cohosh extract for climacteric symptoms. *Obstetrics & Gynocology*. 2005:105:1074-83.
Powell, S., Farnsworth, N. et al. *In vitro* serotonergic activity of black cohosh and identification of N(omega)-methylserotonin as a potential active constituent. *J Agric Food Chem*. 2008 Dec 24;56(24):11718-26.
Reame, N. et al. Black cohosh has central opioid activity in postmenopausal women: evidence from naloxone blockade and positron emission tomography neuroimaging. *Menopause*. Sep-Oct 2008;15(5):832-840.
Rebbeck, T. et al. A retrospective case-control study of the use of hormone-related supplements and association with breast cancer. *Int J Cancer*. 2007;120:1523-1528.
Reid, D. *A Handbook of Chinese Healing Herbs*. Boston, MA: Shambala, 1995;85.
Richard, C., Jurgens, T. Effects of natural health products on blood pressure. *Ann Pharmacother*. April 2005;39:712-20.
Ringer, D. (Ed.). *Physicians' Guide to Nutriceuticals*. Omaha, NE: Nutritional Data Resources LP; 1998.
Ross, S. Menopause: a standardized isopropanolic black cohosh extract (remifemin) is found to be safe and effective for menopausal symptoms. *Holistic Nurse Practitioner*. 2012 Jan-Feb;26(1):58-61.
Seidlova-Wuttke, D. et al. Pharmacology of *Cimicifuga racemosa* extract BNO 1055 in rats: bone, fats and uterus. *Maturitas*. 2003;44(1):S39.

__________________. Osteoprotective effects of *Cimicifuga racemosa* and its triterpene-saponins are responsible for reduction of bone marrow fat. *Phytomedicine*. 2012 Jul 15;19(10):855-60.
Shams, T. et al. Efficacy of black cohosh-containing preparations on menopausal symptoms. *Altern Ther Health Med.* 2010;16(1):36-44.
Soule, D. *The Roots of Healing*. New York, NY: Citadel Press, 1996.
Stolze, H. An Alternative to Treat Menopausal Complaints. *Gynecology*. 1982;3:14-16.
Teschke, R., Schwarzenboeck, A. Suspected hepatotoxicity by *Cimicifuga racemosae* rhizome: Critical analysis and structured causality assessment. *Phytomedicine.* 2009;16:72-84.
____________________ et al. Spontaneous reports of assumed herbal hepatotoxicity by black cohosh: is the liver-unspecific Naranjo scale precise enough to ascertain causality? *Pharmacoepidemiol Drug Safety*. 2011 Jun;20(6):567-82.
____________________ et al. Herb induced liver injury presumably caused by black cohosh: a survey of initially purported cases and herbal quality specifications. *Ann Hepatol*. 2011 Jul-Sep;10(3):249-59.
Warnecke, G. Influencing Menopausal Symptoms with a Phytotherapeutic Agent: Successful therapy with *Cimicifuga* mono-extract. *Med Welt.* 1985;36:871-4.
Wood, M. *Seven Herbs, Plants as Teachers*. Berkeley, CA: North Atlantic Books, 1986.
Wuttke, W. et al. The *Cimicifuga* preparation BNO 1055 vs. conjugated estrogens in a double-blind placebo-controlled study: effects on menopause symptoms and bone markers. *Maturitas*. 2003;44(1):S67-77.
____________. Phytoestrogens: endocrine disruptors or replacement for hormone replacement therapy? *Maturitas*. 2003;44(1):S9-20.
____________. Effects of black cohosh *(Cimicifuga racemosa)* on bone turnover, vaginal mucosa, and various blood parameters in postmenopausal women: a double-blind, placebo-controlled, and conjugated estrogens-controlled study. *Menopause*. 2006:13(2);185-196.
____________. Efficacy and tolerability of the black cohosh (*Actaea racemosa*) ethanolic extract BNO 1055 on climacteric complaints: a double-blind, placebo- and conjugated estrogens-controlled study. *Maturitas*. 2006;55(Suppl 1): S83-S91.
____________. The non-estrogenic alternative for the treatment of climacteric complaints: Black cohosh (*Cimicifuga* or *Actaea racemosa*). *Journal of Steroid Biochemistry & Molecular Biology.* 2014 Jan;139:302-10.
Xi, S., Liske, E., Wang, S. et al. Effects of isopropanolic *Cimicifuga racemosa* extract on uterine fibroids in comparison with tibolone among patients of a recent randomized, double blind, parallel-controlled study in Chinese women with menopausal symptoms. *Evid Based Complement Alternat Med.* 2014:717686
Zava, D. et al. Estrogen and progestin bioactivity of foods, herbs, and spices. *Proc Soc Exp Biol Med.* 1998 Mar;217(3):369-78.

BLACK WALNUT

GENERAL REFERENCES: 1) pp. 227, 381; 2) p. 401; 3) pp. 42, 298; 8) p. 180; 9) p. 491; 12) p. 87; 14) p. 334; 16) pp. 56, 334; 17); 18) p. 328; 19) p. 69; 27) p. 310; 29) p. 1440; 31); 33) p. 842; 37) p. 724; 44) p. 386; 46) p. 65; 49) p. 280; 51) p. 230; 62) p. 389; 64) pp. 169-70, 300, 301; 66) p. 39; 67) pp. 41, 48, 58, 60, 67,73, 96; 79) p. 445; 80) p. 323; 81).
Ali-Shtayeh, M., Aby Ghdeib, S. Antifungal activity of plant extracts against dermatophytes. *Mycoses.* 1999;42(11-12):665-72.
Alkhawajah, A. Studies on the antimicrobial activity of *Juglans regia*. *Am J Chin Med*. 1997;25(2):175-80.
Bensky, D., Gamble, A., Kaptchuk, T. *Chinese Herbal Medicine Materia Medica*. Seattle, WA: Eastland Press, 1993;343.
Bhargava, U., Westfall, B. Antitumor activity of *Juglans nigra* (black walnut) extractives. *Journal of Pharmaceutical Sciences*. 1968;57(10):1674-7.
Brinker, F. *The Eclectic Dispensatory of Botanical Therapeutics*. Sandy, OR: Eclectic Medical Publications,1995.
Brown, D. *Encyclopedia of Herbs and Their Uses.* New York,NY: DK Publishing, Inc. 1995;145,298.
Chae, J. et al. Phosphoinositol 3-kinase, a novel target molecule for the inhibitory effects of juglone on TPA-induced cell transformation. *International Journal of Molecular Medicine.* 2012 Jul;30(1):8-14.
Clark, A. et al. Antimicrobial activity of juglone. *Phytotherapy Research*. 1990;4:11-13.
Fitschen, P. et al. Cardiovascular effects of consumption of Black versus English Walnuts. *J Med Food*. 2011 Sep;14(9):890-898.
Harborne, J., Baxter, H. *Phytochemical Dictionary: A Handbook of Bioactive Compounds from Plants*. Washington: Taylor & Francis. 1993.
Heisey, R., Gorham, B. Antimicrobial effects of plant extracts on *Streptococcus mutans, Candida albicans, Trichophyton rubrum* and other mirco-organisms. *Lett Appl Microbiology*. 1992;14:136-9.
Omar, S. et al. Antimicrobial activity of extracts of eastern North American hardwood trees and relation to traditional medicine. *Journal of Ethnopharmacology*. 2000;73(1-2):161-70.
Owumi, S. et al. Protective effect of *Juglans nigra* on sodium arsenite-induced toxicity in rats. *Pharmacognosy Research*. 2013 Jul;5(3):183-8.
Perusquia, M. et al. Vasoactive effects of aqueous extracts from five Mexican medicinal plants on isolated rat aorta. *Journal of Ethnopharmacology* 1995;46(1):63-9.
Trease, G., Evans, W. *Trease and Evans' Pharmacognosy* (13th ed.). Philadelphia, PA: Bailliere Tindall, 1989.
Tripathi, R. et al. Structure activity relationship amongst some fungitoxic alpha-napthoquinones of angiosperm origin. *Agricul Biol Chemistry*. 1988;44:2483-5.

BLOODROOT

GENERAL REFERENCES: 3) pp. 44, 213, 218, 223, 271; 7) p. 29; 9) p. 678; 13); 14) pp. 262-3, 270, 520, 547; 16) p. 58; 17); 18) p. 242; 19) p. 318; 20) p. 1708; 21) p. 615; 22) p. 84; 23) p. 50; 25) p 58; 27) p. 54; 35) p. 177; 36) p 581; 37); 41) p. 635; 42) p. 208; 43); 44) p. 128; 46) pp. 103, 136, 183; 48) pp. 53, 192, 351; 49) p. 515; 55) p. 42; 62) p. 54; 64) p. 384; 70) p. 354; 74) pp. 116, 129; 76) pp. 37, 269; 79) p. 62; 82) p. 360.
Adhami, V. et al. Sanguinarine causes cell cycle blockade and apoptosis of human prostate carcinoma cells via modulation of cyclin kinase inhibitor-cyclin-cyclin-dependent kinase machinery. *Molecular Cancer Ther*. 2004 Aug;3(8):933-40.
D'Adamo, P. Chelidonium and Sanguinaria alkaloids as anti-HIV therapy. *Journal of Natural Medicine.* 1992;3:31-4.
Dzink, J., Socransky, S. Comparative *in vitro* activity of sanguinarine against oral microbial isolates. *Antimicrob Agents Chemotherapy*. 1985; 27(4):663-5.
Frankos, V. et al. Safety of Sanguinaria extract as used in commercial toothpaste and oral rinse products. *J Canadian Dental Ass*. 1990;7:41-7.
Gladstar, R., Hirsh, P. (Eds.). *Planting the Future: Saving our Medicinal Herbs*. Healing Arts Press, Rochester, VT: 2000;72.
Godowski, K. Antimicrobial action of sanguinarine. *Journal of Clinical Dentisty*. 1989;1(4):96-101.
Han, M., Yoo, Y., Choi, Y. Sanguinarine-induced apoptosis in human leukemia U937 cells via Bcl-2 downregulation and caspase-3 activation. *Chemotherapy*. 2008;54(3):157-65.
Hannah, J. et al. Long-term clinical evaluation of toothpaste and oral rinse containing sanguinaria extract in controlling plaque, gingival inflammation, and sulcular bleeding during orthodontic treatment. *Am Journal Orthod Dentofacial Orthop*. 1989;96(3):199.
Harkrader, R. et al. The history, chemistry, and pharmacokinetics of *Sanguinaria* extract. *J Cananian Dental Association*. 1990;56(7):7-2.
Hussain, A. et al. Sanguinarine-dependent induction of apoptosis in primary effusion lymphoma cells. *Cancer Res*. 2007 Apr 15;67(8):3888-97.
Karlowsky, J. Bloodroot: *Sanguinaria canadensis*. *Canadian Pharmaceutical Journal*. 1991;124(5):260-7.
Kim, S. et al. Sanguinarine-induced apoptosis: generation of ROS, down-regulation of Bcl-2, c-FLIP, and synergy with TRAIL. *J Cell Biochem*. 2008 June 1;104(3):895-907.
Kuftinec, M. et al. Sanguinaria toothpaste and oral rinse regimen clinical efficacy in short- and long-term trial. *J Can Dental Ass*. 1990;56(7):31-3.
Lee, J. et al. Sanguinarine Induces Apoptosis of HT-29 Human Colon Cancer Cells via the Regulation of Bax/Bcl-2 Ratio and Caspase-9-Dependent Pathway. *Int J Toxicol*. 2012 Jan ;31(1):70-7.
Lo Ha Wa Ti An Ka. *Osage Medicine: Ancestral Herbs and the Illnesses that they Treat*. Greyhorse Indian Village, Rt 2 Box 66-1, Fairfax, OK 74637: Scope Publications.
Obiang-Obounou, B. et al. The mechanism of action of sanguinarine against methicillin-resistant *Staphylococcus aureus*. *J Toxicol Sci*. 2011 June; 36(3):277-83.
Southard, G., Boulware, R. et al. Sanguinarine, a New Antiplaque Agent: Retention and Plaque Specificity. *JAMA*. 1984;108:338-341.
Tenenbaum, H., Dahan, M., Soell, M. Effectiveness of a sanguinarine regimen after scaling and root planing. *J Periodontol*. 1999 Mar;70(3):307-11.

BLUE COHOSH

GENERAL REFERENCES: 3) pp. 45, 271; 6) p. 112; 7) p. 41; 8) p. 41; 9) p. 322; 10); 13); 14); 15); 16); 17), 18) p. 480; 19) p. 355; 20) p. 468; 21) p. 282; 22) p. 86; 23) p. 48; 25) p. 60; 27) p. 233; 30) pp. 178, 234; 31) pp. 315-6; 35) p. 177; 37) p. 251; 42) p. 206; 44) p. 129; 46) pp. 24,183; 49) p. 144; 55) p. 82; 60); 62) p. 54; 66) p. 41; 70) p. 291; 71) p. 65; 74) pp. 34, 42; 79) p. 131.

Bergner, P. Cardiotoxic Effects of Blue Cohosh on a fetus. *Medical Herbalism*. 2001;12(1);12-4.
________. Herbal Pairing with Black Cohosh. *Medical Herbalism*. 2002;12(4);17.
Brinker, F. Blue cohosh. *Journal of American Herbalist Guild*. Fall/Winter 2001:4-8.
Costello, L. Estrogenic Substances from Plants. *American Journal Pharm Soc*. 1950;39:177-80.
Crawford, A. *The Herbal Menopause Book*. Berkeley, CA: Crossing Press, 1997.
Fackelmann, K. Medicine for Menopause. *Science News*. 1998.
Finkel, R., Zarlengo, K. Blue cohosh and perinatal stroke. *New England Journal of Medicine*. 2004;351:302-303.
Gladstar, R., Hirsh, P. (Eds.). *Planting the Future: Saving our Medicinal Herbs*. Rochester, VT: Healing Arts Press, 2000;78.
Gunn, T., Wright, I. The use of black and blue cohosh in labor. *New Zealand Medical Journal*. 1996;109(1032):410-1.
Jones, T., Lawson, B. Profound neonatal congestive heart failure caused by maternal consumption of blue cohosh herbal medication. *Journal of Pediatrics*. 1998;132(3):550-2.
Lee ,Y. et al. Anti-Inflammatory Effect of Triterpene Saponins Isolated from Blue Cohosh (*Caulophyllum thalictroides*). *Evidence Based Complementary Alternative Medicine*. 2012;2012:798192.
Low Dog, T. Blue cohosh and neonatal myocardial toxicity. *Journal of American Herbalist Guild*. Fall/Winter 2001:9-10.
McFarlin, B. et al. A national survey of herbal preparations used by nurse-midwives for labor stimulation. Review of the literature and recommendations for practice. *Journal of Nurse Midwifery*. 1999;44(3):205-16.
Moerman, D. *Medicinal Plants of Native America* (Vol. 1). Ann Arbor, MI: University of Michigan Department of Anthropology, 1986;534.
Potterton, D. et al. More on blue cohosh and perinatal stroke. *New England Journal of Medicine*. 2004;351:2239-2241.
Smith, P. *The Indian Doctor's Dispensatory* (Bulletin #2). Cincinnati, OH: Lloyd Library of Botany, Pharmacy and Materia Medica, 1813.
Soule, D. *Roots of Healing*. New York, NY: Citadel Press, 1995.
Tilgner, S. Female Reproductive Herbs Compared. *Medical Herbalism*. 2001;12(3);13-4.

BLUE VERVAIN

GENERAL REFERENCES: 1) p. 380; 3) p. 277; 9) p. 728; 11) p. 189; 12) p. 451; 17); 19) p. 293; 20) p. 2055; 21) p. 693; 27) p. 64; 29) p. 718; 33) p. 831; 37) p. 179; 40) p. 210; 42) p. 233; 44) p. 130; 46) pp. 121, 183; 49) p. 591; 51) pp. 120, 206, 226; 55) p. 263; 62) p. 386; 66) p. 112; 70) p. 386; 79) p. 442; 80) p. 499; 81) pp. 97, 130, 162; 82) pp. 9, 17, 50, 119, 123, 159.
Bingel, A., Farnsworth, N. Higher plants as potential sources of galactagogues. *Ecom Med Plant Research*. 1994;6:1-54.
Casanova, E. Antioxidant and antifungal activity of *Verbena officinalis* L. leaves. *Plant Foods Human Nutrition*. 2008 Sep;63(3):93-7.
Cherkin, D., Street, J. Alternative medicine—the case of herbal remedies [letter]. *New England Journal of Medicine*. 1999;340:565.
De Martino, L. et al. *Verbena officinalis* essential oil and its component citral as apoptotic-inducing agent in chronic lymphocytic leukemia. *Int J Immunopathol Pharmacol*. 2009 Oct-Dec;22(4):1097-104.
_______________. Chemistry, antioxidant, antibacterial and antifungal activities of volatile oils and their components. *Nat Prod Commun*. 2009 Dec;4(12):1741-50.
Deepak, M. Anti-inflammatory activity and chemical composition of extracts of *Verbena officinalis*. *Phytotherapy Research*. 2000;14(6):463-5.
Dudai, N. et al. Citral is a new inducer of caspase-3 in tumor cell lines. *Planta Medica*. 2005 May;71(5):484-8.
Farnsworth, N. Potential value of plants as sources of new antifertility agents. *Journal of Pharmaceutical Science*. 1975;64:535-98.
Grases, F. et al. Urolithiasis and phytotherapy. *Int Urology and Nephrology*. 1994;26(5):507-11.
Inouye, H. et al. Purgative activities of iridoid glucosides. *Planta Medica*. 1974;25(3):285-8.
Lai, S. et al. Novel neuroprotective effects of the aqueous extracts from *Verbena officinalis* Linn. *Neuropharmacology*. 2006 May;50(6):641-50.
Moore, M. *Medicinal Plants of the Mountain West*. Santa Fe, NM: Museum of New Mexico Press, 1979;160.
Oliver-Bever, B. *Medicinal Plants in Tropical West Africa*. Cambridge, MA: Cambridge University Press, 1986.
Owen, N. *Verbena officinalis* L., Vervain. *British Journal of Phytotherapy*. 2002;5(3):114-117.
Sakai, S. Pharmacological Actions of *Verbena Officinalis*. *Gifu Ika Daigaku Kiyo*. 1963;11(1):6-17.
Speroni, E. et al. Effects of differential extraction of *Verbena officinalis* on rat models of inflammation, cicatrization and gastric damage. *Planta Medica*. 2007 Mar;73(3):227-35.
Tehon, L. *The Drug Plants of Illinois*. Illinois Natural History Survey. Circular 44, 1951.

BONESET

GENERAL REFERENCES: 3) pp. 46, 209, 272; 8) p. 224; 9) p. 420; 17); 18) p. 269; 19) pp. 259, 262; 20) p. 738; 21) p. 364; 27) p. 89; 33) pp. 118, 290; 36) p. 549; 37) p. 177; 40) p. 103; 41) p. 636; 43) pp. 41, 42, 105, 402; 44) p. 131; 46) p. 50; 48) pp. 41, 166, 181, 204, 375; 49) p. 229; 55) p. 48; 62) p. 57; 66) p. 42; 70) p. 284; 74) pp. 37, 56; 79) p. 66; 80) p. 259; 81) pp. 43, 61, 352; 82) pp. 23, 51, 69, 79, 111, 117, 187.
Alfs, M. Antiviral Herbs. *Medical Herbalism*. 2005-2006;13(4):15-16.
Bergner, P. Clinical Correspondence. *Medical Herbalism*. 1995;7(4):10-13. Quote reprinted with permission from Paul Bergner.
________. Boneset and Influenza; Historical Notes and Commentary. *Medical Herbalism*. 2003;13(4):16-20.
________. Antiviral Botanicals in Herbal Medicine. *Medical Herbalism*. 2005;14(3):7.
________. Influenza: Treatment of Acute Febrile Disease. *Medical Herbalism*. 2009;16(1):1,18-21.
Brinker, F. Boneset in dyspepsia and febrile infections. *Journal of the American Herbalists Guild*. 2010;9(1):13-23.
Buhner, S. *Herbs for Hepatitis C and the Liver*. North Adams, MA: Storey Publishing, 2000;59-61.
________. *Herbal Antibiotics*. North Adams, MA: Storey Publishing, 2012; 264-8.
Ellingwood, F. *Three Valuable Remedies Used in Grippe and Influenza*. Lloyd Library Archives, 1897.
Greunwald, J., Brendler, T., Jaenicke, C. et al. (Eds.). *PDR for Herbal Medicines*. Montvale, NJ: Medical Economics, 1998;842-43.
Habtemariam, S. MacPherson, A. Cytotoxicity and antibacterial activity of ethanol extract from leaves of a herbal drug, boneset (*Eupatorium perfoliatum*). *Phytotherapy Research*. 2000;14(7):575-7.
Hensel, A., Maas, M., Sendker, J. et al. *Eupatorium perfoliatum* L.: phytochemistry, traditional use and current applications. *Journal of Ethnopharmacology*. December 8, 2011;138(3):641-651.
Lloyd, J., Lloyd, C. A Treatise on *Eupatorium perfoliatum* (Drug Treatise Number XXXI). Cincinnati, OH: Lloyd Brothers Pharmaceutical Company, 1918. Text is available at www.herbaltherapeutics.net/herbal_therapeutics_library.htm.
Lo Ha Wa Ti An Ka. *Osage Medicine: Ancestral Herbs and the Illnesses that they Treat*. Greyhorse Indian Village, Rt 2 Box 66-1, Fairfax, OK 74637: Scope Publications.
Maas, M., Deters, A., Hensel, A. Anti-inflammatory activity of *Eupatorium perfoliatum* L. extracts, eupafolin, and dimeric guaianolide via iNOS inhibitory activity and modulation of inflammation-related cytokines and chemokines. *J Ethnopharmacol*. 2011 Sep 1;137(1):371-81.
Maas, M. et al. An unusual dimeric guaianolide with antiprotozoal [anti-malarial] activity and further sesquiterpene lactones from *Eupatorium perfoliatum*. *Phytochemistry*. 2011 May;72(7):635-44.
Millspaugh, C. *American Medicinal Plants, An Illustrated and Descriptive Guide to the American Plants used as Homeopathic Remedies*. New York, NY: Boericke & Tafel, 1887;314.
Smith, L., Culvenor, C. Plant Sources of Hepatotoxic Pyrrolizidine Alkaloids. *Journal of Natural Products*. 1981;44:129-52.
Wagner, H. et al. Immunostimulating Polysaccharides of Higher Plants. *Arzneimittel Forschung*. 1985;35:1069.
Wagner, H., Jurcic, K. Immunologic studies of plant combination preparations. *In-vitro* and *in-vivo* studies on the stimulation of phagocytosis. *Arzneimittel-forschung*. 1991 Oct;41(10):1072-6.
Woerdenbag, H., Bos, R., Hendricks, H. *Eupatorium perfoliatum*-the boneset. *Z Phytother*. 1992;13:134-9.
Wren, R. *Potter's New Clycopaedia of Botanical Drugs and Preparations*. Saffron Walden, England: C. W. Daniel Company, 1989.

BURDOCK

1) p. 318; 3) pp. 50, 209, 238, 272; 8) p. 64; 9) p. 261; 11) p. 29; 12); 14) pp. 189,328,444; 16) p. 73; 17); 180 p. 378; 20) p. 1118; 21); 22) p. 110; 24) p. 42; 27) pp. 186, 188; 29) p. 809; 31); 33) p. 143; 36) p. 529; 37) p. 730; 44) p. 140; 46) p. 12; 48) pp. 43,243,353; 49) p. 84; 50) p. 94; 51) pp. 3, 57, 249, 279; 55) p. 52; 57) p. 95; 62) p. 63; 65) pp. 162, 310; 66) p. 44; 70) p. 286; 71) p. 87; 74) p. 172; 79) p. 79; 80) p. 137.
Ausubel, K. Tempest in a Tonic Bottle: A Bunch of Weeds? *HerbalGram*. 2000;49:32-43.
Belkin, Hardy, Perrault. Swelling and Vacuolization Induced in Ascites Tumor Cells by Polysaccharides from Higher Plants. *Cancer Research*. 1961;9:330-2.

Bensky, D., Gamble, A., Kaptchuk, T. *Chinese Herbal Medicine Materia Medica*. Seattle, WA: Eastland Press, 1993;41.
Bergner, P. Inulin. *Medical Herbalism*. 1997;9(2):20-1.
________. Adverse effect of the top medicinal herbs. *Medical Herbalism*. 2002;12(4):8.
Bever, B., Zahnd, G. Plants with Oral Hypoglycemic Action. *Quarterly Journal of Crude Drug Research*. 1979;17:139-96.
Bradley, P. (Ed.). *British Herbal Compendium* (Vol. 1). Dorset, England: British Herbal Medicine Association; 1992:46-9.
____________. *British Herbal Pharmacopoeia* (4th ed.). Dorset, England: British Herbal Medicine Association; 1996:47-9.
Cech, R. *Healing with Burdock*. Horizon Herbs, PO Box 69, Williams, OR 97544, 1995.
Chan, Y. et al. A review of the pharmacological effects of *Arctium lappa* (burdock). *Inflammopharmacology*. 2011 Oct;19(5):245-54.
Cho, M. et al. Arctigenin, a phenylpropanoid dibenzylbutyrolactone lignan, inhibits MAP kinases and AP-1 activation. *Int Immunopharm*. 2004;4(10-11):1419-29.
de Almeida, A. et al. Anti-inflammatory intestinal activity of *Arctium lappa L. (Asteraceae)* in TNBS colitis model. *Journal of Ethnopharmacology*. 2013 Mar 7;146(1):300-10.
da Silva, L. et al. Ethanolic extract of roots from *Arctium lappa L.* accelerates the healing of acetic acid-induced gastric ulcer in rats: Involvement of the antioxidant system. *Food Chem Toxicol*. 2013 Jan;51:179-87.
Donbradi, C., Foldeak, S. Screening report on the antitumor activity of purified *Arctium lappa* Extracts. *Tumor*. 1966;52:173-5.
_________. Screening Report on the Antitumor Activity of Purified *Arctium lappa* Extracts. *Tumor*. 1988;53(3):173.
Duke, J. *The Handbook of Edible Weeds*. Boca Raton, FL: CRC Press, 1992.
Eich, E., et al. Arctigenin as a lead structure for inhibitors of human immunodeficiency virus type-1 integrase. *J Med Chem*. 1996 Jan 5;39(1):86-95.
Fan, T. et al. Arctigenin protects focal cerebral ischemia-reperfusion rats by inhibiting neuroinflammation. *Biol Pharm Bull*. 2012;35(11):2004-9.
Ferracane, R. et al. Metabolic profile of the bioactive compounds of burdock (*Arctium lappa*) seeds, roots and leaves. *J Pharm Biomed Anal*. 2010 Jan 20;51(2):399-404.
Foldeak, S., Dombradi, C. Tumor-growth Inhibiting Substances of Plant Origin. *Acta Physiology & Chemistry*. 1964;10:91-3.
Grases, F., et al. Urolithiasis and phytotherapy. *Int Urol Nephrol*. 1994;26(5):507-11.
Hawrelak, J. Prebiotics: What are they and how safe? *Journal of the Australian Traditional Medicine Society*. 2002;8(4):151-155.
Hayashi, K. et al. Therapeutic effect of arctiin and arctigenin in immunocompetent and immunocompromised mice infected with influenza A virus. *Biological and Pharmaceutical Bulletin* 2010;33(7):1199-1205.
Hirose, M, et al. Effects of arctiin on PhIP-induced mammary, colon and pancreatic carcinogenesis in female Sprague-Dawley rats and MeIQx-induced hepatocarcinogenesis in male F344 rats. *Cancer Letters*. 2000 Jul 3;155(1):79-88.
Holetz, F. et al. Screening of some plants used in the Brazilian folk medicine for the treatment of infectious diseases. *Mem Inst Oswaldo Cruz*. 2002 Oct;97(7):1027-31.
Hsieh, C. et al. Arctigenin, a dietary phytoestrogen, induces apoptosis of estrogen receptor-negative breast cancer cells through the ROS/p38 MAPK pathway and epigenetic regulation. *Free Radical Biolog Med*. 2013 Oct 17;67C:159-170.
Hyam, S. et al. Arctigenin ameliorates inflammation *in vitro* and *in vivo* by inhibiting the PI3K/AKT pathway and polarizing M1 macrophages to M2-like macrophages. *European Journal of Pharmacology*. 2013 May 15;708(1-3):21-9.
Kumar, S. et al. Management of skin toxicity during radiation therapy: a review of evidence. *J Med Imaging Radiat Oncol*. 2010 Jun;54(3):264-79.
Lapinina, L., Sisoeva, T. Investigation of Some Plants to Determine their Sugar-Lowering Action. *Farmatsevticcheski Zhurnal*. 1964;19(4):52-8.
Lee, G. et al. Arctiin induces an UVB protective effect in human dermal fibroblast cells through microRNA expression changes. *International Journal of Molecular Medicine*. 2014 Mar;33(3):640-8.
Lee, Y. et al. *Arctium lappa* ameliorates endothelial dysfunction in rats fed with high fat/cholesterol diets. *BMC Complement Altern Med*. 2012 Aug 6;12:116.
Leonard, S. et al. Essiac tea: scavenging of reactive oxygen species and effects on DNA damage. *J Ethnopharmacol*. 2006 Jan 16;103(2):288-96.
Lin, S. et al. Hepatoprotective effects of *Arctium lappa* on carbon tetrachloride- and acetaminophen-induced liver damage. *Am J Chin Med*. 2000;28(2):163-73.
_________. Hepatoprotective effects of *Arctium lappa* Linne on liver injuries induced by chronic ethanol consumption and potentiated by carbon tetrachloride. *Journal of Biomedical Science*. 2002;9(5):401-9.
Liu, J. et al. Comparative analysis of caffeoylquinic acids and lignans in roots and seeds among various burdock (*Arctium lappa*) genotypes with high antioxidant activity. *J Agric Food Chem*. 2012 Apr 25;60(16):4067-75.
Lo Ha Wa Ti An Ka. *Osage Medicine: Ancestral Herbs and the Illnesses that they Treat*. Greyhorse Indian Village, Rt 2 Box 66-1, Fairfax, OK 74637: Scope Publications.
Ma, S. et al. Effect of arctiin on glomerular filtration barrier damage in STZ-induced diabetic nephropathy rats. *Phytotherapy Research*. 2013 Oct; 27(10):1474-80.
Matsumoto, T. et al. Antiproliferative and apoptotic effects of butyrolactone lignans from *Arctium lappa* on leukemic cells. *Planta Med*. 2006 Feb; 72(3):276-8.
Miele, C., Beguinot, F. New expectations from the well-known medicinal properties of *Arctium lappa. Diabetologia*. 2012 May;55(5):1244-6.
Morita, K., Kada, T., Namiki, M. A desmutagenic factor isolated from burdock (*Arctium lappa*). *Mutation Research*. 1984;129:261-78.
Moskalenko, S. Preliminary screening of far-eastern ethno-medical plants for antibacterial activity. *J Ethnopharmacol*. 1986;15:231-59.
Predes, F. et al. Antioxidative and *in vitro* antiproliferative activity of *Arctium lappa* root extracts. *BMC Complement Altern Med*. 2011 Mar 23;11:25.
Reddy, B. et al. Effect of dietary oligofructose and inulin on colonic preneoplastic abberrant crypt foci inhibition. *Carcinogenisis*. 1997;18(7)1371.
Reid, D. *A Handbook of Chinese Healing Herbs*. Boston, MA: Shambala, 1995;73-4.
Schulte, K., Reuker, G., Boehme, R. Polyacetylenes in Burdock Roots. *Arzneimittel-Forschung*. 1967;17(7):829-33.
Spiller, G. *Dietary Fiber in Health and Nutrition*. Boca Raton, FL: CRC Press, 1994.
Sun, Q. et al. Lappaol f, a novel anticancer agent isolated from plant *Arctium lappa L. Molecular Cancer Therapy*. 2014 Jan;13(1):49-59.
Susanti, S. et al. Tumor specific cytotoxicity of arctigenin isolated from herbal plant *Arctium lappa L. J Natural Medicine*. 2012 Oct;66(4):614-21.
___________. Mechanism of arctigenin-mediated specific cytotoxicity against human lung adenocarcinoma cell lines. *Phytomedicine*. 2013 Dec 15;21(1):39-46.
Tezuka, Y. et al. Anti-austeric activity of phenolic constituents of seeds of *Arctium lappa. Nat Prod Commun*. 2013 Apr;8(4):463-6.
Urazova, L. et al. Efficacy of natural L-asparagine in complex therapy for malignant tumors in experimental studies. *Exp Oncol*. 2011 Jun;33(2):90-3.
Vincent, E., Segonzac, G. Higher Plants having Antibiotic Properties. *Toulouse Medicae*. 1948;49:669.
Vlietinck, A. et al. Plant-derived leading compounds for chemotherapy of human immunodeficiency virus (HIV) infection. *Planta Med*. 1998 Mar; 64(2):97-109.
Wegiera, M. et al. Cytotoxic effect of some medicinal plants from *Asteraceae* family on J-45.01 leukemic cell line--pilot study. *Acta Pol Pharm*. 2012 Mar-Apr;69(2):263-8.
Xie, L. et al. Transformation of arctiin to estrogenic and antiestrogenic substances by human intestinal bacteria. *Chemical and Pharmaceutical Bulletin*. 2003;51:4(378-384).
Yance, D. *Herbal Medicine, Healing & Cancer*. Chicago, IL: Keats Publishing, 1999.
Zhao, F., Wang, L., Liu, K. *In vitro* anti-inflammatory effects of arctigenin, a lignan from *Arctium lappa L.*, through inhibition on iNOS pathway. *Journal of Ethnopharmacology*. 2009;(122:3): 457-462.
Zhao, Z. et al. Arctigenin exhibits relaxation effect on bronchus by affecting transmembrane flow of calcium. *Biol Trace Elem Res*. 2013 Dec; 156 (1-3):181-7.

CALENDULA

GENERAL REFERENCES: 1) pp. 100, 318; 2) p. 44; 3) pp. 52, 236, 272; 9) p. 299; 14) pp. 125, 185, 265, 477, 486, 504, 531; 16) p. 77; 17); 18) p. 389; 20) p. 401; 21) p. 262; 22) p. 414; 23) p. 56; 24) p. 40; 25) p. 74; 29) p. 739; 31); 33) p. 517; 36) p. 534; 37) p. 616; 43); 44) p. 143; 46) p. 22; 48) pp. 98, 390; 55) p. 58; 62) p. 70; 66) p. 46; 67); 79) p. 286; 82) pp. 165, 224, 308.
Abdel-Aziem, S. et al. Ameliorative effects of thyme and calendula extracts alone or in combination against aflatoxins-induced oxidative stress and genotoxicity in rat liver. *Cytotechnology*. 2013 Oct 6.
Akihisa, T. et al. Triterpene alcohols from the flowers of compositae and their anti-inflammatory effects. *Phytochemistry*. 1996;43(6):1255-60.
Ali, F. et al. Assessment of Augmented Immune Surveillance and Tumor Cell Death by Cytoplasmic Stabilization of p53 as a Chemopreventive

Strategy of 3 Promising Medicinal Herbs in Murine 2-Stage Skin Carcinogenesis. *Integrative Cancer Therapy*. 2013 Dec 19.
Bashir, S. et al. Studies on spasmogenic and spasmolytic activities of *Calendula officinalis* flowers. *Phytother Res*. 2006 Oct; 20(10):906-10.
Borsuk, O. et al. New promising natural immunocorrective agents. *Vestn Ross Akad Med Nauk*. 2009;(11):9-12.
Boucaud-Maitre, Y. et al. Cytotoxic and antitumoral activity of *Calendula officinalis* extracts. *Pharmizie*. 1988;43(3):220-1.
Brown, D. Herbal Ear Drops Effectively Treat Ear Pain Associated with Acute Otitis Media. *HerbalGram*. 2002;54:23.
Casey-Smith, J. Effect of *Unguentum lymphaticum* on acute experimental lymphedema and other high-protein edemas. *Lymphology*.1983;16:150.
Chakurski,I. et al. Treatment of chronic colitis with an herbal combination of *Taraxacum officinale, Hypericum perforatum, Melissa officinalis, Calendula officinalis* and *Foeniculum vulgare*. *Vutr Boles*. 1981;20(6):51-4.
____________. Treatment of duodenal ulcers and gastroduodenitis with a herbal combination of *Symphytum officinalis* and *Calendula officinalis* with and without antacids. *Vutr Boles*. 1981;20(6):44-7.
Cwikla, C. et al. Investigations into the antibacterial activities of phytotherapeutics against *Helicobacter pylori* and *Campylobacter jejuni*. *Phytother Res*. 2010 May;24(5):649-56.
Danilets, M. at al. Effect of plant polysaccharides on TH1-dependent immune response: screening investigation. *Eksp Klin Farmakol*. 2010;73(6):19.
Duran, V. et al. Results of the clinical examination of an ointment with marigold (*Calendula officinalis*) extract in the treatment of venous leg ulcers. *Int J Tissue React*. 2005;27(3):101-6.
Efstratiou, E. et al. Antimicrobial activity of *Calendula officinalis* petal extracts against fungi, as well as Gram-negative and Gram-positive clinical pathogens. *Complement Ther Clin Pract*. 2012 Aug;18(3):173-6.
Faria, R. et al. Antimicrobial activity of *Calendula officinalis, Camellia sinensis* and chlorhexidine against the adherence of microorganisms to sutures after extraction of unerupted third molars. *J Appl Oral Sci*. 2011 Oct;19(5):476-82.
Foster, S., Leung, A. *Encyclopedia of Common Natural Ingredients Used in Food, Drugs and Cosmetics*. New York, NY: John Wiley & Sons, 1996;113.
Fronza, M. et al. Determination of the wound healing effect of Calendula extracts using the scratch assay with 3T3 fibroblasts. *J Ethnopharmacol*. 2009 Dec 10;126(3):463-7.
Gazim, Z. et al. Antifungal activity of essential oil from *Calendula officinalis L.* (asteraceae) growing in Brazil. *Brazil J Microbiol*. 2008 Jan;39(1):61-3.
Hofbauer, R. et al. Heparin-binding epidermal growth factor expression in KATO-III cells after *Helicobacter pylori* stimulation under the influence of *strychnos Nux vomica* and *Calendula officinalis*. *Homeopathy*. 2010 Jul;99(3):177-82.
Kalvatchev, Z., Walder, R., Garzaro, D. Anti-HIV activity of extracts from *C. officinalis* flowers. *Biomedical Pharmacotherapy*. 1997;51(4);176.
Kiouchek-Popova, E. Influence of physiological regeneration and epithelialization using fractions isolated from *Calendula officinalis*. *Acta Physiol Pharmacol Bulg*. 1982;8(4):63-7.
Krivenko, V., et al. Experience in treating digestive organ diseases with medicinal plants. *Vrach Delo*. 1989;3:76-8.
Loggia, D. et al. Topical Anti-inflammatory activity of *Calendula officinalis* extracts. *Planta Medica*. 1990;56:658.
____________. Role of triterpenoids in topical anti-inflammatory activity of *Calendula officinalis* flowers. *Planta Medica*. 1994;60(6):516-20.
Markvicheva, E. et al. Biodegradable polymer microparticles with entrapped herbal extracts: preparation with super critical carbon dioxide and use for tissue repair. *Biomed Khim*. 2009 Jul-Aug;55(4):479-88.
Matic, I. et al. Chamomile and marigold tea: chemical characterization and evaluation of anticancer activity. *Phytother Res*. 2013 Jun;27(6):852-8.
Ozkol, H. et al. Subacute effect of cigarette smoke exposure in rats: protection by pot marigold (*Calendula officinalis L.*) extract. *Toxicol Ind Health*. 2012 Feb;28(1):3-9.
Parente , L. et al. Angiogenic activity of *Calendula officinalis* flowers L. in rats. *Acta Cir Bras*. 2011 Feb;26(1):19-24.
Patrick, K. et al. Induction of vascularization by an aqueous extract of the flowers of *Calendula officinalis*. *Phytomed*. 1996;3:11-8.
Pommier, P. et al. Phase III randomized trial of *Calendula officinalis* compared with trolamine for prevention of acute dermatitis during irradiation for breast cancer. *Journal of Clinical Oncology*. 2004;22:1447-53.
Preethi, K., Kuttan, R. Wound healing activity of flower extract of *Calendula officinalis*. *J Basic Clin Physiol Pharmacol*. 2009;20(1):73-9.
________________. Hepato and reno protective action of *Calendula officinalis* L. flower extract. *Indian J Exp Biol*. 2009 March;47(3):163-8.
Preethi, K. et al. Inhibition of metastasis of B16F-10 melanoma cells in C57BL/6 mice by an extract of *Calendula officinalis* L flowers. *Asian Pac J Cancer Prev*. 2010;11(6):1773-9.
Ray, D. et al. Amelioration of myocardial ischemic reperfusion injury with *Calendula officinalis*. *Curr Pharm Biotechnol*. 2010 Dec;11(8):849-54.
Sarrell, E. et al. Efficacy of naturopathic extracts in the management of ear pain associated with acute otitis media. *Archives of Pediatric & Adolescent Medicine*. 2001;155(7):796-9.
Shivasharan, B. et al. Protective Effect of *Calendula officinalis L.* Flowers Against Monosodium Glutamate Induced Oxidative Stress and Excitotoxic Brain Damage in Rats. *Indian Journal of Clinical Biochemistry*. 2013 Jul;28(3):292-8.
Smulski, H., Wojcicki, J. Placebo-controlled, Double-blind Trial to Determine the Efficacy of the Tibetan Plant Preparation Padma 28 for Intermittent Claudication. *Alternative Therapies*. 1995;1(3):44-9.
Szakiel, A. et al. Antibacterial and antiparasitic activity of oleanolic acid and its glycosides isolated from marigold (*Calendula officinalis*). *Planta Med*. 2008 Nov;74(14):1709-15.
Wagner, H. et al. Immunostimulating action of polysaccharides from higher plants. *Arzneimittel Forschung*. 1985;35(7):1069-1057.
Yoshikawa, M. et al. Medicinal flowers. Marigold. (1) hypoglycemic, gastric emptying inhibitory, and gastroprotective principles and new oleanane-type triterpene oligoglycosides, calendasaponins A, B, C, and D, from Egyptian *C. officinalis*. *Chem Pharm Bull*. 2001;49(7):863-70.

CATNIP

GENERAL REFERENCES: 3) pp. 56, 236, 272; 5) p. 101; 8) p. 236; 9) p. 858; 11) p. 103; 13); 14) p. 85; 17); 20) p. 465; 21) p. 281; 22) p. 138; 23) p. 60; 25) p. 88; 29) p. 682; 31); 33) p. 173; 36) p. 569; 37) p. 167; 42) p. 215; 43); 44) p. 150; 46) pp. 79, 183; 48) pp. 205, 302; 51) p. 76; 59) p. 39; 62) p. 85; 64) p. 157; 66) p. 48; 68) p. 81; 69) p. 120; 71); 78) p. 153; 79) p. 104; 81).
Abascal, K., Yarnell, E. Herbs and drug resistance. *Alternative and Complementary Therapies*. August 2002:237-41.
Adiguzel, A. et al. Antimicrobial and antioxidant activity of essential oil and methanol extract of *Nepeta cataria*. *Pol J Microbiol*. 2009;58(1):69-76.
Aydin, S. et al. Analgesic activity of *Nepeta italica* L. *Phytotherapy Research*. 1999 Feb;13(1):20-3.
Gilani, A. et al. Chemical composition and mechanisms underlying the spasmolytic and bronchodilatory properties of the essential oil of *Nepeta cataria L. Journal of Ethnopharmacology*. 2009 Jan 30;121(3):405-11.
Greunwald, J., Brendler, T., Jaenicke, C. et al. (Eds.). *PDR for Herbal Medicines*. Montvale, NJ: Medical Economics, 1998.
Hylton, W. (Ed.). *The Rodale Herb Book*. Emmaus, PA: Rodale Press, 1984;398-401.
Nestorovic, J. et al. Nepetalactone content in shoot cultures of three endemic *Nepeta* species and the evaluation of their antimicrobial activity. *Fitoterapia*. 2010 Sep;81(6):621-6.
Nostro, A. et al. The effect of *Nepeta cataria* extract on adherence and enzyme production of *Staphylococcus aureus*. *International Journal of Antimicrobial Agents*. 2001;18(6):583-5.
Prescott, T. et al. Direct inhibition of calcineurin by caffeoyl phenylethanoid glycosides from *Teucrium chamaedrys* and *Nepeta cataria*. *Journal of Ethnopharmacology*. 2011 Oct 11;137(3):1306-10.
Zomorodian, K. et al. Chemical composition and antimicrobial activities of essential oils from *Nepeta cataria L.* against common causes of food-borne infections. *ISRN Pharm*. 2012;2012:591953.
________________. Chemical composition and antimicrobial activities of essential oil of *Nepeta cataria L.* against common causes of oral infections. *Journal of Dentistry* (Tehran). 2013 May;10(4):329-37.

CAYENNE

GENERAL REFERENCES: 1) p. 178; 2) p. 52; 3) pp. 57, 213, 233, 236, 245, 246; 8) p. 406; 9) p. 302; 14); 16) p. 88; 18) p. 163; 20) p. 434; 21) p. 275; 22) p. 123; 23) p. 62; 25) p. 92; 31); 33) p. 175; 36) p. 536; 37) p. 381; 41) p. 640; 42) p. 215; 43); 45) p. 96; 46) p. 23; 51) pp. 12, 19, 40, 48, 84, 102, 159, 242; 53) p. 70; 55) p. 60; 64) p. 241; 66) p. 48; 76); 79) p. 116; 80) p. 187; 81).
Beltran, J. et al. Immunotherapy of tumors with neuroimmune ligand capsaicin. *J Immunol*. 2007 Mar 1;178(5):3260-4.
Brinker, F. Variations in effective botanical products: The case for diversity of forms for herbal preparations as supported by scientific studies. *HerbalGram*. 1999; 46:37,46.
________. Herbs and drugs in the treatment of respiratory allergies. *British Naturopathic Journal*. 2000;17(3).
Capsaicin Study Group. Effect of treatment with capsaicin on daily activities of patients with painful diabetic neuropathy. *Diabetes Care*. 1992,15: 159-65.

Chad, D. et al. Does capsaicin relieve the pain of diabetic neuropathy? *Pain*. 1990;42:387-8.
Chaiyasit, K. et al. Pharmacokinetic and the effect of capsaicin in *Capsicum frutescens* on decreasing plasma glucose level. *J Med Assoc Thailand*. 2009 Jan;92(1):108-13.
Chevallier, A. The Encyclopedia of Medicinal Plants. London, England: DK Publishing Inc., 1996.
Cichewicz, R., Thorpe, P. The antimicrobial properties of chili peppers (*Capsicum* species) and their uses in Mayan medicine. *Journal of Ethnopharmacology*. 1996;52(2):61-70.
Dib, B. Effects of intrathecal capsaicin on autonomic and behavioral heat loss responses in the rat. *J Gastroenterology & Hepatology*. 1992;7:52-6.
Ellis, C. et al. A double-blind evaluation of topical capsaicin in pruritic psoriasis. *J American Academy of Dermatology*, 1993;29:438-42.
Ellison, N. et al. Phase III placebo-controlled trial of capsaicin cream in the management of surgical neuropathic pain in cancer patients. *Journal of Clinical Oncology*. 1997;15(8):2974-80.
Fusco, B., Alessandri, M. Analgesic effect of capsaicin in idiopathic trigeminal neuralgia. *Anesthesia and Analgesia*. 1992;74:375-7.
Gagnier, J. et al. Herbal medicine for low back pain. *Cochrane Database of Systematic Reviews*. 2006, Issue 2. Art. No.: CD004504.
Hernández-Ortega, M. et al. Antioxidant, antinociceptive, and anti-inflammatory effects of carotenoids extracted from dried pepper (*Capsicum annuum L.*). *J Biomed Biotechnol*. 2012;2012:524019.
Hwang, I. et al. Effects of Different Cooking Methods on the Antioxidant Properties of Red Pepper (*Capsicum annuum L.*). *Prev Nutr Food Sci*. 2012 Dec;17(4):286-92.
Iorizzi, M. et al. Antimicrobial furostanol saponins from the seeds of *C. annuum L. var. acuminatum*. *J Agricul Food Chem*. 2002;50(15):310-6.
Jang, H. et al. *Capsicum annuum L.* methanolic extract inhibits ovalbumin-induced airway inflammation and oxidative stress in a mouse model of asthma. *J Med Food*. 2011 Oct;14(10):1144-51.
Jones, N., Shabib, S., Sherman, P. Capsaicin as an inhibitor of the growth of the gastric pathogen *Helicobactor pylori*. *FEMS Microbiology Letters*. 1997;146:223-7.
Kang, J., Yeoh, K., Chia, H. et al. Chili; protective factor against peptic ulcer? *Digestive Diseases and Sciences*. 1995;40(3):576-9.
Kawada, T. et al. Effects of capsaicin on lipid metabolism in rats fed a high fat diet. *Journal of Nutrition*. 1986;116:1272-8.
Keitel, W. et al. Capsicum pain plaster in chronic non-specific low back pain. *Arzneimittelforschung*. 2001 Nov;51(11):896-903.
Keskin, D., Toroglu, S. Studies on antimicrobial activities of solvent extracts of different spices. *J Environ Biol*. 2011 Mar;32(2):251-6.
La, M., Rand, M. Neurogenic vasodilation in isolated perfused segments of rabbit jejunal artery. *Clinical Exp Pharm Physiology*. 1993;20(5):355-8.
Locock, R. Capsicum. *Canadian Pharmaceutical Journal*. 1985;118:517-9.
Loizzo, M. et al. Influence of drying and cooking process on the phytochemical content, antioxidant and hypoglycaemic properties of two bell *Capsicum annum L.* cultivars. *Food Chem Toxicol*. 2013 Mar;53:392-401.
Marks, D., Rapaport, A., et al. A double-blind placebo-controlled trial of intranasal capsaicin for cluster headache. *Cephalalgia*. 1993;13:114-6.
McCarthy, G., McCarty, D. Effect of topical capsaicin in the therapy of painful osteoarthritis of the hands. *J of Rheumatology*. 1992;19:604-7.
________________ et al. Treatment of pain due to fibromyalgia with topical capsaicin: a pilot study. *Seminars in Arthritis and Rheumatism*. 1994;23(6):41-7.
Myers, B. et al. Effect of red pepper and black pepper on the stomach. *American Journal of Gastroenterology*. 1987;82(3):211-4.
Nick, G. The Capsicum Fruit. *Townsend Letter*. 2002;227;128-33.
Partsch, G., Matucci-Cerinin, M. Effect of capsaicin on the release of substance P from rheumatoid arthritis and osteoarthritis synoviocytes *in vitro*. *Annals of the Rheumatic Diseases*. 1990;49(8):653.
____________________ et al. Collagenase synthesis of rheumatoid arthritis synoviocytes: dose dependent stimulation by substance P and capsaicin. *Scandinavian Journal of Rheumatology*. 1991;20(2):98-103.
Pimparkar, B. et al. Effects of commonly used spices on human gastric secretion. *J Assoc Physicians India*. 1972;20:901-10.
Rosa, A. et al. Antioxidant activity of capsinoids. *Journal of Agricultural Food Chemistry*. 2002;50(25):7396-401.
Ross, D., Varipapa, R. Treatment of painful diabetic neuropathy with topical capsaicin. *New England Journal of Medicine*. 1989;321:474-5.
Sambaiah, K. et al. Hypocholesterolemic effect of red pepper and capsaicin. *Indian Journal of Experimental Biology*. 1980;18:898-9.
Scheffler, N., Sheitel, P., Lipton, M. Treatment of painful diabetic neuropathy with capsaicin 0.075%. *J American Ped Med Ass*. 1991;81(6):288-93.
Solanke, T. The Effect of Red Pepper (*Capsicum frutescens*) on Gastric acid Secretion. *Journal of Surgical Research*. 1973;15:385-90.
Takeuchi, K. et al. *Japanese Journal of Pharmacology*. 1991;55:147-155.
Tandan, R. et al. Topical capsaicin in painful diabetic neuropathy-controlled study with long-term follow-up. *Diabetes Care*. 1992;15:8.
Taveira, G. et al. Thionin-like peptides from *Capsicum annuum* fruits with high activity against human pathogenic bacteria and yeasts. *Biopolymers*. 2014 Jan;102(1):30-9.
Toh, C., Lee, T., Kiang, A. The pharmacological actions of capsaicin and analogues. *British Journal of Pharmacology*. 1955;10:175-182.
Tsuchiya. H. Biphasic membrane effects of capsaicin, an active component in Capsicum species. *J Ethnopharmacol*. 2001 May;75(2-3):295-9.
Viranuvatti, V. et al. Effects of Capsicum solution on human gastric mucosa as observed gastroscopically. *Am J Gastroenterology*. 1972;58:225.
Wang, J., Hsu, M., Teng, C. Antiplatelet effect of capsaicin. *Thrombosis Research*. 1984;36:497-507.
Wasantapruek, S. et al. Enhanced fibrinolytic activity after capsaicin ingestion. *New England Journal of Medicine*. 1974;290:1259-60.
Watson, C. et al. Post-herpetic neuralgia and topical capsaicin. *Pain*. 1988;33:333-40.
____________. The post-mastectomy pain syndrome and the effect of topical capsaicin. *Pain*. 1989;38:177-86.
Weber, L. et al. Expression and functionality of TRPV1 in breast cancer cells. *Breast Cancer*. 2016;8:243-252.
Yeoh, K., Kang, J., Yap, I. et al. Chili protects against aspirin-induced gastroduodenal mucosal injury in humans. *Digestive Diseases and Sciences*. 1995;40(3): 580-3.
Zhang, J. et al. Capsaicin inhibits growth of adult T-cell leukemia cells. *Leukemia Research*. 2003;27(3):275-83.

CHAMOMILE

GENERAL REFERENCES: 1); 2) p. 57; 3); 5) p. 108; 8) p. 218; 9) p. 249; 11) p. 32; 14); 16) pp. 93-5; 17); 18) p. 154; 20) p. 1246, 21) pp. 189, 475; 22) p. 151; 23) p. 64; 25) p. 94; 30) p. 235; 33) p. 185, 36); 37) p. 554; 43); 44) p. 144; 45) p. 105; 48) p. 108; 51) pp. 110, 205; 52) p. 185; 55) pp. 69, 72; 57) p. 111; 62) pp. 91, 92; 66) p. 50; 68) p. 83; 68) pp. 11, 57; 75) p 22; 76) pp. 157, 319; 79) pp. 109, 110; 80) p. 201.
Aertgeerts, P. et al. Comparative testing of Kamillosan cream and steroidal (0.25% hydrocortisone, 0.75% fluocortin butyl ester) and non-steroidal (5% bufexamac) dermatologic agents in maintenance therapy of eczematous diseases. *Z Hautkr*. 1985;60(3);270-277.
Agah, S. Taleb, A. et al. Chamomile efficacy in patients of the irritable bowel syndrome. *Der Pharma Chemica*. 2015;7(4):41-5.
Aggag, E., Yousef, R. Study of antimicrobial activity of chamomile oil. *Planta Medica*. 1972;22:140-4.
Ahmad, A., Misra, L. Isolation of Herniarin and Other Constituents from *Matricaria chamomilla* Flowers. *Int J Pharmacognosy*. 1997;5:121-5.
Amsterdam, J. et al. Randomized, double-blind, placebo-controlled trial of *Matricaria recutita* (Chamomile) extract therapy for generalized anxiety disorder. *Journal of Clinical Phsycopharmacology*. 2009;29: 378-382.
Baradari, A. et al. Comparison of antibacterial effects of oral rinses chlorhexidine and herbal mouth wash in patients admitted to intensive care unit. *Bratisl Lek Listy*. 2012;113(9):556-60.
Batista, A. et al. Clinical efficacy analysis of the mouth rinsing with pomegranate and chamomile plant extracts in the gingival bleeding reduction. *Complement Ther Clin Pract*. 2014 Feb;20(1):93-8.
Bhaskaran, N. et al. Chamomile confers protection against hydrogen peroxide-induced toxicity through activation of Nrf2-mediated defense response. *Phytotherapy Research*. 2013 Jan;27(1):118-25.
Bijak, M. et al. The influence of conjugates isolated from *Matricaria chamomilla L.* on platelets activity and cytotoxicity. *Int J Biol Macromol*. 2013 Oct;61:218-29.
Blumenthal, M. et al. (Eds.). *The ABC Clinical Guide to Herbs*. Austin, TX: American Botanical Council; 2003:51-60.
Booth et al. Confusion regarding anticoagulant coumarins in dietary supplements. *Clin Pharmacol Ther*. 2004;26(6):511-16.
Brown, D. Anti-anxiety effects of chamomile compounds. *HerbalGram*. 1997;39:19.
Burns, E. et al. The use of aromatherapy in intrapartum midwifery practice an observational study. *J Altern Complement Med*. 2000 Apr;6(2):141–7.
Carl, W., Emrich, L. Management of oral mucositis during local radiation and systemic chemotherapy: a study of 98 patients. *J Prosthet Dent*. 1991;66(3):361–9.
Carle, R., Isaac, O. Effect and effectiveness. A commentary on the monograph of *Matricaria* flos (chamomile flowers). *Zeitschrift fur Phytotherapie*. 1987;8:67-77.

Darvishi Khezri, H. et al. Comparison of the antibacterial effects of matrica and Persica™ and chlorhexidine gluconate mouthwashes in mechanically ventilated ICU patients: a double blind randomized clinical trial. *Rev Chilena Infectol.* 2013 Aug;30(4):361-73.
de la Motte, S. et al. Double-blind study comparing pectin/chamomile extract with placebo in children with diarrhea. *Arzneimittel-Forschung.* 1997;47(11):1247–9.
Della Loggia, R. et al. Depressive effects of *Chamomilla recutita (L.)*, Rausch, tubular flowers on central nervous system in mice. *Pharmacological Research Communications.* 1982;14(2):153-162.
Der Marderosian, A., Liberti, L. *Natural Products Medicine: A Scientific Guide to Foods, Drugs, Cosmetics.* Philadelphia, PA: George F. Stickley Company, 1998.
Engels, G., Brinckmann, J. Chamomile. *HerbalGram.* 2015;108:8-17.
Farnsworth, N., Morgan, B. Herb Drinks: Chamomile Tea. *JAMA.* 1972;221:410.
Forster, H. et al. Antispasmodic effects of some medicinal plants. *Planta Medica.* 1980;40(4):309-19.
Foster, S. *Chamomile: Matricaria recutita and Chamaemelum nobile. HerbalGram.* Austin, TX: American Botanical Council, 1990;6.
Gould, L. et al. Cardiac effects of chamomile tea. *Journal of Clinical Pharmacology.* 1973;13(11/12):475-9.
Hashempur, M. et al. A pilot, randomized double-blind placebo-controlled trial on topical chamomile (*Matricaria chamomilla* L.) oil for severe carpal tunnel syndrome. *Complementary Therapies in Clinical Practice.* 2015;21:223-8.
Hausen, B., Busker, E., Carle, R. The sensitizing capacity of Compositae Plants VII. Experimental Investigations, with extracts and Compounds of *Chamomilla recutita* (L.) Rauschert and *Anthemis cotula L. Planta Medica.* 1984;50:229-234.
Isaac, O., Thiemer, K. Biochemical studies on chamomile components/III. *In vitro* studies about the antipeptic activity of (-)-alpha-bisabolol. *Arzneimmittel-Forschung.* 1975;25(9):1352-54.
Jakovlev, V., Isacc, O., Thiemer, K., Kunde, R. Pharmacological investigations with compounds of chamomile. New investigations on the antiphlogistic effects of (-)-alpha-bisabolols and bisabolol oxides. *Planta Medica.* 1979;35(2);125-140.
Kogiannou, D. et al. Herbal infusions; their phenolic profile, antioxidant and anti-inflammatory effects in HT29 and PC3 cells. *Food Chem Toxicol.* 2013 Nov;61:152-9.
Kunde, R. et al. Pharmacological investigations with compounds of chamomile. Investigations on the spasmolytic effect of compounds of chamomile and Kamillosan® on isolated guinea pig ileum. *Planta Medica.* 1980;39:38-50.
Kuo, C. et al. Apigenin has anti-atrophic gastritis and anti-gastric cancer progression effects in *Helicobacter pylori*-infected Mongolian gerbils. *J Ethnopharmacol.* 2013 Dec 25(13)844.
Landolfi, R., Mower, R., Steiner, M. Modification of platelet function and arachidonic acid metabolism by bioflavonoids. *Biochemical Pharmacology.* 1984;33(9):1525-1530.
Lefort, E., Blay, J. Apigenin and its impact on gastrointestinal cancers. *Molecular Nutrition Food Research.* 2013 Jan;57(1):126-44.
Mamalis, A. et al. The active natural anti-oxidant properties of chamomile, milk thistle, and halophilic bacterial components in human skin *in vitro. J Drugs Dermatol.* 2013 Jul 1;12(7):780-4.
Mann, C., Staba, E. The chemistry, pharmacology, and commercial formulations of chamomile. *Herbs, Spices, and Medicinal Plants* (Vol. I). Phoenix, AZ: Oryx Press, 1986;235-280.
Roberts, R. et al. Distinct mechanisms of relaxation to bioactive components from chamomile species in porcine isolated blood vessels. *Toxicol Appl Pharmacol.* 2013 Nov 1;272(3):797-805.
Salamon, I. Chamomile: A Medicinal Plant. *The Herb, Spice and Medicinal Plant Digest.* 1992;10(1):1-4.
Sebai, H. et al. Antidiarrheal and antioxidant activities of chamomile (*Matricaria recutita L.*) decoction extract in rats. *J Ethnopharmacol.* 2014 Mar 14;152(2):327-32.
Sharifi, F. et al. Comparison of the effects of *Matricaria chamomila* (Chamomile) extract and mefenamic acid on the intensity of premenstrual syndrome. *Complement Ther Clin Pract.* 2014 Feb;20(1):81-8.
___________. Comparison of the effects of *Matricaria chamomila* (Chamomile) extract and mefenamic acid on the intensity of mastalgia associated with premenstrual syndrome. *Women's Health Bull.* 2014;1(2).
Szelenyi, I. et al. Pharmacological experiments with compounds of chamomile/III. Experimental studies of the ulcer-protective effect of chamomile. *Planta Medica.* 1979;35(2):218-227.
Theimer, K. et al. Biochemical studies of chamomile constituents. I. Anti-peptic effect of chamomile extract and sodium 1,4-dimethyl-7-isopropylazulen sulfonic acid. *Arzneimmittel-Forschung.* 1972;22(6):1086-7.
Tubaro, A. et al. Evaluation of anti-inflammatory activity of a chamomile extract after topical application. *Planta Medica.* 1984;51:359.
Van Rietshoten, K. Plants with anti-inflammatory action. *British Journal of Phytotherapy.* 1990;1:3,4.
Viola, H. et al. Apigenin, a component of *Matricaria recutita* flowers, is a central benzodiazephine receptors-ligand with anxiolytic effects. *Planta Medica.* 1995;61:213-6.
Wagner, V., Proksch, A. et al. Immunostimulating polysaccharides (heteroglycans) of higher plants. *Arzneimettel-Forschung.* 1984;34:659.
Yakolev, V., von Schlichtegroll, A. Anti-inflammatory activity of (-)-alpha-bisabolol, an essential component of chamomile oil. *Arzneimittel-Forschung.* 1969;19(4);615-6.
Zita, C., Stekdova, B. The influence of pure constituents of Camomile oil on thermal burns. *Casopis Lekaru Ceskych.* 1955;94:203-8.

CHASTEBERRY

GENERAL REFERENCES: 1) p. 108; 2) p. 62; 3) p. 64; 4) p. 179; 12) p. 73; 14) pp. 52, 113, 394, 397, 441; 16) p. 96; 17); 22) p. 156; 23) p. 67; 24) p. 204; 25) p. 98; 29) p. 1387; 30) p. 257; 31); 33) p. 188; 34) pp. 21-2, 82, 162; 36) p 595; 37) p. 597; 45) p. 391; 46) pp. 123, 183; 55) p. 19; 62) p. 94; 65) p. 164; 66) p. 51; 73) pp. 13, 15, 45, 69, 107, 133; 75) p. 317; 79) p. 8; 81) pp. 129, 162, 167, 397.
Alakbarov, F. Aromatic Herbal Baths of the Ancients. *HerbalGram.* 2003;57:44.
Amnon, W. Removing an obstipation using Agnolyt. *Therapiewoche Gynakol.* 1965;104:1263-5.
_________. Acne vulgaris and Angus castus. *Z Allg Med.* 1975;51:1645-8.
Bensky, D., Gamble, A., Kaptchuk, T. *Chinese Herbal Medicine Materia Medica.* Seattle, WA: Eastland Press, 1993;44.
Brown, D. *Vitex agnus castus*: clinical monograph. *Quarterly Review of Natural Medicine.* Summer 1994;111-121.
Carmichael, A. Can *Vitex Agnus Castus* be Used for the Treatment of Mastalgia? What is the Current Evidence? *Evid Based Complement Alternat Med.* 2008 Sep;5(3):247-50.
Choudhary, M. et al. Antiinflammatory and lipoxygenase inhibitory compounds from *Vitex agnus-castus. Phytother Res.* 2009 Sep;23(9):1336-9.
Dixon-Shanies, D., Shaikh, N. Growth inhibition of human breast cancer cells by herbs and phytoestrogens. *Oncol Rep.* 1999 Nov-Dec;6(6):1383-7.
Eftekhari, M. et al. Effects of "*Vitex agnus castus*" extract and magnesium supplementation, alone and in combination, on osteogenic and angiogenic factors and fracture healing in women with long bone fracture. *J Res Med Sci.* Jan 2014;19(1):1-7.
Feldmann, H. et al. The treatment of corpus luteum insufficiency and premenstrual syndrome experience in a multicenter study under practice conditions. *Gynecology.* 1990;42:1-5.
Gerhard, I. et al. Mastodynon® for Female Infertility. Randomized, Placebo-Controlled, Clinical Double-Blind Study. *Forsch Komplementarmed.* 1998;5(6):272-278.
Halaska, M. et al. Treatment of cyclical mastalgia with a solution containing a *Vitex agnus castus* extract: results of a placebo-controlled double-blind study. *Breast.* 1999 Aug;8(4):175-81.
Hirobe, C. et al. Cytotoxic Flavonoids from *Vitex agnus-castus. Phytochemistry.* 1997;46:521-4.
Hobbs, C. *Vitex: The Woman's Herb.* Summertown, TN: Healthy Living Publications, 2003.
Ibrahim, N. et al. Gynecological efficacy and chemical investigation of *Vitex agnus-castus* L. fruits growing in Egypt. *Nat Prod Res.* 2008 April 15;22(6):537-46.
Imai, M. et al. Cytotoxic effects of flavonoids against a human colon cancer derived cell line, COLO 201: a potential natural anti-cancer substance. *Cancer Letters.* 2009 Apr 8;276(1):74-80.
Jarry, H. et al. *Agnus castus* as a dopaminergic active constituent in Mastodynon N. *Z Phytother.* 1991;12:77-82.
__________. *In vitro* prolactin but not LH and FSH release is inhibited by compounds in extracts of *Agnus castus*: direct evidence for a dopaminergic principle by the dopamine receptor assay. *Exp Clinical Endocrinology.* 1994;102(6):448-54.
__________. Evidence for estrogen receptor beta-selective activity of *Vitex agnus-castus* and isolated flavones. *Planta Med.* 2003 Oct;69(10):945-7.
Klaus-Jurgen, B. The use of *Vitex agnus castus* for hyperprolactinemia. *Quarterly Review of Natural Medicine.* 1997; spring:19-20.

Lauritzen, C. et al. Treatment of premenstrual tension syndrome with *Vitex agnus castus*. Controlled, double-blind study verses pyridoxine. *Phytomedicine*. 1997;4(3):183-9.
Loch, E., Kayser, E. Diagnosis and treatment of dyshormonal menstrual periods in the general practice. *Gynakol Praxis*. 1990;14:489-95.
Loch, E. et al. Treatment of premenstrual syndrome with a phytopharmaceutical formulation containing *Vitex agnus castus*. *J Womens Health Gender Based Medicine*. 2000 Apr;9(3):315-20.
Mazzio, E., Soliman, K. *In vitro* screening for the tumoricidal properties of international medicinal herbs. *Phytother Res*. 2009 Mar;23(3):385-98.
Mesaik, M. et al. Isolation and immunomodulatory properties flavonoid, casticin from *Vitex agnus-castus*. *Phytother Res*. 2009 Nov;23(11):1516-20.
Milewicz, A. et al. *Vitex agnus castus* extract in the treatment of luteal phase defects due to latent hyperprolactinemia. Results of a randomized placebo-controlled double-blind study. *Arzneimittel-Forschung*. 1993; July 43(7):752-6.
Mohr, H. Clinical investigation of means to increase lactation. *Dtsch Med Wochenschr*. 1954;41:1513-6.
Muhlenstedt, D. et al. Short luteal phase and prolactin. *International Journal of Fertility*. 1978;23:213-7.
Nasri, S. et al. The effects of *Vitex agnus castus* extract and its interaction with dopaminergic system on LH and testosterone in male mice. *Pak J Biol Sci*. 2007 Jul 15;10(14):2300-7.
Ohyama, K. et al. Cytotoxicity and apoptotic inducibility of *Vitex agnus-castus* fruit extract in cultured human normal and cancer cells and effect on growth. *Biol Pharm Bull*. 2003;26(1):10-18.
Oztürk, A. et al. The effects of phytoestrogens on fracture healing: experimental research in New Zealand white rabbits. *Ulus Travma Acil Cerrahi Derg*. 2008 Jan;14(1):21-7.
Peters-Welte, C., Albrecht, M. Menstrual abnormalities and PMS: *Vitex agnus-castus*. *Therapiewoche Gynakologie*. 1994;7:49-52.
Probst, V., Roth, O. On a plant extract with a hormone-like effect. *Dtsch Med Wochenschr*. 1954;79:1271-4.
Propping, D., Katzorke, T. Treatment of corpus luteum insufficiency. *Z Allg Med*. 1987;63:932-3.
Rotem, C. Kaplan, B. Phyto-Female Complex for the relief of hot flushes, night sweats and quality of sleep: randomized, controlled, double-blind pilot study. *Gynecol Endocrinol*. 2007 Feb;23(2):117-22.
Schellenberg, R. et al. Treatment of the premenstrual syndrome with *Agnus-castus* fruit extract: prospective, randomized, placebo-controlled study. *BMJ* 2001;322:134-7
Schultz, V. et al. *Rational Phytotherapy: A Physician's Guide to Herbal Medicine*. New York, NY: Springer, 1998.
Sehmisch, S. et al. *Vitex agnus castus* as prophylaxis for osteopenia after orchidectomy in rats compared with estradiol and testosterone supplementation. *Phytother Res*. 2009 Jun;23(6):851-8.
Sliutz, G. et al. *Agnus castus* extracts inhibit prolactin secretion of rat pituitary cells. *Hormone and Metabolic Research*. 1993;25:253-5.
Turner, S., Mills, S. A double-blind clinical trial on a herbal remedy for premenstrual syndrome: a case study. *Complementary Therapies in Medicine*. 1993;1:73-7.
Wang, J. et al. Purified vitexin compound 1 induces apoptosis through activation of FOXO3a in hepatocellular carcinoma. *Oncol Rep*. 2014 Jan; 31(1):488-96.
Weisskopf, M. et al. A *Vitex agnus-castus* extract inhibits cell growth and induces apoptosis in prostate epithelial cell lines. *Planta Med*. 2005 Oct; 71(10):910-6.
Wuttke, W. et al. Dopaminergic compounds in *Vitex agnus castus*. Loew D., Rietbrock, N. (Eds.). *Phytopharmaka in Forschung and klinischer Anwendung*. Darmstadt: Steinkopff Verlag. 1995;81-91.
____________. Treatment of cyclical mastalgia with a medication containing *Agnus castus*: results of a randomized, placebo-controlled, double-blind study. *Geburtshilfe und Frauenheilkunde*. 1997;57:569-74.
____________. Chaste tree (*Vitex agnus-castus*)–pharmacology and clinical indications. *Phytomedicine*. 2003 May;10(4):348-57.

CHICKWEED

GENERAL REFERENCES: 8) p. 321; 9); 11); 14) p. 98; 20) p. 1834; 22) p. 160; 24) p. 58; 29) p. 615; 31); 33) p. 195; 36) p. 585; 37) p. 458; 44) p. 155; 49) p. 543; 57) p. 120; 62) p. 97; 72) p. 111; 78) pp. 189-91; 79) p. 115; 81) p. 235.
Budzianowski, J. et al. Studies on antioxidative activity of some C-glycosylflavones. *Polish Journal of Pharmacology*. 1991;43:395-401.
Duke, J. Weeds you eat! *Organic Gardening*. December 1996;39-43.
Gorina,Y. et al. Evaluation of hepatoprotective activity of water-soluble polysaccharide fraction of *Stellaria media L. Bull Exp Biol Med*. 2013 Mar; 154(5):645-8.
Ma, L. et al. Anti-hepatitis B virus activity of chickweed [*Stellaria media* Vill.] extracts in HepG2.2.15 cells. *Molecules*. 2012 Jul 18;17(7):8633-46.
Pieroni, A. et al. *In vitro* antioxidant activity of non-cultivated vegetables of ethnic Albanians southern Italy. *Phytother Res*. 2002 Aug;16(5):467-73.
Shan, Y. et al. Purification and characterization of a novel anti-HSV-2 protein with antiproliferative and peroxidase activities from *Stellaria media*. *Acta Biochim Biophys Sin*. 2013 Aug;45(8):649-55.

CINQUEFOIL

GENERAL REFERENCES: 8) p. 167; 9) p. 638; 11) p. 230; 12) p. 435; 19) pp. 283, 467; 20) p. 1991; 22) p. 639; 29) p. 986; 33) p. 316; 35) p. 231; 37) p. 818; 40) p. 271; 44) p. 157; 46) p. 91; 47) p. 45; 48) pp. 70, 271; 49) p. 435; 59) p. 46; 75) p. 124; 79) p. 178; 80) p. 85; 82) pp. 37, 99, 122, 125.
Bos, M. et al. Procyanindins from Tormentil: Antioxidant Properties Toward Lipoeroxidation and Anti-Elastase Activity. *Biology Pharm Bulletin*. 1996; 19:146-8.
Carr, A. et al. *Encyclopedia of Herbs*. Emmaus, PA: Rodale Press, 1987.
Gurbuz, I. et al. Anti-ulcerogenic activity of some plants used in folk medicine of Pinarbasi (Turkey). *J Ethnopharmacol*. 2005;101(1-3):313-8.
Huber, R. et al. Tormentil for active ulcerative colitis: an open-label, dose-escalating study. *Journal of Clinical Gastroenterology*. 2007;41(9):834-38.
Langmead, L. et al. Antioxidant effects of herbal therapies used by patients with inflammatory bowel disease: an *in vitro* study. *Alimentary Pharmacological Therapy*. 2002;16(2):197-205.
Shushunov, S. et al. Determination of acute toxicity of the aqueous extract of *Potentilla erecta* (tormentil) rhizomes in rats and mice. *Journal of Medicinal Food*. 2009;12(5):1173-76.
Subbotina, M. et al. Effect of oral administration of tormentil root extract (*Potentilla tormentilla*) on rotavirus diarrhea in children: a randomized, double blind, controlled trial. *Pediatric Infectious Disease Journal*. 2003;22(8):706-11.
Tunon, H. et al. Evaluation of anti-inflammatory activity of some Swedish medicinal plants. Inhibition of prostaglandin biosynthesis and PAF-induced exocytosis. *Journal of Ethnopharmacology*. 1995;48(2):61-76.
Volodina, E. et al. The combined treatment of lichen ruber planus of the mouth (mucosa). *Stomatologiia*. 1997;76(2):28-32.
Xue, P. et al. Simultaneous determination of 7 flavonoids in *Potentilla multifida* by HPLC. *Journal of Chromatographic Science*. 2007;45(4):216-19.
Yang, J. et al. Anti-diabetic effect of standardized extract of *Potentilla discolor* and identification of its active components. *Drug Development Research*. 2010;71(2):127-32.

COMFREY

GENERAL REFERENCES:1) p. 115; 3) pp. 75, 224, 273, 279; 5) p. 133; 8) p. 308; 9) p. 708; 11) p. 43; 12) p. 407; 14); 16) p. 111; 17; 18) p. 386; 20) p. 1870; 21) p. 670; 23) p. 74; 25) p. 114; 29) p. 805; 31); 33) p. 215; 36) pp. 188, 586; 37) p. 461; 43); 44) p. 162; 46) pp. 111-2, 150, 182, 188; 55) p. 87; 59) p. 50; 64); 67); 75) p. 334; 79) p. 13.
Anderson, P. , McLean, A. Comfrey and liver damage. *Human Toxicology*. 1989;8:55-74.
Araújo, L. et al. *In vivo* wound healing effects of *Symphytum officinale L.* leaves extract in different topical formulations. *Pharmazie*. 2012 April; 67(4):355-60.
Awang, D. Comfrey. *Canadian Pharmaceutical Journal*. 1987;120:100-4.
________. Comfrey Update. *HerbalGram*. 1991;25:20-3.
Barna, M. et al. Wound healing effects of a *Symphytum* herb extract cream (*Symphytum x uplandicum* Nyman): results of a randomized, controlled double-blind study. *Wien Med Wochenschr*. 2007;157(21-22):569-74.
____________. Randomized double-blind study: wound-healing effects of a *Symphytum* herb extract cream (*Symphytum × uplandicum* Nyman) in children. *Arzneimittel-Forschung*. 2012 Jun;62(6):285-9.
Bergner, P. Comfrey, coltsfoot, and pyrrolizidine alkaloids. *Medical Herbalism*. 1989;1(1):1-5.
________. Letter. *Medical Herbalism*. 1993;5(4):3.
________. Hepatotoxicity of pyrrolizidine alkaloids. *Medical Herbalism*. 1994;6(1):10.

________. Silicon in horsetail and comfrey. *Medical Herbalism*. 1998;10(4):10.
________. Adverse effects of herbs. *Medical Herbalism*. 2002;13(1):7.
Bradley, P. (Ed.). *British Herbal Compendium* (Vol. 1). Dorset, England: British Herbal Medicine Association. 1992;66-8.
Culvenor, C. Pyrrolizidine alkaloids: some aspects of the Australian involvement. *Trends Pharmacology Science*. 1985;6:18-22.
Gafar, M. et al. Apiphytotherapeutic original preparations in the treatment of chronic marginal parodontopathies. A clinical and microbiological study. *Rev Chir Oncol Radiol ORL Oftalmol Stomatol Ser Stomatol*. 1989 Apr-Jun;36(2):91-8.
Giannetti, B. et al. Efficacy and safety of a comfrey root extract ointment in the treatment of acute upper or lower back pain: results of a double-blind, randomized, placebo controlled, multicentre trial. *British Journal of Sport Medicine*. 2010;44:637–641.
Goldman, R. et al. Wound healing and analgesic effects of crude extract of *Symphytum officinale*. *Fitoterapia*. 1985;6:323-9.
Gracza, L. et al. Biochemical-pharmacological investigations of medicinal agents of plant origin, I:Isolation of rosmarinic acid from *Symphytum officinale* L. and its anti-inflammatory activity in an *in-vitro* model. *Arch Pharm (Weinheim)*. 1985;318:1090-5.
Grube, B. et al. Efficacy of a comfrey root (*Symphyti offic. radix*) extract ointment in the treatment of patients with painful osteoarthritis of the knee: Results of a double-blind, randomized, bicenter, placebo-controlled trial. *Phytomedicine*. 2007;14:2–10.
Hirono, et al. Carcinogenic activity of *Symphytum officinale*. *Journal of the National Cancer Institute*. 1978;61(3):865-8.
_________. Induction of hepatic tumors in rats by senkirkine and symphytine. *Journal of the National Cancer Institute*. 1979;63(2):469-71.
Kearns, G. et al. Acetaminophen overdose with therapeutic intent. *Journal of Pediatrics*. 1998 Jan;132(1):5-8.
Koll, R. et al. Efficacy and tolerance of a comfrey root extract (*Extr. Rad. Symphyti*) in the treatment of ankle distorsions: results of a multicenter, randomized, placebo-controlled, double-blind study. *Phytomedicine*. 2004 Sep;11(6):470-7.
Kucera, M. et al. Efficacy and safety of topically applied *Symphytum* herb extract cream in the treatment of ankle distortion: results of a randomized controlled clinical double blind study. *Wien Med Wochenschr*. 2004 Nov;154(21-22):498-507.
____________. Topical *symphytum* herb concentrate cream against myalgia: a randomized controlled double-blind clinical study. *Adv Ther*. 2005 Nov-Dec; 22(6):681-92.
Mattocks, A. Toxicity of pyrrolizidine alkaloids. *Nature*. 1968;217:723-9.
Predel, H. et al. Efficacy of a comfrey root extract ointment in comparison to a diclofenac gel in treatment of ankle distortions: results of an observer-blind, randomized, multicenter study. *Phytomedicine*. 2005;12:707–14.
Ridker, P. et al. Hepatic venocclusive disease associated with the consumption of pyrrolizidine-containing dietary supplements. *Gastroenterology*. 1985 Apr;88(4):1050-4.
Shipochliev, T. Uterotonic action of extracts from a group of medicinal plants. *Vet Med Nauki*. 1981;18(4):94-8.
Steuart, G. Growing Alkaloid-Free Comfrey. *The Herb, Spice, and Medicinal Plant Digest*. 1987;5(4):9.
Suciu, G. et al. Pharmaceutical preparations from plant products employed in stomatologic diseases. *Rev Chir Oncol Radiol O R L Oftalmol Stomatol Ser Stomatol*. 1988 Jul-Sep;35(3):191-4.
Yeong, M. et al. Hepatic veno-occlusive disease associated with comfrey ingestion. *J Gastroenterol Hepatol*. 1990 Mar-Apr;5(2):211-4.

CRANESBILL

3) p. 231; 8) p. 151; 9) p. 446; 14) p. 143; 17); 18) p. 347; 20) p. 927; 21) p. 391; 23) p. 195; 29); 33) p. 820; 35) p. 188; 36) p. 553; 37) p. 820; 44) p. 362; 46) p. 57; 48) pp. 216, 252; 49) p. 246; 51) p. 186; 64) pp. 42, 332, 334; 66) p. 66; 67) pp. 52, 61, 119; 70) p. 390; 79) p. 147.
Lo Ha Wa Ti An Ka. *Osage Medicine: Ancestral Herbs and the Illnesses that they Treat*. Greyhorse Indian Village, Rt 2 Box 66-1, Fairfax, OK, 74637: Scope Publications.

DANDELION

GENERAL REFERENCES: 1) p. 8; 2) p. 78; 3) pp. 79-80; 5) p. 143; 9) p. 711; 11) p. 50; 14); 17); 18) p. 326; 20) p. 1914; 21) p. 672; 23) p. 80; 25) p. 130; 28) p. 114; 29) p. 290; 30); 31); 33) p. 249; 36) p. 587; 37) pp. 196, 677; 46) p. 114; 48); 51) pp. 18, 67, 178, 206, 249; 53) p. 86; 55) p. 96; 63); 64) pp. 193, 218; 70) p. 298; 75) pp. 94, 247, 259; 79) p. 153; 80) p. 467; 82).
Alschuler, L. Dandelion: Medicinal Uses. *International Journal of Integrative Medicine*. May/June 2000;2(3):47-9.
Baba, K., Abe, S., Mizuno, D. Antitumor activity of hot water extract of dandelion. *Yakugaku Zasshi*. 1981;101(6):538-43.
Bensky, D., Gamble, A., Kaptchuk, T. *Chinese Herbal Medicine Materia Medica*. Seattle, WA: Eastland Press, 1993;89.
Blanchet, K. Dandelion: Leaves are a Rich Source of Vitamins and Minerals. *Alternative and Complementary Therapies*. 1995, Jan:115.
Bradley, P. (Ed.). *British Herbal Compendium* (Vol. 1). Bournemouth, England: British Herbal Medicine Association, 1992;73-75.
Broda, B., Andrzejewska, E. Choline content in some medicinal plants. *Farm Polska*. 1966;22:181-4.
Chakurski, I. et al. Treatment of chronic colitis with an herbal combination of *Taraxacum officinale, Hypericum perforatum, Melissa officinalis, Calendula officinalis* and *Foeniculum vulgare*. *Vutr Boles*. 1981;20(6):51-4.
Choi, J. et al. Taraxinic acid, a hydrolysate of sesquiterpene lactone glycoside from the *Taraxacum coreanum* NAKAI, induces the differentiation of human acute promyelocytic leukemia HL-60 cells. *Biol Pharm Bull*. 2002;25(11):1446-50.
Choi, U. et al. Hypolipidemic and antioxidant effects of dandelion (*Taraxacum officinale*) root and leaf on cholesterol-fed rabbits. *Int J Mol Sci*. 2010 Jan 6;11(1):67-78.
Clare, B. et al. The diuretic effect in human subjects of an extract of *Taraxacum officinale* folium over a single day. *J Altern Complement Med*. 2009 Aug;15(8):929-34.
Colle, D. et al. Antioxidant properties of *Taraxacum officinale* leaf extract are involved in the protective effect against hepatoxicity induced by acetaminophen in mice. *J Med Food*. 2012 Jun;15(6):549-56.
Domitrovi, R. et al. Antifibrotic activity of *Taraxacum officinale* root in carbon tetrachloride-induced liver damage in mice. *J Ethnopharmacol*. 2010 Aug 9;130(3):569-77.
Engels, G., Brinckmann, J. Dandelion. *HerbalGram*. 2016;109:8-15.
European Scientific Cooperative on Phytotherapy. Monographs on the medicinal uses of plant drugs. *Fascicule* 1, 1996.
Farnsworth, N., Seligman, A. *Hypoglycemic Plants*. Tile and Till. 1971;57:52-5.
González-Castejón, M. et al. Reduction of Adipogenesis and Lipid Accumulation by *Taraxacum officinale* (Dandelion) Extracts in 3T3L1 Adipocytes: An *in vitro* Study. *Phytother Research*. 2013 Aug 18.
Grases, F. et al. Urolithiasis and phytotherapy. *International Urology and Nephrology*. 1994;26(5):507-11.
Heron, S., Yarnell, E. Recurrent kidney stones: a naturopathic approach. *Alternative & Complementary Therapies*. 1998 Feb;60-7.
Hobbs, C. *Dandelion: A Monograph*. Portland, OR: Eclectic Medical Publications, 1985.
Hussan, Z. et al. The effect of medicinal plants of Islamabad and Muree region of Pakistan on insulin secretion for INS-1 cells. *Phytother Res*. 2004;18(1):73-77.
Kim, H. et al. *Taraxacum officinale* restores inhibition of nitric oxide production by cadmium in mouse peritoneal macrophages. *Immunopharmacology & Immunotoxicology*. 1998;20(2):283-97.
_________. Activation of inducible nitric oxide synthase by *T. officinale* in mouse peritoneal macrphages. *Gen Pharmacology*. 1999;32(6):683-8.
Koo, H. et al. *Taraxacum officinale* induces cytotoxicity through TNF-alpha and IL-1alpha secretion in Hep G2 cells. *Life Sci*. 2004;74(9):1149-57.
Liu, J. et al. Effects of taraxasterol on ovalbumin-induced allergic asthma in mice. *J Ethnopharmacol*. 2013 Jul 30;148(3):787-93.
Mahesh, A. et al. Hepatocurative potential of sesquiterpene lactones of *Taraxacum officinale* on carbon tetrachloride induced liver toxicity in mice. *Acta Biol Hung*. 2010 Jun;61(2):175-90.
Modaresi, M., Resalatpour, N. The Effect of *Taraxacum officinale* Hydroalcoholic Extract on Blood Cells in Mice. *Adv Hematol*. 2012;2012:653412.
Moss, R. Dandelion: Bane or Boon? *Townsend Newsletter*. 2002 June;227;34.
Murray, M. Dandelion: A dandy herb for the liver and digestive system. *Health Counselor*. 1996;8(1).
Park, C. et al. TOP 1 & 2, polysaccharides from *Taraxacum officinale*, inhibit NFB-mediated inflammation and accelerate Nrf2-induced antioxidative potential through the modulation of PI3K-Akt signaling pathway in RAW 264.7 cells. *Food Chem Toxicol*. 2014 Jan 18;66C:56-64.
Qian, L. et al. Preparation and antibacterial activity of oligosaccharides derived from dandelion. *Int J Biol Macromol*. 2014 Mar;64:392-4.
Racz-Kotilla, E. et al. Action of *Taraxacum officinale* extracts on the body weight and diuresis of laboratory animals. *Planta Medica*. 1974;26:212-17.
Reid, D. *A Handbook of Chinese Healing Herbs*. Boston, MA: Shambala, 1995;100-2.
Seo, S. et al. *Taraxacum officinale* protects against cholecystokinin-induced acute pancreatitis in rats. *World J Gastroenterol*. 2005;11(4):597-9.
Sigstedt, S. et al. Evaluation of aqueous extracts of *Taraxacum officinale* on growth and invasion of breast and prostate cancer cells. *Int J Oncol*. 2008 May;32(5):1085-90.

Takasaki, M. et al. Anti-carcinogenic activity of *Taraxacum* plant I. and II. *Biol Pharm Bull.* 1999;22(6):602-61.
You, Y. et al. *In vitro* and *in vivo* hepatoprotective effects of the aqueous extract from *Taraxacum officinale* (dandelion) root against alcohol-induced oxidative stress. *Food Chem Toxicol.* 2010 Jun;48(6):1632-7.
Zhang, X. et al. Protective effect of taraxasterol against LPS-induced endotoxic shock by modulating inflammatory responses in mice. *Immunopharmacol Immunotoxicol.* 2014 Feb;36(1):11-6.

ECHINACEA

GENERAL REFERENCES: 1) pp. 122, 391; 2) p. 98; 3) pp. 83, 209, 261; 4) p. 63; 14); 17); 18) p. 358; 20) p. 671; 21) p. 347; 22) p. 232; 23) p. 85; 24) p. 70; 25) p. 138; 36) p. 544; 37) p. 610; 43); 45) p. 128; 46) pp. 43, 137, 150; 48); 49) p. 205; 51) pp. 118, 250; 53) p. 92; 55) p. 101; 63); 66) p. 59; 70); 75) pp. 229, 255, 326, 343; 76); 79) p. 159; 80) p. 242; 82).
Barrett, B. Echinacea: A Safety Review. *HerbalGram.* 2003;57:36-9.
Bauer, R., Wagner, H. Echinacea species as potential immunostimulatory drugs. *Economic & Medicinal Plants Research.* 1991;5:253.
Bauer, R., Lawson, L. (Eds.). Echinacea: biological effects and active principles. *Phytomedicines of Europe.* Washington, DC: American Chemical Society, 1998:141-57.
Bergner, P. Effect of echinacea on the hyaluronidase system. *Medical Herbalism.* 1991;4(2):8.
________. Echinacea myth: Phagocytosis not diminished after ten days. *Medical Herbalism.* 1994;6(1):1.
________. Contraindications for echinacea? *Medical Herbalism.* 1997(a);9(1):1.
________. Cautions with echinacea in auto-immune disease? *Medical Herbalism.* 1997(b);9(2):17.
________. *The Healing Power of Echinacea, Goldenseal and other Immune System Herbs.* Rocklin, CA: Prima Publishing, 1997(c).
________. Echinacea in autoimmunity revisited. *Medical Herbalism.* 2007;15(3):1.
Binns, S. Antiviral activity of characterized extracts from *Echinacea* spp. against herpes simplex virus. *Planta Medica.* 2002;68(9):780-3.
_______. Light-mediated antifungal activity of Echinacea extracts. *Planta Medica.* 2000;66(3):241-4.
Blumenthal, M. Echinacea highlighted as cold and flu remedy. *HerbalGram.* 1993;29:8-9.
Bonadeo, I. et al. Echinacin B: Active polysaccharide of the Echinacea. *Riv Italian Essenze.* 1971;53:281-295.
Bone, K. Long Term Use of Echinacea. *Medical Herbalism.* 1995;1(2):23.
______. Echinacea: What Makes It Work? *Alternative Medicine Review.* 1997;2(2).
______. Echinacea: When Should it be Used? *European Journal of Herbal Medicine.* 1997-8;3(3):13-17.
______. The Best in Phytotherapy in 2004: Solving the Echinacea Puzzle. *Townsend Letter.* 2005;259:41-44.
Braunig, B. et al. Strengthening of the endogenous resistance to influenzal infections. *Zeitschrift fur Phytotherapie.* 1992;13:7-13.
Brinker, F. Variations in effective botanical products. *HerbalGram.* 1999;46:36,41.
________. Echinacea Differences Matter: Traditional Uses of *E. angustifolia* Root Extracts vs. Modern Clinical Trials with *E. purpurea* Fresh Plant Extracts. *HerbalGram.* 2013;97:47-57.
Busing, K. Inhibition of hyaluronidase by Echinacin. *Arzneimittel-Forschung.* 1952;2:467-72.
________. Influence of *Echinacea purpurea* extracts on properdin levels in rabbits. *Z Immun exp ther.* 1958 Mar;115(3):169-76.
Cech, R. *Echinacea: Native American Tonic Roots.* Williams, OR: Horizon Herbs Publication, 1995.
Coeugniet, E. Recurrent candidiasis: Adjutant immunotherapy with different formulations of Echinacin. *Therapiewoche.* 1986;36:3352.
__________ . *Klin Pharmacy.* 1987;8(87):481-5.
Cruz, I. et al. Alkamides from Echinacea disrupt the fungal cell wall-membrane complex. *Phytomedicine.* 2014 Mar 15;21(4):435-42.
Currier, N., Miller, S. The effect of immunization with killed tumor cells, with/without feeding of *Echinacea purpurea* in an erythroleukemic mouse model. *Journal of Alternative & Complementary Medicine.* 2002;8(1):49-58.
Flannery, M. From Rudbeckia to Echinacea: The Emergence of the Purple Coneflower in Modern Therapeutics. *HerbalGram.* 2001;51:28.
Fonseca, F. et al. *Echinacea purpurea* (L.) Moench modulates human T-cell cytokine response. *Int Immunopharmacol.* 2014 Jan 13;19(1):94-102.
Foster, S. *Echinacea Exalted.* Drury, MO: Ozark Beneficial Plant Project, 1984.
_______. *Echinacea: Nature's Immune Enhancer.* Rochester, VT: Healing Arts Press, 1991.
_______. Echinacea: The Cold and Flu Remedy. *Alternative and Complementary Therapies.* 1995 June/July;254.
_______. *Echinacea: The Purple Coneflower.* American Botanical Council, Botanical Series No. 301, 1999.
Gallo, M. et al. Pregnancy outcome following gestational exposure to Echinacea. *Archives of Internal Medicine.* 2000;160:3141-3.
____________. Can herbal products be used safely during pregnancy? Focus on Echinacea. *Canadian Family Physician.* 2001;47:1727-8.
Gilmore, M. *Uses of Plants by the Indians of the Missouri River Region. 33rd Annual Report of the Bureau of American Ethnology.* Washington D.C. Government Printing Office, 1919.
Goel, V. et al. Echinacea stimulates macrophage function in the lung and spleen of normal rats. *J Nutr Biochemistry.* 2002;13(8):487.
__________. Efficacy of a standardized echinacea preparation (Echinilin) for the treatment of the common cold: a randomized, double-blind, placebo-controlled trial. *J Clin Pharm Ther.* 2004;29:75-83.
Hobbs, C. *The Echinacea Handbook.* Portland, OR: Eclectic Medical Publications, 1989.
_______. *Echinacea: The Immune Herb.* Santa Cruz, CA: Botanical Press,1990.
_______. Echinacea: diminished immune stimulation over time? *Medical Herbalism.* 1994;6(2):3-4.
_______. Echinacea: A Literature Review. *HerbalGram.* 1994;30:33-48.
Hoheisel, O. et al. Echinagard treatment shortens the course of the common cold: a double-blind, placebo-controlled trial. *European Journal of Clinical Research.* 1997;9:261-8.
Hou, C. et al. Echinacea alkamides prevent lipopolysaccharide/D-galactosamine-induced acute hepatic injury through JNK pathway-mediated HO-1 expression. *J Agric Food Chem.* 2011 Nov 23;59(22):11966-74.
Lawrence Review of Natural Products. Echinacea. January, 1990.
Lindenmuth, G. The efficacy of echinacea compound herbal tea preparation on the severity and duration of upper respiratory and flu symptoms: a randomized, double-blind placebo-controlled study. *J Alternative & Complementary Medicine.* 2000;6(4):327-34.
Luettig, B. et al. Macrophage Activation by the Polysaccharide Arabinogalactan Isolated from Plant Cell Cultures of *Echinacea purpurea. Journal of the National Cancer Institute.* 1989;89(9):669-675.
McCaleb, R. Echinacea safety confirmed. *HerbalGram.* 1998;42:15.
Mostbeck, A., Studlar, M. Experimental tests of a plant extract from *Echinacea purpurea* M. as a nonspecific stimulant. With special reference to the effects on the adrenal cortex. *Wiener Med Wochenschrift.* 1962;112(13):259-62.
Pohl, P. Therapy of radiation-induced leukopenia by Esberitox. *Med Klin.* 1969;64:1546-7.
Raus, K. et al. Effect of an Echinacea-Based Hot Drink Versus Oseltamivir in Influenza Treatment: A Randomized, Double-Blind, Double-Dummy, Multicenter, Non-inferiority Clinical Trial. *Curr Ther Res Clin Exp.* 2015 Apr 20;77:66-72.
Rodinet, M., Beuscher. Host-Resistance Increasing Activity of Root Extracts from Echinacea Species. *Planta Medica.* 1993;59:A672.
Schapowal, A. et al. Echinacea reduces the risk of recurrent respiratory tract infections and complications: a meta-analysis of randomized controlled trials. *Adv Ther.* 2015 March;32(3):187-200.
Schulte, K. et al. The presence of polyacetylene compounds in *E. purpurea* M and *E.angustifolia* DC. *Arzneimittel-Forschung.* 1967;17(7):825-9.
See, D. et al. *In vitro* effects of echinacea and ginseng on natural killer and antibody-dependent cell cytotoxicity in healthy subjects and chronic fatigue syndrome or AID syndrome patients. *Immunopharmacology.* 1997;35:229-35.
Shah, S. et al. Evaluation of Echinacea for prevention and treatment of the common cold: a meta-analysis. *Lancet Infectious Disease.* 2007;7:473-80.
Stroll, A. et al. Isolation and constitution of echinacoside, a glycoside from roots of *Echinacea angustifolia* DC. *Helv Chim Acta.* 1950;33:1877-93.
Sun, L. et al. American coneflower: a prophylactic role involving nonspecific immunity. *J Alternative & Complementary Med.* 1999;5(5):437-46.
Tsai, Y. et al. Cytotoxic effects of *Echinacea purpurea* flower extracts and cichoric acid on human colon cancer cells through induction of apoptosis. *J Ethnopharmacol.* 2012 Oct 11;143(3):914-9.
Tunnerhoff, F., Schwabe, H. Animal and human studies on tissue changes after gelatin and thrombin implants. *Arzneimittel-Forschung.* 1956;330.
Viehmann P. Results of treatment with an Echinacea-based ointment. *Erfahrungsheilkunde.* 1978;27:353–358.
Wacker, A., Hilbig, W. Virus inhibition by *Echinacea purpurea. Planta Medica.* 1978;33:89-102.
Wagner, H. et al. Immunostimulating polysaccharides of higher plants. *Arzneimittel-Forschung.* 1984;34:659-60.
Wagner, H., Proksch, A. *Economic and Medicinal Plant Research.* Orlando, FL: Academic Press, 1985;113.

ELDERBERRY

GENERAL REFERENCES: 1); 2) p. 103; 3) p. 293; 9); 10) p. 199; 11); 12) p. 574; 13) p. 423; 14) pp. 168, 329, 514; 16) p. 125; 17); 18); 19) pp. 121-5; 20); 21); 22) p. 235; 24) p. 72; 25) p. 150; 29) p. 1421-4; 31); 33) p. 265; 35) p. 191; 36) p. 580; 37) p. 172; 43) p. 418; 44) p. 178; 46) p. 102; 47) p. 38; 48) pp. 14, 227; 49); 55) p. 104; 62) pp. 141, 142; 63) pp. 19, 40, 44, 124; 64) pp. 158, 177; 66) p. 60; 70) p. 301; 71); 73) pp. 59, 65, 184; 74) p. 40; 75) p. 226; 77) pp. 148, 376, 377; 79) p. 161; 80) p. 423; 81) pp. 187, 191, 200, 209; 82).

Abuja, P. et al. Antioxidant and Pro-oxidant activities of Elderberry (*Sambucus nigra*) in low-density lipoprotein oxidation. *J of Ag Food Chem.* 1998;46:4091-96.

Barak, V. et al. The effect of Sambucol, a black elderberry-based, natural product, on the production of human cytokines: I. Inflammatory cytokines. *European Cytokine Network.* 2001;12(2):290-96.

Bergner, P. Elderberry (*Sambucus nigra, S. canadensis*). *Medical Herbalism.* 1996;8(4):1.

Chatterjee, A. et al. Inhibition of *Helicobacter pylori in vitro* by various berry extracts, with enhanced susceptibility to clarithromycin. *Molecular Cell Biochemistry.* 2004;265(1-2):19-26.

Engels, G., Brinckmann, J. European Elder (*Sambucus nigra*). *HerbalGram.* 2013;97:1-7.

Kilham, C. Health Benefits Boost Elderberry. *HerbalGram.* 2000;50:55-6.

Kuts-Chereaux, A. *Naturae Medicina and Naturopathic Dispensatory.* Des Moines, IA: American Naturopathic Physicians and Surgeons Association, 1952.

Mascolo, N. et al. Biological screening of Italian medicinal plants for anti-inflammatory activity. *Phytotherapy Research.* 1987;1:28-31.

Morag, A. et al. Inhibition of sensitive and acyclovir-resistant HSV-1 strains by an elderberry extract *in vitro.* Tenth International Congress of Virology. Jerusalem, Israel; August 1996.

Murkovic, M. et al. Effects of elderberry juice on fasting and postprandial serum lipids and low-density lipoprotein oxidation in healthy volunteers: a randomized, double-blind, placebo-controlled study. *European J Clinical Nutrition.* 2004;58(2):244-9.

Paulo, E. Effect of phytohaemagglutinin (PHA) from the bark of *S. nigra* on embryonic and foetal development in mice. *Folia Biol.* 1976;24:213.

Pool-Zobel, B. et al. Anthocyanins are potent antioxidants in model systems but do not reduce endogenous oxidative DNA damage in human colon cells. *European J Nutrition.* 1999;38:227-34.

Richter, A. Changes in the motor activity of smooth muscles of the rat uterus *in vitro* as the effect of phytohaemagglutinins from *Sambucus nigra. Folia Biol.* 1973;21:33-48.

Roschek, B. et al. Elderberry flavonoids bind to and prevent H1N1 infection *in vitro. Phtyochemistry.* 2009;70(10):1255-61.

Sauter, C., Wolfensberger, C. Anticancer activities as well as antiviral and virus-enhancing properties of aqueous fruit extracts from fifty-six European plant species. *European J Clinical Oncology.* 1989;25(6):987-90.

Serkedjieva, J. et al. Antiviral activity of the infusion (SHS-174) from flowers of *Sambucus nigra* L., aerial parts of *Hypericum perforatum* L., and roots of *Saponaria officinalis* L. against influenza and herpes simplex viruses. *Phytotherapy Research.* 1990;4:97-100.

Shapira-Nahor, O. et al. The effect of Sambucol on HIV infection *in vitro.* Annual Israel Congress of Microbiology, 1995.

Terpin, J. et al. Antiviral evaluation of elderberry extracts & standardized powder. Frederick, MD: Southern Research Institute. Unpublished, 2000.

Watzl, B. et al. Anthocyanins stimulate cytokine production (TNF-alpha, IL-2) in human mononuclear cells. Paper presented at International Workshop on Immunonutrition. June 24-25, 2000 at Schloss Rauischholzhausen, Austria.

Youdim, K. et al. Incorporation of the Elderberry anthocyanins by endothelial cells increases protection against oxidative stress. *Free Radical Biology & Medicine.* 2000;29(1):51-60.

Zakay-Rones, Z. et al. Inhibition of several strains of influenza virus *in vitro* and reduction of symptoms by an elderberry extract (*Sambucus nigra* L) during an outbreak of influenza B Panama. *J Alternative & Complementary Medicine.* 1995;1:361-9.

_________________. Randomized study of the efficacy and safety of oral elderberry extract in the treatment of influenza A and B virus infections. *J Internal Medical Research.* 2004;32(2):132-40.

ELECAMPANE

1) p. 328; 3) pp. 85, 273, 279; 5) p. 155; 8) p. 341; 9) p. 480; 11) p. 232; 12) pp. 22, 293; 14) pp. 224, 369, 372; 16) p. 127; 17); 18) p. 276; 20) p. 1058; 21) p. 426; 22) p. 237; 23) p. 89; 25) p. 140; 28) p. 116; 29) p. 792; 33) p. 278; 35) p. 192; 36) p. 560; 37) p. 292; 42) p. 238; 44) p. 101; 46) pp. 63, 183, 188; 48) pp. 34, 42; 55) p. 106; 59) p. 67; 63) p. 124; 64) p. 298; 65) p. 320; 66) p. 60; 75) p. 205; 79) p. 162; 81) p. 281.

Bensky, D., Gamble, A., Kaptchuk, T. *Chinese Herbal Medicine Materia Medica.* Seattle, WA: Eastland Press, 1993;193.

Blagojevic, P., Radulovic, N. Conformational analysis of antistaphylococcal sesquiterpene lactones from *Inula helenium* essential oil. *Nat Prod Commun.* 2012 Nov;7(11):1407-10.

Cantrell, C. et al. Antimycobacterial eudesmanolides from *Inula helenium* & *Rudbeckia subtomentosa. Planta Medica.* 1999;65(4):351-5.

Chen, C. et al. Isocostunolide, a sesquiterpene lactone, induces mitochondrial membrane depolarization and caspase-dependent apoptosis in human melanoma cells. *Cancer Letters.* 2007 Feb 8;246(1-2):237-52.

Danilets, M. et al. Effect of plant polysaccharides on TH1-dependent immune response: screening investigation. *Eksp Klin Farmakol.* 2010;73(6):19.

Dorn, D. et al. Tumor cell specific toxicity of *Inula helenium* extracts. *Phytotherapy Research.* 2006 Nov;20(11):970-80.

Enqin, Z. (Ed.). *Chinese Materia Medica.* Shanghai, China: Publishing House of Shanghai College of TCM, 1988;144.

Khan, A. et al. Secondary metabolites from *Inula britannica* L. and their biological activities. *Molecules.* 2010 Mar 10;15(3):1562-77.

Liu, S. et al. Design, synthesis, and anti-tumor activity of (2-O-alkyloxime-3-phenyl)-propionyl-1-O-acetylbritannilactone esters. *Bioorg Med Chem.* 2005 Apr 15;13(8):2783-9.

O'Shea, S. et al. *In vitro* activity of *Inula helenium* against clinical *Staphylococcus aureus* strains including MRSA. *Br J Biomed Sci.* 2009;66(4):186-9.

Pal, H. et al. Activation of caspases and poly (ADP-ribose) polymerase cleavage to induce apoptosis in leukemia HL-60 cells by *Inula racemosa. Toxicology In Vitro.* 2010 Sep;24(6):1599-609.

Qiu, J. et al. Isoalantolactone protects against *Staphylococcus aureus* pneumonia. *FEMS Microbiol Lett.* 2011 Nov;324(2):147-55.

Rasul, A. et al. Targeting apoptosis pathways in cancer with alantolactone and isoalantolactone. *Scientific World Journal.* 2013 Oct 27;2013:248532.

Rhee, J. et al. Structural investigation on the effects of the herbs on *Clonorchis sinensis* in rabbits. *Am J Chin Med.* 1985;13(1-4):119-25.

Seo, J. et al. Nrf2-mediated induction of detoxifying enzymes by alantolactone present in *Inula helenium. Phytother Res.* 2008 Nov;22(11):1500-5.

_________. Isoalantolactone from *Inula helenium* caused Nrf2-mediated induction of detoxifying enzymes. *J Med Food.* 2009 Oct;12(5):1038-45.

Stojakowska, A. et al. Antimicrobial activity of 10-isobutyryloxy-8,9-epoxythymol isobutyrate. *Fitoterapia.* 2005 Dec;76(7-8):687-90.

Tripathi, Y., Chaturvedi, P. Assessment of endocrine response of *Inula racemosa* in relation to glucose homeostasis in rats. *Indian Journal of Exp Biology.* 1995;33(9):686-9.

Wu, M. et al. Isoalantolactone inhibits UM-SCC-10A cell growth via cell cycle arrest and apoptosis induction. *PLoS One.* 2013 Sep 30;8(9):e76000.

Zhang, Y. et al. Alantolactone induces apoptosis in RKO cells through the generation of reactive oxygen species and the mitochondrial pathway. *Mol Med Rep.* 2013 Oct;8(4):967-72.

FEVERFEW

GENERAL REFERENCES: 3) p. 95; 5) p. 173; 9) p. 249; 12) p. 381; 13); 14) pp. 40, 53, 284; 17); 20) p. 1438; 21) p. 672; 22) p. 253; 23) p. 93; 25) p. 168; 29) p. 651; 36) pp. 369-70, 587; 37) p. 591; 43); 44) p. 195; 45) p. 157; 46) pp. 113, 183; 47) p. 43; 48) pp. 83, 379; 53) p. 116; 54) pp. 418, 497; 55) p. 110; 64) p. 159; 66) p. 63; 76); 79) p. 174.

Ansari, M. et al. Measurement of melatonin in alcoholic and hot water extracts of *Tanacetum parthenium. Daru.* 2010;18(3):173–178.

Awang, D. Feverfew (*Tanacetum parthenium*). *The Pharmaceutical Journal.* 1987;239:487.

_________. Feverfew Feedback (letter). *HerbalGram.* 1990;22:2,34,42.

_________. Feverfew Fever. *HerbalGram.* 1993;29:34-6,66.

_________. Feverfew Fever: A Headache for the Consumer. *HerbalGram.* 1993;34:34.

Barsby, R. et al. Feverfew and vascular smooth muscle: Extracts from fresh and dried plants show opposing pharmacological profiles, dependent upon sesquiterpene lactone content. *Planta Med.* 1993;59:20–5.

Blakeman, J., Atkinson, P. Antimicrobial properties and possible role in host-pathogen interactions of parthenolide, a sesquiterpene lactone isolated from glands of *Chrysanthemum parthenium. Physiology and Plant Pathology.* 1979;15:183-92.

Blumenthal, M. Testing Botanicals. *HerbalGram.* 1997;40:45.

Capasso, F. The effect of an aqueous extract of *Tanacetum parthenium* L. on arachidonic acid metabolism by rat peritoneal leukocytes. *Journal of*

Pharmacy and Pharmacology. 1986 Jan;38(1):71-2.
Chavez, M., Chavez, P. Parthenolide inhibited the growth of gram-positive bacteria, yeast, and fungi. *Hospital Pharm.* 1999;34:436–61.
Cheng, G., Xie, L. Parthenolide induces apoptosis and cell cycle arrest of human 5637 bladder cancer cells *in vitro. Molecules.* 2011;16(8):6758.
Collier, H. et al. Extracts of feverfew inhibits prostaglandin biosynthesis. *Lancet.* 1980 Oct;2:922-3.
Culpeper, N. *The English Physician Enlarged.* Dublin: Ireland, H. Colbert, 1787.
Diener, H. et al. Efficacy and safety of 6.25 mg t.i.d. feverfew CO2-extract (MIG-99) in migraine prevention: randomized double-blind, multicentre, placebo-controlled study. *Cephalalgia.* 2005;25(11):1031-41.
Fischedick, J. et al. Activation of antioxidant response element in mouse primary cortical cultures with sesquiterpene lactones isolated from *Tanacetum parthenium. Planta Medica.* 2012 Nov;78(16):1725-30.
Foster, S. Feverfew *Tanacetum parthenium. American Botanical Council,* Series No. 310. P.O. Box 201660, Austin, TX 78720, 1991.
Frances, D. Feverfew for acute headaches. *Medical Herbalism.* 1995;7(4):1.
Groenewegen, W., Heptinstall, S. A Comparison of the Effects of an Extract of Feverfew and Parthenolide, a Component of Feverfew, on Human Platelet Activity *In Vitro. Journal of Pharmacy and Pharmacology.* 1990;42(8):553-7.
Gupta, S. et al. Chemical Mediators of Migraine: Preclinical and Clinical Observations. *Headache.* 2011 June;51(6):1029-45.
Hayes, N., Foreman, J. The activity of compounds extracted from feverfew on histamine release from rat mast cells. *Journal of Pharmacy and Pharmacology.* 1987;39(6):466-70.
Heptinstall, S., Awang, D. et. al. Parthenolide content and bioactivity of Feverfew (*Tanacetum parthenium*). *Journal of Pharmacy and Pharmacology.* 1992;44(5):391-5.
Heptinstall, S. et al. Extracts of feverfew inhibit granule secretion in blood platelets and polymorphonuclear leukocytes. *Lancet.* 1985;1:1071-4.
Hobbs, C. Feverfew *Tanacetum parthenium*: A Review. *HerbalGram.* 1989;20:26-36.
Hwang, D. et al. Inhibition of the expression of inducible cyclooxygenase and proinflammatory cytokines by sesquiterpene lactones in macrophages correlates with the inhibition of MAP kinases. *Biochem Biophys Res Commun.* 1996 Sep 24;226(3):810-8.
Johnson, E. Patients Who Chew Chrysanthemum leaves. *MIMS Magazine.* May 15,1983;32-5.
Johnson, E. et al. Efficacy of Feverfew as a Prophylactc Treatment of Migraine. *British Medical Journal.* 1985;291(6495):569-73.
Kang, B. et al. Inhibition of interleukin-12 production in lipopolysaccharide-activated mouse macrophages by parthenolide, a predominant sesquiterpene lactone in *Tanacetum parthenium*: involvement of nuclear factor-kappaB. *Immunol Lett.* 2001 Jul 2;77(3):159-63.
Kim, S. et al. Parthenolide exerts inhibitory effects on angiogenesis through the downregulation of VEGF/VEGFRs in colorectal cancer. *Int J Mol Med.* 2014;33:1261–1267.
Kwok, B. The anti-inflammatory natural product parthenolide from the medicinal herb feverfew directly binds to and inhibits IkappaB kinase. *Chem Biol.* 2001;8:759–66.
LaValle, J. *Cox-2 Connection: Natural Breakthrough Treatments for Arthritis, Alzheimer's and Cancer.* Rochester, VT: Healing Arts Press, 2001.
Li, Y. et al. Parthenolide induces apoptosis and lytic cytotoxicity in Epstein-Barr virus-positive Burkitt lymphoma. *Mol Med Rep.* 2012;6(3):477-82.
Loesche, W. et al. Feverfew-an antithrombotic herb? *Folia Haematol Int Mag Klin Morphol Blutforsch.* 1988;115(1-2):181-4.
Magni, P. et al. Parthenolide inhibits the LPS-induced secretion of IL-6 and TNF-a and NF-kB nuclear translocation in BV-2 microglia. *Phytother Res.* 2012 Sep;26(9):1405-9.
Majdi, M. et al. Biosynthesis and localization of parthenolide in glandular trichomes of feverfew. *Phytochemistry.* 2011 Oct;72(14-15):1739-50.
Makheja, A., Bailey, J. The active principle in feverfew. *Lancet.* Lancet. 1981 Nov;2:1054–7.
_______________. A platelet phospholipase inhibitor from the medicinal herb feverfew. *Prostaglandins Leukot Med.* 1982 June;8(6):653-60.
Murch, S. et. al. Melatonin in feverfew and other medicinal plants. *Lancet.* 1997;350:1598-99.
Murphy, J. et al. Randomized double-blind placebo-controlled trial of feverfew in migraine prevention. *Lancet.* 1988;2:189-92.
O'Neal, L. et al. Extracts of feverfew inhibit mitogen-induced human peripheral blood mononuclear cell proliferation and cytokine mediated responses: a cytotoxic effect. *British Journal of Clinical Pharmacy.* 1987;23(1):81-2.
Pajak, B. Antiapoptotic proteins as targets for bioactive compounds. *Pol J Vet Sci.* 2007;10(2):127-30.
Palevitch, D. et al. Feverfew (*Tanacetum parthenium*) as a prophylactic treatment for migraine: a double-blind placebo-controlled study. *Phytother Res.* 1997;11(7):508-11.
Piela-Smith, T., Liu, X. Feverfew extracts and the sesquiterpene lactone parthenolide inhibit intercellular adhesion molecule-1 expression in human synovial fibroblasts. *Cell Immunol.* 2001 May 1;209(2):89-96.
Ross, J. et al. Low concentrations of the feverfew component parthenolide inhibit *in vitro* growth of tumor lines in a cytostatic fashion. *Planta Med.* 1999;65:126–9.
Sumner, H. et al. Inhibition of 5-lipoxygenase and cyclo-oxygenase in leukocytes by feverfew. Involvement of sesquiterpene lactones and other components. *Biochem Pharmacol.* 1992;43:2313–20.
Tiuman, T. et al.Antileishmanial activity of parthenolide, a sesquiterpene lactone isolated from *Tanacetum parthenium. Antimicrob Agents Chemother.* 2005;49:176–82.
Williams, C. et al. A biologically active lipophilic flavonol from *Tanacetum parthenium. Phytochemistry.* 1995 Jan;38(1):267-70.
Wyrebska, A. Apoptosis-mediated cytotoxic effects of parthenolide and the new synthetic analog MZ-6 on two breast cancer cell lines. *Mol Biol Rep.* 2013 Feb;40(2):1655-63.
Zhao, Z. et al. Parthenolide, an inhibitor of the nuclear factor-kB pathway, ameliorates dextran sulfate sodium-induced colitis in mice. *Int Immunopharmacol.* 2012 Jan;12(1):169-74.

GOLDENROD

GENERAL REFERENCES: 1) p. 139; 2) p. 178; 3) p. 109; 9); 14) pp. 103, 254, 561; 16) p. 160; 17); 18); 19) pp. 387-391; 20); 23) p. 183; 29) p. 439; 33) p. 361; 35) p. 197; 36) p. 585; 43) pp. 66, 76, 114, 161; 44) p. 208; 46) p. 108; 49) p. 536; 60) p. 265; 62) p. 175; 65) p. 302; 66) p. 69; 67) p. 74; 74) pp. 76, 129; 75) p. 241; 79) p. 198; 80) p. 459; 81).
Apati, P. et al. Herbal remedies of *Solidago*--correlation of phytochemical characteristics and antioxidative properties. *J Pharm Biomed Analysis.* 2003;32(4-5):1045-53.
Bigalow, J. *American Medical Botany; being a collection of the native medicinal plants of the United States* (3 vols.). Boston, MA: Cummings & Hilliard, 1817-1820;190.
Borchert, V. et al. Extracts from *Rhois aromatica* and *Solidago virgaurea* inhibit rat and human bladder contraction. *Naunyn Schmiedebergs Arch Pharmacol.* 2004;369(3):281-6.
Cabrera, M. The strange case of Mr. B. *Medical Herbalism.* 1993;5(4):1.
Cai, T. et al. *Solidago,* orthosiphon, birch and cranberry extracts can decrease microbial colonization and biofilm development in indwelling urinary catheter: a microbiologic and ultrastructural pilot study. *World Journal of Urology.* 2014 Aug;32(4):1007-14.
Duarte, M. et al. Anti-Candida activity of Brazilian medicinal plants. *J Ethnopharmacol,* 2005;97(2):305-311.
Frumenzio, E. et al. Role of phytotherapy associated with antibiotic prophylaxis in female patients with recurrent urinary tract infections. *Arch Ital Urol Androl.* 2013 Dec 31;85(4):197-9.
Ghazaly, M. et al. Study of the anti-inflammatory activity of *Populus tremula, Solidago virgaurea* and *Fraxinus excelsior. Arzneimittel-forschung.* 1992;42:333-36.
Gross, S. et al. Antineoplastic activity of *Solidago virgaurea* on prostatic tumor cells in an SCID mouse model. *Nutr Cancer.* 2002;43(1):76-81.
Laurencon, L. et al. Triterpenoid saponins from the aerial parts of *Solidago virgaurea alpestris* with inhibiting activity of Candida albicans yeast-hyphal conversion. *Phytochemistry.* 2013 Feb;86:103-11.
Metzner, J. et al. Antiphlogistic and analgesic effects of leiocarposide, a phenolic bisglucoside of *Solidago virgaurea L. Pharmazie.* 1984;39:869-70.
Schmeda-Hirschmann, G. et al. Gastroprotective activity of the diterpene solidagenone and its derivatives on experimentally induced gastric lesions in mice. *J Ethnopharmacology.* 2002;81(1):111-5.
Vila, R. et al. Composition and antifungal activity of the essential oil of *Solidago chilensis. Planta Med.* 2002;68(2):164-167.
Yarnell, E. Botanical medicines for the urinary tract. *World Journal of Urology.* 2002;20(5):285-93.

GOLDENSEAL

GENERAL REFERENCES: 3); 8) p. 436; 9) p. 472; 14); 16) p. 161; 17); 18) p. 196; 20) p. 1020; 21) p. 417; 23) p. 102; 25) p. 186; 36) p. 558; 37) p. 634; 38) p. 143; 41) p. 655; 42) p. 244; 43); 44) p. 210; 45) p. 221; 46) pp. 62, 136, 183; 48) pp. 45, 54, 100, 192; 49) p. 270; 51) pp. 147, 158,

257, 272; 52); 53) p. 162; 54); 55) p. 151; 64) p. 204; 70) p. 311; 76); 79) p. 199; 80) p. 293; 81).
Abidi, P. et al. The medicinal plant goldenseal is a natural LDL-lowering agent with multiple bioactive components and new action mechanisms. *Journal of Lipid Research.* 2006;47(10):2134-2147.
Babbar, O. et al. Effect of berberine chloride eye drops on clinically positive trachoma patients. *Indian J Medical Research.* 1982;76:83-8.
Bergner, P. Goldenseal and the common cold: The antibiotic myth. *Medical Herbalism.* 1996;8(4):1-6.
Bhide, M. et al. Absorption, distribution and excretion of berberine. *Indian Journal of Medical Research.* 1969;57:2128-31.
Birdsall, T., Kelly, G. Berberine: Therapeutic Potential of Alkaloid Found in Several Medicinal Plants. *Alternative Med Review.* 1997;2(2):94-102.
Brinker, F. Variations in Effective Botanical Products. *HerbalGram.* 1999;46:46.
Buhner, S. *Herbal Antibiotics: Natural Alternatives for Treating Drug-Resistant Bacteria.* North Adams, MA: Storey Books, 2012;158-60,173-5,177-8.
________. *Healing Lyme Disease Coinfections.* Rochester, VT: Healing Arts Press, 2013;192-4.
Cech, N. et al. Quorum quenching and antimicrobial activity of goldenseal (*Hydrastis canadensis*) against methicillin-resistant *Staphylococcus aureus* (MRSA). *Planta Med.* 2012 Sep;78(14):1556-61.
Cecil, C. et al. Inhibition of H1N1 influenza A virus growth and induction of inflammatory mediators by the isoquinoline alkaloid berberine and extracts of goldenseal (*Hydrastis canadensis*). *Int Immunopharmacol.* 2011 Nov;11(11):1706-14.
Chan, M. The effect of berberine on bilirubin excretion in the rat. *Complementary Medicine East West.* 1977;5:161-8.
Chopra, R. et al. Pharmacological action of berberine. *Indian Journal of Medical Research.* 1932;19:1193-1203.
Choudhry, V. et al. Berberine in giardiasis. *Indian Pediatrics.* 1972;9:143-6.
Clement-Kruzel, S. et al. Immune modulation of macrophage pro-inflammatory response by goldenseal and Astragalus extracts. *J Med Food.* 2008 Sep;11(3):493-8.
Farnsworth, N. et al. Potential value of plants as sources of new antifertility agents. *Journal of Pharm Science.* 1975;64:535-98.
Foster, S. *Goldenseal: Hydrastis canadensis.* American Botanical Council, Botanical Series #309. Austin, TX, 1999.
Genest, K., Hughes, D. Natural products in Canadian pharmaceuticals: *H. canadensis. Canadian Journal Pharm Science.* 1969;4:41-5.
Gladstar, R., Hirsh, P. (Eds.). *Planting the Future: Saving our Medicinal Herbs.* Rochester, VT: Healing Arts Press, 2000;111-122.
Gupte, S. Use of berberine in treatment of giardiasis. *American Journal of Diseases of Childhood.* 1975;129:866.
Gurley, B. et al. Clinical assessment of CYP2D6-mediated herb-drug interactions in humans: effects of milk thistle, black cohosh, goldenseal, kava kava, St. John's wort, and Echinacea. *Mol Nutr Food Res.* 2008 Jul;52(7):755-63.
Hahn, F., Ciak, J. Berberine. *Antibiotics.* 1976;3:577-84.
Harborne, J., Baxter, H. *Phytochemical Dictionary.* London, England: Taylor and Francis, 1993.
Huang, W. Ventricular tachyarrhythmias treated with berberine. *Chung Hua Hsin Hsueh Kuan Ping Tsa Chih.* 1990;18:155-6,190.
Huang, W. et al. Beneficial effects of berberine on hemodynamics during acute ischemic left ventricular failure in dogs. *Chinese Medical Journal.* 1992;105(12):1014-9.
Huang, Z. et al. Protective effects of berberine and phentolamine on myocardial reoxygenation damage. *Chinese Med Science J.* 1992;7(4):221-5.
Hwang, B. et al. Antimicrobial constituents from goldenseal (Rhizomes of *H. canadensis*) against selected oral pathogens. *Planta Med.* 2003 Jul; 69(7):623-7.
Kamat, S. Clinical trial with berberine hydrochloride for the control of diarrhea in acute gastroenteritis. *Indian Medical Journal.* 1974;68:19-23.
Kaneda, Y. et al. *In vitro* effects of berberine sulfate on the growth of *Entamoeba histolytica, Giardia lamblia* and *Trichomonas vaginalis. Ann Trop Med Parasitol.* 1991;85:417-25.
Kong, W. et al. Berberine is a novel cholesterol-lowering drug working through a unique mechanism distinct from statins. Nat Med. 2004 Dec; 10(12):1344-51.
Kumazawa, Y. et al. Activation of peritoneal macrophages by berberine-type alkaloids in terms of induction of cytostatic activity. *International Journal of Immunopharmacology.* 1984;6(6):587-92.
Lesnau, A. et al. Antiviral activity of berberine salts. *Pharmazie.* 1990;45(8):638-9.
Lewis, W., Elvin-Lewis, M. *Medical Botany: Plants Affecting Man's Health.* New York, NY: John Wiley & Sons, 1977.
Liu, C. et al. Studies on plant resources, pharmacology and clinical treatment with berberine. *Phytotherapy Research.* 1991;5:228-30.
Mahady, G. et al. *In vitro* susceptibility of *Heliobacter pylori* to isoquinoline alkaloids from *Sanguinaria canadensis* and *Hydrastis canadensis. Phytotherapy Research.* 2003;17(3):217-21.
Martin-Neti, J. et al. Cardiovascular effects of berberine in patients with severe congestive heart failure. *Clinical Cardiology.* 1988;11:253-60.
Mohan, M. et al. Berberine in trachoma. *Indian Journal of Opthalmology.* 1982;30:69-75.
Nishino, H. et al. Berberine sulfate inhibits tumor-promoting activity of teleocidin in two-stage carcinogenesis on mouse skin. *Oncology.* 1986;43: 131-4.
Ohara, M. et al. A review of 12 commonly used medicinal herbs. *Archives of Family Medicine.* 1998;7:523-36.
Pizzorno, J., Murray, M. *Textbook of Natural Medicine.* Seattle, WA: John Bastyr College Publications, 1988.
Preininger, V. The pharmacology and toxicology of the Papavaraceae alkaloids. *The Alkaloids.* 1975;15:207-51.
Rabbani, G. et al. Randomized controlled trial of berberine sulfate therapy for diarrhea due to enterotoxigenic *Escherichia coli* and *Vibrio cholerae. Journal of Infectious Diseases.* 1987;155(5):979-84.
__________. Mechanism and treatment of diarrhoea due to *Vibrio cholerae* and *E. coli*: roles of drugs and prostaglandins. *Dan Med Bull.* 1996;43:173.
Rehman, J. et al. Increased production of antigen-specific immunoglobins G and M following *in vivo* treatment with the medicinal plants *Echinacea angustifolia* and *Hydrastis canadensis. Immunology Letters.* 1999;68:391-5.
Rong-Xun, Z. et al. Laboratory studies of berberine used alone and in combination with 1,3-bis(2-chloroethyl)-1-nitrosourea to treat malignant brain tumors. *Chinese Medical Journal.* 1990;103(8):658-65.
Sabir, M., Bhide, N. Study of some pharmacologic actions of berberine. *Indian Journal of Physiology & Pharmacology.* 1971;15:111-32.
______________. Further studies on pharmacology of berberine. *Indian J Physiol Pharmacol.* 1978 Jan-Mar;22(1):9-23.
Sack, R., Froehlich, J. Berberine inhibits intestinal secretory response of *Vibrio cholerae* toxins and *Escherichia coli* enterotoxins. *Infect Immun.* 1982;35:471-5.
Scazzocchio, F. et al. Antibacterial activity of *Hydrastis canadensis* extract and its major isolated alkaloids. *Planta Medica.* 2001;67:561-564.
Snow. *Hydrastis canadensis:* Goldenseal monograph. *Protocol Journal of Botanical Medicines.* May 6, 1998.
Subbaiah, T., Amin, A. Effect of berberine sulfate on *Entamoeba histolytica. Nature.* 1967;215:527-78.
Sun, D. et al. Berberine sulfate blocks adherence of *Streptococcus pyogenes* to epithelial cells, fibronectin, and hexadecane. *Antimicrobial Agents and Chemotherapy.* 1988 Sept;32:1370-4.
Wagner, H., Proksch, A. Immunostimulatory drugs of fungi and higher plants. *Economic Medicinal Plant Research.* 1985;1:113-53.
Watanabe, A. et al. Berberine therapy of hypertyraminemia in patients with liver cirrhosis. *Acta Med Okayama.* 1982;36:277-81.
Zeng, X. Efficacy and safety of berberine for CHF secondary to ischemic or idiopathic dilated cardiomyopathy. *Am J Cardiology.* 2003;92:173-6.
Zhou, J. Effects of tetrahydroberberine on ischemic and reperfused myocardum in rats. *Chung Kuo Yao Li Hsueh Pao.* 1993;14(2):130.

HOLY BASIL (TULSI)

GENERAL REFERENCES: 3) p. 240; 16); 17); 22) p. 46; 28) p. 102; 36); 62) p. 194; 79) p. 46.
Agrawal, P. et al. Randomized placebo controlled, single-blind trial of Holy Basil leaves in patients with non-insulin-dependent diabetes mellitus. *Int J Clinical Pharmacol Therapies.* 1996;34:406-9.
Aruna, K., Sivaramakrishnan, V. Anticarcinogenic effects of some Indian plant products. *Food Chemistry and Toxicology.* 1992;30(11):953-6.
Balanehru, S., Nagarajan, B. Protective effect of oleanolic acid and ursolic acid against lipid peroxidation. *Biochemistry Int.* 1991;24(5):981-90.
_____________________. Intervention of adriamycin induced free radical damage. *Biochemisty Int.* 1992;28(4):735-44.
Baliga, M. et al. *Ocimum sanctum* L (Holy Basil or Tulsi) and its phytochemicals in the prevention and treatment of cancer. *Nutr Cancer.* 2013;65 Suppl 1:26-35.
Batta, S. Santhakumari, G. The antifertility effect of *Ocimum sanctum* and *Hibiscus rosa sinensis. Indian J of Medical Res.* 1971;59:777.
Bever, B., Zahnd, G. Plants with oral hypoglycaemic action. *Quarterly J of Crude Drug Res.* 1979;17:139-96.
Bhargava, K., Singh, N. Anti-stress activity of *Ocimum sanctum. Indian J Medical Res.* 1981;73:443-51.
________________. Comparative evaluation of anti-stress activity of *Eleutherococcus senticosus, Panax ginseng* and *Ocimum sanctum. Proc 2nd Symp Eleutherococcus Moscow.* 1984:181-9.

__________________. Indian plants as anti-stress agents. *Natural Product College Pharmacy*. University of N. Carolina. 1985; Abstract 202.
Bhattacharyya, D. et al. Controlled programmed trial of *Ocimum sanctum* leaf on generalized anxiety disorders. *Nepal Med Coll J*. 2008;10(3):176.
Das, S. et al. *Ocimum sanctum* in the treatment of viral encephalitis (preliminary clinical study). *The Antiseptic*. 1983;1-5.
Devi, P. et al. A comparative study of radioprotection by *Ocimum* flavonoids and synthetic aminothiol protectors in the mouse. *British J Radiology*. 1998;71(847):782-4.
Dixit, K. et al. Effect of *Ocimum sanctum* on stress induced alterations upon some brain neurotransmitters and enzyme activity. *Proc 17th Annual Conference. I.P.S.*, JIMPER, Pondichery, India. 1985;57.
__________. *Inula racemosa, Terminalia belerica* and *Ocimum sanctum*-A preliminary clinical trial in asthma patients. *Proc Int Seminar Clinical Pharm Dev Count*. Lucknow, India. 1986;2:22-27.
Dixit, K., Singh, N. An assessment of immunomodulator activity of some anti-stress Indian plants. *Proc 10th Int Congress Pharmacology*. Sydney, Australia. 1987;1:265.
Engels, G., Brinckmann, J. Holy Basil. *HerbalGram*. 2013;98:1-5.
Garg, G. *An Encyclopedia of Indian Literature*. New Delhi, India: Mittal Publisher. 1982;313.
Gholap, S. Kar, A. Hypoglycaemic effects of some plant extracts are possibly mediated through inhibition in corticosteroid concentration. *Pharmazie*. 2004;59(11):876-8.
Gupta, K., Vishwanathan. A short note on antitubercular substance from *Ocimum sanctum. Antibiotic and Chemotherapy*. 1955;5:33.
Jalil, A. Clinical trial of *Ocimum sanctum* in peptic ulcer and hyperacidity patients. *J Res Indian Med*. 1970;4(2):238-9.
Jogetia, G. et al. Radiation modifying effects of *Ocimum sanctum* on mouse survival. *Proc Indian Sci Congress* (Jaipur, India). 1986;20.
Kalsi, R. et al. Effects of stress and anti-stress drugs on succinate dehydrogenase enzyme (SDH) in rat brain. *Physiology of Human Performance*. 1987;114-7.
Karthikeyan, K. et al. Chemoprotective effect of *Ocimum sanctum* on DMBA-induced hamster buccal pouch carcinogensis. *Oral Oncology*. 1999;35(1):112-9.
Kolte, A. et al. Immunomodulating effect of dry powder of *Ocimum sanctum* and leaf gall of *Ficus racemosa* leaves in broilers naturally infected with IBD virus. *Indian Vet J*. 1999;76:84-6.
Kumar, P. et al. A clinical assessment of changes in cell-mediated immune response induced by Geriforte. *The Antiseptic*. 1982;10:560.
Lahariya, A., Rao, J. *In vitro* antimicrobial studies of essential oils of *Cyperus scariosus* and *Ocimum basilicum*. *Indian Drugs*. 1979;16(7):150-2.
Majupuria, T. *Religious and Useful Plants of Nepal & India*. Lashkar, India: M. Gupta Publisher, 1989.
Mandal, S. et al. *Ocimum sanctum*-a study on gastric ulceration and gastric secretion in rats. *Ind J Physiol Pharmacol*. 1993;37(1):91-2.
Marles, R. Farnsworth, N. Antidiabetic plants and the active constituents. *Phytomedicine*. 1995;2(2):137-89.
Maulik, G. et al. Evaluation of antioxidant effectiveness of a few herbal plants. *Free Radical Research*. 1997;27(2):221-8.
Mehta, A. et al. Antimicrobial activity of some essential oils against certain pathogenic bacteria. *Bull Bot Soc Univ Saugua*. 1978-9;14:25-6.
Mishra, N. et al. *Evaluation of Ayurvedic herbal drugs on the damage caused by free radicals*. PhD Thesis, Dept Pharm & Therapeutics, Lucknow University; Lucknow, India, 1998.
Misra, N. et al. Plant drugs and biochemical changes during stress reaction. *Physiology of Human Performance*. 1987;104-8.
Mondal, S. et al. Double-blinded randomized controlled trial for immunomodulatory effects of tulsi (*Ocimum sanctum* Linn.) leaf extract on healthy volunteers. *J Ethnopharmacol*. 2011;136(30);452-6.
Newmark, T., Schulick, P. *Beyond Aspirin*. Prescott, AZ: Hohm Press, 2000.
Palit, G. et al. Antiasthmatic potentials of *Ocimum sanctum* and *Terminalia belerica*. *Proc 14th Conv Indian Coll Allergy Immunol*. 1980;10.
__________. Experimental evaluation of antiasthmatic plant drugs from ancient Ayurvedic medicine. *Asp Allergy Appl Immunol*. 1983;16:36-41.
Patel, V., Bhatt, H. Folklore therapeutic indigenous plants in peridontal disorders in India. *Int J Clin Pharm Ther Toxicol*. 1988;26(4):176-84.
Prashar, R. et al. Chemopreventive action by an extract from *Ocimum sanctum* on mouse skin papillomagenesis and its enhancement of skin glutathione S-transferase activity and acid soluble sulfydryl level. *Anticancer Drugs*. 1994;5(5):567-72.
Rajalakshmi, G. et al. Management of viral hepatitis. *J Res Ayurvedic Sid*. 1988;9:118.
Ramaswami, A., Sirsi, M. Antitubercular activity of some natural products. *Indian Journal of Pharmacology*. 1967;29(5):157-9.
Rastogi, R., Mehrotra, B. *Compendium of Indian Medicinal Plants*. New Delhi, India: CSIR,1995;4:510.
Robbins, S. et al. *Disease at the Cellular Level: Free Radical Basic Pathology*. Philadelphia, PA: W.S. Saunders Company, 1982;9.
Saksena, A. et al. Effect of *Ocimum sanctum* on physical endurance during thermal stress. *Physiology of Human Performance. Proc Nat Symp Physiol Hum Perfor*. 1987;109-113.
Samson, J. et al. Oxidative stress in brain and antioxidant activity of *Ocimum sanctum* in noise exposure. *Neurotoxicology*. 2007 May;28(3):679-85.
Sankaran, J. Tefroli in the management of viral hepatitis. *The Antiseptic*. 1980;77:7643.
Sarkar, A. et al. Changes in the blood lipid profile after administration of *Ocimum sanctum* leaves in normal albino rabbits. *Ind J Physiol Pharmacol*. 1994;38(4):311-2.
Sen, P. et al. Mechanism of anti-stress activity of *Ocimum sanctum*, eugenol, and *Tinospora malabarica* in experimental animals. *Ind J Exp Biol*. 1992;30(7):592-6.
Singh, N., Singh, S. Experimental evaluation of adaptogenic properties of *Ocimum sanctum*. *Ind J Pharmacol*. 1978;10:74.
Singh, N. A pharmaco-clinical evaluation of some Ayurvedic crude plant drugs as anti-stress agents and their usefulness in some stress diseases of man. *Ann Nat Acad Ind Med*. 1986b;2(1):14-26.
_______. A comparative evaluation of the effect of some species of *Ocimum sanctum* on anoxia tolerance in albino rats. *36th Ann Cong Med Plant Research*. 1988;28.
Singh, N. et al. Effects of anti-stress plants on biochemical changes during stress reactions. *Ind J Pharmacol*. 1991b;23(3):137-42.
Singh, N., Misra, N. Experimental methods-tools for assessment of anti-stress activity in medicinal plants. *J Bio Chem Res*. 1993;12(182):124-7.
Singh, N., Abbas, S. Effect of *Ocimum sanctum* (Tulsi) in aging patients of arterial hypertension, rheumatoid arthritis, osteoporosis. (Unpublished data). International Institute of Herbal Medicines, Lucknow, U.P., India. 1995b. (Cited in *Tulsi, the Mother Medicine of Nature)*.
_______________. Effect of *Ocimum sanctum* (Tulsi) in sex-related chronic fatigue syndrome in young Indians. *J Bio Chem Sci*. 1995c;14:184-7.
Singh, N., Hoette, Y., Miller, R. *Tulsi, the Mother Medicine of Nature*. Lucknow, India; International Institute of Herbal Medicine. 2002.
Singh, S. et al. *Terminalis belerica* and *Ocimum sanctum*- A preliminary clinical trial in asthma patients. *Proc Int Sem Clin Pharmacol*. Lucknow, India. 1986a;I:18-21.
Singh, S., Agrawal, S. Anti-asthmatic and anti-inflammatory activity of *O. sanctum*. *Int J Pharmacognosy*. 1991a;29:306-10.
Singh, S., Majumdar, D. Analgesic activity of *O. sanctum* and its possible mechanism of action. *Int J Pharmacognosy*. 1995;33:188-92.
Sirtori, A. et al. The saponins of the seed of four lupin species. *J Plant Foods*. 1979;3:181-90.
Srivastava, A. et al. A preliminary clinical trial of *Ocimum sanctum* (Tulsi) extract in stress related hypertensive patients. *Proc Int Sem Clin Pharmacol. Dev Count*. (Saxena, R., Gupta, T., Dixit, K. Eds.). Lucknow, India: K.G.M.C. 1986;11:36-8.
Suri, R., Thind, T. Antibacterial activity of some essential oils. *Ind Drugs Pharmacol*. 1978;13(6):25-8.
_______________. *In vitro* antifungal efficacy of four essential oils. *Ind Perfume*. 1979a;23(2):138-40.
_______________. *In vitro* antifungal efficacy of some essential oils. *East Pharm*. 1979b;22(257):109-110.
Uma, D. et al. *In vivo* radio-protection by *Ocimum* flavonoids: survival of mice. *Radiation Research*. 1999;151(1):74-8.
Upton, R. Holy Basil: *Ocimum Sanctum*. *Herbal Perspectives*. 2006;7(1):2.
Yarnell, E., Abascal, K. Herbs for curbing inflammation. *Alternative & Complementary Therapies*. 2006;Feb:22-28.

HOPS

GENERAL REFERENCES: 1) p. 147; 2) p. 193; 3) pp. 119, 210, 236; 5) p. 212; 8) p. 395; 9);11) p. 75; 17); 18) p. 124; 20) p. 998; 21) p. 407; 22) p. 332; 23) p. 106; 25) p. 212: 29) p. 884; 30) p. 243; 33) p. 411; 36) p. 557; 37) p. 558; 42) p. 248; 43); 44) p. 230; 46) p. 61; 48) pp. 124, 259, 340; 51) pp. 217, 164; 55) p. 162; 66) p 74; 68) p. 175; 70) p. 318; 74) p. 121; 75) p. 285; 78) pp. 228-9; 79) p. 220; 81).
Allsopp, P. et al. A comparison of the anticancer properties of isoxanthohumol and 8-prenylnaringenin using *in vitro* models of colon cancer. *Biofactors*. 2013 Jul-Aug;39(4):441-7.
Aoshima, H. et al. Effects of beer and hop on ionotropic gamma-aminobutyric acid receptors. *J Agric Food Chem*. 2006 Apr 5;54(7):2514-9.
Bhattacharya, S. et al. Inhibition of *Streptococcus mutans* and other oral *Streptococci* by hop constituents. *Economic Botany*. 2003;57(1):118-125.
Butterweck, V. et al. Hypothermic effects of hops are antagonized with the competitive melatonin receptor antagonistic luzindole in mice. *J Pharmacy*

Pharmacol. 2007;59(4):549-52.
Caujolle, et. al. Spasmolytic action of hops (*Humulus lupulus*). *Agressologie*. 1969;10:405-10.
Chadwick, L. et al. The pharmacognosy of *H. lupulus L.* (hops) with an emphasis on estrogenic properties. *Phytomedicine*. 2006 Jan;13(1-2):119-31.
Chakarski, I. et al. Clinical study of a herb combination consisting of *Humulus lupulus, Cichorium intybus, Mentha piperita* in patients with chronic calculous and non-calculous cholecystitis. *Probl Vatr Med*. 1982;10:65-9.
Chang, H., But, P. *Pharmacology and Applications of Chinese Materia Medica*. Philadelphia, PA: World Scientific. 1986;1077-83.
Chung, W. et al. Hop proanthocyanidins induce apoptosis, protein carbonylation, and cytoskeleton disorganization in human colorectal adenocarcinoma cells via reactive oxygen species. *Food Chem Toxicol*. 2009 Apr;47(4):827-36.
Coldham, N., Sauer, M. Identification, quantitation and biological activity of phytoestrogens in a dietary supplement for breast enhancement. *Food Chem Toxicol*. 2001;39:1211–1224.
Colgate, E. et al. Xanthohumol, a prenylflavonoid derived from hops induces apoptosis and inhibits NF-kappaB activation in prostate epithelial cells. *Cancer Lett*. 2007 Feb 8;246(1-2):201-9.
Delmulle, L. et al. Treatment of PC-3 and DU145 prostate cancer cells by prenylflavonoids from hop (*Humulus lupulus* L.) induces a caspase-independent form of cell death. *Phytother Res*. 2008 Feb;22(2):197-203.
Dimpfel, W., Suter, A. Sleep improving effects of a single dose administration of a valerian/hops fluid extract - a double blind, randomized, placebo-controlled sleep-EEG study in a parallel design using electrohypnograms. *Eur J Med Res*. 2008 May 26;13(5):200-4.
Erkkola, R. et al. A randomized, double-blind, placebo-controlled, cross-over pilot study on the use of a standardized hop extract to alleviate menopausal discomforts. *Phytomed*. 2010;17(6):389-396.
Festa, M. et al. Xanthohumol induces apoptosis in human malignant glioblastoma cells by increasing reactive oxygen species and activating MAPK pathways. *J Nat Prod*. 2011 Dec 27;74(12):2505-13.
Fussel, A. et al. Effects of a fixed valerian-hop extract combination (Ze91019) on sleep polygraphy in patients with non-organic insomnia: a pilot study. *European J Medical Research*. 2000;5:385-90.
Hansel, R. et al. The sedative-hypnotic principle of hops. *Planta Medica*. 1982;45:224-8.
Hemachandra, L. et al. Hops (*Humulus lupulus*) inhibits oxidative estrogen metabolism and estrogen-induced malignant transformation in human mammary epithelial cells (MCF-10A). *Cancer Prev Res*. 2012 Jan;5(1):73-81.
Heyerick, A. et al. A first prospective, randomized, double-blind, placebo-controlled study on the use of a standardized hop extract to alleviate menopausal discomforts. *Maturitas*. 2006 May 20;54(2):164-75.
Honma, Y. et al. Induction of differentiation of myelogenous leukemia cells by humulone, a bitter in hop. *Leukemia Research*. 1998;22(7):605-10.
Koch, W., Heim, G. Estrogen hormone in Hops and Beer. *Muench Med Wochenschr*. 1953;95:845.
Koetter, U., Biendl, M. Hops (*Humulus lupulus)*: A Review of its Historic and Medicinal Uses. *Herbalgram*. 2010;87:44-57.
Lee, Y. et al. Xanthohumol, a Prenylated Flavonoid from Hops (*Humulus lupulus)*, Prevents Platelet Activation in Human Platelets. *Evidence Based Complement Alternat Med*. 2012;2012:852362.
Lemay, M. et al. *In vitro* and *ex vivo* cyclooxygenase inhibition by a hops extract. *Asia Pacific journal of clinical nutrition*. 2004; 13(Suppl):S110.
Liu, J. et al. Evaluation of estrogenic activity of plant extracts for the potential treatment of menopausal symptoms. *Journal of Agricultural Food*. 2001;49(5):2472-9.
Matsumura, A. et al. Comparative study of oestrogenic properties of eight phytoestrogens in MCF7 human breast cancer cells. *J Steroid Biochem Mol Biol*. 2005 Apr;94(5):431-43.
McKendree, et al. Mechanics of pain and treatment of dysmenorrhea. *Clinical Med Surg*. 1937;44:536-40.
Milligan, S. et al. The endocrine activities of 8-prenylnaringenin and related Hop flavonoids. *J Clin Endocrinology Metab*. 2000;85(12):4912-5.
_____________. Oestrogenic activity of the hop phyto-oestrogen, 8-prenylnaringenin. *Reproduction*. 2002;123:235–242.
Miranda, C. et al. Antiproliferative and cytotoxic effects of prenylated flavonoids from hops (*Humulus lupulus*) in human cancer cell lines. *Food Chem Toxicol*. 1999 Apr;37(4):271-85.
Miyashita, M., Sadzuka, Y. Effect of linalool as a component of *Humulus lupulus* on doxorubicin-induced antitumor activity. *Food Chem Toxicol*. 2013 Mar;53:174-9.
Mizobuchi, S., Sato, Y. A new flavanone with antifungal activity isolated from hops. *Agric Biol Chem*. 1984;48:2771-5.
_________________. Antifungal activities of hop bitter resins and related compounds. *Agric Biol Chem*. 1985;49:399-405.
Monteiro, R. et al. Modulation of breast cancer cell survival by aromatase inhibiting hop (*Humulus lupulus* L.) flavonoids. *J Steroid Biochem Mol Biol*. 2007 Jun-Jul;105(1-5):124-30.
Morali, G. et al. Open, non-controlled clinical studies to assess the efficacy and safety of a medical device in the form of gel topically and intravaginally used in postmenopausal women with genital atrophy. *Arzneimittel-forschung*. 2006;56(3):230-8.
Morin, C. et al. Valerian-hops combination and diphenhydramine for treating insomnia: a randomized placebo-controlled trial. *Sleep*. 2005;28(11): 1465-71.
Oberbauer, E. et al. Chroman-like cyclic prenylflavonoids promote neuronal differentiation and neurite outgrowth and are neuroprotective. *J Nutr Biochem*. 2013 Nov;24(11):1953-62.
Prokopenko, et al. Pharmacological and chemical properties of hops (*Humulus lupulus*). *Farm. Zh. (Kiev.)*. 1986;1:28-30.
Rad, M. et al. Pharmacokinetics and systemic endocrine effects of the phyto-oestrogen 8-PN after single oral doses to postmenopausal women. *Br J Clinical Pharmacol*. 2006 Sept;62(3):288-96.
Rodenbeck, A. et al. Alterations of the sleep stage structure as a feature of GABAergic effects of a valerian-hop preparation in patients with psychophysiological insomnia. *Somnologie*. 1998;2:26-31.
Rong, H. et al. 8-Prenylnaringenin, the phytoestrogen in hops and beer, upregulates the function of the E-cadherin/catenin complex in human mammary carcinoma cells. *Eur J Cell Biol*. 2001 Sep;80(9):580-5.
Schellenberg, R. et al. Fixed combination of valerian/hops (Ze91019) acts via a central adenosine mechanism. *Planta Medica*. 2004;70(7):594-7.
Schmitz, M., Jackel, M. Comparative study for assessing quality of life of patients with exogenous sleep disorders treated with a hops and valerian preparation and a benzodiazepine drug. *Wien Med Wochenschr*. 1998;148(13):291-8.
Smith, E. *Therapeutic Herb Manual*. Williams, OR: Ed Smith. 1999;38.
Stephan, T. et al. Hexahydrocolupulone and its antitumor cell proliferation activity *in vitro*. *Biochem Pharmacol*. 1998;55(4):505-14.
Teuber, M., Schmalreck, A. Membrane leakage in *Bacillus subtilis* 168 induced by the hop constituents lupulone, humulone, isohumulone and humulinic acid. *Arch Mikrobiology*. 1973;94:159-71.
Tobe, H. et al. Bone resorption inhibitors from hop extract. *Bioscience, Biotechnology, Biochemistry*. 1997;61(1):158-9.
___________. Apoptosis to HL-60 by humulone. *Bioscience, Biotechnology, Biochemistry*. 1997;61(6):1027-9.
Vonderheid-Guth, B. et al. Pharmacodynamic effects of valerian and hops extract combination Ze (91019) on the quantitative-topographical EEG in healthy volunteers. *European J Medical Research*. 2000;5:139-44.
Wang, X. et al. *In vitro* and *in vivo* antioxidant and antimutagenic activities of polyphenols extracted from hops (*Humulus lupulus* L.). *J Sci Food Agric*. 2013 Dec 13.
Wohlfart, R. et al. Detection of sedative-hypnotic hop constituents. *Arch Pharm (Weinheim)*. 1982;315:132-7.
_____________. An investigation of sedative-hypnotic principle of hops. Part 4. *Planta Medica*. 1983;48:120-3.
Yamaguchi, N. et al. *In vitro* evaluation of antibacterial, anticollagenase, and antioxidant activities of hop components (*Humulus lupulus*) addressing acne vulgaris. *Phytomedicine*. 2009 Apr;16(4):369-76.
Yasukawa, K. et al. Humulon, a bitter in the hop, inhibits tumor promotion by 12-0-tetradecanoylphorbol-13-acetate in two-stage carcinogenesis in mouse skin. *Oncology*. 1995;52:156-8.
Zava, D. et al. Estrogen and progestin bioactivity of foods, herbs, and spices. *Proc Soc Exp Biol Med*. 1998;217:369-78.
Zierau, O. et al. Estrogenic activity of the phytoestrogens naringenin, 6-(1,1-dimethylallyl), naringenin and 8-PN. *Planta Med*. 2002;68(5):449-51.

HOREHOUND

GENERAL REFERENCES: 1) p. 148; 2) p. 197, 3) pp. 120, 274; 8) p. 346; 9) p. 556; 11) p. 75; 12) p. 349; 14) pp. 53, 119, 149, 371; 16) p. 307; 17); 20) p. 1240; 21) p. 475; 23) 108; 29) p. 692; 33) p. 415; 37) p. 240; 42) p. 249; 43); 44) p. 231; 46) pp. 74, 183; 48) pp. 123, 198, 331; 51) pp. 131, 242; 55) p. 65; 64) p. 380; 68) p. 177; 69) p. 95; 79) p. 222; 81) pp. 93, 392.
Ahmed, B. et al. A new monoterpene acid from *Marrubium vulgare* with potential antihepatotoxic activity. *Nat Prod Res*. 2010 Nov;24(18):1671-80.

Berrougui, H. et al. *Marrubium vulgare* extract inhibits human-LDL oxidation and enhances HDL-mediated cholesterol efflux in THP-1 macrophage. *Life Sci*. 2006 Dec 14;80(2):105-12.
Boudjelal, A. et al. Compositional analysis and *in vivo* anti-diabetic activity of wild Algerian *Marrubium vulgare* L. infusion. *Fitoterapia*. 2012 Mar; 83(2):286-92.
El Bardai, S. et al. The vasorelaxant activity of marrubenol and marrubiin from *Marrubium vulgare. Planta Med.* 2003 Jan;69(1):75-7.
_____________. Characterisation of marrubenol, a diterpene extracted from *Marrubium vulgare,* as an L-type calcium channel blocker. *Br J Pharmacol*. 2003 Dec;140(7):1211-6.
_____________. Comparative study of the antihypertensive activity of *Marrubium vulgare* and of the dihydropyridine calcium antagonist amlodipine in spontaneously hypertensive rat. *Clin Exp Hypertens*. 2004 Aug;26(6):465-74.
Karryev, M. et al. Some therapeutic properties and phytochemistry of common horehound. *Izvestiya Akademiya Nauk Turkmenskoi SSR, Seriya Biologicheskikh Nauk*. 1976;3:86-8.
Krejci, I., Zadina, R. Die Gallentreibende Wirkung von Marrubiin und Marrabinsaure. *Planta Medica.* 1959;7:1-7.
Meyre-Silva, C. et al. Analgesic potential of marrubiin derivatives, bioactive diterpene present in *M. vulgare. Farmaco.* 2005 Apr;60(4):321-6.
Paula de Oliveira, A. et al. Gastroprotective activity of methanol extract and marrubiin obtained from leaves of *Marrubium vulgare* L. (Lamiaceae). *J Pharm Pharmacol*. 2011 Sep;63(9):1230-7.
Saleh, M. et al. Volatile oil of *Marrubium vulgare* and its anti-schistosomal activity. *Planta Medica*. 1989;55:105.
Yousefi, K. et al. Indian Cardioprotective effect of methanolic extract of *Marrubium vulgare L.* on isoproterenol-induced acute myocardial infarction in rats. *J Exp Bio*l. 2013 Aug;51(8):653-60.
___________. *Marrubium vulgare L.* methanolic extract inhibits inflammatory response and prevents cardiomyocyte fibrosis in isoproterenol-induced acute myocardial infarction in rats. *Bioimpacts*. 2014;4(1):21-7.

HYSSOP

GENERAL REFERENCES: 1) p. 338; 3) pp. 122, 274; 5) p. 222; 8) pp. 128, 231-3; 9) p. 478; 11) p. 75; 12) p. 263; 14) p. 329; 16) p. 182; 17); 20) p. 1039; 21) p. 693; 22) p. 343; 23) p. 110; 24) p. 120; 29) p. 578; 33) p. 426; 42) p. 250; 44) p. 236; 46) pp. 63, 171, 186; 64) p. 150; 66) p. 76; 68) p. 183; 78) p. 152; 79) p. 230; 81) pp. 197, 391; 82) pp. 17, 89, 111, 141.
Bove, M. Botanical medicines for common pediatric conditions. *Medical Herbalism*. 1992;4(4):1.
Gollapudi et al. Isolation of a previously unidentified polysaccharide from *Hyssop officinalis* that exhibits strong activity against human immunodeficiency virus type I. *Biochemical and Biophysical Research Communications*. 1995;210(1):145.
Kaplan, K. et al. Inhibition of HIV replication by *Hyssop officinalis* extracts. *Antiviral Research.* 1990;14(6):323-37.
Lu, M. et al. Muscle relaxing activity of *Hyssopus officinalis* essential oil on isolated intestinal preparations. *Planta Medica*. 2002;68(3):213-6.
Ma, X. et al. Effect of *Hyssopus officinalis L.* on inhibiting airway inflammation and immune regulation in a chronic asthmatic mouse model. *Exp Ther Med*. 2014 Nov;8(5):1371-1374.
Vlase, L. et al. Evaluation of antioxidant and antimicrobial activities and phenolic profile for *Hyssopus officinalis, Ocimum basilicum* and *Teucrium chamaedrys. Molecules.* 2014 Apr 28;19(5):5490-507.

ISATIS

GENERAL REFERENCES: 17); 46) p. 64; 50) p. 128; 64) p. 196; 65) p. 179.
Ahmad, I., Fatima, I. Butyrylcholinesterase, lipoxygenase inhibiting and antifungal alkaloids from *Isatis tinctoria. J Enzyme Inhib Med Chem*. 2008 Jun;23(3):313-6.
Bensky, D., Gamble, A., Kaptchuk, T. *Chinese Herbal Medicine Materia Medica*. Seattle, WA: Eastland Press, 1993;87-88.
Brattström, A. et al. The plant extract *Isatis tinctoria* L. extract (ITE) inhibits allergen-induced airway inflammation and hyper-reactivity in mice. *Phytomedicine*. 2010 Jul;17(8-9):551-6.
Buhner, S. *Herbal Antibiotics: Natural Alternatives for Treating Drug-Resistant Bacteria.* North Adams, MA: Storey Pub. 2012;48,51,57,65,70,75,76.
_______. *Healing Lyme Disease Coinfections*. Rochester, VT: Healing Arts Press, 2013;164-70.
Chang, S. et al. Antiviral Activity of *Isatis indigotica* Extract and Its Derived Indirubin against Japanese Encephalitis Virus. *Complement Alternat Med.* 2012:925830.
Chung, Y. et al. *Isatis indigotica* induces hepatocellular cancer cell death via caspase-independent apoptosis-inducing factor translocation apoptotic pathway *in vitro* and *in vivo. Integr Cancer Ther*. 2011 Jun;10(2):201-14.
Danz, H. et al. Inhibitory activity of tryptanthrin on prostaglandin and leukotrine synthesis. *Planta Medica.* 2002;68(10):875-80.
Enqin, Z. (Ed.). *Chinese Materia Medica*. Shanghai, China: Publishing House of Shanghai College of Traditional Medicine, 1988;128-130.
Fang, J. et al. Antiviral effect of *Folium Isatidis* on herpes simplex virus type I. *Zhongguo Zhong Yao Za Zhi.* 2005 Sep;30(17):1343-6.
Hoessel, R. et al. Indirubin, the active constituent of a Chinese antileukaemia medicine, inhibits cyclin-dependent kinases. *Nat Cell Biolog*. 1999 May;1(1):60-7.
Liu, G. *Chinese Natural Products and New Drugs Pharmaceutical News* (Vol. 2, No. 2). 1995:10-12.
Oberthur, C. et al. A comparative study on the skin penetration of pure tryptanthrin and tryptanthrin in *Isatis tinctoria* extract by dermal microdialysis coupled with isotope dilution ESI-LC-MS. *Planta Medica*. 2003;69(5):385-9.
Qi, C. et al. Clinical research of isatis root eye drops on the acute bacterial conjunctivitis. *Zhong Yao Cai*. 2007 Jan;30(1):120-2.
Roxas, M., Jurenka, J. Colds and influenza: a review of diagnosis and conventional, botanical, and nutritional considerations. *Altern Med Rev.* 2007;12(1):25-48.
Shan, J. et al An a-glucan isolated from root of *Isatis Indigotica,* its structure and adjuvant activity. *Glycoconj Journal*. 2014 May;31(4):317-26.
Sheehan, M. et al. A controlled trial of traditional Chinese medicinal plants in widespread non-exudative atopic eczema. *British Journal of Dermatology*. 1992;340:13-17.
Song, Z. et al. Effects of Chinese medicinal herbs on a rat model of chronic *Pseudomonas aeruginosa* lung infection. *APMIS.* 1996;104(5):350-4.
Suzuki, H. et al. Therapeutic efficacy of the Qing Dai in patients with intractable ulcerative colitis. *World J Gastroenterol*. May 2013;19(17):2718-22.
Wang, X. et al. Chemical constituents from root of *Isatis indigotica*. *Zhongguo Zhong Yao Za Zhi*. 2013 Apr;38(8):1172-82.
Wu, Y. et al. Novel indole C-glycosides from *Isatis indigotica* and their potential cytotoxic activity. *Fitoterapia*. 2011 Mar;82(2):288-92.
Xu, Y., Lu, P. Experimental studies on immuno-stimulatory effects of the *Isatis indigotica* polysaccharide. *Zhong Xi Yi Jie He Za Zhi*. 1991 Jun;11(6): 357-9.
You, W. et al. Effect of extracts from indigowood root (*Isatis indigotica* Fort.) on immune responses in radiation-induced mucositis. *J Altern Complement Med*. 2009 Jul;15(7):771-8.
Zhang, J. et al. Extraction technology of *radix Isatidis*. *Chung Kuo Chung Yao Tsa Chih*. 1990 May;15(5):287-9,318.

LAVENDER

GENERAL REFERENCES: 1) p. 159; 2) p. 226; 3) pp. 129, 237, 274; 6) pp. 47, 163; 9) p. 504; 11) p. 85; 12) p. 265; 14) pp. 130, 423, 456, 537; 16) p. 190; 17); 20) pp. 1123-4, 1362; 21) p. 442; 23) p. 113; 25) p. 114; 29) p. 583; 30) p. 246; 33) p. 467; 36) p. 561; 37) p. 526; 43); 44) p. 251; 45) p. 281; 46) p. 68; 61); 66) p. 79; 79) p. 260.
Alakbarov, F. Aromatic Herbal Baths of the Ancients. *HerbalGram*. 2003;57:47.
Bronfen, J. et al. Inhibition of human pancreatic carcinoma cell proliferation by perillyl alcohol. *Proceedings of the American Association for Cancer Research*. 1994,35:431.
Buchbauer, G. et al. Aromatherapy: evidence for sedative effects of the essential oil of lavender after inhalation. *Zeitschrift fur Naturforschung*. 1991;46c:1067-72.
Dale, A., Cornwell, S. The role of lavender oil in relieving perineal discomfort following childbirth: a blind randomized clinical trial. *Journal of Advanced Nursing*. 1994;19(1):89-96.
Diego, M. et al. Aromatherapy positively affects mood, EEG patterns of alertness and math computations. *International Journal of Neuroscience.* 1998;96(3-4):217-24.
Dunn, C. et al. Sensing an improvement: an experimental study to evaluate the use of aromatherapy, massage and periods of rest in an intensive care unit. *Journal of Advanced Nursing*. 1995;21(1):34-40.
Effati-Daryani, F. et al. Effect of lavender cream with or without foot-bath on anxiety, stress, and depression in pregnancy: a randomized, placebo-controlled trial. *J Caring Sci*. 2015;4(1):63-73.

Engels, G. Lavender. *HerbalGram.* 2007;73:1.
Fißler, M., Quante A. A case series on the use of lavendula oil capsules in patients suffering from major depressive disorder and symptoms of psychomotor agitation, insomnia and anxiety. *Complement Ther Med.* February 2014;22(1):63-69.
Gould, M. Prevention and therapy of mammary cancer by monoterpenes. *Journal of Cellular Biochemistry.* 1995;22:139-144.
Haag, J., Gould, M. Mammary carcinoma regression induced by perillyl alcohol, a hydroxylated analog of limonene. *Cancer Chemotherapy and Pharmacology.* 1994;34:477-83.
Hardy, M. et al. Replacement of drug therapy for insomnia by ambient odor. *Lancet.* 1995;346:701.
Holmes, C. Lavender oil as a treatment for agitated behavior in severe dementia: a placebo controlled study. *International Journal of Geriatric Psychiatry.* 2002;17:305-8.
Inouye, S. et al. Anti-sporulating and respiration-inhibitory effects of essential oils on filamentous fungi. *Mycoses.* 1998;41(9-10):403-10.
Izzo, A. et al. Spasmolytic activity of medicinal plants used for the treatment of disorders involving smooth muscles. *Phytotheraphy Research.* 1996;10:S107-8.
Jager, W. et al. Percutaneous absorption of lavender oil from a massage oil. *Journal of Society of Cosmetic Chemists.* 1992;43:49-54.
Jeffers, L. et al. The effect of perillyl alcohol on the proliferation of human prostatic cell lines. *Proceedings of the American Association for Cancer Research.* 1995;36:303.
Kasper, S. et al. Lavender oil preparation Silexan is effective in generalized anxiety disorder – a randomized, double-blind comparison to placebo and paroxetine. *Int J Neuropsychopharmacol.* January 23, 2014:1-11.
__________. Efficacy of Silexan in mixed anxiety-depression – a randomized, placebo-controlled trial. *Eur Neuropsychopharm.* 2016;26(2):331-40.
Larrondo, J. et al. Antimicrobial activity of essences from labiates. *Microbios.* 1995;82(332):171-2.
Lillehei, AS. et al. Effect of inhaled lavender and sleep hygiene on self-reported sleep issues: a randomized controlled trial. *J Altern Complement Med.* 2015;21(7):430-8.
Lin, P. et al. Efficacy of aromatherapy (*Lavandula angustifolia*) as an intervention for agitated behaviors in Chinese older persons with dementia: a cross-over randomized trial. *Int J Geriatr Psychiatry.* May 2007;22(5):405-410.
Lis-Balchin, M., Hart, S. A preliminary study of the effect of essential oils on skeletal and smooth muscle *in vitro. J of Ethnophar.* 1997;58(3):183-7.
__________________. Studies on the Modes of Action of the Essential Oil of Lavender (*Lavandula angustifolia* P. Miller). *Phyt Res.* 1999;13:540-2.
Loius, M., Kowalski, S. Use of aromatherapy with hospice patients to decrease pain, anxiety, and depression and to promote an increased sense of well-being. *Am J Hospice Palliat Care.* 2002;19(6):381-6.
Lujan, H. et al. Isoprenylation of proteins in the protozoan *Giardia lamblia. Molecular Biochem Parasitology.* 1995;72(1-2):212-7.
Mills, J. et al. Induction of apoptosis in liver tumors by the monoterpene perillyl alcohol. *Cancer Research.* 1995;55:979-83.
Nelson, R. *In vitro* activities of five plant essential oils against methacillin-resistant *Staphylococcus aureus* and vancomycin-resistant *Enterococcus faecium. Journal of Antimicrobology and Chemotherapy.* 1997;40:305-6.
Park, M., Lee, S. The effect of aroma inhalation method on stress responses of nursing students. *Taehan Kanho Hakhoe Chi.* 2004;34(2):344.
Pattnaik, S. et al. Antibacterial and antifungal activity of aromatic constituents of essential oils. *Microbios.* 1997;89:39-46.
Raisi Dehkordi, Z. et al. Effect of lavender inhalation on the symptoms of primary dysmenorrhea and the amount of menstrual bleeding: A randomized clinical trial. *Complement Ther Med.* 2014 Apr;22(2):212-9.
Reddy, B. et al. Chemoprevention of colon carcinogenesis by dietary perillyl alcohol. *Cancer Research.* 1997;57:420-5.
Schulz, V. et al. Clinical trials with phyto-psychopharmacological agents. *Phytomedicine.* 1997;4(4):379-87.
Shi, W., Gould, M. Induction of differentiation in neuro-2A cells by the monoterpene perillyl alcohol. *Cancer Letters.* 1995;95:1-6.
Shiina, Y. et al. Relaxation effects of lavender aromatherapy improve coronary flow velocity reserve in healthy men evaluated by transthoracic Doppler echocardiography. *Int J Cardiol.* August 7, 2007.
Siurin, S. Effects of essential oil on lipid peroxidation and lipid metabolism in patients with chronic bronchitis. *Klin Med (Mosk).* 1997;75(10):43-5.
Soltani, R. et al. Evaluation of the effect of aromatherapy with lavender essential oil on post-tonsillectomy pain in pediatric patients: a randomized controlled trial. *Int J Pediatr Otorhinolaryngol.* 2013 Sep;77(9):1579-81.
Sosa, S. et al. Extracts and constituents of *Lavandula multifida* with topical anti-inflammatory activity. *Phytomed.* 2005;12:271-277.
Stark, M. et al. Chemotherapy of pancreatic cancer with the monoterpene perillyl alcohol. *Cancer Letters.* 1995;96:15-21.
Ulbrict C. Lavender (*Lavandula angustifolia* Miller). *Journal of Herbal Pharmacotherapy.* 2004;4(2):63-78.
Ziegler, J. Raloxifene, Retinoids, and Lavender: "Me Too" Tamoxifen Alternatives Under Study. *Journal of the National Cancer Institute.* 1997.

LEMON BALM

1) pp. 160, 279, 304, 561; 2) p. 230; 3) p. 130; 12) p 348; 14) pp. 257-8, 277-8, 288, 332, 469; 16) p. 192; 17); 20) p. 1252; 23) p. 116; 24) p. 128; 25) p. 226; 29) p. 689; 30) p. 176; 33) p. 76; 36) p. 567; 37) p. 530; 43); 46) p. 75; 66) p. 80; 75) p. 286; 79) p. 39; 81) p. 307.
Akhondzadeh, S. et al. *Melissa officinalis* extract in the treatment of patients with mild to moderate Alzheimer's disease: a double blind, randomized, placebo controlled trial. *J Neurol Neurosurg Psychiatry.* 2003 Jul;74(7):863-6.
Akbarzadeh, M. et al. Effect of *Melissa officinalis* capsule on the intensity of premenstrual syndrome symptoms on high school girl students. *Nurse Midwifery Study.* 2015;4(2):e27001.
Alijaniha, F. et al. Heart palpitation relief with *Melissa officinalis* leaf extract: double-blind, randomized, placebo controlled trial of efficacy and safety. *J of Ethnopharmacology.* 2015;164:378-384.
Auf'mkolk, M. et al. Inhibition by certain plant extracts of the binding and adenylate cyclase stimulatory effect of bovine thyrotropin in human thyroid membranes. *Endocrinology.* 1984;115(2):527-34.
_______________. Extracts and auto-oxidized constituents of certain plants inhibit the receptor-binding and the biological activity of Graves' immunoglobins. *Endocrinology.* 1985;116:1687-93.
Awad, R. et al. Bioassay-guided fractionation of lemon balm (*Melissa officinalis* L.) using an *in vitro* measure of GABA transaminase activity. *Phytother Res.* 2009 Aug;23(8):1075-81.
Ballard, C. et al. Aromatherapy as a safe and effective treatment for agitation associated with dementia. *J Clinical Psychiatry.* 2002;63(7):553-8.
Buchner, K. et al. Double-blind study as evidence of the therapeutic effect of Melissengeist on psycho-vegetative syndromes. *Med Klin.* 1974;69: 1032-6.
Cerny, A., Schmid, K. Tolerability and efficacy of valerian/lemon balm in healthy volunteers (a double-blind, placebo-controlled, multicentre study). *Fitoterapia.* 1999;70:221-8.
Chakurski, I. et al. Treatment of chronic colitis with an herbal combination of *Taraxacum officinale, Hypericum perforatum, Melissa officinalis, Calendula officinalis,* and *Foeniculum vulgare. Vutr Boles.* 1981;20:51-4.
Cohen, R. et al. Antiviral activity of *Melissa officinalis* (lemon balm) extract. *Proc Soc Exp Biol Med.* 1964;117:431-4.
Dastmalchi, K. et al. Acetylcholinesterase inhibitory guided fractionation of *Melissa officinalis L. Bioorg Med Chem.* 2009 Jan 15;17(2):867-71.
Dimitrova, Z. et al. Antiherpes effect of *Melissa officinalis* extracts. *Acta Microbiol Bulg.* 1993;79:65-72.
Dressing, H. et al. Are valerian/Melissa combinations of equal value to benzodiazepine? *Therapiewoche.* 1992;42:726-36.
Drozd, J., Anuszewska, E. The effect of the *Melissa officinalis* extract on immune response in mice. *Acta Pharm.* 2003 Nov-Dec;60(6):467-70.
Forster, H. et al. Antispasmodic effects of some medicinal plants. *Planta Medica.* 1980;40:309-19.
Gromball, J. et al. Hyperactivity, concentration difficulties and impulsiveness improve during seven weeks' treatment with valerian root and lemon balm extracts. *Phytomedicine.* 2014 Jul-Aug;21(8-9):1098-103.
Hamaguchi, T. et al. Phenolic compounds prevent Alzheimer's pathology through different effects on the amyloid-beta aggregation pathway. *Am J Pathol.* 2009 Dec;175(6):2557-65.
Herrmann, E., Kucera, L. Antiviral substances in plants of the mint family (Labiatae): I. Nontannin polyphenols of Melissa officinalis. *Proc Soc Exp Biol Med.* 1967;124:869-74.
Ibarra, A. et al. Effects of chronic administration of *Melissa officinalis* L. extract on anxiety-like reactivity and on circadian and exploratory activities in mice. *Phytomedicine.* 2010 May;17(6):397-403.
Kennedy, D. et al. Modulation of mood and cognitive performance following acute administration of single doses of *Melissa officinalis* with human CNS nicotinic and muscarinic receptor-binding properties. *Neuropsychopharmacology.* 2003;28(10):1871-81.
Kennedy, D., Scholey, A. Psychopharmacology of European herbs with cognition-enhancing properties. *Curr Pharm Des.* 2006;12(35):4613-23.
Koytchev, R. et al. Balm mint extract (Lo-701) for topical treatment of recurring Herpes labialis. *Phytomedicine.* 1999;6(4):225-30.

Kucera, L., Herrmann, E. Antiviral substances in plants of the mint family (*Labiatae*): I. Tannins of *Melissa officinalis*. *Proc Soc Exp Biol Med.*1967; 124:865-9.
Larrondo, J. et al. Antimicrobial activity of essences from labiates. *Microbios*. 1995;82:171-2.
May, V. , Willuhn, G. Antiviral activity of aqueous extracts from medicinal plants in tissue cultures. *Arzneimittel-Forschung*. 1978;28:1-7.
Müller, S., Klement, S. A combination of valerian and lemon balm is effective in the treatment of restlessness and dyssomnia in children. *Phytomedicine*. 2006 Jun;13(6):383-7.
Schulpis, K. et al. 8-hydroxy-2-desoxyguanosine serum concentrations as a marker of NDA damage in patients with classical galactosaemia. *Acta Paediatrica*. 2006 Feb;95(2):164-9.
Soulimani, R. et al. Neurotropic action of the hydroalcoholic extract of *Melissa officinalis* in the mouse. *Planta Medica*. 1991;57:105-9.
Sourgens, H. et al. Antihormonal effects of plant extract. TSH- and prolactin-suppressing properties of *Lithosperum officinale* and other plants. *Planta Medica*. 1982;45:78-86.
Tagashira, M., Ohtake, Y. A new antioxidative 1,3-benzodioxole from *Melissa officinalis*. *Planta Medica*. 1998;64(6):555-8.
Teitelbaum, J. et al. Effective treatment of chronic fatigue syndrome (CFIDS) & fibromyalgia (FMS)-a randomized, double-blind, placebo-controlled, intent to treat study. *Journal of Chronic Fatigue Syndrome*. 2003;8(2):201.
Thompson, A. et al. Comparison of the antibacterial activity of essential oils and extracts of medicinal and culinary herbs to investigate potential new treatments for irritable bowel syndrome. *Complement Altern Med*. 2013 Nov 28;13:338.
Vejdani, R. et al. The efficacy of an herbal medicine, Carmint, on the relief of abdominal pain and bloating in patients with irritable bowel syndrome: a pilot study. *Dig Dis Sci*. 2006 Aug;51(8):1501-7.
Wake, G. et al. CNS acetylcholine receptor activity in European medicinal plants traditionally used to improve failing memory. *Journal of Ethnopharmacology*. 2000;69(2):105-14.
Wolbing, R., Milbradt, R. Clinical and other therapies for herpes simplex. *Therapiewoche*. 1984;34(9):1193-1200.
Wolbing, R., Leonhardt, K. Local therapy of herpes simplex with dried extract of *Melissa officinalis*. *Phytomedicine*. 1994;1(1):25-31.
Zeraatpishe, A. et al. Effects of *Melissa officinalis* L. on oxidative status and DNA damage in subjects exposed to long-term low-dose ionizing radiation. *Toxicol Ind Health*. 2011 Apr;27(3):205-12.

LOBELIA

GENERAL REFERENCES: 3) p. 136; 8) p. 358; 9) p. 519; 17); 18) p. 235; 19) p. 427; 20) p. 1199; 21) p. 455; 23) p. 121; 33) p. 494; 36) pp. 122, 563; 37) p. 505; 40) p. 147; 41) p. 670; 42) p. 253; 43); 44) p. 257; 46) pp. 71, 168-9, 183; 48) pp. 26, 107, 192, 326; 49) p. 312; 53) p. 240; 55) p. 187; 63) p. 135; 64) p. 68; 66) p. 83; 70) p. 330; 71) pp. 28, 58, 66, 74; 77) pp. 295, 311; 78) pp. 99, 154, 184, 231, 309; 79) p. 272; 80) p. 347; 81) pp. 117, 134, 157, 197, 351; 82) pp. 94, 95, 101.
Bensky, D., Gamble, A., Kaptchuk, T. *Chinese Herbal Medicine Materia Medica*. Seattle, WA: Eastland Press, 1993;149.
Bergner, P. Is lobelia toxic? *Medical Herbalism*. 1998;10(1&2):26. Quote reprinted with permission from Paul Bergner.
________.The adverse effects of herbs. *Medical Herbalism*. 2002;13(1):1.
Cambar, P. et al. Bronchopulmonary and gastrointestinal effects of lobeline. *Arch Int Pharmacodyn*. 1969;177:1-27.
Damaj, M. et al. Pharmacology of lobeline, a nicotinic receptor ligand. *J Pharmacol Exp Ther*. 1997;282(1):410-9.
Dean, K. Lobeline compounds as a treatment for psychostimulant abuse and withdrawal, and for eating disorders. *HerbalGram*. 1999;47:32.
Dwoskin, L., Crooks, P. A novel mechanism of action and potential use for lobeline as a treatment for psychostimulant abuse. *Biochem Pharmacology*. 2002;63(2):89-98.
Gilman, A. et al. *The Pharmacological Basis of Therapeutics*. New York, NY: Macmillan Publishing,1980; 212-4.
Gladstar, R., Hirsch, P. (Eds.). *Planting the Future: Saving our Medicinal Herbs*. Rochester, VT: Healing Arts Press, 2000;150-8.
Hobart, F., Melton, G. *A Concise Applied Pharmacology and Therapeutics of More Important Drugs* (3rd ed.). London, England: Leonard Hill, 1949.
Krochmal, A. et al. Plant and lobeline harvest of *Lobelia inflata*. *Economic Botany*. 1972;26(3):216-20.
Laffan, R., Borison, H. Emetic action of nicotine and lobeline. *Journal of Pharmacological and Experimental Therapeutics*. 1957;121:468-76.
Lim, D. et al. Influence of lobeline on catecholamine release from the isolated perfused rat adrenal gland. *Auton Neurosci*. 2004 ;110(1):27-35.
Mansuri, S. et al. Some pharmacological characteristics of ganglionic activity of lobeline. *Arzneimittel-Forschung*. 1973;23:1271-5.
Nickell, J. et al. The vesicular monoamine transporter-2: an important pharmacological target for the discovery of novel therapeutics to treat methamphetamine abuse. *Adv Pharmacol*. 2014;69:71-106.
Osol, A., Farrar, G. *The Dispensatory of the United States of America* (24th ed.). Philadelphia,PA: J. B. Lippencott Company, 1947.
Robinson, T. The biochemical pharmacology of plant alkaloids. *Herbs, Spices, and Medicinal Plants*. 1986;1:135-65.
Subarnas, A. et al. A possible mechanism of antidepressant activity of beta-amyrin palmitate isolated from *Lobelia inflata* leaves in the forced swimming test. *Life Science*. 1993;52(3):289-96.
Tamboli, A. et al. Antiepileptic activity of lobeline isolated from the leaf of *Lobelia nicotianaefolia* and its effect on brain GABA level in mice. *Asian Pac J Trop Biomed*. 2012 Jul;2(7):537-42.
Teng, L. et al. Lobeline displaces (3H) dihydrotetrabenazine binding and releases (3H) dopamine from rat striatal synaptic vesicles: a comparison with d-amphetamine. *Journal of Neurochemistry*. 1998;71(1):258-65.
Terry, A. et al. Lobeline and structurally simplified analogs exhibit differential agonist activity and sensitivity to antagonist blockade when compared to nicotine. *Neuropharmacology*. 1998;37(1):93-102.

MARSHMALLOW

GENERAL REFERENCES: 1) p. 166; 2) pp. 244-8; 3) p. 143; 5) p. 244; 8) pp. 325, 329, 357, 9) p. 236; 11) p. 91; 12) p. 388; 14); 16) p. 202; 18) p. 431; 20) p. 157; 21) p. 178; 23) p. 143; 24) p. 134; 25) p. 244; 28) p. 128; 29) p. 934; 33) p. 507; 35) p. 208; 36) p. 526; 37) p. 464; 41) p. 672; 46) p. 9; 48); 55) p. 188; 57) p. 79; 62) p. 242; 64) p. 323; 66) p. 86; 75) p. 195; 79) p. 290; 81).
Brinckmann, S. et al. Safety and efficacy of a traditional herbal medicine (Throat Coat) in symptomatic temporary relief of pain in patients with acute pharyngitis: a multicenter, prospective, randomized, double-blinded, placebo-controlled study. J Altern Compl Med. 2003;9(2):285-298.
Buechi, S. et al. Open trial to assess aspects of safety and efficacy of a combined herbal cough syrup with ivy and thyme. *Forsch Komplementarmed Klass Naturheilkd*. 2005 Dec;12(6):328-32.
Deters, A. et al. Aqueous extracts and polysaccharides from Marshmallow roots (*Althea officinalis* L.): cellular internalization and stimulation of cell physiology of human epithelial cells *in vitro*. *J Ethnopharmacol*. 2010 Jan 8;127(1):62-9.
Engels, G. Marshmallow. *HerbalGram*. 2007;75:1-5.
Hage-Sleiman, R. et al. Pharmacological evaluation of aqueous extract of *Althaea officinalis* flower grown in Lebanon. *Pharm Biol*. 2011 Mar;49(3): 327-33.
Kolacz, N. et al. The effect of Burns & Wounds (B&W)/burdock leaf therapy on burn-injured Amish patients: a pilot study measuring pain levels, infection rates, and healing times. Amish Burn Study Group. *J Holistic Nursing*. 2014 Dec;32(4):327-40.
Tomoda, M. et al. Hypoglycemic activity of 20 plant mucilages and 3 modified products. *Planta Medica*. 1987;53:8-12.
Recio, M. et al. Antimicrobial activity of selected plants employed in the Spanish Mediterranean area, part II. *Phytotherapy Research*. 1989;3:77.
Rouhi, H., Ganji, F. Effect of *Althaea officinalis* on cough associated with ACE inhibitors. *Pakistan Journal of Nutrition*. 2007;6(3):256-8.

MOTHERWORT

1) p. 172; 2) p. 267; 3) p. 150; 8) p. 297; 9) p. 505; 11) p. 99; 17); 18) p. 483; 20) p. 1125; 21) p. 443; 22) p. 439; 23) p. 151; 29) p. 704; 33) p. 555; 37) p. 572; 46) pp. 68, 170, 183; 49) p. 301; 55) p. 197; 63) p. 139; 65) p. 309; 75) pp. 186, 279; 79) p. 300; 81); 82) pp. 13, 16, 55, 187.
Bensky, D., Gamble, A., Kaptchuk, T. *Chinese Herbal Medicine Materia Medica*. Seattle, WA: Eastland Press, 1993;273.
Bernatoniene, J. et al. The effect of *Leonurus cardiaca* herb extract and some of its flavonoids on mitochondrial oxidative phosphorylation in the heart. *Planta Med*. 2014 May;80(7):525-32.
Bradley, P. (Ed.). *British Herbal Compendium* (Vol. 1). Bournemouth, England: British Herbal Medicine Association, 1992.
Buhner, S. *Healing Lyme Disease Coinfections*. Rochester, VT: Healing Arts Press, 2013; 230-2.
Chang, C., Li, C. Experimental studies on the mechanism of anti-platelet aggregation action of motherwort. *Chung-Hoi-I-Chich-Ho-YSQ Chin*. 1986; 6:39-40.
Chen, C., Kwan, C. Endothelium-independent vasorelaxation by leonurine, a plant alkaloid purified from Chinese motherwort. *Life Science*. 2001; 68(8):953-60.

Enqin, Z. (Ed.). *Chinese Materia Medica*. Shanghai, China: Publishing House of Shanghai College of Traditional Medicine, 1988;128.
Hu, S. A contribution to our knowledge of *Leonurus* L., I-mu-ts'ao, the Chinese motherwort. *Am Journal of Chinese Medicine*. 1976;4(3):219-37.
Kong, Y. et al. Isolation of the uterotonic principle from *Leonurus Artemisia*, the Chinese motherwort. *Am J Chinese Medicine*. 1976;4(4):373-82.
Kuo-Hsiung, L. et al. The cytotoxic principles of *Prunella vulgaris, Psychotria serpens*, and *Hyptis capitata*: Ursolic acid and related derivatives. *Planta Medica*. 1988;(54):308.
Lee, C. et al. Prehispanolone, a novel platelet activating factor receptor antagonist from *L. heterophyllus*. *British J Pharmoc*. 1991;103(3):1719-24.
Matkowski, A., Piotrowska, M. Antioxidant and free radical scavenging activities of some medicinal plants from the *Lamiaceae*. *Fitoterapia*. 2006 July;77(5):346-53.
Nagasawa, H. et al. Further study on the effects of motherwort (*Leonurus sibiricus* L.) on preneoplastic and neoplastic mammary gland growth in multiparous GR/A mice. *Anticancer Research*. 1992;12(1):141-3.
Satoh, M. et al. Studies on the constituents of *Leonurus sibiricus* L. *Chemical Pharmaceutical Bulletin*. Tokyo, Japan. 2003;51(3):341-2.
Shi, M. et al. Stimulating action of *Carthamus tinctorius* L., *Angelica sinensis* (Oliv.) Diels and *Leonurus sibiricus* L. on the uterus. *Zhongguo Zhong Yao Za Zhi*. 1995;20(3):173-5,192.
Shikov, A. et al. Effect of *Leonurus cardiaca* oil extract in patients with arterial hypertension accompanied by anxiety and sleep disorders. *Phytother Res*. 2011 Apr;25(4):540-3.
Song, X., et al. Leonurine exerts anti-inflammatory effect by regulating inflammatory signaling pathways and cytokines in LPS-induced mouse mastitis. *Inflammation*. 2015 Feb;38(1):79-88.
Tokuda, H. et al. Inhibitory effects of ursolic and oleanolic acid on skin tumor promotion by 12-O-tetradecanoylphorbol-13-acetate. *Cancer Letter*. 1986;33(3):279-85.
Xia, Y. The inhibitory effect of motherwort extract on pulsating myocardial cells *in vitro*. *Journal of Traditional Chinese Medicine*. 1983;3:185-8.
Xu, D. et al. Leonurine ameliorates LPS-induced acute kidney injury via suppressing ROS-mediated NF-KB signaling pathway. *Fitoterapia*. 2014 Sep;97:148-55.
Xu, H. et al. Proliferation of lymphocytes T and B by prehispanolone LC-5504 of *L. hereterophyllus* Sweet. *Yao Xue Xue Bao*.1992;27(11):812-6.
Zou, Q. et al. Effect of motherwort on blood viscosity. *Am Journal of Chinese Medicine*. 1989;17(1-2):65-70.

MUGWORT

GENERAL REFERENCES: 1) p. 352; 3) p. 151; 9) p. 269; 11) p. 95; 12) p. 357; 17); 22) p. 441; 23) p. 152; 28) p. 130; 29) p. 1103; 30) p. 249; 33) p. 556; 37) p. 316; 42) p. 285; 46) pp. 16, 184; 49) p. 103; 63) p. 139; 64) p. 264; 79) p. 303; 82) pp. 56, 59, 105, 119, 121, 191.
Abdul, M. et al. Survey of artemisinin production by diverse *Artemisia* species in northern Pakistan. *Malaria J*. 2010;9:310.
Alakbarov, F. Aromatic Herbal Baths of the Ancients. *HerbalGram*. 2003;57:40-9.
Bamunuarachchi, G. et al. *Artemisia vulgaris* L. ethanolic leaf extract reverses thrombocytopenia/thrombocytosis and averts end-stage disease of experimental severe Plasmodium berghei murine malaria. *Journal Vector Borne Diseases*. 2014 Oct-Dec;51(4):286-93.
Bensky, D., Gamble, A., Kaptchuk, T. *Chinese Herbal Medicine Materia Medica*. Seattle, WA: Eastland Press, 1993; 259.
Cardini, F., Weixin, H. Moxibustion for correction of breech presentation: a randomized controlled trial. *JAMA*. 1998;280(18):1580-4.
Efferth, T. et al. The antiviral activities of artemisinin and artesunate. *Clin Infect Dis*. 2008 Sep 15;47(6):804-11.
Ewies, A., Olah, K. Moxibustion in breech presentation-a descriptive review. *Acupuncture Medicine*. 2002;20(1): 26-9.
Gordanian, B. et al. *In vitro* evaluation of cytotoxic activity of flower, leaf, stem and root extracts of five Artemisia species. *Res Pharm Sci*. 2014 Mar-Apr;9(2):91-6.
Romero, M. et al. Effect of artemisinin/artesunate as inhibitors of hepatitis B virus production in an "in vitro" replicative system. *Antiviral Res*. 2005 Nov;68(2):75-83.
Saleh, A. et al. *In vitro* cytotoxicity of *Artemisia vulgaris* L. essential oil is mediated by a mitochondria-dependent apoptosis in HL-60 leukemic cell line. *BMC Complement Altern Med*. 2014 Jul 7;14:226.
Tigno, X., Gumila, E. *In vivo* microvascular actions of *Artemisia vulgaris* L. in a model of ischemia-reperfusion injury in the rat intestinal mesentery. *Clin Hemorheol Microcirc*. 2000;23(2-4):159-65.
Tigno, X. et al. Phytochemical analysis and hemodynamics of *Artemisia vulgaris* L. *Clin Hemorheol Microcirc*. 2000;23(2-4):167-75.

MULLEIN

1); 2) p. 270; 3) p. 151; 5) p. 265; 8) p. 315; 9) p. 726; 11) p. 96; 12) p. 500; 14) pp. 118, 170, 181, 221, 372; 17); 18) p. 397; 20) pp. 2054-5; 21) p. 693; 24) p. 140; 25) p. 254; 28) p. 131; 29) p. 774; 33) p. 562; 35) p. 211; 36) pp. 417, 512, 592; 37) p. 470; 42) p. 286; 44) p. 285; 46) p. 121; 48) p. 327; 49) p. 590; 62) p. 259; 63) p. 140; 64) p. 389; 66) p. 89; 70) p. 341; 74) pp. 20, 46; 75) p. 197; 78) p. 188; 79) p. 305; 80) p. 491.
Ali, N. et al. Anthelmintic and relaxant activities of *Verbascum Thapsus* Mullein. *BMC Complement Altern Med*. 2012 Mar 30;12:29.
Alipieva, K. et al. Verbascoside-a review of its occurrence, (bio)synthesis and pharmacological significance. *Biotechnol Adv*. 2014;32(6):1065-76.
Fitzpatrick, F. Plant substances active against *mycobacterium tuberculosis*. *Antibiotics and Chemotherapy*. 1954;4(5):528.
Saracoglu, I. et al. Studies on components with cytotoxic and cytostatic activity of two Turkish medical plants. *Biology & Pharmacology Bulletin*. 1995;18:1396-1400.
Sarrell, E. et al. Efficacy of naturopathic extracts in the management of ear pain associated with acute otitis media. *Arch Pediatr Adolesc Med*. 2001 July;155(7):796-9.
__________. Naturopathic treatment for ear pain in children. *Pediatrics*. 2003;111(5):574-579.
Sepahi, S. et al. *In Vitro* Study to Evaluate Antibacterial and Non-haemolytic Activities of Four Iranian Medicinal Plants. *West Indian Med J*. 2014 Feb 24;63(4):293-297.
Sinadinos, C. Medicinal Uses of Mullein Root. *Medical Herbalism*. 2009;16(2):1,12-15.
Slagowska, A. et al. Inhibition of herpes simplex virus replication by Flos verbasci infusion. *Pol J Pharmacol Pharm*. 1987;39(1):55-61.
Turker, A., Camper, N. Biological activity of common mullein, a medicinal plant. *Journal of Ethnopharmacology*. 2002;82(2-3):117-25.
Winston, D. Little Known Uses of Common Plants. *Medical Herbalism*. 2001;12(3):1-2.
Zgorniak-Nowosielska, I. et al. Antiviral activity of *Flos verbasci* infusion against influenza and herpes simplex viruses. *Arch Immunol Ther Exp (Warsz)*. 1991;39(1-2):103-8.
Zheng, R. et al. Inhibition of the auto-oxidation of linoleic acid by phenylpropanoid glycosides from *Pedicularis* in micelles. *Chem Phys Lipids*. 1993;65:151-4.

PASSION FLOWER

GENERAL REFERENCES: 1) pp. 179, 279, 305; 2) p. 293; 3); 5) p. 284; 14) p. 429; 16) p. 230; 17); 18) p. 1439; 20); 21) p. 515; 23) p. 159; 24) p. 152; 25) p. 280; 33) p. 618; 35) p. 215; 36) p. 570; 37) p. 839; 44) p. 303; 46) p. 82; 51) pp. 109, 215; 52) p. 159; 55) p. 206; 64) p. 355; 65) p. 314; 66) p. 93; 68) p. 237; 75) p. 287; 76) p. 226 79) p. 328, 81).
Aarons, D. et al. Cardiovascular actions of three harmala alkaloids: Harmine, harmaline, and harmalol. *J Pharm Sci*. 1977;66:1244-8.
Akhondzadeh, S. et al. Passionflower in the treatment of generalized anxiety: a pilot double-blind randomized controlled trial with oxazepam. *Journal of Clinical Pharmacology and Therapeutics*. 2001;26(5):363-7.
_______________. Passionflower in the treatment of opiates withdrawal: a double-blind randomized controlled trial. *Journal of Clinical Pharmacology and Therapeutics*. 2001;26(5):369-73.
_______________. *Passiflora incarnata* in the treatment of attention-deficit hyperactivity disorder in children and adolescents. *Therapy*. 2005; 2(4):609-14.
Aoyagi, N. et al. Studies on *Passiflora incarnata* dry extract. I. Isolation of maltol and pharmacological action of maltol and ethyl maltol. *Chemical & Pharmaceutical Bulletin*. 1974;22:1008-13.
Appel, K. et al. Modulation of the γ-aminobutyric acid (GABA) system by *Passiflora incarnata* L. *Phytother Res*. 2011 Jun;25(6):838-43.
Aslanargun, P. *Passiflora incarnata* Linneaus as an anxiolytic before spinal anesthesia. *J Anesth*. 2012 Feb;26(1):39-44.
Bergner, P. Passionflower. *Medical Herbalism*. 1995;7(1-2):13-14,26.
Berrougui, H. et al. Vasorelaxant effects of harmine and harmaline extracted from *Peganum harmala* L. seeds in isolated rat aorta. *Pharmacol Res*. 2006;54:150-7.
Borrelli, F. et al. Anti-inflammatory activity of *Passiflora incarnata* L. in rats. *Phytotherapy Research*. 1996;10:S104-6.
Brinker, F. *Formulas for Healthful Living*. Sandy, OR: Eclectic Medical Publications, 1998;99,120.

Brown, E. et al. Evaluation of the anxiolytic effects of chrysin, a *Passiflora incarnata* extract, in the laboratory rat. *AANA J.* 2007 Oct;75(5):333-7.
Cott, J. Medicinal plants and dietary supplements: sources for innovative treatments or adjuncts? *Psychopharmacology Bulletin.* 1995;31:131-7.
Dong, L, et al. Cardioprotection of vitexin on myocardial ischemia/reperfusion injury in rat via regulating inflammatory cytokines and MAPK pathway. *Am J Chin Med.* 2013;41(6):1251-66.
Engels, G., Brinckmann, J. Passionflower. *HerbalGram.* 2017;112:8-18.
Ergene, E., Schoener, E. Effects of harmane (1-methyl-beta-carboline) on neurons in the nucleus accumbens of the rat. *Pharmacological & Biochemical Behavior.* 1993;44(4):951-7.
Farnsworth, N. et al. Potential value of plants as sources of new antifertility agents. *J Pharmaceutical Science.* 1975;64:535-98.
Geiger. H., Markham, K. The C-glycosylflavone pattern of *Passiflora incarnata. L Z Naturforsch.* 1990;41c:949-50.
Grundmann, O. et al. Anxiolytic activity of a phytochemically characterized *Passiflora incarnata* extract is mediated via the GABAergic system. *Planta Med.* 2008 Dec;74(15):1769-73.
Kaviani, N. et al. The efficacy of *Passiflora incarnata* linnaeus in reducing dental anxiety in patients undergoing periodontal treatment. *Journal of Dentistry.* 2013 Jun;14(2):68-72.
Kimura, R. et al. Central depressant effects of maltol analogs in mice. *Chemical & Pharmaceutical Bulletin.* 1980;28:2570-9.
Leiter, E. The Passionflowers. *Herbalgram.* 1994;32:52-5.
Lu, C. et al. Vitexin protects against cardiac hypertrophy via inhibiting calcineurin and CaMKII signaling pathways. *Naunyn Schmiedebergs Arch Pharmacol.* 2013 Aug;386(8):747-55.
Lutomski, J. *Alkaloidy Pasiflora incarnata L.* Dissertation. Institute for Medicinal Plant Research, Poznan, Poland: 1960.
Lutomski, J., Wrocinski, T. Pharmacodynamic properties of *Passiflora incarnata* preparations. The effect of alkaloid and flavonoid components on pharmacodynamic properties of the raw material. *Biul Inst Roslin Leczniczych.* 1960;6:176-184.
Lutomski, J. et al. Pharmacological investigation of the raw materials from the passiflora genus. 2. Pharmacochemical estimation of juices from the fruits of *Passiflora edulis* and *Passiflora edulis* forma *flavicarpa*. *Planta Medica.* 1975;27:112.
_____________. The meaning of Passion Flower in the medicine. *Pharmazie in Unserer Zeit.* 1981;10(2):45-8.
Meier, B. et al. *Passiflora incarnata* L.- Passion flower: portrait of a medicinal plant. *Zeitschrift fur Phytotherapie.* 1995;16:115-26.
Movafegh, A. et al. *Passiflora incarnata* reduces anxiety in ambulatory surgery patients: a double-blind, placebo-controlled study. *Anesth Analg.* 2008 Jun;106(6):1728-32.
Nicholls, J. et al. Passicol, an antibacterial and antifungal agent produced by *Passiflora* plant species: qualitative and quantitative range of activity. *Antimicrobial Agents Chemotherapy.* 1973;3(1):110-17.
Quimin, L. et al. Mass spectral characterization of C-glycosidic flavonoids isolated from a medicinal plant (*Passiflora incarnata*). *Journal of Chromatography.* 1991;562:435-6.
Rommelspacher. H. et al. Harman (1-methyl-beta-carboline) is a natural inhibitor of monoamine oxidase type A in rats. *European Journal of Pharmacology.* 1994;252(1):51-9.
Shi, C. et al. Comparative study on the vasorelaxant effects of three harmala alkaloids *in vitro. Jpn J Pharmacol.* 2001;85:299–305.
Singh, B. et al. Dual protective effect of *Passiflora incarnata* in epilepsy and associated post-ictal depression. *J Ethnopharmacology.* 2012;139(1): 273-9.
Soulimani, R. et al. Behavioral effects of *Passiflora incarnata* L. and its indole alkaloid and flavonoid derivatives and maltol in the mouse. *Journal of Ethnopharmacology.* 1997;57(1):11-20.
Speroni, E., Minghetti, A. Neuropharmacological activity of extracts from *Passiflora incarnata. Planta Medica.* 1988;54(6):488-91.
Speroni, E., Billi, R. Sedative effects of crude extract of *Passiflora incarnata* after oral administration. *Phytotherapy Research.* 1996;10:S92-4.
Trompetter, I. et al. Herbal triplet in treatment of nervous agitation in children. *Wien Med Wochenschr.* 2013 Feb;163(3-4):52-7.
Valli, M. et al. Euphytose and association of plant extracts with anxiolytic activity: investigation of its mechanism of action by an *in vitro* binding study. *Phytotherapy Research.* 1991;5:241-9.
Wahling, C. et al. Triple herbal combination: An effective alternative to benzodiazepines. *Zeitschrift fur Phytotherapie.* 2009;30:69-72.
Wang, X. et al. Effects of Vitexin on the Pharmacokinetics and mRNA Expression of CYP Isozymes in Rats. *Phytother Res.* 2014 Dec 1.
Zanoli, P. et al. Behavioral characterisation of the flavonoids apigenin and chrysin. *Fitoterapia.* 2000 Aug;71 Suppl 1:S117-23.
Zhai, K. et al. Chrysin induces hyperalgesia via the GABA receptor in mice. *Planta Med.* 2008 Aug;74(10):1229-34.

PEPPERMINT

GENERAL REFERENCES: 1); 2) pp. 297-303; 3); 5) p. 253; 8) p. 417; 9) p. 562; 14); 16) p. 235; 18) p. 280; 20) p. 1254; 21) p. 478; 23) p. 148; 24) p. 156; 25) p. 286; 28) p. 129; 29) p. 681; 32); 33) p. 537; 35) p. 216; 36); 37) p. 155; 42) p. 293; 43); 44) p. 275; 46) p. 75; 48) pp. 21, 139; 49); 50) p. 145; 51) p. 75; 53) p. 280; 57) p. 209; 62) p. 291; 64) p. 156; 66) p. 94; 68) p. 246; 69) p. 56; 71) pp. 25, 117; 75) p. 28; 77) pp. 229, 250; 78) p. 133; 79) p. 337; 81).
Akhavan, A. et al. The effect of peppermint oil on symptomatic treatment of pruritus in pregnant women. *Iran J Pharmocol Res.* 2012 Fall;11(4): 1073-7.
Alves, J. et al. Effectiveness of *Mentha piperita* in the treatment of infantile colic: a crossover study. *Evid Based Complementary Alternat Med.* 2012:981352.
Atta, A., Alkofahi, A. Anti-nociceptive and anti-inflammatory effects of some Jordanian medicinal plant extracts. *J. Ethnopharmacology.* 1998;60(2): 117-124.
Bell, G., Doran, J. Gallstone dissolution in man using an essential oil preparation. *British Medical Journal.* 1979;278:24.
Briggs, C. Peppermint: Medicinal herb and flavoring agent. *Canadian Pharm Journal.* 1993;129:89-92.
Brinker, F. *Formulas for Healthful Living.* Sandy, OR: Eclectic Medical Publications, 1998; 52,65,123,152.
Davies, S. et al. A novel treatment of postherpetic neuralgia using Peppermint oil. *Clinical Journal of Pain.* 2002;17(3):200-2.
Doran, J. et al. Rowachol - a possible treatment for cholesterol gallstones. *Gut.* 1979;20:312-17.
Duband, F. et al. The aromatic and polyphenolic composition of peppermint (*Mentha piperita*) tea. *Ann Pharm France.* 1992;50:146-55.
Ellis, W., Bell, G. Treatment of biliary duct stones with a terpene preparation. *British Medical Journal.* 1981;282:611.
Foster, S. *Peppermint.* Botanical Series #306. Austin,TX: American Botanical Council, 1999.
Gobel, H. et al. Effect of peppermint and eucalyptus oil preparations on neurophysiological and experimental algesimetric headache parameters. *Cephalagia.* 1994;14:228-34.
_____________. Essential plant oils and headache mechanisms. *Phytomedicine.* 1995;2(2):93-102.
Grigoleit, H., Grigoleit, P. Peppermint oil in irritable bowel syndrome. *Phytomedicine.* 2005;12(8):601-6.
Hawthorne, M. et al. The actions of peppermint oil and menthol on calcium channel dependent processes in intestinal, neuronal, and cardiac preparations. *J Aliment Pharmacol Therap.* 1988;2:101-8.
Herrman, E., Kucera, L. Antiviral substances in plants of the mint family (*Labiatae*). III. Peppermint (*Mentha piperita*) and other mint plants. *Proceedings of the Society of Experimental Biology and Medicine.* 1967;124:874-5.
Hiki, N. et al. Peppermint oil reduces gastric spasm during upper endoscopy: a randomized, double-blind, double-dummy controlled trial. *Gastrointestinal Endoscopy.* 2003 Apr;57(4):475-82.
Hills, J., Aaronaon, P. Mechanism of action of peppermint oil and menthol in gastrointestinal smooth muscle. *Gastroenterology.* 1991;101:55-6.
Hordinsky, B. Terpenes in the treatment of gallstones. *Minnesota Medicine.* 1971;54:649-51.
Imai, H. et al Inhibition by the essential oils of peppermint and spearmint of the growth of pathogenic bacteria. *Microbios.* 2001;106(1):31-9.
Kline, R. et al. Enteric-coated, pH-dependent peppermint oil capsules for treatment of irritable bowel in children. *J Pediatrics.* 2001;138:125–8.
Lech, U. et al. Treatment of irritable bowel syndrome with peppermint oil. A double-blind study with a placebo. *Ugeskr Laeger.* 1988;150:2388.
Leicester, R., Hunt, R. Peppermint oil to reduce colonic spasm during endoscopy. *Lancet.* 1982;2:989.
Madisch, A. et al. Treatment of functional dyspepsia with a fixed peppermint oil and caraway oil combination preparation as compared to cisapride. A multicenter, reference-controlled double-blind equivalence study. *Arzneimittel-Forschung.* 1999;49(11):925-32.
Mimica-Dukic, N. et al. Antimicrobial and antioxidant activities of three *Mentha* species essential oils. *Planta Medica.* 2003;69(5):413-9.
Pittler, M., Ernst, E. Peppermint oil for irritable bowel syndrome: A critical review and meta-analysis. *American J Gastroenterology.* 1998;93:1131-1135.
Pizsolitto, A. et al. Determination of antibacterial activity of essential oils officialized by the Brazillian Pharmacopeia, 2nd Edition. *Revista da*

Faculdade de Famacia e Odontologia de Araragwara. 1975;9(1):55-61.
Rees, W. et al. Treating irritable bowel syndrome with peppermint oil. *British Medical Journal*. 1979;2:835-6.
Schuhmacher, A. et al. Virucidal effect of peppermint oil on the enveloped viruses *herpes simplex* virus type 1 and type 2 *in vitro*. *Phytomedicine*. 2003;10(6-7):504-10.
Shipochliev, T. Pharmacological study of several essential oil. I. Effect on the smooth muscle. *Vet Med*. (Prague). 1968;13(8-9):63-9.
Sigmond, C., Macnally, E. The action of a carminative on the lower oesophageal sphincter. *Gastroenterology*. 1969;56:13-18.
Somerville, K. et al. Delayed release peppermint oil capsules (Colpermin) for the spastic colon syndrome: a pharmacokinetic study. *British Journal of Clinical Pharmacology*. 1984;18:638-40.
Taylor, B. et al. Inhibitory effect of peppermint oil on gastrointestinal smooth muscle. *Gut*. 1983;24:992.
Trabace, L. et al. Choleretic activity of some typical components of essential oils. *Planta Medica*. 1992;58:A650-1.
Weizman, Z. et al. Efficacy of herbal tea preparation in infantile colic. *Journal of Pediatrics*. 1993;122:650-2.
Westfall, R. Use of anti-emetic herbs in pregnancy: women's choices, and the question of safety and efficacy. *Complementary Therapies Nurse Midwifery*. 2004;10(1):30-6.

PLEURISY ROOT

GENERAL REFERENCES: 3) p. 163; 8) p. 221; 9); 10) p. 124; 16) p. 245; 19) pp. 431, 434; 20); 21); 23) p. 166; 32) p. 197; 33) p. 647; 35) p. 218; 36) pp. 488, 512, 531; 37) p. 238; 40) p. 53; 42) p. 297; 44) p. 313; 46) p. 17; 48) pp. 167, 195, 204; 55) p. 213; 62) p. 249; 64) p. 161; 66) p. 96; 70) p. 287; 74) p. 29; 78) p. 195; 79) p. 349; 80) p. 158.
Abe, F., Yamauchi, T. Pregnane glycosides from the roots of *Asclepias tuberosa*. *Chem Pharm Bull*. 2000 Jul;48(7):1017-22.
Cheatham, S., Johnston, M., Marshall, L. *The Useful Wild Plants of Texas, the Southeastern and Southwestern United States, the Southern Plains, and Northern Mexico* (Vol. 2). Austin, TX: Useful Wild Plants, Inc., 2000.
Conway, G., Slocumb, J. Plants used as abortifacients and emmenagogues by Spanish New Mexicans. *J Ethnopharmacology*. 1979;1:241-61.
Costello, C., Butler, C. The estrogenic and uterine-stimulating activity of *Asclepias tuberosa*. *J Am Pharm Ass Sci Ed*. 1949;39:233-7.
Hassan, W., Reed, H. Studies on species of Asclepias VI. Toxicology, pathology and pharmacology. *J Am Pharm Ass Sci Ed*. 1952;41:298-300.
Lo Ha Wa Ti An Ka. *Osage Medicine: Ancestral Herbs and the Illnesses that they Treat*. Greyhorse Indian Village, Rt 2 Box 66-1, Fairfax, OK 74637: Scope Publications.
Mader, L. Milkweed: Medicine of Monarchs and Humans. *HerbalGram*. 2014;101:38-47.
Millspaugh, C. *American Medicinal Plants, and Illustrated and Descriptive Guide to the American Plants Used as Homeopathic Remedies*. New York, NY: Boericke & Tafel, 1887.
Moerman, D. *Geraniums for the Iroquois: A Field Guide to American Indian Medicinal Plants*. Algonac, MI: Reference Publications, Inc., 1981.
Warashina, T., Noro, T. 8,14-Secopregnane glycosides from the aerial parts of *Asclepias tuberosa*. *Phytochemistry*. 2009 Jul;70(10):1294-304.
__________________. 8,12;8,20-Diepoxy-8,14-secopregnane glycosides from the aerial parts of *Asclepias tuberosa*. *Chem Pharm Bull*. 2010 Feb;58(2):172-9.
Wood, G., Bache, F. *The Dispensatory of the United States of America* (16th ed.). Philadelphia, PA: J. B. Lippincott Company; 1892.
Yarnell, E. *Phytochemistry and Pharmacy for Practitioners of Botanical Medicine*. Wenatchee, WA: Healing Mountain Publishing; 2004.

SAGE

GENERAL REFERENCES: 1) p. 198; 2) p. 330; 3) p. 171; 5) p. 317; 9) p. 676; 11) p. 147; 12) p. 274; 14) pp. 50, 142-3, 154, 264-5, 513, 561; 16) p. 265; 20) p. 1705; 21) p. 614; 23) p. 170; 24) p. 176; 25) p. 318; 29); 31); 33) p. 700; 36) p. 580; 37) p. 771; 42) p. 306; 43); 44) p. 342; 46) p. 102; 55) p. 231; 62) p. 327; 63) p. 96; 64) p. 150; 66) p. 102; 68) p. 271; 69) p. 164; 73) p. 111; 75); 77) p. 250; 79) p. 384; 81).
Akhondzadeh, S. et al. *Salvia officinalis* extract in the treatment of patients with mild to moderate Alzheimer's disease: a double blind, randomized and placebo-controlled trial. *J Clin Pharm Ther*. 2003 Feb;28(1):53-9.
Amin, A., Hamza, A. Hepatoprotective effects of Hibiscus, Rosmarinus and Salvia on azathioprine-induced toxicity in rats. *Life Science*. 2005;77(3): 266-78.
Behradmanesh, S. et al. Effect of *Salvia officinalis* on diabetic patients. *J Renal Inj Prev*. 2013 Jun 1;2(2):51-4.
Berger, F. *Handbuch der Drogenkunde* (Vol. 2). Vienna, Austria: Verlag Wilhelm Maudrich, 1950;292-505.
Bommer, S. et al. First time proof of sage's tolerability and efficacy in menopausal women with hot flushes. *Adv Ther*. 2011 Jun;28(6):490-500.
Caceres, et al. Plants used in Guatemala for the treatment of respiratory diseases. Screening of 68 plants against gram-positive bacteria. *Journal of Ethnopharmacology*. 1991;31:193-208.
Capek, P., Hribalova, V. Water-soluble polysaccharides from *Salvia officinalis* L. possessing immunomodulatory activity. *Phytochemistry*. 2004;65(13): 1983-92.
De Leo, V. et al. Treatment of neurovegetative menopausal symptoms with a phytotherapeutic agent. *Minerva Ginecol*. 1998;50(5):207-11.
Durrafourd, C. et al. *Cahiers de phytotherapie clinique* (Vol. 4). Paris, France; 1982.
Eidi, M. et al. Effect of *S. officinalis* L. leaves on serum glucose and insulin in healthy and streptozotocin-induced diabetic rats. *J Ethnopharmacol*. 2005;100(3):310-3.
Engels, G. Sage. *HerbalGram*. 2011;89:1-4.
Houghton, P. Activity and constituents of Sage relevant to the potential treatment of symptoms of Alzheimer's disease. *HerbalGram*. 2004;61:48.
Hubbert, M. et al. Efficacy and tolerability of a spray with *Salvia officinalis* in the treatment of acute pharyngitis - a randomized, double-blind, placebo-controlled study with adaptive design and interim analysis. *Eur J Med Res*. 2006 Jan 31;11(1):20-6.
Kennedy, D. et al. Effects of cholinesterase inhibiting Sage (*Salvia officinalis*) on mood, anxiety and performance on a psychological stressor battery. *Neuropsychopharmacology*. 2006;31:845-52.
Kianbakht, S., Dabaghian, F. Improved glycemic control and lipid profile in hyperlipidemic type 2 diabetic patients consuming *Salvia officinalis* L. leaf extract: a randomized placebo-controlled clinical trial. *Complement Ther Med*. 2013 Oct;21(5):441-6.
Lima, C. et al. The drinking of a *S. officinalis* infusion improves liver antioxidant status in mice and rats. *J Ethnopharmacology*. 2005;97(2):383-9.
Masterova, I. et al. Royleanones in the roots of *Salvia officinalis* L. of domestic provenance and their antimicrobial activity. *Ceska Slov Farm*. 1996; 45:242-5.
Pereira, R. et al. Antibacterial activity of essential oils on microorganisms isolated from urinary tract infection. *Rev Saude Publica*. 2004;38(2):326.
Perry, N. et al. European herbs with cholinergic activities: potential in dementia therapy. *Int J Geriatric Psychiatry*. 1996;11:1063-9.
___________. *In vitro* inhibition of human erythrocyte acetylcholine esterase by *Salvia lavandulifolia* essential oil and constituent terpenes. *J Pharm Pharmacol*. 2000;52:895-902.
___________. *In vitro* activities of *S. lavandulifolia* relevant to treatment of Alzheimer's disease. *J Pharm Pharmacol*. 2001;53:1347-56.
___________. *S. lavandulifolia* essential oil inhibits cholinesterase *in vivo*. *Phytomedicine*. 2002;9:48-51.
Rahte, S. et al. *S. officinalis* for hot flashes: towards determination of mechanism of activity and active principles. *Planta Med*. 2013;79(9):753-60.
Recio, M. et al. Antimicrobial activity of selected plants employed in the Spanish Mediterranean area. Part II. *Phytotherapy Research*. 1989;3:77.
Schnitzler, P. et al. Comparative *in vitro* study on the anti-herpetic effect of phytochemically characterized aqueous and ethanolic extracts of *Salvia officinalis* grown at two different locations. *Phytomedicine*. 2008 Jan;15(1-2):62-70.
Scholey, A. et al. An extract of *Salvia* (sage) with anticholinesterase properties improves memory and attention in healthy older volunteers. *Psychopharmacology*. 2008 May;198(1):127-39.
Tildesley, N. et al. *Salvia lavandulifolia* (Spanish lavender) enhances on memory in healthy young volunteers. *Pharmacology, Biochemistry and Behavior*. 2003;75:669-74.
Vandecasteele, K. et al. Evaluation of the efficacy and safety of *Salvia officinalis* in controlling hot flashes in prostate cancer patients treated with androgen deprivation. *Phytother Res*. 2012 Feb;26(2):208-13.
Vogl, S. et al. Ethnopharmacological *in vitro* studies on Austria's folk medicine-an unexplored lore *in vitro* anti-inflammatory activities of 71 Austrian traditional herbal drugs. *J Ethnopharmacology*. 2013 Oct;149(3):750-71.

SAINT JOHN'S WORT

GENERAL REFERENCES: 1) p. 214; 2) p. 359; 3); 4) p. 159; 5) p. 321; 11) p. 80; 12) p. 396; 14); 16) pp. 266, 304; 17); 18) p. 152; 20) pp. 1038-9; 21) p. 424; 23) p. 173; 24) p. 192; 25) p. 338; 29); 31); 36); 37) p. 565; 41) p. 692; 44) p. 344; 45) p. 365; 46) p. 62; 53) p. 294; 55) p. 250; 62) p. 359; 64) p. 199; 66) p. 103; 68) p. 275; 69) p. 122; 70) p. 307; 71); 73); 75); 76); 79) p. 414; 80) p. 307; 81).

Barbagallo, C., Chisari, G. Antimicrobial activity of three Hypericum species. *Filoterapia*. 1987;58:175-7.
Baureithel, K. et al. Inhibition of benzodiazepine binding *in vitro* by amentoflavone, a constituent of various species of Hypericum. *Pharm Acta Helv*. 1997;72(3):153-7.
Bone, T. Safety issues in herbal medicine. *Townsend Letter*. 2001;Oct:144-8.
Brondz, T. et al. The relative stereochemistry of hyperforin-an antibiotic from *Hypericum perforatum* L. *Tetrahedron Letter*. 1982;23:1299-1300.
Butterweck, V. Mechanism of action of St. John's Wort in depression: what is known? *CNS Drugs*. 2003;17:539-62.
Chatterjee, S. et al. Hyperforin as a possible antidepressant component of Hypericum extracts. *Life Sciences*. 1998;63(6):499-510.
Cott, J. *In vitro* receptor binding and enzyme inhibition by *Hypericum perforatum* extract. *Pharmacopsychiatry*. 1997;30(2):108-112.
Couldwell, T. et al. Hypericin: a potential antiglioma therapy. *Neurosurgery*. 1994;35:705-10.
Darbinian-Sarkissian, N. et al. P27(SJ) novel protein in St John's Wort that suppresses expression of HIV-1 genome. *Genetic Ther*. 2006;13(4):288.
Demisch, L. et al. Influence of subchronic Hyperforat administration on melatonin production. *Pharmacopsychiatry*. 1991;24.
Dona, M. et al. Hyperforin inhibits cancer invasion and metastasis. *Cancer Research*. 2004;64(17):6225-32.
Fava, M. et al. A double-blind, randomized trial of St. John's wort, fluoxetine, and placebo in major depressive disorder. *J Clin Phychopharmacol*. 2005;25(5):441-7.
Franklin, M. et al. Sub-chronic treatment with an extract of *Hypericum perforatum* (St John's wort) significantly reduces cortisol and corticosterone in the rat brain. *European Neuropsychopharmacology*. 2004;14(1):7-10.
Gastpar, M. et al. Efficacy and tolerability of hypericum extract STW3 in long-term treatment with a once-daily dosage in comparison with sertraline. *Pharmacopsychiatry*. 2005;38(2):78-86.
Geller, S., Studee, L. Botanical and dietary supplements for menopausal symptoms. *J Women's Health*. 2005;14(7):634-49.
Gilani, A. et al. Antispasmodic and bronchodilator activities of St. John's wort are putatively mediated through dual inhibition of calcium influx and phosphodiesterase. *Fundamental Clinical Pharmacology*. 2005;19(6):695-705.
Grube, B. et al. St. John's wort extract: efficacy for menopausal symptoms of psychological origin. *Advances in Therapy*. 1999;16(4):177-86.
Gulick, R. et al. Phase I studies of hypericin, the active compound in St. John's wort, as an antiretroviral agent in HIV-infected adults. AIDS Clinical Trials Group Protocols 150 and 258. *Ann Intern Med*. 1999 Mar 16;130(6):510-4.
Hall, S. et al. The interaction between St. John's wort and an oral contraceptive. *Clinical Pharmacology Ther*. 2003;74(6):525-35.
Herold, A. et al. Antioxidant properties of some hydroalcoholic plant extracts with anti-inflammatory activity. *Roumanian Arch Microbial Immunology*. 2003;62(3-4):217-2.
James, J. *AIDS Treatment News*. 1989;74:91.
Jobst, K. et al. Safety of St. John's wort (*Hypericum perforatum*). *Lancet*. 2000;355(9203):575.
Kapsokalyvas, D. et al. Does *Hypericum perforatum* L. extract show any specificity as photosensitizer for HL-60 leukemic cells and cord blood hemopoietic progenitors during photodynamic therapy? *J Photochem Photobiol B*. 2005;80(3):208-16.
Kerb, R. et al. Single-dose and steady-state pharmacokinetics of hypericin and pseudohypericin. *Antimicrob Agents Chemother*. 1996;40(9):2087.
Lavie, G. et al. Studies of the mechanisms of action of the antiretroviral agents hypericin and pseudohypericin. *Proceedings of the National Academy of Science USA*. 1989;86:5963-7.
___________. The chemical and biological properties of hypericin-a compound with a broad spectrum of biological activities. *Medicinal Research Reviews*. 1995;15:111-119.
Lee, A. et al. The safety of St. John's wort (*Hypericum perforatum*) during breast-feeding. *J Clin Psychiatry*. 2003;64(8):966-8.
Linde, K. et al. St. John's wort for depression-an overview and meta-analysis of randomized clinical trials. *British Medical Journal*. 1996;313:253-8.
____________. St. John's wort for major depression. *Cochrane Database Syst Rev*. 2008 Oct 8;(4):CD000448.
Lopez-Bazzocchi, I. et al. Antiviral activity of the photoactive plant pigment hypericin. *Phytochem Photobiol*. 1991;54:95-98.
Lu, Y. et al. Neuroprotective effects of *H. perforatum* on trauma induced by hydrogen peroxide in PC12 cells. *Am J Chinese Med*. 2004;32(3):397.
Madabushi, R. et al. Hyperforin in St. John's wort drug interactions. *European J Clin Pharmacology*. 2006 Feb 14;1-9.
Mannel, M. et al. Oral hypericum extract LI 160 is an effective treatment of recurrent herpes genitalis and herpes labialis. Paper presented at the 3rd International Congress on Phytomedicine in Munich, Germany. Oct. 11-13, 2000.
Martinez, B. et al. Hypericum in the treatment of seasonal affective disorders. *J Geriatric Psychiatry and Neurology*. 1994;7(1):S29-33.
Martinez-Poveda, B. Hyperforin, a bio-active compound of St. John's Wort, is a new inhibitor of angiogenesis targeting several key steps of the process. *Int J Cancer*. 2005;117(5):775-80.
Meruelo, D. et al. Therapeutic agents with dramatic antiretroviral activity and little toxicity at effective doses: aromatic polycyclic diones hypericin and pseudohypericin. *Proc National Academy of Science. USA*. 1988;85:5230-4.
Moretti, M. et al. Evaluating the safety of St. John's Wort in human pregnancy. *Reprod Toxicol*. 2009 Jul;28(1):96-9.
Muller, W. et al. Effects of Hypericum extract LI 160 on neurotransmitter uptake systems and adrenergic receptor density. 2nd International Congress on Phytomedicine. Munich, Germany; 1996.
____________. Effects of Hypericum extract (LI 160) in biochemical models of antidepressant activity. *Pharmacopsychiatry*. 1997;30(2):102-7.
Mulry, M. St. John's Wort: Conference Report. *HerbalGram*. 1999;45:65.
Murch, S. et al. Melatonin in feverfew and other medicinal plants. *Lancet*. 1997;350:1598-9.
Nahrstedt, A., Butterweck, V. Biologically active and other chemical constituents of the herb of *Hypericum perforatum*. *Pharmacopsychiatry*. 1997; 30:129-34.
Neary, J., Bu, Y. Hypericum LI 160 inhibits uptake of serotonin and norepinepherine in astrocytes. *Brain Research*. 1999;816:358-63.
Pabuccuoglu, A. The *in vitro* effects of Hypericum species on human leukocyte myeloperoxidase activity. *J Ethnopharmacol*. 2003;87(1):89-92.
Pal, D., Mitra, A. MDR- and CYP3A4-mediated drug-herbal interactions. *Life Science*. 2006 Mar 27;78(18):2131-45.
Panossian, A. et al. Immunosuppressive effects of hypericin on stimulated human leukocytes: inhibition of arachidonic acid release, leukotriene B4, and interleukin-1 production and activation of nitric oxide formation. *Phytomedicine*. 1996;3:19-28.
Pfrunder, A. et al. Interaction of St. John's wort with low-dose oral contraceptive therapy: a randomized controlled trial. *Br J Clin Pharmacology*. 2003;56(6):683-90.
Philipp, M. et al. Hypericum extract versus imipramine or placebo in patients with moderate depression: randomized multicenter study of treatment for 8 weeks. *British Medical J*. 1999;319:1534-9.
Piscitelli, S. et al. Indinavir concentrations and St. John's wort. *Lancet*. 2000;355(9203):548.
Roder, C. et al. Meta-analysis of effectiveness and tolerability of treatment of mild to moderate depression with St. John's Wort. *Fortschr Neurol Psychiatr*. 2004;72(6):330-43.
Roscetti, G. et al. Cytotoxic activity of *Hypericum perforatum* L. on K562 erythroleukemic cells: differential effects between methanolic extract and hypericin. *Phytotherapy Research*. 2004;18(1):66-72.
Sakar, M., Tamer, A. Antimicrobial activity of different extracts from some Hypericum species. *Fitoterapia*. 1990;61:464-6.
Saljic, J. Ointment for the treatment of burns. *Geriatric Offen*. 1975;2:406-452.
Samadi, S. et al. The effect of *Hypericum perforatum* on the wound healing and scar of cesarean. *J Alternative Complementary Med*. 2010;16(1): 113-7.
Schempp, C. et al. Topical treatment of atopic dermatitis with St. John's wort cream-a randomized, placebo controlled, double blind half-side comparison. *Phytomedicine*. 2003;10(4):31-7.
Schrader, E. et al. Equivalence of St. John's wort extract (Ze 117) and fluoxetine: a randomized, controlled study in mild-moderate depression. *Int Clinical Psychopharm*. 2000;15:61-8.
Schroeder, C. Influence of St. John's wort on catecholamine turnover and cardiovascular regulation in humans. *Clin Pharmac Ther*. 2004;76(5):480-9.
Schulz, V. Safety of St. John's Wort extract compared to synthetic antidepressants. *Phytomedicine*. 2006;13(3):199-204.
Silva, B. et al. Neuroprotective effect of *H. perforatum* extracts on beta-amyloid-induced neurotoxicity. *Neurotox Res*. 2004;6(2):119-30.
Skalkos, D. et al. The lipophilic extract of *Hypericum perforatum* exerts significant cytotoxic activity against T24 and NBT-II urinary bladder tumor cells. *Planta Medica*. 2005 Nov;71(11):1030-5.
Steinbeck, K., Wernet, P. Successful long-term treatment over 40 months of HIV-patients with intravenous hypericin. International Conference on AIDS in Germany. 1993: Abstract #PO-B26-2012.
Stock, S., Holzl, J. Pharmacokinetic tests of [C]-labeled hypericin and pseudohypericin from *Hypericum perforatum* and serum kinetics of hypericin in man. *Planta Medica*. 1991;57(2):A61.

Szegedi, A. et al. Acute treatment of moderate to severe depression with hypericum extract WS 5570 (St John's wort): randomized controlled double-blind non-inferiority trial versus paroxetine. *British Medical J.* 2005;330(7490):503.
Taylor, L., Kobak, K. An open-label trial of St. John's wort (*H. perforatum*) in obsessive-compulsive disorder. *J Clin Psychiatry.* 2000;61(8):575.
Tedeschi, E. et al. Anti-inflammatory actions of St. John's wort: inhibition of human inducible nitric-oxide synthase expression by down-regulating signal transducer and activator of transcription-1alpha (STAT-1alpha) activation. *J Pharmacol Exp Ther.* 2003;307(1):254-61.
Thiele, B. et al. Modulation of cytokine expression by *Hypericum* extract. *J Geriatric Psychiatry Neurology.* 1994;7(1):S60-62.
Uebelhack, R. et al. Black Cohosh and St. John's Wort for Climacteric Complaints: A Randomized Trial. *Obstetrics Gynecology.* 2006 Feb;107(2): 247-55.
Upton, R. (Ed.). Monograph: St. John's Wort. American Herbal Pharmacopoeia. *HerbalGram.* 1997;40:S1-32.
Volz, H. et al. St. John's wort extract (LI 160) in somatoform disorders: results of a placebo-controlled trial. *Psychopharmacology.* 2002;164(3):294.
Vorbach, E. et al. Efficacy and tolerability of St. John's wort extract LI 160 verses imipramine in patients with severe depressive episodes according to ICD-10. *Pharmacopsychiatry.* 1997;30(2):81-5.
Weber, N. et al. The antiviral agent hypericin has *in vitro* activity against HSV-1 through non-specific associations with viral and cellular membranes. *Antiviral Chemistry & Chemotherapy.* 1994;5:83-90.
Wheatley, D. LI 160, an extract of St. John's wort, verses amitriptyline in mildly to moderately depressed outpatients: A controlled 6-week study. *Pharmacopsychiatry.* 1997;30(2):77-80.
Wilasrusmee, C. et al. *In vitro* immunomodulatory effects of ten commonly used herbs on murine lymphocytes. *J Alternative & Complementary Med.* 2002;8(4):467-475.
Winkler, C. et al. St. John's wort counteracts cytokine-induced tryptophan catabolism *in vitro. Biol Chem.* 2004;385(12):1197-202.
Woelk, H. et al. Benefits and risks of the hypericum extract LI 160: drug monitoring study with 3250 patients. *J Geriatr Psychiatry Neurol.* 1994 Oct;7(1):S34-8.
Wood, S. et al. Antiviral activity of naturally occurring anthraquinones and anthraquinone derivatives. *Planta Medica.* 1990;56:651-2.
Zou, Y. et al. Hypocholesterolemic effects of a flavonoid-rich extract of *Hypericum perforatum* L. in rats fed a cholesterol-rich diet. *J Agric Food Chem.* 2005;53(7):2462-6.

SCULLCAP

GENERAL REFERENCES: 3) p. 237; 5) p. 339; 8) p. 269; 9) p. 687;10) p. 396; 16) p. 281; 17);18) p. 123; 19) p. 291; 20) p. 390; 21) p. 625; 25) p. 330; 28) p. 147; 31); 33) p. 724; 35); 36) pp. 465, 494, 515-7, 582; 37) p. 533; 40) p. 279; 41) p. 693; 42) p. 313; 44) p. 356; 46) p. 105; 47) p. 113; 48); 51) pp. 165, 217, 225; 55) p. 239; 57) p. 229; 62) p. 346; 64); 66) p. 107; 71); 74) p. 90; 79) p. 396; 81).
Awad, R. et al. Phytochemical and biological analysis of skullcap (*Scutellaria lateriflora* L.): a medicinal plant with anxiolytic properties. *Phytomedicine.* 2003;10(8):640-9.
Bergner, P. Scullcap (*Scutellaria lateriflora*). *Medical Herbalism.* 2002;13(2):15-17.
Brock, C. et al. American Scullcap (*Scutellaria lateriflora*): A randomized, double-blind placebo-controlled crossover study of its effects on mood in healthy volunteers. *Phytotherapy Res.* 2014 May;28(5):692-8.
Cole, I. et al. Comparisons of *Scutellaria baicalensis, Scutellaria lateriflora* and *Scutellaria racemosa*: genome size, antioxidant potential and phytochemistry. *Planta Med.* 2008 Mar;74(4):474-81.
Gafner, S. et al. Inhibition of [3H]-LSD binding to 5-HT7 receptors by flavonoids from *Scutellaria lateriflora. J Nat Prod.* 2003 Apr;66(4):535-7.
____________. Analysis of *Scutellaria lateriflora* and its adulterants *Teucrium canadense* and *Teucrium chamaedrys* by LC-UV/MS, TLC, and digital photomicroscopy. *J AOAC Int.* 2003 May-Jun;86(3):453-60.
Huang, Y. et al. Biological properties of baicalein in cardiovascular system. *Curr Drug Targets Cardiovasc Haematol Disord.* 2005 Apr;5(2):177-84.
Lim, B. Effects of wogonin, wogonoside, and 3,5,7,2,6-pentahydroxyflavone on chemical mediator production in peritoneal exudate cells and immunoglobulin E of rat mesenteric lymph node lymphocytes. *J Ethnopharmacology.* 2003;84(1):23–9.
Lohani, M. et al. Anti-oxidative and DNA protecting effects of flavonoids-rich *Scutellaria lateriflora. Nat Prod Commun.* 2013 Oct;8(10):1415-8.
Millspaugh, C. *American Medicinal Plants, an illustrated and descriptive guide to the American plants used as homeopathic remedies.* New York,NY: Boericke & Tafel, 1887.
Peigen, X., Keji, C. Recent advances in clinical studies of Chinese medicinal herbs. 1. Drugs affecting the cardiovascular system. *Phytotherapy Research.* 1987;1:53-7.
Peredery, O., Persinger, M. Herbal treatment following post-seizure induction in rat by lithium pilocarpine: *Scutellaria lateriflora* (Skullcap), *Gelsemium sempervirens* (Gelsemium) and *Datura stramonium* (Jimson Weed) may prevent development of spontaneous seizures. *Phytother Res.* 2004;18(9):700-5.
Shi, X. et al. Scutellarein inhibits cancer cell metastasis *in vitro* and attenuates the development of fibrosarcoma *in vivo. Int J Mol Med.* 2015 Jan; 35(1):31-8.
Wojcikowski, K. et al. An *in vitro* investigation of herbs traditionally used for kidney and urinary system disorders: potential therapeutic and toxic effects. *Nephrology.* 2009 Feb;14(1):70-9.
Wolfson, P., Hoffmann, D. An investigation into the efficacy of *Scutellaria lateriflora* in healthy volunteers. *Alternative Therapies in Health and Medicine.* 2003 March-April;9(2):74-8.

SENNA

1) p. 204; 2) p. 341; 8) p. 188; 14) p. 277; 16) p. 174; 17); 20); 21); 24) p. 184; 25) p. 328; 33) p. 734; 36) p. 582; 37) p. 210; 42) p. 312; 43) p. 459; 44) p. 351; 46) pp. 106, 178, 184; 55) p. 243; 62) p. 343; 64) p. 168; 66) p. 106; 68) p. 297; 69) p. 49; 75) p. 107; 79) 400; 81) p. 167.
Agarwal, V., Bajpai, M. Pharmacognostical and biological studies on senna and its products: an overview. *Int J Pharma and Bio Sciences.* 2010; 1(2):1-10.
Agra, Y. Efficacy of senna versus lactulose in terminal cancer patients treated with opioids. *J Pain Symptom Manage.* 1998;15(1):1-7.
Bailey, S. et al. A trial to assess the effectiveness of bowel preparation prior to intravenous urography. *Clinical Radiology.* 1991;44(5):335-7.
Bensky, D., Gamble, A., Kaptchuk, T. *Chinese Herbal Medicine Materia Medica.* Seattle, WA: Eastland Press, 1993;118.
Brouwers, J. et al. A controlled trial of senna preparations and other laxatives used for bowel cleansing prior to radiological examination. *Pharmacology.* 1980;20(1):58-64.
Kinnunen, O. et al. Safety and efficacy of a bulk laxative containing senna versus lactulose in the treatment of chronic constipation in geriatric patients. *Pharmacology.* 1993 Oct;47(1):253-5.
Sonmez, A. et al. Subacute cholestatic hepatitis likely related to use of senna for chronic constipation. *Acta Gastroenterol Belg.* 2005;68(3):385-7.
Valverde, A. Senna vs polyethylene glycol for mechanical preparation the evening before elective colonic or rectal resection: a multicenter controlled trial. French Association for Surgical Research. *Arch Surg.* 1999;134(5):514-9.
Vanderperren, B. et al. Acute liver failure with renal impairment related to the abuse of senna anthraquinone glycosides. *Ann Pharmacother.* 2005;39(7-8):1353-1357.
Vradelis, S. et al. Addition of senna improves quality of colonoscopy preparation with magnesium citrate. *World J Gastroenterol.* 2009;15(14): 1759-1763.
Wang, X. et al. Screening and identification of proteins mediating senna induced gastrointestinal motility enhancement in mouse colon. *World J Gastroenterol.* 2002;8(1):162-7.
Ziegenhagen, D. et al. Senna vs. bisacodyl in addition to Golytely lavage for colonscopy preparation-a prospective randomized trial. *Z Gastroenterology.* 1992;30(1):17-19.

STINGING NETTLE

GENERAL REFERENCES: 1) pp. 216, 217; 2) p. 367; 3) p. 184; 5) p. 271; 9) p. 721; 11) p. 106; 14); 16) p. 217; 18) p. 355; 20) p. 2032; 21) p. 684; 23) p. 153; 25) p. 340; 27) p. 239; 28); 30); 31); 33) p. 574; 36); 37) p. 439; 42) p. 288; 43); 44) p. 308; 45) p. 307; 46) p. 119; 48); 49) p. 579; 55) p. 201; 62) p. 265; 63) p. 142; 64) p. 333; 66) p. 89; 67); 69) p. 84; 72) p 165; 79) p. 313; 80) p. 479; 81).
Berges, R. et al. Randomized, placebo-controlled, double-blind clinical trial of beta-sitosterol in patients with BPH. *Lancet.* 1995;345:1529-32.
Broncano, J. et al. A study of different preparations of *Urtica dioica* L sobre SNC. *An R Acad Farm.* 1987;53:284-91.
Collier, H., Chesher, G. Identification of 5-hydroxytryptamine in the sting of the nettle (*Urtica dioica*). *British J Pharmacology.* 1956;11:186-9.
Dean, K. Saw Palmetto, Nettles, and Pygeum for male pattern baldness. *HerbalGram.* 2000;49:31.

Engelman, U. et al. Efficacy and safety of a combination of Sabal and Urtica extract in lower urinary tract symptoms. A randomized, double-blind study versus tamsulosin. *Arzneimittel-Forschung.* 2006;56(3):222-9.
Engels, G., Brinckmann, J. Stinging Nettle. *HerbalGram.* 2016;100:8-17.
Hartman, R. et al. Inhibition of 5-a-reductase and aromatase by PHL-00801 (Prostatonin), a combination of PY 102 (*Pygeum africanum*) and UR 102 (*Urtica dioica*) extracts. *Phytomedicine.* 1996;3(2):121-128.
Hiermann, A. The contents of sabal fruits and testing of their anti-inflammatory effect. *Archiv der Pharmazie.* 1989;322:111-114.
Khajeh-Mehrizi, R. et al. The effects of *Uticaria dioica* extract on glycemic control and insulin resistance indices in patients with type 2 diabetes: a randomized double-blind clinical trial. *Iranian Journal of Diabetes and Obesity.* 2014;6(4):149-155.
Kirchhoff, H. Brennesselsaft als diuretikum. *Z Phytother.* 1983;4:621-6.
Kraus, R. et al. (10-E, 12Z)-9-hydroxy-10,12-octadecadienic acid, an aromatase inhibiting substance from the root extract of *Urtica dioica. Liebigs Ann Chem.* 1991;19:335-339.
Krzeski, T. et al. Combined extracts of *Urtica dioica* and *Pygeum africanum* in the treatment of BPH: double-blind comparison of two doses. *Clinical Therapeutics.* 1993;15(6):1011-20.
Lopatkin, N. et al. Long-term efficacy and safety of a combination of Sabal and Urtica extract for lower urinary tract symptoms: a placebo-controlled, double-blind, multicenter trial. *World Journal of Urology.* 2005;23(2):139-146.
Maitai, C. et al. Effect of extract of hairs from the herb *Urtica massaica* in smooth muscle. *Toxicon.* 1980;18:225-9.
Mittman, P. Randomized, double-blind study of freeze-dried *Urtica dioica* in the treatment of allergic rhinitis. *Planta Medica.* 1990;56(1):44-7.
Namazi, N. et al. Effect of hydroalcoholic Nettle (*Urtica dioica*) extract on some cardiovascular risk factors in patients with type 2 diabetes. *J Med Science.* 2011-a;11(3):138-144.
_____________. The effect of hydro alcoholic Nettle (*Urtica dioica*) extracts on insulin sensitivity and some inflammatory indicators in patients with type 2 diabetes: a randomized double-blind control trial. *Pakistan J Biol Sci.* 2011-b. Aug 1;14(15):775-9.
_____________. The effect of hydro alcoholic nettle (*Urtica dioica*) extract on oxidative stress in patients with type 2 diabetes: a randomized double-blind clinical trial. *Pakistan J Biol Sci.* 2012 Jan 15;15(2):98-102.
Obertreis, B. et al. Anti-inflammatory effect of *Urtica dioica folia* extract in comparison to caffeic malic acid. *Arzneimittel-Forsch.* 1996;46(1):52-6.
______________. *In-vivo in-vitro* inhibition of lipopolysaccharide-stimulated tumor necrosis factor and interleukin-1 secretion in human whole blood extractum *Urticae dioicae folium. Arzneimittel-Forschung.* 1996;46(4):389-94.
Ramm, S., Hansen, C. Brennessel-Extrakt bei rheumatischen Beschwerden. *Dtsch Apoth Ztg.* 1995;135:3-8.
Randell, C. Stinging nettles for osteoarthritis pain of the hip (letter). *British Journal of General Practice.* 1994;44:533-4.
________. Nettle sting of *Urtica dioica* for joint pain-an exploratory study of this complementary therapy. *Complementary Therapies in Medicine.* 1999;7(3):126-31.
________. Randomized controlled trial of nettle sting for treatment of base-of-thumb pain. *J Royal Society Medicine.* 2000;93(6):305-9.
Safarinejad, M. *Urtica dioica* for treatment of benign prostatic hyperplasia: prospective, randomized, double-blind, placebo-controlled, crossover study. *J Herb Pharmacotherapy.* 2005;5(4):1-11.
Saxena, P. et al. Identification of pharmacologically active substances in the Indian stinging nettle, *Urtica Parviflora* (Roxb.) *Canadian Journal of Physiol Pharmaco.* 1965;43:869-76.
Schneider, H. et al. Treatment of benign prostatic hyperplasia: results of a treatment study with phytogenic combination of Sabal extract WS 1473 and Urtica extact WS 1031 in urologic specialty practices. *Fortschritte der Medizin.* 1995;113(3):37-40.
Schottner, M. et al. Lignans from roots of *U. dioica* and their metabolites bind to human sex hormone bonding globulin. *Planta Medica.* 1997;63:529.
Sokeland, J., Albrecht, J. Combination of Sabal and Urtica extract vs. finasteride in benign prostatic hyperplasia (Aiken stages I to II). Comparison of therapeutic effectiveness in a one-year double-blind study. *Urologe A.* 1997;36(4):327-33.
Sokeland, J. Combined sabal and urtica extract compared with finasteride in men with benign prostatic hyperplasia: analysis of prostate volume and therapeutic outcome. *British J Urology.* 2000:(86);439-42.
Stahl, H. Treatment of prostatic nocturia with standardized extract of *Radix Urticae. Zeitschrift Allgemeiner Medizin.* 1984;60:128-32.
Sturdivant, L., Blakley, T. *Medicinal Herbs in the Garden, Field & Marketplace.* Friday Harbor, WA: San Juan Naturals, 1999;225.
Testai, L. et al. Cardiovascular effects of *Urtica dioica* root extract. *Journal of Ethnopharmacology.* 2002;81(1):105-9.
Wagner, H. et al. Search for the antiprostatic principle of stinging nettle (*Urtica dioica*) roots. *Phytomedicine.* 1994;1:213-24.
_____________. Studies on the binding of *Urtica dioica* agglutinin (UDA) and other lectins in an *in vitro* epidermal growth factor receptor test. *Phytomedicine.* 1995;4:287-90.

THYME

GENERAL REFERENCES: 1) p. 219; 2) p. 376; 3) p. 64; 5) p. 351; 8) p. 228; 9) p. 715; 11) p. 183; 12) p. 278; 14); 16) p. 297; 17); 20) p. 1936; 21) p. 674; 23) p. 189; 24) p. 198; 25) p. 358; 29) p. 570; 33) p. 808; 35); 36) p. 589; 37) p. 219; 42) p. 320; 43) p. 464; 44) p. 378; 46) p. 116; 55) p. 256; 57) p. 239; 62) p. 372; 63); 64) p. 386; 66) p. 109; 69) pp. 90, 96; 75) pp. 208-9, 219, 267, 348; 79) p. 430; 81).
Agbor, G. Antioxidant capacity of some herbs/spices from Cameroon comparative study of two methods. *J Agric Food Chem.* 2005;53(17):6819.
Bahadoran, P. et al. Investigating the therapeutic effect of vaginal cream containing garlic and thyme compared to clotrimazole cream for the treatment of mycotic vaginitis. *Iran J Nurs Midwifery Res.* 2010 Dec;15(1):343-9.
Bonjar, G. Inhibition of Clotrimazole-resistant *Candida albicans* by plants used in Iranian folkloric medicine. *Fitoterapia.* 2004;75(1):74-6.
Boskabady, M. et al. Relaxant effect of *T. vulgaris* on guinea-pig tracheal chains and its possible mechanism(s). *Phytother Res.* 2006;(1):28-33.
Bozin, B. et al. Characterization of the volatile composition of essential oils of some *Lamiaceae* spices and the antimicrobial and antioxidant activities of the entire oils. *J Agric Food Chem.* 2006;54(5):1822-8.
Direkvand-Moghadam, A., Khosravi, A. The impact of a novel herbal Shirazi *Thymus Vulgaris* on primary dysmenorrhea in comparison to the classical chemical Ibuprofen. *J Res Med Sci.* 2012 Jul;17(7):668-70.
Engels, G. Thyme (*Thymus vulgaris*). *HerbalGram.* 2008;80:1-2.
Ernst, E. et al. A controlled multi-center study of herbal versus synthetic secretolytic drugs for acute bronchitis. *Phytomedicine.* 1997;4(4):287-93.
Giorgani, R. et al. Antifungal effect of various essential oils against *Candida albicans.* Potentiation of antifungal action of amphotericin B by essential oil from *Thymus vulgaris. Phytother Res.* 2004;18(12):990-5.
Grande, S. et al. Vasomodulating potential of Mediterranean wild plant extracts. *J Agric Food Chem.* 2004;52(16):5021-6.
Hersch-Martinez, P. et al. Antibacterial effects of commercial essential oils over locally prevalent pathogenic strains in Mexico. *Fitoterapia.* 2005; 76(5):453-7.
Kemmerich, B. et al. Efficacy and tolerability of a fluid extract combination of thyme herb and ivy leaves and matched placebo in adults suffering from acute bronchitis with productive cough. A prospective, double-blind, placebo-controlled clinical trial. *Arzneimittel-Forschung.* 2006;56(9):652-60.
_______________. Evaluation of efficacy and tolerability of a fixed combination of dry extracts of thyme herb and primrose root in adults suffering from acute bronchitis with productive cough. A prospective, double-blind, placebo-controlled multicentre clinical trial. *Arzneimittel-Forschung.* 2007;57(9):607-15.
Mohsin, A. et al. Analgesic, antipyretic activity and phytochemical screening of some plants used in traditional Arab system of medicine. *Fitoterapia.* 1989;60:174.
Nguefack, J. et al. Five essential oils from aromatic plants of Cameroon: their antibacterial activity and ability to permeabilize the cytoplasmic membrane of *Listeria innocua* examined by flow cytometry. *Lett Appl Microbiol.* 2004;39(5):395-400.
Nolkemper, S. et al. Antiviral effect of aqueous extracts from species of the *Lamiaceae* family against *Herpes simplex* virus type 1 and type 2 *in vitro. Planta Med.* 2006 Dec;72(15):1378-82.
Okazaki, K. et al. Human platelet aggregation inhibitors from thyme (*Thymus vulgaris* L.). *Phytother Res.* 2002;16(4):398-9.
Penalver, P. Antimicrobial activity of five essential oils against origin strains of the *Enterobacteriaceae* family. *APMIS.* 2005 Jan;113(1):1-6.
Pina-Vaz, C. et al. Antifungal activity of Thymus oils and their major compounds. *J Eur Acad Dermatol Venereol.* 2004;18(1):73-8.
Priestley, C. et al. Thymol, a constituent of thyme essential oil, is a positive allosteric modulator of human GABA(A) receptors and a homo-oligomeric GABA receptor from *Drosophila melanogaster. Br J Pharmacol.* 2003;140(8):1363-72.
Proestos, C. et al. RP-HPLC analysis of the phenolic compounds of plant extracts. Investigation of their antioxidant capacity and antimicrobial activity. *J Agric Food Chem.* 2005;53(4):1190-5.

Rasooli, I., Owlia, P. Chemoprevention by thyme oils of *Aspergillus parasiticus* growth and aflatoxin production. *Phytochem.* 2005;66(24):2851.
Rota, C. *In vitro* antimicrobial activity of essential oils from aromatic plants against selected foodborne pathogens. *J Food Prot.* 2004;67(6):1252-6.
Salmalian, H. et al. Comparative effect of *Thymus vulgaris* and ibuprofen on primary dysmenorrhea: A triple-blind clinical study. *Caspian J Intern Med.* 2014 Spring;5(2):82-8.
Tabak, M. et al. *In vitro* inhibition of *H. pylori* by extracts of thyme. *J Applied Bacteriology.* 1996;80:667-72.
Van Den Broucke, C., Lemli, J. Spasmolytic activity of the flavonoids from *Thymus vulgaris*. *Pharm Week Sci.* 1983 Feb 25;5(1):9-14.
Yamamoto, J. et al. Testing various herbs for antithrombotic effect. *Nutrition.* 2005;21(5):580-7.

VALERIAN

GENERAL REFERENCES: 1); 2) p. 394; 3); 4) p. 173; 5) p. 362; 8) p. 375; 9); 11) p. 188; 10) p. 434; 14) pp. 150, 312, 346, 358; 16); 17); 18); 20); 23) p. 192; 24) p. 202; 25) p. 362; 30) p. 256; 31); 33) p. 824; 35) p. 232; 36) p. 592; 37) p. 522; 42) p. 322; 43) p. 467; 44) p. 199; 45) p. 382; 46) p. 120; 51) pp. 12, 164, 215; 52) pp. 123-4, 149-58, 314-16; 53) p. 339; 54) p. 393; 55) p. 260; 57) p. 245; 62) p. 384; 63) p. 158; 66) p. 111; 68) p. 315; 69) p. 117; 73); 74) p. 17; 75) pp. 281-5; 76) pp. 32, 212, 226-9; 78) p. 229; 79) p. 440; 81).
Abourashed, E. et al. *In vitro* binding experiments with a Valerian, hops and their fixed combination extract (Ze91019) to selected central nervous system receptors. *Phytomedicine.* 2004 Nov;11(7-8):633-8.
Ammer, K., Melnizky, P. Medicinal baths for treatment of generalized fibromyalgia. *Forsch Komplementarmed.* 1999;6(2):80-5.
Benke, D. et al. GABA A receptors as *in vivo* substrate for the anxiolytic action of valerenic acid, a major constituent of valerian root extracts. *Neuropharmacology.* 2009 Jan;56(1):174-81.
Busanny-Caspari, E. et al. Indikationen: Funktionelle Herzbeschwerden Hyponie and Wetterfuhligkeit. *Therapiewoche.* 1986;(36):2545-50.
Cech, R. *Middle Earth Cultivation of Medicinals from the English Tradition.* Williams, OR. Horizon Herbs Publication, 1995.
Cerny, A., Schmid, K. Tolerability and efficacy of valerian/lemon balm in healthy volunteers (a double-blind, placebo-controlled, multicenter study). *Fitoterapia.* 1999;70:221-8.
De Feo, V., Faro, C. Pharmacological effects of extracts from *Valeriana adscendens* Trel. II. Effects on GABA uptake and amino acids. *Phytotherapy Research.* 2003 Jun;17(6):661-4.
Dietz, B. et al. Valerian extract and valerenic acid are partial agonists of the 5-HT5a receptor *in vitro*. *Molecular Brain Res.* 2005 Aug 18;138(2):191-7
Fields, A. et al. Analysis of responses to valerian root extract in the feline pulmonary vascular bed. *J Altern Complement Med.* 2003 Dec;9(6):909-18.
Frances, A., Dempster, R. Effect of valerian, *Valeriana edulis*, on sleep difficulties in children with intellectual deficits: randomized trial. *Phytomedicine.* 2002;9:273-9.
Fussel, A. et al. Effect of a fixed Valerian-Hop extract combination (Ze 91019) on sleep polygraphy in patients with non-organic insomnia: a pilot study. *European J Med Res.* 2000 Sep 18;5(9):385-90.
Granger, R. et al. (+)- And (-)-borneol: efficacious positive modulators of GABA action at human recombinant alpha 1 beta 2 gamma 2 L-GABA(A) receptors. *Biochem Pharmacol.* 2005 Apr 1;69(7):1101-11.
Gromball, J. et al. Hyperactivity, concentration difficulties and impulsiveness improve during seven weeks' treatment with valerian root and lemon balm extracts in primary school children. *Phytomed.* 2014;21(8-9):1098-1103.
Hazelhoff, B. et al. Antispasmodic effects of valeriana compounds: an *in-vivo* and *in-vitro* study on the guinea-pig ileum. *Arch Int Pharmacodyn Ther.* 1982 Jun;257(2):274-87.
Hobbs, C. *Valerian: The Relaxing and Sleep Herb.* Capitola, CA: Botanica Press, 1993.
Holst, L. et al. Use of herbal drugs during early pregnancy in relation to maternal characteristics and pregnancy outcome. *Pharmacoepidemiol Drug Safety.* 2008 Feb;17(2):151-9.
Holzl, J., Godau, P. Receptor binding studies with *Valeriana officinalis* on the benzodiazepine receptor. *Planta Medica.* 1989;55:642.
Kamm-Kohl, A. et al. Modern valerian therapy of nervous disorders in elderly patients (in German). *Medwelt.* 1984;35:1450-54.
Kneibel, R., Burchard, J. The treatment of depressive moods in medical practice (in German). *Zeitschrift Allgemeiner Medizin.* 1988;64:689-96.
Kuhlmann, J. et al. The influence of Valerian treatment on reaction time, alertness and concentration in volunteers. *Pharmacopsychiatry.* 1999;32(6): 235-41.
Leathwood, P. et al. Aqueous extract of valerian root improves sleep quality in man. Reduces sleep latency to fall asleep in man. *Pharmacol Biochem & Behav.* 1982 July;17(1):65-71.
Malva, J. et al. Neuroprotective properties of *Valeriana officinalis* extracts. *Neurotox Res.* 2004;6(2):131-40.
Mennini, T. et al. *In vitro* study on the interaction of extracts and pure compounds from *Valeriana officinalis* roots with GABA, benzodiazepine and barbiturate receptors in rat brain. *Fitoterapia.* 1993;54(4):291-300.
Morin, C. et al. Valerian-hops combination and diphenhydramine for treating insomnia: a randomized placebo-controlled clinical trial. *Sleep.* 2005 Nov 1;28(11):1465-71.
Muller, S., Klement, S. A combination of valerian and lemon balm is effective in the treatment of restlessness and dyssomnia in children. *Phytomedicine.* 2006 Jun;13(6):383-7.
Ortiz, J. et al. Effects of *Valeriana officinalis* extracts on [3H]flunitrazepam binding, synaptosomal [3H]GABA uptake, and hippocampal [3H]GABA release. *Neurochem Res.* 1999 Nov;24(11):1373-8.
Pakseresht, S. et al. Extract of valerian root (*Valeriana officinalis* L.) vs. placebo in treatment of obsessive-compulsive disorder: a randomized double-blind study. *J Complement Integr Med.* 2011 Oct 11;8.
Panijel, M. Die behandlung mittelschwerer angstzustande. *Therapiewoche.* 1985;41:4659-68.
Piccinelli, A. et al. New lignans from the roots of *Valeriana prionophylla* with antioxidative and vasorelaxant activities. *J Nat Prod.* 2004 Jul;67(7): 1135-40.
Santos, M. et al. An aqueous extract of Valerian influences transport of GABA in synaptosomes. *Planta Medica.* 1994;60:278-9.
____________. The amount of GABA present in aqueous extracts of Valerian is sufficient to account for [3H]GABA release in synaptosomes. *Planta Medica.* 1994;60:475-6.
Schellenberg, R. et al. Fixed combination of valerian and hops (Ze91019) acts via a central adenosine mechanism. Planta Med. 2004;70(7):594-7.
Schulz, V. et al. Clinical trials with phyto-psychopharmacological agents. *Phytomedicine.* 1997;4(4):379-87.
Takeda, S. et al. Pharmacological studies on iridoid compounds. III. The choleretic mechanism of iridoid compounds. *J Pharm Dyn.* 1981;4:612.
Vorbach, E. et al. Therapy for insomnia: efficacy and tolerability of a valerian preparation (in German). *Psychopharmakotherapie.* 1996;3(3):109.
Willey, L. Valerian Overdose: a Case Report. *Veterinary and Human Toxicology.* 1995;37(4):364-5.
Yang, G., Wang, W. Clinical studies on the treatment of coronary heart disease with *Valeriana officinalis* var *latifolia*. *Zhongguo Zhong Xi Yi Jie He Za Zhi.* 1994 Sep;14(9):540-2.
Ziegler, G. et al. Efficacy and tolerability of valerian extract LI 156 compared with oxazepam in the treatment of non-organic insomnia- a randomized, double-blind, comparative clinical study. *European J Med Res.* 2002 Nov 25;7(11):480-6.

WOOD BETONY

GENERAL REFERENCES: 8) p. 389; 11) p. 17; 12) p. 399; 14) p. 53; 16) p. 315; 29) p. 714; 33) p. 97; 35) pp. 29, 65, 72-3, 141; 36) pp. 122, 517, 585; 37) p. 538; 42) p. 331; 44) p. 116; 46) p. 109; 51) pp. 208, 216, 224-5; 63) pp. 14, 46, 161; 64) pp. 123, 355; 62) p. 45; 66) p. 37; 68) p. 43; 79) p. 455; 80) pp. 165; 81) pp. 211, 396; 82) pp. 13, 15, 54, 98, 159, 187, 209-11.
Háznagy-Radnai, E. et al. Anti-inflammatory activities of Hungarian *Stachys* species and their iridoids. *Phytother Res.* 2012 Apr;26(4):505-9.
Lazarevi, J. et al. Chemical composition and antimicrobial activity of the essential oil of *Stachys officinalis* (L.) Trevis. (*Lamiaceae*). *Chem Biodivers.* 2013 Jul;10(7):1335-49.
Matkowski, A., Piotrowska, M. Antioxidant and free radical scavenging activities of some medicinal plants from the *Lamiaceae*. *Fitoterapia.* 2006;77(5):346-53.
Miyase, T. et al. Phenylethanoid glycosides from Stachys officinalis. *Phytochemistry.* 1996;43(2):475-9.
Zinchenko, T., Fefer, I. Investigation of glycosides from *Betonica officinalis*. *Farmatsevt Zhurnal.* 1962;17(3):35-8.

YARROW

1) p. 233; 2) p. 419; 3) pp. 137, 146, 147, 171, 181; 5) p. 378; 8) p. 213; 9); 10) p. 462; 11) p. 204; 12) p. 508; 13) p. 10; 14) pp. 53, 399; 16) p. 318; 17); 18); 19) pp. 397, 400; 20); 21); 23) p. 202; 25) p. 376; 29) p. 1072; 30); 31); 33) p. 863; 35) p. 237; 36) p. 523; 37) p. 748; 40) p. 17; 41); 42) p. 332; 43); 44) p. 271; 46) pp. 171, 184; 48) pp. 122, 166, 229, 251; 49); 52) p. 285; 55) p. 271; 62) p. 398; 63) p. 162; 64) p. 161; 66) p. 116;

67); 70); 73) pp. 13, 44, 49, 143; 74) pp. 32, 55, 145; 78) pp. 134, 148, 149, 168; 79) p. 462; 81); 82) pp. 48, 50-1, 98, 117, 122, 125.
Benedek, B. et al. Choleretic effects of yarrow (*Achillea millefolium* s.l.) in the isolated perfused rat liver. *Phytomedicine*. 2006 Nov;13(9-10):702-6.
Benedek, B., Kopp, B. *Achillea millefolium* s.l. revisited: recent findings confirm the traditional use. *Wien Med Wochenschr*. 2007;157(13-14):312-4.
Borrelli, F. et al. Prokinetic effect of a standardized yarrow (*Achillea millefolium*) extract and its constituent choline: studies in the mouse and human stomach. *Neurogastroenterol Motil*. 2012 Feb;24(2):164-71.
Candan, F. et al. Antioxidant and antimicrobial activity of the essential oil and methanol extracts of *Achillea millefolium* subsp. *millefolium Afan. (Asteraceae)*. *Journal of Ethnopharmacology*. 2003;87(2-3):215-20.
Cavalcanti, A. et al. Safety and antiulcer efficacy studies of *Achillea millefolium* L. after chronic treatment in Wistar rats. *J Ethnopharmacol*. 2006 Sep 19;107(2):277-84.
Chandler, R. et al. Herbal remedies of the Maritime Indians: sterols and triterpenes of *Achillea millefolium* L. (Yarrow). *Journal of Pharm Science*. 1982 June;71(6):690-3.
Chou, S. et al. *Achillea millefolium* L. Essential Oil Inhibits LPS-Induced Oxidative Stress and Nitric Oxide Production in RAW 264.7 Macrophages. *Int J Mol Sci*. 2013 Jun 24;14(7):12978-93.
Goldberg, A. et al. Isolation of anti-inflammatory principles from *Achillea millefollium (Compositae)*. *J Pharm Sci*. 1969;58:938-41.
Haidara, K. et al. The flavonoid Casticin has multiple mechanisms of tumor cytotoxicity action. *Cancer Lett*. 2006 Oct 28;242(2):180-90.
Innocenti, G. et al. *In vitro* estrogenic activity of *Achillea millefolium* L. *Phytomedicine*. 2007 Feb;14(2-3):147-52.
Konyalioglu, S., Karamenderes, C. The protective effects of *Achillea* L. species native in Turkey against H(2)O(2)-induced oxidative damage in human erythrocytes and leucocytes. *Journal of Ethnopharmacology*. 2005;102(2):221-7.
Kudrzycka-Bieloszabska, F., Glowniak, K. Pharmacodynamic properties of oleum chamomillae and oleum millefolii. *Diss Pharm Pharmacol*. 1966;18:449-54.
Lemmens-Gruber, R. et al. Investigation of the spasmolytic activity of the flavonoid fraction of *Achillea millefolium* s.l. on isolated guinea-pig ilea. *Arzneimittel-Forschung*. 2006;56(8):582-8.
Miller, F., Chow, L. Alkaloids of *Achillea millefolium* L.I. Isolation and characterization of Achilleine. *J Am Chem Soc*. 1954;76:1353-4.
Molochko, V. et al. The antistaphylococcal properties of plant extracts in relation to their prospective use as therapeutic and prophylactic formulations for the skin. *Vestn Dermatol Venerol*. 1990;(8):54-6.
Molokovskii, D. et al. The action of adaptogenic plant preparations in experimental alloxan diabetes. *Probl Endokrinol* (Moskow). 1989 Nov-Dec;35(6):82-7.
Shipochliev, T., Fournadjiev, G. Spectrum of the anti-inflammatory effect of *Arctostaphylos uva ursi* and *Achillea milefolium*. *Probl Vutr Med*. 1984; 12:99-107.
Stojanovic, G. et al. *In vitro* antimicrobial activity of extracts of four *Achillea* species: the composition of *Achillea clavennae* L. (*Asteraceae*) extract. *Journal of Ethnopharmacology*. 2005;101(1-3):185-90.
Vahid, S. et al. Effect of herbal medicine *Achillea millefolium* on plasma nitrite and nitrate levels in patients with chronic kidney disease: a preliminary study. *Iran J Kidney Dis*. 2012 Sep;6(5):350-4.
Wood, M. *The Book of Herbal Wisdom*. Berkeley, CA: North Atlantic Books, 1997;70.
Yaeesh, S. et al. Studies on hepatoprotective, antispasmodic and calcium antagonist activities of the aqueous-methanol extract of *Achillea millefolium*. *Phytother Res*. 2006 Jul;20(7):546-51.

YELLOW DOCK

GENERAL REFERENCES: 3); 8) p. 93; 9); 10) p. 192; 11); 12); 14) p. 537; 16) p. 319; 17); 18) p. 378; 19) p. 223; 20); 24) p. 214; 25) p. 378; 28) p. 153; 29) p. 387; 30) p. 81-3; 31); 33) p. 258; 35); 36); 37) p. 682; 42) p. 333; 43); 44) p. 411; 46) pp. 100, 149, 157; 48) pp. 244, 354; 49) p. 496; 51) pp. 19, 207, 250; 55) p. 274; 57) p. 259; 62) p. 133; 63); 64) p. 194; 65) p. 301; 66) p. 116; 68) p. 325; 71); 73); 74) p. 27; 79) p. 463; 81).
Buhner, S. *Sacred Plant Medicine: The Wisdom in Native American Herbalism*. Rochester, VT: Bear & Company, 2006;141.
Erichsen-Brown C. *Medicinal and Other Uses of North American Plants: A Historical Survey with Special Reference to the Eastern Indian Tribes*. Dover Publications, Inc., New York,NY. 1979;223-224.
Miyazawa, M., Kameoka, H. Constituents of essential oil from *Rumex crispus*. *Yakagaku*. 1983;32:45-7.
Panciera, R. et al. Acute oxalate poisoning attributable to ingestion of curly dock (*Rumex crispus*) in sheep. *J Am Vet Med Assoc*. 1990 Jun 15; 196(12):1981-4.
Reig, R. et al. Fatal poisoning by *Rumex crispus* (curled dock): pathological findings and application of scanning electron microscopy. *Vet Hum Toxicol*. 1990 Oct;32(5):468-70.

HERBS FOR PREGNANCY, CHILDBIRTH AND LACTATION

GENERAL REFERENCES: 8) pp. 141-3, 238-40, 277-8, 391-3, 402-5; 25) pp. 38-9, 54-7, 60-1,180-1, 368-9; 30) pp. 165-204; 34) pp. 167-72; 45) pp. 186, 194-8, 391-6; 46); 48) pp. 107, 211-13, 383-4, 386; 55) pp. 15-6, 23-4, 52-3, 60-1, 69- 70, 80-1, 82, 96-7, 110-12, 129-32, 135-7, 188, 226, 227,248, 263, 274; 66) pp. 36, 37-8, 41, 93, 100, 114-5, 237, 245-7; 71) pp. 17-75; 78) pp. 232-3, 264-5; 81) pp. 155-69.
Christopher, J., Gileadi, C. *Every Woman's Herbal*. Springville, UT: Christopher Publications, 1987;26-86.
Circosta, C. et al. Estrogenic activity of standardized extracts of *Angelica sinensis*. *Phytother Res*. 2006 Aug;20(8):665-9.
Frye, A. *Holistic Midwifery: A Comprehensive Textbook for Midwives in Homebirth Practice* (Vol 1). Portland, OR: Labrys Press, 2010.
Gallo, M. et al. Pregnancy outcome following gestational exposure to Echinacea. *Archives of Internal Medicine*. 2000;160:3141-3.
___________. Can herbal products be used safely during pregnancy? Focus on Echinacea. *Canadian Family Physician*. 2001;47:1727-8.
Hudson, T. *Gynecology and Naturopathic Medicine*. Aloha, OR: TK Publications, 1992.
Nagabhushan, M. et al. Mutagenicity of gingerol and shogaol and antimutagenicity of zingerone in Salmonella/microsome assay. *Cancer Lett*. 1987;36(2):221-223.
Namakura, H., Yamamoto, T. Mutagen and anti-mutagen in ginger, *Zingiber officinale*. *Mutat Res*. 1982;103(2):119-126.
Parsons, M., Simpson, M., Ponton, T. Raspberry leaf and its effect on labour: safety and efficacy. *Aust Coll Midwives Inc J*. 1999;12(3):20-25.
Parvati, J. *Hygieia: A Woman's Herbal*. Monroe, UT: Freestone Press, 1978.
Romm, A. *Natural Healing for Babies and Children*. Freedom, CA: The Crossing Press, 1996.
________. Naturally Healthy Babies and Children: A Commonsense Guide to Herbal Remedies, Nutrition and Health. New York, NY: Celestial Arts, 2003.
________. *The Natural Pregnancy Book*. New York, NY: Ten Speed Press, 2014.
Simpson, M., Parsons, M. et al. Raspberry leaf in pregnancy: its safety and efficacy in labor. *J Midwifery Womens Health*. 2001;46(2):51-59.

General Index

In addition to this General Index, the **"Index of Health Issues and Herbal Recommendations"** on pages 553-598 in Section Three can be used to locate specific illnesses and diseases.

About the Author

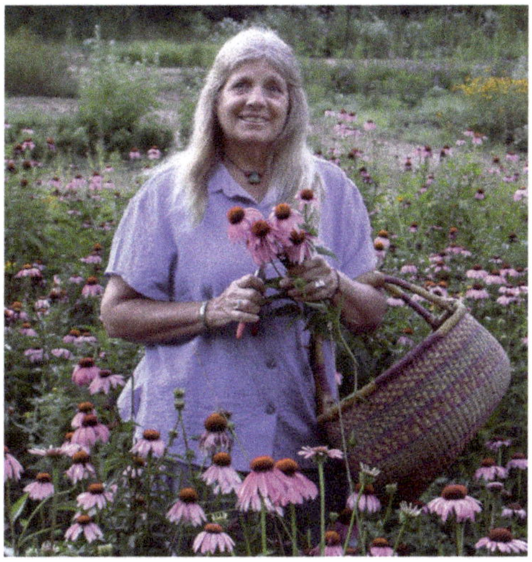

Susan Clearwater, RN, BSN, is a private-practice holistic nurse, clinical herbalist, and cultivator of medicinal herbs. She attended Indiana University School of Nursing in Bloomington, Indiana, motivated by the vision of becoming a holistic nurse, and graduated in 1988 with a Bachelor of Science degree in Nursing. Expanding her experience, she enjoyed working as a medical/surgical charge nurse at Bloomington Hospital until she started her private practice Holistic Nursing Service in 1993. She was certified as a Holistic Nurse Practitioner by the American Holistic Nursing Association in 1999.

Susan also developed and maintains Green Turtle Botanical Sanctuary where she organically cultivates medicinal herbs and processes freshly harvested plants into teas, tinctures, salves and other preparations for family, friends, clients, and local health food stores. She has taught many aspects of medicinal herbalism and holistic healing to a multitude of students and apprentices over the years. She continues to enjoy serving and empowering clients in their healing at her office located at Green Turtle Botanical Sanctuary outside Nashville, Indiana.

Living in her log cabin home on the Botanical Sanctuary grounds in the hilly woodlands of Brown County in southern Indiana, Susan is continually grateful and inspired to live in nature with her cat, an amazing community of friends and family, and amidst the wild critters and the beautiful, bountiful plants.

www.ingramcontent.com/pod-product-compliance
Lightning Source LLC
LaVergne TN
LVHW070844210926
848482LV00016B/862